Lecture Notes in Computer Science　　　9123

Commenced Publication in 1973
Founding and Former Series Editors:
Gerhard Goos, Juris Hartmanis, and Jan van Leeuwen

More information about this series at http://www.springer.com/series/7412

Sebastien Ourselin · Daniel C. Alexander
Carl-Fredrik Westin · M. Jorge Cardoso (Eds.)

Information Processing in Medical Imaging

24th International Conference, IPMI 2015
Sabhal Mor Ostaig, Isle of Skye, UK, June 28 – July 3, 2015
Proceedings

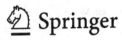 Springer

Editors

Sebastien Ourselin
Centre for Medical Image Computing
University College London
London
UK

Daniel C. Alexander
Centre for Medical Image Computing
University College London
London
UK

Carl-Fredrik Westin
Dept. of Radiology
Harvard Medical School Brigham
  and Women's Hospital
Boston, MA
USA

M. Jorge Cardoso
Centre for Medical Image Computing
University College London
London
UK

ISSN 0302-9743   ISSN 1611-3349   (electronic)
Lecture Notes in Computer Science
ISBN 978-3-319-19991-7   ISBN 978-3-319-19992-4   (eBook)
DOI 10.1007/978-3-319-19992-4

Library of Congress Control Number: 2015940972

LNCS Sublibrary: SL6 – Image Processing, Computer Vision, Pattern Recognition, and Graphics

Springer International Publishing AG Switzerland is part of Springer Science+Business Media
(www.springer.com)

Preface

The 24th biennial international conference on Information Processing in Medical Imaging (IPMI 2015) was held at the Sabhal Mor Ostaig College on the Isle of Skye, UK, June 28 – July 3, 2015. The conference was the latest in a series of biennial scientific meetings, the last being held in July of 2013 at the Asilomar Conference Grounds near Pacific Grove, California, USA, during which new developments in acquisition, formation, analysis, and display of medical images are presented, discussed, dissected, and extended.

IPMI is one of the longest running conferences devoted to these topics in medical imaging. Over the last five decades, IPMI has evolved with the medical imaging community it serves. The first IPMI conference was held in 1969, when a group of young scientists working in nuclear medicine gathered to discuss the current problems in their field. Since that time the conference has expanded into other medical imaging acquisition modalities, including ultrasound, optics, magnetic resonance, and x-ray imaging techniques. IPMI is now widely recognized as one of the most exciting and influential meetings in medical imaging, with a unique emphasis on active participation from all attendees and a strong commitment to vigorous discussion and open debate.

A wide variety of topics are covered at IPMI meetings, all within a single-track format. This year 195 full-length manuscripts were submitted to the conference. Of these, 22 papers were selected for oral presentation and 41 were accepted as posters. Submissions were carefully reviewed by four members of the Scientific Review Committee, who evaluated the novelty, methodological development, and scientific rigor of each manuscript. The Paper Selection Committee, along with the co-chairs, took on the difficult task of creating a meeting program. Using the rankings and detailed comments of the reviewers of each manuscript, and adding to that their own judgment of the merits of each manuscript, they designed the meeting program represented in this volume. The many high-quality manuscripts submitted for consideration made the selection process extremely difficult, and many excellent papers did not make it into the final program. This is an unfortunate inevitability of the high selectivity for which IPMI is known.

One of the key goals of IPMI is to encourage participation of the most promising and talented young researchers in the field, allowing them to explore new ideas with some of the leading researchers in this area. Active involvement is stimulated by preparation before the sessions in small study groups, in which everyone participates. After reading the papers of their session, the study group members meet to discuss the papers before they are presented, and to formulate questions and comments to kick off the discussions. The study groups thus lead off the discussion of each paper, ensuring a lively and vigorous dialog. The prestigious Francois Erbsmann Prize for first-time IPMI presenters adds an extra stimulus for young researchers for active involvement in the meeting. The Francois Erbsmann Prize is awarded for the best contribution by a young scientist who is the first author of a paper and a first-time IPMI oral presenter. This year 16 (of 22) oral presenters were eligible for the Erbsmann Prize.

IPMI 2015 featured a keynote talk describing the Allen Brain atlas and its impact in neuroimaging research by Boudewijn Lelieveldt, Professor of Biomedical Imaging at Leiden University Medical Center, and Delft University of Technology, The Netherlands.

The conference features the traditions that past IPMI attendees have come to expect as part of the unique character of the meeting. Most importantly, each oral presentation has unlimited time for discussion to give the audience the opportunity to resolve all questions regarding the methods and results. IPMI discussions can go on for hours, involving virtually every attendee in the room! Session chairs play a key role at IPMI as they strive to ensure that these extended discussions are productive and continuing to add to the group's understanding of the nature and significance of each presentation's original contribution.

This year, also for the first time, the conference featured an elective oral session. Meeting attendees voted for the poster presentations they would most like to see presented orally. The IPMI board selected several poster presenters from those most popular among the attendees. The selected presenters gave their oral presentation during the closing session of the conference providing extra exposure to work of key interest to the community.

IPMI is traditionally held in a small and sometimes remote location. This year's venue, the Sabhal Mor Ostaig on the Isle of Skye, Scotland, is a unique venue, situated above the shoreline of the picturesque Sound of Sleat in Scotland, known worldwide as the University for Gaelic Language. Sabhal Mor Ostaig is spread over two campuses, Arainn Ostaig and Arainn Chaluim Chille. The two are interlinked by a well-lit pathway and are only a short walk apart. The venue itself is conveniently located just two miles north-east from the main ferry terminal at Armadale village. The venue has great facilities: The Talla Dhonaidh Caimbeul lecture theater can seat up to 190 people, there are two additional board rooms that can accommodate up to 25 people each, and the restaurant consists of a glass-fronted dining room that offers magnificent views over the Sound of Skye and the nearby Knoydart peninsula.

Conference delegates relaxed and enjoyed various group excursions on the afternoon of day 3 of the conference. The excursions made the most of the unique location and culture ranging from whale-spotting in the Sound of Skye, through axe-throwing competitions, to visiting the Talisker distillery (the most famous of Skye's malt whiskies). The afternoon of day 4 of the conference saw the traditional IPMI soccer match, pitting the American team against "the rest of the world." After the disappointing 0-0 draw in 2013, "the rest of the world" are still looking to avenge their first-ever defeat in the history of IPMI in 2011 – an embarrassment that still scars deep.

These proceedings contain the IPMI 2015 papers in the order presented at the meeting. We hope that this volume serves as a valuable source of information for the participants, as well as a reminder of the great conference experience. For those who were not able to attend the conference, we hope that these proceedings provide you with an excellent summary of the latest research contributions to the medical imaging field. We look forward to the next IPMI.

The organization of the 24th IPMI conference was only possible through the efforts and contributions of several organizations and many individuals. First of all, the IPMI 2015 co-chairs would like to thank the members of the Scientific Review Committee for providing so many high-quality reviews within a very limited time frame; because of these reviews, we were able to make a fair selection of the best papers for the final program. We also express our gratitude to the Paper Selection Committee members, who each read many papers and their reviews and travelled to London for a marathon organizational meeting that resulted in an outstanding final program.

Thanks also to Microsoft Corporation for assistance with their excellent CMT conference management system, which we used for the automation of submissions and review of manuscripts. We also thank Jerry Prince for providing the template for this front matter. Finally, we thank Ron Gaston and Dominique Drai for their invaluable administrative support, without which the conference would most certainly not have happened, and the many local organizers at Sabhal Mor Ostaig for their dedicated support.

June 2015

Sebastien Ourselin
Daniel C. Alexander
Carl-Fredrik Westin
M. Jorge Cardoso

Organization

Conference Chairs

Sebastien Ourselin   University College London, UK
Daniel C. Alexander   University College London, UK
Carl-Fredrik Westin   Harvard University, USA

Organizing Committee

Ron Gaston   University College London, UK
Dominique Drai   University College London, UK

Paper Selection Committee

Chris Taylor   Manchester University, UK
Marleen de Bruijne   Copenhagen University, Denmark
Marc Niethammer   University of North Carolina, USA
Sarang Joshi   University of Utah, USA
M. Jorge Cardoso   University College London, UK

Committee

Simon Arridge   University College London, UK
John Ashburner   University College London, UK
Suyash Awate   University of Utah, USA
Christian Barillot   IRISA/CNRS, France
Pierre-Louis Bazin   Max Planck Gesellschaft, Germany
Ismail Ben Ayed   Western University, USA
Sylvain Bouix   BWH Harvard, USA
Djamal Boukerroui   Mirada Medical, UK
Michael Brady   University of Oxford, UK
Owen Carmichael   University of California - Davis, USA
Gary Christensen   University of Iowa, USA
Albert Chung   HKSUT, HK
Ela Claridge   The University of Birmingham, UK
Olivier Commowick   Inria Rennes, France
Tim Cootes   Manchester University, UK
Sune Darkner   DIKU, Denmark
Benoit Dawant   Vanderbilt University, USA
Rachid Deriche   Inria Sophia Antipolis, France

Maxime Descoteaux	Sherbrooke, Canada
Jim Duncan	Yale University, USA
Stanley Durrleman	Inria/ICM, France
Yong Fan	University of Pennsylvania, USA
Aaron Fenster	Robarts Research Institute, USA
Aasa Feragen	DIKU, Denmark
Thomas Fletcher	University of Utah, USA
Alejandro Frangi	University of Sheffield, UK
James Gee	University of Pennsylvania, USA
Guido Gerig	University of Utah, USA
Ben Glocker	Imperial College, UK
Polina Golland	Massachusetts Institute of Technology, USA
Michael Goris	Stanford University School of Medicine, USA
Matthias Guenther	Fraunhofer MEVIS, Germany
Horst Hahn	Fraunhofer MEVIS, Germany
Justin Haldar	University of Southern California, USA
Dave Hawkes	University College London, UK
Mattias Heinrich	University of Lübeck, Germany
Joachim Hornegger	University of Erlangen, Germany
Brian F. Hutton	University College London, UK
Juan E. Iglesias	Basque Center on Cognition, Brain and Language, Spain
Ivana Isgum	University Medical Center Utrecht, The Netherlands
Anand Joshi	University of Southern California, USA
Enrico Kaden	University College London, UK
Nico Karssemeijer	Radboud University, The Netherlands
Boklye Kim	University of Michigan, USA
Andy King	King's College London, UK
Ender Konukoglu	Massachusetts General Hospital, USA
Frithjof Kruggel	University of California Irvine, USA
Sebastian Kurtek	The Ohio State University, USA
Jan Kybic	Czech Technical University, Czech Republic
Georg Langs	Medical University of Vienna, Austria
Tobias Lasser	Technical University of Munich, Germany
Richard Leahy	University of Southern California, USA
Boudewijn Lelieveldt	Leiden University Medical Center, The Netherlands
Marco Lorenzi	University College London, UK
Frederik Maes	Katholieke Universiteit Leuven, Belgium
Stephen Marsland	Massey University, New Zealand
Bernard Ng	Stanford University, USA
Mads Nielsen	University of Copenhagen, Denmark
Wiro Niessen	Erasmus Medical Center Rotterdam, The Netherlands
Marc Niethammer	UNC Chapel Hill, USA
Alison Noble	University of Oxford, UK
Lauren O'Donnell	Harvard Medical School, USA
Evren Ozarslan	Harvard University, USA

Xavier Pennec	Inria, France
Jens Petersen	University of Copenhagen, Denmark
Dzung Pham	Center for Neuroscience and Regenerative Medicine, USA
Stephen Pizer	The University of North Carolina at Chapel Hill, USA
Kilian Pohl	SRI/Stanford, USA
Marcel Prastawa	University of Utah, USA
Jerry Prince	Johns Hopkins University, USA
Jinyi Qi	University of California Davis, USA
Anqi Qiu	National University of Singapore, Singapore
Yogesh Rathi	BWH Harvard, USA
Joseph Reinhardt	University of Iowa, USA
Emma Robinson	Oxford University, UK
Karl Rohr	University of Heidelberg, Germany
Daniel Rueckert	Imperial College London, UK
Mert Sabuncu	Massachusetts General Hospital, USA
Benoit Scherrer	Boston Children's Hospital, USA
Julia Schnabel	University of Oxford, UK
Christof Seiler	Stanford University, USA
Pengcheng Shi	Rochester Institute of Technology, USA
Kaleem Siddiqi	McGill University, Canada
Nikhil P. Singh	University of North Carolina Chapel Hill, USA
Lawrence Staib	Yale University, USA
Colin Studholme	Washington University, USA
Martin Styner	University of North Carolina at Chapel Hill, USA
Gabor Szekely	ETH Zurich, Switzerland
Maxime Taquet	Boston Children's Hospital, USA
Bertrand Thirion	Inria, France
Matthew Toews	Harvard Medical School, USA
Carole Twining	The University of Manchester, UK
Koen Van Leemput	Harvard Medical School/Massachusetts General Hospital, USA
Gael Varoquaux	Inria, France
Baba Vemuri	University of Florida, USA
Tom Vercauteren	University College London, UK
Hongzhi Wang	IBM Almaden Research Center, USA
Simon Warfield	Harvard Medical School and Children's Hospital, USA
Demian Wassermann	Inria, France
William M. Wells	BWH Harvard, USA
Ross Whittaker	University of Utah, USA
Pew-Thian Yap	The University of North Carolina at Chapel Hill, USA
Paul Yushkevich	University of Pennsylvania, USA
Gary Zhang	University College London, UK
Kevin Zhou	Siemens Corporate Research, USA
Lilla Zollei	Harvard Medical School, USA

IPMI Board

Contents

Multi-atlas Fusion

Fast Image Registration

Deformation Models

Poster Papers

Probabilistic Graphical Models

Colocalization Estimation Using Graphical Modeling and Variational Bayesian Expectation Maximization: Towards a Parameter-Free Approach

Suyash P. Awate[✉] and Thyagarajan Radhakrishnan

Computer Science and Engineering Department, Indian Institute of Technology (IIT)
Bombay, Mumbai, India
suyash@cse.iitb.ac.in

Abstract. In microscopy imaging, *colocalization* between two biological entities (e.g., protein-protein or protein-cell) refers to the (stochastic) dependencies between the spatial locations of the two entities in the biological specimen. Measuring colocalization between two entities relies on fluorescence imaging of the specimen using two fluorescent chemicals, each of which indicates the presence/absence of one of the entities at any pixel location. State-of-the-art methods for estimating colocalization rely on post-processing image data using an adhoc sequence of algorithms with many free parameters that are tuned visually. This leads to loss of reproducibility of the results. This paper proposes a brand-new framework for estimating the nature and strength of colocalization directly from corrupted image data by solving a single unified optimization problem that automatically deals with noise, object labeling, and parameter tuning. The proposed framework relies on probabilistic graphical image modeling and a novel inference scheme using variational Bayesian expectation maximization for estimating *all* model parameters, including colocalization, from data. Results on simulated and real-world data demonstrate improved performance over the state of the art.

Keywords: Microscopy · Colocalization · Probabilistic graphical models · Expectation maximization · Variational Bayesian inference · Mean field · Pseudo likelihood

1 Introduction

Colocalization [10,20] between two biological entities refers to the (stochastic) *dependencies between the spatial locations of the two entities* in the specimen. For instance, the presence of a protein at a specific location may be codependent with the presence of a specific cell type in the spatial neighborhood [14].

We thank funding via the IIT Bombay Seed Grant 14IRCCSG010 and T. Liou for the data.

S. Ourselin et al. (Eds.): IPMI 2015, LNCS 9123, pp. 3–16, 2015.
DOI: 10.1007/978-3-319-19992-4_1

The degree of codependence in the spatial distributions of two proteins can reveal details about their dynamic interaction and help understand several biochemical processes [4,8]. Such studies are crucial in understanding the mechanisms of several debilitating diseases, including cancer.

The semantics of colocalization has two aspects: (i) co-occurrence, i.e., the presence of the two entities within a spatial neighborhood, and (ii) correlation or *codependence*, where the two entities co-occur *and* their local quantities exhibit a functional relationship. This paper focuses on the latter, more general, aspect and proposes a framework to automatically estimate the nature and strength of such colocalization from image data.

In microscopy, the *measurement* of colocalization typically relies on fluorescence imaging that involves simultaneous or successive detection of multiple fluorescent chemicals in the same biological specimen, where each fluorescent chemical is designed to bind to exactly one of the biological entities. Thus, the imaging produces multiple images, lying in the same physical coordinate space, where the intensity at each pixel in an image is indicative of the presence/absence of the corresponding biological entity at that pixel location. This paper proposes to estimate a quantitative measure of colocalization directly from noisy image data involving two fluorescence microscopy images.

The literature describes several different strategies for formulating and estimating quantitative measures of colocalization [10,11,20,23]. However, none of these measure colocalization directly from image data, but only from a post-processed version of the data. This post-processing is typically performed manually and in an adhoc manner, i.e., via an adhoc sequence of algorithms with several free parameters tuned visually. This leads to loss of reproducibility of the results. In contrast, this paper proposes a brand new framework for colocalization estimation directly from unprocessed data, by *solving a single optimization problem* with *data-driven parameter optimization for all model parameters*. This framework includes (i) a novel quantitative measure of colocalization, incorporated as a model parameter, and (ii) a novel scheme for statistical inference.

2   Related Work

Quantification of the nature and strength of colocalization is challenging and continues to be an area of active research [1,6,8,9,11,18,22,23,28]. Conventional colocalization techniques were typically qualitative and, thereby, highly prone to random error and bias stemming from inter-rater and intra-rater variability [28].

Colocalization measures involving *pixelwise analysis* [1,6,8,9,18] typically rely on (i) cross-correlation (CC) of the intensities in the two images or (ii) clustering of the joint intensity histogram of the two images. Such methods, however, severely fail to account for long-range spatial dependencies when the two entities occur in close proximity but (almost) never occur in the same pixel. Furthermore, background pixels artificially inflate CC because both image intensities are significantly below their average levels [10]. Some methods [10,27] address this effect by excluding a background region from the analysis, but the background detection uses an adhoc sequence of semi-supervised algorithms, thereby making it highly inconsistent across experts.

On the other hand, *objectwise analysis* [11,22,23] involves a two-step process that first detects and delineates entities/objects represented in the images and then, independently, quantifies colocalization by measuring overlaps or nearest-neighbor distances. However, these methods (i) rely on hard segmentations, (ii) use segmentation methods involving several disconnected algorithms and free parameters (e.g., thresholds, smoothing levels, filter parameters, etc.) that are difficult to tune, and (iii) fail to improve segmentation by feeding back knowledge of the estimated colocalization. Lack of data-driven parameter tuning typically leads to reported results that are inconsistent and irreproducible [28]. On the other hand, the proposed framework in this paper (i) treats segmentation labels as hidden random variables and, thereby, accounts for the uncertainty in the optimal segmentation, (ii) automatically estimates all crucial parameters in a data-driven manner, and (iii) integrates the tasks of segmentation and colocalization estimation as a single unified estimation problem given noisy data.

The noise model underlying fluorescence microscopy involves a complicated combination of several statistical distributions. While the intrinsic noise obeys the Poisson process, several sources of extrinsic noise are characterized by Poisson, Gaussian, and uniform distributions [25]. Indeed, denoising fluorescence microscopy images is an active research area [12,17]. Many state-of-the-art methods approximate the noise model by an independent and identically-distributed (i.i.d.) additive Gaussian model to achieve numerical tractability without significant loss of efficacy [25]. This approximation hold good when the signal-to-noise ratio is high. We follow the same strategy.

In broader contexts, some segmentation methods involve estimation with (hidden) Markov random field (MRF) modeling and expectation maximization (EM) [2,3,7,13,16,19,21,24,26]. However, virtually all such works manually tune the MRF smoothness parameter, unlike the proposed approach that estimates all MRF parameters from the data. Moreover, while some methods [26] employ adhoc gross approximations for evaluating the E step, others [13] evaluate the E step via Gibbs sampling that is computationally expensive and that poses well-known theoretical problems of selecting optimal burn-in periods and detecting sampler convergence. In contrast, the proposed approach employs principled and efficient variational inference to evaluate the E step.

This paper makes several contributions. *First*, it proposes a brand new framework for estimating colocalization directly from image data by solving a single optimization problem that automatically deals with noise, object labeling, and parameter tuning. Consequently, unlike previous works, the proposed framework eliminates (i) adhoc pipelines of disconnected algorithms and (ii) adhoc tuning of parameters, thereby enabling reproducible results. *Second*, the proposed framework relies on (i) a novel probabilistic graphical model for image data and (ii) a novel efficient inference scheme using variational Bayesian expectation maximization (VBEM) [5] for data-driven estimation of *all* model parameters. Specifically, it derives a novel combination of mean-field theory and pseudo-likelihood estimation for parameter inference. *Third*, the results on simulated and real-world data demonstrate that the proposed method estimates colocalization more accurately and consistently, compared to the state of the art.

3   Methods

We first formulate the problem of quantifying colocalization strength and nature (positive/negative codependence) as a Bayesian estimation problem. Then, we describe a novel VBEM inference algorithm that estimates *all* model parameters from data.

3.1   Bayesian Random-Field Image Modeling

We present a generative model for a pair of fluorescence microscopy images to measure colocalization of two objects, relying on probabilistic graphical modeling (Fig. 1).

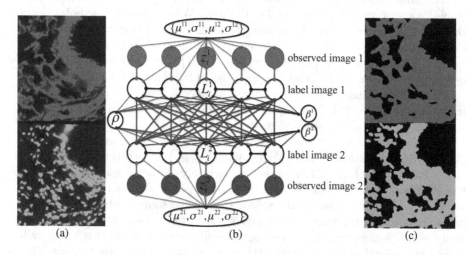

Fig. 1. (a) Real-world fluorescence microscopy images z^1 (top) and z^2 (bottom), depict the presence of protein and cell nuclei, respectively. **(b) Proposed Probabilistic Graphical Model for Colocalization Estimation.** Filled circles denote observed image data $\{z^1, z^2\}$. Label images $\{L^1, L^2\}$ are hidden random variables. We estimate *all* parameters θ from data. The nature and strength of colocalization is modeled by parameter ρ. Parameters β^1, β^2 model spatial smoothness of the labels in l^1, l^2. In this paper, for simplicity, we use a single $\beta = \beta^1 = \beta^2$. Means and standard deviations $\mu^{\cdot\cdot}, \sigma^{\cdot\cdot}$ model image intensities of objects and backgrounds in z^1, z^2. **(c)** MAP label images l^{1*}, l^{2*}, indicating object presence /absence, computed after optimal parameters θ^* are found by VBEM. *Note:* this paper focuses on estimating colocalization ρ using VBEM, which is crucial to several clinical and scientific studies; the MAP label images are unused by VBEM and are shown only to provide additional insights into the proposed approach.

Let $L := \{L^1, L^2\}$ denote a random field modeling the pixel *labels* of the two objects. Specifically, let L^1 be a binary label image with I pixels $\{L_i^1\}_{i=1}^I$ with possible label values $\in \{+1, -1\}$, where $l_i^1 = +1$ indicates the object's presence at pixel i in l^1; similarly, $l_i^1 = -1$ indicates the object's absence at pixel i in l^1. We follow similar notations and semantics for L^2. We assume that the spatial distributions of objects are (i) smooth within each image and (ii) codependent between images. To model these properties, each pixel has intra-image and inter-image neighbors.

We introduce a *neighborhood system* $\mathcal{N} := \{N_i^{\text{self}}, N_i^{\text{other}}\}_{i=1}^I$, where N_i^{self} and N_i^{other} denote sets of neighbors of pixel i in the same image (to which pixel i belongs) and the other image, respectively. To have isotropic neighborhoods, we employ Gaussian-weighted masks w where the ij-th element $w_{ij} := \exp(- \parallel x_j - x_i \parallel^2 / \alpha^2)$, where x_i and x_j are physical coordinates of pixels i and j, respectively. We use two such masks, i.e., w^{self} (for intra-image smoothness) and w^{other} (for inter-image colocalization) with underlying parameters α^{self} and α^{other}, respectively. We set $\alpha^{\text{self}} := 2/3$ pixels to restrict the neighborhood to 2 neighbors along each dimension (we restrict the neighborhood so that $w_{ij} > 10^{-3}$ for neighbors i, j); we found that this level of smoothness suffices for the data used in this paper. We set α^{other} to be large enough to be able to model the longest-range *direct* spatial interactions between the biological entities; this is application dependent and informed by prior knowledge, but the results are fairly robust to the choice of this parameter. In this paper, $\alpha^{\text{other}} := 2$ pixels.

We model the *prior* probability mass function (PMF) of the label image pair L as

$$P(l) := \frac{1}{Z(\rho, \beta)} \exp \left(\sum_{i=1}^I \sum_{j \in N_i^{\text{self}}} \beta \left(l_i^1 l_j^1 + l_i^2 l_j^2 \right) w_{ij}^{\text{self}} + \sum_{i=1}^I \sum_{j \in N_i^{\text{other}}} \rho l_i^1 l_j^2 w_{ij}^{\text{other}} \right),$$
(1)

where the normalization constant (partition function) $Z(\rho, \beta)$ is a function of the smoothness parameter $\beta \in \mathbb{R}^+$ and the colocalization parameter $\rho \in \mathbb{R}$. The motivation for this model is as follows. The terms involving β are derived from a standard Ising model of smoothness on the label images. The term involving ρ is novel and carefully designed as follows. *First,* $\rho = 0$ decouples the two label images such that $P(l)$ can be written as $P(l_1)P(l_2)$; this indicates absence of colocalization. *Second,* because the labels are designed to be ± 1, a positive $\rho \gg 0$ forces the interacting labels in the two images l^1, l^2 (i.e., labels in neighborhoods of each other) towards being equal (i.e., both $+1$ or both -1) to produce a high label image probability. This implies that the neighboring labels in the two images both likely indicate the presence of the objects or both indicate the absence of the objects. *Third,* similarly, a negative $\rho \ll 0$ forces the interacting labels in the two images to be negative of each other, i.e., the presence of the object on one image indicates the absence of the other object in the other image.

Let $Z := \{Z^1, Z^2\}$ denote a random field modeling the *intensities* of the two objects and the backgrounds. We assume that the intensities of each object are

Gaussian distributed as a result of natural intensity variation, partial-volume effects, minor shading artifacts, etc. We assume that the data is corrupted by i.i.d. additive Gaussian noise. Let the intensities of the object and the background in the observed image z^k, where $k \in \{1, 2\}$, be Gaussian distributed with parameters $\{\mu^{k1}, \sigma^{k1}\}$ and $\{\mu^{k2}, \sigma^{k2}\}$, respectively. Then, the *likelihood* of observing data z, given labels l, is

$$P(z|l) := \prod_{i=1}^{I} G(z_i^1 | \mu^{1t_i^1}, \sigma^{1t_i^1}) \prod_{i=1}^{I} G(z_i^2 | \mu^{2t_i^2}, \sigma^{2t_i^2}), \qquad (2)$$

where t_i^1 maps the label value l_i^1 to the object number, i.e., $t_i^1 := 1$ if $l_i^1 = -1$ and $t_i^1 := 2$ if $l_i^1 = +1$; similarly for t_i^2.

Let the set of *parameters* be $\theta := \theta_P \cup \theta_L$, where the prior parameters are $\theta_P := \{\rho, \beta\}$ and the likelihood parameters are $\theta_L := \{\mu^{11}, \sigma^{11}, \mu^{12}, \sigma^{12}, \mu^{21}, \sigma^{21}, \mu^{22}, \sigma^{22}\}$. We propose to *formulate colocalization estimation* as the following maximum-a-posteriori Bayesian estimation problem over all parameters θ:

$$\arg\max_{\rho} \left(\max_{\theta - \{\rho\}} P(z|\theta) \right), \text{ where } P(z|\theta) = \sum_l P(z, l|\theta) = \sum_l P(z|l, \theta_L) P(l|\theta_P). \tag{3}$$

A novelty in our approach is that we estimate ρ (as well as β) automatically from the data. We observe that the optimization of the parameters ρ and β is non-trivial because of their involvement in the partition function $Z(\rho, \beta)$ that is intractable to evaluate. Furthermore, we optimize *all* parameters underlying the model directly from the data.

3.2   Expectation Maximization for Parameter Estimation

We treat the labels L as *hidden variables* and solve the parameter-estimation problem using EM. EM is an iterative optimization algorithm, each iteration comprising an E step and an M step. Consider that after iteration n, the parameter estimate is θ^n. Then, in iteration $n + 1$, the updated parameter estimate θ^{n+1} is obtained as follows.

The E step involves constructing the $Q(\cdot)$ function

$$Q(\theta; \theta^n) := E_{P(L|z, \theta^n)}[\log P(z, L|\theta)] \tag{4}$$

that is intractable to evaluate analytically. Furthermore, a Monte-Carlo simulation-based approximation of the expectation leads to challenges in reliable and efficient sampling; e.g., while Gibbs sampling of the label fields is computationally expensive, determining an appropriate burn-in period and detecting convergence of the Gibbs sampler pose serious theoretical challenges. Thus, we opt for variational inference and choose to approximate the posterior PMF $P(L|z, \theta^n)$ by a factorizable analytical model

$$P(L|z, \theta^n) \approx F(L|z, \theta^n) := \prod_{i=1}^{I} F_i^1(L_i^1) F_i^2(L_i^2), \tag{5}$$

where we optimize the per-pixel factors, i.e., PMFs, $F_i^1(L_i^1), F_i^2(L_i^2)$ to best fit the posterior. This factorized approximation for the posterior makes the $Q(\theta; \theta^n)$ function more tractable. We describe this strategy in the next section.

The M step subsequently maximizes the $Q(\theta; \theta^n)$ function over parameters θ. The E and M steps are repeated until convergence; we observe that a few iterations are suffice.

3.3 E Step: Variational Inference of the Factorized Posterior

Within each EM iteration, we use variational inference to optimize the factors underlying $F(L|z, \theta^n)$. To simplify notation, we omit θ where it is obvious. We rewrite

$$\log P(Z|\theta) = \mathcal{L}(F(L), \theta) + \mathrm{KL}\Big(F(L) \parallel P(L|z, \theta)\Big), \text{ where} \qquad (6)$$

$$\mathcal{L}(F(L), \theta) := \sum_l F(l) \log \Big(P(z, l|\theta)/F(l)\Big) \qquad (7)$$

and $\mathrm{KL}(A \parallel B) \geq 0$ denotes the Kullback-Leibler (KL) divergence between distributions A and B. Our goal is to find the maximal lower bound $\mathcal{L}(F(L))$ of the data log-probability $\log P(Z)$, under the factorization constraint on $F(L)$. We do this by maximizing $\mathcal{L}(F(L))$, because $\mathrm{KL}(\cdot) \geq 0$ guarantees $\mathcal{L}(F(L))$ to be a lower bound. We perform this functional optimization by iterative optimization of each of the factor functions; this is possible because the factors are designed to be independent of each other. We now incorporate the factorized form of $F(L)$ and, without loss of generality, separate terms involving F_j^1 from the other terms. This yields

$$\mathcal{L}(F(L)) = \sum_{l_j^1} F_j^1(l_j^1) \log \widetilde{P}(z, l_j^1) - \sum_{l_j^1} F_j^1(l_j^1) \log F_j^1(l_j^1) + \text{ constant}, \quad (8)$$

$$\text{where } \log \widetilde{P}(z, l_j^1) := \sum_{l_{i:i\neq j}^1} \sum_{l^2} \log P(z, l) \prod_{i:i\neq j} F_i^1(l_i^1) \prod_i F_i^2(l_i^2) + \text{constA}, \quad (9)$$

where (i) the first term on the right hand side is an expectation of the log complete-data probability $\log P(z, l)$ over all the factors in $F(L)$ except $F_j^1(\cdot)$ and (ii) constA is the normalization factor for $P(z, L_j^1)$. We see that $\mathcal{L}(F(L))$ is the negative KL divergence between the distributions $F_j^1(L_j^1)$ and $\log \widetilde{P}(z, L_j^1)$. Thus, fixing the set of functions $\{F_{i\neq j}^1(\cdot), F_i^2(\cdot)\}_{i=1}^I$, the optimal function $F_j^1(\cdot)$ that maximizes $\mathcal{L}(F(L))$ is

$$F_j^1(l_j^1) := \widetilde{P}(z, l_j^1) = \frac{1}{\eta} \exp\left(\sum_{l_{i:i\neq j}^1} \sum_{l^2} \log P(z, l) \prod_{i:i\neq j} F_i^1(l_i^1) \prod_i F_i^2(l_i^2)\right), \quad (10)$$

where η is the normalization constant. The expectation inside the exponent on the right hand side is easy to evaluate for the following reasons. First, because we designed $P(z, l)$ to be in the exponential class, $\log P(z, l)$ gives us the terms in its exponent. *Second*, because we are estimating a PMF solely on the label l_j^1, we only need to consider terms involving l_j^1. *Third*, by our design, all terms in $\log P(z, l)$ involving the label l_j^1 are linear functions of other labels $l_{i:i\neq j}^1$ and l_i^2. Thus, the optimal $F_j^1(\cdot)$ is similar to the conditional PMF of label l_j^1 given (i) its neighboring labels in both images and (ii) data z_j^1, but a crucial difference is that the contributions of the neighboring labels are through their expectations under the corresponding factors, instead of their values themselves. This variational inference scheme is also called mean-field approximation [15].

Within the n-th EM iteration, we propose the following algorithm for variational optimization of the factors:

1. *Input:* Observed data z and the current parameter estimates θ^n.
2. Initialize the expectations of all labels $\{l_i^1, l_i^2\}_{i=1}^I$. This can be taken to be the (i) maximum-a-posteriori estimate given θ^n and z or (ii) empirically-computed expectation using Gibbs sampling of the labels from the posterior PMF. We have found the former strategy to be effective as well as computationally efficient.
3. Iterate over all pixels (order column by column) in both the label images. At each pixel, perform the next step.
4. Without loss of generality, consider pixel j in the first image. Analytically evaluate the optimal PMF $F_j^1(\cdot)$, given the expected values of the interacting labels and data; as described previously in this section. Analytically evaluate the expectation of l_j^1 over this optimal PMF $F_j^1(\cdot)$ and update it.
5. Repeat the last two steps, until convergence of the expected label images and thereby the factorized approximation $F(L|z, \theta^n)$.
6. *Output:* The factorized posterior $F(L|z, \theta^n)$ in terms of the factors $\{F_i^1(\cdot), F_i^2(\cdot)\}_{i=1}^I$.

After obtaining the factorized posterior $F(L|z, \theta^n)$, we evaluate the $Q(\theta; \theta^n)$ function efficiently as follows.

1. *Input:* Observed data z, the current parameter estimates θ^n, and the optimal factorized posterior $F(L|z, \theta^n)$.
2. Sample a large number S of label image pairs $\{l^s := (l^{s1}, l^{s2})\}_{s=1}^S$ from $F(L|z, \theta^n)$ by independent sampling at each pixel from the label distribution. This is straightforward (unlike Gibbs sampling) and computationally cheap because sampling at each pixel is sampling from a binomial (factor) distribution. Thus, we can easily generate a large sample size to ensure a high-quality approximation.
3. Closely approximate the $Q(\theta; \theta^n)$ function as follows:

$$Q(\theta; \theta^n) \approx \widehat{Q}(\theta; \theta^n) := \frac{1}{S} \sum_{s=1}^S \log P(z, l^s | \theta) \tag{11}$$

4. *Output:* The function $\widehat{Q}(\theta; \theta^n)$.

The next section describes the M step for optimizing parameters θ using $\widehat{Q}(\theta; \theta^n)$.

3.4 M Step: Parameter Updates

The M step in the n-th EM iteration updates the parameter estimates θ as

$$\theta^{n+1} := \arg\max_{\theta} \widehat{Q}(\theta; \theta^n) = \arg\max_{\theta} \sum_{s=1}^{S} \log P(z, l^s | \theta). \qquad (12)$$

We perform alternating minimization over the set of parameter estimates as follows.

The optimal likelihood parameters θ_L maximize the data likelihood given labels:

$$\arg\max_{\theta_L} \sum_{s=1}^{S} \log P(z, l^s | \theta) = \arg\max_{\theta_L} \sum_{s=1}^{S} \log P(z | l^s, \theta_L). \qquad (13)$$

These updates, for the means and variances of the object-specific and background-specific Gaussians, are obtained in closed form.

The optimal prior parameters θ_P maximize the label prior probability:

$$\arg\max_{\theta_P} \sum_{s=1}^{S} \log P(z, l^s | \theta) = \arg\max_{\theta_P} \sum_{s=1}^{S} \log P(l^s | \theta_P). \qquad (14)$$

The optimization of the prior parameters θ_P is more difficult because they appear as part of the intractable partition function $Z(\theta_P)$. Nevertheless, we have found an effective strategy for estimating θ_P, which relies on the principles underlying maximum pseudo-likelihood (MPL) estimation [15] that obtains parameter estimates by maximizing a pseudo-likelihood function instead of the true likelihood function (Note: in the context of MPL, the "likelihood" is the probability of observing a label image given the MRF model and underlying parameters). The key idea is that the pseudo-likelihood function (i) is simpler to optimize because it eliminates the partition function and, (ii) for sufficiently large data, mimics the true likelihood function well.

The classic MPL strategy for estimation of MRF parameters relies on a *single* observed (label) image, where the MPL estimator is known to be consistent [15]. In our case, we have a *set of sampled label images* $\{l^s\}_{s=1}^{S}$. This image set can be considered similar to data obtained by cutting out images from a much larger image. In a statistical sense, observing one large image drawn from a MRF model is equivalent to observing many smaller images drawn from the same model (i.e., with same potential functions and parameters). Thus, we propose to apply the MPL strategy to the entire set of images by replacing each $P(l^s | \theta_P)$ by its pseudo-likelihood analog to optimize θ_P as:

$$\max_{\theta_P} \sum_{s=1}^{S} \log P(l^s | \theta_P) \approx$$

$$\max_{\theta_P} \sum_{s=1}^{S} \log \left(\prod_{i=1}^{I} P(l_i^{s1} | l_{N_i^{\text{self}}}^{s1}, l_{N_i^{\text{other}}}^{s2}, \theta_P) \prod_{i=1}^{I} P(l_i^{s2} | l_{N_i^{\text{self}}}^{s2}, l_{N_i^{\text{other}}}^{s1}, \theta_P) \right) =$$

$$\max_{\theta_P} \sum_{s=1}^{S} \left(\sum_{i=1}^{I} \log P(l_i^{s1}|l_{N_i^{\text{self}}}^{s1}, l_{N_i^{\text{other}}}^{s2}, \theta_P) + \sum_{i=1}^{I} \log P(l_i^{s2}|l_{N_i^{\text{self}}}^{s2}, l_{N_i^{\text{other}}}^{s1}, \theta_P) \right).$$

(15)

We optimize θ_P by alternately optimizing ρ and β. We optimize each parameter by iterative gradient descent using adaptive step sizes and initialized using previous parameter estimates. We observe that a few iterations are sufficient for convergence.

4   Validation on Simulated Data

We validate the proposed algorithm using simulated data. First, we choose several values of $\rho \in \{-0.2, -0.1, -0.05, 0, 0.05, 0.1, 0.2\}$, where $|\rho| = 0.2$ indicates very strong colocalization. For each ρ value, we choose several values of $\beta \in \{0.05, 0.1, 0.15, 0.2\}$, indicating low to high spatial smoothness. Then, we Gibbs sample 5 label image pairs $l = (l^1, l^2)$ from the prior model per (ρ, β) pair; each image is 200×200 pixels. Subsequently, we select two sets of likelihood parameters θ_L (to mimic high and low contrast-to-noise ratios) and generate observed image pairs $z = (z^1, z^2)$. Thus, for every ρ, we generate 40 different data z instances. We give the data z as input to our algorithm and estimate all parameters θ, including the colocalization parameter ρ.

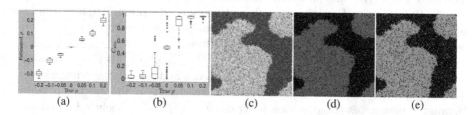

(a)   (b)   (c)   (d)   (e)

Fig. 2. Colocalization Estimation on Simulated Data using **(a)** proposed algorithm and **(b)** Squassh [23]. **(c)** Simulated noisy data (z^1, z^2) for $\beta = 0.1, \rho = 0.05$ shown as a 2-channel (red-green) color image and **(d)-(e)** its MAP label images l^{1*}, l^{2*} for each channel (computed after optimal parameters θ^* are found by VBEM), which are virtually identical to ground truth.

We compare the proposed algorithm with Squassh (`fiji.sc/Squassh`) [23] relying on objectwise analysis that first segments the objects and then computes a colocalization measure, namely $Csize \in [0, 1]$, which detects spatial overlaps of the segmented objects. The underlying segmentation pipeline involves 5-6 stages (with ≈ 10 free parameters) involving several crucial parameters (e.g., for background detection, regularization, thresholding) that are tuned visually. We evaluate this method by (i) using the same 40 data instances generated before and (ii) varying only two of the visually-tuned parameters for thresholding and regularization over a reasonable range (0.4–$2.5\times$ around the central value;

3 values per parameter) to mimic inter-expert and intra-expert usage variability. Thus, for every ρ, we evaluate Squassh 360 times.

Estimated colocalization ρ values using the proposed algorithm (Fig. 2(a)) are very close to the ground-truth values, for both (i) $\rho > 0$ cases, i.e., both kinds of objects promote each other's presence, and (ii) $\rho < 0$ cases, i.e., both kinds of objects inhibit each other's presence. After VBEM produces the optimal parameter values θ^*, we compute the MAP estimate l^* for the label images, i.e., $\arg\max_l P(l|z, \theta^*)$, and find them to be indistinguishable from the ground truth label images for all (ρ, β) combinations.

Results using Squassh (Fig. 2(b)) (i) produces estimates $Csize$ with very high variability, despite only small changes in manually-tuned parameter values, (ii) fails to distinguish between some cases with sufficiently different colocalization strengths, by producing average $Csize$ estimates that are too close, and (iii) incorrectly produces close-to-zero $Csize$ estimates (indicating mutually inhibiting object behavior) when the two objects actually co-occur in close proximity but with little spatial overlap.

Lack of colocalization is represented (i) in the proposed framework by $\rho = 0$ and (ii) in Squassh by $Csize = 0.5$ indicating pure-chance overlaps between the spatial locations of the two objects. Similarly, negative colocalization $\rho < 0$ corresponds to $Csize < 0.5$ and positive colocalization $\rho > 0$ corresponds to $Csize > 0.5$.

5   Results on Real-World Data

We evaluate the proposed algorithm and Squassh [23] on two real-world datasets.

First, we evaluate on the openly available Colocalization Benchmark Source (www.colocalization-benchmark.com) [28]. We take datasets depicting five increasing strengths/levels of colocalization. We have 3 image pairs per level; 1024×1024 images; we split each image into 16 smaller 256×256 images, producing 48 different z instances per level. We run Squassh [23], varying only two of the approximately ten visually-tuned parameters for thresholding and regularization over a reasonable range (as described in previous section) to mimic inter-expert and intra-expert usage variability. The results (Fig. 3) show that for the five increasing colocalization strengths (denoted by $1 \rightarrow 5$), the proposed colocalization estimates ρ (Fig. 3(a)) have clearly separable medians and low variability, unlike $Csize$ estimates by Squassh (Fig. 3(b)).

Second, we evaluate on a laboratory dataset (Fig. 1(a)), imaged during a biopsy. Expert visual assessment indicates the spatial locations of these two entities to be positively codependent, i.e., both objects promote each other's presence. The proposed algorithm correctly indicates a positive colocalization $\rho = 0.08 > 0$. Perturbing $\alpha^{self}, \alpha^{other}$ by 0.5–2× around the central value maintains ρ to be positive and within $[0.06, 0.09]$. However, for Squassh, similar perturbations in the manually-tuned parameters produce widely varying colocalization $Csize$ estimates: 25-th, 50-th, and 75-th percentiles are 0.33, 0.54, and 0.77, respectively. Moreover, $Csize$ estimates < 0.5 indicate mutually inhibiting colocalization that is inconsistent with expert visual evaluation.

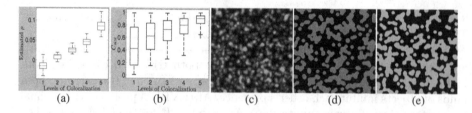

Fig. 3. Colocalization Estimation on Real-World Benchmark Data using **(a)** proposed algorithm and **(b)** Squassh [23]. **(c)** Example data (z^1, z^2) for colocalization level 1 $(\equiv \rho < 0)$ shown as a red-green image with **(d), (e)** MAP label images l^{1*}, l^{2*}, indicating object presence, computed after optimal parameters θ^* are found by VBEM (Colour figure online).

6 Conclusions

This paper proposes a brand-new framework for estimating the nature and strength of colocalization directly from corrupted image data by solving a single unified optimization problem that automatically deals with noise, object detection, and parameter tuning. The proposed framework relies on probabilistic graphical image modeling and a novel inference scheme using variational Bayesian expectation maximization for estimating *all* model parameters, including colocalization, from data. It achieves this by deriving a novel combination of mean-field and pseudo-likelihood theory.

To avoid pitfalls of the state of the art, the proposed colocalization measure ρ quantifies the spatial proximity of the two objects, instead of measuring (some form of) object overlap. Moreover, the proposed algorithm optimizes all parameters in a data-driven manner, thereby avoiding severe problems faced by the state of the art leading to high variability in results because of inter/intra-expert subjectivity in parameter tuning. The results on simulated data, real-world benchmark data, and laboratory data clearly demonstrate the advantages of the proposed framework. We also evaluated an alternative colocalization measure *Cnum* in Squassh, but that yielded poorer results than *Csize*.

Future work can incorporate a more sophisticated imaging model that includes artifacts like blurring and shading. To employ the proposed framework in a clinical application, calibration of the computed measure may be needed for suitable interpretation.

References

1. Adler, J., Parmryd, I.: Quantifying colocalization by correlation: the Pearson correlation coefficient is superior to the Mander's overlap coefficient. Cytometry A **77**(8), 733–42 (2010)
2. Awate, S.P., Whitaker, R.T.: Multiatlas segmentation as nonparametric regression. IEEE Trans. Med. Imaging **33**(9), 1803–1817 (2014)

3. Awate, S.P., Zhang, H., Gee, J.C.: A fuzzy, nonparametric segmentation framework for DTI and MRI analysis: with applications to DTI tract extraction. IEEE Trans. Med. Imaging **26**(11), 1525–1536 (2007)
4. Batada, N., Shepp, L., Siegmund, D.: Stochastic model of protein-protein interaction: why signaling proteins need to be colocalized. Proc. Nat. Acad. Sci. **101**(17), 6445–6449 (2004)
5. Beal, M., Ghahramani, Z.: The variational Bayesian EM algorithm for incomplete data: with application to scoring graphical model structures. Bayesian Stat. **7**, 453–465 (2003)
6. Bolte, S., Cordelieres, F.: A guided tour into subcellular colocalization analysis in light microscopy. J. Microsc. **224**(3), 213–32 (2006)
7. Chang, M., Sezan, M., Tekalp, A., Berg, M.: Bayesian segmentation of multislice brain magnetic resonance imaging using 3-D Gibbsian priors. Opt. Eng. **35**(11), 97–106 (1996)
8. Costes, S., Daelemans, D., Pavlakis, G., Lockett, S.: Automatic and quantitative measurement of protein-protein colocalization in live cells. Biophys. J. **86**(6), 3993–4003 (2004)
9. Demandolx, D., Davoust, J.: Multicolour analysis and local image correlation in confocal microscopy. J. Microsc. **185**(1), 21–36 (2003)
10. Dunn, K., Kamocka, M., McDonald, J.: A practical guide to evaluating colocalization in biological microscopy. Am. J. Physiol. Cell Physiol. **300**, C723–C742 (2011)
11. Helmuth, J., Paul, G., Sbalzarini, I.: Beyond co-localization: inferring spatial interactions between sub-cellular structures from microscopy images. BMC Bioinf. **11**(372), 1–12 (2010)
12. Jezierska, A., Talbot, H., Pesquet, J., Engler, G.: Poisson-Gaussian noise parameter estimation in fluorescence microscopy imaging. In: IEEE International Symposium on Biomedical Imaging (ISBI), pp. 1663–1666 (2012)
13. Leemput, K.V., Maes, F., Vandermeulen, D., Suetens, P.: A unifying framework for partial volume segmentation of brain MR images. IEEE Trans. Med. Imaging **22**(1), 105–119 (2003)
14. Lew, M., Lee, S., Ptacin, L., Lee, M., Twieg, R., Shapiro, L., Moerner, W.: Three-dimensional superresolution colocalization of intracellular protein superstructures and the cell surface in live Caulobacter crescentus. Proc. Nat. Acad. Sci. **108**(46), E1102–E1110 (2011)
15. Li, S.Z.: Markov Random Field Modeling in Image Analysis. Advances in Pattern Recognition. Springer, London (2009)
16. Liu, W., Awate, S.P., Anderson, J., Fletcher, P.T.: A functional networks estimation method of resting-state fMRI using a hierarchical Markov random field. NIMG **100**, 520–34 (2014)
17. Luisier, F., Blu, T., Unser, M.: Image denoising in mixed Poisson-Gaussian noise. IEEE Trans. Imaging Process **20**(3), 696–708 (2011)
18. Manders, E., Verbeek, F., Aten, J.: Measurement of co-localisation of objects in dual-colour confocal images. J. Microsc. **169**(3), 375–382 (1993)
19. Ng, B., Hamarneh, G., Abugharbieh, R.: Modeling brain activation in fMRI using group MRF. IEEE Trans. Med. Imaging **31**(5), 1113–1123 (2012)
20. Oheim, M., Li, D.: Quantitative colocalisation imaging: concepts, measurements, and pitfalls. In: Frischknecht, F., Shorte, S.L. (eds.) Imaging Cellular and Molecular Biological Functions. Principles and Practice, pp. 117–155. Springer, Heidelberg (2007)

21. Pham, D.L., Prince, J.L.: A generalized EM algorithm for robust segmentation of magnetic resonance images. In: Proceedings of Conference on Information Science and Systems, pp. 558–563 (1999)

22. Ramirez, O., Garcia, A., Couve, A., Hartel, S.: Confined displacement algorithm determines true and random colocalization in fluorescence microscopy. J. Microsc. **239**, 173–183 (2010)

23. Rizk, A., Paul, G., Incardona, P., Bugarski, M., Mansouri, M., Niemann, A., Ziegler, U., Berger, P., Sbalzarini, I.: Segmentation and quantification of subcellular structures in fluorescence microscopy images using Squassh. Nat. Protoc. **9**(3), 586–596 (2014)

24. Roche, A., Ribes, D., Bach-Cuadra, M., Kruger, G.: On the convergence of EM-like algorithms for image segmentation using Markov random fields. Med. Imaging Anal. **15**(6), 830–839 (2011)

25. Sarder, P., Nehorai, A.: Deconvolution methods for 3-D fluorescence microscopy images. IEEE Signal Process. Mag. **23**(3), 32–45 (2006)

26. Zhang, Y., Brady, M., Smith, S.: Segmentation of brain MR images through a hidden Markov random field model and the expectation maximization algorithm. IEEE Trans. Med. Imaging **20**, 45–57 (2001)

27. Zinchuk, V., Zinchuk, O.: Quantitative colocalization analysis of confocal fluorescence microscopy images. Curr. Protoc. Cell Biol. **62**(4.19), 1–14 (2008)

28. Zinchuk, V., Wu, Y., Grossenbacher-Zinchuk, O.: Bridging the gap between qualitative and quantitative colocalization results in fluorescence microscopy studies. Nature: Sci. Rep. **3**(1365), 1–5 (2013)

Template-Based Multimodal Joint Generative Model of Brain Data

M. Jorge Cardoso[1,2]([✉]), Carole H. Sudre[1,2], Marc Modat[1,2],
and Sebastien Ourselin[1,2]

[1] Centre for Medical Image Computing (CMIC), University College London,
London, UK
m.jorge.cardoso@ucl.ac.uk
[2] Dementia Research Centre (DRC), University College London, London, UK

Abstract. The advent of large of multi-modal imaging databases opens up the opportunity to learn how local intensity patterns covariate between multiple modalities. These models can then be used to describe expected intensities in an unseen image modalities given one or multiple observations, or to detect deviations (e.g. pathology) from the expected intensity patterns. In this work, we propose a template-based multi-modal generative mixture-model of imaging data and apply it to the problems of inlier/outlier pattern classification and image synthesis. Results on synthetic and patient data demonstrate that the proposed method is able to synthesise unseen data and accurately localise pathological regions, even in the presence of large abnormalities. It also demonstrates that the proposed model can provide accurate and uncertainty-aware intensity estimates of expected imaging patterns.

1 Introduction

Neuroimaging studies have become increasingly multimodal, as different imaging techniques (e.g. CT, T1- and T2-weighted MRI, FLAIR, DWI, etc.) contain complementary information about the underlying anatomy, its microstructure and/or its function. However, different modalities also share a large amount of information. As an example, it is possible to predict how a T2 MRI image of a subject should look like given the subject's T1 MRI and a model of image formation [1]. This process, known in the medical image community as image/modality synthesis, has been recently exploited for the purpose of improving multimodal image registration and tissue segmentation [1], synthesising DTI-FA images [2] and PET attenuation-map reconstruction [3], using techniques such as nearest-neighbour patch propagation [1], iterative region-restricted patch-search [2], local similarity-weighted voting [3] and sparse patch-match [4].

One limitation of current synthesis strategies is the lack of knowledge about the uncertainty of the generative process. By generating only one single image estimate, one is assuming that the process of image synthesis is deterministic, or at least that it's uncertainty is non-spatially variant. This is an erroneous assumption that can overestimate the confidence in the synthesis

S. Ourselin et al. (Eds.): IPMI 2015, LNCS 9123, pp. 17–29, 2015.
DOI: 10.1007/978-3-319-19992-4_2

process, possibly propagating large errors to other steps of the image processing pipeline. These uncertainty estimates are especially important in regions where there is no one-to-one intensity correspondence between medical images, e.g. skull/sinus/brain/eye region in CT synthesis from MRI data [3]. In these specific regions, the sinus and skull have highly distinguishable intensities, making the CT probability density function multi-modal. The process of sample averaging seen in [1–4], equivalent to estimating the expectation of the probability density function, is not a good approximation of the MAP estimate, thus producing unrealistic and improbable estimates of the target intensities.

Another limitation of image synthesis methodologies is that one can only reproduce a target modality from a source modality if they share common information or if the missing information can be obtained *a priori* from a population. For example, if a lesion visible in a T2-FLAIR MRI is not visible in a T1 MRI, then this lesion will not appear if one tries to synthesise a T2-FLAIR from a T1 MRI. This limitation has been exploited in the context of pathology detection by synthesising a T2-FLAIR MRI from an observed T1-weighted MRI [2,4], as the pathology is hardly visible in the T1 image. By subtracting the real T2 MRI with a tumour from the T1-derived synthetic T2 MRI, one can obtain a region of interest localising the pathological areas. However, as the synthesis process is considered deterministic (i.e. no estimates of uncertainty), this subtraction process has the same limitations as above - the subtraction process generates edge effects, mis-localising pathological areas when the model does not fit.

From a generative model point-of-view, another strategy to localise intensity outliers in an image is through the process of image clustering [5]. This class of models assume an underlying number of healthy brain tissue classes, normally white-matter (WM), grey-matter and cerebrospinal fluid (CSF), and detects deviations from them. However, any intensity pattern that deviates from these three healthy tissue intensity distributions would be considered as an outlier, even though they commonly appear in healthy brains (e.g. T2 hypo-intensity due to accumulation of cysteine-iron complex in the globus pallidus and substantia nigra). This requires extra empirical pathology-specific post-processing to select a subset of the outliers [5].

With the problem in mind, this work proposes a template-based generative model of brain data and applies it to both the problem image synthesis and inlier/outlier pattern classification for the localisation of image abnormalities. We build on the preliminary idea of [2] but instead of applying a deterministic method, the proposed model describes the full joint probability distribution of a pair of observed images given a set of previously observed templates, making the algorithm robust to edge effects and uncertainty in the model. Furthermore, by describing the process probabilistically, it becomes trivial to further extend the proposed model to an hierarchical segmentation approach.

2   Methods

Image synthesis can be seen as the process of generating an expected image $E[\tilde{y}]$ given an observed image $\tilde{x}$ from a different imaging modality and a database of N previously observed image pairs $\mathcal{X} = \{y_n, x_n\}$, indexed by n. Note that the technique can be easily extended to more than 2 modalities. The process of collapsing all the available information from $\mathcal{X}$ into one single estimate $E[\tilde{y}]$ ignores both the fact that generating $\tilde{y}$ is an uncertain process an that $p(\tilde{y})$ can be multimodal. Thus, contrary to [2,4], where only the expected image $E[\tilde{y}]$ is generated, we characterise $p(\tilde{y}, \tilde{x} | \mathcal{X}, \theta)$, i.e. the joint probability of observing the image pair $\{\tilde{y}, \tilde{x}\}$ given a set of N previously observed templates $\mathcal{X}$ and the model parameters $\theta = \{\sigma_x^2, \sigma_y^2, \Sigma_{j_n}, \mu_{j_n}, G, w\}$.

From an intuitive point of view, the main difference between the proposed method and previous approaches pertains with the idea that the process of image synthesis is uncertain. Thus, rather than trying to find the expected observation y from an observation x, we estimate what is the probability of observing different values of y when observing x.

2.1   The Observation Model

In order to estimate $p(\tilde{y}, \tilde{x} | \mathcal{X}, \theta)$ one has to first note that, due to the presence of pathology or imaging artefacts, not all intensity pairs $\{\tilde{y}, \tilde{x}\}$ will be likely given a certain set of previously observed images. Thus, it is important to model the possible presence of outliers - intensity pairs that deviate from previous templates. This does not mean that one would be able to predict unseen pathological intensity pairs. Instead, the model assumes that imaging data can fall outside the predictable intensity patterns.

With this aim in mind, the proposed generative model assumes that the observed data is generated from a mixture of $K = 2$ classes labeled by l_i^k, i.e. an inlier class, derived from previous observations, and an outlier class, modelled by a uniform distribution. The probability $p(\tilde{y}_i, \tilde{x}_i, j, l_i |, \mathcal{X}, \theta)$ of observing an intensity pair $\{\tilde{y}_i, \tilde{x}_i\}$, a transformation j and label l at location i, is then defined as

$$p(\tilde{y}_i, \tilde{x}_i, j | l_i, \mathcal{X}, \theta)p(l_i^k) = w \underbrace{p(\tilde{y}_i, \tilde{x}_i, j | l_i^I, \mathcal{X}, \theta)p(l_i^I)}_{\text{inlier model}} + (1 - w) \underbrace{p(\tilde{y}_i, \tilde{x}_i | l_i^O)p(l_i^O)}_{\text{outlier model}}$$

In this model, the distribution of the pair $\{\tilde{y}, \tilde{x}\}$ for the outlier class (l^O) is given by an uniform distribution $p(\tilde{y}_i, \tilde{x}_i | l_i^O) = \mathcal{U}$, an inlier class (l^I) describing the similarity between the observed pair $\{\tilde{y}_i, \tilde{x}_i\}$ and the previously observed pairs $\mathcal{X} = \{y_n, x_n\}$, a coordinate mapping j_n, a prior distribution $p(l_i^I)$ and $p(l_i^O)$ over the labelling l_i^k, and a global mixing weight w.

In this work, given N previously observed images, the inlier model is defined as a mixture model given by

$$p(\tilde{y}_i, \tilde{x}_i, j | l_i^I, \mathcal{X}, \theta) = \frac{1}{N} \sum_{n=1}^{N} p(\tilde{y}_i, \tilde{x}_i | l_i^I, j_n, \mathcal{X}_n, \theta)p(j_n | l_i^I, \theta).$$

i.e., the probability of observing a certain pair of intensities $\{\tilde{y}_i, \tilde{x}_i\}$ is a equally-weighted mixture of the N probabilities of observing the pair given a previously observed pair $\mathcal{X}_n$.

As in the Non-Local STAPLE algorithm [6], we assume that j_n is unknown, or at least uncertain, as the coordinate mapping problem is *ill posed* [7]. As in Simpson *et al.* [7], $p(j_n|l_i^I, \theta)$ is a multivariate Gaussian distribution with parameters $\theta = \{\mu_j^n, \Sigma_j\}$. Here, the expectation of the mapping j_n, i.e. μ_j^n, is estimated using a multimodal pairwise b-spline parameterised registration between the observed image pair and the n-th image pair. A multichannel locally normalised cross correlation is used as an image similarity for registration purposes. In addition, the precision matrix Σ_{ji}^{-1} at location i, represents the inverse of the local directional estimate of registration uncertainty as described in [7]. In this work, Σ_{ji}^{-1} is approximated using the local second-moment matrix, also known as the structure tensor [8], of the observed image $\tilde{x}$ in a cubic convolution region of size $s \times s \times s$ (empirically set to $s = 7$ voxels). This covariance uncertainty approximation assumes that the registration in more uncertain along the edges of the image than across them. Thus, j_n is less likely if it deviates from μ_j^n in a direction orthogonal to the image edges. In future work, this approximation will be replaced by a local covariance estimate as provided by Simpson *et al.* [7].

Similarly to [6], as j_n is unknown, $p(\tilde{y}_i, \tilde{x}_i|l_i^I, j_n, \mathcal{X}, \theta)p(j_n|l_i^I, \theta)$ is approximated by its expected value given a multivariate Gaussian distribution on the patch L_2 norm and a multivariate Gaussian distribution over the mapping j_n

$$p(\tilde{y}_i, \tilde{x}_i|l_i^I, j_n, \mathcal{X}, \theta)p(j_n|l_i^I, \theta) \approx E[p(\tilde{y}_i, \tilde{x}_i|l_i^I, j_n, \mathcal{X}, \theta)p(j_n|l_i^I, \theta)]$$

$$= \sum_{j^* \in \mathcal{N}_s} p(\tilde{y}_i, \tilde{x}_i|l_i^I, j_n^*, \mathcal{X}, \theta)p(j_n^*|l_i^I, \theta). \quad (1)$$

Under this approximation and under the assumption of conditional independence between $\tilde{y}$ and $\tilde{x}$, then $p(\tilde{y}_i, \tilde{x}_i|l_i^I, j_n^*, \mathcal{X}, \theta)$ is defined as

$$p(\tilde{y}_i, \tilde{x}_i|l_i^I, j_n^*, \mathcal{X}, \theta) = p(\tilde{x}_i|l_i^I, j_n^*, \mathcal{X}, \theta)p(\tilde{y}_i|l_i^I, j_n^*, \mathcal{X}, \theta)$$

$$= e^{-\frac{||\mathcal{N}_p(y_i) - \mathcal{N}_p(y_{nj_n^*})||_2^2}{\sigma_{y_{in}}^2} - \frac{||\mathcal{N}_p(x_i) - \mathcal{N}_p(x_{nj_n^*})||_2^2}{\sigma_{x_{in}}^2}} \quad (2)$$

under the assumption of conditional independence between x and y, and

$$p(j_n^*|l_i^I, \theta) = \frac{1}{Z_{j^*}}e^{-D\Sigma_j^{-1}D^T} \quad (3)$$

In Eq. (1), $\mathcal{N}_s$ is an integration neighbourhood of size $s \times s \times s$ (again with $s = 7$ voxels) of an image similarity component (Eq. 2) and the registration uncertainty distance component (Eq. 3). In Eq. 2, $\mathcal{N}_p(\varkappa)$ is a patch of size $p \times p \times p$ (with $p = 5$ voxels) centred at location $\varkappa$, and in Eq. 3, $D = j_n^* - \mu_n$ is a 1×3 vector characterising the 3-dimensional components of a displacement from μ_n. Both the parameters $\sigma_{y_n}^2$ and $\sigma_{x_n}^2$ denote the sum of a local and a global normally distributed noise model (*iid*) between the observation $\tilde{y}$ and the template y_n, defined as

$$\sigma_{y_{in}}^2 = \sigma(y - y_{n\mu_n})^2 + \sigma(\mathcal{N}_s(y_i) - \mathcal{N}_s(y_{n\mu_n}))^2$$

and equivalently for $\sigma^2_{x_{in}}$, with $\sigma(\varkappa)$ representing the standard deviation of $\varkappa$. Note that the L_2 of the patch can here be used as all images $\mathcal{X}$ have been histogram matched to $\{\tilde{y}_i, \tilde{x}_i\}$ using a 3rd order polynomial fit after non-rigid registration. Finally, Z_{xj^*} is a partition function enforcing

$$\sum_{j^* \in \mathcal{N}_s} p(\tilde{x}_i, j_n^* | l_i^2, x_n, \theta) = 1.$$

The generative model is depicted in Fig. 1. Also of note is the fact that the model extends naturally to more imaging modalities by converting the intensity pairs to K dimensional vectors. In this scenario, the extension of Eq. 2 provides extra complementary information.

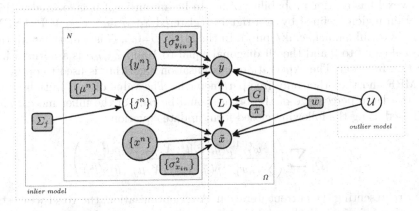

Fig. 1. Generative model of the observed data, with the observed values represented by shaded circles, parameters by shaded rounded-rectangles, and hidden/integrated variables as white circles. Boxes represent replication plates, while the dashed-line boxes annotates the components of the inlier and outlier models.

2.2 Outlier Mixing-Coefficient Prior Estimates

Given the above observation model, one can then estimate the most probable label L, characterising if a certain location belongs to the inlier or outlier class, given by

$$\hat{L} \approx \underset{L}{\mathrm{argmax}} \, p(l | \tilde{y}, \tilde{x}, j, \mathcal{X}, \theta)$$

$$\propto \underset{L}{\mathrm{argmax}} \, p(\tilde{y}, \tilde{x}, j | l, \mathcal{X}, \theta) p(l | \theta) p(\theta)$$

$$= \underset{L}{\mathrm{argmax}} \prod_{i \in \Omega} p(\tilde{y}_i, \tilde{x}_i, j | l_i, \mathcal{X}, \theta) p(l_i | \theta) p(\theta),$$

where $p(\theta)$ is the prior distribution of the parameters θ, here assumed to be non-informative, and

$$p(l_i^k|\theta) = \pi_k \frac{1}{Z_{MRF}} e^{-\beta U_{MRF}(l_i^k, G)}$$

is the combination of a population prior given the location of the brain and smoothness prior given by a probabilistic extension of a Potts-model-based Markov Random Field (MRF), optimised using a mean field theory approximation, as described in [9]. As we are only interested in outliers within the brain, then

$$\pi_O = 0.5 * (\pi_{GM} + \pi_{WM}) \qquad \pi_I = 1 - \pi_O,$$

i.e. a voxel has a prior probability of 0.5 to be an outlier if it is located within the brain region, defined by non-rigidly registered π_{WM} and π_{GM} ICBM SPM priors (www.fil.ion.ucl.ac.uk/spm/). In the MRF, $\beta=0.5$, G is a matrix with the diagonal equal to 0 and the off diagonal equal to 1 and Z_{MRF} is a normalising partition function. The expectation-maximisation algorithm is used to optimise the MRF and the other only free parameter w. The value of w is initialised to 0.9, as a large percentage of the brain should be part of the inlier model, and optimised using the following closed-form update equation

$$w_I^t = \frac{1}{|\Omega|} \sum_i \left(\frac{w_I^{t-1} p(\tilde{y}_i, \tilde{x}_i | l_i^I, \mathcal{X}, \mu_{j_n}, \theta) p(l_i^I)}{\sum_k^K w_k^{t-1} p(\tilde{y}_i, \tilde{x}_i | l_i^k, \mathcal{X}, \mu_{j_n}, \theta) p(l_i^k)} \right)$$

with t representing the current iteration. After optimisation, the voxel-wise estimate of $p(l_i | \tilde{y}_i, \tilde{x}_i, j, \mathcal{X}, \theta)$ provides information about the location of outlier regions as it represents the probability that the voxel in the patch centred at i belong to either the inlier $p(In)_i$ or outlier $p(Out)_i$ classes. This probability can then be used as an estimate of the prior probability that voxel i is an outlier.

2.3   Outlier Segmentation

Given a pair of observed images $\{\tilde{y}, \tilde{x}\}$ and the estimate of $p(l_i | \tilde{y}_i, \tilde{x}_i, j, \mathcal{X}, \theta)$, a voxel-wise segmentation of the outliers of an image can be obtained using a multivariate Gaussian mixture model approach [9] where

$$\pi_i = \{\pi_{WM_i} . p(In)_i, \pi_{GM_i} . p(In)_i, \pi_{CSF_i} . p(In)_i, p(Out)_i\}$$

is a prior distribution for $K = 4$ classes at location i, with π_{WM_i}, π_{GM_i} and π_{CSF_i} representing the healthy population's prior probability to belong to white matter, grey matter and cerebrospinal fluid respectively. Note that any other probabilistic segmentation algorithm can be used at this stage.

2.4 Modality Synthesis

While the proposed generative model enables one to segment and localise out-of-model patterns, a simplified version of the model can also be used for image synthesis. As the process of image synthesis cannot generate more information than the one provided by the observed image $\tilde{x}$ and the priors, we can only look at the inlier part of the described generative model

$$p(\tilde{y}_i, \tilde{x}_i, j_n | l_i^I, \mathcal{X}, \theta).$$

By integrating j_n and assuming that $\tilde{x}_i$ is known but $\tilde{y}_i$ is unknown, one obtains a mixture of mono-modal probability density functions. One can then see this distribution $p(\tilde{y}_i | l_i^I, \mathcal{X}, \theta)$ as a non-parametric probabilistic estimate of $\tilde{y}_i$ using a Gaussian kernel support function, or conversely, a weighted kernel density estimate with the weight given by the $\{\tilde{x}, x_n\}$ patch similarity. Under this model, one can then:

- take random samples from $p(\tilde{y} | \mathcal{X}, \theta)$,
- estimate its expected value $E_{\tilde{y}}[p(\tilde{y} | \mathcal{X}, \theta)]$, which is approximately what is being estimated in [3] but with a different local image similarity,
- calculate the most likely mode of the distribution (i.e. $\hat{y} = \text{argmax}_{\tilde{y}} \, p(\tilde{y} | \mathcal{X}, \theta)$), which provides the most likely intensity given the obtained distribution,
- or make use of the full distribution, providing estimates of the uncertainty of the synthesis process,

all under the assumption of voxel-wise independence.

3 Experiments and Results

3.1 Quantitative Assessment of Image Synthesis in MRI-CT Data

Attenuation correction is an essential requirement for quantification of Positron Emission Tomography (PET) data. In PET/CT acquisition systems, attenuation maps are derived from Computed Tomography (CT) images. However, in hybrid PET/MR scanners, Magnetic Resonance Imaging (MRI) images do not directly provide a patient-specific attenuation map. Current state-of-the-art techniques generate a synthetic CT image from MRI data, either by mapping a tissue segmentation to specific attenuation values, or by directly synthesising the CT image from T1 MRI data [3]. Both these techniques assume that the process of synthesis is deterministic. However, due to the lack of one-to-one mapping between T1 and CT data, some regions can actually have more than one possible cluster of intensities, i.e. the pseudoCT intensity distribution is voxel-wise bimodal. In order to test the advantage of modelling the pseudoCT distribution as a full mixture of Gaussians rather than generating a deterministic intensity, a set of T1-weighted MRI and CT pairs was acquired for 20 elderly subjects with multiple forms of dementia. We compared the state-of-the-art method by Burgos *et al.* [3] to the proposed model. For the proposed model,

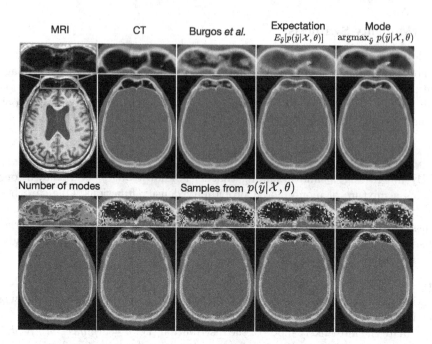

Fig. 2. Top row, from left to right: the original T1-weighted MRI and the patient CT, followed by the output of the method by Burgos et al. and the proposed model's expectation and mode. Bottom row, from left to right: the number of modes of $p(\tilde{y}|\mathcal{X}, \theta)$ (1 mode = transparent, 2 modes = red, 3 modes = yellow), followed by four samples of the same distribution. Note the sharp sinus region in the mode image. Also note the number of modes of the distribution increases in uncertain or boundary regions (Colour figure online).

we estimated the expected value $E_{\tilde{y}}[p(\tilde{y}|\mathcal{X}, \theta)]$, which should provide a result similar to the averaging process of Burgos et al., and the mode of the distribution (i.e. $\hat{y} = \mathrm{argmax}_{\tilde{y}}\, p(\tilde{y}|\mathcal{X}, \theta)$), which should be beneficial in regions where the pseudoCT distribution is bimodal. For the sake of completeness, we also estimate voxel-wisely the number of modes of the estimated distribution, i.e. the number of peaks in the distribution, and also took a few samples from the posterior predictive distribution to demonstrate that the samples vary more in regions with more modes. Results are presented in Fig. 2. Note the sharper intensity in the sinus region, an are which is prone to bimodal intensity distributions. Also note that the four samples of $p(\tilde{y}|\mathcal{X}, \theta)$ are less compact in the sinus region. In order to quantitatively assess the accuracy of the proposed methodology, we estimate the mean squared error (MSE) between the real CT and the pseudo CT using [3], and the *per* voxel expectation and the highest mode of $p(\tilde{y}|\mathcal{X}, \theta)$. The MSE is defined as $\mathrm{MSE} = \frac{1}{|\Omega|}\sum_i(\mathrm{pseudoCT}_i - \mathrm{realCT}_i)^2$. The mean (std) MSE was found to be 40767.4 (3118.3), 39205.9 (2884.1) and 37216.2 (2179.9) for [3], the expectation and the mode respectively. Due to the non Gaussian nature of the pairwise differences in MSE, a Wilcoxon Signed-Rank paired test was used for all statistical comparisons. The voxel-wise mode of $p(\tilde{y}|\mathcal{X}, \theta)$ performed statistically significant better ($p < 0.05$) in terms of MSE when compared to [3]. On the other side, no significant different was found between the expectation $E_{\tilde{y}}[p(\tilde{y}|\mathcal{X}, \theta)]$ and [3]. Furthermore, to test the presence of bias in the synthesis process we also estimated the mean error (ME), defined as $\text{ME} = \frac{1}{|\Omega|}\sum_i(\text{pseudoCT}_i - \text{realCT}_i)$. The mean (std) error for the proposed method was 3.2 (25.5) HU and did not significantly differ from zero, supporting the idea that the current synthesis approach is unbiased.

3.2 Quantitative Assessment of the Outlier Segmentation Using Brainweb

The 3 multiple sclerosis (MS) datasets (mild, moderate and severe models) and one normal anatomy dataset were generated using the BrainWeb MR image simulator. Each dataset had both a simulated T1 and T2 MRI images, and for the 3 MS datasets, an associated ground truth probabilistic lesion segmentation. The simulated data was generated using a FLASH sequence with TR = 18 ms, TE = 10 ms, $\alpha = 30°$ for the T1-weighted MRI, and using a spoiled DSE_LATE sequence with TR = 3300 ms, TE = 35, 120 ms, $\alpha = 90°$ for the T2-weighted MRI, both with a 1-mm isotropic voxel size with simulated 3 % noise [10].

As this experiment is solely testing the feasibility of the proposed methodology for the purpose of locating MS lesions under ideal conditions, the normal anatomy T1 and T2 MRIs are used as a single pair $\mathcal{X}$, i.e. N = 1. The method pro-

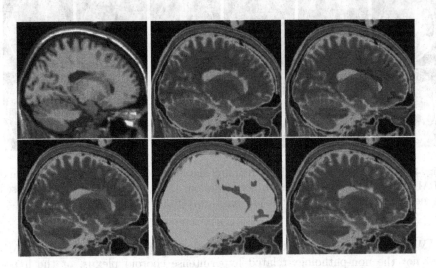

Fig. 3. Brainweb moderate MS model. Left to right) T1 and T2 MRI, groundtruth lesion segmentation and the proposed lesion segmentation, folowed by the inlier observation model $p(\tilde{y}_i, \tilde{x}_i, j_n | l_i^I, \mathcal{X}, \theta)$ and the outlier prior $p(l_i^O | \tilde{y}_i, \tilde{x}_i, j, \mathcal{X}, \theta)$. Note that the outlier prior combines $p(\tilde{y}_i, \tilde{x}_i, j_n | l_i^I, \mathcal{X}, \theta)$ and the label priors.

posed at the end of Sect. 2.2 is here compared to the classical EM-based outlier segmentation method (OSM) [5] with $\kappa = 3$ as recommended. A representative example of both the OSM and proposed methods' results is presented in Fig. 3. OSM obtained a Dice overlap of 3.8, 22.0 and 43.0, for the mild, moderate and severe MS lesion loads respectively, and equivalently, a Dice overlap of 41.8, 51.6 and 65.5 for the proposed method. Note the dramatic increase in accuracy, mainly for the mild MS model. No statistical comparison was performed for this experiment because only three MS models are available in Brainweb.

3.3   Quantitative Assessment of the Outlier Segmentation Using Diabetes Data

This validation aims to determine quantitatively the accuracy of type 2 diabetes white matter lesion (WML) segmentation using the proposed segmentation algorithm and the classical OSM method [5]. For this study, the 20 brain images from the MRBrainS2013 challenge, comprised of both controls and Type 2 diabetes patients (mean age 71 ± 4 years) with WML, were acquired on a 3T Philips scanner with a 3D T1 ($1 \times 1 \times 1$ mm), and fluid attenuated inversion recovery (FLAIR) image ($0.96 \times 0.95 \times 3$ mm) were obtained. Further details about the acquisition and data preprocessing (bias field correction and T1-FLAIR registration) is described in [11] and in the MRBrainS2013 website. Manual WML segmentation was performed on FLAIR images.

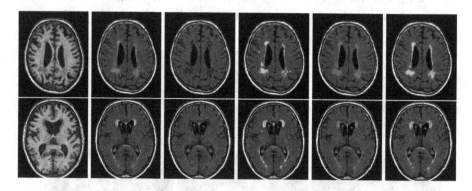

Fig. 4. Subject 4 and 18 of the MRBrainS database. (From left to right) T1 and FLAIR MRI, gold standard lesion segmentation, OMS segmentation, the proposed segmentation and the outlier prior $p(l_i^O | \tilde{y}_i, \tilde{x}_i, j, \mathcal{X}, \theta)$.

With the aim of segmenting only pathological FLAIR hyperintense WML and not the non-pathology-related hyperintense choroid plexus, or the hypo-intense iron accumulation in the globus pallidus (see the manual segmentation in Fig. 4), the template observations $\mathcal{X}$ should contain some non-pathological intensity outliers but no WML. This was achieved by lesion filling [12] the 20 datasets using the manual WML segmentations, which replaces the WML hyper intensities with normal WM intensities. A leave-one-out cross validation was then used to segment the lesions, where for each one of the 20 subjects, the remaining $N = 19$ lesion filled T1-FLAIR pairs were used as templates $\mathcal{X}$, avoiding bias due towards a subject's morphology.

Example results are depicted in Fig. 4. Using both the Dice score and lesion volume as accuracy measures, the proposed method obtained a Dice score of 0.45 and a volume R^2 between estimated and the gold standard volume of 0.94, while the OSM [5] method obtained a mean Dice score of 0.38 and a R^2 of 0.55. As the Dice score errors were Gaussian distributed (tested using the one-sample Kolmogorov-Smirnov test on the residuals), a one-tailed T-test was chosen to assess the presence of statistical significant differences in the Dice score. Under this test statistic, the proposed method achieved statistically significantly higher $(p < 10^{-4})$ Dice overlap when compared to the OSM technique.

3.4 Proof-of-Concept Localisation of Anatomically Abnormal Regions in Anatomical Oncology Data

In order to test the feasibility of the proposed algorithm to detect pathologies with extreme presentation in anatomical imaging and to assess the robustness of the algorithm to variations in image quality, structural contrast, and the amount of outliers in the histogram matching approach, the proposed algorithm was applied to the localisation of high grade tumours from the BRATS 2013 database. The 20 lesion filled T1 and FLAIR images from Sect. 3.3 were used as the templates of non-pathological datasets $\mathcal{X}$. As a proof-of-concept, results for the first two subjects (0301 and 0302) of the training database are presented in Fig. 5. Even with large differences in image contrast, the presence of large lesions and large deformations and low contrast in both T1 and FLAIR images,

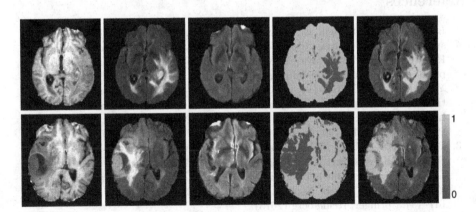

Fig. 5. Tumour localisation using MICCAI BRATS2013 data. Left to right) T1 and FLAIR MRI, synthetic FLAIR using the mode of $p(\tilde{y}_i, \tilde{x}_i, j_n | l_i^I, \mathcal{X}, \theta)$ assuming $\tilde{x}$ is observed, the inlier model $p(\tilde{y}_i, \tilde{x}_i, j_n | l_i^I, \mathcal{X}, \theta)$ and outlier segmentation $p(l_i^O | \tilde{y}_i, \tilde{x}_i, j, \mathcal{X}, \theta)$.

the proposed algorithm was able to localise the non-healthy regions of the image without any pathology specific knowledge about a tumour appearance. Also, for the sake of completeness, a synthetic image was generated using the mode of the distribution. Note that even given a low quality T1 image, the synthetic image is detailed in non-pathological areas.

3.5   Conclusions

This paper proposed a generative model of brain data based from a set of pre-acquired templates. The algorithm enables not only a principled and extensible solution to the problem of modality synthesis, but also a robust way to identify abnormal patterns in medical images. As future work, the proposed framework will be extended to more modalities, allowing it to make use of complementary imaging contrasts to jointly estimate the intensity distributions of multiple modalities. We will also apply the algorithm to the localisation of inhomogeneous pathologies, such as MS and vascular dementia, and other extreme abnormalities, such as traumatic brain injury and cystic lesions. All software will be made available at the time of publication.

Acknowledgments. MJC receives funding from EPSRC (EP/H046410/1). MM and CS are supported by the UCL Leonard Wolfson Experimental Neurology Centre (PR/ylr/18575). SO receives funding from the EPSRC (EP/H046410/1, EP/J020990/1, EP/K005278), the MRC (MR/J01107X/1), the EU-FP7 project VPH-DARE@IT (FP7-ICT-2011-9-601055), the NIHR Biomedical Research Unit (Dementia) at UCL and the National Institute for Health Research University College London Hospitals Biomedical Research Centre (NIHR BRC UCLH/UCL High Impact Initiative - BW.mn.BRC10269).

References

1. Iglesias, J.E., Konukoglu, E., Zikic, D., Glocker, B., Van Leemput, K., Fischl, B.: Is synthesizing MRI contrast useful for inter-modality analysis? In: Mori, K., Sakuma, I., Sato, Y., Barillot, C., Navab, N. (eds.) MICCAI 2013, Part I. LNCS, vol. 8149, pp. 631–638. Springer, Heidelberg (2013)
2. Ye, D.H., Zikic, D., Glocker, B., Criminisi, A., Konukoglu, E.: Modality propagation: coherent synthesis of subject-specific scans with data-driven regularization. In: Mori, K., Sakuma, I., Sato, Y., Barillot, C., Navab, N. (eds.) MICCAI 2013, Part I. LNCS, vol. 8149, pp. 606–613. Springer, Heidelberg (2013)
3. Burgos, N., Cardoso, M.J., Modat, M., Pedemonte, S., Dickson, J., Barnes, A., Duncan, J.S., Atkinson, D., Arridge, S.R., Hutton, B.F., Ourselin, S.: Attenuation correction synthesis for hybrid PET-MR scanners. In: Mori, K., Sakuma, I., Sato, Y., Barillot, C., Navab, N. (eds.) MICCAI 2013, Part I. LNCS, vol. 8149, pp. 147–154. Springer, Heidelberg (2013)
4. Roy, S., Carass, A., Prince, J.: Magnetic resonance image example based contrast synthesis. IEEE Trans. Med. Imaging **32**(12), 2348–2363 (2013)
5. Van Leemput, K., Maes, F., Vandermeulen, D., Colchester, A., Suetens, P.: Automated segmentation of multiple sclerosis lesions by modeloutlier detection. IEEE Trans. Med. Imaging **20**(8), 677–688 (2001)

6. Asman, A.J., Landman, B.A.: Non-local STAPLE: an intensity-driven multi-atlas rater model. In: Ayache, N., Delingette, H., Golland, P., Mori, K. (eds.) MICCAI 2012, Part III. LNCS, vol. 7512, pp. 426–434. Springer, Heidelberg (2012)
7. Simpson, I.J.A., Woolrich, M.W., Cardoso, M.J., Cash, D.M., Modat, M., Schnabel, J.A., Ourselin, S.: A bayesian approach for spatially adaptive regularisation in non-rigid registration. In: Mori, K., Sakuma, I., Sato, Y., Barillot, C., Navab, N. (eds.) MICCAI 2013, Part II. LNCS, vol. 8150, pp. 10–18. Springer, Heidelberg (2013)
8. Knutsson, H., Westin, C.-F., Andersson, M.: Representing local structure using tensors II. In: Heyden, A., Kahl, F. (eds.) SCIA 2011. LNCS, vol. 6688, pp. 545–556. Springer, Heidelberg (2011)
9. Cardoso, M.J., Melbourne, A., Kendall, G.S., Modat, M., Robertson, N.J., Marlow, N., Ourselin, S.: AdaPT: an adaptive preterm segmentation algorithm for neonatal brain MRI. NeuroImage **65**, 97–108 (2013)
10. Aubert-Broche, B., Griffin, M., Pike, G.B., Evans, A.C., Collins, D.L.: Twenty new digital brain phantoms for creation of validation image data bases. IEEE Trans. Med. Imaging **25**(11), 1410–1416 (2006)
11. Prados, F., Cardoso, M.J., MacManus, D., Wheeler-Kingshott, C.A.M., Ourselin, S.: A modality-agnostic patch-based technique for lesion filling in multiple sclerosis. In: Golland, P., Hata, N., Barillot, C., Hornegger, J., Howe, R. (eds.) MICCAI 2014, Part II. LNCS, vol. 8674, pp. 781–788. Springer, Heidelberg (2014)
12. Battaglini, M., Jenkinson, M., De Stefano, N.: Evaluating and reducing the impact of white matter lesions on brain volume measurements. Hum. Brain Mapp. **33**(9), 2062–2071 (2012)

Generative Method to Discover Genetically Driven Image Biomarkers

Nematollah K. Batmanghelich[1][(✉)], Ardavan Saeedi[1], Michael Cho[2],
Raul San Jose Estepar[2], and Polina Golland[1]

[1] Computer Science and Artificial Intelligence Lab, MIT, Cambridge, USA
`kayhan@csail.mit.edu`
[2] Harvard Medical School, Brigham and Womens Hospital, Boston, USA

Abstract. We present a generative probabilistic approach to discovery of disease subtypes determined by the genetic variants. In many diseases, multiple types of pathology may present simultaneously in a patient, making quantification of the disease challenging. Our method seeks common co-occurring image and genetic patterns in a population as a way to model these two different data types jointly. We assume that each patient is a mixture of multiple disease subtypes and use the joint generative model of image and genetic markers to identify disease subtypes guided by known genetic influences. Our model is based on a variant of the so-called topic models that uncover the latent structure in a collection of data. We derive an efficient variational inference algorithm to extract patterns of co-occurrence and to quantify the presence of heterogeneous disease processes in each patient. We evaluate the method on simulated data and illustrate its use in the context of Chronic Obstructive Pulmonary Disease (COPD) to characterize the relationship between image and genetic signatures of COPD subtypes in a large patient cohort.

1 Introduction

We propose and demonstrate a joint model of image and genetic variation associated with a disease. Our goal is to identify disease-specific image biomarkers that are also correlated with side information, such as the genetic code or other biologically relevant indicators. Our approach targets diseases that can be thought of as a superposition of different processes, or subtypes, that are subject to genetic influences and are often present simultaneously in the same patient. Our motivation comes from a study of the Chronic Obstructive Pulmonary Disease (COPD), but the resulting model is applicable to a wide range of heterogeneous disorders.

COPD is a lung disease characterized by chronic and progressive difficulty in breathing; it is one of the leading causes of death in the United States [11]. COPD is often associated with emphysema, i.e., the destruction of lung air sacs, and an airway disease, which is caused by inflammation of the airways. In this

---

N.K. Batmanghelich and A. Saeedi—equal contribution.

© Springer International Publishing Switzerland 2015
S. Ourselin et al. (Eds.): IPMI 2015, LNCS 9123, pp. 30–42, 2015.
DOI: 10.1007/978-3-319-19992-4_3

paper, we focus on modeling emphysema based on lung CT images. Emphysema exhibits many subtypes. It is common for several subtypes to co-occur in the same lung [13]. Genetic factors play an important role in COPD [11], and it is believed that variability of COPD is driven by genetics [5]. We therefore aim to quantify the lung tissue heterogeneity that is associated with the genetic variations in the patient cohort.

CT imaging is used to measure the extent of COPD, and particularly of emphysema. The standard approach to quantifying emphysema is to use the volume of sub-threshold intensities in the lung as a surrogate measure for the volume of emphysema [6]. More recently, histograms [10], texture descriptors [15], and combination of both [16] have been proposed to classify subtypes of emphysema based on training sets of CT patches labeled by clinical experts. While histograms and intensity features have been shown to be important for emphysema characterization, the clinical definitions of disease subtypes are based on visual assessment of CT images by clinicians and are not necessarily genetically driven. In prior studies, association between image and genetic variants was established as a separate stage of analysis and was not taken into account when extracting relevant biomarkers from images.

Most methodological innovations in joint analysis of imaging and genetics have used image data as an intermediate phenotype to enhance the discovery of relevant genetic markers in the context of neuro-degenerative diseases [3]. In the context of COPD, Castaldi et al. [5] used local histograms to measure distinct emphysema patters and performed genome-wide association study (GWAS) to validate their results. In contrast to prior research in imaging genetics, we use the results of genetic analysis to help us characterize image patterns associated with the disease, in effect reversing the direction of analysis for disorders with high anatomical heterogeneity and available information on genetic influences. We model image and genetic variations jointly, and demonstrate efficient inference of co-occurrence pattern, as indicated by our results.

In this paper, we assume that a few important genetic markers associated with the disease are available. We build a generative model that captures the commonly occurring image and genetic patterns in a population. Each subject is modeled as a sample from the population-wide collection of joint image and genetic patterns. This abstraction at the population level reveals the associations between image-based and genetic subtypes and uses genetic information to guide the definition of image biomarkers for distinct disease subtypes. Our method is based on a non-parametric topic modeling [17], originally developed in machine learning for characterizing structure of documents. We build an analogy between topics contributing words to a document and disease subtypes contributing local image patterns and minor alleles to a patient. The closest work to our approach is by Batmanghelich et al. [2] who developed a topic model for global histograms of the lung intensity values. The model did not include local image patterns; genotype data was not considered as part of the model. In contrast, our topic model builds on rich local descriptors and integrates image and genetic information into a single framework. Our approach can be readily extended to include other clinical or demographic data.

We evaluate the method on a synthetic data set that matches our clinical assumptions, demonstrating substantial benefits of using a hierarchical population model to capture common patterns of heterogeneity in the image phenotype and in the genetic code. We also show that the genetic data as side information boosts the performance of the method compared to the baselines and a variant of our model without the genetic data. Finally, we illustrate an application of our method to a study of COPD and identify common emphysema subtypes associated with genetic factors implicated in COPD.

Table 1. Model variables and Variational Bayes (VB) estimates used throughout the paper.

Model Variables	
I_{sn}	image descriptor of supervoxel n in subject s
G_{sm}	genetic location of minor allele m in subject s
z_{sn}^{I}	subject-specific topic that generates super-voxel n in subject s, $1 \leq z_{s,n}^{I} \leq T$
z_{sm}^{G}	subject-specific topic that generates minor allele m in subject s, $1 \leq z_{s,m}^{G} \leq T$
c_{st}	population-level topic that serves as subject-specific topic t in subject s, $1 \leq c_{st} \leq K$
v	parameter vector that determines the stick-breaking proportions of topics in a population template
π_s	parameter vector that determines the stick-breaking proportions of topics in subject s
(μ_k, Σ_k)	mean and covariance matrix of image descriptors for population-level topic k
β_k	frequency of different locations in genetic signatures for population-level topic k
ω	hyper-parameters of the Beta prior for v
α	hyper-parameters for the Beta prior for π_s
η^{I}	hyper-parameters of the Normal-Inverse-Wishart prior for (μ_k, Σ_k)
η^{G}	hyper-parameters of the Dirichlet prior for β_k
VB Estimates	
$(\hat{\mu}_k, \hat{\Sigma}_k)$	mean and covariance of image descriptors for population-level topic k
$\hat{\beta}_k$	frequency of different locations in genetic signatures for population-level topic k

2   Model

In this section, we describe the generative model for image and genetic data based on a population-wide common patterns that are instantiated in each subject. Our notation is summarized in Table 1 and the generative process is illustrated in Fig. 1.

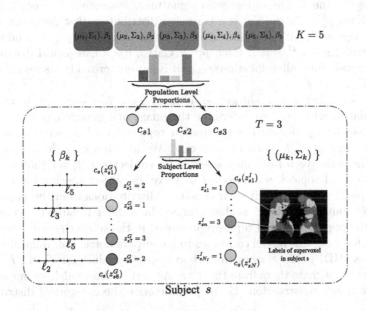

Fig. 1. Subject s draws a subset of T topics from K population-level topics. Indices of the subject-level topics are stored in $c_{s1}, .., c_{sT}$ drawn from a categorical distribution. At the subject level, indices of the supervoxels $\{z_{sn}^I\}$ and locations of minor alleles $\{z_{s,m}^G\}$ are drawn from the subject-specific categorical distribution. Vector c_s acts as a map from subject-specific topics to the population-level topics (i.e., $c_s(z_{sm}^G)$ or $c_s(z_{sn}^I)$).

Image and Genetic Data. We assume each subject in a study is characterized by an image and a genetic signature for the loci in the genome *previously* implicated in the disease. Based on the analogy to the "bag-of-words" representation [14], we assume that an image domain is divided for each subject into relatively homogeneous spatially contiguous regions (i.e., "supervoxels"). We let $I_{sn} \in \mathbb{R}^D$ denote the D-dimensional descriptor of supervoxel n in subject s that summarizes the intensity and texture properties of the supervoxel. The genetic data in our problem comes in a form of minor allele counts (0, 1 or 2) for a set of L loci. Our representation for genetic data is inspired by the commonly used additive model in GWAS analysis [4]. In particular, we assume that the risk of the disease increases monotonically by the minor allele count. We let $G_{sm} \in \{1, \cdots, L\}$ denote minor allele m in genetic signature of subject s.

For example, suppose $L = 2$, and subject s has one and two minor alleles in locations ℓ_1 and ℓ_2 respectively. This subject is represented by a list of 3 elements $G_s = \{\ell_1, \ell_2, \ell_2\}$.

Population Model. Our population model is based on the Hierarchical Dirichlet Process (HDP) [17]. The model assumes a collection of K "topics" that are shared across subjects in the population. We let p_k^I and p_k^G denote the distributions for the image and genetic signatures, respectively, associated with topic k. Each $p_k^I = \mathcal{N}(\mu_k, \Sigma_k)$ is a Gaussian distribution that generates supervoxel descriptors I_{sn}; it is parameterized by its mean vector $\mu_k \in \mathbb{R}^D$ and covariance matrix $\Sigma_k \in \mathbb{R}^D \times \mathbb{R}^D$. Each $p_k^G = \text{Cat}(\beta_k)$ is a categorical distribution that generates minor allele locations G_{sm}; it is parameterized by its weight vector $\beta_k \in (0, 1)^L$.

When sampling a new subject s, at most $T < K$ topics are drawn from the population-wide pool to determine the image and genetic signature of this subject. We let c_{st} denote the population topic selected to serve as subject-specific topic t ($1 \leq t \leq T$) in subject s. We also use $c_s = [c_{s1}, \ldots, c_{sT}]$ to refer to the entire vector of topics selected for subject s. $c_s[t] = k$ indicates that population-level topic k was selected to serve as subject-specific topic t. The subject-specific topics inherit their signature distributions from the population prototypes, but each subject is characterized by a different subset and proportions of the population-level topics represented in the subject-specific data.

As $T, K \to \infty$, this model converges to a non-parametric Hierarchical Dirichlet Process (HDP) [17]. Rather than choose specific values for T and K, HDP enables us to estimate them from the data. As part of this model, we employ the "stick-breaking" construction [17] to parameterize the categorical distribution for c_{st}:

$$c_{st} \sim \text{Cat-SB}(v), \tag{1}$$

where $\text{Cat-SB}(v)$ is a categorical distribution whose weights are generated through the stick-breaking process from the (potentially infinite) parameter vector v whose components are in the interval $(0, 1)$. Formally, if we define a random variable $x \sim \text{Cat-SB}(v)$, then

$$p(x) \triangleq v_x \prod_{i=1}^{x-1} (1 - v_i) \quad \text{for } x = 1, \ldots. \tag{2}$$

This parameterization accepts infinite alphabets. The stick-breaking construction penalizes high number of topics hence encouraging parsimonious representation of data. A similar construction enables an automatic selection of the number of topics at the population level and at the subject level. We employ a truncated HDP variant that uses finite values for T and K [9]. In this setup, $v \in (0, 1)^{K-1}$. In contrast to finite (fixed) models, we set K to high enough value, and the estimation procedure uses as many topics as needed but not necessarily all K topics to explain the observations.

Subject-Specific Data. To generate an image descriptor for supervoxel n in subject s, we sample random variable $z_{sn}^I \sim \text{Cat-SB}(\pi_s)$ from a categorical distribution parameterized by the vector of stick-breaking proportions $\pi_s \in (0, 1)^{T-1}$. $z_{sn}^I = t$ indicates that the subject-specific topic t generates image descriptor I_{sn}:

$$I_{sn}|z_{sn}^I, c_s \sim \mathcal{N}\left(\mu_{c_s[z_{sn}^I]}, \Sigma_{c_s[z_{sn}^I]}\right). \tag{3}$$

Similarly, to generate minor allele location m in subject s, we sample random variable $z_{sm}^G \sim \text{Cat-SB}(\pi_s)$ and draw G_{sm} from the corresponding genetic signature of subject-specific topic z_{sm}^G:

$$G_{sm}|z_{sm}^G, c_s \sim \text{Cat}\left(\beta_{c_s[z_{sm}^G]}\right). \tag{4}$$

Priors. Following the Bayesian approach, we define priors for the remaining latent variables $\{v_k, \pi_{st}\}$ and the parameters of the likelihood distributions $\{\mu_k, \Sigma_k, \beta_k\}$. For the computational reasons, we choose the priors from the exponential family. Specifically, we use the Beta distribution as the prior of the parameter vectors v and π_s that determine the stick-breaking proportions at the population-wide and subject-specific levels, respectively:

$$v_k \sim \text{Beta}(1, \omega), \quad k = 1, \ldots, K - 1, \tag{5}$$
$$\pi_{st} \sim \text{Beta}(1, \alpha), \quad t = 1, \ldots, T - 1, \tag{6}$$

where $\omega > 0$ and $\alpha > 0$ are the corresponding shape parameters of the Beta distribution. For computational reasons, we also assume priors for image and genetic signature parameters that are conjugate for the corresponding likelihood distributions (3) and (4):

$$\mu_k, \Sigma_k \sim \text{NIW}(\eta^I) \quad \text{and} \quad \beta_k \sim \text{Dir}(\eta^G),$$

where $\text{NIW}(\eta)$ is the Normal-Inverse-Wishart distribution with parameters η and $\text{Dir}(\eta)$ is the Dirichlet distributions with parameters η.

3 Inference

Given a study of S subjects with their respective image descriptors $\{I_{sn}\}$ and genetic signatures $\{G_{sm}\}$, we seek posterior distributions of the model parameters. Since exact computation of the posterior quantities is computationally intractable, we resort to an approximation. Due to the size of data and its dimensionality, sampling is computationally impractical. We therefore derive a Variational Bayes (VB) approximation [9]. For notational convenience, we define $\mathcal{D} = \{I_{sn}, G_{sm}\}_{s=1}^S$ to be all image and genetic data, $\mathcal{S} = \{z_{sn}^I, z_{s,m}^G, c_s, \pi_s\}_{s=1}^S$ to be all subject-specific latent variables, and $\mathcal{P} = \{\mu_k, \Sigma_k, \beta_k, v_k\}_{k=1}^K$ to be all population-based latent variables. We omit fixed hyper-parameters to simplify the notation. Variational Bayes inference selects an approximating distribution $q(\mathcal{S}, \mathcal{P})$ for the true posterior distribution $p(\mathcal{S}, \mathcal{P}|\mathcal{D})$ by minimizing the cost functional

$$F(q) = \mathbb{E}_q\left[\ln p(\mathcal{D}, \mathcal{S}, \mathcal{P})\right] - \mathbb{E}_q\left[\ln q(\mathcal{S}, \mathcal{P})\right], \tag{7}$$

where $\mathbb{E}_q$ is the expectation with respect to the probability measure q and Eq. (7) can be thought of as the KL divergence between the approximating distribution and the true posterior distribution. Additional details and the update rules of the iterative inference algorithm can be found in the Appendix.

We use the parameters of the approximating distribution $q(\mathcal{S}, \mathcal{P})$ to construct estimates of the relevant model parameters. Specifically, we seek the estimates $(\hat{\mu}_k, \hat{\Sigma}_k)$ of the image descriptors and the estimates $\hat{\beta}_k$ of the associated genetic signatures for each population-level topic k. Moreover, for each subject s we estimate a distribution over the population topics for each supervoxel to visualize the spatial distributions of disease subtypes for clinical assessment.

4   Experiments

In this section, we demonstrate and evaluate the algorithm on simulated and real data. We use simulated data to study the advantages offered by the hierarchical model and investigate the effects of the side information (genetic data in our case) on the accuracy of recovering the latent topics. We also investigate the behavior of the model with respect to the hyper-parameters. We illustrate the method on a subset of a large-scale study of lung based on CT images of COPD patients. In this experiment, we characterize co-occurring image and genetic patterns in the data.

4.1   Simulation

To evaluate the performance of the method, we sampled the data from the proposed hierarchical model. In particular, we generated image and genetic signatures for $S = 100$ subjects from 20 population-level topics while limiting the number of subject-specific topics to 5. We used Beta(1, 8) and Beta(1, 1) for population-level and subject-specific stick-breaking proportions that govern the relative frequencies of the topics. Such choice generates higher variability of weights at the population level than those at the subject level. We drew the image signature parameters for population topics from a 2-dimensional NIW distribution with a zero mean vector, identity covariance matrix, and the shape and scale parameters set to 5 and 0.5. The subject-specific image signatures ($N = 75$ for all s) are drawn from Gaussian distributions whose parameters are determined by the corresponding image parameters of the population topic. The weights of the genetic signatures for each population-level topic are drawn from a Dirichlet distribution with all parameters set to one. The subject-specific genetic signatures ($M = 65$ for all s) are drawn from a categorical distributions determined by the weights of the corresponding genetic signature of the topic model.

Hyper-parameters ω and α control the model size, i.e., the number of topics at the population level and the subject level respectively. Of the two, the population-level parameter ω has a stronger influence on how well the model explains subject-specific data. We sweep a range (0.5, 5.0) for both parameters.

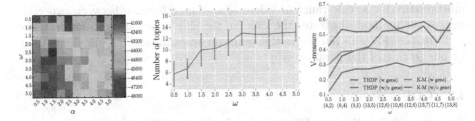

Fig. 2. Simulated data results. Left: variational lower bound $F(q^*)$ for different values of (α, ω). Middle: the number of topics discovered by the model as a function of ω averaged over α. Right: normalized mutual information between the true and the discovered topics for our method and for k-means clustering (K-M) applied to pooled data. The number of discovered topics is reported in brackets under the corresponding value of ω (w gene, w/o gene). Two variants of our method are denoted by THDP.

Figure 2(Left) reports the value of the lower bound $F(q^*)$ for each pair of the parameter settings which we use for model selection. We observe that the algorithm's performance depends smoothly on the parameter values. In subsequent experiments, we set α to the optimal values based on $F(q^*)$ and study the behavior of the model for a range of values of ω. Figure 2(Middle) reports the number of population topics estimated by the model as a function of ω. Not surprisingly, the model size grows with ω, but is quite stable for a wide range of values of ω.

To evaluate the effects of the hierarchical model and of joint modeling of image and genetic information, we compare our approach (with and without genetic data) to a k-means algorithm applied to the pooled data from all subjects. We apply the baseline k-means clustering to image data only, and also to the data set of image signatures of all supervoxels concatenated with the entire genetic signature of the same subject. Figure 2(Right) compares our method with the two k-means variants using a standard measure of normalized mutual information (v-measure) [12] between the true and discovered topics. The measure varies between 0 and 1; 1 corresponds to the perfect match. While adding genetic information to image features boosts the performance of our method and clustering on pooled data, our hierarchical model outperforms both baseline methods

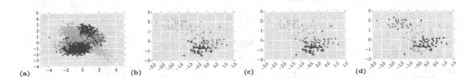

Fig. 3. Example simulated image data using 2D features. (a) Features from all subjects pooled into one set. Colors correspond to true topics, unavailable to the algorithm. (b) Image features for a single subject in a set. (c) Topics recovered by our algorithm (with genetic data) for the same subject based on the whole data set. (d) Topics recovered by k-means clustering applied to the pooled data in (a) (Colour figure online).

substantially for a wide range of values of ω. The difference between two variants of our method illustrates the value of the side information to improve the performance. Figure 3 illustrates this point on an example from our simulations for one setting of the parameters.

4.2   COPD Study

We apply the method to CT images of lung in 2399 subjects from a the COPDGene study [11]. After automatic segmentation of the lung, we employ a modified version of super-voxelization method [1] to subdivide the lungs into coherent, spatially contiguous regions. From each supervoxel, we extract local histogram of the intensity (CT number) as a local descriptor. We choose to work with this particular descriptor because it has been shown to be highly informative for emphysema sub-typing [5]. Furthermore, working with such a straightforward image descriptor removes the confounding parameters introduced by more complex image descriptors and helps us to quantify the contribution of the model. For each supervoxel, we use PCA to map the local intensity histogram to a 30-dimensional vector, i.e., $I_{sn} \in \mathbb{R}^{30}$. The 30 principal components explain more than 99 % of variance in the entire data. Moreover, we complied a list of SNPs previously identified in genome-wide association studies for COPD or lung function measurements that define COPD (FEV1 and FEV1/FVC) [7]. Based on our experience with the simulated data and the expected number of disease subtypes, we set $K = 30$ and $T = 10$. Furthermore, we set $\alpha = 1$, $\omega = 5$ and set uninformative priors for the image and genetic signature parameters.

The method summarizes the population into 23 population-level topics. The number of topics per patient varies from one to four. Figure 4 visualizes the top four topics where each topic is an intensity distribution. The tables on the right are the top six minor alleles in the genetic signature of each topic. We observe that the genetic signatures (relative weights or rankings) vary across topics, suggesting variable genetic patterns that give rise to different image properties. To visualize the spatial distribution of the topics, we computed the membership

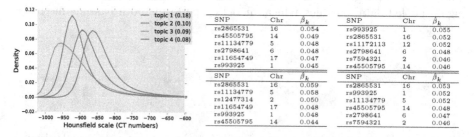

SNP	Chr	$\hat{\beta}_k$		SNP	Chr	$\hat{\beta}_k$
rs2865531	16	0.054		rs993925	1	0.055
rs45505795	14	0.049		rs2865531	16	0.052
rs11134779	5	0.048		rs11172113	12	0.052
rs2798641	6	0.048		rs2798641	6	0.048
rs11654749	17	0.047		rs7594321	2	0.046
rs993925	1	0.045		rs45505795	14	0.046
SNP	**Chr**	$\hat{\beta}_k$		**SNP**	**Chr**	$\hat{\beta}_k$
rs2865531	16	0.059		rs2865531	16	0.053
rs11134779	5	0.058		rs993925	1	0.052
rs12477314	2	0.050		rs11134779	5	0.052
rs11654749	17	0.048		rs45505795	14	0.048
rs993925	1	0.048		rs2798641	6	0.047
rs45505795	14	0.044		rs7594321	2	0.046

Fig. 4. Four first topics, ranked according to their proportions. Each histogram density is one topic. The values inside of the brackets are the overall proportion computed from the posterior. The tables on the right report the top six SNPs for each topic with their estimated relative weights. We observe that the genetic signatures vary across topics.

value of the supervoxel in the population-level topics (i.e., $\sum_t \phi^I_{sn}(t)\xi_{st}$), which yields one image per topic for each subject. Then, we warped the resulting probability maps to a common coordinate frame (i.e., lung atlas). Figure 5 demonstrates average distributions of the three topics that tend to localize around the boundary of the lung.

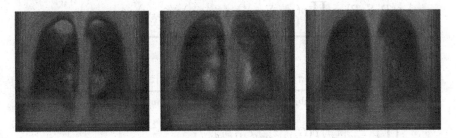

Fig. 5. Spatial average distribution of three topics. The color indicates the posterior probability. The higher the intensity of the color, the higher the probability (Colour figure online).

5   Conclusions

We proposed and demonstrated a generative model based on the truncated Hierarchical Dirichlet Process to identify common image and genetic patterns in a population. The underlying assumption of our model is that every subject is a superposition of few topics. Our main contribution is to model side information- in this case, genetic variants - jointly with imaging data. We demonstrated the method on synthesized data and reported preliminary results for the COPD study (Fig. 5).

Once population-wide template of image and genetic variability has been constructed, it enables us to answer many interesting questions about the heterogeneity of the disease in the population and in individual subjects. In particular, investigating the variability of topic representation in different subjects and using subject-specific topic proportions promise to provide a handle on how the disease varies in a population and suggest numerous interesting directions for future work.

Acknowledgements. This work was supported by NIH NIBIB NAMIC U54-EB005149, NIH NCRR NAC P41-RR13218 and NIH NIBIB NAC P41-EB015902, NHLBI R01HL089856, R01HL089897, K08HL097029, R01HL113264, 5K25HL104085, 5R01HL116931, and 5R01HL116473. The COPDGene study (NCT00608764) is also supported by the COPD Foundation through contributions made to an Industry Advisory Board comprised of AstraZeneca, Boehringer Ingelheim, Novartis, Pfizer, Siemens, GlaxoSmithKline and Sunovion.

Appendix: Variational Bayes Inference Procedure

Combining all components of the model defined in Sect. 2, we construct the joint distribution of all variables in the model (Fig. 6):

$$p(\mathcal{D}, \mathcal{S}, \mathcal{P}) = \underbrace{\prod_{k=1}^{K} p(\mu_k, \Sigma_k; \eta^I)\, p(\beta_k; \eta^G)\, p(v_k; \omega)}_{\text{population-level topics}} \times$$

$$\prod_{s=1}^{S} \prod_{t=1}^{T} \underbrace{p(c_{st}|v_k) p(\pi_{st}; \alpha)}_{\text{topics for subject } s} \prod_{n=1}^{N} \underbrace{p(z_{sn}^I|\pi_{st})}_{\text{image topic}} \underbrace{p(I_{sn}|z_{sn}^I, c_{st}, \{\mu_k, \Sigma_k\})}_{\text{image likelihood}}$$

$$\prod_{m=1}^{M} \underbrace{p(z_{sm}^G|\pi_{st})}_{\text{genetic topic}} \underbrace{p(G_{sm}|z_{sm}^G, c_{st}, \beta_k)}_{\text{genetic likelihood}},$$

where N and M are the number of supervoxels and minor alleles, respectively, identified for subject s.

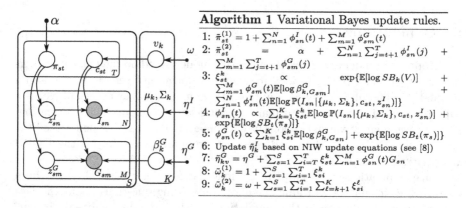

Algorithm 1 Variational Bayes update rules.

1: $\tilde{\pi}_{st}^{(1)} = 1 + \sum_{n=1}^{N} \phi_{sn}^I(t) + \sum_{m=1}^{M} \phi_{sm}^G(t)$
2: $\tilde{\pi}_{st}^{(2)} = \alpha + \sum_{n=1}^{N} \sum_{j=t+1}^{T} \phi_{sn}^I(j) + \sum_{m=1}^{M} \sum_{j=t+1}^{T} \phi_{sm}^G(j)$
3: $\xi_{st}^k \propto \exp\{\mathbb{E}[\log SB_k(V)] + \sum_{m=1}^{M} \phi_{sm}^G(t)\mathbb{E}[\log \beta_{k,G_{sm}}^G] + \sum_{n=1}^{N} \phi_{sn}^I(t)\mathbb{E}[\log \mathbb{P}(I_{sn}|\{\mu_k, \Sigma_k\}, c_{st}, z_{sn}^I)]\}$
4: $\phi_{sn}^I(t) \propto \sum_{k=1}^{K} \xi_{st}^k \mathbb{E}[\log \mathbb{P}(I_{sn}|\{\mu_k, \Sigma_k\}, c_{st}, z_{sn}^I)] + \exp\{\mathbb{E}[\log SB_t(\pi_s)]\}$
5: $\phi_{sn}^G(t) \propto \sum_{k=1}^{K} \xi_{st}^k \mathbb{E}[\log \beta_{k,G_{sn}}^G] + \exp\{\mathbb{E}[\log SB_t(\pi_s)]\}$
6: Update $\tilde{\eta}_k^I$ based on NIW update equations (see [8])
7: $\tilde{\eta}_{kv}^G = \eta^G + \sum_{s=1}^{S} \sum_{i=T}^{T} \xi_{st}^k \sum_{n=1}^{M} \phi_{sn}^G(t) G_{sn}$
8: $\tilde{\omega}_k^{(1)} = 1 + \sum_{s=1}^{S} \sum_{i=1}^{T} \xi_{si}^k$
9: $\tilde{\omega}_k^{(2)} = \omega + \sum_{s=1}^{S} \sum_{i=1}^{T} \sum_{\ell=k+1}^{K} \xi_{si}^\ell$

Fig. 6. Left: Graphical model that represents the joint distribution. The open gray and white circles correspond to the observed and the latent random variables, respectively. The full circles represent fixed hyper-parameters. Superscript I and G denote image and genetic parts of the model respectively. Right: Update rules for the variational parameters.

We choose a factorization for the distribution q that captures most model assumptions and yet is computationally tractable:

$$q(\mathcal{S}, \mathcal{P}) = \underbrace{\prod_{k=1}^{K} \text{NIW}(\mu_k, \Sigma_k; \tilde{\eta}_k^I) \, \text{Dir}(\beta_k; \tilde{\eta}_k^G) \, \text{Beta}(\upsilon_k; \tilde{\omega}_k) \times}_{\text{population-level topics}}$$

$$\prod_{s=1}^{S} \prod_{t=1}^{T} \underbrace{\text{Cat}(c_{st}; \xi_{st}) \, \text{Beta}(\pi_{st}; \tilde{\alpha}_{st})}_{\text{topics for subject } s} \prod_{n=1}^{N} \underbrace{\text{Cat}(z_{sn}^I; \phi_{sn}^I)}_{\text{image topic}} \prod_{m=1}^{M} \underbrace{\text{Cat}(z_{sm}^G; \phi_{sm}^G)}_{\text{genetic topic}},$$

where we choose an appropriate approximating distribution for each latent variable and use ˜ to denote parameters of the approximating distributions. The optimization is defined in the space of the variational parameters $\{\tilde{\eta}^I, \tilde{\eta}^G, \tilde{\omega}, \xi, \tilde{\alpha}, \phi^I, \phi^G\}$. We omit the derivation of the updates due to space constraints; Algorithm 1 provides pseudocode for the resulting updates. We run the algorithm five times starting from different random initializations and report the result with the highest lower bound $F(q)$.

Once the algorithm converges, we estimate the population-level quantities of interest as means of the corresponding approximating distributions:

$$\hat{\mu}_k = \mathbb{E}\left[\mu_k | \mathcal{D}\right] \approx \mathbb{E}_q\left[\mu_k; \tilde{\eta}_k^I\right], \quad \hat{\Sigma}_k = \mathbb{E}\left[\Sigma_k | \mathcal{D}\right] \approx \mathbb{E}_q\left[\Sigma_k; \tilde{\eta}_k^I\right],$$

$$\hat{\beta}_k = \mathbb{E}\left[\beta_k | \mathcal{D}\right] \approx \mathbb{E}_q\left[\beta_k^G; \tilde{\eta}_k^G\right].$$

Each expectation above can be easily evaluated from the parameters of the corresponding distribution. In addition, we construct spatial maps that display the posterior probability of each population topic for each supervoxel in a particular subject s to visually evaluate the disease structure in that subject.

References

1. Achanta, R., Shaji, A., Smith, K., Lucchi, A., Fua, P., Susstrunk, S.: Slic superpixels compared to state-of-the-art superpixel methods. IEEE Trans. Pattern Anal. Mach. Intell. **34**(11), 2274–2282 (2012)
2. Batmanghelich, K.N., Cho, M., Jose, R.S., Golland, P.: Spherical topic models for imaging phenotype discovery in genetic studies. In: Cardoso, M.J., Simpson, I., Arbel, T., Precup, D., Ribbens, A. (eds.) BAMBI 2014. LNCS, vol. 8677, pp. 107–117. Springer, Heidelberg (2014)
3. Batmanghelich, N.K., Dalca, A.V., Sabuncu, M.R., Golland, P.: Joint modeling of imaging and genetics. In: Gee, J.C., Joshi, S., Pohl, K.M., Wells, W.M., Zöllei, L. (eds.) IPMI 2013. LNCS, vol. 7917, pp. 766–777. Springer, Heidelberg (2013)
4. Bush, W.S., Moore, J.H.: Genome-wide association studies. PLoS Comput. Biol. **8**(12), e1002822 (2012)
5. Castaldi, P.J., et al.: Genome-wide association identifies regulatory loci associated with distinct local histogram emphysema patterns. Am. J. Respir. Crit. Care Med. **190**(4), 399–409 (2014)

6. Castaldi, P.J., San José Estépar, R., Mendoza, C.S., Hersh, C.P., Laird, N., Crapo, J.D., Lynch, D.A., Silverman, E.K., Washko, G.R.: Distinct quantitative computed tomography emphysema patterns are associated with physiology and function in smokers. Am. J. Respir. Crit. Care Med. **188**(9), 1083–1090 (2013)
7. Cho, M.H., et al.: Risk loci for chronic obstructive pulmonary disease: a genome-wide association study and meta-analysis. Lancet Respir. Med. **2**(3), 214–225 (2014)
8. Guan, Y., Dy, J.G., Niu, D., Ghahramani, Z.: Variational inference for nonparametric multiple clustering. In: MultiClust Workshop, KDD 2010 (2010)
9. Hoffman, M.D., Blei, D.M., Wang, C., Paisley, J.: Stochastic variational inference. J. Mach. Learn. Res. **14**(1), 1303–1347 (2013)
10. Mendoza, C.S., et al.: Emphysema quantification in a multi-scanner hrct cohort using local intensity distributions. In: 2012 9th IEEE International Symposium on Biomedical Imaging (ISBI), pp. 474–477. IEEE (2012)
11. Regan, E.A., Hokanson, J.E., Murphy, J.R., Make, B., Lynch, D.A., Beaty, T.H., Curran-Everett, D., Silverman, E.K., Crapo, J.D.: Genetic epidemiology of copd (copdgene) study design. COPD: J. Chronic Obstructive Pulm. Dis. **7**(1), 32–43 (2011)
12. Rosenberg, A., Hirschberg, J.: V-measure: a conditional entropy-based external cluster evaluation measure. In: EMNLP-CoNLL, vol. 7, pp. 410–420. Citeseer (2007)
13. Satoh, K., Kobayashi, T., Misao, T., Hitani, Y., Yamamoto, Y., Nishiyama, Y., Ohkawa, M.: CT assessment of subtypes of pulmonary emphysema in smokers. CHEST J. **120**(3), 725–729 (2001)
14. Sivic, J., Zisserman, A.: Efficient visual search of videos cast as text retrieval. IEEE Trans. Pattern Anal. Mach. Intell. **31**(4), 591–606 (2009)
15. Song, Y., Cai, W., Zhou, Y., Feng, D.D.: Feature-based image patch approximation for lung tissue classification. IEEE Trans. Med. Imaging **32**(4), 797–808 (2013)
16. Sorensen, L., Shaker, S.B., De Bruijne, M.: Quantitative analysis of pulmonary emphysema using local binary patterns. IEEE Trans. Med. Imaging **29**(2), 559–569 (2010)
17. Teh, Y.W., Jordan, M.I., Beal, M.J., Blei, D.M.: Hierarchical dirichlet processes. J. Am. Stat. Assoc. **101**(476), 1566–1581 (2006)

MRI Reconstruction

A Joint Acquisition-Estimation Framework for MR Phase Imaging

Joseph Dagher[✉]

Department of Medical Imaging, The University of Arizona,
Tucson, AZ, USA
jdagher@email.arizona.edu

Abstract. Measuring the phase of the MR signal is faced with fundamental challenges such as phase aliasing, noise and unknown offsets of the coil array. There is a paucity of acquisition, reconstruction and estimation methods that rigorously address these challenges. This reduces the reliability of information processing in phase domain. We propose a joint acquisition-processing framework that addresses the challenges of MR phase imaging using a rigorous theoretical treatment. Our proposed solution acquires the multi-coil complex data without any increase in acquisition time. Our corresponding estimation algorithm is applied optimally voxel-per-voxel. Results show that our framework achieves performance gains up to an order of magnitude compared to existing methods.

1 Introduction

The vast majority of MRI methods have historically retained the magnitude of the reconstructed image and ignored its complex phase. The main usage of the MR phase signal has focused on estimating *globally* varying field inhomogeneities [1]. Recently, however, the *local* phase has been showing its promise in quantifying underlying physiology such as blood flow, electro-magnetic tissue property, tissue elasticity, and temperature [1,3,5,11]. While currently utilized MR pulse sequences and algorithms are optimized for magnitude-domain contrast or SNR, current methods for acquisition of the tissue-dependent phase do not guarantee any optimality criteria. Furthermore, existing phase reconstruction methods are inherently limited by ambiguities due to phase-wrapping, phase-noise and parallel channels' phase-offset. We present here a novel framework for MR phase imaging and formulate the phase estimation problem rigorously using a joint acquisition-processing approach. We consider the problem associated with imaging MR phase originating as a response to a Gradient-Echo (GRE) sequence using an array of receive coils. The measurement obtained using such a sequence at channel (receive coil) element c and echo time TE_k could be written as:

$$\mathbf{m}_{k,c}(x,y) = \rho_{k,c}(x,y) \exp\left\{i(\phi_{0,c}(x,y) + 2\pi\Delta B(x,y)\text{TE}_k)\right\} + \mathbf{w}(x,y) \quad (1)$$

where $\rho_{k,c}(x,y)$ is the decayed magnitude at echo time TE_k modulated by the sensitivity of channel c, $2\pi\Delta B(x,y)\text{TE}_k$ is the underlying tissue phase value and

© Springer International Publishing Switzerland 2015
S. Ourselin et al. (Eds.): IPMI 2015, LNCS 9123, pp. 45–56, 2015.
DOI: 10.1007/978-3-319-19992-4_4

$\phi_{0,c}(x, y)$ is the channel-dependent phase offset of channel c. $\phi_{0,c}(x, y)$ varies spatially due to factors such as the distance between the excited spins and the coil, the length of the coil's cables, and electronic delay [9]. Strictly speaking, $\phi_{0,c}(x, y)$ also varies with time due to drifts in frequency synthesizer and/or imperfections in the centering of k-space [5]. The term $\Delta B(x, y)$ accounts for all deviations from the main magnetic field at location (x, y) which are due to both, inherent local tissue properties (which induce such local changes), as well as global object coil-loading effects. We refer here to $\Delta B(x, y)$ as "tissue frequency." Finally, the noise term $\mathbf{w}(x, y)$ in each voxel is drawn i.i.d. from a complex Gaussian Random Variable (RV), i.e. $\mathbf{w} = \mathbf{w}_R + i\mathbf{w}_I$, $\mathbf{w}_R, \mathbf{w}_I \sim \mathcal{N}(0, \sigma_w)$. Quantitation from MR phase requires the extraction of the term $\Delta B(x, y)$ from the measurements $\mathbf{m}_{k,c}(x, y)$. However, instead of the absolute phase, we are restricted to measuring the numerically computed angle of $\mathbf{m}_{k,c}(x, y)$, namely,

$$\mathbf{\Psi}_{k,c}(x, y) = \phi_{0,c}(x, y) + 2\pi \Delta B(x, y)\mathrm{TE}_k + \mathbf{\Omega}_{k,c}(x, y) + 2\pi \mathbf{r}_{k,c}(x, y), \qquad (2)$$

where $\mathbf{\Omega}_{k,c}(x, y)$ is the phase contribution of the additive noise term and $\mathbf{r}_{k,c}(x, y)$ is a phase wrapping integer which forces the sum of the first three terms on the right side of (2) to be in the range $[-\pi, \pi)$. Note that, because the noise's contribution in the phase depends on $\rho_{k,c}(x, y)$, both $\mathbf{\Omega}_{k,c}(x, y)$ and $\mathbf{r}_{k,c}(x, y)$ are a function of TE_k and channel c. It is clear from (2) that there are four unknowns in the angle measurements $\mathbf{\Psi}_{k,c}(x, y)$: the parameter of interest $\Delta B(x, y)$, and 3 additional sources of ambiguity (phase offset, noise and phase-wrapping integer).

Phase Offsets $\phi_{0,c}$: Existing methods attempt to address this challenge by either (a) referencing $\mathbf{m}_{k,c}$ to a known coil or given location (equalization) [4,7], (b) estimating then eliminating $\phi_{0,c}$ [6,8] or (c) inverting the sensitivity profile of the coil-array [10,12]. Equalization methods are sensitive to coil geometry, often resulting in severe artifacts in areas of low SNR, or areas of ΔB variations. Cancelation methods suffer from an inherent SNR penalty, and require separate "reference" scans which assume that $\phi_{0,c}$ are temporally invariant [5]. Finally, inversion methods suffer from substantial errors/artifacts in areas of noise/poor regularization.

Phase Noise and Wrapping: The authors in [1] have shown that imaging the MR phase signal inherently trades off two types of errors: noise and phase wrapping. There, the authors have identified three phase imaging regimes: (I) a regime dominated by phase-wrapping, with reduced levels of noise, (II) a regime dominated by noise, with no phase-wrapping and (III) a regime where the phase signal needs to be disambiguated from both phase-wrapping and noise contributions. Most phase imaging methods operate in Regime III [1] where post-processing is relied on in order to perform phase unwrapping and denoising. As carefully documented in [9], phase unwrapping methods are not robust and often require expert-user intervention. Other methods proposed in [2] use a combination of short (Regime II) and long (Regime I) echo times in order to recover the phase signal using an ML framework. However, as shown in [1], such methods are suboptimal because (a) long echo acquisitions rely on short echo acquisitions

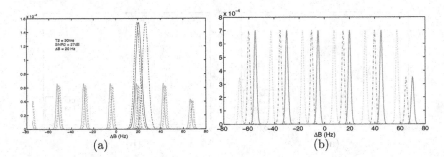

Fig. 1. (a) Example likelihood functions, with $\phi_{0,c} = 0$, in a voxel where $\Delta B = 20\,\mathrm{Hz}$, SNR0=22 (27 dB) and T2*=30 ms. The family of blue lines correspond to $\mathcal{L}_{k,c}(\Delta B)$ for different $\psi_{k,c}$ realizations, at TE = 5 ms. The red lines are $\mathcal{L}_{k,c}(\Delta B)$ obtained at TE = 40 ms. (b) $\mathcal{L}_{k,c}(\Delta B)$ for the same voxel as (a), at TE=40 ms, but obtained through 3 channels each with different phase offsets.

(which induces error propagation) and (b) the phase is computed using echo referencing (which induces noise amplification). Furthermore, the method in [2] relies on spatial regularization which biases the estimate.

2   MAGPI: A Maximum-Likelihood Framework

2.1   Problem Formulation

The task here is to estimate ΔB from $\mathbf{\Psi}_{k,c}$. The ML estimator is popular due to its optimality properties such as efficiency, sufficiency, consistency and invariance. We can show that the likelihood function for our problem, $\mathcal{L}_{k,c}$, is given by:

$$\mathcal{L}_{k,c}(\Delta B) \triangleq \mathrm{pr}\left(\mathbf{\Psi}_{k,c} = \psi_{k,c}/\Delta B\right) = \mathrm{pr}\left(\mathbf{\Omega}_{k,c} + 2\pi\mathbf{r}_{k,c} = \psi_{k,c} - 2\pi\Delta B \mathrm{TE}_k - \phi_{0,c}\right) \quad (3)$$

where $\psi_{k,c}$ is a realization of the random variable (RV) $\mathbf{\Psi}_{k,c}$. Note that, because the phase wrapping integer $\mathbf{r}_{k,c}$ depends on the phase noise RV $\mathbf{\Omega}_{k,c}$, this implies that $\mathbf{r}_{k,c}$ is also a (discrete) RV. Using the total probability theorem, and carrying on derivations not shown here, we can write:

$$\mathcal{L}_{k,c}(\Delta B) = \sum_r P(\mathbf{r}_{k,c} = r) f_{\mathbf{\Omega}_{k,c}}(\psi_{k,c} - 2\pi\Delta B \mathrm{TE}_k - 2\pi r - \phi_{0,c}) \quad (4)$$

where $P(\mathbf{r}_{k,c} = r)$ is the probability of obtaining a given wrapping integer r and $f_{\mathbf{\Omega}_{k,c}}$ is the PDF of the noise in channel c, at echo time k, each given by:

$$P(\mathbf{r} = r) = \frac{\sigma_{k,c}\sqrt{2}}{4\zeta_{\max}}\left[\frac{e^{-b_2^2} - e^{-a_2^2}}{\sqrt{\pi}} - a_2\mathrm{erf}(a_2) + b_2\mathrm{erf}(b_2) - \frac{e^{-b_1^2} - e^{-a_1^2}}{\sqrt{\pi}} + a_1\mathrm{erf}(a_1) - b_1\mathrm{erf}(b_1)\right] \quad (5)$$

$$\text{where} \quad a_1 = \frac{\left(\frac{2r-1}{2\mathrm{TE}_k} - \zeta_{\max}\right)}{\sqrt{2}\sigma_{k,c}}; \quad b_1 = \frac{\left(\frac{2r+1}{2\mathrm{TE}_k} - \zeta_{\max}\right)}{\sqrt{2}\sigma_{k,c}}; \quad a_2 = \frac{\left(\frac{2r-1}{2\mathrm{TE}_k} + \zeta_{\max}\right)}{\sqrt{2}\sigma_{k,c}}; \quad b_2 = \frac{\left(\frac{2r+1}{2\mathrm{TE}_k} + \zeta_{\max}\right)}{\sqrt{2}\sigma_{k,c}} \quad (6)$$

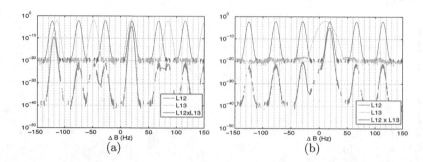

Fig. 2. Example system likelihood functions obtained from individual dual-echo likelihoods. Note that the system likelihoods (red) are not subject to the same noise-phase wrapping trade offs as the dual-echo likelihoods (green and blue) (Color figure online).

and ζ_{max} is the maximum value of $\Delta B + (\phi_{0,c}/2\pi TE_k)$, and,

$$f_{\Omega_{k,c}}(\Omega) = \frac{\exp\left(-snr_{k,c}^2/2\right)}{2\pi}\left\{1 + snr_{k,c}\sqrt{\frac{\pi}{2}}\cos\Omega\exp\left(snr_{k,c}^2\cos^2\Omega/2\right)\left[1 + \mathrm{erf}\left(\frac{snr_{k,c}\cos\Omega}{\sqrt{2}}\right)\right]\right\} \quad (7)$$

and $snr_{k,c}$ is the magnitude-domain SNR in channel c at TE_k. Note that our phase signal model does not assume any specific magnitude-decay model. We validated these theoretical predictions using numerical simulations and observed a close match (not shown here). We focus here on the dependence of the likelihood functions on TE_k, ΔB, T2* and $SNR_{0,c}$. We plot in Fig. 1(a) two families of likelihood functions obtained at two different values of TE_k. We ignore the channel offsets ($\phi_{0,c} = 0, \forall c$) in this figure. We note the following: First, depending on the choice of TE_k, the likelihood functions exhibit either sharp but multiple maxima (wrapping-dominated regimes), or a broad unimodal peak (noise-dominated regimes). Therefore, the likelihood function captures the inherent trade-offs between noise and phase wrapping with respect to the choice of TE_k. Second, we note that repeated measurements (dashed family of lines) yield randomly shifted $\mathcal{L}_{k,c}(\Delta B)$. Measurements at the larger TE_k result in a family of likelihood functions that are more tightly centered around the true ΔB, as compared to the shorter TE_k. We include the effects of the unknown phase offset in Fig. 1(b), where we plot example $\mathcal{L}_{k,c}(\Delta B)$ for different channels c. Note that likelihoods in the same voxel are shifted with respect to one another by an unknown amount, $\phi_{0,c}$. This example illustrates that maximizing the likelihood is not trivial due to: (1) the function either having multiple maxima or one maximum whose location is sensitive to noise and (2) the unknown $\phi_{0,c}$.

2.2   Proposed Solution: MAGPI

Our proposed framework, coined MAGPI (**M**aximum **A**mbi**G**uity distance for **P**hase **I**maging), acquires Multi-Echo Gradient Echo (MEGE) measurements from a collection of K echoes, and N_c channels, within a single TR. The estimation step is described using the 3-pass process detailed below.

Pass I: *Find the most likely ΔB that explains the angle buildup between echoes.*
We can show that the angle buildup between any two echoes is:

$$\Delta\Psi_{2:1,c} \triangleq \angle\left\{\mathbf{m}_{2,c}\mathbf{m}_{1,c}^*\right\} = 2\pi\Delta B\Delta\mathrm{TE}_{2:1} + \Delta\Omega_{2:1,c} + 2\pi\mathbf{r}_{2:1,c}, \qquad (8)$$

where $\Delta\mathrm{TE}_{2:1} \triangleq \mathrm{TE}_2 - \mathrm{TE}_1$, $\Delta\Omega_{2:1,c} \triangleq \Omega_{2,c} - \Omega_{1,c}$ and $\mathbf{r}_{2:1,c}$ is a phase wrapping integer which forces the sum of the first two terms on the right side of (8) to be in the range $[-\pi, \pi)$. We note two differences in (8) as compared to (2). First, the relative phase buildup does not depend on $\phi_{0,c}$. The second important difference is a reduced tissue phase amplification (due to multiplication with a smaller term, $\Delta\mathrm{TE}_{2:1}$) accompanied by noise amplification (two contributions from noise RVs). We will address this shortcoming in pass III below. The likelihood function, denoted by $\mathcal{L}_{2:1,c}(\Delta B) \triangleq \mathrm{pr}(\Delta\Psi_{2:1,c}/\Delta B)$, is now given by:

$$\mathcal{L}_{2:1,c}(\Delta B) = \sum_{r=-R}^{R} P(\mathbf{r}_{2:1,c} = r)f_{\Delta\Omega_{2:1,c}}(\Delta\psi_{2:1,c} - 2\pi\Delta B\Delta\mathrm{TE}_{2:1} - 2\pi r) \qquad (9)$$

where the noise and wrapping PDFs $f_{\Delta\Omega_{2:1,c}}$ and $P(\mathbf{r}_{2:1,c})$ could be readily obtained in closed-form, similar to (5) and (7). Note that, since there is no $\phi_{0,c}$ ambiguity in this dual-echo likelihood, all the peaks of $\mathcal{L}_{2:1,c}^{(\Delta B)}$ are now exactly co-aligned. We can then seek the maximum of the product of the dual-echo likelihoods over all channels c, $\prod_c \mathcal{L}_{2:1,c}(\Delta B)$, as the solution to the ML problem. This product assumes that the angle measurements over all the channels are conditionally independent. This assumption may not be exact, due to noise correlation across channels, but we ignore any inter-channel dependence in this treatment. Nevertheless, the resulting dual-echo likelihood is not guaranteed to have a single maximum: we still face here the same unimodal vs multimodal trade-offs as single-echo likelihoods. To address this inherent limitation, we make use of (at least) one additional echo, $k = 3$, and compute a second set of likelihood functions $\mathcal{L}_{3:1,c}^{(\Delta B)}$. We can then ask the following question: what value of ΔB most-likely explains both angle buildups from echo pairs (1,2) and (1,3)? Approximating both angle build-ups as conditionally independent RVs, we can formally write this question as:

$$\widehat{\Delta B}_{(\mathrm{I})} = \arg\max_{\Delta B} \prod_{k,k_0;k\neq k_0} \prod_c \mathcal{L}_{k:k_0,c}(\Delta B). \qquad (10)$$

The product of likelihoods $\mathcal{L}_{\delta k}(\Delta B) \triangleq \prod_{k,k_0} \prod_c \mathcal{L}_{k:k_0,c}(\Delta B)$ is defined as the "system likelihood." We claim that system likelihoods are not subject to the same multimodal vs unimodal tradeoffs as individual likelihood functions. To illustrate this, we plot in Fig. 2 example $\mathcal{L}_{\delta k}(\Delta B)$ having a single sharp maximum, despite the underlying individual likelihoods having multimodal peaks (Fig. 2(a)) or both unimodal and multimodal peaks (Fig. 2(b)).

Nevertheless, not all system likelihoods are of equal value. For a given ΔB, T2* and $\mathrm{SNR}_{0,c}$ in a voxel, it is obvious that there exists a large number of system likelihood functions (selected by TE_k) that one could choose from, each with its own corresponding performance, given by the asymptotic Minimum Variance Unbiased (MVU) bound. A careful design procedure would pick $\mathcal{L}_{\delta k}(\Delta B)$ which achieves the lowest MVU bound amongst all possible bounds. This is the key to our method: the design of acquisition parameters (TE_k) such as the corresponding estimation (MLE) achieves the best (MVU) estimate. We formalize the optimizer below. Although the 1D search of system likelihoods (10) still possesses local maxima, the guaranteed global maximum can be obtained with "brute force" as the likelihoods are given by an analytical expression. Furthermore, it is important to emphasize that this step can be solved one voxel at a time, substantially reducing the complexity.

Pass II: *Estimate the channel-dependent phase offsets* $\phi_{0,c}$. After obtaining an ML estimate of ΔB in Pass I, the remaining data in the original measurements (2) that is "unexplained" by the Pass I model (8) can be attributed to $\phi_{0,c}$ and errors in the ΔB estimate. The task in this step is to extract $\phi_{0,c}$ from the remainder terms: $\phi_{k,c}^{\text{rem}} = \angle\left(\mathbf{m}_{k,c}e^{-i\widehat{\Delta B}_{(\text{I})}}\right)$. To achieve this, we take advantage of the following distinct features of $\phi_{0,c}$: smooth variation over space and channel dimensions (x, y, c), and invariance with echo times. Using this prior knowledge, we can use various signal-separation techniques (such as PCA, Wavelet decomposition, Spectral Decomposition methods, Fractional-Fourier methods) to extract $\phi_{0,c}$ from $\phi_{k,c}^{\text{rem}}$. We resort here to a simple and fast technique: spatio-temporal linear low-pass filtering using an operator $\widehat{\phi}_{0,c} = \mathcal{LPF}\left\{\phi_{k,c}^{\text{rem}}\right\}$. We omit details here on this filter for brevity.

Pass III: *Find the most likely* ΔB *that explains the angle of all* K *echoes.* We use here the estimate of $e^{i\widehat{\phi}_{0,c}}$, obtained from Pass II, to rewrite the single-echo likelihood functions without any channel-offset ambiguity, namely:

$$\mathcal{L}_{k,c}(\Delta B) \triangleq \text{pr}\left(\mathbf{\Psi}_{k,c}' = \psi_{k,c}'/\Delta B\right) = \sum_r P_{(\mathbf{r}_{k,c}=r)} f_{\mathbf{\Omega}_{k,c}}(\psi_{k,c}'-2\pi\Delta B\text{TE}_k-2\pi r) \quad (11)$$

$$\text{where} \qquad \psi_{k,c}' = \angle m_{k,c}e^{-i\widehat{\phi}_{0,c}}. \quad (12)$$

That is, in this pass, we can directly solve the following estimation problem: What is the most likely ΔB that could explain the angle as given by (12)? Formally, we solve this MLE problem:

$$\widehat{\Delta B}_{(\text{III})} = \arg\max_{\Delta B} \prod_{k=1}^{K} \prod_c \mathcal{L}_{k,c}(\Delta B). \quad (13)$$

We define (another) system likelihood, given by the product of the K individual likelihoods: $\mathcal{L}(\Delta B) \triangleq \prod_{k=1}^{K} \prod_c \mathcal{L}_{k,c}(\Delta B)$. Similar to Pass I, the system likelihood of Pass III is not subject to the unimodal vs multimodal trade-offs of individual likelihoods. Furthermore, $\mathcal{L}(\Delta B)$ could be designed (by choice of TE_k) to yield the lowest MVU bound possible. The optimizer thus needs to optimize 2 system likelihoods, $\mathcal{L}_{\delta k}(\Delta B)$ for Pass I and $\mathcal{L}(\Delta B)$ for Pass III.

2.3 Optimizer

The solution to MLE problems (10) and (13) are not guaranteed to achieve the "best" tissue phase estimate for arbitrary choices of echo times. The quality of the estimation here is measured using the asymptotic MVU bound. We denote $\sigma_\mathrm{I}(\Delta B)$ and $\sigma_\mathrm{III}(\Delta B)$ the MVUs associated with MLE problems (10) and (13), respectively. Each of these MVUs is given by the inverse of their distribution's Fisher Information, $I^{-1}(\Delta B)$. In this work, we make use of the closed form of the likelihood functions to obtain an approximate numerical estimate of $I(\Delta B)$. Ideally, we need to minimize both $\sigma_\mathrm{I}(\Delta B)$ and $\sigma_\mathrm{III}(\Delta B)$, for all possible values of ΔB. Clearly, this may not be possible. Instead, we propose the following alternative: minimize the average $\sigma_\mathrm{III}(\Delta B)$ subject to an upper bound constraint on the average $\sigma_\mathrm{I}(\Delta B)$. Formally, this optimization problem could be written as:

$$[\mathrm{TE}_1^\mathrm{opt}, \mathrm{TE}_2^\mathrm{opt}, \ldots, \mathrm{TE}_K^\mathrm{opt}] = \underset{[\mathrm{TE}_1, \mathrm{TE}_2, \ldots, \mathrm{TE}_K]}{\arg\min} \; \mathbb{E}\left[\sigma_\mathrm{III}(\Delta B)\right]_{\Delta B} \qquad (14)$$

$$\text{such that,} \quad \mathbb{E}\left[\sigma_\mathrm{I}(\Delta B)\right]_{\Delta B} <= \epsilon_I \; \& \; [\mathrm{TE}_1, \mathrm{TE}_2, \ldots, \mathrm{TE}_K] \in \mathcal{C}_\mathrm{TE}.$$

We make the following notes about this optimizer:

(1) $\mathcal{C}_\mathrm{TE}$ is the set of echo times that are physically achievable with the pulse sequence of choice. This constraint set takes into account pulse sequence parameters known *a priori* such as the minimum echo time spacing and the minimum or maximum echo times.
(2) We assume ΔB to be uniformly distributed in the expectations of (14). The range of the distribution can be easily determined based on the strength of the main magnetic field and the anatomy of interest.
(3) Note that both $\sigma_\mathrm{I}(\Delta B)$ and $\sigma_\mathrm{III}(\Delta B)$ are a function of $\mathrm{SNR}_{0,c}$ and T2*, both of which are spatially-varying quantities. In order to address this challenge, we only optimize echoes for the minimum expected $\mathrm{SNR}_{0,c}$ and T2* of interest. The design would thus target the "worst-case imaging scenario." Since the optimizer is run offline, once, various imaging scenarios corresponding to different $\mathrm{SNR}_{0,\mathrm{min}}$, $\mathrm{T2}^*_\mathrm{min}$ and echo time constraint sets $\mathcal{C}_\mathrm{TE}$ could be tabulated and used at acquisition time.

3 Results

In all our acquisitions below, the set of echo times $\mathcal{C}_\mathrm{TE}$ was constrained such that the *acquisition time is no longer* than traditional single-echo GRE. Also, ϵ_I in (14) was set to 1 Hz. In post-processing, the estimation procedures of (10) and (13) were independently solved for every voxel in the image. *No spatial averaging/smoothing* was ever employed with our method.

3.1 Numerical Phantom

We validated the performance of our proposed MAGPI framework on a modified Shepp-Logan phantom which consists of a 128×128 tissue frequency map

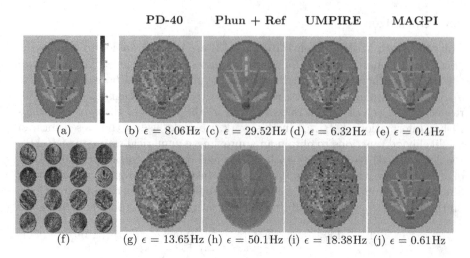

Fig. 3. (a) Original ΔB and (f) angle of measurements $\psi_{k,c}$ at SNR=27 dB. (Columns 2–4) Example ΔB estimates using a collection of methods for 2 different SNR=30 dB (row 1) and SNR = 27 dB (row 2). RMSE of each estimate is shown in sub-captions.

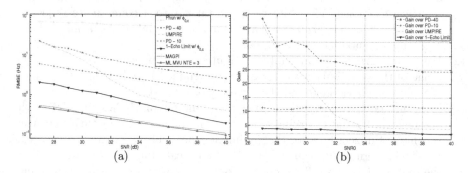

Fig. 4. (a) RMSE (Hz) averaged over random realizations of noise, ΔB and $\phi_{0,c}$. Result in log-scale. (b) RMSE reduction achieved with MAGPI over other methods.

(Fig. 3(a)) and a corresponding magnitude image. The tissue frequency values are randomly chosen between ±125 Hz, corresponding to the range of values found in the brain at 1.5T. We simulated GRE acquisitions of this complex-domain object using an array of 16-channel receive coils at different SNRs. The resulting angle of the measurements $\psi_{k,c}$ (2) at $TE_k = 40$ ms are shown in Fig. 3(f) for an SNR= 27 dB. In all the numerical simulations, the object was assumed to have a T2* of 40 ms. Figure 3 shows the estimated ΔB from $\psi_{k,c}$ using a variety of methods, for different values of SNR_0 (SNR at TE=0). **Column 1 (PD-40)** is the Phase Difference method [6] which uses an echo pair, TE={36, 40} ms, with phase conjugation (similar to (8)) to cancel $\phi_{0,c}$ and estimate ΔB. One of the echoes is constrained at 40 ms for its utility as a magnitude contrast, and the 3.5 ms echo step is chosen to be just small enough to avoid phase wrapping. **Column 2 (Phun+ref)** is a single-echo phase unwrapping method (TE = 40 ms) [8]. Single-echo methods require knowledge of $\phi_{0,c}$ in order to combine the complex measurements from all the channels. Phun+ref here assumes perfect knowledge of $\phi_{0,c}$. **Column 3 (UMPIRE)** uses a triple-echo method, TE = $\{6.67, 21.67, 40\}$ms. This recently proposed method [9] was shown to vastly outperform phase unwrapping algorithms, particularly when the spatial pattern of ΔB is complex. The UMPIRE echoes were chosen here according to the prescription in [9], whereby the smallest difference between the echo steps is able to unwrap a maximum tissue frequency buildup of 150 Hz. **Column 4** is our proposed **MAGPI**, which uses the following optimized echoes: TE = $\{26.56, 35, 40.91\}$ms for $SNR_0 = 30$ dB (Fig. 3(e)) and TE = $\{16.4, 22.27, 36.83\}$ms for $SNR_0 = 27$ dB (Fig. 3(j)). We note the following from Fig. 3: phase unwrapping fails to recover the underlying tissue frequency for this ΔB pattern. PD-40 and UMPIRE are not robust in the presence of noise, and exhibit noise-induced phase wrapping at low SNRs. MAGPI clearly outperforms all these methods and achieves RMSE reductions by a factor of 15.8X over UMPIRE (at 30 dB) and 22.37X over PD-40 at 27 dB. We repeat this experiment for different random selections of ΔB, $\phi_{0,c}$ and noise and plot in Fig. 4(a) the RMSE of the ΔB estimate as a function of SNR_0, for all methods. We also include an additional PD method (PD-10) with the same echo time step as PD-40, but without the 40 ms echo time constraint (TE = $\{6.5, 10\}$ms). The black lines in the figure constitute theoretical performance bounds. The first bound, 1-Echo-Limit, is the lower bound on the RMSE obtained with a single echo scan which (a) has perfect knowledge of $\phi_{0,c}$ and (b) only operates on values of ΔB that induce no phase wrapping. Thus, the only ambiguity with this method would be due to noise. The second bound, ML-MVU, is the minimum MVU bound as predicted from our theoretical derivations, with K=3 echoes. We note the substantial performance gain (Fig. 4(b)) obtained with MAGPI over other methods. In particular, MAGPI achieves an RMSE reduction by an order of magnitude (11X) over PD-10 at all SNRs. MAGPI's gain over UMPIRE increases as SNR decreases, from 3.83X at 40 dB to 41X at 27 dB. Furthermore, MAGPI outperforms the lower bound derived for ideal single echo methods by a factor of 1.81X at 40 dB up to 3.9X at 27 dB. The RMSE obtained with MAGPI also closely matches the MVU predicted by theory, thereby suggesting the rapid convergence of our ML-based approach.

3.2   Real Phantom

We also validated the performance of MAGPI in real phantom experiments. A water phantom was acquired at 1.5T on a Siemens Aera scanner using a 20-channel head coil and a voxel size of $0.9 \times 0.9 \times 0.9$ mm^3 (Fig. 5, first column). Figure 5 (top row) shows the resulting ΔB estimates for each of the following methods (along columns): PD-10 x20Avgs, Phun + Ref scan, UMPIRE and MAGPI, respectively. The PD-10 method (TE = $\{4, 10\}$ms) was averaged over 20 acquisitions in order to form a wrapping-free reduced-noise reference.

SSQ   PD-10 x20avgs Phun + Ref   UMPIRE   MAGPI

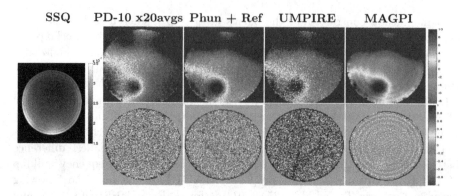

Fig. 5. (First Column) Magnitude image combined using standard sum of squares (SSQ) method. (Top Row) ΔB estimate in a water phantom. (Bottom row) Remainder after removing background phase from top row: result measures noise content. All units in Hz. Note that the circular truncation artifacts visible in the SSQ image are only detectable with MAGPI which shows that (i) MAGPI substantially reduces the noise floor and (ii) MAGPI does not use spatial smoothing and preserves pixel resolution (Color figure online).

The Phun+ Ref method uses the phase offsets derived from one of the reference PD-10 scans in order to coherently sum the aligned complex data, then unwrap its phase (TE = 40 ms, TR = 46 ms, TA = 5 min 30 s). UMPIRE (TR = 46 ms, TA = 3 min 09 s) and MAGPI (TR = 42 ms, TA = 2 min 45 s) used the same echoes as in simulations. MAGPI's echoes were optimized for $SNR_{0,min} = 28$ dB, $T2^*_{min} = 40$ ms. The inter-echo spacing with the optimizer was constrained to be 5.82 ms, to accommodate flow-compensation and monopolar readout at a bandwidth of 240 Hz/pxl. We note the overall agreement between these methods. We note from the figure the clear phase SNR improvement obtained with MAGPI's estimate, despite having the shortest acquisition time. In order to quantify this phase SNR gain over the other methods, we removed the smooth background phase in each ΔB estimate. Since this is a water-only phantom, the result of such filtering process (bottom row of Fig. 5) is mainly the residual noise image. The reduction in noise with MAGPI is clear. We computed the standard deviation in the residual images and noted the following reduction in standard deviation (or gain in phase SNR) with MAGPI: a gain of **3.95X** over the 20-time averaged PD-10, a **3.661X** gain over Phun+Ref and a **7.7X** gain over UMPIRE. These gains are consistent with our simulations (Fig. 4(a)), given that SNR_0 in this water phantom was 33 dB.

3.3   In-Vivo

The brain of healthy volunteers was imaged after approval was obtained from our Institutional Review Board and informed consent was given by the subjects. The first set of scans was done on a Siemens Aera 1.5T with a 20-channel

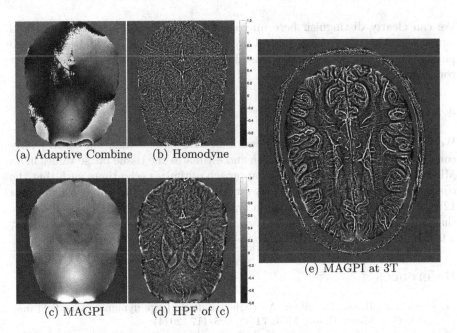

(a) Adaptive Combine   (b) Homodyne

(c) MAGPI   (d) HPF of (c)

(e) MAGPI at 3T

Fig. 6. *in-vivo* ΔB estimates at 1.5T, at in-plane resolution of 0.49 mm, obtained with (a,b) traditional single echo methods and (c,d) MAGPI. Images in (b) and (d) are the high-pass counterparts of (a) and (c). (e) *in-vivo* ΔB at 3T, at in-plane resolution 0.39 mm obtained using MAGPI.

head coil: 3D GRE, FOV = 220(read out) $\times$ 200 mm^2, $N_x = 448$, $N_y = 406$, slice thickness 2 mm, FA = 15°, BW= 240 Hz/pxl. The voxel size in this scan is thus $0.49 \times 0.49 \times 2$ mm^3. Figure 6(a) shows the ΔB image reconstructed by a Siemens product sequence (Adaptive Combine method [12]), from a traditionally utilized single-echo scan (TE = 40 ms, TR = 45 ms, TA = 6 min 10 s). The artifacts in this method originate from phase wrapping errors and phase-offset alignment errors. In order to mitigate these artifacts, a technique known as "Homodyne Filtering" adds the channels' complex data directly in high pass domain (Fig. 6(b)) [3]. The high-pass filter is used here to reduce large values of ΔB, and reduce impact of $\phi_{0,c}$. Note the predominantly noisy image in Fig. 6(b), as expected at high resolutions not traditionally utilized at 1.5T. Finally, we applied our MAGPI framework, optimized for SNR$_{0,\min} = 26.5$ dB, T2$^*_{\min} = 40$ ms: TE = $\{16.18, 27.98, 35.37\}$ms, TR = 40 ms, and TA = 5 min 20 s (i.e., 87 % of the time of the traditional single echo scan). The resulting images are shown in Figs. 6(c) (ΔB) and 6(d) (high-pass filtered ΔB). Consistent with our simulations and phantom results, we note substantially improved phase SNR with our proposed technique. This is particularly apparent in the homodyne domain, where we see venous structures not seen with the traditional method. Finally, we show in Fig. 6(e) a tissue frequency image in homodyne domain obtained at 3T using MAGPI, at an impressive in-plane resolution of 390 μm.

We can clearly distinguish here microstructures such as perforator veins and laminar pattern of cerebral cortical layers. To the best of our knowledge, such phase images displaying high-contrast high-resolution anatomical details are not commonly seen at 3T.

4   Conclusion

We presented here a unifying framework for MR phase estimation which jointly combines the complex channels' data and estimates the tissue phase values in an ML-optimal fashion. The proposed approach optimizes echo times such that the corresponding MLE achieves the lowest MVU bound possible. Reconstructing a 128×128 phase image took $\sim$1 min on a personal computer. Our results show that our proposed MAGPI framework achieves gains in phase SNR by at least a factor of 3.5X (and up to a factor of 40X), compared to other methods.

References

1. Dagher, J., Reese, T., Bilgin, A.: High-resolution, large dynamic range field map estimation. Magn. Reson. Med. **71**(1), 105–117 (2014)
2. Funai, A., Fessler, J., Yeo, D., Noll, D.: Regularized field map estimation in MRI. IEEE Trans. Med. Imaging **27**(10), 1484–1494 (2008)
3. Haacke, E.M., Reichenbach, J.R.: Susceptibility Weighted Imaging in MRI: Basic Concepts and Clinical Applications. Wiley-Blackwell, New Jersey (2011)
4. Hammond, K.E., Lupo, J.M., Xu, D., Metcalf, M., Kelley, D.A.C., Pelletier, D., Chang, S.M., Mukherjee, P., Vigneron, D.B., Nelson, S.J.: Development of a robust method for generating 7.0 T multichannel phase images of the brain with application to normal volunteers and patients with neurological diseases. NeuroImage **39**(4), 1682–1692 (2008)
5. Huber, K.M., Roland, J., Schoepfer, J., Biber, S., Martius, S.: Using MR thermometry for SAR verification in local pTX applications. In: International Society for Magnetic Resonance in Medicine, vol. 21 (2013)
6. Lu, K., Liu, T.: Optimal phase difference reconstruction: comparison of two methods. Magn. Reson. Imaging **26**(1), 142–145 (2008)
7. Parker, D.L., Payne, A., Todd, N., Hadley, J.R.: Phase reconstruction from multiple coil data using a virtual reference coil. Magn. Reson. Med. **72**(2), 563–569 (2013)
8. Robinson, S., Grabner, G., Witoszynskyj, S., Trattnig, S.: Combining phase images from multi-channel RF coils using 3D phase offset maps derived from a dual-echo scan. Magn. Reson. Med. **65**(6), 1638–1648 (2011)
9. Robinson, S., Schodl, H., Trattnig, S.: A method for unwrapping highly wrapped multi-echo phase images at very high field: UMPIRE. Magn. Reson. Med. **72**(1), 80–92 (2014)
10. Roemer, P.B., Edelstein, W.A., Hayes, C.E., Souza, S.P., Mueller, O.M.: The NMR phased array. Magn. Reson. Med. **16**(2), 192–225 (1990)
11. Schweser, F., Deistung, A., Lehr, B.W., Reichenbach, J.R.: Quantitative imaging of intrinsic magnetic tissue properties using MRI signal phase: an approach to in vivo brain iron metabolism? NeuroImage **54**(4), 2789–2807 (2011)
12. Walsh, D.O., Gmitro, A.F., Marcellin, M.W.: Adaptive reconstruction of phased array MR imagery. Magn. Reson. Med. **43**(5), 682–690 (2000)

A Compressed-Sensing Approach
for Super-Resolution Reconstruction
of Diffusion MRI

Lipeng Ning[1]([✉]), Kawin Setsompop[2], Oleg Michailovich[3], Nikos Makris[2],
Carl-Fredrik Westin[1], and Yogesh Rathi[1]

[1] Harvard Medical School, Brigham and Women's Hospital, Boston, USA
lning@bwh.harvard.edu
[2] Harvard Medical School, Massachusetts General Hospital, Boston, USA
[3] University of Waterloo, Waterloo, Canada

Abstract. We present an innovative framework for reconstructing high-spatial-resolution diffusion magnetic resonance imaging (dMRI) from multiple low-resolution (LR) images. Our approach combines the twin concepts of compressed sensing (CS) and classical super-resolution to reduce acquisition time while increasing spatial resolution. We use sub-pixel-shifted LR images with down-sampled and non-overlapping diffusion directions to reduce acquisition time. The diffusion signal in the high resolution (HR) image is represented in a sparsifying basis of spherical ridgelets to model complex fiber orientations with reduced number of measurements. The HR image is obtained as the solution of a convex optimization problem which can be solved using the proposed algorithm based on the alternating direction method of multipliers (ADMM). We qualitatively and quantitatively evaluate the performance of our method on two sets of in-vivo human brain data and show its effectiveness in accurately recovering very high resolution diffusion images.

1 Introduction

Diffusion-weighted MRI is a key technique in studying the neural architecture and connectivity of the brain. It can be utilized as imaging-based biomarkers for investigating several brain disorders such as Alzheimer's disease, schizophrenia, mild traumatic brain injury, etc. [1]. In many clinical applications such as neurosurgical planning and deep brain stimulation, it is critically important to use high-spatial-resolution diffusion images to accurately localize brain structures, especially those that are very small (such as substantia nigra and sub-thalamic nucleus). Moreover, HR images are critical for tracing small white-matter fiber bundles and to reduce partial volume effects. Further, with high spatial resolution, gray-matter and white-matter structures can be better resolved, especially

The authors would like to acknowledge the following grants which supported this work: R01MH099797 (PI: Rathi), R00EB012107 (PI: Setsompop), P41RR14075 (PI: Rosen), R01MH074794 (PI: Westin), P41EB015902 (PI: Kikinis) and Swedish Research Council (VR) grant 2012-3682.

© Springer International Publishing Switzerland 2015
S. Ourselin et al. (Eds.): IPMI 2015, LNCS 9123, pp. 57–68, 2015.
DOI: 10.1007/978-3-319-19992-4_5

in neonate and infant brains. The typical voxel size of a dMRI image acquired from a clinical scanner is about 1.7^3 to 2^3 mm^3 which is too large to study certain brain structures that are a few millimeters thick. Due to signal loss from T_2 decay with longer echo times, reducing the voxel size leads to a proportionate decrease in the signal-to-noise ratio (SNR). Though SNR could be enhanced by averaging multiple acquisitions, the total acquisition time may be too long to apply this approach in clinical settings.

Existing techniques that obtain high-resolution (HR) dMRI can be classified into two categories based on their data acquisition scheme. The first group of methods obtain HR data using a single LR image via intelligent interpolations or regularizations. These types of methods have been investigated in structural MRI [2] and in dMRI to enhance anatomical details as in [3]. However, as pointed out in [3], the performance of some of these methods still largely relies on the information contained in the original LR image. The second group of methods require multiple LR images acquired according to a specific sampling scheme to reconstruct a HR image. Each of the LR image is modeled as the measurement of an underlying HR image via a down-sampling operator. Then the HR image is estimated by solving a linear inverse problem with suitable regularization. These methods use the classical concept of super-resolution reconstruction (SRR) [4]. In dMRI, these methods were used in [5,6] to reconstruct each diffusion weighted volume independently. A different acquisition scheme with the LR images having orthogonal slice acquisition direction was proposed in [7]. However, the distortions from LR scans with different slice directions need to be corrected prior to applying the SRR algorithm, which involves complex non-linear spatial normalization. Moreover, each diffusion-weighted image (DWI) volume is reconstructed independently, requiring the LR images to be acquired or interpolated on the same dense set of gradient directions. Thus, these methods require the same number of measurements (e.g., 60 gradient directions) for each LR acquisition. To address this problem, more recently, [8] introduced a method that used the diffusion tensor imaging (DTI) technique to model the diffusion signal in q-space. However, a very simplistic diffusion tensor model was assumed, which is not appropriate for modeling more complex diffusion phenomena (crossing fibers). A similar method has been proposed in [9] to improve distortion corrections for DWI's using interlaced q-space sampling.

Our Contributions: We propose a compressed-sensing-based super-resolution reconstruction (CS-SRR) approach for reconstructing HR diffusion images from multiple sub-pixel-shifted thick-slice acquisitions. As illustrated in Fig. 1, we use three LR images with anisotropic voxel sizes that are shifted in the slice acquisition direction. **Each LR image is acquired with a different (unique) set of gradient directions** to construct a single HR image with isotropic voxel size and a combined set of gradient directions. This is in contrast to classical SRR techniques which require each LR scan to have the same set of gradient directions. In the proposed framework, only a subset (one-third) of the total number of gradient directions are acquired for each LR scan, which reduces scan time significantly while making the technique robust to head motion. To account

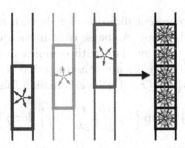

Fig. 1. An illustration of the CS-SRR scheme: a high-resolution image is reconstructed using three overlapping thick-slice volumes with down-sampled diffusion directions.

for the correlation between diffusion signal along different gradients, we represent the signal in the HR image in a sparsifying basis of spherical ridgelets. To obtain the HR image, we propose a framework based on the ADMM algorithm, where we enforce sparsity in the spherical-ridgelet domain and spatial consistency using total variation regularization. We perform quantitative validation of our technique using very high resolution data acquired on a clinical 3 T scanner.

2   Background

We consider diffusion images acquired on single spherical shell in q-space [10]. Hence, the problem of super resolution reduces to that of reconstructing the spherical signal at each voxel of the HR image. Before introducing the proposed method, we provide a brief note on the concepts of compressed sensing and spherical ridgelets that are used to model and estimate the diffusion signals.

Compressed Sensing: The theory of compressed sensing provides the mathematical foundation for accurate recovery of signals from set of measurements far fewer than that required by the Nyquist criteria [11]. In the CS framework, a signal of interest $s \in \mathbb{R}^n$ is represented in an over-complete basis $\Phi \in \mathbb{R}^{n \times m}$ with $n \ll m$ such that $s = \Phi c$ with $c \in \mathbb{R}^m$ being a sparse vector, i.e. c only has few non-zero elements. Let $y \in \mathbb{R}^p$ denote a measurement vector given by $y = \Psi s + \mu = \Psi \Phi c + \mu$ where μ is the noise component and $\Psi \in \mathbb{R}^{p \times n}$ is a down-sampling operator. If the matrix $\Psi \Phi$ satisfies certain incoherent properties, then the CS theory [11] asserts that the sparse vector c can be robustly recovered by solving the ℓ_1-norm regularized problem

$$\min_{c} \frac{1}{2} \|y - \Psi \Phi c\|^2 + \lambda \|c\|_1 \tag{1}$$

for a suitable $\lambda \geq 0$. Hence, the signal s can be accurately recovered as Φc using the lower dimensional measurement y. This CS methodology has been used to estimate the dMRI signal from reduced number of measurements [12–14] with the basis given by the spherical ridgelets.

Spherical Ridgelets: Spherical ridgelet functions were introduced in [12] as a frame to represent L_2 functions on the sphere. Each spherical ridgelet function is specially designed to represent diffusion signals with a particular orientation and certain degree of anisotropy. A sparse combination of such basis functions is suitable to model the diffusion data with complex fiber orientations [13,14]. Specifically, the spherical ridgelets are constructed as follows: For $x \in \mathbb{R}_+$ and $\rho \in (0,1)$, let $\kappa(x) = \exp\{-\rho x(x+1)\}$ be a Gaussian function. Further, we let

$$\kappa_j(x) = \kappa(2^{-j}x) = \exp\left\{-\rho\frac{x}{2^j}\left(\frac{x}{2^j}+1\right)\right\} \text{ for } j = 0,1,2,\ldots.$$

Then the spherical ridgelets with their energy spread around the great circle supported by a unit vector $\boldsymbol{v} \in \mathbb{S}^2$ is given by

$$\psi_{j,\boldsymbol{v}}(\boldsymbol{u}) = \frac{1}{2\pi}\sum_{n=0}^{\infty}\frac{2n+1}{4\pi}\lambda_n(\kappa_{j+1}(n) - \kappa_j(n))P_n(\boldsymbol{u}\cdot\boldsymbol{v}), \forall \boldsymbol{u} \in \mathbb{S}^2 \qquad (2)$$

where P_n denotes the Legendre polynomial of order n, $\kappa_{-1}(n) = 0$, $\forall n$ and $\lambda_n = 2\pi(-1)^{n/2}\frac{1.3...(n-1)}{2.4...n}$ if n is even, otherwise $\lambda_n = 0$.

To construct a finite over-complete dictionary, we follow the method in [13,14] and restrict the values for the resolution index j to the set $\{-1,0,1\}$. For each resolution index j, the set of all possible orientations $\boldsymbol{v} \in \mathbb{S}^2$ is discretized to a set of M_j directions on the unit sphere with $M_{-1} = 25$, $M_0 = 81$ and $M_1 = 289$. To this end, the set of over-complete spherical ridgelets is given by $\Psi_{\mathrm{SR}} = \left\{\phi_{j,\boldsymbol{v}_j^i} \mid j = -1,0,1, i = 1,2,\ldots,M_j\right\}$. Since the spherical ridgelets are anisotropic, the isotropic diffusion signal in the CSF areas is not efficiently modeled as a sparse combination of the basis functions. To resolve this issue, we expand the basis functions by adding one isotropic element as $\Psi := \{\psi_{\mathrm{iso}}, \Psi_{\mathrm{SR}}\}$ where ψ_{iso} denotes a constant function on the unit sphere. For convenience, we denote the functions in Ψ as $\psi_1, \psi_2, \ldots, \psi_M$ with $\psi_1 = \psi_{\mathrm{iso}}$. Given the diffusion signal measured along N diffusion directions $\{\boldsymbol{u}_n\}_{n=1}^N$, we construct a basis matrix A with $A_{nm} = \psi_m(\boldsymbol{u}_n)$ for $m = 1,\ldots,M$ and $n = 1,\ldots,N$.

3   Method

Let L_k, $k = 1,\ldots,K$, denote the K low-resolution diffusion weighted imaging (DWI) volumes. For each L_k, the diffusion signal is acquired along a set of gradient directions $U_k = \{\boldsymbol{u}_1^{(k)}, \ldots, \boldsymbol{u}_{N_k}^{(k)}\}$ at the same b-value. The set of gradient directions for each LR image L_k is assumed to be different, i.e. $U_k \cap U_\ell = \emptyset$ for $k \neq \ell$. The HR image that has $n_x \times n_y \times n_z$ voxels and $N = \sum_{k=1}^K N_k$ gradient directions is denoted by a matrix H of size $n_x n_y n_z \times N$. Then, each LR image L_k is given by

$$L_k = D_k B_k H Q_k^T + \mu_k \text{ for } k = 1,\ldots,K, \qquad (3)$$

where D_k denotes the down-sampling matrix that averages neighboring slices, B_k denotes the blurring (or point-spread function) and Q_k is the sub-sampling matrix in q-space. The main difference between the above model and the one used in [6,15] is given by the Q_k's that allow the LR images to have different sets of gradient directions. Further, we use the spherical ridgelets basis to model the diffusion signal at each voxel of H. To this end, H is assumed to satisfy $H = VA^T$ with A being the basis matrix of spherical ridgelets (SR) constructed along the set of gradient directions $\{U_1, \ldots, U_K\}$ and each row vector of V being the SR coefficients at the corresponding voxel. Since each basis function is designed to model a diffusion signal with certain degree of anisotropy, a nonnegative combination of spherical ridgelets provides more robust representation for diffusion signals especially when the SNR is low. Hence, the coefficients V are restricted to be non-negative. Following (1), we estimate H by solving

$$\min_{H, V \geq 0} \left\{ \frac{1}{2} \sum_{k=1}^{K} \|L_k - D_k B_k H Q_k^T\|^2 + \lambda \|W \circ V\|_1 \right\} \text{ s.t. } H = VA^T \quad (4)$$

where $\circ$ denotes the element-wise multiplication, $\|M\|^2$ is the squared Frobenius norm of a matrix M and $\|M\|_1$ is the summation of the absolute values of all the entries of M. W is the weighting matrix with each row having the form $[w, 1, \ldots, 1]$ where w is used to adjust the penalty for choosing the isotropic basis function in a voxel. The value of w can be obtained a-priori from a probabilistic segmentation of the T1-weighted image of the brain. Thus, w is small in the CSF and large in white and gray-matter areas.

3.1 Total-Variation (TV) Regularization

Let $h_r(u_n)$ denote the diffusion signal along the direction u_n at the voxel $r \in \Omega$ with Ω being the set of all voxels of the HR image. The diffusion signal along the gradient u_n in all voxels forms a 3D image volume denoted by H_n. The correlation of the diffusion signal in neighboring voxels implies that H_n is spatially smooth. A standard technique to utilize this fact is to minimize the TV semi-norm of H_n defined as $\|H_n\|_{\text{TV}} = \sum_{r \in \Omega} \left[\sum_{p \in \mathcal{N}(r)} |h_r(u_n) - h_p(u_n)|^2 \right]^{1/2}$, where $\mathcal{N}(r)$ denotes a set of neighbors around r. For a collection of image volumes $H = \{H_n\}_{n=1}^{N}$, the TV semi-norm of H is defined as the sum of the TV semi-norm of each image volume H_n, i.e. $\|H\|_{\text{TV}} = \sum_{n=1}^{N} \|H_n\|_{\text{TV}}$. By adding a regularization term for $\|H\|_{\text{TV}}$ in (4), we rewrite the optimization problem as

$$\min_{V \geq 0, H} \left\{ \frac{1}{2} \sum_{k=1}^{K} \|L_k - D_k B_k H Q_k^T\|^2 + \lambda_1 \|W \circ V\|_1 + \lambda_2 \|H\|_{\text{TV}} \right\} \text{ s.t. } H = VA^T$$

$$(5)$$

where the positive parameters λ_1, λ_2 determine the relative importance of the data fitting terms versus the sparsity and the total regularization terms. Next, we introduce an efficient algorithm for solving (5) based on the alternating directions method of multipliers (ADMM) [16].

3.2 Optimization Algorithm

The optimization problem (5) typically involves high dimensional optimization variables. A suitable implementation of the ADMM algorithm may distribute the computational cost and decompose the optimization into a sequence of simpler problems. First, we note that (5) can be equivalently written as

$$\min_{V \geq 0, H, Z} \left\{ \frac{1}{2} \sum_{k=1}^{K} \|L_k - D_k B_k H Q_k^T\|^2 + \lambda_1 \|W \circ V\|_1 + \lambda_2 \|Z\|_{\mathrm{TV}} \right.$$
$$\left. + \frac{\rho_1}{2} \|H - V A^T\|^2 + \frac{\rho_2}{2} \|H - Z\|^2 \right\} \text{ s.t. } H - V A^T = 0, \ H - Z = 0,$$

where Z is an auxiliary variable that equals to H, and the augmented terms $\frac{\rho_1}{2}\|H - V A^T\|^2 + \frac{\rho_2}{2}\|H - Z\|^2$ with $\rho_1, \rho_2 \geq 0$ do not change the optimal value. Let Λ_1, Λ_2 be the multipliers for $H - V A^T = 0$ and $H - Z = 0$, respectively. Then, each iteration of the ADMM algorithm consists of several steps of alternately minimizing the augmented Lagrangian $\left\{ \frac{1}{2}\sum_{k=1}^{K} \|L_k - D_k B_k H Q_k^T\|^2 + \lambda_1 \|W \circ$ $V\|_1 + \lambda_2 \|Z\|_{\mathrm{TV}} + \frac{\rho_1}{2}\|H - V A^T + \Lambda_1\|^2 + \frac{\rho_2}{2}\|H - Z + \Lambda_2\|^2 \right\}$ over H, V, Z and one step of updating Λ_1, Λ_2. More specifically, let V^t, H^t, Z^t and Λ_1^t, Λ_2^t denote the values of these variables at iteration t. Then, iteration $(t+1)$ consists of two steps of estimating $\{V^{t+1}, Z^{t+1}\}$ and H^{t+1} by solving

$$\min_{V \geq 0, Z} \left\{ \lambda_1 \|W \circ V\|_1 + \lambda_2 \|Z\|_{\mathrm{TV}} + \frac{\rho_1}{2}\|H^t - V A^T + \Lambda_1^t\|^2 + \frac{\rho_2}{2}\|H^t - Z + \Lambda_2^t\|^2 \right\} \quad (6)$$

$$\min_{H} \left\{ \frac{1}{2} \sum_{k=1}^{K} \|L_k - D_k B_k H Q_k^T\|^2 + \frac{\rho_1}{2}\|H - V^{t+1} A^T + \Lambda_1^t\|^2 + \frac{\rho_2}{2}\|H - Z^{t+1} + \Lambda_2^t\|^2 \right\}$$
$$(7)$$

and one step of updating the multipliers as

$$\Lambda_1^{t+1} = \Lambda_1^t + (H^{t+1} - V^{t+1} A^T), \ \Lambda_2^{t+1} = \Lambda_2^t + (H^{t+1} - Z^{t+1}).$$

A typical stopping criteria is to check if Λ_1^t and Λ_2^t have "stopped changing", i.e. $\|\Lambda_1^{t+1} - \Lambda_1^t\|^2 \leq \epsilon_1$ and $\|\Lambda_2^{t+1} - \Lambda_2^t\|^2 \leq \epsilon_2$ for some user defined choice of ϵ_1, ϵ_2.

We point out some important notes for the above iterative algorithm: (1) Problem (6) can be decomposed into two independent optimization problems on V and Z, respectively. The update for V^t is obtained by solving an ℓ_1-minimization problem. In particular, the solution for each voxel can be obtained independently (parallely). We have also developed an ADMM-based algorithm for solving the non-negative weighted ℓ_1-regularization problem, which is not presented here due to page limitations. (2) The update for Z^t is a standard TV denoising problem. (3) Problem (7) is a least-squared problem which needs a matrix inversion to compute the closed-form solution. Though, in general a huge matrix needs to be inverted, in this particular situation where the LR images are sub-pixel-shifted scans with B_k's representing a blurring operation along the slice-selection direction and $[Q_1^T, \ldots, Q_K^T]$ is a permutation matrix, the computation reduces to inverting K matrices of size $n_z \times n_z$, i.e. $(B_k^T D_k^T D_k B_k + (\rho_1 + \rho_2)I)$ for $k = 1, \ldots, K$, which can be easily done on standard workstations. We also note that in extreme situations, when the matrix size is too large, the steepest descent iterative method in [6] or the conjugate gradient method can be used alternatively.

4   Experiments

We tested the performance of the proposed method using two experiments. In the first one, we used artificially generated thick-slice acquisitions based on the high resolution data set from the Human Connectome Project (HCP) while the second experiment consisted of an actual validation setup where both the LR and HR images were acquired on a 3T Siemens clinical scanner. We compared the recovered CS-SRR result with the corresponding gold-standard (GS) HR data using the following metrics:

- FA and Trace difference: Whole brain multi-tensor tractography [17] was computed on the GS and the reconstructed data, and several fiber bundles were extracted. The average fractional anisotropy (FA) and trace for tensors along the fiber bundles were computed.
- Fiber-bundle overlap: The Bhattacharyya coefficient described in [18] was used to compare the fiber bundle overlap. This measure ranges between [0, 1], with 0 being no overlap, while 1 being complete overlap of fibers.

4.1   Evaluation on HCP Data

In this experiment, we used HCP data, which has spatial resolution of $1.25 \times 1.25 \times 1.25$ mm^3 with 90 gradient directions at $b = 2000$ s/mm^2. To construct LR images, we first artificially blurred the DWI volumes along the slice direction using a Gaussian kernel with full width at half maximum (FWHM) of 1.25 mm. Then the data was down-sampled by averaging three contiguous slices to obtain a single thick-slice volume with spatial resolution of $1.25 \times 1.25 \times 3.75$ mm^3. Similarly, two additional LR volumes were obtained so that all the three LR volumes were slice-shifted in physical space (see Fig. 1). The thick-slice volumes were also sub-sampled in q-space so that each set had 30 unique gradient directions. We also obtained a segmentation of the brain into three tissue types, namely, gray, white and CSF, from the T_1-weighted MR images. This tissue classification was used as a prior to set $w = 10^{-4}$ in CSF and $w = 1$ in gray and white matter areas. The auxiliary parameter ρ_1 was set to $\rho_1 = 1$.

To compare the tractography results, we first obtained the whole-brain tractography using the method in [17] for the GS and the reconstructed data sets, respectively. Next, we extracted the cingulum bundle (CB), the corticospinal tract (CST), the superior longitudinal fasiculus II (SLF-II) and a sub-part of the corpus callosum called caudal middle frontal bundle (CC-CMF), respectively, using the white matter query language (WMQL) [19] which uses Freesurfer cortical parcellations. The four pairs of fiber bundles are shown in Fig. 2a to d, respectively. The fiber-bundle overlap measure is very close to one, indicating

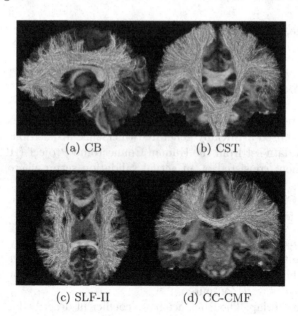

(a) CB   (b) CST

(c) SLF-II   (d) CC-CMF

Fig. 2. (a), (b) (c) and (d) are the tractography results for the cingulum bundle (CB), the corticospinal tract (CST), the superior longitudinal fasciculus II (SLF-II) and the corpus callosum caudal middle frontal (CC-CMF) bundle (with red and yellow tracts obtained using the GS and CS-SRR data sets respectively). The comparison metrics for the tractography results are shown in the following table.

	GS FA	CS-SRR FA	GS Trace	CS-SRR Trace	Fiber-bundle overlap
CB	0.54	0.52	2.1×10^{-3}	2.0×10^{-3}	0.97
CST	0.69	0.66	2.0×10^{-3}	2.0×10^{-3}	0.97
SLF-II	0.63	0.60	2.0×10^{-3}	2.0×10^{-3}	0.95
CC-CMF	0.63	0.61	2.2×10^{-3}	2.1×10^{-3}	0.95

a significant overlap between the fiber bundles obtained using the GS and CS-SRR data. Further, the estimated average FA and trace are very similar for both data sets.

Another important goal of this work is to demonstrate the advantage of using high-resolution DWI image in studying small white-matter fascicles. For this purpose, we generated a low-resolution DWI volume by averaging every $2 \times 2 \times 2$ neighboring voxels from the GS data to obtain a LR dMRI data with isotropic voxel size of 2.5^3 mm^3. Figure 3a–c shows the single tensor glyphs color coded by the direction of the dominant eigenvector for the GS, LR and SRR data sets in the same brain region from a coronal slice. Linear interpolations were used to increase the spatial resolution of the LR image. The background of the glyphs is the corresponding T_1 weighted image. As pointed out in the rectangular area in

Fig. 3b, due to partial-volume effects, the LR image was not able to capture the fine curvature of of fiber bundles near the gray matter areas. Figure 3d–f show the tractography results for tracts originating from the sub-thalamic nucleus with fibers being color-coded by orientation. While the tracts obtained from the GS and CS-SRR data are very similar, as pointed out by the arrow in Fig. 3e, most of the green fibers are missing in the LR image, though the number of seeds in the LR image is 8 times higher than the HR images.

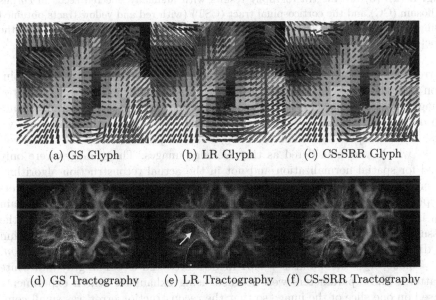

(a) GS Glyph   (b) LR Glyph   (c) CS-SRR Glyph

(d) GS Tractography   (e) LR Tractography   (f) CS-SRR Tractography

Fig. 3. (a), (b) and (c) show the single tensor glyphs for the GS, LR and CS-SRR HCP data sets, respectively. The rectangle in (b) shows the partial-volume effects in the LR image where the orientations of the glyphs are not estimated correctly. (d), (e) and (f) are the fiber tracts, color-coded with tract orientation for the three data sets with seeds in sub-thalamic nucleus. The arrow points out some missing fiber tracts in the LR image.

4.2   True CS-SRR Scenario

The second experiment was based on a data set acquired on a 3T Siemens clinical scanner. We acquired three overlapping thick-slice scans with spatial resolution $1.2 \times 1.2 \times 3.6$ mm^3. The DWI volumes were sub-pixel shifted by 1.2 mm along the slice-selection direction. Each LR DWI had a set of 30 unique gradient directions with $b = 1000$. For comparison, we also acquired 9 acquisitions (with 90 gradient directions each) of the same subject with a spatial resolution of $1.2 \times 1.2 \times 1.2$ mm^3, which was used as the "gold standard" data. Due to time limitations, these high resolution scans had partial brain coverage (it took about 1.5 hours to obtain these 9 scans). The average of these 9 scans (after motion

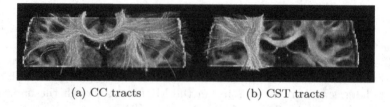

(a) CC tracts   (b) CST tracts

Fig. 4. (a), (b) are the tractography results with manually selected seeds in corpus callosum (CC) and the corticospinal tract (CST) (with red and yellow tracts obtained using the GS and CS-SRR data sets respectively). The comparison metrics for the tractography results are shown in the following table.

correction) was considered as the gold standard. We also acquired a high resolution B_0 image, i.e. the $b = 0$ image with no diffusion encoding, and a T_1-weighted image to obtain tissue classifications for prior-information used in our algorithm. To ensure that the LR DWI's were in the same spatial co-ordinate system, we first down-sampled the whole-brain B_0 image to produce three thick-slice volumes which were considered as the reference images. These images were only used for spatial normalization and not in the actual reconstruction algorithm. Then, the three acquired thick-slice LR DWI scans were registered to the corresponding reference volumes. The T_1 image was registered to the whole-brain B_0 image using a nonlinear transformation. From the registered T_1 image, the tissue brain segmentation was used for adjusting the parameters of the algorithm in different tissue types. We set the FWHM of the blurring kernel to 1.2 mm, $\lambda_1 = 0.005$, $\lambda_2 = 0.05$, and $w = 0.01$ in CSF area and $w = 1$ in gray and white matters. These parameters were learned using exhaustive search experiments based on one slice of the image so that the reconstruction error was small compared with the gold-standard. For computing quantitative metrics, we registered the reconstructed whole-brain data to the partial-brain GS data set.

We first obtained the tractography results from the reconstructed (CS-SRR) and GS partial-brain data sets using the method in [17]. Since whole-brain Freesurfer cortical parcellation was not available, we could not employ WMQL for tract extraction. Consequently, we use manually selected ROI's to extract fiber bundles in the corpus callosum (CC) and the corticospinal tract (CST), respectively. The extracted fiber bundles are shown in Fig. 4a and b, respectively. We note that there is minor difference between FA and Trace obtained from both the data sets. The value of the Bhattacharyya coefficient also indicates a significant overlap between the fiber bundles.

	GS FA	CS-SRR FA	GS Trace	CS-SRR Trace	Fiber-bundle overlap
CC	0.64	0.65	2.2×10^{-3}	2.4×10^{-3}	0.96
CST	0.62	0.64	2.0×10^{-3}	2.2×10^{-3}	0.94

To demonstrate the difference between HR and LR images, we also generated a LR image by averaging every $2 \times 2 \times 2$ neighboring voxel in the GS data set to obtain a LR dMRI data set with isotropic voxel size of 2.4^3 mm^3. Figure 5 shows the single tensor glyphs color coded by direction for the GS, LR and the CS-SRR data sets in the same brain region from a coronal slice. The background of the glyphs is the corresponding T_1 weighted image. As pointed out in the rectangular region in Fig. 5b, due to partial-volume effects, the LR image was not able to capture the correct fiber orientations near the gray matter areas. Figure 5c is similar to Fig. 5a, indicating that the proposed method was able to correctly reconstruct the fiber orientations near gray-matter areas.

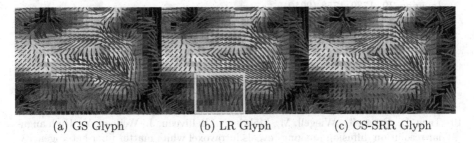

(a) GS Glyph   (b) LR Glyph   (c) CS-SRR Glyph

Fig. 5. (a), (b) and (c) show the single tensor glyphs colored coded by fiber orientation for the GS, LR and CS-SRR data sets, respectively. The rectangle in (b) points out the partial-volume effects in the LR image where the directions of the glyphs are not estimated correctly (shown by different colors from the GS glyphs).

5   Conclusion

We introduced a novel method for reconstructing very high-resolution diffusion data on a standard clinical scanner. By combining the concepts of compressed sensing and super-resolution, we were able to with significantly reduce scan time while increasing the spatial resolution. Preliminary results show that the our method is capable of accurately recovering complex fiber orientations in white and gray matter regions at a high spatial resolution, similar to a physically acquired gold-standard data. Future work involves doing extensive validation on several subjects in different brain regions.

References

1. Shenton, M., Hamoda, H., Schneiderman, J., Bouix, S., Pasternak, O., Rathi, Y., Vu, M.A., Purohit, M., Helmer, K., Koerte, I., et al.: A review of magnetic resonance imaging and diffusion tensor imaging findings in mild traumatic brain injury. Brain Imaging Behav. **6**, 137–192 (2012)
2. Manjón, J.V., Coupé, P., Buades, A., Fonov, V., Louis Collins, D., Robles, M.: Non-local MRI upsampling. Med. Image Anal. **14**, 784–792 (2010)
3. Dyrby, T.B., Lundell, H., Burke, M.W., Reislev, N.L., Paulson, O.B., Ptito, M., Siebner, H.R.: Interpolation of diffusion weighted imaging datasets. NeuroImage **103**, 202–213 (2014)

4. Irani, M., Peleg, S.: Motion analysis for image enhancement: resolution, occlusion, and transparency. J. Vis. Commun. Image Represent. **4**, 324–335 (1993)
5. Peled, S., Yeshurun, Y.: Superresolution in MRI: application to human white matter fiber tract visualization by diffusion tensor imaging. Magn. Reson. Med. **45**, 29–35 (2001)
6. Scherrer, B., Gholipour, A., Warfield, S.K.: Super-resolution reconstruction to increase the spatial resolution of diffusion weighted images from orthogonal anisotropic acquisitions. Med. Image Anal. **16**, 1465–1476 (2012)
7. Gholipour, A., Estroff, J.A., Warfield, S.K.: Robust super-resolution volume reconstruction from slice acquisitions: application to fetal brain MRI. IEEE Trans. Med. Imaging **29**, 1739–1758 (2010)
8. Steenkiste, G., Jeurissen, B., Veraart, J., den Dekker, A.J., Parizel, P.M., Poot, D.H., Sijbers, J.: Super-resolution reconstruction of diffusion parameters from diffusion-weighted images with different slice orientations. Magn. Reson. Med. (2015). doi:10.1002/mrm.25597
9. Bhushan, C., Joshi, A.A., Leahy, R.M., Haldar, J.P.: Improved b_0-distortion correction in diffusion MRI using interlaced q-space sampling and constrained reconstruction. Magn. Reson. Med. **72**, 1218–1232 (2014)
10. Tuch, D., Reese, T., Wiegell, M., Makris, N., Belliveau, J., Wedeen, V.: High angular resolution diffusion imaging reveals intravoxel white matter fiber heterogeneity. Magn. Reson. Med. **48**, 577–582 (2002)
11. Candès, E.J., Romberg, J., Tao, T.: Robust uncertainty principles: exact signal reconstruction from highly incomplete frequency information. IEEE Trans. Inf. Theory **52**, 489–509 (2006)
12. Michailovich, O., Rathi, Y.: On approximation of orientation distributions by means of spherical ridgelets. IEEE Trans. Image Process. **19**, 461–477 (2010)
13. Michailovich, O., Rathi, Y., Dolui, S.: Spatially regularized compressed sensing for high angular resolution diffusion imaging. IEEE Trans. Med. Imaging **30**, 1100–1115 (2011)
14. Rathi, Y., Michailovich, O., Setsompop, K., Bouix, S., Shenton, M.E., Westin, C.-F.: Sparse multi-shell diffusion imaging. In: Fichtinger, G., Martel, A., Peters, T. (eds.) MICCAI 2011, Part II. LNCS, vol. 6892, pp. 58–65. Springer, Heidelberg (2011)
15. Greenspan, H., Oz, G., Kiryati, N., Peled, S.: MRI inter-slice reconstruction using super-resolution. Magn. Reson. Imaging **20**, 437–446 (2002)
16. Boyd, S., Parikh, N., Chu, E., Peleato, B., Eckstein, J.: Distributed optimization and statistical learning via the alternating direction method of multipliers. Found.Trends Mach. Learn. **3**, 1–122 (2011)
17. Malcolm, J.G., Shenton, M.E., Rathi, Y.: Filtered multi-tensor tractography. IEEE Trans. Med. Imaging **29**, 1664–1675 (2010)
18. Rathi, Y., Gagoski, B., Setsompop, K., Michailovich, O., Grant, P.E., Westin, C.-F.: Diffusion propagator estimation from sparse measurements in a tractography framework. In: Mori, K., Sakuma, I., Sato, Y., Barillot, C., Navab, N. (eds.) MICCAI 2013, Part III. LNCS, vol. 8151, pp. 510–517. Springer, Heidelberg (2013)
19. Wassermann, D., Makris, N., Rathi, Y., Shenton, M., Kikinis, R., Kubicki, M., Westin, C.-F.: On describing human white matter anatomy: the white matter query language. In: Mori, K., Sakuma, I., Sato, Y., Barillot, C., Navab, N. (eds.) MICCAI 2013, Part I. LNCS, vol. 8149, pp. 647–654. Springer, Heidelberg (2013)

Accelerated High Spatial Resolution Diffusion-Weighted Imaging

Benoit Scherrer$^{(\boxtimes)}$, Onur Afacan, Maxime Taquet, Sanjay P. Prabhu, Ali Gholipour, and Simon K. Warfield

Department of Radiology Boston Children's Hospital, Computational Radiology Laboratory, 300 Longwood Avenue, Boston, MA 02115, USA
`benoit.scherrer@childrens.harvard.edu`

Abstract. Acquisition of a series of anisotropically oversampled acquisitions (so-called anisotropic "snapshots") and reconstruction in the image space has recently been proposed to increase the spatial resolution in diffusion weighted imaging (DWI), providing a theoretical 8x acceleration at equal signal-to-noise ratio (SNR) compared to conventional dense k-space sampling. However, in most works, each DW image is reconstructed separately and the fact that the DW images constitute different views of the same anatomy is ignored. In addition, current approaches are limited by their inability to reconstruct a high resolution (HR) acquisition from snapshots with different subsets of diffusion gradients: an isotropic HR gradient image cannot be reconstructed if one of its anisotropic snapshots is missing, for example due to intra-scan motion, even if other snapshots for this gradient were successfully acquired. In this work, we propose a novel multi-snapshot DWI reconstruction technique that simultaneously achieves HR reconstruction and local tissue model estimation while enabling reconstruction from snapshots containing different subsets of diffusion gradients, providing increased robustness to patient motion and potential for acceleration. Our approach is formalized as a joint probabilistic model with missing observations, from which interactions between missing snapshots, HR reconstruction and a generic tissue model naturally emerge. We evaluate our approach with synthetic simulations, simulated multi-snapshot scenario and *in vivo* multi-snapshot imaging. We show that (1) our combined approach ultimately provides both better HR reconstruction and better tissue model estimation and (2) the error in the case of missing snapshots can be quantified. Our novel multi-snapshot technique will enable improved high spatial characterization of the brain connectivity and microstructure *in vivo*.

Keywords: Diffusion-weighted imaging · High spatial resolution · Model-based · Joint model

1 Introduction

Increasing the spatial resolution in diffusion-weighted magnetic resonance imaging (DW-MRI) enables substantial reduction of the intra-voxel microstructural

---

This work was supported in part by NIH grants R01 EB018988, R01 LM010033, U01 NS082320, R01 NS079788 and BCH CTREC K-to-R Merit Award.

S. Ourselin et al. (Eds.): IPMI 2015, LNCS 9123, pp. 69–81, 2015.
DOI: 10.1007/978-3-319-19992-4_6

complexity. This has been shown to enable better delineation of the trajectory of white matter (WM) fascicles [1,10,11] and to decrease the impact of partial voluming, critical in population studies [14] and when imaging brain structures prone to partial volume effect such as the cerebellum. However, because the SNR is directly proportional to the voxel volume, reducing the voxel size directly increases the noise of each measurement which strongly impacts the precision of estimated model parameters. High spatial resolution imaging with constant SNR can be achieved by repeating the measurements, but requires a quadratic imaging time increase. Moreover, enhancing the resolution in the slice direction requires the acquisition of additional slices to cover the same area which also increases the duration of the scans. To illustrate, reducing the resolution from $2 \times 2 \times 2 \, \mathrm{mm}^3$ to $1 \times 1 \times 1 \, \mathrm{mm}^3$ requires 128 times more imaging time at equal SNR; a 5 min. acquisition would thus become a 10.7 h. acquisition, which is not realistic.

Enhancing the spatial resolution requires sampling of higher frequencies in k-space which is very challenging to accomplish with high SNR and short acquisition duration time. Instead of acquiring high frequencies along all the axes simultaneously, [8] demonstrated that high-resolution (HR) k-space sampling for a diffusion gradient can be achieved by imaging this diffusion gradient with a series of anisotropically oversampled acquisitions (so-called "snapshots") that each densely samples more frequencies along a limited number of axes (one or two). Compared to full, dense HR sampling, this multi-snapshot non-Cartesian sampling reduces the spatial encoding burden and provides substantially increased SNR for each snapshot due to the larger voxel size. In [8], an image generation model was then employed to describe how the anisotropic low resolution (LR) snapshots are observations of the unknown, underlying HR isotropic DW images we aim to recover (forward model), and the corresponding HR DW images recovered by inversing this forward model. A similar technique was later employed in [6]. A particular strength of this approach is that it only requires a conventional DW-MRI sequence and is therefore straightforward to implement. When using three orthogonal snapshots for each diffusion gradient, this effectively enhances spatial resolution along all the axes (x,y,z) while providing an 8x theoretical reduction in imaging time compared to conventional sampling at equal SNR [8].

A major limitation in [6,8] is that each DW image was reconstructed separately. First, the fact that the DWIs constitute different views of the same anatomy was ignored. DW images are coupled and this correlation of information can be leveraged by introducing in the reconstruction the knowledge of the local tissue microstructure. Second, an isotropic HR gradient image could not be recovered if one of its snapshots was missing, for example because of intra-scan motion, even if other snapshots for this gradient were successfully acquired.

Tobisch *et al.* [12] built upon the work in [6,8] and proposed to introduce an ad-hoc coupling between HR reconstruction and tissue model estimation to capture the coupling between DW images. They considered the ball-and-stick tissue model at each voxel, thereby assuming (1) the presence of a single fascicle in each voxel; (2) the absence of radial diffusivity; and (3) a prefixed axial diffusivity value constant for the entire brain. This model, however, poorly represents *in vivo* brain tissues. This is critical because, when HR reconstruction and tissue model estimation are coupled, the ability of the tissue model to accurately predict the DW signal for a diffusion gradient *conditions* the ultimate HR reconstruction accuracy. In [12], only results with synthetic simulations were reported, but no evidence of the technical efficacy of the technique was reported with *in vivo* data. More importantly, and similarly to [6,8], this technique required the successful acquisition of *all the snapshots* for a diffusion gradient to reconstruct the corresponding HR gradient image.

In this work, we propose a novel multi-snapshot DWI reconstruction technique that simultaneously achieves HR reconstruction and tissue model estimation while enabling reconstruction with missing snapshots. Instead of an ad-hoc coupling [12], our approach is formalized as a joint probabilistic model with missing observations, from which interactions between missing snapshots, HR reconstruction and a generic tissue model naturally emerge. We describe the tissue microstructure at a voxel with a diffusion compartment imaging (DCI) tissue model that reflects the presence of tissue compartments in each voxel, providing a model-based description of the signal attenuation for any diffusion gradient orientation and strength. Our novel Simultaneous multi-snapsHot highresOlution ReconsTruCtion and diffUsion comparTment imaging (SHORTCUT) approach enables reconstruction from snapshots with different subsets of gradients, providing increased robustness to patient motion and potential for acceleration. We evaluate SHORTCUT with synthetic simulations, simulated multi-snapshot scenario and *in vivo* multi-snapshot imaging. We investigate the robustness to missing snapshots. We show that SHORTCUT enables both better reconstruction of each DW image and better estimation of the tissue parameters.

2 Theory

2.1 The SHORTCUT Framework

We formalize SHORTCUT as a joint probabilistic model synthetized in Fig. 1. We consider G unique diffusion gradients and a maximum of K snapshots per gradient. We denote by $\mathbf{y}_{g,s}$ the DW image for the snapshot s of the diffusion gradient g and by $\mathbf{y} = (\mathbf{y}_{1,1}, \ldots, \mathbf{y}_{1,K}, \; \cdots \;, \mathbf{y}_{G,1}, \ldots, \mathbf{y}_{G,K})$ the images of the KG snapshots in which only $\mathbf{y} = (\mathbf{y}_{1,1}, \ldots, \mathbf{y}_{1,K_1}, \; \cdots \;, \mathbf{y}_{G,1}, \ldots, \mathbf{y}_{G,K_G})$ have been acquired and $(\mathbf{y}_{1,K_1+1}, \ldots, \mathbf{y}_{1,K}, \; \cdots \;, \mathbf{y}_{G,K_G+1}, \ldots, \mathbf{y}_{G,K})$ are missing. We denote by $\mathbf{x} = (\mathbf{x}_1, \ldots, \mathbf{x}_G)$ the unknown HR DW images we aim to recover. We also consider a generic DCI tissue model dependent on some parameters $\mathbf{t}$ that describes the DW signal attenuation at a voxel i for a diffusion gradient g by $S_g(\mathbf{t}_i)$. We aim at recovering (1) the series of missing snapshots; (2) the series of unknown HR DW images $\mathbf{x}$; (3) the parameters $\mathbf{t}$ of the tissue model at each voxel. The simultaneous estimation of $\mathbf{x}, \mathbf{t}, \mathbf{y}$ is performed according to the maximum *a posteriori* principle, by maximizing:

$$\widehat{\mathbf{x}}_{\mathrm{MAP}}, \widehat{\mathbf{t}}_{\mathrm{MAP}}, \widehat{\mathbf{y}}_{\mathrm{MAP}} = \arg\max_{\mathbf{x},\mathbf{t},\mathbf{y}} p(\mathbf{x},\mathbf{t}|\mathbf{y}) = \arg\max_{\mathbf{x},\mathbf{t},\mathbf{y}} p(\mathbf{y}|\mathbf{x},\mathbf{t})p(\mathbf{x}|\mathbf{t})p(\mathbf{t}). \qquad (1)$$

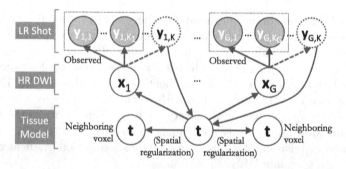

Fig. 1. Graphical representation of the SHORTCUT joint model in which we consider that some gradients may not be acquired in all snapshots.

Factor $p(\mathbf{y}|\mathbf{x}, \mathbf{t})$. The likelihood $p(\mathbf{y}|\mathbf{x}, \mathbf{t})$ describes the probability of observing the snapshots $\mathbf{y}$ given a realization of $\mathbf{x}$ and $\mathbf{t}$ and relates to HR reconstruction. Assuming conditional independence we can show that:

$$p(\mathbf{y}|\mathbf{x}, \mathbf{t}) \propto \prod_{g=1}^{G} \prod_{k=1}^{K_g} p(\mathbf{y}_{g,k}|\mathbf{x}_g, \mathbf{t}) \prod_{k=K_g+1}^{K} p(\mathbf{y}_{g,k}|\mathbf{t}, \mathbf{x}_g).$$

For *acquired* DW images (i.e., $k \in [1, K_g]$), we consider that all the information about $\mathbf{y}_{g,k}$ is contained in the HR image $\mathbf{x}_g$. The term $p(\mathbf{y}_{g,k}|\mathbf{x}_g, \mathbf{t})$ then describes how each snapshot constitutes an observation of the unknown $\mathbf{x}$. Similarly to [8], we consider an *image generation model* that describes how the LR snapshots are obtained from the unknown underlying HR volumes. Specifically, for each diffusion gradient g, we consider that $\mathbf{x}_g$ goes through geometric and signal modifying operations to generate the K acquired LR volume: $\mathbf{y}_{g,k} = \mathbf{W}_{g,k}\mathbf{x}_g + \epsilon_{g,k}$, where $\mathbf{y}_{g,k}$ and $\mathbf{x}_{g,k}$ are expressed as column vectors by a lexicographical reordering of the pixels. We consider $\mathbf{W}_{g,k} = \mathbf{D}_{g,k}\mathbf{B}_{g,k}\mathbf{M}_{g,k}$ where $\mathbf{D}_{g,k}$ is the down-sampling matrix, $\mathbf{M}_{g,k}$ is the warping matrix that maps the HR volume $\mathbf{x}$ to the LR volume $\mathbf{y}_{g,k}$, $\mathbf{B}_{g,k}$ describes the point spread function (PSF) of the MRI signal acquisition process and $\epsilon_{g,k}$ is the vector of residual noise. We assume that, conditionally on $\mathbf{x}$, the LR data $\mathbf{y}$ are normally distributed around the unknown HR intensities with variance σ_A^2, so that:

$$\forall k \le K_g, \; p(\mathbf{y}_{g,k}|\mathbf{x}_g, \mathbf{t}) = \frac{1}{\sigma_A \sqrt{2\pi}} \exp\left(-\frac{||\mathbf{y}_{g,k} - \mathbf{W}_{g,k}\mathbf{x}_g||^2}{2\sigma_A^2}\right). \qquad (2)$$

For *non-acquired* images (i.e., $k \in [K_g+1, K]$) the term $p(\mathbf{y}_{g,k}|\mathbf{t}, \mathbf{x}_g)$ describes the agreement between the missing snapshot $\mathbf{y}_{g,k}$ and the signal arising from the DCI model for the unobserved k^{th} snapshot of the gradient g. This term relates to the missing snapshot recovery using the tissue model. We consider that all the information about $\mathbf{y}_{g,k}$ is contained in $\mathbf{t}$ and assume that, conditionally on $\mathbf{y}_{g,k}$, the intensities of the missing snapshot $\mathbf{y}_{g,k}$ are normally distributed around the intensities of the recovered LR snapshot $\mathbf{W}_{g,k}S_g(\mathbf{t})$ with variance σ_B^2:

$$\forall k > K_g,\ p(\mathbf{y}_{g,k}|\mathbf{t},\mathbf{x}_g) = \frac{1}{\sigma_B\sqrt{2\pi}}\exp\left(-\frac{||\mathbf{y}_{g,k} - \mathbf{W}_{g,k}S_g(\mathbf{t})||^2}{2\sigma_B^2}\right) \qquad (3)$$

Factor $p(\mathbf{x}|\mathbf{t})$. The term $p(\mathbf{x}|\mathbf{t})$ describes the agreement between the series of DW images $\mathbf{x}$ and the HR signal modeled by the tissue model and relates to the DCI model estimation. We consider that the HR image domain V^{HR} is a regular 3-dimensional (3D) grid and denote by $\mathbf{x}_{g,i}$ the ith voxel of the gth HR DW image $\mathbf{x}_g$. We assume that, conditionally on $\mathbf{t}$, the HR DW images $\mathbf{x}$ are normally distributed around the unknown modeled signal $S_g(\mathbf{t}_i)$ with variance σ_C^2:

$$p(\mathbf{x}|\mathbf{t}) = \prod_{i\in V^{HR}}\prod_{g=1}^{G}\frac{1}{\sigma_C\sqrt{2\pi}}\exp\left(-\frac{||\mathbf{x}_{g,i} - S_g(\mathbf{t}_i)||^2}{2\sigma_C^2}\right). \qquad (4)$$

Factor $p(\mathbf{t})$. The term $p(\mathbf{t})$ enables us to incorporate a prior knowledge on the tissue model parameters. It can be used to introduce a regularization prior that exploits spatial homogeneity (see Sect. 2.3).

2.2   SHORTCUT-DTI and SHORTCUT-MTM

The SHORTCUT approach derived in Sect. 2.1 is independent of the choice of tissue model. The simplest solution is to consider a diffusion tensor at each voxel (DTI). This amounts to modeling the signal by $S_g(\mathbf{t}_i) = S_{0,i}\exp\left(-b_g\mathbf{g}_g^T\mathbf{D}_i\mathbf{g}_g\right)$ where $S_{0,i}$ is the non-attenuated signal, $\mathbf{D}_i$ is the diffusion tensor at voxel i and b_g and $\mathbf{g}_g$ are the gth b-value and unit-norm diffusion gradient direction. The parameters to estimate are $\mathbf{t}_i = \{S_{0,i},\mathbf{D}_i\}$ and the corresponding HR reconstruction approach referred to as SHORTCUT-DTI.

We also considered a diffusion compartment imaging model that reflects the presence of tissue compartments in each voxel and captures the non-monoexponential decay of the diffusion observed in voxels. More precisely, we considered that each compartment is in slow exchange and modeled the signal arising from each of them with a diffusion tensor. We considered in each voxel a multi-tensor model (MTM) [13] with 1) an isotropic diffusion compartment to model the diffusion of free water; and 2) a series of anisotropic cylindrical diffusion compartments to model the combined contribution of hindered and intra-axonal diffusion arising from each WM fascicle, leading to the attenuation DW signal:

$$S_g(\mathbf{t}_i) = S_0\left[f_{0,i}\exp(-D_{iso}b_g) + \sum_{j=1}^{N_i^f}f_{j,i}\exp(-b_g\mathbf{g}_g^T\mathbf{D}_{j,i}\mathbf{g}_g)\right], \qquad (5)$$

where N_i^f is the number of WM fascicles, $\{f_{j,i}, j = 1,\ldots,N_i^f\}$ are the volumic fractions of occupancy of each compartment and sum to one, D_{iso} is the diffusivity of free water and $\{\mathbf{D}_{j,i}, j = 1,\ldots,N_i^f\}$ are tensors describing each compartment. In this case, the parameters to estimate are $\mathbf{t}_i = \{S_{0,i}, N_i^f, (f_{j,i},\mathbf{D}_{j,i}), j = 1,\ldots,N_i^f\}$ and we refer to this HR reconstruction approach to as SHORTCUT-MTM.

2.3   Estimation of the Model Parameters

We considered a regularization prior $p(\mathbf{t})$ that exploits spatial homogeneity between tensors by setting $p(\mathbf{t}) \propto \prod_{i \in V} \prod_{j=1}^{N_i^f} \exp\left(-\alpha_{\mathrm{reg}}\phi(\|\nabla \log(\mathbf{D}_{j,i})\|)\right)$ (considering $N_i^f = 1$ for SHORTCUT-DTI), where $\|\nabla \log(\mathbf{D}_{j,i})\|$ is the norm of the spatial gradient of $\mathbf{D}_{j,i}$ taken in the log-euclidean space and α_{reg} is a parameter controlling the regularization strength. As in [9], we chose the regularization function $\phi(s) = \sqrt{1 + s^2/K_{\mathrm{reg}}^2}$, K_{reg} being a normalization factor, to account for *anisotropic* regularization and to preserve sharp contours.

The maximization (1) was achieved by adopting a relaxation approach, by iteratively maximizing for $\mathbf{t}$, for $\mathbf{y}$ and for $\mathbf{x}$, resulting in a novel algorithm that iteratively achieves (1) DCI tissue model estimation; (2) recovery of the DWIs for the unobserved snapshots; and (3) HR reconstruction. In this work, we considered equal constant noise variances, leading to the update rules:

$$\mathbf{t}^{(n+1)} = \arg\min_{\mathbf{t}} \sum_{i \in V^{\mathrm{HR}}} \left[\sum_{g=1}^{G} \|\mathbf{x}_i^{(n)} - S_g(\mathbf{t}_i)\|^2 + \sum_{g=1}^{G} \sum_{k=K_g+1}^{K} \|\mathbf{y}_{(g,k)_i}^{(n)} - \mathbf{W}_{g,k} S_g(\mathbf{t}_i)\|^2 \right.$$

$$\left. + \alpha_{\mathrm{reg}} \sum_{j=1}^{N_i^f} \sqrt{1 + \|\nabla \log(\mathbf{D}_{0,i}^j)\|^2/K_{\mathrm{reg}}^2} \right] \tag{6}$$

$$\forall k \in [K_g + 1, K] : \mathbf{y}_{g,k}^{(n+1)} = \mathbf{W}_{g,k} S_g(\mathbf{t}^{(n+1)}) \tag{7}$$

$$\forall g \in [1, G] : \mathbf{x}_g^{(n+1)} = \arg\min_{\mathbf{x}} \sum_{k=1}^{K_g} \|\mathbf{y}_{g,k}^{(n+1)} - \mathbf{W}_{g,k}\mathbf{x}\|^2 + \|\mathbf{x} - S_g(\mathbf{t}^{(n+1)})\|^2 \tag{8}$$

This iterative algorithm is initialized by computing the mean of the observed LR snapshots. The number N_i^f of fascicle at each voxel was estimated by minimizing the generalization error [2]. We chose to estimate it only a single time after initialization of the HR reconstruction to reduce the computational burden. The steps (6), (7), (8) were achieved until the average root-mean squared difference (RMSD) between consecutive reconstructed $\mathbf{x}^{(n-1)}$ and $\mathbf{x}^{(n)}$ is lower than a threshold θ. The joint HR reconstruction and tissue model reconstruction is synthesized by the pseudo-code:

```
n <- 0; Initialize each x_g^(n=0),g  =  1,...,G to the mean of the
y_g,.'s
Compute N_i^f at each voxel from x^(0) (model selection)
DO
   t^(n+1) <- Update tissue model (6)
   y^(n+1) <- Recover missing snapshots (7)
   x^(n+1) <- Update HR reconstruction (8)
   n <- n+1
WHILE 1/K ∑_{k=1}^{K} RMSD(x^(n),x^(n-1)) > θ
t^(n+1) <- Update tissue model
```

3   Methods

Algorithm Settings. SHORTCUT was implemented in C++. The tissue model estimation was parallelized over the image space and the DW HR reconstruction was parallelized over the space of diffusion gradients. The model-based HR reconstruction (8) was computed voxelwise by implementing the image generation model with a functional that maps a HR voxel to the LR space k accounting for downsampling, warping and sinc PSF. In SHORTCUT-MTM, the tensor representing each WM fascicle was constrained to be cylindrical. The minimizations (8) and (6) were achieved with Bobyqa [7], a derivative-free bound-constrained iterative algorithm that computes at each iteration a quadratic approximation for the objective function. We found that Bobyqa provided lower cost-function minima than using a levenberg-marquardt scheme with estimation of the Jacobian via finite differences. The model parameters were set to $\alpha_{reg} = 0.8$, $K_{reg} = 0.01$, $D_{iso} = 3 \times 10^{-3} \, \text{mm}^2/\text{s}$ the diffusivity of free water at $37°$ [5] and $\theta = 0.1$.

Numerical Phantom. We first evaluated our approach with a numerical phantom for which a noise-free ground truth could be generated. We simulated the diffusion signal arising from 1000 tensors (FA = 0.8) crossing with various angles (Fig. 2d). We considered a CUSP65 gradient encoding set [9] which achieves multiple non-zero b-values between $1000 \, \text{s/mm}^2$ and $3000 \, \text{s/mm}^2$ with low echo time (TE) and therefore high SNR. The DW images were corrupted with Rician noise (SNR on the b = $0 \, \text{s/mm}^2$ image: 25 dB). We simulated dense undersampling of k-space by removing half of the high frequencies along a single axis in Fourier space and by recovering the corresponding image in image space. This was achieved for the X, Y and Z axes and led to three orthogonal anisotropic acquisitions with a slice thickness twice the size of the in-plane resolution. We compared SHORTCUT-DTI and SHORTCUT-MTM to HR reconstruction alone (DwI with Separate high resolution reCOnstRuction and Diffusion model estimation, DISCORD) [6,8] by assessing the reconstruction accuracy (peak signal-to-noise ratio, PSNR) with the noise-free DW images. We also investigated the convergence of SHORTCUT and assessed the estimation accuracy of tissue model parameters for increasing number of iterations. This was achieved by comparing the compartment fractional anisotropy (cFA) of the first compartment to that of the ground truth (0.8).

Simulated Multi-snapshot Scenario with *in vivo* Data. We considered an *in vivo* CUSP65 scan acquired on a Siemens 3T Trio scanner with a 32-channel head coil and the following parameters : FOV = 240 mm, matrix = 128×128, resolution = $1.88 \times 1.88 \times 2 \text{mm}^3$. The Rician-noise corrected SNR in the WM measured in a $b = 0 \, \text{s/mm}^2$ was $\frac{296}{4.3} \sqrt{\frac{4-\pi}{2}} = 68.8$ (33 dB). Similarly as above, we simulated three dense undersamplings of k-space by removing half of the high frequencies in Fourier space along a single axis for consecutively the axial, sagittal, and coronal orientations. We compared SHORTCUT-DTI and

SHORTCUT-MTM by computing the PSNR of HR reconstructed DWIs with the original densely sampled HR DWIs (reference standard). Because the reference standard contains noise, the PSNR does not reflect the true HR reconstruction accuracy of the underlying anatomy. However, this enables investigation of the impact of the tissue model on the HR reconstruction. We compared the MTM tissue model estimated by SHORTCUT-MTM to the MTM tissue model estimated when using the original HR acquisition (HR-MTM). We assessed the relative error between the highest cFA at each voxel between SHORTCUT-MTM and HR-MTM, HR-MTM being considered as the reference standard. The maximum cFA was used as a proxy to identify at each voxel the same fascicle between the multi-tensor fields. We also compared to the relative error when estimating the MTM model after SHORTCUT-DTI reconstruction (SHORTCUT-DTI-MTM).

In-vivo **Multi-snapshot Imaging.** We acquired three orthogonal CUSP65 scans on a healthy volunteer using a Siemens 3T Trio scanner with a 32-channel head coil and the following parameters : FOV = 220 mm, matrix = 176 × 176, resolution = 1.25 × 1.25 × 2 mm^3. For each orientation, two $b = 0$ s/mm^2 images were also scanned with opposite phase encoding directions and used to correct the images for geometric and intensity distortions using *topup* (FSL). The Rician-noise corrected SNR in the WM measured in a $b = 0$ s/mm^2 was 26.4 (24.7 dB). The average Rician-noise corrected SNRs in the WM for DW images at $b = 1000$ s/mm^2, $b = 1500$ s/mm^2, $b = 2000$ s/mm^2 and $b = 3000$ s/mm^2 were respectively 14.0 (19.2 dB), 12.9 (18.5 dB), 10.8 (17.0 dB) and 9.4 (15.8 dB), above SNR > 3 for which the Rician distribution can be accurately approximated by a Gaussian distribution [3]. We achieved HR reconstruction and compared HR reconstruction alone (DISCORD), SHORTCUT-DTI and SHORTCUT-MTM (computational time: 20 h for full brain reconstruction with a double Intel Xeon E5 processor, 8 cores each).

Robustness to Missing Snapshots. Finally, we investigated with *in vivo* data the impact of missing snapshots. We considered the aforementioned three *in vivo* CUSP65 scans and quantified the impact of discarding an increasing number M of snapshots on the estimated MTM parameters. For each number $M \in [1, 120]$, we randomly discarded M DW snapshots among the 195 available and computed SHORTCUT-MTM. This was repeated 100 times. We assessed the average error between the 100 estimated MTM models and the MTM estimated by SHORTCUT-MTM with full gradient sampling, considered as reference standard. This was achieved by assessing in two single fascicle regions 1) the average relative error of cFA; and 2) the average minimum angle (AMA) error [13].

4   Results

Numerical Phantom. Figure 2a shows that the RMSD between consecutive DW images reconstructions monotonically decreases toward zero, experimentally showing the convergence of the algorithm. Figure 2b shows that the average

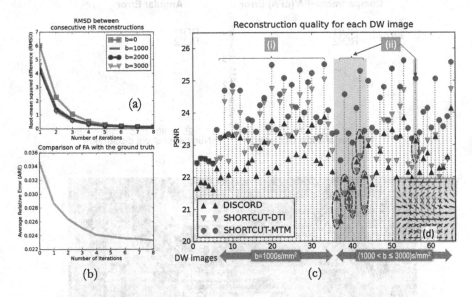

Fig. 2. Simulations with a synthetic phantom. (a) RMSD between consecutive DW images with SHORTCUT-MTM (for various b-value DW images). (b) Average Relative Error of the highest cFA with that of the ground truth. (c) Reconstruction accuracy for *each* DW image (PSNR). Highlighted are DWIs for which SHORTCUT-DTI provides lower PSNR than DISCORD. (d) Illustration of a slice of the numerical phantom.

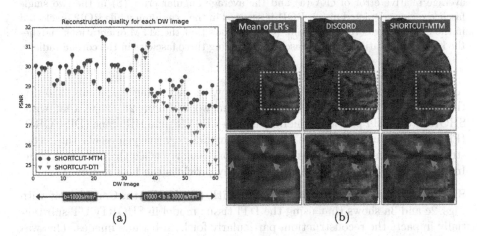

Fig. 3. (a) Simulated multi-snapshot scenario: impact of the tissue model on the HR reconstruction. (b) *In vivo* multi-snapshot imaging: for a $b=1000s/mm^2$ image, qualitative evaluation of the mean of the orthogonal snapshots; the HR reconstruction alone (DISCORD); and SHORTCUT-MTM. (see electronic version for better grayscale visualization).

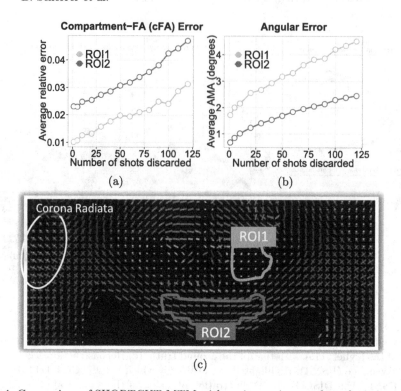

Fig. 4. Comparison of SHORTCUT-MTM with an increasing number of missing snapshots to SHORTCUT-MTM with full sampling (reference standard). Are shown the average relative error of cFA (a) and the average angular error (b) in the two single fascicle regions depicted in (c). ROI1 is selected in the cyngulum while ROI2 is selected in the body of the corpus callosum. (c) also shows that the MTM orientations matches the known orientations of WM fascicles, including three fascicles in the corona radiata.

relative error of cFA gradually decreases with increasing iterations, showing the benefits of the joint SHORTCUT framework. Figure 2c shows that while SHORTCUT-DTI provides generally a higher PSNR than HR alone (DISCORD) (Fig. 2c i), the over-simplistic DTI tissue model negatively impacts the reconstruction for some DW images (Fig. 2c ii), particularly when the b-value is large. In contrast, SHORTCUT-MTM consistently provides the best results.

Simulated Multi-snapshot Scenario with *in vivo* Data. Consistently with Figs. 2c and 3a shows that using the DTI tissue model in SHORTCUT substantially impacts the reconstruction, particularly for high b-value images. This was also verified by comparing MTM model parameters of SHORTCUT-MTM and SHORTCUT-DTI-MTM to HR-MTM over the entire white matter : the average relative error of the highest cFA at each voxel was $0.018 \pm 7.27 \times 10^{-2}$ with SHORTCUT-MTM and $0.031 \pm 1.35 \times 10^{-1}$ with SHORTCUT-DTI-MTM.

In-vivo **Multi-snapshot Imaging.** Figure 3b reports the results from *in vivo* multi-snapshot imaging. It qualitatively shows that the mean of the three orthogonal snapshots for a diffusion gradient is blurred and that the HR reconstruction alone (DISCORD) is highly impacted by noise. In contrast, incorporation of the tissue model in SHORTCUT-MTM provides a regularized solution that preserves edges, qualitatively leading to a better HR reconstruction.

Robustness to Missing Snapshots. Figure 4a shows the relative error of cFA in the cyngulum (ROI1) and in the body of the corpus callosum (ROI2). It shows that a relative error lower than 3 % is ensured when a maximum of 50 gradients (i.e., 25 % of the snapshots) is discarded. Figure 4b reports the average minimumm angular error The corresponding maximum angular error is on the order of 3°.

5 Discussion

We propose a novel algorithm to achieve HR reconstruction from multi-snapshot DW imaging. Instead of performing the reconstruction of each DW image independently [6,8], we account for the correlations between DW images by incorporating the knowledge of a local tissue model. Instead of an ad-hoc coupling [12], we formalize the simultaneous HR reconstruction and tissue model estimation with a joint probabilistic model from which interactions between the two processes naturally emerge. Importantly, and unlike [6,8,12], our framework enables reconstruction from snapshots with different subsets of diffusion gradients. This enables reconstruction from acquisitions in which snapshots are missing, for example due to corruption by intra-scan motion. This also provides potential for (1) scan time acceleration for a fixed gradient set or (2) increased *q*-space sampling for a fixed acquisition time.

We provided experimental evidence of the convergence of our novel SHORT-CUT algorithm (Fig. 2a) and quantitatively assessed its performance (Fig. 2b-c). Importantly, we demonstrated that incorporating an over-simplistic tissue model (DTI) substantially impacts the reconstruction (Figs. 2c.ii and 3a). This was especially observed for high b-value images, which is consistent with the known non-monoexponential decay of the DW signal for high b-values in voxels. We also showed that with *in vivo* acquisitions, HR reconstruction alone produces noisy results (Fig. 3b). This is probably due to slight local misalignment of the orthogonal acquisitions caused by imperfect susceptibility distortion correction. In contrast, SHORTCUT enables regularization of the reconstruction by introducing the knowledge of the local microstructure in each voxel, providing better results. Finally, we quantified the expected relative error when snapshots are not acquired (e.g., due to motion or to accelerate the acquisition) compared to full gradient sampling.

In the literature, a popu lar multi-*shot* technique is read-out segmented EPI [4] (rosEPI), which relies on the read-out of k-space with several adjacent segments and on their recombination in k-space. While rosEPI offers a slight SNR increase due to the shorter read-out of each segment (leading to lower

TE), rosEPI does not benefit from increased SNR due to the larger voxel size. Moreover, phase inconsistencies in k-space resulting from even minimal physiological motion during the application of the gradients remain challenging to correct. In contrast, our multi-snapshot high resolution technique provides, for each snapshot, a substantial SNR boost due to the larger voxel size and performs reconstruction in the image space. Similarly to rosEPI, reduced distortion can be obtained by using snapshots with low resolution in the phase encoding direction, reducing the number of phase encodes and, in the aggregate, the amount of T2* relaxation-induced distortion.

It is important to note that, with multi-snapshot imaging and reconstruction in the image space, employing at least three *orthogonal* scans is necessary to ultimately recover high frequencies along all the dimensions. However, with only three scans, the frequencies in the corners of k-space are missing. In future work, we will evaluate the impact of this approximation by experimentally assessing the effective spatial resolution by imaging a physical phantom. We will also evaluate the impact of (1) non-Gaussian noise modeling when using high SNR DW data (SNR on $b = 0 s/mm^2 \geq 25\,dB$); and (2) various PSF modeling strategies.

References

1. Bach, M., Fritzsche, K.H., Stieltjes, B., Laun, F.B.: Investigation of resolution effects using a specialized diffusion tensor phantom. Magn Reson Med **71**, 1108–1116 (2013)
2. Efron, B.: Estimating the error rate of a prediction rule: improvement on cross-validation. J. Am. Stat. Assoc. **78**(382), 316–331 (1983)
3. Gudbjartsson, H., Patz, S.: The Rician distribution of noisy MRI data. Magn Reson Med **34**(6), 910–914 (1995)
4. Holdsworth, S.J., Skare, S., Newbould, R.D., Guzmann, R., Blevins, N.H., Bammer, R.: Readout-segmented EPI for rapid high resolution diffusion imaging at 3T. Eur J Radiol **65**(1), 36–46 (2008)
5. Mills, R.: Self-diffusion in normal and heavy water in the range 1–45.deg. J. Phys. Chem. **77**(5), 685–688 (1973)
6. Poot, D.H., Jeurissen, B., Bastiaensen, Y., Veraart, J., Van Hecke, W., Parizel, P.M., Sijbers, J.: Super-resolution for multislice diffusion tensor imaging. Magn Reson Med **69**(1), 103–113 (2013)
7. Powell, M.J.D.: The BOBYQA algorithm for bound constrained optimization without derivatives. In: Technical report NA2009/06. Department of Applied Mathematics and Theoretical Physics, Cambridge, England (2009)
8. Scherrer, B., Gholipour, A., Warfield, S.K.: Super-resolution reconstruction to increase the spatial resolution of diffusion weighted images from orthogonal anisotropic acquisitions. Med Imag Anal. **16**(7), 1465–1476 (2012)
9. Scherrer, B., Warfield, S.K.: Parametric representation of multiple white matter fascicles from cube and sphere diffusion MRI. PLoS ONE **7**(11), e48232 (2012)
10. Song, A.W., Chang, H.C., Petty, C., Guidon, A., Chen, N.K.: Improved delineation of short cortical association fibers and gray/white matter boundary using whole-brain three-dimensional diffusion tensor imaging at submillimeter spatial resolution. Brain Connect **4**(9), 636–640 (2014)

11. Sotiropoulos, S.N., Jbabdi, S., Xu, J., Andersson, J.L., Moeller, S., Auerbach, E.J., Glasser, M.F., Hernandez, M., Sapiro, G., Jenkinson, M., Feinberg, D.A., Yacoub, E., Lenglet, C., Van Essen, D.C., Ugurbil, K., Behrens, T.E.: WU-Minn HCP Consortium: advances in diffusion MRI acquisition and processing in the human connectome project. Neuroimage **80**, 125–143 (2013)
12. Tobisch, A., Neher, P., Rowe, M., Maier-Hein, K., Zhang, H.: Model-based super-resolution of diffusion MRI. In: Schultz, T., Nedjati-Gilani, G., Venkataraman, A., O'Donnell, L., Panagiotaki, E. (eds.) Computational Diffusion MRI and Brain Connectivity Workshop, pp. 25–34. Springer, Heidelberg (2014)
13. Tuch, D.S., Reese, T.G., Wiegell, M.R., Makris, N., Belliveau, J.W., Wedeen, V.J.: High angular resolution diffusion imaging reveals intravoxel white matter fiber heterogeneity. Magn Reson Med **48**(4), 577–582 (2002)
14. Vos, S.B., Jones, D.K., Viergever, M.A., Leemans, A.: Partial volume effect as a hidden covariate in DTI analyses. Neuroimage **55**(4), 1566–1576 (2011)

Clustering

Joint Spectral Decomposition
for the Parcellation of the Human Cerebral
Cortex Using Resting-State fMRI

Salim Arslan[✉], Sarah Parisot, and Daniel Rueckert

Biomedical Image Analysis Group, Department of Computing,
Imperial College London, London, UK
s.arslan13@imperial.ac.uk

Abstract. Identification of functional connections within the human brain has gained a lot of attention due to its potential to reveal neural mechanisms. In a whole-brain connectivity analysis, a critical stage is the computation of a set of network nodes that can effectively represent cortical regions. To address this problem, we present a robust cerebral cortex parcellation method based on spectral graph theory and resting-state fMRI correlations that generates reliable parcellations at the single-subject level and across multiple subjects. Our method models the cortical surface in each hemisphere as a mesh graph represented in the spectral domain with its eigenvectors. We connect cortices of different subjects with each other based on the similarity of their connectivity profiles and construct a multi-layer graph, which effectively captures the fundamental properties of the whole group as well as preserves individual subject characteristics. Spectral decomposition of this joint graph is used to cluster each cortical vertex into a subregion in order to obtain whole-brain parcellations. Using rs-fMRI data collected from 40 healthy subjects, we show that our proposed algorithm computes highly reproducible parcellations across different groups of subjects and at varying levels of detail with an average Dice score of 0.78, achieving up to 9% better reproducibility compared to existing approaches. We also report that our group-wise parcellations are functionally more consistent, thus, can be reliably used to represent the population in network analyses.

1 Introduction

The human cerebral cortex is assembled into subregions that interact with each other in order to coordinate the neural system. Identification of these subregions is critical for a better understanding of the functional organization of the human brain and to reveal the connections of underlying subsystems [19]. Functional connectivity studies have identified several subsystems, each of which is spanned across different cortical areas and associated with a specific functional ability [16]. This has further advanced the analysis of the functional architecture of the brain by constructing graphical models of the connections within individual subsystems and their interactions with each other at different levels of detail [14,25]. Analysis of these networks is also important for

© Springer International Publishing Switzerland 2015
S. Ourselin et al. (Eds.): IPMI 2015, LNCS 9123, pp. 85–97, 2015.
DOI: 10.1007/978-3-319-19992-4_7

deriving biomarkers of neurological disorders such as Alzheimer's disease [20] and schizophrenia [1].

In this paper, our main motivation is to identify functionally homogeneous and spatially continuous cortical subregions which can be used as the network nodes for a whole-brain connectivity analysis. In a typical network analysis, nodes are usually represented by the average signal within each cortical subregion, which is further beneficial to improve the SNR [9]. A good parcellation framework should be capable of grouping cortical regions with similar functional patterns together, thus the average signal can effectively represent each part of the subregion. It is also highly critical to generate a reliable group-wise representation that reflects the common functional characteristics of the community, yet is tolerant to changes in the functional organization at the single-subject level that may emerge due to functional and anatomical differences across subjects.

Our proposed method is based on connectivity patterns captured from resting-state functional magnetic resonance imaging (rs-fMRI) data. Rs-fMRI records neurocognitive activity by measuring the fluctuations in the blood oxygen level signals (BOLD) in the brain while the subject is at wakeful rest. Since the brain is still active in the absence of external stimuli, these fluctuations can be used to identify the cerebral functional connections [4]. On the other hand, task-based fMRI parcellations driven by neuropsychological studies, e.g. language task [12], target specific subregions in the cortex in order to investigate their functional organization, but ignores the activation from the non-target areas, which makes them incapable for the whole-brain network analyses. Similarly, anatomical parcellations generated from cytoarchitectonic atlases [22] are not able to capture the functional organization of the brain. This can be attributed to the fact that cytoarchitecture of the cerebral cortex does not necessarily require to be consistent with the functional connectivity patterns [12,21] and arbitrary parts of the same cytoarchitectonic region can exhibit structural and functional variability [6]. Nevertheless, parcellating the cerebral cortex based on resting-state correlations can potentially identify functional organization of the cerebral cortex without the knowledge of the cytoarchitecture and an external stimulus or a cognitive process [18].

The rs-fMRI-based cortical parcellation literature consists of methods that subdivide the cerebral cortex into different number of subregions according to the requirements of the applications and topological network features across the cerebral cortex [15]. These methods are based on but not limited to independent component analysis (ICA) [2], region growing [5,24], spectral graph theory [6,14,17], boundary mapping [9], k-means clustering [3,8] and hierarchical clustering [11,23]. Some of these techniques [2,3,14,25] parcellate the cortex at a very coarse level (less than hundred subregions), with the aim of identifying resting-state networks spanning across the cortex or some fractions of it. Because of the aforementioned risks of having non-uniform functional patterns within subregions, these parcellations cannot be reliably used for network node identification. Other methods typically generate a few hundred clusters without losing the ability of representing the functional organization of the cortex.

The most critical issue that is not addressed by these techniques is the adaptability of group representation to individual single subjects. The group-wise parcellations generated from a set of subjects are generally assumed to represent the whole group. However, due to functional and structural variations at the single-subject level, it is very unlikely that a group parcellation would highly match with single-level parcellations [9].

We address this problem and introduce a new parcellation framework which is capable of both generating group-wise and single-level parcellations from a joint graphical model. To this end, we make use of spectral graph decomposition techniques and represent the population in a multi-layer graph which effectively captures the fundamental properties of the whole group as well as preserves individual subject characteristics. We show that the parcellations obtained in this setting are (a) more reproducible across different groups of subjects and (b) better reflect functional and topological features shared by multiple subjects in the group compared to other parcellation methods. These aspects of the proposed method differentiate it from the previous parcellation algorithms and constitute our main contributions in this paper. Finally, our framework can be used to generate parcellations with different number of subregions, allowing users to conduct a network analysis at different levels of detail.

2 Methodology

2.1 Data Acquisition and Preprocessing

We evaluate our algorithm using data from the WU-Minn Human Connectome Project (HCP). We conducted our experiments on the rs-fMRI datasets, containing scans from 40 different unrelated subjects (22 female, 18 male healthy adults, ages 22–35). The data for each subject was acquired in two sessions, divided into four runs of approximately 15 min each. During the scans, subjects were presented a fixation crosshair, projected against a dark background, which prevented them from falling asleep. The dataset was preprocessed and denoised by the HCP structural and functional minimal preprocessing pipelines [7]. The final result of the pipeline is a standard set of cortical time courses which have been registered across subjects to establish correspondences. This was achieved by mapping the cortical gray matter voxels to the native cortical surface and registering them onto the 32k standard triangulated mesh. Following the preprocessing step, each time course was temporally normalized to zero-mean and unit-variance. We concatenated the time courses of each scan, obtaining an almost 60-minute rs-fMRI data for each of the 40 subjects and used them to evaluate our approach.

2.2 Joint Spectral Decomposition

We propose a clustering approach based on spectral decomposition to identify whole-cortex parcellations that can effectively capture the functional associations across multiple subjects. At the single-subject level, the cerebral cortex is represented as an adjacency matrix, in which the functional correlations are encoded as edge weights. Each adjacency matrix is transformed to the spectral domain via an eigenspace decomposition. The corresponding eigenvectors are combined into a multi-layer graph, which is capable of representing the fundamental properties of the underlying functional organization of individual subjects. Similar to the single-level graph decomposition, this joint multi-layer graph can then be decomposed into its eigenvectors, creating a feature matrix in the spectral domain that can be fed into a clustering algorithm, e.g. k-means, for grouping each vertex into a subregion, hence producing the final parcellations. A visual summary of the approach is given in Fig. 1.

Sparse Adjacency Matrix. The cerebral cortex of the brain is represented as a smooth, triangulated mesh with no topological defects. We model the mesh vertices and their associations as a weighted graph $G = (V, E)$, where V is the set of vertices (nodes) and E is the set of edges connecting them. Here we enforce a spatial constraint and construct an edge between two vertices if and only if they are adjacent to each other. This spatial constraint results in a sparse adjacency matrix with two benefits: (a) it ensures that resulting clusters are spatially continuous and (b) it reduces the computational overhead during the spectral decomposition of the graph. Finally, the edge weights between the adjacent vertices are set to the Pearson product-moment correlation coefficients of their rs-fMRI time courses (after discarding negative correlations and applying Fisher's z-transformation) and represented as an $n \times n$ weighted adjacency matrix W, where n is the number of vertices on the cortex.

Spectral Decomposition. Given the adjacency matrix W, the graph Laplacian can be computed as $L = D - W$, where $D = diag(\sum_j w_{ij})$ is the degree matrix of W. L is a diagonalizable matrix which can be factorized as $L = U \Lambda U^{-1}$, where $U = (u_1, u_2, ..., u_n)$ is the eigensystem, with u_i representing each eigenvector and Λ is a diagonal matrix that contains the eigenvalues, represented as $\Lambda_{ii} = \lambda_i$. Eigenvectors are powerful tools in terms of encapsulating valuable information extracted from the decomposed matrix in a lower dimension. In particular, after sorting the eigenvalues as $0 = \lambda_1 \leq \lambda_2 \leq \cdots \leq \lambda_n$ and organizing the corresponding eigenvectors accordingly, the first k eigenvectors denoted as the *spectral feature matrix* $F = (u_1, u_2, \cdots, u_k)$ are capable of representing the most important characteristics of the decomposed matrix. Thus, each vertex on the cortical surface can be represented by its corresponding row in F, without losing any critical information.

Spectral Matching. The idea of spectral matching is finding the closest vertex pairs in two eigensystems by comparing their eigenvectors in the spectral feature matrices [13]. The observations on the cortical surfaces transformed to the spectral domain revealed that eigenvectors show very similar characteristics across

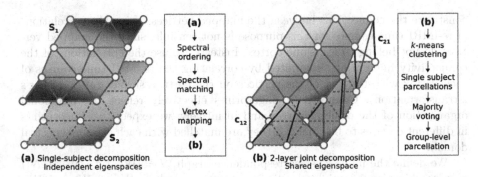

Fig. 1. Visual representation of the parcellation pipelines with an emphasis on (a) single-subject and (b) joint spectral decomposition, illustrated on the patches cropped from the cortical surfaces S_1 and S_2. The red and blue edges correspond to the mappings c_{12} and c_{21}, obtained by matching the closest vertices in S_1 and S_2, respectively (Color figure online).

subjects. This attribute can be utilized to obtain a common eigensystem that reflects structural and functional features shared by the subjects in the group, while also preserving individual subject characteristics.

Notably, the same cortical information represented with the eigenvector u_i in F_1 can be decoded in the eigenvector u_j in F_2, without the necessity of being in the same order or having the same sign. Therefore, an additional correction must be carried out in order to find the corresponding eigenvectors on both cortical surfaces before applying spectral matching. To this end, we make use of a simple spectral ordering technique, where for each eigenvector u_i in F_1 we compute its closest eigenvector u_j in F_2 using Euclidean distance and if $i \neq j$ we mark u_j for re-ordering. We then take another iteration and repeat the same process after flipping the signs of each eigenvector in F_2 and if a closer match is found, the new eigenvector is marked and its new sign is preserved throughout the sequential processes. Finally, the marked eigenvectors in F_2 are re-ordered accordingly.

After spectral ordering, we use only the first 8 eigenvectors for spectral matching, since our experiments showed that increasing the number of eigenvectors do not change the mappings between corresponding vertices, thus has no effect on the final parcellations. The spectral matching problem can be solved by mapping the closest vertices x and y on cortex S_1 and cortex S_2 with respect to their re-ordered spectral feature matrices F_1 and F_2 as illustrated in Fig. 1. The mappings $c_{12} : x_i \mapsto y_{c_{12}(i)}$ and $c_{21} : y_i \mapsto x_{c_{21}(i)}$ for $i = 1, \cdots, n$ can be identified with a nearest-neighbor search applied on F_1 and F_2.

Multi-layer Correspondence Graph. The use of spectral matching to find the mappings between pairs of cortical surfaces can be extended to generate a multi-layer correspondence graph for representing the whole group of subjects. The most critical part in such a setting is the definition of edge weights that constitute the connections between the mapped vertices. Using the correlations of rs-fMRI time courses for this purpose is not sensible, since the mapped vertices do not belong to the same cortex. Instead, we use the correlations of the connectivity fingerprints, computed by correlating the rs-fMRI time courses of each vertex with the rest of the vertices on the cortical surface (after Fisher's z-transformation). Connectivity fingerprints effectively reflect the functional organization of the cerebral cortex and intuitively, we expect two fingerprints in different cortices to be similar if they are matched with each other in spectral domain.

We define the multi-layer correspondence graph $\mathbb{W} = (W_{ij} \mid \forall \ i, j \in [1, N])$ as a combination of weighted adjacency matrices, where $W_{ii} = W_i$ and W_{ij} $(i \neq j)$ is the set of edges between cortical surfaces S_i and S_j with respect to their mappings c_{ij} and c_{ji}, weighted by the connectivity fingerprint correlations. $\mathbb{W}$ is an N-layer graph, with a size of $(n \times N) \times (n \times N)$ where N is the number of subjects in the group. A small patch taken from a 2-layer graph is illustrated as an example in Fig. 1(b).

Generation of Group-wise and Single Subject Parcellations. The spectral decomposition of $\mathbb{W}$ is performed similarly as described in the Spectral Decomposition section. The corresponding eigenvectors provide us with a shared feature matrix $\mathbb{F}$, representing every subject in the group with a combined parametrization. That is, each eigenvector can be separated into sub-vectors and used to characterize the underlying subjects. Similarly, each row in $\mathbb{F}$ can be used to describe its corresponding cortical vertex, thus can be used in a clustering setting. Here, we use k-means clustering for its simplicity and applicability, however it can be replaced by any other technique. We set the number of eigenvectors k to the desired number of subregions K, into which we would like to parcellate the cortical surfaces.

The output of the clustering approach is a label vector $\mathbb{L}$ of length $n \times N$ that assigns a parcel to each vertex on all cortical surfaces used to define $\mathbb{W}$. By dividing $\mathbb{L}$ into sequential sub-vectors of length n, we can obtain a parcellation for each subject. A simple majority voting across the single parcellations can then be used to generate the group parcellation. Hence, our method is capable of computing both a group-wise parcellation and single subject parcellations from the same graphical model.

3 Results

We compare our algorithm with a state-of-the-art parcellation approach based on spectral clustering [6]. This method decomposes subject specific adjacency matrices and makes use of the corresponding eigenvectors to obtain single-level parcellations with the help of normalized cut clustering. In order to be consistent in comparisons, we used the same adjacency matrices initially computed in our approach. The single level clustering is followed by a second level clustering, in which a coincidence matrix is computed [10]. This is a special adjacency matrix where an edge between two vertices is weighted by the number of times they appear in the same parcel across all individual parcellations and used to obtain a group-level parcellation. Alternatively, a group-wise parcellation can be performed by averaging the individual adjacency matrices (after Fisher's z-transformation) and then submitting the average to the normalized cut clustering algorithm. These methods will be referred as two-level and group-mean clustering, respectively, throughout the rest of the paper.

We assess the performance of the methods in two ways: (a) parcellation reproducibility across different groups of subjects and (b) functional consistency between single-level parcellations and the group-wise parcellation.

3.1 Reproducibility

We measure the reproducibility using the Dice similarity measure [5, 17]. We first identify overlapping parcels in two parcellations and compute their Dice scores. The overlapping parcels with the highest Dice score constitute a match and both are excluded from the parcellations. The algorithm iteratively continues to match the remaining parcels until all overlapping pairs are identified. The average Dice score of all pairs is used to measure the reproducibility of the parcellations. We also include overlap scores of 0 for non-matching parcels to the average calculation in order to penalize parcellations with non-overlapping parcels.

We present the group-wise reproducibility results obtained by our proposed algorithm as well as the comparison methods in Fig. 2. In this experiment, we separated all subjects in the dataset into two equally-sized, mutually exclusive groups by random selection and computed group-level parcellations for each group by running the algorithms separately on the left and right hemispheres. This process was repeated for 10 times, each time setting new groups and

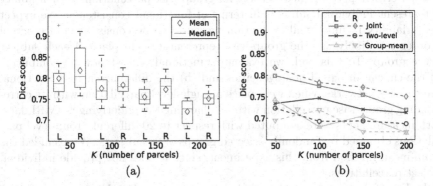

Fig. 2. Group-wise parcellation reproducibility results for different number of parcels obtained on different groups of subjects by running each method separately on the left and right hemispheres (indicated by L and R, respectively). (a) Dice scores of the proposed method, boxes indicating the range within different runs. (b) Dice scores of each method, averaged across all runs.

generating the corresponding group-wise parcellations for each method. Results indicate that our joint spectral decomposition approach is able to obtain more reproducible parcellations at each level of resolution, with at least an average Dice score of 0.72. The right hemisphere is slightly more reproducible than its left conjugate, which can be attributed to the topological differences between two hemispheres. There is a general decreasing trend in all methods with the increasing parcellation resolution. Dice scores for $K > 200$ were even lower, which might indicate that larger resolutions are not appropriate for parcellation. This can be attributed to the fact that, as K gets larger, the functional variability across subjects gets more prominent, thus, reducing the similarity between the common characteristics within different groups and leading to less reproducible group parcellations.

In Fig. 3, we present the group-wise parcellations obtained by our approach from one group of 20 randomly selected subjects with different number of parcels and visualize the reproducibility of each group-level parcel across single subject parcellations. Cross-subject reproducibility is measured by the same Dice similarity based method. For each group-level parcel we find its match in a single-level parcellation and record their Dice score. We repeat the same process for all subjects and average the Dice scores to get the reproducibility measure for that group-parcel. Darker colors indicate a high reproducibility across single-subject parcellations. Due to high functional inter-variability between different individuals and the varying levels of SNR in the rs-fMRI data, it is not possible to obtain high Dice scores for each part of the cerebral cortex [9]. Nevertheless, our approach is robust enough to achieve an average Dice score of at least 0.5 for each group-wise parcel.

3.2   Functional Consistency

Another critical performance measure for group-wise parcellations is their ability to represent individual subjects in terms of functional consistency. We expect the variability in functional evaluation measures to be consistent and minimal in order to reliably use the group-wise representation in place of each subject in the group. To this end, we evaluate functional consistency by computing (a) the change in parcel homogeneities and (b) the difference across functional connectivity networks, when we replace a single-level parcellation with its corresponding group-wise parcellation without changing the underlying rs-fMRI data. Both measurements were computed with respect to 20 different group-level parcellations obtained by randomly selected groups of 20 subjects. We excluded the group-mean method from this experiment, since it does not provide individual subject parcellations.

In Fig. 4(a), we present the whole-brain homogeneity changes for different number of parcels. Homogeneity of a parcel is measured by summing the Euclidean distances between the constituent rs-fMRI time courses and their average. A homogeneous parcellation consists of subregions with alike time courses, thus the sum of distances is expected to be low across the parcellated brain. The results indicate that the homogeneity levels between group- and single-level

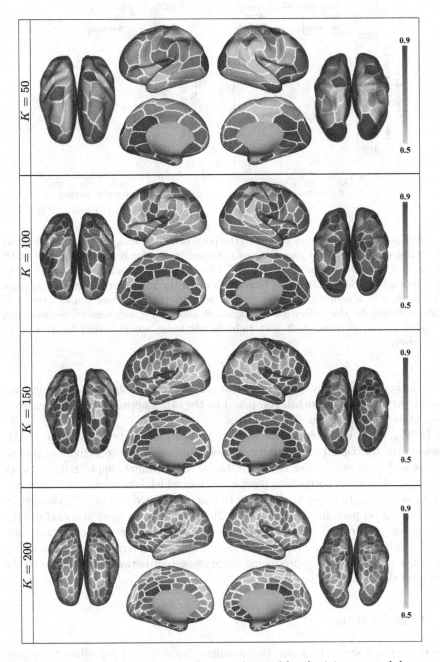

Fig. 3. Group-wise whole-brain parcellations obtained by the joint spectral decomposition method, run on each hemisphere separately for the number of parcels $K = 50$, 100, 150, and 200. The color of the parcellations indicates the average reproducibility score of each parcel across single-level parcellations (Color figure online).

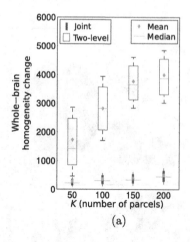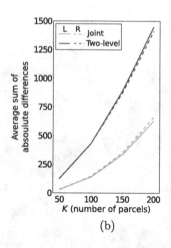

(a)   (b)

Fig. 4. Functional consistency results of the proposed and two-level method computed for 20 different group-level parcellations obtained by randomly selected groups of 20 subjects at different resolution levels. (a) The change in parcel homogeneities averaged throughout the whole brain, boxes indicating the range across different groups. (b) The sum of absolute differences (SAD) between the functional connectivity networks obtained by the individual parcellations and their group-wise representations, averaged across all runs. Left and right hemispheres are indicated by L and R, respectively.

parcellations obtained by our approach are highly consistent across different runs and at varying levels of detail compared to the other approach, which performs even worse for higher number of parcels.

In Fig. 4(b), we present the average sum of absolute differences (SAD) between the functional connectivity networks obtained by the individual parcellations and their group-wise representations. A functional connectivity network is computed by cross-correlating parcels, each of which is represented by its average time course. In order to compare two networks, we first match the single- and group-level parcellations using the Dice similarity method and exclude the non-matching parcels from the comparison in order to allow an objective comparison of both methods. SAD results show a similar pattern as the homogeneity results, with our approach producing more consistent networks compared to the two-level clustering.

4   Conclusions

We presented a spectral graph decomposition approach to parcellate the entire human cerebral cortex using resting-state fMRI data. Our experiments demonstrated that the proposed algorithm can produce robust parcellations with higher reproducibility and can better reflect functional and topological features shared by multiple subjects compared to other parcellation methods. The functional consistency of our parcellations can be attributed to the graphical model we propose, which combines individual functional features with the general functional tendency of the group. Group-wise parcellations obtained by our approach can be reliably used to represent the individual subjects in the group as well as to identify the nodes in a network analysis. In order to show the effectiveness of our approach, a planned future work is to conduct a network analysis using parcellations derived from different age groups and demonstrate how connectivity changes though aging.

One bottleneck of the proposed approach is the high computational space and time requirements in order to decompose the multi-layer graph. To overcome this, we are working on an initial clustering stage for grouping highly correlated and spatially close vertices into pre-parcels represented by their average time course, thus reduce the dimensionality of the graph and improve the SNR levels across the cerebral cortex.

Acknowledgments. The research leading to these results has received funding from the European Research Council under the European Union's Seventh Framework Programme (FP/2007-2013) / ERC Grant Agreement no. 319456. Data were provided by the Human Connectome Project, WU-Minn Consortium (Principal Investigators: David Van Essen and Kamil Ugurbil; 1U54MH091657).

References

1. Bassett, D.S., Bullmore, E., Verchinski, B.A., Mattay, V.S., Weinberger, D.R., Meyer-Lindenberg, A.: Hierarchical organization of human cortical networks in health and schizophrenia. J. Neurosci. **28**(37), 9239–9248 (2008)
2. Beckmann, C., Smith, S.: Probabilistic independent component analysis for functional magnetic resonance imaging. IEEE Trans. Med. Imaging **23**(2), 137–152 (2004)
3. Bellec, P., Rosa-Neto, P., Lyttelton, O.C., Benali, H., Evans, A.C.: Multi-level bootstrap analysis of stable clusters in resting-state fMRI. NeuroImage **51**(3), 1126–1139 (2010)
4. Biswal, B., Yetkin, F.Z., Haughton, V.M., Hyde, J.S.: Functional connectivity in the motor cortex of resting human brain using echo-planar MRI. Magn. Reson. Med. **34**(4), 537–541 (1995)
5. Blumensath, T., Jbabdi, S., Glasser, M.F., Van Essen, D.C., Ugurbil, K., Behrens, T.E., Smith, S.M.: Spatially constrained hierarchical parcellation of the brain with resting-state fMRI. NeuroImage **76**, 313–324 (2013)
6. Craddock, R.C., James, G., Holtzheimer, P.E., Hu, X.P., Mayberg, H.S.: A whole brain fMRI atlas generated via spatially constrained spectral clustering. Hum. Brain Mapp. **33**(8), 1914–1928 (2012)
7. Glasser, M.F., Sotiropoulos, S.N., Wilson, J.A., Coalson, T.S., Fischl, B., Andersson, J.L., Xu, J., Jbabdi, S., Webster, M., Polimeni, J.R., Van Essen, D.C., Jenkinson, M.: The minimal preprocessing pipelines for the Human Connectome Project. NeuroImage **80**, 105–124 (2013)
8. Golland, Y., Golland, P., Bentin, S., Malach, R.: Data-driven clustering reveals a fundamental subdivision of the human cortex into two global systems. Neuropsychologia **46**(2), 540–553 (2008)

9. Gordon, E.M., Laumann, T.O., Adeyemo, B., Huckins, J.F., Kelley, W.M., Petersen, S.E.: Generation and evaluation of a cortical area parcellation from resting-state correlations. Cereb. Cortex (2014)

10. van den Heuvel, M., Mandl, R., Hulshoff Pol, H.: Normalized cut group clustering of resting-state fMRI data. PLoS ONE **3**(4), e2001 (2008)

11. Jenatton, R., Gramfort, A., Michel, V., Obozinski, G., Bach, F., Thirion, B.: Multiscale mining of fMRI data with hierarchical structured sparsity. In: IEEE International Workshop on Pattern Recognition in NeuroImaging, pp. 69–72. IEEE Computer Society, Washington (2011)

12. Langs, G., Sweet, A., Lashkari, D., Tie, Y., Rigolo, L., Golby, A.J., Golland, P.: Decoupling function and anatomy in atlases of functional connectivity patterns: language mapping in tumor patients. NeuroImage **103**, 462–475 (2014)

13. Lombaert, H., Sporring, J., Siddiqi, K.: Diffeomorphic spectral matching of cortical surfaces. In: Gee, J.C., Joshi, S., Pohl, K.M., Wells, W.M., Zöllei, L. (eds.) IPMI 2013. LNCS, vol. 7917, pp. 376–389. Springer, Heidelberg (2013)

14. Power, J.D., Cohen, A.L., Nelson, S.M., Wig, G.S., Barnes, K.A., Church, J.A., Vogel, A.C., Laumann, T.O., Miezin, F.M., Schlaggar, B.L., Petersen, S.E.: Functional network organization of the human brain. Neuron **72**(4), 665–678 (2011)

15. de Reus, M.A., van den Heuvel, M.P.: The parcellation-based connectome: limitations and extensions. NeuroImage **80**, 397–404 (2013)

16. Salvador, R., Suckling, J., Coleman, M.R., Pickard, J.D., Menon, D., Bullmore, E.: Neurophysiological architecture of functional magnetic resonance images of human brain. Cereb. Cortex **15**(9), 1332–1342 (2005)

17. Shen, X., Tokoglu, F., Papademetris, X., Constable, R.T.: Groupwise whole-brain parcellation from resting-state fMRI data for network node identification. NeuroImage **82**, 403–415 (2013)

18. Smith, S.M., Vidaurre, D., Beckmann, C.F., Glasser, M.F., Jenkinson, M., Miller, K.L., Nichols, T.E., Robinson, E.C., Salimi-Khorshidi, G., Woolrich, M.W., Barch, D.M., Ugurbil, K., Van Essen, D.C.: Functional connectomics from resting-state fMRI. Trends Cogn. Sci. **17**(12), 666–682 (2013)

19. Sporns, O., Tononi, G., Ktter, R.: The human connectome: a structural description of the human brain. PLoS Comput. Biol. **1**(4), e42 (2005)

20. Supekar, K., Menon, V., Rubin, D., Musen, M., Greicius, M.D.: Network analysis of intrinsic functional brain connectivity in alzheimer's disease. PLoS Comput. Biol. **4**(6), e1000100 (2008)

21. Thirion, B., Flandin, G., Pinel, P., Roche, A., Ciuciu, P., Poline, J.B.: Dealing with the shortcomings of spatial normalization: multi-subject parcellation of fMRI datasets. Hum. Brain Mapp. **27**(8), 678–693 (2006)

22. Tzourio-Mazoyer, N., Landeau, B., Papathanassiou, D., Crivello, F., Etard, O., Delcroix, N., Mazoyer, B., Joliot, M.: Automated anatomical labeling of activations in SPM using a macroscopic anatomical parcellation of the MNI MRI single-subject brain. NeuroImage **15**(1), 273–289 (2002)

23. Varoquaux, G., Gramfort, A., Pedregosa, F., Michel, V., Thirion, B.: Multi-subject dictionary learning to segment an atlas of brain spontaneous activity. In: Székely, G., Hahn, H.K. (eds.) IPMI 2011. LNCS, vol. 6801, pp. 562–573. Springer, Heidelberg (2011)

24. Wig, G.S., Laumann, T.O., Cohen, A.L., Power, J.D., Nelson, S.M., Glasser, M.F., Miezin, F.M., Snyder, A.Z., Schlaggar, B.L., Petersen, S.E.: Parcellating an individual subject's cortical and subcortical brain structures using snowball sampling of resting-state correlations. Cereb. Cortex **24**(8), 2036–2054 (2013)

25. Yeo, B.T., Krienen, F.M., Sepulcre, J., Sabuncu, M.R., Lashkari, D., Hollinshead, M., Roffman, J.L., Smoller, J.W., Zollei, L., Polimeni, J.R., Fischl, B., Liu, H., Buckner, R.L.: The organization of the human cerebral cortex estimated by intrinsic functional connectivity. J. Neurophysiol. **106**(3), 1125–1165 (2011)

Joint Clustering and Component Analysis of Correspondenceless Point Sets: Application to Cardiac Statistical Modeling

Ali Gooya[1]([⊠]), Karim Lekadir[1,2], Xenia Alba[1,2], Andrew J. Swift[3], Jim M. Wild[3], and Alejandro F. Frangi[1]

[1] Centre for Computational Imaging and Simulation Technologies in Biomedicine (CISTIB), The University of Sheffield, Sheffield, UK
a.gooya@sheffield.ac.uk
http://www.cistib.org/
[2] CISTIB, Universitat Pompeu Fabra, Barcelona, Spain
[3] Unit of Academic Radiology, University of Sheffield, Sheffield, UK

Abstract. Construction of Statistical Shape Models (SSMs) from arbitrary point sets is a challenging problem due to significant shape variation and lack of explicit point correspondence across the training data set. In medical imaging, point sets can generally represent different shape classes that span healthy and pathological exemplars. In such cases, the constructed SSM may not generalize well, largely because the probability density function (pdf) of the point sets deviates from the underlying assumption of Gaussian statistics. To this end, we propose a generative model for unsupervised learning of the pdf of point sets as a mixture of distinctive classes. A Variational Bayesian (VB) method is proposed for making joint inferences on the labels of point sets, and the principal modes of variations in each cluster. The method provides a flexible framework to handle point sets with no explicit point-to-point correspondences. We also show that by maximizing the marginalized likelihood of the model, the optimal number of clusters of point sets can be determined. We illustrate this work in the context of understanding the anatomical phenotype of the left and right ventricles in heart. To this end, we use a database containing hearts of healthy subjects, patients with Pulmonary Hypertension (PH), and patients with Hypertrophic Cardiomyopathy (HCM). We demonstrate that our method can outperform traditional PCA in both generalization and specificity measures.

Keywords: Statistical shape models · Variational bayes · Model selection

1 Introduction

Statistical shape models (SSMs) from point sets, proposed by Cootes *et al.* in [2], are powerful tools in medical imaging to encode the natural variability of anatomical structures. To construct an SSM, traditionally, points are selected on

© Springer International Publishing Switzerland 2015
S. Ourselin et al. (Eds.): IPMI 2015, LNCS 9123, pp. 98–109, 2015.
DOI: 10.1007/978-3-319-19992-4_8

training surfaces and point-to-point correspondences are required. By consistently concatenating the points on each training data set, shapes are represented as high-dimensional vectors and assumed to be sampled from a Gaussian distribution; under this hypothesis the major modes of variation are then extracted by PCA. In reality, however, the training data can have a multi-modal distribution and represent various classes of shapes. As a result, no particular class is fully represented by the mean model and the constructed SSM often does not generalize well. To alleviate this problem, Zhang et al. [15] proposed sparse non-parametric shape description, and Cootes et al. [3] used a Gaussian Mixture Model (GMM) to represent the pdf of the training sets; the shape space is first partitioned and then PCA is applied in each cluster. But, it is likely that clustering of point sets and the estimation of variation modes may mutually benefit from each other. In addition, this approach requires having point-to-point correspondences, and a user-selected a priori number of components, which is difficult.

Establishing point-to-point correspondences across training point sets is a major challenge that undermines the practicality of the SSMs. Manually specifying correspondences over landmarks could be an ambiguous subjective task. 3D automatic techniques based on image registration [5] or minimizing the description length [4] have a varying performance, in particular for complex structures such as the heart. EM-ICP based methods [7,11] offer more flexibility by computing probabilistic matchings between points and are shown to be robust to the matching errors. Recently, Hufnagel et al. [8] proposed a generative model for estimating modes of variation in point sets without resourcing to PCA from point sets with no correspondences. This method, however, still assumes that the distribution is a monomodal Gaussian distribution.

We present a hierarchical clustering scheme to estimate pdfs of unstructured, rigidly aligned, point sets having no point-to-point correspondences. Points at each set are regarded as samples from a low dimensional GMM, whose means are concatenated to form higher dimensional vector. This vector is considered to be a sample drawn from a Mixture of Probabilistic Principal Component Analyzers (PPCA) [13]. The latter is essentially a higher dimensional GMM, where the covariance matrices of its clusters can be decomposed to subspaces of local principal components. An inference algorithm based on variational Bayes (VB) [1] is proposed for unsupervised learning of class labels and variations.

Thanks to this hierarchical structure, the proposed method estimates probabilistic point matchings across the training data sets; and handles mixtures of different shape classes. Another important advantage of the proposed VB approach is that the number of clusters is automatically learned from data. It is noteworthy that, in machine learning, VB has been successfully applied for inferring mixtures of subspace analyzers [6] from training vectors having equal lengths. However, adopting the framework for point sets, as order-less random variables having different cardinalities (point counts), is a challenging problem. In the rest of this paper, we first present our generative model, derive an efficient inference algorithm and finally compare the method to the standard PCA model using cardiac data with different pathologies.

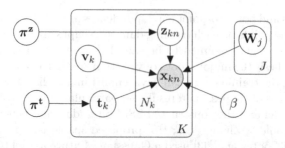

Fig. 1. The graphical representation of the proposed model; shaded and hollow circles represent observed and latent variables, respectively, arrows imply the dependencies and plates embrace numbered incidences of events.

2   Methods

2.1   Probabilistic Generative Model

Our observation consists of K point sets, denoted as $\mathcal{X}_k = \{\mathbf{x}_{kn}\}_{n=1}^{N_k}$, $1 \leq k \leq K$, where $\mathbf{x}_{kn}$ is a D dimensional feature vector corresponding to the nth landmark in the kth point set. The model can be explained as two interacting layers of mixture models. In the first (lower-dimension) layer, $\mathcal{X}_k$ is assumed to be a collection of D-dimensional samples from a GMM with M Gaussian components. Meanwhile, by concatenating the means of the GMM (with a consistent order), a vector representation for $\mathcal{X}_k$ can be derived in $M \cdot D$ dimension. Clustering and linear component analysis for $\mathcal{X}_k$ takes place in this space.

More specifically, we consider a mixture of J probabilistic principal component analyzers (MPPCA). A PPCA is essentially an $M \cdot D$-dimensional Gaussian specified by a mean vector, $\bar{\boldsymbol{\mu}}_j \in \mathcal{R}^{MD}$, $1 \leq j \leq J$, and a covariance matrix having a subspace component in the form of $\mathbf{W}_j\mathbf{W}_j^T$ [13]. Here, $\mathbf{W}_j$ is a $MD \times L$ dimensional matrix, whose column l, $i.e.$ $\mathbf{W}_j^{(l)}$, represents one mode of variation for the cluster j. Let $\mathbf{v}_k$ be an L dimensional vector of loading coefficients corresponding to $\mathcal{X}_k$ and let us define: $\boldsymbol{\mu}_{jk} = \mathbf{W}_j\mathbf{v}_k + \bar{\boldsymbol{\mu}}_j$. These vectors can be thought of as variables that bridge the two layers of our model: In the higher dimension, $\boldsymbol{\mu}_{jk}$ is a $re\text{-}sampled$ representation of $\mathcal{X}_k$ in the space spanned by principal components of the jth cluster; meanwhile, if we partition $\boldsymbol{\mu}_{jk}$ into a series of M subsequent vectors, and denote each as $\boldsymbol{\mu}_{jk}^{(m)}$, we obtain the means of D dimensional Gaussians of the corresponding GMM.

Let $\mathcal{Z}_k = \{\mathbf{z}_{kn}\}_{n=1}^{N_k}$ be a set of N_k, 1-of-M coded latent membership vectors for the points in $\mathcal{X}_k$. Each $\mathbf{z}_{kn} \in \{0,1\}^M$ is a vector of zeros, whose mth component equals one ($z_{knm} = 1$) indicates that $\mathbf{x}_{kn}$ is a sample from the D dimensional Gaussian m. The precision (inverse of the variance) of Gaussians is globally denoted by $\beta\mathbf{I}_{D \times D}$. Similarly, let $\mathbf{t}_k \in \{0,1\}^J$ be a latent, 1-of-J coded vector whose component j being one ($t_{kj} = 1$) indicates the membership of the $\mathcal{X}_k$ to cluster j. The conditional pdf of $\mathbf{x}_{kn}$ is then given by:

$$p(\mathbf{x}_{kn}|\mathbf{z}_{kn}, \mathbf{t}_k, \beta, \mathbb{W}, \mathbf{v}_k) = \prod_{j=1}^{J} \prod_{m=1}^{M} \left(\mathcal{N}(\mathbf{x}_{kn}|\boldsymbol{\mu}_{jk}^{(m)}, \beta^{-1}\mathbf{I}_{D \times D})^{z_{knm}} \right)^{t_{kj}} \quad (1)$$

where $\mathbb{W} = \{\mathbf{W}_j\}_{j=1}^{J}$ is the set of principal component matrices. To facilitate our derivations, we introduce the following prior distributions over $\mathbf{W}_j$, $\mathbf{v}_k$, and β, which are conjugate to the normal distribution in Eq. (1):

$$p(\mathbf{W}_j) = \prod_{l=1}^{L} \mathcal{N}(\mathbf{W}_j^{(l)}|\mathbf{0}, \alpha_{jl}^{-1}\mathbf{I}), \quad p(\mathbf{v}_k) = \mathcal{N}(\mathbf{v}_k|\mathbf{0}, \mathbf{I}), \quad p(\beta) = \Gamma(\beta|a_0, b_0) \quad (2)$$

The hyper-parameters of the Gamma distribution in the last line are set to $a_0 = 10^{-3}$ and $b_0 = 1$ to have a flat prior over β. Next, we respectively denote the mixture weights of GMMs and MPPCA by $\boldsymbol{\pi}^z$ and $\boldsymbol{\pi}^t$ vectors, each having a Dirichlet distribution as priors: $p(\boldsymbol{\pi}^z) = \text{Dir}(\boldsymbol{\pi}^z|\lambda_0^z)$, $p(\boldsymbol{\pi}^t) = \text{Dir}(\boldsymbol{\pi}^t|\lambda_0^t)$. where we set $\lambda_0^z = \lambda_0^t = 10^{-3}$. The conditional distributions of membership vectors of $\mathbf{z}_{kn}$ (for points) and $\mathbf{t}_k$ (for point sets) given mixing weights are specified by two multi-nomial distributions: $p(\mathbf{z}_{kn}|\boldsymbol{\pi}^z) = \prod_{m=1}^{M} (\pi_m^z)^{z_{knm}}$, and $p(\mathbf{t}_k|\boldsymbol{\pi}^t) = \prod_{j=1}^{J} (\pi_j^t)^{t_{kj}}$, where $0 \leq \pi_m^z$, $0 \leq \pi_j^t$ are the components m, j of $\boldsymbol{\pi}^z$, $\boldsymbol{\pi}^t$, respectively. We now construct the joint pdf of the sets of all random variables, by assuming (conditional) independence and multiplying the pdfs where needed. Let $\mathbb{X} = \{\mathcal{X}_k\}_{k=1}^{K}$, $\mathbb{Z} = \{\mathcal{Z}_k\}_{k=1}^{K}$, $\mathbb{V} = \{\mathbf{v}_k\}_{k=1}^{K}$, and $\mathbb{T} = \{\mathbf{t}_k\}_{k=1}^{K}$, then the distributions of these variables can be written as:

$$p(\mathbb{W}) = \prod_j p(\mathbf{W}_j|\alpha_j), \quad p(\mathbb{Z}|\boldsymbol{\pi}^z) = \prod_k p(\mathcal{Z}_k|\boldsymbol{\pi}^z) = \prod_k \prod_n p(\mathbf{z}_{kn}), \quad p(\mathbb{T}|\boldsymbol{\pi}^t) = \prod_k p(\mathbf{t}_k|\boldsymbol{\pi}^t)$$

$$p(\mathbb{V}) = \prod_k p(\mathbf{v}_k), \quad p(\mathbb{X}|\mathbb{Z}, \mathbb{T}, \mathbb{W}, \mathbb{V}, \beta) = \prod_k p(\mathcal{X}_k|\mathcal{Z}_k, \mathbf{t}_k, \beta, \mathbb{W}, \mathbf{v}_k), \quad (3)$$

$$p(\mathcal{X}_k|\mathcal{Z}_k, \mathbf{t}_k, \beta, \mathbb{W}, \mathbf{v}_k) = \prod_{n=1}^{N_k} p(\mathbf{x}_{kn}|\mathbf{z}_{kn}, \mathbf{t}_k, \beta, \mathbb{W}, \mathbf{v}_k) \quad (4)$$

Having defined the required distributions through Eqs. (1)-(3), the distribution of the *complete* observation is given as

$$p(\mathbb{X}, \mathbb{Z}, \mathbb{T}, \mathbb{W}, \mathbb{V}, \boldsymbol{\pi}^t, \boldsymbol{\pi}^z, \beta) = p(\mathbb{X}|\mathbb{Z}, \mathbb{T}, \mathbb{W}, \mathbb{V}, \beta)p(\mathbb{Z}|\boldsymbol{\pi}^z)p(\mathbb{T}|\boldsymbol{\pi}^t)p(\boldsymbol{\pi}^z)p(\boldsymbol{\pi}^t)p(\mathbb{W})p(\mathbb{V})p(\beta) \quad (5)$$

Figure 1 is a graphical representation for the generative model considered in this paper. Given observations (colored dark gray) as D dimensional points, our problem is to estimate the posterior distributions of all the latent random variables (hollow circles) and hyper-parameters, which include the discrete cluster and the continuous variables (*e.g.* means and modes of variations).

2.2 Approximated Inference

If we denote the set of latent variables as $\theta = \{\mathbb{Z}, \mathbb{T}, \mathbb{W}, \mathbb{V}, \boldsymbol{\pi}^t, \boldsymbol{\pi}^z, \beta\}$, direct inference of $p(\theta|\mathbb{X})$ (as our objective) is analytically intractable thus an approximated distribution, $q(\theta)$, is sought. Owing to the dimensionality of the data, we prefer Variational Bayes (VB) over sampling based methods. The VB principle for obtaining $q(\boldsymbol{\theta})$ is explained briefly. The model evidence, *i.e.* $p(\mathbb{X})$ [1], can be decomposed as $p(\mathbb{X}) = \mathcal{L} + \mathrm{KL}(p(\boldsymbol{\theta}|\mathbb{X})||q(\boldsymbol{\theta}))$, where $0 \leq \mathrm{KL}(\cdot||\cdot)$ denotes the Kullback-Leilber divergence, and

$$\mathcal{L} = \int q(\boldsymbol{\theta}) \ln \frac{p(\mathbb{X}, \boldsymbol{\theta})}{q(\boldsymbol{\theta})} d\boldsymbol{\theta} \leq p(\mathbb{X}) \tag{6}$$

is a lower bound on $p(\mathbb{X})$. To obtain $q(\boldsymbol{\theta})$, the KL divergence between the true and the approximated posterior should be minimized. However, this is not feasible because the true posterior is not accessible to us. Thus, $q(\boldsymbol{\theta})$ can be computed by maximizing $\mathcal{L}$. We approximate the true posterior as a factorized form, *i.e.*, $q(\boldsymbol{\theta}) = \prod_i q(\theta_i)$, where θ_i refers to any of our latent variables. This factorization leads to the following tractable result: let ε be the variable of interest in $\boldsymbol{\theta}$, and $\xi = \boldsymbol{\theta} - \varepsilon$, then the variational posterior of ε is given by $\ln q(\varepsilon) = \langle \ln p(\mathbb{X}, \boldsymbol{\theta}) \rangle_{\xi} +$ const, where $p(\mathbb{X}, \boldsymbol{\theta})$ is given in Eq. (5), $\langle \cdot \rangle_{\xi}$ denotes the expectation w.r.t. to the product of $q(\cdot)$ of all variable in ξ.

2.3 Update of Posteriors and Hyper-Parameters

In this section, we provide equations to update the variational posteriors. Thanks to conjugacy of priors to likelihoods, these derivations are done by inspecting expectations of logarithms and matching posteriors to their corresponding likelihood template forms. Detailed proof of our derivations is skipped for brevity. Starting from $\mathbb{Z}$ variables we have $q(\mathbb{Z}) = \prod_k q(\mathcal{Z}_k) = \prod_{k,m,n} (r_{knm})^{z_{knm}}$ Under this equation, we have $\langle z_{knm} \rangle = r_{knm}$, where the right hand side can be computed using the following relationships:

$$r_{knm} = \frac{\rho_{knm}}{\sum_{m'} \rho_{knm'}}, \quad \ln \rho_{knm} = -\frac{\langle \beta \rangle}{2} \sum_j \langle t_{kj} \rangle \langle |\mathbf{x}_{kn} - \boldsymbol{\mu}_{jk}^{(m)}|^2 \rangle + \langle \ln \pi_m^{\mathbf{z}} \rangle \tag{7}$$

The first term can be directly computed using the expectations of $\mathbb{W}$ and $\mathbb{V}$ as follows: $\langle |\mathbf{x}_{kn} - \boldsymbol{\mu}_{jk}^{(m)}|^2 \rangle = |\mathbf{x}_{kn} - \langle \boldsymbol{\mu}_{jk}^{(m)} \rangle|^2 + \mathrm{Tr}[\mathrm{Cov}[\boldsymbol{\mu}_{jk}]^{(m,m)}]$, where the super indexes $(\cdot)$, $(\cdot, \cdot)$ specify the D and $D \times D$ dimensional block numbers of the vector $\langle \boldsymbol{\mu}_{jk} \rangle = \langle \mathbf{W}_j \rangle \langle \mathbf{v}_k \rangle + \bar{\boldsymbol{\mu}}_j$ and the matrix defined by:

$$\mathrm{Cov}[\boldsymbol{\mu}_{jk}] = \langle \mathbf{W}_j \rangle \langle \mathbf{v}_k \mathbf{v}_k^T \rangle \langle \mathbf{W}_j \rangle^T + \sum_l \langle \mathbf{v}_k \mathbf{v}_k^T \rangle_{ll} \mathrm{Cov}[\mathbf{W}_j^{(l)}] \tag{8}$$

To simplify the rest our notations, we introduce the following auxiliary variables:

$$\mathbf{R}_k = \mathrm{Diag}(\underbrace{R_{k1} \cdots R_{k1}}_{D \text{ copies}}, \cdots, \underbrace{R_{kM} \cdots R_{kM}}_{D \text{ copies}}), \quad \bar{\mathbf{x}}_k = [\bar{\mathbf{x}}_{k1}^T, \cdots, \bar{\mathbf{x}}_{kM}^T]^T \tag{9}$$

---

[1] More precisely, $p(\mathbb{X})$ is conditioned on parameters with no prior distribution. Hence, it is equivalently referred to as marginal likelihood.

where: $R_{km} = \sum_n r_{knm}$, and $\bar{\mathbf{x}}_{km} = \sum_n r_{knm}\mathbf{x}_{kn}$. Under these definitions, the posteriors of $\mathbb{T}$ is given by $q(\mathbb{T}) = \prod_k q(\mathbf{t}_k) = \prod_{k,j}(r'_{kj})^{t_{kj}}$ where, in analogy to Eq. (7), we have: $\langle t_{kj}\rangle = r'_{kj}$ and

$$r'_{kj} = \frac{\rho'_{kj}}{\sum_{j'}\rho'_{kj'}}, \quad \ln\rho'_{kj} = \langle\beta\rangle\mathrm{Tr}[-\frac{1}{2}\mathbf{R}_k\langle\boldsymbol{\mu}_{jk}\boldsymbol{\mu}_{jk}^T\rangle + \boldsymbol{\mu}_{jk}\bar{\mathbf{x}}_k^T] + \langle\ln\pi_j^{\mathbf{t}}\rangle \quad (10)$$

The posterior of the principal components is given by

$$q(\mathbb{W}) = \prod_{j,l}q(\mathbf{W}_j^{(l)}), \quad q(\mathbf{W}_j^{(l)}) = \mathcal{N}(\mathbf{W}_j^{(l)}|\langle\mathbf{W}_j^{(l)}\rangle, \mathrm{Cov}[\mathbf{W}_j^{(l)}]) \quad (11)$$

where the means and covariance matrices are specified as:

$$\mathrm{Cov}[\mathbf{W}_j^{(l)}] = [\alpha_{jl}\mathbf{I} + \langle\beta\rangle\sum_k\langle t_{kj}\rangle\langle\mathbf{v}_k\mathbf{v}_k^T\rangle_{ll}\mathbf{R}_k]^{-1}$$

$$\langle\mathbf{W}_j^{(l)}\rangle = \langle\beta\rangle\mathrm{Cov}[\mathbf{W}_j^{(l)}](\sum_k\langle t_{kj}\rangle\mathbf{Q}_{kj}^{(l)}) \quad (12)$$

Here, the auxiliary matrix $\mathbf{Q}_{kj}$ is defined as

$$\mathbf{Q}_{kj} = (\bar{\mathbf{x}}_k - \mathbf{R}_k\bar{\boldsymbol{\mu}}_j)\langle\mathbf{v}_k\rangle^T - \mathbf{R}_k\langle\mathbf{W}_j\rangle\left[\langle\mathbf{v}_k\mathbf{v}_k^T\rangle - \mathrm{Diag}(\mathrm{diag}\langle\mathbf{v}_k\mathbf{v}_k^T\rangle)\right] \quad (13)$$

where the inner diag operator copies the main diagonal of $\langle\mathbf{v}_k\mathbf{v}_k^T\rangle$ into a vector, and the outer Diag transforms the vector back into a diagonal matrix. The posterior of $\mathbf{v}_k$ vectors is given by

$$q(\mathbb{V}) = \prod_k q(\mathbf{v}_k) = \mathcal{N}(\mathbf{v}_k|\langle\mathbf{v}_k\rangle, \mathrm{Cov}[\mathbf{v}_k]), \quad \mathrm{Cov}[\mathbf{v}_k] = \left[\mathbf{I} + \langle\beta\rangle\sum_j\langle t_{kj}\rangle\langle\mathbf{W}_j^T\mathbf{R}_k\mathbf{W}_j\rangle\right]^{-1}$$

$$\langle\mathbf{W}_j^T\mathbf{R}_k\mathbf{W}_j\rangle = \langle\mathbf{W}_j\rangle^T\mathbf{R}_k\langle\mathbf{W}_j\rangle + \mathrm{Diag}\left(\mathrm{Tr}[\mathbf{R}_k\mathrm{Cov}[\mathbf{W}_j^{(1)}]], \cdots, \mathrm{Tr}[\mathbf{R}_k\mathrm{Cov}[\mathbf{W}_j^{(L)}]]\right)$$

$$\langle\mathbf{v}_k\rangle = \langle\beta\rangle\mathrm{Cov}[\mathbf{v}_k]\sum_j\langle t_{kj}\rangle\langle\mathbf{W}_j\rangle^T(\bar{\mathbf{x}}_k - \mathbf{R}_k\bar{\boldsymbol{\mu}}_j) \quad (14)$$

The posterior of the precision β is a Gamma distribution specified by:

$$q(\beta) = \Gamma(\beta|a,b), \quad a = a_0 + \frac{DN}{2}, \quad b = b_0 + \frac{1}{2}\sum_{k,n,m,j}\langle z_{knm}\rangle\langle t_{kj}\rangle\langle|\mathbf{x}_{kn} - \boldsymbol{\mu}_{jk}^{(m)}|^2\rangle \quad (15)$$

Under these definitions, we have $\langle\beta\rangle = a/b$ and $\langle\ln\beta\rangle = \psi(a) - \ln(b)$, where ψ is the *Digamma* function. Finally, the posteriors of the mixing coefficients are Dirichlet distributions:

$$q(\boldsymbol{\pi}^{\mathbf{t}}) = \mathrm{Dir}(\boldsymbol{\pi}^{\mathbf{t}}|\boldsymbol{\lambda}^{\mathbf{t}}), \lambda_j^{\mathbf{t}} = \lambda_0^{\mathbf{t}} + \sum_k\langle t_{kj}\rangle, \quad q(\boldsymbol{\pi}^{\mathbf{z}}) = \mathrm{Dir}(\boldsymbol{\pi}^{\mathbf{z}}|\boldsymbol{\lambda}^{\mathbf{z}}), \lambda_m^{\mathbf{z}} = \lambda_0^{\mathbf{z}} + \sum_{k,n}\langle z_{knm}\rangle \quad (16)$$

Using Eq. (16), the expectations related to the mixing coefficients are computed as $\langle \pi_m^{\mathbf{z}} \rangle = \lambda_m^{\mathbf{z}} / \sum_{m'} \lambda_{m'}^{\mathbf{z}}$, and $\langle \ln \lambda_j^{\mathbf{t}} \rangle = \psi(\lambda_j^{\mathbf{t}}) - \psi(\sum_{j'} \lambda_{j'}^{\mathbf{t}})$. Finally, by maximizing Eq. (6) with regard to $\bar{\mu}_j$ and α_{jl}, we obtain:

$$\bar{\mu}_j = \left[\sum_k \langle t_{kj} \rangle \mathbf{R}_k \right]^{-1} \left[\sum_k \langle t_{kj} \rangle (\bar{\mathbf{x}}_k - \mathbf{R}_k \langle \mathbf{W}_j \rangle \langle \mathbf{v}_k \rangle) \right], \tag{17}$$

$$\alpha_{jl} = MD / \left[|\langle \mathbf{W}_j^{(l)} \rangle|^2 + \mathrm{Tr}[\mathrm{Cov}[\mathbf{W}_j^{(l)}]] \right] \tag{18}$$

2.4   Predictive Distribution

For a new test point set $\mathcal{X}_r = \{\mathbf{x}_{rn}\}_{n=1}^{N_r}$, with $K < r$, we can obtain a model projected point set as $\hat{\mathcal{X}}_r = \{\langle \hat{\mathbf{x}}_{rn} \rangle\}_{n=1}^{N_r}$, where $\langle \hat{\mathbf{x}}_{rn} \rangle = \int \hat{\mathbf{x}}_{rn} p(\hat{\mathbf{x}}_{rn} | \mathcal{X}_r, \mathbb{X}) d\hat{\mathbf{x}}_{rn}$. Here, the predictive distribution should be computed by marginalizing the corresponding latent and model variables by

$$p(\hat{\mathbf{x}}_{rn} | \mathcal{X}_r, \mathbb{X}) = \sum_{\mathbf{z}_{rn}, \mathbf{t}_r} \int p(\hat{\mathbf{x}}_{rn} | \mathbf{z}_{rn}, \mathbf{t}_r, \beta, \mathbb{W}, \mathbf{v}_r) p(\mathbf{z}_{rn}, \mathbf{t}_r, \beta, \mathbb{W}, \mathbf{v}_r | \mathcal{X}_r, \mathbb{X}) d\mathbb{W} d\mathbf{v}_r d\beta$$

Because this integral is analytically intractable, we use an approximation for the posterior using $p(\mathbf{z}_{rn}, \mathbf{t}_r, \beta, \mathbb{W}, \mathbf{v}_r | \mathcal{X}_r, \mathbb{X}) \approx q(\mathbf{z}_{rn}) q(\mathbf{t}_r) q(\mathbf{v}_r) q(\beta) q(\mathbb{W})$. Thus, having $\mathcal{X}_r$ we iterate over updating $q(\mathbf{z}_{rn}), q(\mathbf{t}_r)$ and $q(\mathbf{v}_r)$, and replace $q(\beta)$ and $q(\mathbb{W})$ from the training step.

2.5   Initialization and Computational Burden

To initialize the model, a GMM with M Gaussians is fit to the set of all points. Next, for the Gaussian component m in the GMM, a corresponding point from $\mathcal{X}_k$ is identified having the maximum posterior probability in $\mathcal{X}_k$. Iterating over M Gaussian components, all the corresponding points from point set k are identified and concatenated to form an MD dimensional vector. This procedure is then repeated over K training point sets and the obtained vectors are clustered using k-means. Next, by applying PCA at each cluster, we identify the mean $\bar{\mu}_j$, $\mathbf{W}_j$ as the first L components, and $\mathbf{v}_k$ as the projections of the original vectors to these components. Finally, β is initialized as the component wise average L2 difference of the original and the PCA projected vectors. In practice, we have observed that for a set of fifty point sets each having 4000 points, sufficient convergence is achieved by 50 VB iterations in nearly an hour.

3   Results

We evaluate our method on both synthetic and real data sets of cardiac MRI as follows. The reliability of the lower bound as a criterion to select the number of clusters of point sets is evaluated in both data types. We also measure generalization and specificity errors, and compare them to the standard PCA based SSM

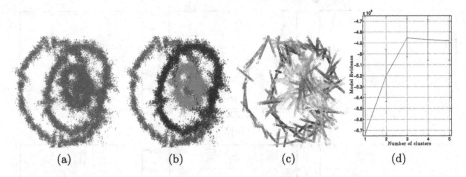

Fig. 2. Clustering and mode estimation of synthetic point sets. (a) overlay of 750 point sets, (b) corresponding color separated ground true clusters, (c) estimated labels (colors), GMM centroids showing local modes of variations, (d) lower bound $\mathcal{L}$ on the model evidence versus number of clusters, indicating $J = 3$ as the optimal number (Color figure online).

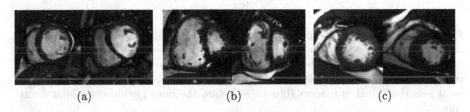

Fig. 3. Short axis MR images from normal (a), PH (b), and HCM patients (c).

on the real data sets. Generalization ability is the error between the actual and the model projected point sets. Specificity is related to the ability of the model to instantiate correct samples resembling the training data. We randomly divide the available point sets into the testing and training subsets and trained the model using latter. Next, we measure the generalization and specificity using the testing, and model generated point sets as explained in [4]. To measure the distances between point sets, we considered: $d(\mathcal{X}_k, \hat{\mathcal{X}}_k) = 1/N_k \sum_x \min_{y \in \hat{\mathcal{X}}_k} \|\mathbf{x} - \mathbf{y}\|_2$. Here, N_k is the number of points in $\mathcal{X}_k$, and $\hat{\mathcal{X}}_k$ denote the model projected point set. Furthermore, since d is asymmetric, we also compute $\hat{d}(\mathcal{X}_k, \hat{\mathcal{X}}_k) = d(\hat{\mathcal{X}}_k, \mathcal{X}_k)$ and report both.

3.1 Synthetic Dataset

We investigate the problem of selecting a proper number of clusters, J, from the data by generating synthetic point sets using ancestral sampling [1]. We expect the model evidence, *i.e.* $p(\mathbb{X}|J)$, to reach a maximum for the proper number of clusters used to generate data, due to the marginalization of the latent variables. Three distinctive 2D point set patterns are generated as the cluster means. To help visualization, by setting $L = 1$, a single mode of variation per cluster is considered and sampled from $p(\mathbf{W}_j)$. Next, a set of 250 point

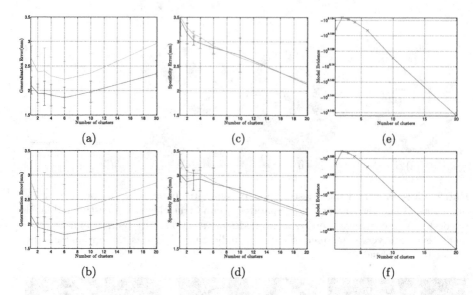

Fig. 4. Quantitative results for models trained by clustering normal-HCM (top row) and normals-PH (bottom row) cases versus number of clusters, (a-b) Generalization errors as distances between the model projected and original test sets (red), and vice versa (blue), (c-d) Specificity errors as distances between model generated and training point sets (red), and vice versa (blue). (e-f) show the model evidecene (Color figure online).

sets for each cluster is generated by sampling from $p(\mathbf{v}_k)$ and by applying the corresponding variations at each point (local Gaussians in Fig. 2), by adding the measurement noise (by the precision of $\beta = 1$). The number of points in each point set is around 100, but this is variable over the population and thus no correspondence is assumed. For $1 \leq J \leq 5$, we repeated 15 rounds of experiments with variable patterns (one shown in Fig. 2), and recorded the mean and one standard deviation on $\mathcal{L}$ (Fig. 2(d)). As shown, for $J = 3$ a maximum for the model evidence is correctly found, and the color match between (b)-(c) indicates correct clustering of point sets. In addition, the linear patterns of GMM means, i.e. $\boldsymbol{\mu}_{jk}^{(m)}$, in (c) match the local structures of the points in (d), showing that variation modes are estimated reasonably.

Table 1. Generalization and Specificity errors (in *mm*) for PCA and the proposed method at $J = 2, 6$. Significant differences between results of PCA and our method are indicated in bold (p-value < 0.001). Double lines separate $d|\hat{d}$ distances computed from the models trained by clustering PH or HCM patients versus normals.

	Generalization				Specificity			
	PH		HCM		PH		HCM	
PCA	2.9±0.4	2.9±0.4	3.1±0.4	3.2±0.5	3.2±0.3	3.2±0.3	3.5±0.4	3.5 ± 0.6
$J = 2$	**2.5±0.5**	**1.9±0.2**	**2.4±0.3**	**1.9±0.2**	3.0±0.1	**2.8±0.2**	3.3±0.1	3.2±0.2
$J = 6$	**2.2±0.5**	**1.7±0.2**	**2.2±0.3**	**1.8±0.2**	2.8±0.1	2.8±0.3	2.9±0.1	2.8±0.1

3.2   Cardiac Datasets

We apply the proposed approach to the analysis of cardiac data sets, which are known to display significant variability and geometrical complexity. We consider three groups of individuals, 36 normal cases, 20 subjects with Pulmonary Hypertension (PH), and 20 subjects with Hypertrophic Cardiomyopathy (HCM). The data acquisition of these data sets were done using a balanced Steady State Free Precession protocol under various brands of 1.5 MR scanners, resulting in image matrices of 256×256 in short axial direction and slice thicknesses of $8 - 10$ mm.

These subjects differ in the properties of the cardiac shapes. For PH patients, which are associated with pulmonary vascular proliferation [12], complex shape remodeling of both the left and right ventricles occurs (see Fig. 3). As a result, the RV becomes very dilated, pushing onto the LV, which deforms and loses its roundness [14]. On the other hand, HCM [9] is a condition in which the muscle of the heart shows an excessive thickening, and the most characteristic feature is a hypertrophied LV (asymmetric thickening prominently involving the ventricular septum) without abnormal enlargement of the ventricular cavities.

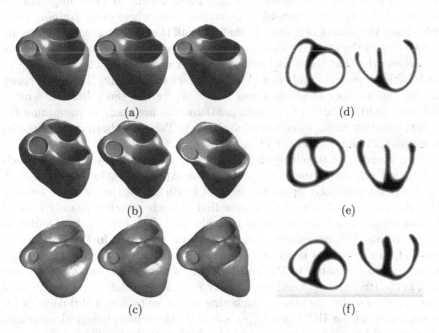

(a)   (d)

(b)   (e)

(c)   (f)

Fig. 5. Means and variation modes for normal (a), PH (b), and HCM (c) cases, with mean models in the middle and variations in opposite directions at two sides, (d-f) axial and coronal cross sections of the mean models for each population.

To derive cardiac surfaces, the initial shape was obtained by labeling the MRI slices, thus obtaining binary masks, then a volume mesh was generated form the binary images, finally, we extracted a surface mesh and considered vertices of the mesh as a point set. Next, we registered the point sets removing scaling, rotation the translation effects. Because we want to compare our method to standard PCA, point correspondences between training sets was needed and established using the projection method proposed in [10]. However, to implement our proposed method we ignore this information.

We cluster mixtures of normal-PH and normal-HCM cases in two sets of experiments. We randomly pick 33 (20 normals and 13 pathological) cases, ignore the labels and perform clustering. We then sample random point sets from the trained generative model and compute specificity. To quantify generalization on the test point sets, we use Eqn. (19) to compute model projected point sets for the test set. The number of clusters, $i.e.$ J, is varied from 1 to maximum 20. At each number, we compare both measures to the PCA model, taking 13-15 number of modes to cover 95 % of the full trace of the covariance matrix.

Figure 4 shows the quantitative results obtained as described above. It can be seen that the generalization distances, $i.e.$, d (blue) and $\hat{d}$ (red), are minimum at $J = 6$. Compared to PCA, both generalization and specificity improve (indicated in Table 1). Also, note that as the number of clusters increases and the variations within each cluster are eliminated, specificity error improves. To understand this behavior, consider an extreme case, where every training point set becomes the cluster of it own. In that case, all the intra-cluster variations are eliminated and the trained model becomes strictly specific to the training data. It is noteworthy that the model evidence is maximized at $J = 2$ (see Fig. 4(c)), which is the expected number of clusters at each experiment. The discrepancy between this number of clusters and $J = 6$ where the generalization error is minimum could be due to the approximations that are made in computing the predictive distribution. Nevertheless, as shown in Table 1, at both $J = 2, 6$ results are significantly improved over PCA model.

Next, we evaluate the clustering efficiency by comparing the estimated labels of the point sets to ground truths. For these experiments, by setting $L = 2$, $J = 2$, we independently apply the method to cluster all the available normal-PH and normal-HCM cases. We observe that at both experiments only 2 out of 53 cases are clustered incorrectly as normals cases. The first mode of variation both in 3D and in longitudinal cross sections are visualized in Fig. 5. It can be seen that, in the normal heart (see (a) and (d)), LV is significantly larger than RV, and when compared to PH and HCM, it is more spherical. On the other hand, in the PH heart ((b) and (e)), the RV is evidently dilated and the LV loses it roundness. Finally, significant thickening of the septum and shrinkage of LV are noticeable in the HCM heart ((c) and (f)). These morphological variations in the normal heart have been reported for both pathologies [9,14].

4   Conclusion

We proposed a unified framework for joint clustering and component analysis of point sets. We modeled the pdf of point sets as a mixture of principal component analyzers, where the labels of the point sets and variations of clusters are derived through a Variational Bayesian framework. The method is flexible to handle point sets with no point-to-point correspondences. We showed that the method can identify the number of clusters automatically, and outperform traditional PCA based SSMs in generalization and specificity. Application of the proposed framework to heart data sets shows successful clustering of normal and pathological cases, as well as extraction of their intra-cluster variations.

Acknowledgement. This project was funded by the Marie Skodowska-Curie Individual Fellowship (Contract Agreement 625745).

References

1. Bishop, C.M.: Pattern Recognition and Machine Learning. Springer, Heidelberg (2009)
2. Cootes, T.F., Taylor, C.J.: Active shape models-their training and application. Comput. Vis. Image Underst. **61**(10), 38–59 (1995)
3. Cootes, T.F., Taylor, C.J.: A mixture model for representing shape variation. Image Vis. Comput. **17**(8), 567–574 (1999)
4. Davis, R.H., Twinning, C.J., Cootes, T.F., Taylor, C.J.: Building 3D statistical shape models by direct optimization. IEEE Trans. Med. Imaging **29**(4), 961–982 (2010)
5. Frangi, A.F., Rueckert, D., Schnabel, J.A., Niessen, W.J.: Automatic construction of multiple-object three-dimensional statistical shape models: application to cardiac modeling. IEEE Trans. Med. Imaging **21**(9), 1151–1165 (2002)
6. Ghahramani, Z., Beal, M.J.: Variational inference for bayesian mixtures of factor analysers. In: Advances in Neural Information Processing Systems 12, pp. 449–455. MIT Press (2000)
7. Granger, S., Pennec, X.: Multi-scale EM-ICP: a fast and robust approach for surface registration. In: Heyden, A., Sparr, G., Nielsen, M., Johansen, P. (eds.) ECCV 2002. LNCS, vol. 2353, pp. 418–432. Springer, Heidelberg (2002)
8. Hufnagel, H.: A Probabilistic Framework for Point-Based Shape Modeling in Medical Image Analysis. Springer, Heidelberg (2011)
9. Maron, B., et al.: Hypertrophic cardiomyopathy. Interrelations of clinical manifestations, pathophysiology, and therapy. N. Engl. J. Med. **316**, 780–844 (1987)
10. Pereanez, M., Lekadir, K., Butakoff, C., Hoogendoorna, C., Frangi, A.F.: A framework for the merging of pre-existing and correspondenceless 3D statistical shape models. Med. Image Anal. **18**(7), 1044–1058 (2014)
11. Rasoulian, A., Rohling, R., Abolmaesumi, P.: Group-wise registration of point sets for statistical shape models. IEEE Trans. Med. Imaging **31**(11), 2025–2033 (2012)
12. Swift, A.J., et. al.: Diagnostic accuracy of cardiovascular magnetic resonance imaging of right ventricle morphology and function in assessment of suspected pulmonary hypertension results from the ASPIRE registry. J. Cardiovasc. Magn. Reson. 14(40) (2012)
13. Tipping, M.E., Bishop, C.M.: Mixtures of probabilistic principal component analyzers. Neural Comput. **11**(2), 443–482 (1999)
14. Voelkel, N., Quaife, R., Leinwand, L., Barst, R., et al.: Right ventricular function and failure: a report. Circ. **114**, 1883–1891 (2006)
15. Zhang, S., Zhan, Y., Dewan, M., Metaxas, D.N., Zhou, X.S.: Towards robust and effective shape modeling: sparse shape composition. Med. Image Anal. **16**, 265–277 (2012)

Statistical Methods

Bootstrapped Permutation Test
for Multiresponse Inference on Brain
Behavior Associations

Bernard Ng[1,2]([✉]), Jean Baptiste Poline[2], Bertrand Thirion[2],
Michael Greicius[1], and IMAGEN Consortium

[1] Functional Imaging in Neuropsychiatric Disorders Lab, Stanford University,
Stanford, CA, USA
bernardyng@gmail.com
[2] Parietal Team, Neurospin, INRIA Saclay, Palaiseau, France

Abstract. Despite that diagnosis of neurological disorders commonly involves a collection of behavioral assessments, most neuroimaging studies investigating the associations between brain and behavior largely analyze each behavioral measure in isolation. To jointly model multiple behavioral scores, sparse multiresponse regression (SMR) is often used. However, directly applying SMR without statistically controlling for false positives could result in many spurious findings. For models, such as SMR, where the distribution of the model parameters is unknown, permutation test and stability selection are typically used to control for false positives. In this paper, we present another technique for inferring statistically significant features from models with unknown parameter distribution. We refer to this technique as bootstrapped permutation test (BPT), which uses Studentized statistics to exploit the intuition that the variability in parameter estimates associated with relevant features would likely be higher with responses permuted. On synthetic data, we show that BPT provides higher sensitivity in identifying relevant features from the SMR model than permutation test and stability selection, while retaining strong control on the false positive rate. We further apply BPT to study the associations between brain connectivity estimated from pseudo-rest fMRI data of 1139 fourteen year olds and behavioral measures related to ADHD. Significant connections are found between brain networks known to be implicated in the behavioral tasks involved. Moreover, we validate the identified connections by fitting a regression model on pseudo-rest data with only those connections and applying this model on resting state fMRI data of 337 left out subjects to predict their behavioral scores. The predicted scores significantly correlate with the actual scores, hence verifying the behavioral relevance of the found connections

Keywords: Bootstrapping · Brain behavior associations · Connectivity · fMRI · Multiresponse regression · Permutation test · Statistical inference

1 Introduction

Diagnosis of neurological disorders generally entails assessments of multiple behavioral domains. For instance, Attention Deficit Hyperactivity Disorder (ADHD) is commonly diagnosed based on a collection of criteria related to inattention,

© Springer International Publishing Switzerland 2015
S. Ourselin et al. (Eds.): IPMI 2015, LNCS 9123, pp. 113–124, 2015.
DOI: 10.1007/978-3-319-19992-4_9

hyperactivity, and impulsivity as specified in the Diagnostic and Statistical Manual of Mental Disorders (DSM). Thus, for most cases, it is the aggregate of multiple criteria that characterizes a neurological disorder. Past neuroimaging studies investigating brain behavior relationships typically analyze each behavioral measure independently [1]. One of the state-of-the-art approaches for jointly modeling multiple response variables is to incorporate a group least absolute shrinkage and selection operator (LASSO) penalty into the regression model [2] to promote selection of features associated with all response variables. However, directly applying this sparse multi-response regression (SMR) technique and assuming that all features corresponding to nonzero regression coefficients are relevant could result in many spurious findings, since SMR alone does not control for false positives [3]. Another approach is to find linear combinations of features and responses that best correlate with each other using partial least square (PLS) or canonical correlation analysis (CCA), which can be cast as a reduced rank regression (RRR) problem [4]. In limited sample settings, especially when the number of features exceeds the number of samples, sparse variants of PLS, CCA, and RRR are often used [5], but these sparse variants in their raw forms suffer the same limitation as SMR in terms of false positives not being controlled.

The growing feature dimensionality of today's problems warrants caution in controlling for false positives [6]. A number of techniques have been put forth for addressing this critical concern in the context of sparse regression [7]. The key idea behind these techniques is to de-bias the sparse regression coefficient estimates, so that parametric inference can be applied to generate approximate p-values. How to de-bias the parameter estimates of SMR as well as sparse variants of PLS, CCA, and RRR is currently unclear. For models with unknown parameter distribution, a widely-used technique is permutation test (PT) [8], which is applicable to any statistics generated from the model parameters since PT requires no assumptions on the underlying parameter distribution. Another flexible technique is stability selection (SS) [9], which operates under the rationale that if we subsample the data many times and perform feature selection on each subsample using e.g. SMR, relevant features will likely be selected over a large proportion of subsamples, whereas irrelevant features will unlikely be repeatedly selected. Importantly, SS has a theoretical threshold that bounds the expected number of false positives. Also, SS eases the problem of regularization level selection in penalized models, such as SMR, in which only a range of regularization levels needs to be specified without having to choose a specific level. However, as we will show in Sects. 2.2 and 4, the choice of threshold and regularization range has a major impact on the results.

Further complicating statistical inference on multi-feature models is the problem of multicollinearity [3]. In the face of correlated features, small perturbations to the data can result in erratic changes in the parameter estimates. In particular, sparse models with a LASSO penalty tends to arbitrarily select one feature from each correlated set [3]. One way to deal with this problem is to perturb the data e.g. by subsampling as employed in SS, and examine which features are consistently selected. Complementing this strategy is a technique called Randomized LASSO, which involves deweighting a random subset of features for each subsample. This combined technique is shown to improve relevant feature identification over pure subsampling [9]. Another strategy is to cluster the features to moderate their correlations, which has the additional advantage of reducing the feature dimensionality [3].

In this paper, we present a technique that combines bootstrapping with permutation test for inferring significant features from models with unknown parameter distribution. We refer to this technique as bootstrapped permutation test (BPT). BPT is originally proposed for inferring significant features from classifier weights [10], but as discussed here and in the next section, BPT is in fact applicable to arbitrary models with a number of properties that makes it advantageous over PT and SS. Bootstrapping is traditionally used for assessing variability in model parameters. In BPT, the variability differences in parameter estimates with and without permutation are exploited. The intuition is that parameter estimates of relevant features are presumably more variable when responses are permuted. Thus, dividing the parameter estimates with and without permutation by their respective standard deviation should magnify their magnitude differences. This intuition is incorporated by using Studentized statistics, as generated by taking the mean of bootstrapped parameter estimates and dividing it by the standard deviation. The Studentized statistics is known to be approximately normally-distributed [11]. Thus, we can generate a null distribution by fitting a normal distribution to Studentized statistics derived from the permuted responses, thereby enabling parametric inference, which is statistically more powerful than pure PT [12]. Also, BPT is more flexible than SS, since it can directly operate on parameter estimates from any models without the need for feature selection, which could be nontrivial for certain non-sparse models that do not possess an inherent feature selection mechanism. In this work, we focus on the SMR model for drawing associations between brain connectivity estimated from functional magnetic resonance imaging (fMRI) data and multiple behavioral measures related to attention deficit hyperactivity disorder (ADHD). Functional connectivity is typically estimated by computing the Pearson's correlation between fMRI time series of brain region pairs, which are highly inter-related. To reduce the correlations between these connectivity features, we cluster them based on the network to which each brain region belongs, thereby accounting for the similarity between time series of brain regions within the same network. To compare BPT against PT and SS, we generate synthetic behavioral scores using network-level connectivity estimates derived from real fMRI data. We also apply these techniques on pseudo-rest fMRI data from 1139 fourteen year olds in identifying significant connections that are relevant to ADHD behavioral measures. The identified connections are validated on resting state fMRI data from 337 left out subjects by comparing their predicted and actual scores.

2 Methods

We first briefly review SMR (Sect. 2.1) and describe how stability selection (Sect. 2.2) can be incorporated to control for false positives. We then discuss the properties of PT, and how BPT improves upon PT via the use of Studentized statistics as generated by bootstrapping (Sect. 2.3).

2.1   Sparse Multiresponse Model

Let $\mathbf{Y}$ be a $n \times q$ matrix, where n is the number of samples, and q is the number of response variables. Further, let $\mathbf{X}$ be a $n \times d$ matrix, where d is the number of features. The standard way for assessing associations between $\mathbf{Y}$ and $\mathbf{X}$ is via regression:

$$\min_{\boldsymbol{\beta}} \|\mathbf{Y} - \mathbf{X}\boldsymbol{\beta}\|_2^2, \tag{1}$$

where $\boldsymbol{\beta}$ is the $d \times q$ regression coefficient matrix. The optimal $\boldsymbol{\beta}$ obtained by solving (1) is equivalent to regressing each column of $\mathbf{Y}$ on $\mathbf{X}$ independently. Thus, the relations between columns of $\mathbf{Y}$ are ignored. To incorporate this information in estimating $\boldsymbol{\beta}$, one of the state-of-the-art approaches is to employ the SMR model [2]:

$$\min_{\boldsymbol{\beta}} \|\mathbf{Y} - \mathbf{X}\boldsymbol{\beta}\|_2^2 + \lambda \|\boldsymbol{\beta}_g\|_{2,1}, \text{ s.t. } \|\boldsymbol{\beta}_g\|_{2,1} = \sum_{i=1}^{d} \|\boldsymbol{\beta}_{i,:}\|_2 = \sum_{i=1}^{d} \sqrt{\sum_{j=1}^{q} \boldsymbol{\beta}_{ij}^2} \tag{2}$$

where $\|\boldsymbol{\beta}_g\|_{2,1}$ is the group LASSO penalty and each row of $\boldsymbol{\beta}$, denoted as $\boldsymbol{\beta}_{i,:}$, corresponds to a feature. With elements of each $\boldsymbol{\beta}_{i,:}$ taken as a group, only features associated with all q response variables would be selected with the corresponding $\boldsymbol{\beta}_{i,j} \neq 0$ for all j. To set λ, we search over 100 λ's in $[\lambda_{\max}, \lambda_{\min}]$, where $\lambda_{\max} = max_j \|\mathbf{X}_{:,j}^T \mathbf{Y}\|_2$ and $\lambda_{\min} = c\lambda_{\max}, c < 1$. Optimal λ is defined as the one that minimizes the prediction error over 1000 subsamples with the data randomly split into 80 % for model training and 20 % for error evaluation. A fast solver of (2) can be solved with GLMNET [13].

2.2   Stability Selection

A problem with assuming features associated with nonzero $\boldsymbol{\beta}_{i,:}$ in SMR are all relevant is that this property is true only under very restricted conditions, which are largely violated in most real applications [3]. In particular, this guarantee on correct feature selection does not hold when features are highly correlated, which is often the case for real data [3]. With correlated features, perturbations to the data can result in drastic changes in the features that are selected. Based on this observation, an intuitive approach to deal with correlated features is to perturb the data and declare features that are consistently selected over different perturbations as relevant, which is the basis of SS. We describe here SS in the case of SMR, but SS can generally be applied to any models that are equipped with a feature selection mechanism. Given $\mathbf{X}$, $\mathbf{Y}$, and $[\lambda_{\max}, \lambda_{\min}]$, SS combined with Randomized LASSO proceeds as follows [9]:

1. Multiply each column of $\mathbf{X}$ by 0.5 or 1 selected at random.
2. Randomly subsample $\mathbf{X}$ and $\mathbf{Y}$ by half to generate $\mathbf{X}^s$ and $\mathbf{Y}^s$.
3. For each λ in $[\lambda_{\max}, \lambda_{\min}]$, apply SMR to generate $\boldsymbol{\beta}^s(\lambda)$. Let $\mathbf{S}^s(\lambda)$ be a $d \times 1$ vector with elements corresponding to selected features, i.e. nonzero $\boldsymbol{\beta}^s(\lambda)$, set to 1.
4. Repeat steps 2 and 3 S times, e.g. with $S = 1000$.

5. Compute the proportion of subsamples, $\pi_i(\lambda)$, that each feature i is selected for each λ in $[\lambda_{max}, \lambda_{min}]$.
6. Declare feature i as significant if $max_\lambda \pi_i(\lambda) > \pi_{th}$.

A π_{th} that controls for the expected number of false positives, $E(V)$, is given by [9]:

$$E(V) \le \frac{1}{2\pi_{th} - 1} \frac{\gamma^2}{d}, \tag{3}$$

where V is the number of false positives and γ is the expected number of selected features, which can be approximated by: $1/S \cdot \sum_s \sum_i (U_\lambda S_i^s(\lambda))$. U_λ denotes the union over λ. We highlight two insights on (3) that have major implications on applying SS in practice. First, (3) is a conservative bound on the family-wise error rate (FWER) = $P(V \ge 1)$, since $E(V) = \sum_{v=1}^{\infty} P(V \ge v) > P(V \ge 1)$. To control FWER at $\alpha = 0.05$ with multiple comparison correction (MCC), i.e. $P(V \ge 1) \le \alpha/d$, even for $\gamma = 1$, π_{th} based on (3) is >1. Since $\pi_i(\lambda) \in [0,1]$, π_{th} should be clipped at 1, but whether FWER is still controlled is unclear. Second, a key property of SS is that it does not require choosing a specific λ. However, for $n/2 > d$, a "small enough" λ_{min} could lead to all features being selected in all subsamples, resulting in $max_\lambda \pi_i(\lambda) = 1$. Hence, all features would be declared as significant. λ selection is thus translated into λ_{min} selection, which warrants caution. An example from real data (Sect. 3.2) illustrating the impact of λ_{min} and π_{th} is shown in Fig. 1(a). Even with λ_{min} set to 0.1, i.e. a λ range that would strongly encourage sparsity, a π_{th} of 0.9 (strictest π_{th} in the suggested range of [0.6, 0.9] in [9]) declares >40 % of the features as significant, i.e. fails to control for false positives.

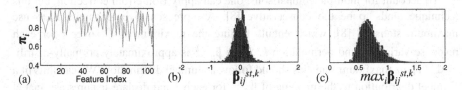

Fig. 1. Behavior of SS and BPT on real data. (a) $\pi_i(\lambda)$ at $\lambda = 0.1$ (for SS). (b) Gaussian fit on Studentized statistics (for BPT). (c) Gumbel fit on maxima of Studentized statistics (for BPT).

2.3   Bootstrapped Permutation Testing

For models with unknown parameter distribution, including those with no intrinsic feature selection mechanisms, PT is often used to perform statistical inference. PT involves permuting responses a large number of times (e.g. 10000 in this work) and relearning the model parameters for each permutation in generating null distributions of the parameters. Features with original parameter values greater than (or less than) a certain percentile of the null, e.g. >100·(1 0.025/d)th percentile (or <100·(0.025/d)th percentile), are declared as significant. Equivalently, one can count the number of permutations with parameter values exceeding/below the original parameter values to generate approximate p-values. A key attribute of PT is that it does not impose any distributional assumptions on the parameters, but the cost of this flexibility is the need for a large number of permutations to ensure the resolution of the approximate p-values are fine enough for proper statistical testing, i.e. the smallest p-value attainable from N permutation is $1/N$. Also, if the underlying parameter distribution is known, the associated parametric test is statistically more powerful [12].

The central idea behind BPT is to generate Studentized statistics via bootstrapping to exploit how the variability of the parameter estimates associated with relevant features are likely higher with responses permuted. Similar to PT, BPT can be applied to any models. We describe here BPT in the context of SMR, which proceeds as follows.

Estimation of Studentized statistics, $\beta_{ij}{}^{st}$:

1. Bootstrap $\mathbf{X}$ and $\mathbf{Y}$ with replacement for $B = 1000$ times, and denote the bootstrap samples as $\mathbf{X}^b$ and $\mathbf{Y}^b$.
2. Multiply each column of $\mathbf{X}^b$ by 0.5 or 1 selected at random.
3. Select the optimal λ for SMR by repeated random subsampling on $\mathbf{X}$ and $\mathbf{Y}$, and apply SMR on $\mathbf{X}^b$ and $\mathbf{Y}^b$ for each bootstrap b with this λ to estimate β^b.
4. Compute Studentized statistics, $\beta_{ij}{}^{st} = 1/B \cdot \sum_b \beta_{ij}{}^b / std(\beta_{ij}{}^b)$ where $/std(\beta_{ij}{}^b)$ is the standard deviation over bootstrap samples.

Estimation of the null distribution of $\beta_{ij}{}^{st}$:

5. Permute $\mathbf{Y}$ for $N = 500$ times.
6. For each permutation k, compute $\beta_{ij}{}^{st,k}$ with the same λ, samples, and feature weighting used in each bootstrap b as in the non-permuted case.
7. $p-value = 2 \cdot \min(1 - \Phi(\beta_{ij}{}^{st} | 1/N \cdot \sum_k \beta_{ij}{}^{st,k}, std(\beta_{ij}{}^{st,k})), \Phi(\beta_{ij}{}^{st} | 1/N \sum_k \beta_{ij}{}^{st,k}, std(\beta_{ij}{}^{st,k})))$, where $\Phi(\cdot)$ = the normal cumulative distribution function.

To account for multiple comparisons, one can apply Bonferroni correction, but this technique tends to be too conservative [8]. A more sensitive technique is to use maximum statistics [8], which entails finding the maximum $\beta_{ij}{}^{st,k}$ over i for each response variable j and permutation k. Since $\beta_{ij}{}^{st,k}$ is approximately normally-distributed [11], its maximum statistics should follow a Gumbel distribution. We can thus fit a Gumbel distribution to the maxima of $\beta_{ij}{}^{st,k}$ for each j and declare features associated with $\beta_{ij}{}^{st,k}$ exceeding a certain percentile of the fitted Gumbel distribution as significant. Negative can be similarly tested with maximum replaced by minimum. An example from real data (Sect. 3.2) illustrating a Gaussian and a Gumbel distribution fit to the empirical distribution of $\beta_{ij}{}^{st,k}$ and its maxima, respectively, for an exemplar feature and response is shown in Fig. 1(b) and (c). Another sensitive MCC technique is false discovery rate (FDR) correction [8], which involves sorting the p-values in ascending order, and testing the lth p-value against $l \cdot \alpha/d$, e.g. $\alpha = 0.05$.

We highlight here properties of BPT that make it advantageous over PT and SS. First, $std(\beta_{ij}{}^b)$ of relevant features are likely larger with responses permuted. By using Studentized statistics, i.e. dividing the bootstrapped mean of β_{ij} by $std(\beta_{ij}{}^b)$, the magnitude differences in β_{ij} between the permuted and non-permuted cases would be magnified. Second, Studentized statistics approximately follows a normal distribution [11], hence justifying the use of parametric inference, which is more powerful than PT. It is worth noting that normal approximation on Studentized statistics is more accurate than on conventional mean [11]. Lastly, in contrast to SS, BPT does not require a feature selection mechanism. Instead, BPT can directly operate on the parameter estimates, which additionally accounts for the magnitude of β_{ij}. Also, BPT facilitates greater flexibility in the choice of statistical inference procedures, e.g. MCC with maximum statistics cannot be easily incorporated into SS.

3 Materials

3.1 Synthetic Data

To generate synthetic data, we used the network connectivity matrix, X_{real}, estimated from pseudo-rest fMRI data (Sect. 3.2), which comprised 1139 subjects and 105 features. This way, the feature correlations present in the real data would be retained to enable method evaluation under more realistic settings. Two scenarios were considered: $n = 50 < d = 105$ and $n = 200 > d = 105$. For each scenario, we generated 50 $n \times 3$ response matrices, Y_{syn}. Each Y_{syn} was created by randomly selecting n out of 1139 subjects and 10 out of 105 features taken as ground truth. Denoting the resulting $n \times 10$ feature matrix as X_{syn}, we generated Y_{syn} as $X_{syn}\beta_{syn} + \varepsilon$, where β_{syn} is a $d \times 3$ matrix with each element randomly drawn from a uniform distribution, $U(0.01, 0.1)$, and ε corresponds to Gaussian noise. Each Y_{syn} and the corresponding n rows of X_{real} (i.e. with all features kept, not X_{syn}) constituted as one synthetic dataset.

3.2 Real Data

Neuroimaging and behavioral data from $\sim$ 1,000 fourteen year olds were obtained from the IMAGEN database [14]. Details on data acquisition can be found in [14]. In this work, we focused on 3 behavioral measures of the Cambridge Neuropsychological Test Automated Battery (CANTAB) associated with ADHD [15]. Specifically, we examined the between error and strategy scores of the spatial working memory (SWM) task as well as the response accuracy score of the rapid visual information processing (RVP) task. For estimating connectivity, we used fMRI data acquired during a localizer task (140 volumes) as well as at rest (187 volumes) for model training and validation, respectively. For the task fMRI data, slice timing correction, motion correction, and spatial normalization to MNI space were performed using SPM8. Motion artifacts, white matter and cerebrospinal fluid confounds, principal components of high variance voxels found using CompCor [16], and their shifted variants as well as task paradigm convolved with the canonical hemodynamic response and discrete cosine functions (for highpass filtering at 0.008 Hz) were regressed out from the task fMRI time series. The task regressors were included to decouple co-activation from connectivity in generating pseudo-rest data. The resting state fMRI data were similarly preprocessed except a bandpass filter with cutoff frequencies of 0.01 Hz and 0.1 Hz was used. Taking the intersection of subjects with all 3 behavioral scores and task fMRI data, while excluding those who also have resting state fMRI data to ensure that subjects for model training and validation are independent, 1139 subjects were available for model training. For validation, 337 subjects with all 3 behavioral scores and rest data were

available. To estimate connectivity, we generated brain region time series by averaging
the voxel time series within the 90 regions of interest (ROIs) of a publicly available
functional atlas that span 14 large-scale networks [17]. The Pearson's correlation
between ROI time series was taken as estimates of connectivity. Since time series of
ROIs within the same network would be similar, the magnitude of their correlation with
other ROIs would also be similar. To reduce the correlations between these connectivity features, we computed the within and between network connectivity from the
90 × 90 Pearson's correlation matrix. For estimating within network connectivity, we
averaged the Pearson's correlation values between all ROI pairs within each network,
which resulted in 14 features. For estimating between network connectivity, we
averaged the Pearson's correlation values of all between network ROI connections for
each network pair, which resulted in 91 features. Age, sex, scan site, and puberty
development scores were regressed out from both the behavioral scores and the network connectivity features (separately for the training and validation subjects), which
were further demeaned and scaled by the standard deviation.

4 Results and Discussion

On synthetic (Sect. 4.1) and real data (Sect. 4.2), we compared BPT at $p < 0.05$ with
maximum statistics-based MCC and FDR correction against SMR with features
associated with non-zero regression coefficients assumed significant, SS at $p < 0.05/$
d with π_{th} set based on (3) and $\pi_{th} = 0.75$ (midpoint of suggested range of [0.6, 0.9] in
[9], and PT at $p < 0.05$ with maximum statistics-based MCC and FDR correction.
Central to applying SMR is the choice of λ. We thus examined results for $\lambda_{min} = 0.001$,
0.01 and 0.1. Setting λ_{min} to 0.1 produces a very narrow λ range that tends to generate
overly-sparse β. This value of λ_{min} was considered due to SS's failure to control for
false positives for smaller λ_{min} in our real data experiments.

4.1 Synthetic Data

We evaluated the contrasted techniques by computing the average true positive rate
(TPR) and average false positive rate (FPR) over the 50 synthetic datasets for each $n/$
d scenario. TPR was defined as the proportion of ground truth significant features that
were correctly identified, and FPR was defined as the proportion of ground truth non-
significant features that were incorrectly found. Results for $n/d = 50/105$ and $n/d = 200/$
105 are shown in Figs. 2 and 3. PT declared all features as non-significant, hence its
results were not displayed. Also, $\lambda_{min} = 0.1$ led to degraded performance for all
techniques, which was likely due to the resulting λ range enforcing overly-sparse
solutions. We thus focused our discussion on results for $\lambda_{min} = 0.001$ and 0.01.

For $n/d = 50/105$, SMR achieved a TPR close to 1, but also included many false
positives. Using SS with π_{th} set based on (3) had FPR well controlled, but TPR was
merely 0.1. Note that π_{th} was >1 in all cases even without MCC, and was thus clipped
at 1. By relaxing π_{th} to 0.75, SS's TPR increased to ~0.9, and FPR was <0.04, despite
FPR control was not guaranteed. Using BPT with maximum statistics-based MCC,
which exerts strong control over FPR, attained a TPR of ~0.8 with FPR being close to

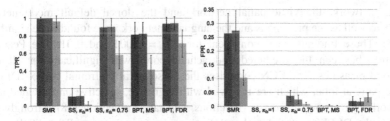

Fig. 2. Synthetic data results for $n/d = 50/105 < 1$. Each set of three bars (left to right) correspond to $\lambda_{min} = 0.001, 0.01$, and 0.1, respectively. MS = maximum statistics.

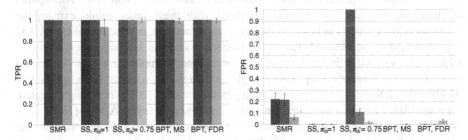

Fig. 3. Synthetic data results for $n/d = 200/105 > 1$. Each set of three bars (left to right) correspond to $\lambda_{min} = 0.001, 0.01$, and 0.1, respectively. MS = maximum statistics.

0. Relaxing the control on FPR using FDR correction resulted in TPR of ~ 0.94 and FPR < 0.02, which is half the FPR of SS with $\pi_{th} = 0.75$. Thus, for similar control on FPR, BPT provides higher sensitivity than SS. For $n/d = 200/105$, all contrasted techniques (except PT) achieved a TPR of ~ 1, but FPR was not well controlled with SMR and SS. In particular, SS with $\pi_{th} = 0.75$ resulted in a FPR of 1 for $\lambda_{min} = 0.001$ due to all features being selected for small λ's near λ_{min} across all subsamples. Thus, declaring features as significant if $\pi_i(\lambda) \geq \pi_{th}$ for any λ could be erroneous for small λ_{min} in $n > d$ settings. Also worth noting was the lack of sensitivity with PT, which clearly demonstrates the enhanced sensitivity gained by using Studentized statistics in BPT. Nevertheless, PT with $n = 1139$ attained a TPR of ~ 1 and FPR close to 0.

4.2 Real Data

We applied the contrasted techniques to the pseudo-rest fMRI data of 1139 subjects to identify the significant network connections associated with ADHD behavioral measures. Since the ground truth is unknown, we validated the identified connections by first fitting a regression model (1) to the pseudo-rest data but with only the identified connections retained. We then applied these models to the resting state fMRI data of 337 left out subjects to predict their behavioral scores. The Pearson's correlation between the predicted and actual scores of these subjects was computed with significance declared at the nominal α level of 0.05.

Using BPT with FDR correction, connections between the right executive control network (ECN) and the anterior salience network (ASN), the language network and the auditory network, the visuospatial network and the dorsal default mode network (DMN), as well as the precuneus and the language network were found to be significant (Fig. 3). These findings were consistent for $\lambda_{\min} = 0.001$ and 0.01. The Pearson's correlation between the predicted and actual scores was significant for all three behavioral measures. The ECN comprises the dorsolateral prefrontal cortex (DLPFC) and the parietal lobe, which are involved with vigilance, selective and divided attention, working memory, executive functions, and target selection [18]. Strongly connected to the DLPFC is the dorsal anterior cingulate cortex (part of the ASN), which plays a major role in target and error detection [18]. Hence, the finding of the connection between the ECN and the ASN to be significant matches well with the cognitive processes required for the SWM and RVP tasks. Also, the visuospatial manipulation and memory demands involved with these tasks would explain the detection of the connection between the visuospatial network and the dorsal DMN. The detection of the connection between the precuneus and the language network might relate to the variability in the level of linguistic strategy employed by the subjects to process spatial relations [19]. Interestingly, although all subjects have subclinical ADHD scores, there is moderate variability in their values [20], which might explain the resemblance between the found networks and those affected by ADHD [18, 21, 22]. We note that BPT with the stricter maximum statistics-based MCC detected only the connection between the Precuneus and the language network.

SMR found connections between the visuospatial network and the language network as well as connections within the left ECN to be behaviorally relevant, in addition to those found by BPT. These extra connections, although seem relevant, resulted in the Pearson's correlation for the RVP task to fall below significance. As for SS, $\pi_{\mathrm{th}} > 1$ based on (3) for all $\lambda_{\min}$ tested, even for $E(V) < 0.05$ instead of $0.05/d$, i.e. no MCC. Setting $\lambda_{\min}$ to 0.001 and 0.01 resulted in almost all network connections declared as significant for $\pi_{\mathrm{th}} = 1$. For $\lambda_{\min} = 0.1$, only one connection survived with $\pi_{\mathrm{th}} = 1$, and $>1/3$ of the connections declared significant with $\pi_{\mathrm{th}} = 0.9$ (Fig. 1(a)). To obtain sensible results, we used $\pi_{\mathrm{th}} = 1$ with $\lambda_{\min} = 0.05$, which declared the connections between the language network and the auditory network, the primary visual network and the precuneus, as well as connections within the left ECN as significant. With these connections, only the Pearson's correlation for the RVP task was significant. Using PT detected connections between the Precuneus and the language network as well as the language network and the auditory network, which constitutes a subset of the connections found by BPT, and the Pearson's correlations obtained were similar.

We highlight here several notable observations. First, our results show that models built from pseudo-rest data can generalize to true rest data. This finding provides further support for the hypothesis that intrinsic brain activity is sustained during task performance [23]. The correlations between the predicted and actual scores, however, are rather small in absolute terms, which might limit practical applications. Second, SS is gaining popularity due to its generality and claimed robustness to regularization settings. Our results show that SS is actually sensitive to the choice of threshold and regularization range, especially for $n > d$. Thus, SS should be applied with caution. Third, applying BPT with $1/B \cdot \sum_b \beta_{ij}{}^b$ without diving by $std(\beta_{ij}{}^b)$ resulted in degraded performance (similar to PT's), which indicates that modeling differences in variability between the permuted and non-permuted cases is key to BPT's superior

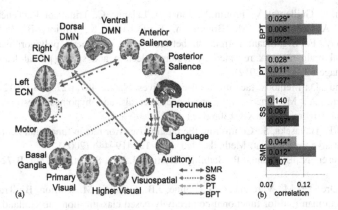

Fig. 4. Real data results. $\lambda_{min} = 0.001$, except SS where $\lambda_{min} = 0.05$ used. (a) Significant network connections found on pseudo-rest fMRI data. (b) Pearson's correlation between predicted and actual scores with p-values noted. Each set of three bars (top to bottom) correspond to SWM strategy, SWM between errors, and RVP accuracy scores. *Significance declared at $p < 0.05$.

sensitivity. Lastly, Studentized bootstrap conference intervals are known to have lower coverage errors than its empirically derived counterpart [24]. Improvements with BPT over PT could partly be attributed to this property of Studentized statistics (Fig. 4).

5 Conclusions

We presented BPT for statistical inference on models with unknown parameter distributions. Superior performance over PT and SS was shown on both synthetic and real data. The resemblance of the found networks with those implicated in ADHD suggests the associated network connections might be promising for ADHD classification, which currently has accuracy < 70% with most neuroimaging-based classifiers.

Acknowledgements. Bernard Ng is supported by the Lucile Packard Foundation for Children's Health, Stanford NIH-NCATS-CTSA UL1 TR001085 and Child Health Research Institute of Stanford University. Jean Baptiste Poline is partly funded by the IMAGEN project (E.U. Community's FP6, LSHM-CT-2007-037286).

References

1. Seeley, W.W., Menon, V., Schatzberg, A.F., Keller, J., Glover, G.H., Kenna, H., Reiss, A.L., Greicius, M.D.: Dissociable intrinsic connectivity networks for salience processing and executive control. J. Neurosci. **27**, 2349–2356 (2007)
2. Simon, N., Friedman, J., Hastie, T.: A Blockwise descent algorithm for group-penalized multiresponse and multinomial regression. arXiv:1311.6529 (2013)
3. Varoquaux, G., Gramfort, A., Thirion, B.: Small-sample brain mapping: sparse recovery on spatially correlated designs with randomization and clustering. In: Int. Conf. Mach. Learn. (2012)
4. De la Torre, F.: A least-squares framework for component analysis. IEEE Trans. Patt. Ana. Mach. Intell. **34**, 1041–1055 (2012)

5. Le Floch, E., Guillemot, V., Frouin, V., Pinel, P., Lalanne, C., Trinchera, L., Tenenhaus, A., Moreno, A., Zilbovicius, M., Bourgeron, T., Dehaene, S., Thirion, B., Poline, J.B., Duchesnay, E.: Significant correlation between a set of genetic polymorphisms and a functional brain network revealed by feature selection and sparse partial least squares. NeuroImage **63**, 11–24 (2012)

6. MacArthur, D.: Methods: face up to false positives. Nature **487**, 427–428 (2012)

7. Javanmard, A., Montanari, A.: Confidence intervals and hypothesis testing for high-dimensional regression. arXiv:1306.3171 (2013)

8. Nichols, T., Hayasaka, S.: Controlling the familywise error rate in functional neuroimaging: a comparative review. Stat. Methods Med. Res. **12**, 419–446 (2003)

9. Meinshausen, N., Bühlmann, P.: Stability selection. J. Roy. Statist. Soc. Ser. B **72**, 417–473 (2010)

10. Ng, B., Dressler, M., Varoquaux, G., Poline, J.B., Greicius, M., Thirion, B.: Transport on riemannian manifold for functional connectivity-based classification. In: Golland, P., Hata, N., Barillot, C., Hornegger, J., Howe, R. (eds.) MICCAI 2014, Part II. LNCS, vol. 8674, pp. 405–412. Springer, Heidelberg (2014)

11. Delaigle, A., Hall, P., Jin, J: Robustness and accuracy of methods for high dimensional data analysis based on student's t-statistic. arXiv:1001.3886 (2010)

12. Tanizaki, H.: Power comparison of non-parametric tests: small-sample properties from monte carlo experiments. J. Appl. Stat. **24**, 603–632 (1997)

13. http://www.stanford.edu/~hastie/glmnet_matlab/

14. Schumann, G., et al.: The IMAGEN study: reinforcement-related behaviour in normal brain function and psychopathology. Mol. Psychiatr. **15**, 1128–1139 (2010)

15. Chamberlain, S.R., Robbins, T.W., Winder-Rhodes, S., Müller, U., Sahakian, B.J., Blackwell, A.D., Barnett, J.H.: Translational approaches to frontostriatal dysfunction in attention-deficit/hyperactivity disorder using a computerized neuropsychological battery. Biol. Psychiatry **69**, 1192–1203 (2011)

16. Behzadi, Y., Restom, K., Liau, J., Liu, T.T.: A component based noise correction method (CompCor) for BOLD and perfusion based fMRI. NeuroImage **37**, 90–101 (2007)

17. Shirer, W.R., Ryali, S., Rykhlevskaia, E., Menon, V., Greicius, M.D.: Decoding subject-driven cognitive states with whole-brain connectivity patterns. Cereb. Cortex **22**, 158–165 (2012)

18. Bush, G., Valera, E.M., Seidman, L.J.: Functional neuroimaging of attention-deficit/hyperactivity disorder: a review and suggested future directions. Biol. Psychiatry **57**, 1273–1284 (2005)

19. Wallentin, M., Weed, E., Østergaard, L., Mouridsen, K., Roepstorff, A.: Accessing the mental space-spatial working memory processes for language and vision overlap in precuneus. Hum. Brain Mapp. **29**, 524–532 (2008)

20. Whelan, R., et al.: Adolescent impulsivity phenotypes characterized by distinct brain networks. Nat. Neurosci. **15**, 920–925 (2012)

21. Westerberg, H., Hirvikoski, T., Forssberg, H., Klingberg, T.: Visuo-spatial working memory span: a sensitive measure of cognitive deficits in children with ADHD. Child Neuropsychol. **10**, 155–161 (2004)

22. Ghanizadeh, A.: Sensory processing problems in children with Adhd, a systematic review. Psychiatry Investig. **8**, 89–94 (2011)

23. Fox, M.D., Raichle, M.E.: Spontaneous fluctuations in brain activity observed with functional magnetic resonance imaging. Nat. Rev. Neurosci. **8**, 700–711 (2007)

24. Kuonen, D.: Studentized bootstrap confidence intervals based on M-estimates. J. Appl. Stats. **32**, 443–460 (2005)

Controlling False Discovery Rate in Signal Space for Transformation-Invariant Thresholding of Statistical Maps

Junning Li[✉], Yonggang Shi, and Arthur W. Toga

Laboratory of Neuro Imaging (LONI), Institute for Neuroimaging
and Informatics (INI), Keck School of Medicine of USC, Los Angeles, USA
{Junning.Li,yshi,toga}@loni.usc.edu

Abstract. Thresholding statistical maps with appropriate correction of multiple testing remains a critical and challenging problem in brain mapping. Since the false discovery rate (FDR) criterion was introduced to the neuroimaging community a decade ago, various improvements have been proposed. However, a highly desirable feature, transformation invariance, has not been adequately addressed, especially for voxel-based FDR. Thresholding applied after spatial transformation is not necessarily equivalent to transformation applied after thresholding in the original space. We find this problem closely related to another important issue: spatial correlation of signals. A Gaussian random vector-valued image after normalization is a random map from a Euclidean space to a high-dimension unit-sphere. Instead of defining the FDR measure in the image's Euclidean space, we define it in the signals' hyper-spherical space whose measure not only reflects the intrinsic "volume" of signals' randomness but also keeps invariant under images' spatial transformation. Experiments with synthetic and real images demonstrate that our method achieves transformation invariance and significantly minimizes the bias introduced by the choice of template images.

1 Introduction

Mapping functional activation or genetic influence to brain anatomy involves hypothesis tests carried out at numerous voxel locations. Due to its stochastic nature, it is impossible to completely eliminate statistical errors, but at best to keep an appropriate balance between false positives and false negatives. If the threshold is too conservative, then true hints may be overlooked; if it is too liberal, then spurious claims may flood in, and accompanied with publication bias [16] towards positive results they will later mislead the research community to spend extra resources on hypotheses that do not exist in the first place.

A good threshold should be selected according to the amount of simultaneously conducted tests and an error rate criterion. Though an arbitrary uncorrected threshold may yield more "promising" results, its misgauged uncertainty

This work is supported by grants P41EB015922, U54EB020406, R01MH0974343, and K01EB013633 from the National Institutes of Health (NIH).

© Springer International Publishing Switzerland 2015
S. Ourselin et al. (Eds.): IPMI 2015, LNCS 9123, pp. 125–136, 2015.
DOI: 10.1007/978-3-319-19992-4_10

may turn into pitfalls. A functional study in 2009 [5] illustrated that "significant" activation can be "detected" with uncorrected thresholds even in a dead salmon's brain. Two widely used criteria are (1) the family wise error rate (FWER) [11] which is the probability that at least one error occurs in the results, and (2) the false discovery rate (FDR) [2,19] which, roughly speaking, is the expected portion of false discoveries among reported discoveries. Rather than prohibiting even a single error, the FDR provides a direct trade-off between detection power and error ratio, so since its debut in 1995 [2] it has been actively adopted.

Though multiple testing affects a broad range of modern science, from hunting genetic causes of complex diseases to correlating social factors with economic decisions, its application in statistical mapping is uniquely challenging because it involves both randomness and geometry. First, it essentially involves an infinite and uncountable number of tests residing on a continuous space, unlike a finite number of tests in genetic scans. Second, geometric operations and topological properties, such as spatial transformation and connected components, stand as important concerns. Moreover, spatial dependence among signals makes the problem highly complicated.

In this paper, we are particularly interested in transformation invariance in FDR control, especially for voxel-based FDR. We find it closely related to another important issue, spatial correlation, as discussed in Sect. 4. It is a popular practice to warp subjects' images to a template space for statistical mapping, for example, the Talairach atlas [12], the LPBA40 atlas [18], the ICBM152 atlas [8] or customized atlases built with various software, such as ANTS, AIR, ART, Diffeomorphic Demons, FNIRT. As statistical mapping may take place in so many possible image spaces, it naturally raises a question: if we threshold a statistical map in two homogeneous spaces with the same FDR level, will their results be consistent under spatial transformation? If our methods are transformation variant, then our results may include the bias introduced by our arbitrary choice of atlases or registration software and parameters.

Since Genovese, Lazar, and Nichols [9] introduced the FDR to the neuroimaging community a decade ago, various adaptations and improvements have been made. However, transformation invariance, this highly desirable feature, has not been adequately addressed. To the best of our knowledge, this is the first paper dedicated to this topic. In Genovese et al.'s work (2002) [9], the FDR is the defined as the volumetric ratio of false positive regions again positive regions, and controlled by Benjamini and Hochberg's step-up procedure [2,4] applied to voxel p-values. Nguyen et. al. (2014) [14] revisited Genovese et al.'s method [9], and reduced speckles with Markov random field. This voxel-based FDR definition has an obvious problem: if the image is spatially transformed, its volumetric measure will change and so does the FDR.

Pacifico et al. (2004) [15] pioneered to control the FDR for the number of clusters (which formally are connected excursion sets), instead of the volumetric ratio. He classified a cluster as false positive if its false positive volume exceeds a pre-defined ratio. Heller et. al. (2006) [10] then proposed a two-stage method: in the first stage, functional activated clusters are segmented with pilot data; then in the second stage, FDR control is applied to p-values derived from clusters' average signals. Benjamini and Heller (2007) [1] later extended the method in [10] by weighting each cluster with its volumetric size. Though the number of clusters does not change under spatial transformation, these methods all partially rely on volumetric measure which is transformation variant: classification of false positive clusters by volumetric ratio in Pacifico et al.'s method [15], taking clusters' average signals in Heller et. al.'s method [10], and weighting clusters with their sizes in Benjamini and Hochberg's method [1].

Chumbley and Friston (2009) [7] and Chumbley et. al. (2010) [6] worked on random field theory. According to Gaussian random field theory, they calculated cluster p-values by either their sizes [7] or peak signals [6], and then they applied Benjamini and Hochberg's step-up procedure [2,4] for FDR correction. Though these methods enjoy transformation invariance in their cluster-based FDR definition and p-value calculation, they introduced another problem: the number of clusters entering into the FDR stage, even pre-screened with a fixed threshold, becomes a random variable, while Benjamini and Hochberg's methods [2,4] demand a fixed number of clusters. These methods then require the number of pre-screened clusters to be independent of cluster p-values, an assumption whose proof is unclear.

To achieve transformation invariance, we shall either define the FDR based on topological indices such as the number of clusters, or local properties such as local maximas, or if volumetric integration is involved, use a measure that does not change under transformation. Here we explore defining the measure in the signal space instead of the native image space. Although it is natural to define the measure directly in the image's Euclidean space, spatial transformation and atlas choice affect this measure. Rather, the signal space is intrinsic and unaffected. We find that normalized residuals of a Gaussian multi-variate linear regression model uniformly distribute on a unit hyper-sphere independent of its regression statistics such as the t-statistics, F-statistics and p-values. Therefore, the image and the normalized residuals form a mapping from a Euclidean space to a unit hyper-sphere. We can define the volumetric measure as the "area" spanned by signals on the unit hyper-sphere. Because volumetric measure is involved in many aforementioned FDR methods [1,9,10,14,15], embedding our hyper-spherical measure could equip them with this highly desirable transformation-invariance feature.

In Sect. 2, we elaborate our method, including the unit hyper-sphere of normalized residuals, the weighted FDR, and the voxel-based FDR using signal space measure. In Sect. 3, we demonstrate with synthetic and real images that our method significantly reduces the bias introduced by spatial transformation. In Sect. 4, we discuss transformation invariance and signal's spatial dependence.

2   Methods

2.1   Intrinsic Spherical Signal Space

We consider a linear model $Y = X\beta + \varepsilon$ where X is an m-by-n $(m > n)$ full column-rank matrix, Y is a column vector of length m, β is a column vector of length n, and ε_is $(i = 1, \cdots, m)$ are identical and independently distributed (i.i.d.) variables following a Gaussian distribution $N(0, \sigma^2)$. In research applications, Y may be an fMRI time serials at a voxel location and X may be the design matrix of functional tasks, or in a tensor-based morphometry (TBM) study Y may be subjects' Jacobian determinant at a voxel location and X may be a factor matrix of age, gender or disease states, etc. Please note:

– We assume that X is full column-rank so that the inverse of $X^\mathsf{T} X$ exists.
– We assume that $m > n$ so that it is possible to estimate σ^2.

The maximum-likelihood and unbiased estimate of β is

$$\hat{\beta} \equiv (X^\mathsf{T} X)^{-1} X^\mathsf{T} Y = \beta + (X^\mathsf{T} X)^{-1} X^\mathsf{T} \varepsilon.$$

The residuals and the unbiased estimate of σ^2 are

$$\begin{cases} \hat{\varepsilon} & = Y - X\hat{\beta} = \left[I - X (X^\mathsf{T} X)^{-1} X^\mathsf{T} \right] \varepsilon, \\ \hat{\sigma}^2 & \equiv \frac{\hat{\varepsilon}^\mathsf{T} \hat{\varepsilon}}{df}, \text{ where } df = m - n. \end{cases}$$

Let us focus on the probabilistic and geometric properties of $\hat{\varepsilon}$.

1. It follows a σ^2-variance isotropic multi-variate Gaussian distribution embedded in the null space of X's columns. More specifically, there exists an m-by-df matrix Z which satisfies $X^\mathsf{T} Z = 0$ and $Z^\mathsf{T} Z = I$, such that $\tilde{\varepsilon} \equiv Z^\mathsf{T} \hat{\varepsilon} \sim N(0, \sigma^2 I_{df \times df})$ and $\hat{\varepsilon} = Z\tilde{\varepsilon}$.
2. It is independent of $\hat{\beta}$.
3. Its normalized vector $\hat{u} = \hat{\varepsilon}/|\hat{\varepsilon}|$ uniformly distributes on a unit hyper-sphere in the null space of X's columns, independent of σ^2 and $\hat{\sigma}^2$.

Property 1 is the most insightful and it easily derives properties 2 and 3. We outline its proof as follows:

1. Because X is a full column-rank m-by-n matrix, its column null space has $df = m - n$ dimensions.
2. Define Z as an m-by-df matrix whose columns are a set orthonormal bases of the null space of X's columns. By definition, Z satisfies $X^\mathsf{T} Z = 0$ and $Z^\mathsf{T} Z = I$.
3. Define $\tilde{\varepsilon} \equiv Z^\mathsf{T} \hat{\varepsilon}$, then this df-element random vector follows a Gaussian distribution $N(0, \sigma^2 I_{df \times df})$, because:
   – $\tilde{\varepsilon} \equiv Z^\mathsf{T} \hat{\varepsilon} = Z^\mathsf{T} \left[I - X (X^\mathsf{T} X)^{-1} X^\mathsf{T} \right] \varepsilon = Z^\mathsf{T} \varepsilon$, as a linear combination of ε, follows a multi-variate Gaussian distribution;
   – The expected value of $\tilde{\varepsilon}$ is $E\tilde{\varepsilon} = Z^\mathsf{T} E\varepsilon = 0$;
   – The variance of $\tilde{\varepsilon}$ is $E\tilde{\varepsilon}\tilde{\varepsilon}^\mathsf{T} = E[Z^\mathsf{T} \varepsilon \varepsilon^\mathsf{T} Z] = Z^\mathsf{T} E[\varepsilon \varepsilon^\mathsf{T}] Z = I\sigma^2$.
4. Z also satisfies $ZZ^\mathsf{T} = I - X (X^\mathsf{T} X)^{-1} X^\mathsf{T}$ because:
   – Both $ZZ^\mathsf{T} [X \ Z]$ and $\left[I - X (X^\mathsf{T} X)^{-1} X^\mathsf{T} \right] [X \ Z]$ equal $[0 \ Z]$;
   – $[X \ Z]$ is a full-rank m-by-m matrix so its inverse exists;
   – Both ZZ^T and $\left[I - X (X^\mathsf{T} X)^{-1} X^\mathsf{T} \right]$ equal $[0 \ Z] [X \ Z]^{-1}$.
5. $\hat{\varepsilon}$ equals $Z\tilde{\varepsilon}$ because

$$\hat{\varepsilon} = \left[I - X (X^\mathsf{T} X)^{-1} X^\mathsf{T} \right] \varepsilon = ZZ^\mathsf{T} \varepsilon = Z\tilde{\varepsilon}.$$

2.2 Weighted FDR in Volume

Let R_{pos} denote the detected region, R_{tru} the underlying truth, and $|\bullet|$ the volume of a region. The volume-based FDR is defined as follows

$$FDR \equiv E\left[\frac{|R_{pos} \setminus R_{tru}|}{|R_{pos}|}\right] \quad \text{where} \quad \frac{|R_{pos} \setminus R_{tru}|}{|R_{pos}|} \equiv 0 \text{ if } |R_{pos}| = 0. \quad (1)$$

Genovese, Lazar, and Nichols [9] defined the volumetric measure in the image space, and consequently it can be translated as the number of voxels in voxel-based analysis. Benjamini and Hochberg's step-up procedure [2] was applied to control the FDR. The step-up procedure finds

$$k^* = \max\{k|\frac{p_{(k)}N}{k} \leqslant q\},$$

where q is the user specified FDR level, $p_{(k)}$ is the k-th smallest voxel p-value, and N is the number of voxels. This step-up procedure is able to handle positive dependence among tests, as Benjamini and Yekutieli discussed in [4]. For more general dependence among tests, please refer to [4].

Benjamini and Hochberg (1997) [3] upgraded it to a weighted version whose FDR and control procedure are

$$FDR \equiv E\left[\frac{\sum_{i \in R_{pos} \setminus R_{tru}} w_i}{\sum_{i \in R_{pos}} w_i}\right], \quad k^* = \max\{k|\frac{p_{(k)} \sum_{i=1}^{N} w_{(i)}}{\sum_{i=1}^{k} w_{(i)}} \leqslant q\}, \quad (2)$$

where w_i is the weight associated with a voxel.

2.3 FDR in Signal Space

If an image is spatially transformed, some voxels will expand and some will shrink, so does the volumetric measure of the positive and false positive regions. The weighted FDR provides us a way to exploit the signal space volumetric measure for transformation invariance. The normalized residual image $u = f(x)$ (where x is a point and u is a normalized residual vector) defines a mapping from $\mathcal{R}^D$ to $\mathcal{S}^{df-1}$ (where D is the image's dimension). Instead of defining $|R_{pos}|$ and $|R_{tru}|$ in $\mathcal{R}^D$, we define them in the unit $\mathcal{S}^{df-1}$ space:

$$|R|_{sig} = \int_{x \in R} \sqrt{\det[J^\intercal(x)J(x)]}dx,$$

where R stands for either R_{pos} or R_{tru}, and $J(x)$ is the Jacobian matrix of the mapping at x. For voxel-based FDR implementation, we can assign each voxel i a weight $w_i = \sqrt{J^\intercal J}$ and then apply the weighted step-up procedure (2). For the calculation of $J(x)$, instead of directly taking linear difference between a center u and its neighboring voxel value $u^\dagger$, we first map $u^\dagger$ to u's tangent plane:

$$v^\dagger \equiv \log(u^\dagger) \equiv \frac{u^\dagger - u\cos\varphi}{\|u^\dagger - u\cos\varphi\|}\varphi, \text{ where } \varphi = \arccos\left(\langle u, u^\dagger \rangle\right).$$

The length of $v^\dagger$ is the length of the geodesic connecting u and $u^\dagger$ on $\mathcal{S}^{df-1}$ and its direction is same as the initial velocity from u to $u^\dagger$.

3   Experiments

The proposed method is tested with synthetic 2D brain images and real 3D brain images, in comparison with Genovese, Lazar, and Nichols' [9] voxel-based FDR method using the image space measure. For convenience, we denote the two methods as sigFDR and volFDR respectively. We choose the method in [9] for comparison because it is the most straight-forward adaptation of FDR to statistical maps. In this way, we minimize influence introduced by other factors, such as Markov Random Field smoothing [14] or cluster pre-screening [10], but solely focus on the use of difference volumetric measures.

The experiments are performed in the following framework: vector-valued images are generated in its original space which we call the fixed image space, and then warped with linear interpolation to a new space which we call the moving image space. After FDR thresholding is applied at the 5 % level in both the fixed and moving image spaces, the results in the two image spaces are compared. To evaluate the FDR, positive signals are added to some regions, so the ground truth is known in the image generation stage and the evaluation stage, but blind to the FDR thresholding stage. This procedure randomly repeats several times to estimate the expected value and standard deviation of performance indices. We span the signal to noise ratio (SNR) in a range to provide a broad view of the performance. The evaluation indices include:

- Image-wise consistency: Let P_{fix} and P_{mov} respectively denote the detected binary-valued image (where 1 stands for positive and 0 for negative) in the fixed and moving image spaces, and $P_{mov} \circ \Phi$ the transformation of P_{mov} to the fixed image space with linear interpolation followed by thresholding at 0.5. Image-wise consistency, measured with the Dice index between P_{fix} and $P_{mov} \circ \Phi$, is

$$Dice \equiv \frac{2\sum_{i\in brain} P_{fix}(i) \wedge P_{mov} \circ \Phi(i)}{\sum_{i\in brain}[P_{fix}(i) + P_{mov} \circ \Phi(i)]}.$$

- Image-wise detection power: Let T denote the binary image of the ground truth, and P a detection result in the same space. Image-wise detection power is

$$Power = \frac{\sum_{i\in brain} P(i) \wedge T(i)}{\sum_{i\in brain} T(i)}.$$

P_{fix} and $P_{mov} \circ \Phi$ are respectively used as P and the truth image in the fixed image space is used as T.

- FDR: For P_{fix} and $P_{mov} \circ \Phi$, their FDR is calculated with Eq. (1).
- Voxel-wise consistency: The detection of a voxel in repetitive trials builds a binary vector. The detection consistency at a voxel location is the Dice index between the two binary vectors derived from P_{fix} and $P_{mov} \circ \Phi$.
- Voxel-wise detection power: The detection power at a voxel location is the ratio of its detection in the repetitive trials.

3.1 Experiment with Synthetic 2D Images

50 T1-weighted MR images are selected from the Philadelphia Neurodevelopmental Cohort (PNC) [17] to construct an 3D atlas. An axial slice of the atlas is extracted as the fixed image, and spatially transformed to generate the moving image. In each trial, 40 images filled with unit-variance white noises are simulated and then smoothed with a 4-voxel wide Gaussian kernel. Then, signals are added in the regions shown in Fig. 1. The SNR ranges from 0.1 to 0.2. Voxel p-values are calculated with the two-sided t-test. 50 random trials are repeated.

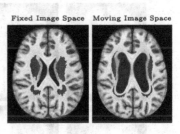

Fixed Image Space   Moving Image Space

Fig. 1. Truth images

The image-wise FDR, detection power and consistency are shown in Fig. 2. Both the sigFDR (green) and the volFDR (red) methods control the FDR, as measured in the fixed image space, around the target 5 %. However, the volFDR shows considerable difference in its FDR and detection power between detection

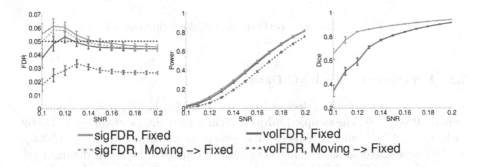

—sigFDR, Fixed   —volFDR, Fixed
···sigFDR, Moving –> Fixed   ···volFDR, Moving –> Fixed

Fig. 2. Image-wise performances evaluated in the fixed image space. Green and red curves respectively show the performance of the sigFDR and volFDR methods. In the FDR and Power plots, solid curves are for detection directly in the fixed image space, and dashed curves (except the black one) are for detection in the moving image space later warped back to the fixed image space. The dashed black curve is the target FDR value 5 %. In the Dice plot, curves show the consistency between the detection taking place in the two image spaces (Color figure online).

directly in the fixed image space (solid curves) and that warped back from the moving image space (dashed curves). On the other hand, the sigFDR shows much less difference. This is also evidenced by the Dice index plot.

The voxel-wise detection power and consistency at SNR = 0.16 are shown in Fig. 3. The power images of the volFDR method show considerable difference between the two image spaces, while the sigFDR results are much more consistent. The Dice images show clear evidence of the sigFDR method's improved consistency.

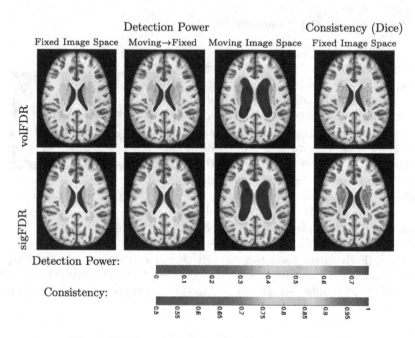

Fig. 3. Voxel-wise performances (Color figure online)

3.2   Experiment with PNC Data

50 subjects are randomly selected from the Philadelphia Neurodevelopmental Cohort (PNC) [17]. The sampled subjects include 29 males (average age = 14.069 with std. = 3.741), and 21 females (average age = 15.4286 with std. = 3.9060). A 3D T1-weighted atlas is constructed and normalized Jacobian determinant maps are derived from TBM analysis for each subject. To build null hypotheses, we remove the linear effects contributed by both age and gender from the normalized Jacobian maps, but just utilize the residual images. Please note that the residual images still hold the non-homogeneous spatial dependence in the real data. 50 random trials are generated with bootstrap as follows. In each trial, 50 subjects are randomly re-sampled to replace the original residuals, and then signals (SNR=0.1~0.2) correlated with their ages are added to the hippocampus

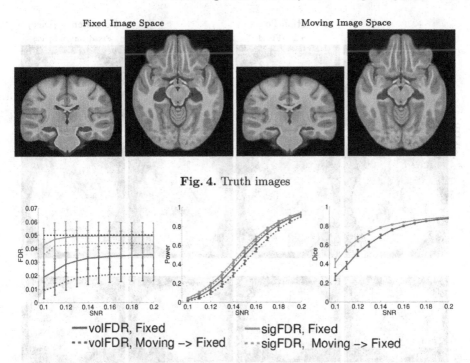

Fig. 4. Truth images

Fig. 5. Image-wise performances evaluated in the fixed image space. Green and red curves respectively show the performance of the sigFDR and volFDR methods. In the FDR and Power plots, solid curves are for detection directly in the fixed image space, and dashed curves (except the black one) are for detection in the moving image space later warped back to the fixed image space. The dashed black curve is the target FDR value 5 %. In the Dice plot, curves show the consistency between the detection taking place in the two image spaces (Color figure online).

region, as shown in Fig. 4. Voxel p-values are calculated with two-sided t-test to detect the effect of age. The hippocampus region is shrinked to produce moving images.

The image-wise FDR, detection power and consistency are shown in Fig. 5. The sigFDR (green) controls the FDR more close to the target value 5 % than the volFDR (red) does. The detection power of the volFDR decreases by about 7 % in the moving image space (dashed curves), while that of the sigFDR only changes slightly. The sigFDR also gains 7 %~20 % absolute increase in the Dice consistency. The reader should note that it is possible for the volFDR to acheive higher detection power if the regions of interest expand instead of shrink. The key advantage of the sigFDR is its consistency under spatial transformation.

The voxel-wise detection power and consistency at SNR=0.15 are shown in Fig. 6. The detection power of the volFDR decreases considerably in the moving image space, while the sigFDR method does not show significant changes. The sigFDR also achieves high voxel-wise consistency than the volFDR.

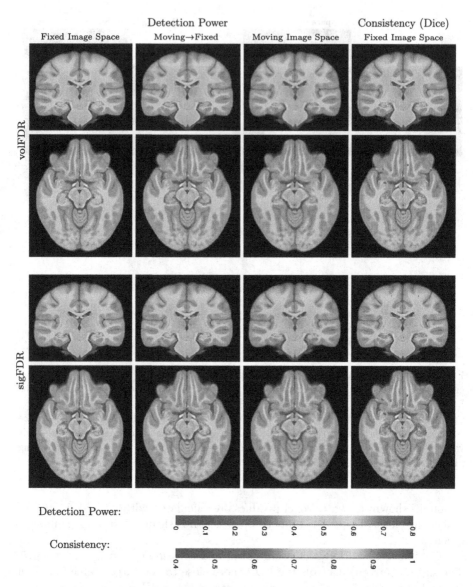

Fig. 6. Voxel-wise performances (Colour figure online)

4   Discussions and Conclusions

We have shown in theory that defining volumetric measure in the intrinsic signal space can achieve transformation invariance in FDR control. Our experiments evidence the significant gain in consistency across thresholding taking place in different image spaces. (It should be noted that interpolation error may still affect consistency.) As volumetric measure is a fundamental component in

FDR control, it can benefit many variations of spatial FDR control methods, for instance, those in [1,10,14,15], as we have already shown with Genovese, Lazar, and Nichols' method [9]. Therefore, the relationship between our method and other methods are complementary rather than competitive.

Volumetric measure in the intrinsic signal space is also closely related to signals' "effective volume of randomness". Generally, the more tests are conducted simultaneously, the more stringent the p-values should be adjusted. Due to dependence among the tests, it may be over-conservative to adjust with the number of tests, but more suitable with the effective number of independent tests, as successfully demonstrated in many genetic studies [13]. In statistical mapping, the volumetric measure in signal space indicates the dispersion of signals on the unit hyper-sphere, and adjusts dynamically with signals's spatial dependence.

Worsley (1999) [20] used resels to adjust the FWER of cluster sizes in random field theory. He assumed that the image space can be "flattened" to make signals' spatial dependence homogeneous. It is unclear how to prove this assumption in general cases. Our method does not rely on such an assumption, but consider the normalized residual image as a mapping from a Euclidean space to a unit hyper-sphere. Worsley's work was dedicated to signals' spatial dependence and the FWER, while ours is for transformation invariance and the FDR, and also provides a thorough examination on the statistical and geometric properties of residuals. Putting these two works together, it is very clear that transformation invariance and spatial dependence are two closely related issues.

References

1. Benjamini, Y., Heller, R.: False discovery rates for spatial signals. J. Am. Stat. Assoc. **102**(480), 1272–1281 (2007)
2. Benjamini, Y., Hochberg, Y.: Controlling the false discovery rate: a practical and powerful approach to multiple testing. J. Roy. Stat. Soc.: Ser. B (Method.) **57**(1), 289–300 (1995)
3. Benjamini, Y., Hochberg, Y.: Multiple hypotheses testing with weights. Scand. J. Stat. **24**(3), 407–418 (1997)
4. Benjamini, Y., Yekutieli, D.: The control of the false discovery rate in multiple testing under dependency. Ann. Stat. **29**(4), 1165–1188 (2001)
5. Bennett, C.M., Miller, M.B., Wolford, G.L.: Neural correlates of interspecies perspective taking in the post-mortem atlantic salmon: an argument for multiple comparisons correction. NeuroImage **47**, S125 (2009)
6. Chumbley, J., Worsley, K., Flandin, G., Friston, K.: Topological FDR for neuroimaging. Neuroimage **49**(4), 3057–3064 (2010)
7. Chumbley, J.R., Friston, K.J.: False discovery rate revisited: FDR and topological inference using Gaussian random fields. Neuroimage **44**(1), 62–70 (2009)
8. Fonov, V.S., Evans, A.C., McKinstry, R.C., Almli, C.R., Collins, D.L.: Unbiased nonlinear average age-appropriate brain templates from birth to adulthood. NeuroImage **47**, S102 (2009)
9. Genovese, C.R., Lazar, N.A., Nichols, T.: Thresholding of statistical maps in functional neuroimaging using the false discovery rate. Neuroimage **15**(4), 870–878 (2002)

10. Heller, R., Stanley, D., Yekutieli, D., Rubin, N., Benjamini, Y.: Cluster-based analysis of FMRI data. NeuroImage **33**(2), 599–608 (2006)
11. Hochberg, Y., Tamhane, A.C.: Multiple Comparison Procedures. Wiley Series in Probability and Statistics. Wiley, Hoboken (1987)
12. Lancaster, J.L., Woldorff, M.G., Parsons, L.M., Liotti, M., Freitas, C.S., Rainey, L., Kochunov, P.V., Nickerson, D., Mikiten, S.A., Fox, P.T.: Automated talairach atlas labels for functional brain mapping. Hum. Brain Mapp. **10**(3), 120–131 (2000)
13. Li, J., Ji, L.: Adjusting multiple testing in multilocus analyses using the eigenvalues of a correlation matrix. Heredity **95**(3), 221–227 (2005)
14. Nguyen, H.D., McLachlan, G.J., Cherbuin, N., Janke, A.L.: False discovery rate control in magnetic resonance imaging studies via Markov random fields. IEEE Trans. Med. Imaging **33**(8), 1735–1748 (2014)
15. Perone Pacifico, M., Genovese, C., Verdinelli, I., Wasserman, L.: False discovery control for random fields. J. Am. Stat. Assoc. **99**(468), 1002–1014 (2004)
16. Rosenthal, R.: The file drawer problem and tolerance for null results. Psychol. Bull. **86**(3), 638–641 (1979)
17. Satterthwaite, T.D., Elliott, M.A., Ruparel, K., Loughead, J., Prabhakaran, K., Calkins, M.E., Hopson, R., Jackson, C., Keefe, J., Riley, M., et al.: Neuroimaging of the Philadelphia neurodevelopmental cohort. NeuroImage **86**, 544–553 (2014)
18. Shattuck, D.W., Mirza, M., Adisetiyo, V., Hojatkashani, C., Salamon, G., Narr, K.L., Poldrack, R.A., Bilder, R.M., Toga, A.W.: Construction of a 3D probabilistic atlas of human cortical structures. NeuroImage **39**(3), 1064–1080 (2008)
19. Storey, J.D.: A direct approach to false discovery rates. J. Roy. Stat. Soc.: Ser. B (Stat. Method.) **64**(3), 479–498 (2002)
20. Worsley, K.J., Andermann, M., Koulis, T., MacDonald, D., Evans, A.C.: Detecting changes in nonisotropic images. Hum. Brain Mapp. **8**(2–3), 98–101 (1999)

Longitudinal Analysis

Group Testing for Longitudinal Data

Yi Hong[1]([✉]), Nikhil Singh[1], Roland Kwitt[2], and Marc Niethammer[1]

[1] Department of Computer Science, UNC Chapel Hill, Chapel Hill, NC, USA
yihong@cs.unc.edu
[2] Department of Computer Science, University of Salzburg,
Salzburg, Austria

Abstract. We consider how to test for group differences of shapes given longitudinal data. In particular, we are interested in differences of *longitudinal models* of each group's subjects. We introduce a generalization of principal geodesic analysis to the tangent bundle of a shape space. This allows the estimation of the variance and principal directions of the distribution of *trajectories* that summarize shape variations within the longitudinal data. Each trajectory is parameterized as a point in the tangent bundle. To study statistical differences in two distributions of trajectories, we generalize the Bhattacharyya distance in Euclidean space to the tangent bundle. This not only allows to take second-order statistics into account, but also serves as our test-statistic during permutation testing. Our method is validated on both synthetic and real data, and the experimental results indicate improved statistical power in identifying group differences. In fact, our study sheds new light on group differences in longitudinal corpus callosum shapes of subjects with dementia versus normal controls.

Keywords: Longitudinal data · Distribution of trajectories · Tangent bundle · Group testing · Bhattacharyya distance

1 Introduction

Longitudinal data designs frequently arise in medical research that involves repeated measurements during follow-up studies. Analysis of such longitudinal data often involves constructing statistical models to summarize growth, aging and disease progression over time. For example, longitudinal studies in new-borns and young children use imaging at multiple follow-up visits to understand the process of early brain development [6]. Similarly, recent collective efforts have enabled longitudinal data collection to facilitate the study of neurodegeneration due to aging and age-related neurological disorders, such as the Alzheimer's disease [11]. Conventional cross-sectional models of regression that do not take into account the temporal dependencies of measurements are inappropriate for modeling such longitudinal data designs.

Recent methods for analyzing longitudinal, manifold-valued data have enabled modeling and even detection of changes over time [4,7,13]. These methods allow for the estimation of trajectories, *i.e.*, smooth paths estimated from

© Springer International Publishing Switzerland 2015
S. Ourselin et al. (Eds.): IPMI 2015, LNCS 9123, pp. 139–151, 2015.
DOI: 10.1007/978-3-319-19992-4_11

the longitudinal data of subjects. Building upon these methods, Riemannian approaches for computing averages of trajectories have been proposed [12,16]. The registration and comparison of trajectories has also been studied in [3,17,18]. In general, statistical methods for longitudinal manifold-valued data focus on first-order statistics, such as computing the mean, which only captures limited information of the data distribution. Capturing higher-order statistics on the trajectories themselves would be useful for a more comprehensive description of the underlying distributions and for designing test-statistics that go beyond a simple comparison of means; an example would be testing differences in variances.

Motivated by this, we develop an approach that leverages second-order statistics of shape trajectories for group testing. In particular, we propose a generalization of principal component analysis (PCA) and principal geodesic analysis (PGA) [5] to the tangent bundle [9] of a shape space. Similar to PCA/PGA, the first principal direction characterizes the dominant variability in a *population of trajectories*, and each point along this principal direction is a trajectory. This differs from previous studies which have focused on computing averages on the tangent bundle. Incorporating second-order statistics additionally allows to identify differences between groups of trajectories in situations where the average longitudinal trend over time is similar (or equal) between two groups. We refer to this approach as *principal geodesic analysis on the tangent bundle*.

Contribution. We extend principal geodesic analysis to the tangent bundle of a shape to estimate both variance and principal directions of shape trajectories. We then introduce a generalization of the Bhattacharyya distance to manifold-valued data, which enables the assessment of statistical differences between groups of trajectories. We validate our approach on both synthetic and real shapes. The results indicate improved statistical power in distinguishing groups with different distributions, especially for cases with similar means but different variances.

Organization. The paper is organized as follows: Sect. 2 discusses the basic principles of our approach in Euclidean space. Section 3 then generalizes these concepts to manifolds and discusses group testing on the tangent bundle. Section 4 presents our experimental study and Sect. 5 concludes the paper with a summary of the main points, open problems and an outlook on future work.

2   Distribution of Trajectories in Euclidean Space

We first illustrate the concept of analyzing populations of trajectories in Euclidean space, which is a trivial case of a Riemannian manifold.

Consider the case of two groups of subjects such that each subject is measured at multiple points in time. Such a data configuration is also referred to as a *staggered longitudinal design*, see Fig. 1(b). If we ignore the within-subject correlations and model the data with a cross-sectional design, illustrated in Fig. 1(a), the two groups cannot be separated using statistical tests that rely on a comparison of means only (*cf.* Table 1). Hence, to leverage longitudinal information, we

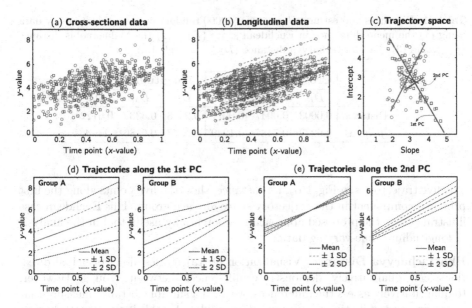

Fig. 1. A toy example in Euclidean space. *Top*: (a) Cross-sectional data of two groups, illustrated as red circles and blue squares; (b) the same data *with* longitudinal information (middle) where points on the same line are observations from one subject; (c) the trajectory space, represented by a slope and an intercept. Every point in this space corresponds to a straight line in (b). *Bottom*: (d) Trajectories generated by points along the 1st principal component (PC) of standard PCA in trajectory space with $\{0, \pm1, \pm2\}$ standard deviations (SD); (e) trajectories generated along the 2nd PC (best-viewed in color) (Colour figure online).

first estimate linear regression models on each subject to summarize its trend. The regression line, a smooth trajectory approximating a subject's data points, is parameterized the tuple of *slope* and *intercept*, which can be represented as a point in the space of trajectories. As shown in Fig. 1(c), representing the data in this trajectory space separates the populations (at least visually) in this example. In fact, Table 1 indicates that including longitudinal information allows us to identify differences between the two groups statistically.

To further analyze the group differences, we explore the distribution of trajectories within the (slope, intercept) space, *i.e.*, the trajectory space. Under a Gaussian assumption, principal component analysis (PCA) is a standard tool to estimate the variance and principal directions of a sample. By applying PCA to (slope, intercept) data, we obtain a representation of the population of trajectories, namely their variances and their principal components. For example, the solid lines with different colors in Fig. 1(c) show the principal components of the two groups, respectively. By moving along these two principal components, we generate new points in the trajectory space such that each point represents a straight line in the original space of the data points. Figure 1(d) and (e) visualize the trajectories along the principal components for different standard deviations.

Table 1. Distances and estimated p-values (10000 random permutations) on toy data using (1) the mean difference in Euclidean space ($\bar{D}_E$), (2) the Mahalanobis distance ($\bar{D}_M$), and (3) the Bhattacharyya distance (D_B) as a test-statistic.

	Cross-sectional data			Longitudinal data		
	$\bar{D}_E$	$\bar{D}_M$	D_B	$\bar{D}_E$	$\bar{D}_M$	D_B
Distance	0.0003	0.0047	0.0077	0.2438	0.3332	0.6722
p-value	0.9232	0.7487	0.1249	0.0347	0.0186	**1e-4**

The five trajectories in Fig. 1(d), for instance, show the five points along the first principal component in the trajectory space for each group. This Euclidean case illustrates that the proposed approach is a potentially useful tool in the analysis of longitudinal time-varying data.

Bhattacharyya Distance. Visualization of trajectories along principal directions can qualitatively demonstrate differences between groups. However, to quantitatively assess the differences, we need a suitable distance measure that serves as a test-statistic. An appropriate candidate for this is the Bhattacharyya distance [1], which measures the similarity of two probability distributions. Given two multivariate Gaussians, with means (μ_1, μ_2) and covariance matrices (Σ_1, Σ_2), the Bhattacharyya distance D_B has the closed-form expression

$$D_B((\mu_1, \Sigma_1), (\mu_2, \Sigma_2)) = \frac{1}{8}(\mu_1 - \mu_2)\Sigma^{-1}(\mu_1 - \mu_2)^\top + \frac{1}{2}\ln\left(\frac{|\Sigma|}{\sqrt{|\Sigma_1| \cdot |\Sigma_2|}}\right), \quad (1)$$

where $\Sigma = (\Sigma_1 + \Sigma_2)/2$, and $|\cdot|$ denotes the matrix determinant. The first term in Eq. (1) measures the separability of the distributions w.r.t. their means. It is related to the squared Mahalanobis distance [10], which can be considered a special case of Eq. (1) when the difference between the covariances (as measured by the second term in the summation) is not considered. This additional term makes D_B more suitable, compared to the Mahalanobis distance, in cases where the distributions differ in variances. In particular, the Mahalanobis distance is zero when two distributions have equal means. However, as D_B only satisfies three conditions of a distance metric (non-negativity, identity of indiscernibles, and symmetry), but lacks the triangle inequality, it is only a semi-metric.

In fact, Eq. (1) allows us to compute a distance between the two distributions (assuming Gaussianity) in Fig. 1(c), and thereby to define a test-statistic to test for group differences in a permutation testing setup. The null-hypothesis H_0 of the permutation test is that the two distributions (say P, Q) to be tested are the same, i.e., $H_0 : P = Q$. We estimate the empirical distribution of the test-statistic under H_0 by repeatedly permuting the group labels of the points in Fig. 1(c), and re-computing D_B between the two groups that result from the permuted labels. The p-value under H_0 then is the proportion of the area under the empirical distribution of samples for which the distance is less than the one estimated for the original (unpermuted) label assignments. In Table 1, D_B, tested on the longitudinal data, exhibits the best performance in separating the groups with an estimated p-value of $<$1e-4 under 10000 permutations.

3 Distribution of Trajectories on Manifolds

To explore the distribution of trajectories for manifold-valued data, *e.g.*, images or shapes, we need to generalize the statistical test of the previous section from Euclidean space to manifolds. Specifically, let $\{P_{i,j,k}\}$ be a population of longitudinal data on the same manifold, where i is the group identifier, j is the subject identifier, and k identifies the time point. Further assume we have N groups: group i has S_i subjects ($i = 1, \ldots, N$), and each subject has multiple time points, $\{t_{i,j,k}\}, k = 1, \ldots, T_{i,j}$. Our objective is to characterize the distribution of trajectories for each group, $\{D_i\}$, *i.e.*, to estimate its variance and principal directions, and to assess whether two groups are significantly different.

Individual Trajectories for Longitudinal Data. To perform statistical tests on subjects with associated longitudinal data, our first step is to summarize the variations within a subject as a smooth trajectory. The parametric geodesic regression approaches for data in Kendall's shape space [4], or images [7,13], which generalize linear regression in Euclidean space, provide a compact representation of the continuous trajectory for each subject. The trajectory of subject j from group i is parametrized by the initial point $\hat{p}_{i,j}$ and the initial velocity $\hat{u}_{i,j}$. This trajectory minimizes the sum-of-squared geodesic distances between the observations and their corresponding points on the trajectory, *i.e.*,

$$(\hat{p}_{i,j}, \hat{u}_{i,j}) = \arg \min_{(p_{i,j}, u_{i,j})} \sum_{k=1}^{T_{i,j}} d_g^2(\text{Exp}(p_{i,j}, t_{i,j,k} \cdot u_{i,j}), P_{i,j,k}), \qquad (2)$$

where $d_g(\cdot, \cdot)$ is the geodesic distance and $\text{Exp}(\cdot, \cdot)$ denotes the exponential map on some manifold $\mathcal{M}$ [4]. This compact representation, $(\hat{p}_{i,j}, \hat{u}_{i,j})$, is a point in the tangent bundle $T\mathcal{M}$ of $\mathcal{M}$. $T\mathcal{M}$ is also a smooth manifold, which can be equipped with a Riemannian metric, such as the *Sasaki metric* [15]. Since each subject's longitudinal data is represented as a point on $T\mathcal{M}$, we work in this space, instead of the space of the data points, to perform group testing.

Principal Geodesic Analysis (PGA) for Trajectories. We generalize principal geodesic analysis to estimate the variance and the principal directions of trajectories on the tangent bundle for each group. We follow the definitions of the exponential- and the log-map on $T\mathcal{M}$ in [12] and use the Sasaki metric. Specifically, given two points $(p_1, u_1), (p_2, u_2) \in T\mathcal{M}$, the log-map outputs the tangent vector such that $(v, w) = \text{Log}_{(p_1, u_1)}(p_2, u_2)$. The exponential map enables us to shoot forward with a given base point and a tangent vector, *i.e.*, $(p_2, u_2) = \text{Exp}_{T\mathcal{M}}((p_1, u_1), (v, w))$. Furthermore, using the log-map, the geodesic distance on $T\mathcal{M}$ can be computed as $d_{T\mathcal{M}}((p_1, u_1), (p_2, u_2)) = \| \text{Log}_{(p_1, u_1)}(p_2, u_2) \|$.

Before computing the variance and the principal directions, we first need to estimate the mean of the trajectories for each group. This is done by minimizing the sum-of-squared geodesic distances, for each group, on $\mathcal{TM}$ as

$$\forall i : (\bar{p}_i, \bar{u}_i) = \arg\min_{(p_i, u_i)} \sum_{j=1}^{S_i} d^2_{\mathcal{TM}}((p_i, u_i), (\hat{p}_{i,j}, \hat{u}_{i,j})). \tag{3}$$

Then, following the PGA algorithm of [5], we compute the variance and principal directions w.r.t. the estimated mean of the trajectories. Specifically, we first compute the tangent vector from the mean of group i to the trajectory of its subject j, $(v_{i,j}, w_{i,j}) = \mathrm{Log}_{(\bar{p}_i, \bar{u}_i)}(\hat{p}_{i,j}, \hat{u}_{i,j})$ and then calculate the covariance matrix $\Sigma_i = \frac{1}{S_i - 1} \sum_{j=1}^{S_i} (v_{i,j}, w_{i,j})(v_{i,j}, w_{i,j})^\top$. The principal decomposition of Σ_i results in the eigenvalues $\lambda_{i,q} \in \mathbb{R}_0^+$ and eigenvectors $(v_{i,q}, w_{i,q}) \in \mathcal{T}_{(\bar{p}_i, \bar{u}_i)}\mathcal{M}$ with $q = 1, \ldots, Q_i$ for group i. As a result, we can identify the distribution of trajectories for each group by $D_i = \{(\bar{p}_i, \bar{u}_i), \Sigma_i\}$ with $i = 1, \ldots, N$. By moving along a principal direction, we can generate points on $\mathcal{TM}$, which correspond to trajectories on the manifold of the data points.

Generalized Bhattacharyya Distance. Since we can characterize the distribution of trajectories on $\mathcal{TM}$ for each group, to measure the distance between them, we generalize the Bhattacharyya distance from Euclidean space to $\mathcal{TM}$. Again, the distribution D_i on $\mathcal{TM}$, is identified by a mean $\mu_i = (\bar{p}_i, \bar{u}_i) \in \mathcal{TM}$, and a covariance matrix Σ_i with respect to the mean μ_i.

Generalizing the first term of the Bhattacharyya distance in Eq. (1), i.e., the pooling of covariance matrices $\Sigma = (\Sigma_1 + \Sigma_2)/2$, is not as straightforward on $\mathcal{TM}$ as it is in Euclidean space because the covariance matrices Σ_1 and Σ_2 of the two groups reside in tangent spaces at different points on $\mathcal{TM}$. Hence, we follow the strategy in [12], and replace the first term with the average of two squared-Mahalanobis distances, i.e., $(\mathrm{Log}_{\mu_1} \mu_2 \Sigma_1^{-1} \mathrm{Log}_{\mu_1} \mu_2^\top + \mathrm{Log}_{\mu_2} \mu_1 \Sigma_2^{-1} \mathrm{Log}_{\mu_2} \mu_1^\top)/2$. Furthermore, because most manifold-valued data in medical applications is high dimensional and low sample size, the resulting covariance matrix is usually semi-positive-definite (SPD) with zero eigenvalues. This means that in many applications Σ_1 and Σ_2 are not invertible[1]. To address this issue, we approximate the covariance matrix via eigen-decomposition by dropping the eigenvalues that are smaller than a cutoff value, ϵ^2. In this way, the covariance matrix can be decomposed approximately as $\Sigma_i \approx U_{i,Q_i} \Lambda_{i,Q_i} U_{i,Q_i}^\top$, where $\lambda_{i,q} < \epsilon$ if $q > Q_i$, resulting in $\Sigma_i^{-1} \approx U_{i,Q_i} \Lambda_{i,Q_i}^{-1} U_{i,Q_i}^\top$ [14].

To generalize the second term of the Bhattacharyya distance, which involves the computation of the determinant of a covariance matrix, we use the pseudo-determinant, i.e., the product of all non-zero eigenvalues of a square matrix. For consistency, the same number of eigenvalues as for the first term is used, i.e., $|\Sigma_i| = \prod_{q=1}^{Q_i} \lambda_{i,q}$. Since it is non-trivial to compute the pooled covariance

---

[1] A better estimate of the covariance matrix may be obtained, e.g., by using [8] or [2].

[2] The threshold ϵ varies with the application. In our experiments, we set it to 1e-6. Usually, the eigenvalues larger than ϵ cover almost 99 % of the variances.

matrix Σ, we replace its determinant in Eq. (1) with the averaged determinants of Σ_1 and Σ_2. While this changes the original definition of the Bhattacharyya distance, its properties are kept (see Appendix A). Also, it can be shown that the value of the second term increases as the difference in the determinants gets larger. Hence, the generalized second term can serve as a distance measure of generalized variances of covariance matrices on $\mathcal{TM}$. In summary, we define the *generalized Bhattacharyya distance* between two Gaussians D_1, D_2 on $\mathcal{TM}$ as

$$D_B^{\mathcal{TM}}(D_1, D_2) = \frac{1}{16}(D_M^{\mathcal{TM}}(\mu_1, D_2) + D_M^{\mathcal{TM}}(\mu_2, D_1)) + \frac{1}{2}\ln\left(\frac{(|\Sigma_1| + |\Sigma_2|)}{2\sqrt{|\Sigma_1| \cdot |\Sigma_2|}}\right) \quad (4)$$

where $D_M^{\mathcal{TM}}$ is a generalized version of the squared Mahalanobis distance, given by $D_M^{\mathcal{TM}}(\mu_i, D_j) = \langle \mathrm{Log}_{\mu_j} \mu_i, U_{j,Q_j} \rangle \Lambda_{j,Q_j}^{-1} \langle \mathrm{Log}_{\mu_j} \mu_i, U_{j,Q_j} \rangle^{\top}$, and $\langle \cdot, \cdot \rangle$ is the inner product on the tangent bundle. $D_B^{\mathcal{TM}}$ is a *pseudo-semimetric*, *i.e.*, it satisfies (1) non-negativity, (2) symmetry, and (3) $D_B^{\mathcal{TM}}(D_i, D_i) = 0$ for all D_i (required for the identity of indiscernibles); see Appendix A for a detailed proof of these properties. As shown in the proof, although Eq. (4) does not satisfy the positivity property, *i.e.*, for all $D_1 \neq D_2$, $D_B^{\mathcal{TM}}(D_1, D_2) > 0$, only the distance between two distributions with equal mean *and* generalized variance is zero. Consequently, we can distinguish two distributions of trajectories that have different means and/or different determinants of the covariance matrices.

We use Eq. (4) as our test-statistic in the same permutation testing setup as described in Sect. 2. The null-hypothesis H_0 is that the samples of trajectories from the two groups were drawn from the same underlying distribution. The distribution of test-statistics under H_0 is estimated by randomly permuting the group label assignments. We then count the number of times that the distance is larger than the one computed without permutation to obtain a p-value estimate. Compared to the Hotelling T^2 statistic used in [12], which tests for difference in sample means (based on the squared Mahalanobis distance), our permutation test is based on Eq. (4), which is more appropriate in situations where two distributions have similar means but different variances.

4 Experiments

We demonstrate our method on (1) a toy example in Euclidean space, (2) a 2D example with synthetic shapes, and (3) real corpus callosum shapes. All shapes are represented in (2D) Kendall's shape space.

Toy Example in Euclidean Space. Figure 1 shows the generated toy data and the qualitative comparison between two groups using PCA in the trajectory space. Both groups have 50 subjects each, measured at 3 to 7 time points. Table 1 reports the quantitative comparison, *i.e.*, permutation testing with 10000 permutations and three different distances: the Euclidean distance $\bar{D}_E$ (*i.e.*, the squared mean differences), the Mahalanobis distance $\bar{D}_M$ (*i.e.*, the squared mean difference based on the pooled covariance matrix), and the Bhattacharyya distance D_B. The results of the cross-sectional *vs.* longitudinal tests indicate that

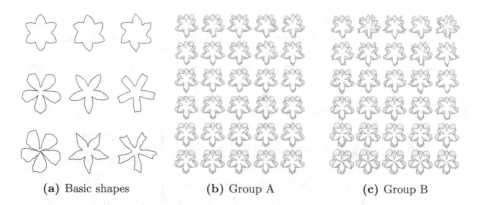

(a) Basic shapes   (b) Group A   (c) Group B

Fig. 2. Synthetic shapes: (a) Basic shapes used to generate the population on the right; (b) and (c) show the two groups of trajectories (best-viewed in color) (Colour figure online).

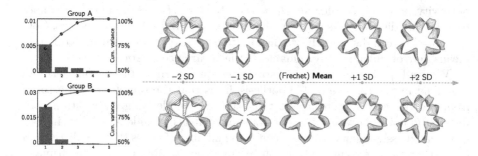

Fig. 3. Visualization of the variances (left) and principal directions (right) of trajectory distributions for the synthetic data (best-viewed in color) (Colour figure online).

leveraging the longitudinal information greatly improves our ability to identify differences, as indicated by low p-values. Besides, among the three evaluated distance measures, the Bhattacharyya distance most clearly highlights this difference with a p-value of <1e-4 (given the number of permutations).

Synthetic Shapes in Kendall's Shape Space. To verify the advantage of the generalized Bhattacharyya distance over the generalized Mahalanobis distance, we generate two groups of 2D shapes with similar mean trajectories but different variances, see Fig. 2(b) and (c). Hence, the distributions are different by design. In particular, we use the three shapes in the first row of Fig. 2(a) to uniformly sample 60 shapes within the triangle region in Kendall's shape space, spanned by the three shapes[3]. We call them the *base shapes*. In the same way, the shapes

---

[3] We use two geodesics to connect three given shapes and uniformly sample points on these two geodesics. Then, by connecting opposing points, we obtain new geodesics which are located within the triangle region to sample a population of shapes.

Table 2. Distances and estimated p-values (10000 random permutations) on synthetic shapes using the averaged Mahalanobis distance ($\bar{D}_M^{\mathcal{TM}}$) and the generalized Bhattacharyya distance ($D_B^{\mathcal{TM}}$). The last two columns report the test results when dropping one of the initial conditions.

	$(\hat{p}, \hat{u})$		$(\hat{p}, 0)$		$(0, \hat{u})$	
	$\bar{D}_M^{\mathcal{TM}}$	$D_B^{\mathcal{TM}}$	$\bar{D}_M^{\mathcal{TM}}$	$D_B^{\mathcal{TM}}$	$\bar{D}_M^{\mathcal{TM}}$	$D_B^{\mathcal{TM}}$
Distance on $\mathcal{TM}$	0.7212	2.2833	0.0232	0.0152	0.7439	2.3057
p-value	0.1817	**0.0234**	0.8486	0.6801	0.1650	**0.0297**

in the second and third row are used to sample 30 shapes each; we refer to these shapes as the *target shapes*. In summary, we have 60 base shapes from the same distribution and two groups of target shapes from two different distributions. By splitting the 60 base shapes into two subsets of equal size and connecting each base shape with one target shape (via a geodesic), we obtain 30 trajectories per group. Assuming every base shape is at time 0 and every target shape is at time 1, we sample 5 shapes along each trajectory to represent one subject. To make sure these two groups of trajectories have similar means, the shapes in the third row of Fig. 2(a) are not picked randomly, but generated using the shapes in the second row. This is done by computing the mean of the shapes in the second row, then shooting a geodesic from the mean to each of the three shapes and continuing to move beyond time 1 (for two times) to generate the shapes in the third row. Essentially, this has the effect that the means of the trajectories of both groups are similar, but the variances differ.

Figure 3 shows the results of PGA in trajectory space for the synthetic shapes. The largest eigenvalue of the trajectories in *Group A* is 0.005 at 72 % cumulative variance, compared to the largest eigenvalue of 0.02 at 85 % cumulative variance in *Group B*. Also, as expected, the trajectories visualized by 10 shapes in Fig. 3 show that the shapes of *Group B* change faster than in *Group A*. Table 2 reports the quantitative measures of the difference between the two groups. Since, by design, the mean trajectories are similar, it is difficult to identify significant deviations from the null-hypothesis H_0 using the generalized Mahalanobis distance; this is indicated by the relatively high p-values of $\bar{D}_M^{\mathcal{TM}}$ in Table 2[4]. As desired, $D_B^{\mathcal{TM}}$ is sensitive w.r.t. differences in variance, indicated by the relatively low p-value. This would allow to reject H_0 at the customary significance level of 0.05.

Furthermore, since all base shapes are uniformly sampled from within the shape triangle spanned by the first row of Fig. 2(a), *i.e.*, the initial points of the two groups have similar means, it is *not* possible to only use the initial points to separate the two groups; this is confirmed by the high p-values for both distance measures in the $(\hat{p}, 0)$ column of Table 2. In fact, even when specifically testing for differences in the initial velocity, the generalized Bhattacharyya distance

---

[4] The average of two generalized squared-Mahalanobis distances is related to the first term of the generalized Bhattacharyya distance in Eq. (4).

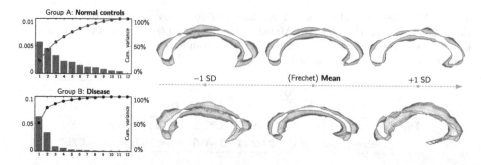

Fig. 4. Visualization of the variances (left) and principal directions (right) of trajectory distributions for the *normal control* (top) and *disease* group (bottom) of corpus callosum shapes (best-viewed in color, blue to red: young to old) (Colour figure online).

Table 3. Distances and estimated p-values (10000 random permutations) on corpora callosa using the averaged Mahalanobis distance ($\bar{D}_M^{\mathcal{TM}}$) and the generalized Bhattacharyya distance ($D_B^{\mathcal{TM}}$). The last two columns report the test results of dropping one of the initial conditions during the distance computation.

	$(\hat{p}, \hat{u})$		$(\hat{p}, 0)$		$(0, \hat{u})$	
	$\bar{D}_M^{\mathcal{TM}}$	$D_B^{\mathcal{TM}}$	$\bar{D}_M^{\mathcal{TM}}$	$D_B^{\mathcal{TM}}$	$\bar{D}_M^{\mathcal{TM}}$	$D_B^{\mathcal{TM}}$
Distance on $\mathcal{TM}$	3.1817	4.0029	3.7377	3.6863	4.1537	4.3765
p-value	0.0241	**0.0054**	0.2014	0.0654	0.0319	**0.0046**

exhibits better behavior than the generalized Mahalanobis distance in terms of lower p-values (*cf.* column $(0, \hat{u})$ of Table 2).

Corpora Callosa in Kendall's Shape Space. The longitudinal corpus callosum dataset used in [12], contains 23 subjects, 11 of which are males with dementia, and the rest are normal controls. Every subject has been measured at three time points within the age range of 60 to 92 years old, and each corpus callosum shape is represented by 64 2D boundary landmarks.

Figure 4 demonstrates the variances and the principal directions of the trajectories from the normal controls and the disease group. As shown in Fig. 4, the largest eigenvalue of the normal control group only accounts for 24 % variability with a numeric value of 0.006, while the largest eigenvalue of the disease group accounts for 52 % variability with a numeric value of 0.06. Figure 4 (right) further shows the trajectories of each group along the first principal direction with standard deviations changing from -1 to 1. The plots indicate that the corpora callosa with dementia degenerate faster than the normal controls.

Table 3 reports the quantitative measures of the group tests on the corpus callosum shapes with 10000 permutations. Compared to the generalized squared-Mahalanobis distance, the generalized Bhattacharyya distance consistently exhibits better behavior in identifying the group differences. Similar to the experiments on the synthetic shapes, during the distance computation we drop one term of the initial conditions to measure which one plays a more important role in the group tests. As shown in Table 3, regardless of the distance measure, the initial velocity is most relevant in identifying group differences; this is consistent with [12]. If we declare the statistical significance at the level of 0.01, the p-value of the generalized Bhattacharyya distance, either using both initial conditions or only the initial velocity, indicates that the disease group of corpus callosum shapes is significantly different from the normal control group.

5 Discussion

We have proposed an approach for studying group differences in the distributions of shape *trajectories*, estimated from longitudinal data. By means of a generalized version of the Bhattacharyya distance, we demonstrated, on both real and toy data, that taking second-order statistics into account can be beneficial in assessing group differences. However, the proposed approach also has limitations. For instance, although the compact representation of a trajectory is an efficient way to summarize longitudinal data, its accuracy inevitably influences the test-statistics. Currently, the adopted regression approach for estimating a trajectory is a generalization of linear regression in Euclidean space. Hence, we expect poor fitting performance on data that cannot be represented by a geodesic. For that reason, our test-statistic may not be appropriate under such a model. Furthermore, our real dataset only contains a limited number of subjects, which does not allow strong conclusions and requires to interpret results in the context of the low sample size. A potential direction for future work is to apply our method to other types of longitudinal data, *e.g.*, images, which is straightforward but slightly more involved due to the complexity of the tangent bundle.

Acknowledgements. This work was supported by NSF EECS-1148870 and NSF EECS-0925875.

Appendix

A Properties of the Generalized Bhattacharyya Distance

Non-negativity. In the first term of Eq. (4), D_M^{TM} is the generalized squared-Mahalanobis distance which is non-negative; consequently, the first term in Eq. (4) is non-negative. Furthermore, the determinant of a covariance matrix in the second term is also non-negative, since it is the product of all non-negative eigenvalues. Besides, it is easy to demonstrate that $(|\Sigma_1|+|\Sigma_2|)/(2\sqrt{|\Sigma_1||\Sigma_2|}) \geq 1$, indicating the second term is non-negative. Hence, $D_B^{TM}(D_1, D_2) \geq 0$.

Identity of Indiscernibles. If $D_1 = D_2$, *i.e.*, $\mu_1 = \mu_2$ and $\Sigma_1 = \Sigma_2$, we see that (1) $\mathrm{Log}_{\mu_1} \mu_2$ and $\mathrm{Log}_{\mu_2} \mu_1$ are zero tangent vectors, and (2) $|\Sigma_1| = |\Sigma_2|$. Hence, $D_M^{TM}(\mu_1, D_2) = D_M^{TM}(\mu_2, D_1) = 0$, *i.e.*, the first term of Eq. (4)

is 0; also, the second term is 0. Now, if $D_1 = D_2$ then $D_B^{\mathcal{TM}}(D_1, D_2) = 0$. On the other hand, assuming $D_B^{\mathcal{TM}}(D_1, D_2) = 0$, we can only obtain $\mu_1 = \mu_2$ and $|\Sigma_1| = |\Sigma_2|$, because of the non-negativity properties of the two terms in Eq. (4). But, we *cannot* draw the conclusion that the two covariance matrices are equal. Therefore, if $D_1 = D_2$ then $D_B^{\mathcal{TM}}(D_1, D_2) = 0$, but it is possible that $D_B^{\mathcal{TM}}(D_1, D_2) = 0$ for some $D_1 \neq D_2$, if $\mu_1 = \mu_2$ and $|\Sigma_1| = |\Sigma_2|$.

Symmetry. Because both terms of Eq. (4) are symmetric, the sum of them is also symmetric, *i.e.*, $D_B^{\mathcal{TM}}(D_1, D_2) = D_B^{\mathcal{TM}}(D_2, D_1)$.

Triangle Inequality. Since, Eq. (1) in $\mathbb{R}^n$ does not satisfy the triangle inequality, our generalized variant will not satisfy it either.

References

1. Bhattacharyya, A.: On a measure of divergence between two multinomial populations. Sankhyā Indian J. Stat. **7**(4), 401–406 (1946)
2. Bickel, P.J., Levina, E.: Covariance regularization by thresholding. Ann. Stat. **36**(6), 2577–2604 (2008)
3. Durrleman, S., Pennec, X., Trouvé, A., Braga, J., Gerig, G., Ayache, N.: Toward a comprehensive framework for the spatiotemporal statistical analysis of longitudinal shape data. IJCV **103**(1), 22–59 (2013)
4. Fletcher, P.T.: Geodesic regression and the theory of least squares on Riemannian manifolds. IJCV **105**(2), 171–185 (2013)
5. Fletcher, P.T., Lu, C., Pizer, S.M., Joshi, S.: Principal geodesic analysis for the study of nonlinear statistics of shape. IEEE TMI **23**(8), 995–1005 (2004)
6. Gilmore, J.H., Shi, F., Woolson, S.L., Knickmeyer, R.C., Short, S.J., Lin, W., Zhu, H., Hamer, R.M., Styner, M., Shen, D.: Longitudinal development of cortical and subcortical gray matter from birth to 2 years. Cereb. Cortex **22**(11), 2478–2485 (2012)
7. Hong, Y., Joshi, S., Sanchez, M., Styner, M., Niethammer, M.: Metamorphic geodesic regression. In: Ayache, N., Delingette, H., Golland, P., Mori, K. (eds.) MICCAI 2012, Part III. LNCS, vol. 7512, pp. 197–205. Springer, Heidelberg (2012)
8. Ledoit, O., Wolf, M.: A well-conditioned estimator for large-dimensional covariance matrices. J. Multivar. Anal. **88**(2), 365–411 (2004)
9. Lee, J.: Introduction to Smooth Manifolds. Springer, New York (2012)
10. Mahalanobis, P.C.: On the generalized distance in statistics. Proc. Natl. Inst. Sci. (Calcutta) **2**, 49–55 (1936)
11. Marcus, D.S., Fotenos, A.F., Csernansky, J.G., Morris, J.C., Buckner, R.L.: Open access series of imaging studies: longitudinal mri data in nondemented and demented older adults. J. Cogn. Neurosci. **22**(12), 2677–2684 (2010)
12. Muralidharan, P., Fletcher, P.T.: Sasaki metrics for analysis of longitudinal data on manifolds. In: CVPR, pp. 1027–1034 (2012)
13. Niethammer, M., Huang, Y., Vialard, F.-X.: Geodesic regression for image time-series. In: Fichtinger, G., Martel, A., Peters, T. (eds.) MICCAI 2011, Part II. LNCS, vol. 6892, pp. 655–662. Springer, Heidelberg (2011)
14. Oliver, D.S.: Calculation of the inverse of the covariance. Math. Geol. **30**(7), 911–933 (1998)
15. Sasaki, S.: On the differential geometry of tangent bundles of riemannian manifolds. TMJ **10**(3), 338–354 (1958)

16. Singh, N., Hinkle, J., Joshi, S., Fletcher, P.T.: A hierarchical geodesic model for diffeomorphic longitudinal shape analysis. In: Gee, J.C., Joshi, S., Pohl, K.M., Wells, W.M., Zöllei, L. (eds.) IPMI 2013. LNCS, vol. 7917, pp. 560–571. Springer, Heidelberg (2013)

17. Su, J., Kurtek, S., Klassen, E., Srivastava, A.: Statistical analysis of trajectories on riemannian manifolds: bird migration, hurricane tracking and video surveillance. Ann. Appl. Stat. 8(1), 530–552 (2014)

18. Su, J., Srivastrava, A., de Souza, F., Sarkar, S.: Rate-invariant analysis of trajectories on riemannian manifolds with application in visual speech recognition. In: CVPR, pp. 620–627 (2014)

Spatio-Temporal Signatures to Predict Retinal Disease Recurrence

Wolf-Dieter Vogl[1,2]($\boxtimes$), Sebastian M. Waldstein[2], Bianca S. Gerendas[2],
Christian Simader[2], Ana-Maria Glodan[2], Dominika Podkowinski[2],
Ursula Schmidt-Erfurth[2], and Georg Langs[1]

[1] Computational Imaging Research Lab,
Department of Biomedical Imaging and Image-guided Therapy,
Medical University Vienna, Vienna, Austria
{wolf-dieter.vogl,georg.langs}@meduniwien.ac.at
[2] Christian Doppler Laboratory for Ophthalmic Image Analysis,
Vienna Reading Center, Department of Ophthalmology and Optometry,
Medical University Vienna, Vienna, Austria

Abstract. We propose a method to predict treatment response patterns
based on spatio-temporal disease signatures extracted from longitudinal
spectral domain optical coherence tomography (SD-OCT) images. We
extract spatio-temporal disease signatures describing the underlying retinal structure and pathology by transforming total retinal thickness maps
into a joint reference coordinate system. We formulate the prediction as
a multi-variate sparse generalized linear model regression based on the
aligned signatures. The algorithm predicts if and when recurrence of the
disease will occur in the future. Experiments demonstrate that the model
identifies predictive and interpretable features in the spatio-temporal signature. In initial experiments recurrence vs. non-recurrence is predicted
with a ROC AuC of 0.99. Based on observed longitudinal morphology
changes and a time-to-event based Cox regression model we predict the
time to recurrence with a mean absolute error (MAE) of 1.25 months,
comparing favorably to elastic net regression (1.34 months), demonstrating the benefit of a spatio-temporal survival model.

1 Introduction

Biomarkers derived from medical imaging data are an essential tool for diagnosis, therapeutic decisions, and evaluation of treatment response. They provide
valuable insight by quantifying informative changes in anatomic, physiological,
biochemical or molecular processes [1]. In a clinical setting predictive biomarkers
that estimate future disease development and treatment response are exception-
ally beneficial, since they allow to personalize treatment, and to optimize its

W.-D. Vogl—The financial support by the Austrian Federal Ministry of Economy,
Family and Youth and the National Foundation for Research, Technology and Development, the EU (FP7-ICT-2009-5/318068, VISCERAL), and OeNB (15929) is gratefully acknowledged.

S. Ourselin et al. (Eds.): IPMI 2015, LNCS 9123, pp. 152–163, 2015.
DOI: 10.1007/978-3-319-19992-4_12

effect. We propose a data-driven algorithm to identify spatio-temporal predictive imaging biomarkers or *signatures* in longitudinal medical imaging data. The algorithm localizes these markers in a joint reference space shared across individuals after anatomical alignment, and predicts treatment response using sparse learning methods. We demonstrate the effectiveness of the proposed method on a longitudinal ophthalmic imaging dataset of patients with macular edema secondary to Retinal Vein Occlusion (RVO). The algorithm predicts two variables: based on morphology observed in the early stage of treatment, it predicts if edema will recur in an individual patient after treatment. Secondly, it predicts the time-point of the first recurrence of edema.

Challenges in the Treatment of Retinal Diseases. Retinal vein occlusion is the second most common sight-threatening retinal vascular disorder after diabetic retinopathy with an estimated 16.4 million adults suffering from RVO worldwide [2]. In most cases a consequence of RVO is an exudation of fluid into the macula, a so-called macular edema. Left untreated, this edema inevitably leads to irreversible vision loss. An effective treatment for macular edema is an intraocular injection of anti-vascular endothelial growth factor (anti-VEGF) agents. However, without frequent treatment a recurrence of edema often occurs. The high treatment burden on a patient, the variable response to the anti-VEGF agent, the risk of complications as well as the very high cost of the drug ($2000 per injection) and the possible side-effects of frequent treatments make a solid pro re nata (PRN, as needed) regimen on an individualized basis with the smallest amount of anti-VEGF injections given while remaining effective, a vital necessity. In current clinical practice, PRN treatment is guided by the presence or absence of cystic retinal and subretinal fluid visible in Spectral-Domain Optical Coherence Tomography (SD-OCT) images acquired at monthly intervals. SD-OCT acquires 3-dimensional scans of the retina on a micrometer resolution and enables a visualization and quantification of microstructural changes in the eye. In Fig. 1 a SD-OCT reconstruction from a healthy retina and a retina with macular edema are shown, where in the diseased eye the retinal structure is disrupted by a spongy cystic fluid structure, causing a swelling of the retina, i.e. macular edema (Fig. 1c). The prediction of individual disease paths enables a personalized treatment with the potential reduction in the frequency of both monitoring visits and particularly injections, which provides the urgently needed relief of the current burden on both patients and healthcare systems in a high-frequency, high-cost therapy [2].

Contribution. In this paper we propose a method to predict treatment outcome based on observations made during early stages of treatment. We identify interpretable biomarkers in longitudinal imaging data for prediction. To compare features through follow-up examinations, and across patients, we obtain a joint coordinate reference space from retinal OCT images by intra-patient and inter-patient registration using fundus and OCT image landmarks. From pixel-wise features extracted from the initial three months within the reference frame coordinate system we predict the treatment response of *recurrence vs. non-recurrence*

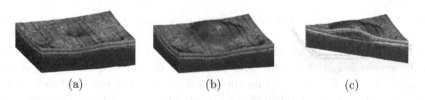

(a)   (b)   (c)

Fig. 1. 3D SD-OCT reconstruction of a (a) healthy retina with the foveal pit in the center, and (b) a retina with edema, where the swelling of the retina is caused by cystic and subretinal fluid (c).

of macular edema in a 12 month follow-up using elastic net regularized generalized linear models. Furthermore, we predict the *time-point of the first recurrence of edema*. Cross-validation experiments demonstrate that the proposed method yields good prediction accuracy and interpretable results. Furthermore, we show that longitudinal features together with time-to-event survival statistics in the Cox proportional hazard model increase time-to-recurrence prediction accuracy.

Related Work. We pose the prediction of treatment response as a multivariate regression problem. In the following, we briefly review relevant related approaches. By treating each pixel/voxel or small groups of pixels as a single feature we are operating in a high-dimension-low-sample-size setting, where the feature dimension size p is several orders of magnitude larger than the number of patients n $(p \gg n)$. Multivariate sparse linear regression methods, for instance Lasso [3] or elastic net [4] as well as non-linear regression methods such as Random Forests [5] are able to provide a prediction in such a setting [6,7]. In addition, they compute measures of feature-importance enabling insight into disease mechanisms. Such feature selection methods are used for instance in gene expression studies [8], fMRI network analysis [9] or predictions in structural neuroimages [10]. Most of these studies focus on prediction of the *present* condition from images, not dealing with the prediction of the *future*.

Sabuncu [11] proposed a sparse Bayesian multivariate prediction model combined with a survival model for studying longitudinal follow-up data. He demonstrated that an image based time-to-event prediction improves the result compared to a binary classification of converter/non-converter. Bogunović et al. [12] proposed a machine learning approach to predict the treatment response from retinal OCT in patients with age-related macular degeneration by classifying quantitative features extracted from the fovea center aligned image data.

To compensate for the anatomical variation in imaging studies the individual data is usually mapped to a common coordinate system or atlas [13]. Spatial variations in retinal images arise from different scanning positions and the varying anatomy of the retina across subjects. To ensure spatial consistency across the retinal data Abràmoff et al. [14] described a method to normalize eye fundus images by using visible landmarks such as the optic disc center, the fovea, and the main vessel arcades. Due to the smaller field of view of clinical OCT images compared to fundus images not all of these landmarks are available in OCT.

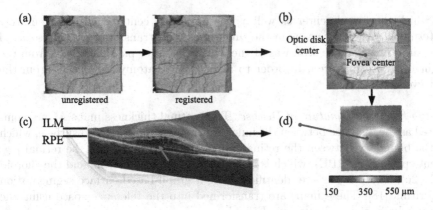

Fig. 2. Steps to get spatio-temporal signatures in a joint reference space: (a) Intra-patient registration via vessel structure. For illustration purpose 2D projections from OCTs of two time-points are overlayed and colored blue resp. red. The steps in the projections come from the motion-correction. (b) Inter-patient alignment via fovea center and optic disk center. (c) Disease features as total retinal thickness maps are obtained by measuring the distance between the ILM layer and RPE layer. The cut through the retina reveals the pathological cystic structure causing edema (green arrow). (d) Transformation of the thickness maps into the reference frame (Color figure online).

2   Spatio-Temporal Features in a Joint Reference Space

We normalize the retinal OCT images by transforming the data into a joint reference coordinate system using intra-patient follow-up registration based on the vessel structure, and inter-patient alignment via landmarks visible in OCT and fundus images.

First, we reduce motion artefacts introduced by patient movement during acquisition by the method described in [15]. To obtain landmarks for the intra-patient follow-up registration, automatic vessel segmentation is performed on the OCT images. Parameters for the affine registration are generated by applying Coherent Point Drift [16] to the segmented retinal vessel point sets, as described in [17] (Fig. 2a). The inter-patient affine registration is performed by aligning the fovea center and the optic disk center within patients (Fig. 2b). Due to the limited field of view of the macular centered OCT the optic disk is only visible in the corresponding fundus image. Hence, a registration of the fundus image to OCT is performed using the projection of the OCT image, registered rigidly to the fundus image by minimizing the normalized cross-correlation of the intensity values. The foveal center landmark (center of the foveal pit) (Fig. 1a), was set manually by expert readers. The optic disk center was identified by applying circular Hough transformation with varying radii on the binary threshold fundus image, and picking the circle showing the highest response. The optic disk center position is the center of the circle. Since the quality of the fundus images obtained by the OCT-scanner varies substantially, and the fovea center is sometimes hard to identify in cases with heavy pathology, we chose as reference scan the time-point at which the foveal center as well as the optic disc center could be accurately determined. All other scans in the time-series were transformed to the selected one, and the reference scan was aligned with the other patients. Scans from the right eye were mirrored, in order to align their anatomy with scans from the left eye.

Spatio-temporal Signature of Disease. Total retinal thickness maps M are computed as the distance between the inner limiting membrane (ILM) surface, which is the boundary between the retina and the vitreous body, and the retinal pigment epithelium (RPE), which is the border between the retina and the choroid (Fig. 2c). These layers are identified using a graph-based surface segmentation algorithm [18]. These maps are transformed into the reference space using the obtained affine transformation (Fig. 2d).

Let $v^{(m)} = (x_1, x_2, ..., x_k)$ be the vectorized pixel values from the transformed thickness map M for the month m. By concatenating the thickness map vectors and the change of thickness over time up to month m, a spatio-temporal signature vector is obtained for each individual: $x^{(m)} = (v^{(0)}, v^{(1)}, ..., v^{(m)}, v^{(1)} - v^{(0)}, v^{(2)} - v^{(1)}, ..., v^{(m)} - v^{(m-1)})$. These signatures are pooled in a matrix $X \in \mathbb{R}^{n \times p}$, where each row represents a signature vector of a subject and each column is a distinct spatio-temporal anatomical position in the retina. $x_i^{(m)} \in \mathbb{R}^p$ is the signature vector for subject i.

3   Prediction of Recurrence

We predict the treatment response based on data up to the initial loading phase of three monthly injections. Specifically, we predict for an individual based on the corresponding spatio-temporal signature $x_i^{(m)}$ covering the three month loading phase, if a treated edema will recur in the future. In a second task we predict at which time-point the first recurrence happens for patients with recurring edema. For notational clarity, we drop the time-index $^{(m)}$ in the following explanation.

3.1   Prediction by Sparse Linear Regression

We assume that the continuous response variable y_i for an individual i is a weighted linear combination of the input variables x_i: $y_i = w_0 + w_1 x_1 + ... + w_p x_p = x_i w$. The coefficients (or weights) w are estimated for a training-set X in a regularized way by minimizing the following objective function:

$$\underset{w}{argmin} \frac{1}{2n} \| X w - y \|_2^2 + \lambda P(w) \tag{1}$$

Since in our case the system is strongly underdetermined $(p \gg n)$, a regularization function P is necessary, where λ controls the amount of regularization. Recently, sparsity has been proposed as property of the coefficients [3,8], where only a few but relevant coefficients w are non-zero, highlighting predictive anatomical regions and time-points. Sparsity can be obtained by applying the ℓ_1 norm on $\boldsymbol{w}$, known as Lasso regularization [3]. When features are strongly correlated, Lasso tends to pick only one of these features at random. Thus, Zou and Hastie proposed elastic net regularization [4] to overcome the limitation of Lasso regularization, by combining the ℓ_1 norm with a ridge regularization (ℓ_2 norm):

$$P(\boldsymbol{w}) = \rho \|\boldsymbol{w}\|_1 + \frac{(1-\rho)}{2} \|\boldsymbol{w}\|_2^2, \tag{2}$$

where ρ defines the ratio of the convex combination of ℓ_1 and ℓ_2 regularization.

The features x_i with non-zero coefficients w_i represent anatomical locations and time-points whose characteristics are informative for the prediction. They enable interpretation by ophthalmologists.

3.2 Categorical Variable Prediction

Using a generalized version of the sparse linear regression, where the outcome variable y is replaced by a function, categorical variables can be predicted using logistic regression. The probabilities of the binary outcomes are modeled as logit function (log of the odds): $\text{logit}(p_i) = ln(\frac{p_i}{1-p_i}) = \boldsymbol{x}_i \boldsymbol{w}$, where $p_i = \text{Pr}(y_i = 1|\boldsymbol{x}_i)$. To obtain the coefficients Eq. 1 is modified such that:

$$\underset{\boldsymbol{w},c}{\text{argmin}} \sum_{i=1}^{n} (\log(\exp(y_i(\boldsymbol{x}_i \boldsymbol{w} + c)) + 1)) + \lambda P(\boldsymbol{w}) \tag{3}$$

The class probability p_i for a new case with covariates $\boldsymbol{x}$ can be predicted from the trained weights via the inverse logit: $p_i = \text{logit}^{-1}(\boldsymbol{x}\boldsymbol{w})$.

We compute the coefficients $\boldsymbol{w}$ by training an elastic net regularized logistic regression model using the spatio-temporal signature matrix $\boldsymbol{X}$ and the binary outcome labels $\boldsymbol{y}$ of non-recurring/recurring edema within 12 months. By applying the trained model on an unseen case we obtain the probability of recurrence p_i. Finally, we threshold the probability in order to obtain a binary outcome.

3.3 Temporal Variable Prediction

We predict the time to the first recurrence of edema using survival analysis, where the recurrence is modeled as a time duration T until an event happens. A common tool in survival analysis is the Cox proportional hazards (PH) model [19]. The model assumes a log-linear relationship of the covariates to a baseline hazard h_0, which describes how the risk of event changes over time based on baseline covariates. The time-parameterized hazard function is then:

$$h(t|\boldsymbol{x}_i) = h_0(t) \exp(\boldsymbol{x}_i \boldsymbol{w}) \tag{4}$$

A generalized linear model is obtained by formalizing the model as a hazard ratio: $\log \frac{h(t|\boldsymbol{X})}{h_0(t)} = \boldsymbol{X}\boldsymbol{w}$. Inference can be performed using partial likelihood [19]

$$L(\boldsymbol{w}) = \prod_{r \in D} \frac{\exp(\boldsymbol{x}_r \boldsymbol{w})}{\sum_{j \in R_i} \exp(\boldsymbol{x}_j \boldsymbol{w})} \tag{5}$$

where D is the set of indices of patient events and R_i is the set of indices of individuals which are at risk at time t_i. The coefficients are obtained by minimizing the regularized negative partial log-likelihood:

$$\operatorname*{argmin}_{w} - \sum_{r \in D} (x_r w - \log(\sum_{j \in R_i} \exp(x_j w))) + \lambda P(w) \qquad (6)$$

Predictions of hazards for a new individual with covariates x can be obtained by using Eq. 4 with the new covariates. In that case the baseline hazard h_0 has to be estimated by using the Breslow estimator:

$$h_0(t_i) = \frac{d_i}{\sum_{j \in R_i} \exp(x_j w)} \qquad (7)$$

where d_i is the number of events at t_i. Furthermore, we can estimate the individual survival function $S_i(t)$, which is defined as $S_i(t) = Pr(T > t)$, describing the probability that the time of event is later than some specified time t. The function can be estimated from the individual relative risk, the cumulative hazard Λ_0 and the baseline survival function $S_0(t)$ [20]:

$$S_i(t) = S_0(t) \exp(x_i w), \quad \text{with} \qquad (8)$$

$$\Lambda_0(t) = \sum_{j:t_j \leq t} h_0(t_j), \quad \text{and} \quad S_0(t) = exp(-\Lambda_0(t)) \qquad (9)$$

We obtain the coefficients w by training an elastic net regularized Cox PH model on the spatio-temporal signature matrix X and the time-points of events in month. For an unseen case we estimate from the covariates x the baseline hazard h_0 using Eq. 7 and the individual survival function $S_i(t)$ using Eq. 9. By computing the survival function for all time-points we determine the time-point of recurrence where the survival function drops below a given threshold.

A description of how to optimize the objective functions using coordinate descent can be found in [21] and [22]. We used the implementation from the package glmnet of the statistics software R for our computation.

4   Evaluation and Results

We evaluated the proposed method in two prediction experiments, (1) predicting recurrence vs. non-recurrence of edema within 12 months, and (2) predicting the time to the first recurrence of edema. Baseline SD-OCT scans and 12 monthly follow-up scans of 44 patients with central retinal vein occlusion (CRVO) were included. All patients received initial ranibizumab (anti-VEGF) injections for three months followed by a PRN regimen. Total retinal thickness maps were computed for all scans, and were transformed into the joint coordinate system as described in Sect. 2. All maps were smoothed with a Gaussian kernel with $\sigma = 1$. Figure 3 shows the aligned total retinal thickness maps for two patients with resp. without recurring edema.

Recurrence

Non-Recurrence

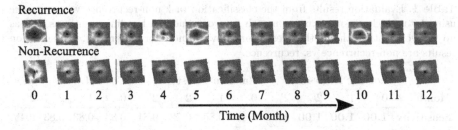

0   1   2   3   4   5   6   7   8   9   10   11   12

Time (Month)

Fig. 3. 12 month follow-up series of aligned total retinal thickness maps for two patients with recurring edema at month 5 and 10 resp. without recurring edema.

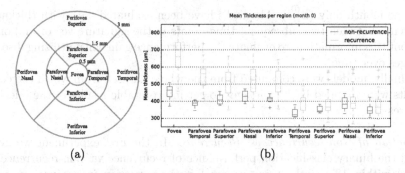

(a)   (b)

Fig. 4. (a) Division of macula in nine regions of interest defined by ETDRS [23]. (b) Mean retinal thickness of the baseline (month 0) per region stratified by patients with non-recurrence and recurrence of edema.

The time-point of a recurrence was determined algorithmically for each patient to serve as a standard-of-reference for evaluation. First, the total thickness maps were divided into nine circular regions of interest within three concentric circles with diameters of 1 mm, 3 mm and 6 mm, centered at the fovea (Fig. 4a) as defined by the Early Treatment Diabetic Retinopathy Study (ETDRS) design [23]. From each region the mean thickness was computed. A recurrence was defined as an increase of the mean thickness by 15 pixels ($= 29 \,\mu m$) of two subsequent time-points in any region. 6 of the 44 patients showed no recurring edema within 12 months.

We used two-level nested five-fold cross-validation (CV) on patient level, where in the inner loop we conduct a grid search to tune the sparsity parameters ρ and λ, as well as the optimal threshold for the probability outcomes in terms of maximizing the F-score on the training set (harmonized mean of sensitivity and specificity). In the outer CV loop we measure the performance of the trained model on the test fold. All evaluations were repeated 20 times with random stratified CV partitioning, with at least one non-recurrence case in each fold.

To evaluate the benefit of using longitudinal data, we performed the training and testing on thickness maps up to month two ($x_i^{(2)}$), one ($x_i^{(1)}$), resp. the

Table 1. Evaluation results from the classification task non-recurrence vs. recurrence using total thickness maps up to month two, one and the baseline month, as well as up to two month with the thickness change over time information (2'). Classification results are non-recurrence vs. recurrence.

	Logistic Regression				Random Forest				Cox PH			
Month	0	1	2	2'	0	1	2	2'	0	1	2	2'
Sensitivity	**1.00**	**1.00**	**1.00**	**1.00**	0.88	0.85	0.78	0.81	0.83	0.83	0.83	0.45
Specificity	0.92	0.90	0.90	0.82	0.98	0.98	0.98	**1.00**	0.99	0.90	0.94	0.96
ROC AuC	**0.99**	**0.99**	**0.99**	**0.99**	**0.99**	**0.99**	**0.99**	**0.99**	**0.99**	0.91	0.93	0.96

baseline month only ($x_i^{(0)}$). The tasks have been evaluated once with thickness difference between two subsequent time-points in the signature vector and once without this information, to evaluate the performance gain when utilizing disease changes over time.

Finally, models were computed from the whole dataset, from which the coefficients were mapped back to images to get interpretable results of the selected features.

Prediction of Non-recurrence vs. Recurrence. In the first experiment we evaluated the binary classification performance of recurrence vs. non-recurrence of edema within 12 months using sparse logistic regression in comparison to a Random Forest classification. As error measures we computed the sensitivity, specificity and the Receiver-Operating-Curve (ROC) Area-under-Curve (AuC), where the AuC was obtained from the predicted probabilities within the outer cross-validation loop, and a mean AuC has been computed from these. The classification results are listed in Table 1. In the classification task the baseline month is already enough to obtain predictive results with an AuC of 0.99 for logistic regression and Random Forest classification (note that at this point due to the small amount of patients with non-recurrence the confidence interval for sensitivity/specificity is large. For a sensitivity/specificity of 1.00/0.92 the 95 % confidence intervals are 0.52-1.00 / 0.78-0.98). When mapping the coefficients back to the reference frame (Fig. 5a) it can be observed that almost all features were selected from the fovea center and the parafovea temporal area at month zero. By comparing the mean thickness for each region between the two groups, as done in Fig. 4b, it can be observed that there is a (significant) difference of the mean thickness between the groups in these two areas, as well as almost no overlap of the mean thickness in the parafovea temporal area. The sparse feature selection correctly identified these areas and used them for prediction.

Prediction of time to Recurrence. In the second experiment we predicted the time to the first recurrence of edema for patients with recurring edema. We trained an elastic net regularized regression model, as well as Random Forest regression model with the thickness maps as input and the time-to-recurrence as outcome variables. To evaluate the benefit of using a survival model in comparison to a

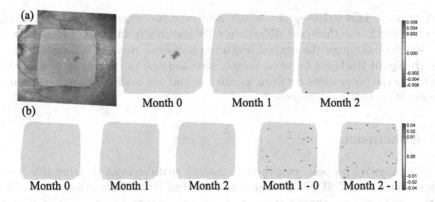

Fig. 5. Sparse coefficients mapped into the common reference coordinate system. (a): An exemplary fundus image mapped into the reference frame, overlaid by the retained coefficients from a single month and coefficients retained from the sparse logistic regression for month zero to two. (b) Coefficients retained from the Cox PH model for month zero, one and two as well as from the thickness differences between month one and zero resp. month two and one.

regression model, we furthermore trained a Cox PH model on the same dataset, where patients with no recurrence were set to censored after 12 months, since we do not know if edema recurred afterwards. For each patient we estimated the survival function $S_i(t)$ as described in Sect. 3.3. The time at which the survival function dropped below 0.5 has been set as the time at which an recurrence of edema is estimated. Patients with a survival function > 0.5 after twelve month got the non-recurrence label. Hence, the Cox PH model was used for both tasks, the binary classification and the time-point of recurrence estimation.

Mean absolute error (MAE) between predicted and true month of recurrence are reported in Table 2. The Cox PH model showed superior results compared to linear regression and Random Forest regression, with an MAE of 1.25 for Cox PH model resp. 1.34 for linear regression and 1.38 for Random Forest. Furthermore, the addition of thickness changes over time as features improved the performance for Cox and elastic net regression. By looking at the coefficients for the Cox PH model (Fig. 5b) it can be observed that almost only thickness difference features are picked. Features from the difference between month one

Table 2. Evaluation results of the time to recurrence prediction task. The mean absolute error (MAE) and the standard deviation (SD) is computed as the absolute difference between predicted and true time to recurrence in months.

	Elastic Net				Random Forest				Cox PH			
Month	0	1	2	2'	0	1	2	2'	0	1	2	2'
MAE [month]	1.37	1.40	1.43	1.34	1.39	1.38	1.54	1.46	1.30	1.26	1.29	**1.25**
SD	1.10	1.12	1.10	1.01	1.11	1.12	1.12	1.06	1.28	1.27	1.27	1.26

and zero are selected over the whole field of view, whereas from the month two to month one thickness difference only features from the perifoveal areas are selected, skipping the central and the parafoveal area. This indicates that the change of thickness between month zero and one in general as well as the change in the outer areas between month two and one are informative regarding the duration until recurrence.

5 Conclusion

In this paper we propose a method to extract spatio-temporal signatures from longitudinal retinal SD-OCT images transformed into a joint reference coordinate system, and use these features to predict the *future* development of disease under treatment. In particular we predicted two variables from image acquisitions during the initial three monthly treatments, (1) the non-recurrence vs. recurrence of edema within twelve months, and (2) the time to recurrence of edema. We demonstrated that sparse feature selection via elastic net in a multivariate generalized linear model setting yields accurate prediction and interpretable results. Furthermore, we showed that using survival models in terms of the Cox proportional hazards model increases the accuracy when predicting the temporal variable. The proposed methodology is an important step towards image-based individualization of patient treatment and disease management.

References

1. Smith, J.J., Sorensen, A.G., Thrall, J.H.: Biomarkers in imaging: Realizing radiology's future. Radiology **227**(3), 633–638 (2003)
2. Laouri, M., Chen, E., Looman, M., Gallagher, M.: The burden of disease of retinal vein occlusion: review of the literature. Eye **25**(8), 981–988 (2011)
3. Tibshirani, R.: Regression shrinkage and selection via the lasso. J. Roy. Stat. Soc. Ser. B (Methodol.) **58**, 267–288 (1996)
4. Zou, H., Hastie, T.: Regularization and variable selection via the elastic net. J. Roy. Stat. Soc. Ser. B (Methodol.) **67**(2), 301–320 (2005)
5. Breiman, L.: Random forests. Machine learning **45**(1), 5–32 (2001)
6. Hastie, T.J., Tibshirani, R.J., Friedman, J.H.: The Elements of Statistical Learning: Data Mining, Inference, and Prediction. Springer, Heidelberg (2011)
7. Rasmussen, P.M., Hansen, L.K., Madsen, K.H., Churchill, N.W., Strother, S.C.: Model sparsity and brain pattern interpretation of classification models in neuroimaging. Pattern Recogn. **45**(6), 2085–2100 (2012). Brain Decoding
8. Zou, H., Hastie, T.: Regression shrinkage and selection via the elastic net, with applications to microarrays. J. Roy. Stat. Soc. B. **67**, 301–320 (2003)
9. Langs, G., Menze, B.H., Lashkari, D., Golland, P.: Detecting stable distributed patterns of brain activation using gini contrast. NeuroImage **56**(2), 497–507 (2011)
10. Kandel, B.M., Wolk, D.A., Gee, J.C., Avants, B.: Predicting cognitive data from medical images using sparse linear regression. In: Gee, J.C., Joshi, S., Pohl, K.M., Wells, W.M., Zöllei, L. (eds.) IPMI 2013. LNCS, vol. 7917, pp. 86–97. Springer, Heidelberg (2013)

11. Sabuncu, M.R.: A Bayesian algorithm for image-based time-to-event prediction. In: Wu, G., Zhang, D., Shen, D., Yan, P., Suzuki, K., Wang, F. (eds.) MLMI 2013. LNCS, vol. 8184, pp. 74–81. Springer, Heidelberg (2013)

12. Bogunović, H., Abràmoff, M.D., Zhang, L., Sonka, M.: Prediction of treatment response from retinal oct in patients with exudative age-related macular degeneration. In: Chen, X., Garvin, M.K., L.J., (ed.) Proceedings of the Ophthalmic Medical Image Analysis First International Workshop, OMIA 2014, Held in Conjunction with MICCAI 2014, Boston, Massachusetts, September 14, 2014, pp. 129–136 Iowa Research Online (2014)

13. Reuter, M., Schmansky, N.J., Rosas, H.D., Fischl, B.: Within-subject template estimation for unbiased longitudinal image analysis. Neuroimage $61(4)$, 1402–1418 (2012)

14. Abràmoff, M.D., Garvin, M.K., Sonka, M.: Retinal imaging and image analysis. IEEE Rev. Biomed. Eng. 3, 169–208 (2010)

15. Montuoro, A., Wu, J., Waldstein, S., Gerendas, B., Langs, G., Simader, C., Schmidt-Erfurth, U.: Motion artefact correction in retinal optical coherence tomography using local symmetry. In: Golland, P., Hata, N., Barillot, C., Hornegger, J., Howe, R. (eds.) MICCAI 2014, Part II. LNCS, vol. 8674, pp. 130–137. Springer, Heidelberg (2014)

16. Myronenko, A., Song, X.: Point set registration: Coherent point drift. IEEE Trans. Pattern Anal. Mach. Intell. $32(12)$, 2262–2275 (2010)

17. Wu, J., Gerendas, B.S., Waldstein, S.M., Langs, G., Simader, C., Schmidt-Erfurth, U.: Stable registration of pathological 3D-oct scans using retinal vessels. In: Chen, X., Garvin, M.K., Liu, J.J. (eds.) Proceedings of the Ophthalmic Medical Image Analysis First International Workshop, OMIA 2014, Held in Conjunction with MICCAI 2014, pp. 1–8. Iowa Research Online (2014)

18. Garvin, M.K., Abràmoff, M.D., Wu, X., Russell, S.R., Burns, T.L., Sonka, M.: Automated 3-D intraretinal layer segmentation of macular spectral-domain optical coherence tomography images. IEEE Trans. Med. Imaging $28(9)$, 1436–1447 (2009)

19. Cox, D.: Regression models and life tables (with discussion). J. Roy. Stati. Soc. B 34, 187–220 (1972)

20. Cox, D.R., Oakes, D.: Analysis of survival data. vol. 21. CRC Press (1984)

21. Friedman, J., Hastie, T., Tibshirani, R.: Regularization paths for generalized linear models via coordinate descent. J. Stat. Softw. $33(1)$, 1 (2010)

22. Simon, N., Friedman, J., Hastie, T., Tibshirani, R.: Regularization paths for cox's proportional hazards model via coordinate descent. J. Stat. Softw. $39(5)$, 1–13 (2011)

23. Chew, E.Y., Klein, M.L., Ferris, F.L., Remaley, N.A., Murphy, R.P., Chantry, K., Hoogwerf, B.J., Miller, D.: Association of elevated serum lipid levels with retinal hard exudate in diabetic retinopathy: Early treatment diabetic retinopathy study (etdrs) report 22. Arch. Ophthalmol. $114(9)$, 1079–1084 (1996)

Microstructure Imaging

A Unifying Framework for Spatial and Temporal Diffusion in Diffusion MRI

Rutger Fick[✉], Demian Wassermann, Marco Pizzolato,
and Rachid Deriche

Athena Project-Team, Inria Sophia Antipolis - Méditerranée,
Valbonne, France
rutger.fick@inria.fr

Abstract. We propose a novel framework to simultaneously represent the diffusion-weighted MRI (dMRI) signal over diffusion times, gradient strengths and gradient directions. Current frameworks such as the 3D Simple Harmonic Oscillator Reconstruction and Estimation basis (3D-SHORE) only represent the signal over the spatial domain, leaving the temporal dependency as a fixed parameter. However, microstructure-focused techniques such as Axcaliber and ActiveAx provide evidence of the importance of sampling the dMRI space over diffusion time. Up to now there exists no generalized framework that simultaneously models the dependence of the dMRI signal in space and time. We use a functional basis to fit the 3D+t spatio-temporal dMRI signal, similarly to the 3D-SHORE basis in three dimensional 'q-space'. The lowest order term in this expansion contains an isotropic diffusion tensor that characterizes the Gaussian displacement distribution, multiplied by a negative exponential. We regularize the signal fitting by minimizing the norm of the analytic Laplacian of the basis, and validate our technique on synthetic data generated using the theoretical model proposed by Callaghan et al. We show that our method is robust to noise and can accurately describe the restricted spatio-temporal signal decay originating from tissue models such as cylindrical pores. From the fitting we can then estimate the axon radius distribution parameters along any direction using approaches similar to AxCaliber. We also apply our method on real data from an ActiveAx acquisition. Overall, our approach allows one to represent the complete 3D+t dMRI signal, which should prove helpful in understanding normal and pathologic nervous tissue.

1 Introduction

One of the unsolved quests of diffusion-weighted imaging (DW-MRI) is the reconstruction of the complete four-dimensional ensemble average propagator (EAP) describing the diffusion process of water molecules over three-dimensional space

---

Rutger Fick and Demian Wassermann contributed equally to this work.

This work was partially supported by the MOSIFAH ANR (France) Grant.Marco Pizzolato thanks Olea Medical and the PACA Regional council for support.

© Springer International Publishing Switzerland 2015
S. Ourselin et al. (Eds.): IPMI 2015, LNCS 9123, pp. 167–178, 2015.
DOI: 10.1007/978-3-319-19992-4_13

and diffusion time (3D+t) in biological tissues. To the best of our knowledge, most recent imaging techniques focus on reconstructing the three-dimensional (3D) EAP using a fixed diffusion time. However, methods like Axcaliber [1] show the added value of incorporating different diffusion times when estimating the axon diameter in white matter tissue. Thus, a 3D+t representation of the EAP may provide means to infer diffusion contrasts sensitive to axon diameters and other tissue characteristics. To our knowledge, no such representation has been proposed. We therefore propose an analytic model that enables the reconstruction of the complete 3D+t EAP.

To relate the observed diffusion signal to the underlying tissue microstructure, we need to understand how the diffusion signal is influenced by the tissue geometry and properties. Starting from the concept of a single particle moving by Brownian motion, the movements of this particle over time are obstructed by surrounding tissue structures such as cell walls. Then considering a large group (ensemble) of particles, the average propagation of these particles will, depending on the length of the diffusion time, be more or less restricted by surrounding tissues. This ensemble average propagator (EAP) is denoted as $P(\mathbf{R}, \tau)$ with $\mathbf{R}$ the real displacement vector and τ the diffusion time.

In DW-MRI the EAP is estimated by obtaining diffusion-weighted images (DWIs). A DWI is obtained by applying two sensitizing diffusion gradients of pulse length δ to the tissue, separated by separation time Δ. The resulting signal is 'weighted' by the average particle movements in the direction of the applied gradient. When these gradients are considered infinitely short ($\delta \approx 0$), the relation between the measured signal $S(\mathbf{q}, \tau)$ and the EAP $P(\mathbf{r}, \tau)$ is given by an inverse Fourier transform (IFT) [2] as

$$P(\mathbf{R}, \tau) = \int_{\mathbb{R}^3} E(\mathbf{q}, \tau) e^{-2\pi i \mathbf{q} \cdot \mathbf{r}} d\mathbf{q} \quad \text{with} \quad \mathbf{q} = \frac{\gamma \delta \mathbf{G}}{2\pi} \tag{1}$$

where $E(\mathbf{q}, \tau) = S(\mathbf{q}, \tau)/S_0$ is the normalized signal attenuation measured at position $\mathbf{q}$, and S_0 is the baseline image acquired without diffusion sensitization ($q = 0$). We denote $\tau = (\Delta - \delta/3)$, $q = |\mathbf{q}|$, $\mathbf{q} = q\mathbf{u}$ and $\mathbf{R} = R\mathbf{r}$, where $\mathbf{u}$ and $\mathbf{r}$ are 3D unit vectors and $q, R \in \mathbb{R}^+$. The wave vector $\mathbf{q}$ on the right side of Eq. (1) is related to pulse length δ, nuclear gyromagnetic ratio γ and the applied diffusion gradient vector $\mathbf{G}$. Furthermore, the clinically used b-value is related to q as $b = 4\pi^2 q^2 \tau$. In accordance with the Fourier theory, measuring $E(\mathbf{q}, \tau)$ at higher $\mathbf{q}$ makes one sensitive to more precise details in $P(\mathbf{R}, \tau)$, while measuring at longer τ makes the recovered EAP more specific to the white matter structure.

The relation between the EAP and white matter tissue is often modeled by representing different compartments as pores [10]. Examples of these are parallel cylinders for aligned axon bundles and spherical pores for cell bodies and astrocytes. Several techniques exist to infer the properties of these pores such as their orientation or radius. Of these techniques many sample the 3D diffusion signal exclusively in q-space with one preset diffusion time [3–5]. Among the most used methods is diffusion tensor imaging (DTI) [3]. However, DTI is limited by its assumption that the signal decay is purely Gaussian over $\mathbf{q}$

and purely exponential over τ. These assumptions cannot account for *in-vivo* observed phenomena such as restriction, heterogeneity or anomalous diffusion. Approaches that overcome the Gaussian decay assumption over $\mathbf{q}$ include the use of functional bases to represent the 3D EAP [4,5]. These bases reconstruct the radial and angular properties of the EAP by fitting the signal to a linear combination of orthogonal basis functions $E(\mathbf{q}) = \sum_i c_i \Xi_i(\mathbf{q})$ with $\mathbf{c}$ the fitted coefficients. In the case of [5], these basis functions are eigenfunctions of the Fourier transform, allowing for the directly reconstruction of the EAP as $P(\mathbf{R}) = \sum_i c_i \Psi(\mathbf{R})$, where $\Psi = \mathrm{IFT}(\Xi)$. However, these approaches are not designed to include multiple diffusion times, and therefore cannot accurately model the complete 3D+t signal.

The 3D EAP can be related to the mean pore (axon) sizes, e.g. mean volume, diameter and cross-sectional area, by assuming the q-space signal was acquired at a long diffusion time. In this case the diffusing particles have fully explored the tissue structure and thus the shape of the EAP is indicative of the shape of the tissue. This concept was proven in 1D-NMR [7–9] and extended to *3D* with the 3D Simple Harmonic Oscillator Reconstruction and Estimation (3D-SHORE) and Mean Apparent Propagator (MAP)-MRI [5] basis. However, this long diffusion time requirement is hard to fulfill in practice as the scanner noise begins to dominate the signal at higher diffusion times.

In contrast, in 1D+t space, Axcaliber [1] samples both over q and τ to estimate axon radius distribution. This allows it to overcome the long diffusion time constraint. However, though a 3D-Axcaliber was briefly proposed [6], it is essentially a 1D technique that needs to fit a parametric model to a signal that is sampled exactly perpendicular to the axon direction. While this limits its applicability in clinical settings, this method thickly underlines the importance of including τ in the estimation of axon diameter properties.

Our main contribution in this paper is the generalization of the 3D-SHORE model to include diffusion times. Our new model allows us to obtain analytic representations of the complete 3D+t diffusion space from sparse samples of the diffusion signal attenuation $E(\mathbf{q}, \tau)$. In other words, our representation simultaneously represents the 3D+t signal and EAP for any interpolated diffusion time. This allows the *time-dependent* computation of the orientation distribution function (ODF) previously proposed scalar measures such as the return-to-origin probability (RTOP) and return-to-axis probability (RTAP) [5].

While our new 3D+t framework opens the door to many new ideas, in this work we consider an initial application of this framework by implementing the Axcaliber model to be used in 3D. In our procedure we first fit our model to a sparsely sampled synthetic 3D+t data set consisting of cylinders with Gamma distributed radii. We then sample an Axcaliber data set from the 3D+t representation perpendicular to the cylinder direction and fit Axcaliber to the resampled data. We compare this method with a previously proposed version of 3D-Axcaliber [6] that uses the composite and hindered restricted model of diffusion (CHARMED) model to interpolate the data points in 3D+t space.

All contributions from this paper are publicly available on the Diffusion Imaging in Python (DiPy) toolkit [19]. http://nipy.org/dipy/.

2   Theory

We propose an appropriate basis with respect to the dMRI signal by studying its theoretical shape over diffusion time τ. The effect of diffusion time on the dMRI signal for different pore shapes has been extensively studies by Callaghan et al. [10]. In general, the equations for restricted signals in planar, cylindrical and spherical compartments can be formulated as:

$$E(q, \tau) = \sum_k \beta_k e^{-\alpha_k \tau} \cdot f_k(q) \tag{2}$$

where α_k and β_k depend on the order of the expansion. Here $f_k(q)$ is a function that depends on the expansion order and value of q. The exact formulations can be found in Eqs. (9), (13) and (17) in [10]. As Eq. (2) shows, every expansion order is given as a product of two functions: A negative exponential on τ with some order dependent scaling and a function $f_k(q)$ depending only on q. Therefore, an appropriate basis to fit the signal described in Eq. (2) should be a similar product of an exponential basis over τ and another spatial basis over $\mathbf{q}$. We provide the formulation of our basis in the next section.

2.1   Specific Formulation of the 3D+t Basis

In accordance with the theoretical model presented in Sect. 2 we fit the 3D+t space with a functional basis that is both separable and orthogonal over both $\mathbf{q}$ and τ. For the temporal aspect of the signal we choose to use an exponential modulated by a Laguerre polynomial, which together form an orthogonal basis over τ. Then, following the separability of the signal, we are free to choose any previously proposed spatial basis to complete our 3D+t functional basis. We choose to use the well-known 3D-SHORE basis [5] as it robustly recovers both the radial and angular features from sparse measurements [11]. Our combined basis finally describes the 3D+t diffusion signal as

$$E(\mathbf{q}, \tau) = \sum_{\{jlm\}}^{N_{\max}} \sum_{o=0}^{O_{\max}} c_{jlmo} \, S_{jlm}(\mathbf{q}) T_o(\tau) \tag{3}$$

where $T_o(\tau)$ is our temporal basis with basis order o and $S_{jlm}(\mathbf{q})$ is the 3D-SHORE basis with basis orders jlm. Here $N_{\max}$ and $O_{\max}$ are the maximum spatial and temporal order of the bases, which can be chosen independently. We formulate the bases themselves as

$$S_{jlm}(\mathbf{q}, u_s) = \sqrt{4\pi} i^{-l} (2\pi^2 u_s^2 q^2)^{l/2} e^{-2\pi^2 u_s^2 q^2} L_{j-1}^{l+1/2}(4\pi^2 u_s^2 q^2) Y_l^m(\mathbf{u}) \tag{4}$$

$$T_o(\tau, u_t) = \exp(-u_t \tau / 2) L_o(u_t \tau)$$

where u_s and u_t are the spatial and temporal scaling factors. Here $\mathbf{q} = q\mathbf{u}$, $L_n^{(\alpha)}$ is a generalized Laguerre polynomial and Y_l^m is the real spherical harmonics basis [12]. Here j, l and m are the radial order, angular order and angular moment of the 3D-SHORE basis which are related as $2j + l = N + 2$ with $N \in \{0, 2, 4 \ldots N_{\max}\}$ [5].

Furthermore, we require data-dependent scaling factors u_s and u_t to efficiently fit the data. We calculate u_s by fitting a tensor $e^{-2\pi^2 q^2 u_s^2}$ to the signal values $E(\mathbf{q}, \cdot)$ for all measured $\mathbf{q}$. Similarly, we compute u_t by fitting an exponential $e^{-u_t \tau}$ to $E(\cdot, \tau)$ for all measured τ. Lastly, for a symmetric propagator in our 3D+t basis (as is the case in dMRI) we give the total number of estimated coefficients N_{coef} as

$$N_{\text{coef}} = (O_{\max} + 1)(N_{\max}/2 + 1)(N_{\max}/2 + 2)(4N_{\max}/2 + 3). \qquad (5)$$

For notation convenience, we use a linearized indexing of the basis functions in the rest of the paper. We denote $\Xi_i(\mathbf{q}, \tau, u_s, u_t) = S_{jlm(i)}(\mathbf{q}, u_s)T_{o(i)}(\tau, u_t)$ with $i \in \{1 \ldots N_{\text{coef}}\}$.

2.2   Signal Fitting and Regularization

As the measured signal always contains noise we need to regularize the coefficient estimation. Therefore, as our second contribution in this work, we provide the analytic form of the Laplacian regularization of our basis.

Following Eq. (3), we fit our basis using regularized least squares by first constructing a design matrix $\mathbf{Q} \in \mathbb{R}^{N_{\text{data}} \times N_{\text{coef}}}$ with $\mathbf{Q}_{ik} = \Xi_k(\mathbf{q}_i, \tau_i, u_s, u_t)$. We then fit the signal as

$$\mathbf{c} = \operatorname{argmin}_{\mathbf{c}} \|\mathbf{y} - \mathbf{Q}\mathbf{c}\|^2 + \lambda U(\mathbf{c}) \qquad (6)$$

where $\mathbf{y}$ is the measured signal, $\mathbf{c}$ are the fitted coefficients and λ is the weight for our Laplacian regularization $U(\mathbf{c})$. We define $U(\mathbf{c})$ as

$$U(\mathbf{c}) = \int_{\mathbb{R}} \|\nabla^2 E_{\mathbf{c}}(\mathbf{q}, \tau)\|^2 d\mathbf{q} d\tau \qquad (7)$$

with $\nabla^2 E_{\mathbf{c}}(\mathbf{q}, \tau) = \sum_i c_i \nabla^2 \Xi_i(\mathbf{q}, \tau, u_s, u_t)$ the Laplacian of the reconstructed signal. $U(\mathbf{c})$ can be rewritten in quadratic form as

$$\mathbf{U}_{ik} = \int_{\mathbb{R}} \nabla^2 \Xi_i(\mathbf{q}, \tau, u_s, u_t) \cdot \nabla^2 \Xi_k(\mathbf{q}, \tau, u_s, u_t) d\mathbf{q} d\tau \qquad (8)$$

where the subscript ik indicates the ik^{th} position in the regularization matrix. We use the orthogonality of the basis functions to compute the values of the regularization matrix to a closed form depending only on the basis orders and scale factors. For brevity here we give the formulation of $\mathbf{U}$ in the Appendix A. We finally estimate the coefficients using regularized least squares

$$\mathbf{c} = (\mathbf{Q}^\mathsf{T}\mathbf{Q} + \lambda \mathbf{U})^{-1}\mathbf{Q}^\mathsf{T}\mathbf{y}. \qquad (9)$$

We find the weight λ through generalized cross-validation (GCV) [13]. We fit our model on both synthetic data generated using the theoretical signal model and real data. We describe the theoretical signal model in more detail in the next section.

2.3   Synthetic Data Generation and Axcaliber Model

To validate our method we generate synthetic data using the Callaghan model [10]. In the case of a cylindrical (axonal) compartment this model simulates the restricted component perpendicular to the cylinder walls as:

$$
E_r(q,\tau) = \sum_k 4\exp(-\beta_{0k}^2 D\tau/a^2) \times \frac{\left((2\pi qa)J_0'(2\pi qa)\right)^2}{\left((2\pi qa)^2 - \beta_{0k}^2\right)^2}
$$
$$
+ \sum_{nk} 8\exp(-\beta_{nk}^2 D\tau/a^2) \times \frac{\beta_{nk}^2}{(\beta_{nk}^2 - n^2)} \times \frac{\left((2\pi qa)J_n'(2\pi qa)\right)^2}{\left((2\pi qa)^2 - \beta_{nk}^2\right)^2}
\tag{10}
$$

where J_n' are the derivatives of the nth-order Bessel function, β_{nk} are the arguments that result in zero-crossings and the cylinders are of radius a. As Eq. (10) models diffusion for a single fiber population, this expression is extended as in Axcaliber to include contributions from a Gamma distribution of fiber diameters [1]. In fact, Eq. (10) is exactly the model that is fitted to the 1D+t signal in Axcaliber. Following Eq. (3) in [16] we complete the model for a cylindrical compartment by adding a free diffusion component as

$$
E(\mathbf{q},\tau) = E_r(q_\perp,\tau) \cdot E_{\text{free}}(q_\parallel,\tau).
\tag{11}
$$

where $q_\parallel = \langle \mathbf{q}, \mathbf{f} \rangle$ with $\langle \cdot \rangle$ the inner product and $\mathbf{f}$ the orientation of the cylinder. Using the free water diffusivity $D = 3 \cdot 10^{-9} \text{m/s}^2$, the parallel compartment is given as

$$
E_{\text{free}}(q_\parallel,\tau) = e^{-4\pi^2\mathbf{q}^2 D\tau}.
\tag{12}
$$

3   Experiments

In this section we first validate our method using synthetic data generated using the theoretical Callaghan model [10]. We then apply our method on real data acquired for ActiveAx [14].

3.1   Synthetic Data Experiments

Using the theoretical model outlined in Sect. 2.3 we generate two axon populations with Gamma distributed radii. We choose the shape and scale parameters of the Gamma distribution similar to the optic nerve and sciatic nerve distributions presented in the Axcaliber paper [1]. We show the shapes of the Gamma distributions and corresponding restricted signal attenuations in Fig. 1.

We sample Eq. (11) in q-points distributed according to [17]. For every diffusion time τ we sample different q-space shells at $q = \{0, 2, 5, 10, 30, 50, 70\} \text{ mm}^{-1}$. Each shell is sampled with $\{3, 10, 10, 10, 20, 20, 20\}$ samples, respectively. This acquisition is repeated for every diffusion time $\tau = \{10, 20, 40, 60\}$ ms, leading to a total of 372 samples. We compute this data for both Gamma distributions for the signal fitting and Axcaliber experiments in the next sections.

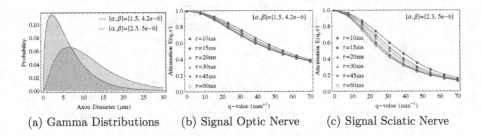

(a) Gamma Distributions   (b) Signal Optic Nerve   (c) Signal Sciatic Nerve

Fig. 1. Signals generated using the Callaghan model.

3.2   Signal Fitting and Effect of Regularization

In our first experiment we test how many spatial or temporal basis functions we need to fit a 3D+t diffusion signal. We choose to study in the case of restricted diffusion in a cylindrical compartment, since this is a good model for white matter tissue in highly organized areas. We generate the noiseless signal as described in Sect. 2.3 with the sampling scheme we described in Sect. 3.1. We then fit the signal with increasing maximum order for the spatial and temporal basis. We then compute the mean squared error (MSE) of the fitted signal compared to the ground truth. We show a heat map of the results in Fig. 2a where we see that the signal fitting in this specific signal model only improves very little after a spatial order of 6 and a temporal order of 5. Using Eq. (5) this means we fit 300 coefficients to accurately represent the 3D+t signal.

Using these settings for the maximum radial and temporal order we then study the effectiveness of our proposed Laplacian regularization when we (1) remove samples or (2) add noise to the data. In (1) we add a typical amount of noise to the data such that SNR=20 and remove samples from the data in steps of 12 samples. We then compare the MSE of the fitted signal with the noiseless *whole* signal of 372 samples. We present the results in Fig. 2b, where you can see that the regularized 3D+t basis (in red) has significantly lower MSE than the unregularized basis. You can also see that the MSE error starts to increase when the number of samples is reduced below 300. In (2) we set the number of samples to 300 and increase the noise from SNR=5 to SNR=50. In Fig. 2c you can again see that our regularized basis has lower MSE values.

3.3   Three Dimensional Axcaliber from 3D+t

With this experiment we explore an application of our 3D+t basis by including Axcaliber [1]. Axcaliber is a method that can estimate the parameters of the Gamma distribution of the fiber radii by fitting the Gamma distributed version of Eq. (10) to the signal over both q and τ. However, it requires that the data is sampled exactly perpendicular to the axon population, which makes it impractical for clinical use.

An advantage of our model is that we can apply Axcaliber in any direction by first fitting the entire 3D+t signal with Eq. (9) and then sampling the data

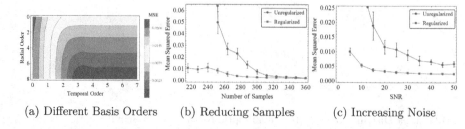

(a) Different Basis Orders   (b) Reducing Samples   (c) Increasing Noise

Fig. 2. (a) A heat map representing the mean squared error (MSE) of the basis fitting for different maximum radial and temporal orders. (b) The effect of reducing the number of samples on the MSE. (c) The effect of increasing the noise in the data on the MSE.

again perpendicular to the observed fiber direction. We compare our approach with a similar proposal [6] previously made using the composite and hindered restricted model of diffusion (CHARMED) model [15]. In contrast to our method, which assumes no a-priori shape on the EAP, the CHARMED model fits specific hindered and restricted compartments to the signal [16].

In this experiment we simulate 300 signal samples at SNR=20 using Eq. (11) for both Gamma distributions presented in Fig. 1. In this experiment we, without loss of generality, fix the axon direction along the z-axis and only consider the intra-axonal signal (i.e. no hindered compartment). We then fit our model with a radial order of 6 and temporal order of 5. We fit CHARMED using 3 restricted compartments. Then, as the signal in a cylindrical compartment should be axially symmetric, we sample 10 different directions on the plane perpendicular to z and average the signals to reduce the effects of noise. The Axcaliber data set consists of $q = \{0, 10, 20, 30, 40, 50, 60, 70\}$ at $\tau = \{10, 20, 30, 40, 50, 60\}$, resulting in 42 samples. We repeat the experiment 100 times.

Figure 3 shows box plots of the recovered shape and scale parameters α and β from the optic and sciatic nerve data sets for both our 3D+t method and CHARMED. The blue box contains values that are within the first and third quartile of the obtained values, while the horizontal line in the middle is the median value. On the right we also show the estimated mean radius, which can be directly estimated from the gamma distribution as $\langle R \rangle = \alpha\beta$. The green line represents the ground truth. It can be seen that the ground truth is always within the first and third quartile for our method, while CHARMED typically overestimates β and underestimates α.

3.4   Axon Diameter from Monkey Data

As a real data experiment we apply our model to an ActiveAx data set [14,18] of an ex-vivo monkey brain. The data set consists of four shells with 93 samples each, and uses gradient strengths $G = \{.14, .14, .14, .13\}$T/m, separation times $\Delta = \{35.78, 16.7, 16.7, 45.9\}$ms and pulse lengths $\delta = \{17.74, 10.15, 10.17, 7.17\}$ms, respectively. As you can see the pulse lengths δ are comparable to Δ and differ between acquisition shells, which makes it not

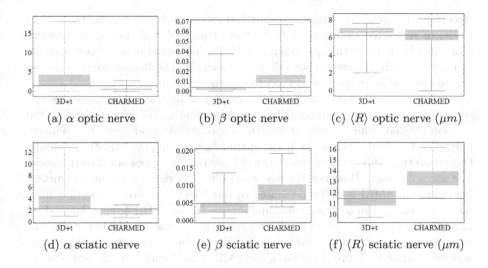

(a) α optic nerve   (b) β optic nerve   (c) $\langle R \rangle$ optic nerve (μm)

(d) α sciatic nerve   (e) β sciatic nerve   (f) $\langle R \rangle$ sciatic nerve (μm)

Fig. 3. The recovered shape α, scale β and average axon radius $\langle R \rangle$ for the optic nerve (top row) and sciatic nerve (bottom row) data sets. The green line is the ground truth.

ideal for our method. However, it is the only data set publicly available that has different measurements in Δ.

We use the provided mask of the corpus callosum [14] and fit Eq. (9) to the data using a radial order of 6 and a temporal order of 3. We then use the approach in Sect. 3.3 and compute the mean axon radii. We present these results in Fig. 4. We can see that, while the results are somewhat noisy, we find smaller radii near the splenium and genu (around 2–3 μm) and bigger near the midbody (around 3–4 μm). This trend roughly follows what was found in [14], showing that our method obtains reasonable results even in this data.

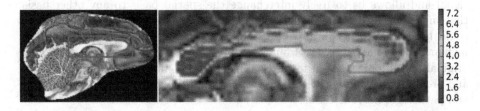

Fig. 4. A fractional anisotropy (FA) map of the ex-vivo monkey brain (left) and the estimated axon radii in the corpus callosum (right).

4   Discussion and Conclusions

Our main contribution in this work is a novel framework to simultaneously represent the diffusion-weighted MRI (dMRI) signal over diffusion times, gradient strengths and gradient directions. Our framework is based on the theoretical model of restricted diffusion by Callaghan et al. [10] and uses an orthogonal functional basis to fit the spatio-temporal diffusion signal over q-space and diffusion times, which together we call 3D+t space. To the best of our knowledge, we are the first to propose a method to represent the 3D+t space using a functional basis. In accordance with the separability of our functional basis, we can choose our spatial and temporal basis independently. We proposed to fit the temporal signal using a basis of negative exponentials modulated by Laguerre polynomials, while we chose to fit the spatial signal using the 3D-SHORE basis. One theoretical limitation of this choice of basis is that it does not directly model free water diffusion. However, the free water diffusion signal with the parameters found in WM dMRI is well-represented by our basis, hence the theoretical limitation does not seem to represent a major issue in our dMRI applications. More importantly, this formulation retains all properties of the 3D-SHORE basis, but with the added information over diffusion time. These benefits include a *time-dependent* analytic representation of the dMRI signal and diffusion propagator.

Our formulation also allows for the efficient regularization of the basis in the form of the minimization of the Laplacian. We provide the analytic solution of this Laplacian regularization depending only on the basis order and scaling factors, allowing for instant computation of the regularization matrix for any combination of basis order. We show on synthetic data that it effectively regularizes the basis fitting.

Furthermore, we explored a possible application of our 3D+t framework by including Axcaliber [1]. We showed on synthetic data that by first fitting our basis to a sparse 3D+t sampling, we can accurately interpolate an Axcaliber data set along any direction. This allowed us to estimate the axon radius distribution parameters despite not sampling directly perpendicular to the axon orientation. We compared this approach with a similar proposal using CHARMED [15] and we showed that our approach is more appropriate to fit the 3D+t signal.

In its current form our framework effectively represents the 3D+t diffusion signal and allows us to freely interchange the spatial basis to any other basis that more readily fits anisotropic data. For instance, the MAP-MRI basis [5] could be used, which can also be extended to include the analytic Laplacian regularization. Therefore, the framework presented in this work is meant as an original and important step towards complete 3D+t imaging in diffusion MRI, and provides great potential to better understand the diffusion signal in normal and pathologic nervous tissue.

A   Analytic Laplacian Regularization

Here we compute the analytic form of the Laplacian regularization matrix in Eq. (8). As our basis is separable in $\mathbf{q}$ and τ, we can separate the Laplacian over our basis function Ξ_i in a the spatial and temporal Laplacian as

$$\nabla^2 \Xi_i(\mathbf{q}, \tau, u_s, u_t) = \left(\nabla_{\mathbf{q}}^2 S_i(\mathbf{q}, u_s)\right) T_i(\tau, u_t) + S_i(\mathbf{q}, u_s) \left(\nabla_{\tau}^2 T_i(\tau, u_t)\right) \quad (13)$$

with $\nabla_{\mathbf{q}}^2$ and ∇_τ^2 the Laplacian to either $\mathbf{q}$ or τ. We then rewrite Eq. (8) as

$$
\mathbf{U}_{ik} = \overbrace{\int_{\mathbb{R}} (\nabla_{\mathbf{q}}^2 S_i)(\nabla_{\mathbf{q}}^2 S_k) d\mathbf{q} \int_{\mathbb{R}} T_i T_k d\tau}^{\mathbf{U}_{ik}^{\mathrm{I}}} + \overbrace{\int_{\mathbb{R}} (\nabla_{\mathbf{q}}^2 S_i) S_k d\mathbf{q} \int_{\mathbb{R}} T_i (\nabla_\tau^2 T_k) d\tau}^{\mathbf{U}_{ik}^{\mathrm{IIa}}}
$$

$$
+ \underbrace{\int_{\mathbb{R}} S_i (\nabla_{\mathbf{q}}^2 S_k) d\mathbf{q} \int_{\mathbb{R}} (\nabla_\tau^2 T_i) T_k d\tau}_{\mathbf{U}_{ik}^{\mathrm{IIb}}} + \underbrace{\int_{\mathbb{R}} S_i S_k d\mathbf{q} \int_{\mathbb{R}} (\nabla_\tau^2 T_i)(\nabla_\tau^2 T_k) d\tau}_{\mathbf{U}_{ik}^{\mathrm{III}}}
$$

where $\mathbf{U}_{ik}^{\mathrm{IIa}} = \mathbf{U}_{ki}^{\mathrm{IIb}}$. In all cases the integrals over $\mathbf{q}$ and τ can be calculated to a closed form using the orthogonality of the spherical harmonics, and Laguerre polynomials with respect to weighting function e^{-x}. The closed form of $\mathbf{U}^{\mathrm{I}}$ is

$$
\mathbf{U}_{ik}^{\mathrm{I}} = \frac{u_s}{u_t} \delta_{o(k)}^{o(i)} \delta_{l(k)}^{l(i)} \delta_{m(k)}^{m(i)}
\begin{cases}
\delta_{(j(i),j(k)+2)} \dfrac{2^{2-l}\pi^2 \Gamma(\frac{5}{2}+j(k)+l)}{\Gamma(j(k))} \\[2mm]
\delta_{(j(i),j(k)+1)} \dfrac{2^{2-l}\pi^2(-3+4j(i)+2l)\Gamma(\frac{3}{2}+j(k)+l)}{\Gamma(j(k))} \\[2mm]
\delta_{(j(i),j(k))} \dfrac{2^{-l}\pi^2\left(3+24j(i)^2+4(-2+l)l+12j(i)(-1+2l)\right)\Gamma(\frac{1}{2}+j(i)+l)}{\Gamma(j(i))} \\[2mm]
\delta_{(j(i),j(k)-1)} \dfrac{2^{2-l}\pi^2(-3+4j(k)+2l)\Gamma(\frac{3}{2}+j(i)+l)}{\Gamma(j(i))} \\[2mm]
\delta_{(j(i),j(k)-2)} \dfrac{2^{2-l}\pi^2\Gamma(\frac{5}{2}+j(i)+l)}{\Gamma(j(i))}
\end{cases}
$$

where δ is the Kronecker delta. Similarly computing $\mathbf{U}_{ik}^{\mathrm{II}} = \mathbf{U}_{ik}^{\mathrm{IIa}} + \mathbf{U}_{ki}^{\mathrm{IIb}}$ gives

$$
\mathbf{U}_{ik}^{\mathrm{II}} = \frac{u_t}{u_s} \delta_{l(k)}^{l(i)} \delta_{m(k)}^{m(i)}
\begin{cases}
\delta_{(j(i),j(k)+1)} \dfrac{2^{-l}\Gamma(\frac{3}{2}+j(k)+l)}{\Gamma(j(k))} \\[2mm]
\delta_{(j(i),j(k))} \dfrac{2^{-(l+1)}(1-4j(i)-2l)\Gamma(\frac{1}{2}+j(i)+l)}{\Gamma(j(i))} \\[2mm]
\delta_{(j(i),j(k)-1)} \dfrac{2^{-l}\Gamma(\frac{3}{2}+j(i)+l)}{\Gamma(j(i))}
\end{cases}
$$

$$
\times \left(\tfrac{1}{2}\delta_{o(i)}^{o(k)} + (1 - \delta_{o(i)}^{o(k)}) \cdot |o(i) - o(k)| \right)
$$

where $|\cdot|$ is the absolute sign. We now denote the operator $M_{x_1}^{x_2} = \min(x_1, x_2)$ for the minimal value of x_1, x_2 and H_x the Heaviside step function with $H_x = 1$ iff $x \geq 0$. The last term $\mathbf{U}_{ik}^{\mathrm{III}}$ evaluates to

$$
\mathbf{U}_{ik}^{\mathrm{III}} = \frac{u_t^3}{u_s^3} \delta_{j(k)}^{j(i)} \delta_{l(k)}^{l(i)} \delta_{m(k)}^{m(i)} \frac{2^{-(l+2)}\Gamma(j(i)+l+1/2)}{\pi^2\Gamma(j)} \times \left(\tfrac{1}{4}|o(i) - o(k)| + \tfrac{1}{16}\delta_{o(i)}^{o(k)} + M_{o(i)}^{o(k)} \right.
$$

$$
+ \sum_{p=1}^{M_{o(i)}^{o(k)}+1} (o(i) - p)(o(k) - p) H_{M_{o(i)}^{o(k)}-p} + H_{o(i)-1} H_{o(k)-1} \left(o(i) + o(k) + 2 \right.
$$

$$
\left. \left. + \sum_{p=0}^{M_{o(i)-1}^{o(k)-2}} p + \sum_{p=0}^{M_{o(i)-2}^{o(k)-1}} p + M_{o(i)-1}^{o(k)-1} \left(|o(i) - o(k)| - 1\right) H_{(|o(i)-o(k)|-1)} \right) \right)
$$

We finally compute the complete 3D+t Laplacian regularization matrix as

$$
\mathbf{U} = \mathbf{U}^{\mathrm{I}} + \mathbf{U}^{\mathrm{II}} + \mathbf{U}^{\mathrm{III}} \tag{14}
$$

References

1. Assaf, Y., Katzir, T.B., Yovel, Y., Basser, P.: AxCaliber: a method for measuring axon diameter distribution from diffusion MRI. Mag. Reson. Med. **59**(6), 1347–1354 (2008)
2. Stejskal, E.: Use of spin echoes in a pulsed magnetic field gradient to study anisotropic, restricted diffusion and flow. J. Chem. Phys. **43**(10), 3597–3603 (1965)
3. Basser, P., Mattiello, J., LeBihan, D.: Estimation of the effective self-diffusion tensor from the NMR spin echo. J. Mag. Reson. Ser. B **103**(3), 247–254 (1994)
4. Merlet, S., Deriche, R.: Continuous diffusion signal, EAP and ODF estimation via compressive sensing in diffusion MRI. Med. Im. Anal. **17**(5), 556–572 (2013)
5. Özarslan, E., Koay, C., Shepherd, T., Komlosh, M., İrfanoğlu, M., Pierpaoli, C., Basser, P.: Mean apparent propagator (map) MRI: a novel diffusion imaging method for mapping tissue microstructure. NeuroImage **78**, 16–32 (2013)
6. Barazanyand, D., Jones, D., Assaf, Y.: Axcaliber 3D. In: ISMRM (2011)
7. Bar-Shir, A., Avram, L., Özarslan, E., Basser, P., Cohen, Y.: The effect of the diffusion time and pulse gradient duration ratio on the diffraction pattern and the structural information estimated from q space diffusion MR: experiments and simulations. J. Mag. Reson. **194**(2), 230–236 (2008)
8. Özarslan, E., Shemesh, E., Koay, N., Cohen, C., Basser, P.: Nuclear magnetic resonance characterization of general compartment size distributions. New J. Phys. **13**(1), 015010 (2011)
9. Sanguinetti, G., Deriche, R.: Mapping average axon diameters under long diffusion time. In: ISBI (2014)
10. Callaghan, P.: Pulsed-gradient spin-echo NMR for planar, cylindrical, and spherical pores under conditions of wall relaxation. JMR Ser. A **113**(1), 53–59 (1995)
11. Sparse Reconstruction Challenge for Diffusion. http://projects.iq.harvard.edu/sparcdmri/challenge
12. Descoteaux, M., Angelino, E., Fitzgibbons, S., Deriche, R.: Regularized, fast, and robust analytical Qball imaging. MRM **58**(3), 497–510 (2007)
13. Craven, P., Wahba, G.: Smoothing noisy data with spline functions. Numer. Math. **31**(4), 377–403 (1978)
14. Alexander, D., Hubbard, P., Hall, M., Moore, E., Ptito, M., Parker, G., Dyrby, T.: Orientationally invariant indices of axon diameter and density from diffusion MRI. Neuroimage **52**(4), 1374–1389 (2010)
15. Assaf, Y., Basser, P.: Composite hindered and restricted model of diffusion (CHARMED) MR imaging of the human brain. Neuroimage **27**(1), 48–58 (2005)
16. Assaf, Y., Freidlin, R., Rohde, G., Basser, P.: New modeling and experimental framework to characterize hindered and restricted water diffusion in brain white matter. MRM **52**(5), 965–978 (2004)
17. Caruyer, E., Lenglet, C., Sapiro, G., Deriche, R.: Design of multishell sampling schemes with uniform coverage in diffusion MRI. MRM **69**(6), 1534–1540 (2013)
18. Dyrby, T., Baaré, W., Alexander, D., Jelsing, J., Garde, E., Søgaard, L.: An ex vivo imaging pipeline for producing high quality and high resolution diffusion weighted imaging datasets. HBM **32**(4), 544–563 (2011)
19. Garyfallidis, E., Brett, M., Amirbekian, B., Rokem, A., van der Walt, S., Descoteaux, M., Nimmo-Smith, I., Contributors, D.: Dipy, a library for the analysis of diffusion MRI data. Front. Neuroinformatics **8**(8), 1–17 (2014)

Ground Truth for Diffusion MRI in Cancer: A Model-Based Investigation of a Novel Tissue-Mimetic Material

Damien J. McHugh[1,2,3](✉), Fenglei Zhou[1,3,4],
Penny L. Hubbard Cristinacce[1,2], Josephine H. Naish[1,2],
and Geoffrey J.M. Parker[1,2,3]

[1] Centre for Imaging Sciences, The University of Manchester,
Manchester, UK
damien.mchugh@manchester.ac.uk
[2] Biomedical Imaging Institute, The University of Manchester,
Manchester, UK
[3] CRUK and EPSRC Cancer Imaging Centre in Cambridge and Manchester,
Manchester, UK
[4] Materials Science Centre, The University of Manchester,
Manchester, UK

Abstract. This work presents preliminary results on the development, characterisation, and use of a novel physical phantom designed as a simple mimic of tumour cellular structure, for diffusion-weighted magnetic resonance imaging (DW-MRI) applications. The phantom consists of a collection of roughly spherical, micron-sized core–shell polymer 'cells', providing a system whose ground truth microstructural properties can be determined and compared with those obtained from modelling the DW-MRI signal. A two-compartment analytic model combining restricted diffusion inside a sphere with hindered extracellular diffusion was initially investigated through Monte Carlo diffusion simulations, allowing a comparison between analytic and simulated signals. The model was then fitted to DW-MRI data acquired from the phantom over a range of gradient strengths and diffusion times, yielding estimates of 'cell' size, intracellular volume fraction and the free diffusion coefficient. An initial assessment of the accuracy and precision of these estimates is provided, using independent scanning electron microscope measurements and bootstrap-style simulations. Such phantoms may be useful for testing microstructural models relevant to the characterisation of tumour tissue.

Keywords: Tumour microstructure · Diffusion MRI · Biomimetic phantoms · Core–shell microspheres · Coaxial electrospraying

1 Introduction

The dependence of the DW-MRI signal on tissue microstructural properties underpins the use of DW-MRI in investigating cellular changes in a variety of pathological conditions, such as stroke [1] and cancer [2]. While the apparent

© Springer International Publishing Switzerland 2015
S. Ourselin et al. (Eds.): IPMI 2015, LNCS 9123, pp. 179–190, 2015.
DOI: 10.1007/978-3-319-19992-4_14

diffusion coefficient (ADC) derived from DW-MRI can provide sensitivity to microstructural changes, it lacks specificity as it is potentially affected by a range of tissue properties without directly characterising them. This has motivated the use of microstructural models that describe the DW-MRI signal as a function of sequence parameters and specific tissue properties. Such models typically represent tissue in terms of intra- and extra-cellular compartments, with cells modelled as idealised shapes with impermeable or permeable membranes. These models can be fitted to acquired data to estimate parameters such as cell size, compartment volume fractions and diffusivities. For example, optic nerve has been modelled as a combination of ellipsoids (axons), spheres (glial cells), and an extracellular space, with a multi-compartment exchange model used to estimate the size, volume fraction, diffusivities and permeabilities of the compartments [3]. Axons have also been modelled as impermeable cylinders with a distribution of diameters, enabling axon size distributions to be estimated in fixed tissue [4] and in vivo [5]. A model comprising monodisperse impermeable cylinders has also been used to estimate indices of axonal diameter and density in human brains [6]. Recently, impermeable spheres have been used to model tumour tissue, allowing cell size and volume fractions to be estimated in vivo [7]. The increasing interest in using such model-based analyses to extract specific microstructural information from DW-MRI data motivates the development of model systems where the ground truth can be independently determined and used to validate microstructural models.

Such model systems range from in silico geometries [8,9] and synthetic physical phantoms [10–12], through to plant [13] and fixed biological tissue [3,4]. Synthetic physical phantoms provide a system where ground truth properties can potentially be characterised and varied more easily than with biological tissue, but less easily than in silico models, and where the experimental methods more closely reflect those used when investigating real tissue than when using in silico approaches. A number of studies have used synthetic phantoms to test DW-MRI methods developed for applications in white matter. Fibre phantoms with variable packing density have been used to study extracellular diffusion [10], while silica microcapillaries have been used to mimic intra-axonal diffusion and test microstructural modelling methods [12]. Recently, coaxial electrospinning has been used to develop axon-mimicking hollow fibres whose orientation and size can be controlled [14,15], with intracellular diffusivity measurements showing sensitivity to fibre size [11]. In contrast to these white matter phantoms that seek to mimic specific microstructural properties, phantom studies in oncology have focussed on free-diffusion phantoms for validation of ADC values. For example, ice-water phantoms have been investigated as a way of validating ADC measurements in multi-centre clinical trials [16]. While such phantoms are useful for assessing the repeatability and reproducibility of ADC measurements, they are not suitable for studying the specific tissue properties that underlie tumour ADC measurements.

The present work describes in silico and experimental investigations undertaken to validate an analytic model of the DW-MRI signal relevant to the characterisation of tumour tissue. This model was initially investigated through

Monte Carlo diffusion simulations, allowing a comparison between analytic and simulated signals. The model was then applied to experimental DW-MRI data obtained from a novel physical phantom designed as a simple mimic of tumour tissue. The phantom was developed using coaxial electrospraying [17] to generate a collection of roughly spherical, micron-sized hollow polymer particles, mimicking cells. Scanning electron microscope (SEM) imaging was used to obtain a ground truth measurement of the mean sphere size, which was compared with the size estimated from modelling the DW-MRI data. The paper starts with a description of the model and the Monte Carlo simulations used for in silico validation. Details of the phantom construction and characterisation are then presented, followed by a description of the MR experiments and the results.

2   Microstructural Model

The microstructural model considered here consists of diffusion in two non-exchanging compartments: a restricted intracellular compartment with volume fraction f_i and diffusion coefficient D_i, and a hindered extracellular compartment with volume fraction $f_e = 1 - f_i$ and diffusion coefficient D_e. The DW-MRI signal, S, is given by

$$S = f_i S_i + (1 - f_i) S_e, \tag{1}$$

where

$$S_i = \exp\left(-2\gamma^2 G^2 \sum_{m=1}^{\infty} \frac{1}{\alpha_m^2(\alpha_m^2 R^2 - 2)}\left[\frac{2\delta}{\alpha_m^2 D_i}\right.\right.$$
$$\left.\left.+\frac{2e^{-\alpha_m^2 D_i \delta} + 2e^{-\alpha_m^2 D_i \Delta} - e^{-\alpha_m^2 D_i(\Delta-\delta)} - e^{-\alpha_m^2 D_i(\Delta+\delta)} - 2}{\alpha_m^4 D_i^2}\right]\right), \tag{2}$$

$$S_e = \exp\left(-\gamma^2 \delta^2 G^2 (\Delta - \delta/3)\frac{D_e}{1 + f_i/2}\right). \tag{3}$$

Equation (2) is the pulsed gradient spin-echo (PGSE) signal for diffusion restricted inside an impermeable sphere of radius R [18] (assuming a Gaussian phase distribution [19]), and (3) gives the signal for hindered extracellular diffusion with the diffusion coefficient reduced by a tortuosity factor, $1 + f_i/2$ [20]. The α_m in (2) is obtained from the mth root of $\alpha_m R J'_{3/2}(\alpha_m R) - \frac{1}{2}J_{3/2}(\alpha_m R) = 0$, where $J_{3/2}$ is the Bessel function of the first kind, order 3/2 [18,19]. The signals calculated analytically from (1)–(3) were compared with synthetic signals generated from Monte Carlo diffusion simulations. The Camino toolkit [8] was used to perform random walk simulations in a 3D geometry of monodisperse, packed impermeable spheres. All simulations had spatial and temporal resolutions of $0.655\,\mu m$ and $0.0357\,ms$, respectively, used 195000 walkers and had intra- and extra-cellular diffusion coefficients set to $2 \times 10^{-3}\,mm^2/s$. Models with different cell sizes ($R = 7$–$30\,\mu m$) and intracellular volume fractions ($f_i = 0.16$–0.71) were used in separate simulations. For each combination of R and f_i, synthetic signals were generated for PGSE sequences with a range of gradient strengths, $G = 0$–$263\,\mathrm{mT/m}$, and separations, $\Delta = 12$–$45\,\mathrm{ms}$, with the gradient duration $\delta = 4\,\mathrm{ms}$. These sequence parameters can be obtained on preclinical scanners, and match the range used in the phantom MR experiments (see below). Figure 1 shows an example of the geometry used in these simulations, and plots synthetic (circles) and analytic (dashed lines) signals as a function of G and Δ for different combinations of R and f_i. In general, good agreement was found between the synthetic and analytic signals over a range of tissue properties and sequence parameters, with a maximum difference between simulated and analytic signals of 0.02. This suggests that (1)–(3) provide an accurate description of this simple tissue model.

3   Phantom Construction and Characterisation

Coaxial electrospraying was performed using polyethylene glycol (PEG) dissolved in chloroform for the core, and polycaprolactone (PCL) dissolved in chloroform for the shell. The PEG solution was injected into the inner needle of a coaxial spinneret at a flow rate of $1\,\mathrm{ml/h}$, while the PCL solution was injected into the outer needle at $3\,\mathrm{ml/h}$. A voltage of $9\,\mathrm{kV}$ was applied between the spinneret and a ground electrode (a thin aluminium plate) placed $20\,\mathrm{cm}$ below.

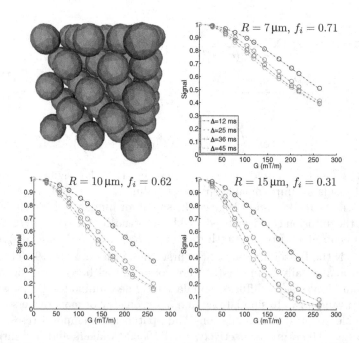

Fig. 1. Spherical cell geometry used in the simulations, along with synthetic (circles) and analytic (dashed lines) signals plotted as a function of G and Δ for different combinations of R and f_i.

The core–shell spheres, which form as the liquid jet emerging from the spinneret breaks up, were collected on a copper wire placed on the ground electrode, forming a bulk sample over a period of 1 − 2 h. The wire was then removed, leaving a bulk sample structured as a hollow cylinder. Two parts of the bulk phantom were used for SEM and MR characterisation, respectively. For the MR experiments the phantom was placed in an NMR tube (5 mm outer diameter), which was filled with cyclohexane approximately one week before scanning. Cyclohexane provides the MR signal in these experiments and was chosen instead of water as PCL is hydrophobic and therefore prevents water molecules reaching the intracellular space. The potential for using other polymers is currently being investigated, which may allow water to be used instead of cyclohexane.

From the part of the bulk sample set aside for SEM analysis, ten subsamples were taken and imaged with a Phenom G2 Pro desktop SEM. These ten SEM images were then used to estimate the size of the spheres. Analysis was carried out using ImageJ (National Institutes of Health, Bethesda, Maryland, USA, http://imagej.nih.gov/ij/), and began by selecting which spheres in each image would be measured. In order to avoid potential bias in choosing spheres manually, a grid was placed on each SEM image, and spheres which contained a grid intersection were chosen as potential candidates for measurement. Not all of these spheres could be measured, however, as spheres in the foreground could obstruct those behind. As such, candidate spheres were selected for measurement if two perpendicular lines could be drawn from one edge to another, approximately through the sphere centre, without other spheres occluding the edges. In some cases the edges merged with another sphere, making the boundary less well defined. In this way, two diameter measurements were made for each chosen sphere, with the final estimate taken as the mean of these two lengths. At least ten spheres per image were chosen for measurement, and the process was performed independently by two observers after deciding which spheres were to be analysed. The mean difference and limits of agreement were calculated to compare the two observers' measurements [21]. For consistency with the MR analysis, the measurements are reported as sphere radii, as opposed to diameters. It should be noted that these measurements provide an estimate of the outer radius of the spheres, which is larger than the internal radius due to the non-zero thickness of the sphere walls.

4 MR Methods

4.1 MR Acquisition

MR experiments were carried out on a 7 T Bruker system (Bruker BioSpin, Ettlingen, Germany), using a transmit/receive volume coil. Data were acquired using four separate PGSE sequences, each with a different gradient separation: $\Delta = 12, 25, 36, 45$ ms. For each Δ scan, images were acquired at seven gradient strengths: $G = 0, 28.5, 78.1, 119, 147, 202, 263$ mT/m; δ was fixed at 4 ms for each scan. In order to maximise signal to noise ratio (SNR), the lowest possible echo time (TE) was chosen for each Δ, giving TE = 21.2, 34.2, 45.2, 54.2 ms for $\Delta = 12$, 25, 36, 45 ms, respectively. Each scan acquired images with three diffusion gradient directions, using a spin-echo readout with a 30 mm × 30 mm field of view, 128 × 128 matrix, 1 mm slice thickness and a 2500 ms repetition time.

4.2   MR Analysis

The phantom ROI was defined by thresholding the $G = 0$ mT/m images to leave only the voxels within the phantom, excluding those containing the free cyclohexane. The equivalent voxels in each diffusion-weighted image were found, and the mean signal intensity taken for each G value to boost SNR. Repeating this for each Δ scan therefore gave ROI-averaged signal intensities as a function of G and Δ, which were then normalised to the unweighted signal for their respective Δ scans. The two-compartment analytic expression given by (1)–(3) was then fitted to these normalised signals. The free diffusivities in the intra- and extra-cellular spaces were assumed to be equal, $D_i = D_e = D$. Two methods of performing the fitting were investigated. First, the full four-parameter fit was carried out, yielding estimates of each model parameter (cell radius, R, intracellular volume fraction, f_i, free diffusivity, D, and unweighted signal, S_0) directly from the ROI-averaged phantom signals. Second, D was fixed during the optimisation, with the fit returning estimates of R, f_i and S_0 only. In this case, D was fixed at the value of the diffusion coefficient measured in the free cyclohexane, which serves as a ground truth measurement of the free diffusion coefficient. This value was obtained by averaging the median ADC values from a ROI in the free cyclohexane, over the different Δ experiments and gradient directions. The ADC fits were performed on a voxel-wise basis using maximum likelihood (ML) fitting [22], with the full range of G for each Δ experiment. The ML method used a single Rician probability density function (PDF) in the objective function and was appropriate here as the signals used in the ADC fitting were not averaged [23].

For the microstructural estimates, the fitting procedure was repeated for a range of starting values, and the final result taken as the fit which gave the lowest value of the objective function. Three starting values were picked at random for each parameter, within a wide range of possible values: $R = 1$–35 µm, $f_i = 0$–1, $D = 0.1$–3.1 ×10^{-3} mm^2/s. The fitting was then repeated for each combination of these randomly chosen values, giving $3^3 = 27$ different fits; only one starting value was used for S_0, which was 1. Picking 2, 3, 4, 5 or 6 starting values for each parameter (giving 8, 27, 64, 125 and 216 repeated fits, respectively) was observed to have negligible effect on the final results. Different random selections within the same range also had negligible effect on the results, suggesting that the values of the fitted parameters were not an artefact of the starting values. Apart from fixing D in the second fitting method, no constraints were applied to any of the fitted parameters. In contrast to the non-averaged signals used for the free cyclohexane ADC calculations, the fits to the two-compartment model used averaged signals, making the use of a single Rician PDF for ML fitting no longer appropriate [23]. As the PDF for averaged Rician-distributed signals has no closed-form expression, the ML method used above cannot be employed, and least squares (LS) fitting was used instead.

Bootstrap-style simulations were performed to investigate the precision of the parameter estimates. Specifically, propagation of errors was used to calculate the errors on the normalised signals from the phantom ROI, according to:

$$\sigma'(G_i, \Delta) = S'(G_i, \Delta) \sqrt{\left(\frac{\sigma(G_i, \Delta)}{S(G_i, \Delta)}\right)^2 + \left(\frac{\sigma(G_1, \Delta)}{S(G_1, \Delta)}\right)^2}, \quad (4)$$

where $\sigma'(G_i, \Delta)$ is the standard deviation (SD) of the normalised signal for the ith gradient strength, $S'(G_i, \Delta)$ is the normalised mean signal for the ith gradient strength, $\sigma(G_i, \Delta)$ and $S(G_i, \Delta)$ are the SD and mean of the unnormalised ith gradient strength ROI-averaged signal and $\sigma(G_1, \Delta)$ and $S(G_1, \Delta)$ are the SD and mean of the unnormalised $G = 0\,\mathrm{mT/m}$ ROI-averaged signal. The $\sigma'(G_i, \Delta)$ values were then used to construct 95 % confidence intervals, ci, for each $S'(G_i, \Delta)$. A new set of signals, $S'_{\mathrm{new}}(G, \Delta)$, was generated by adding or subtracting a random amount from $S'(G, \Delta)$, such that 95 % of $S'_{\mathrm{new}}(G, \Delta)$ lay within $S'(G, \Delta) \pm ci$. Parameter estimates from the new set of signals were then obtained using the fitting described above, and this process was repeated for 10000 sets of synthetic signals. Histograms of the resulting parameter estimates were then plotted. All model fitting was performed using the Nelder-Mead simplex algorithm in MATLAB 2010a (The MathWorks, Natick, MA, USA).

5   Results and Discussion

5.1   Microstructure Characterisation

An example SEM image is shown in Fig. 2a, illustrating the grid placement and labelling of the spheres chosen for measurement. There is a tendency for the

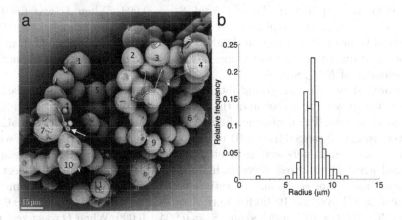

Fig. 2. (a) One of the ten SEM images used for the sphere size measurements, illustrating grid placement and the spheres chosen to measure. **(b)** Histogram of 160 radii measurements made by one observer; mean $\pm$ SD $= (7.9 \pm 1.1)\,\mu\mathrm{m}$.

spheres to merge together, indicating that the bulk phantom is not simply a collection of individual spheres. Also note the presence of one much smaller sphere, with a radius of approximately 1.8 μm; this is visible in Fig. 2a (labelled with the number 8 and indicated by the white arrow), along with three other similarly sized spheres. While such spheres broaden the size distribution, there appear to be few of them and their low volume fraction means they would be expected to contribute little to the measured signal. Diameter measurements were made for a total of 160 spheres. The histogram of the corresponding radii measured by one observer is shown in Fig. 2b. There was good agreement between the measurements made by the two observers; mean difference between the radii estimates: 0.01 μm, with 95 % limits of agreement: −0.5 μm to 0.6 μm, and 95 % confidence interval for the mean difference: −0.03 μm to 0.06 μm. Both observers' measurements had a mean ± SD of (7.9 ± 1.1) μm, which was taken as the ground truth outer radius.

5.2   MR Experiments

Figure 3a shows the $G = 0$ mT/m, $\Delta = 12$ ms image, where the red circle defines the free cyclohexane ROI, and the lower-signal annulus corresponds to the phantom region. The free cyclohexane ADC results are shown in Fig. 3b, where the cyclohexane ADC is shown to be independent of Δ and direction, as expected for fluid undergoing free diffusion. The mean ± SD ADC over all Δ and directions was $(1.36 \pm 0.03) \times 10^{-3}$ mm^2/s; D was therefore fixed to this value when fitting to the phantom data using the second method described above. At high G and high Δ the phantom signal was almost completely attenuated, resulting in very low SNR. For the ROI-averaged phantom signals, the highest G for $\Delta = 36$ ms, and the two highest G for $\Delta = 45$ ms gave SNR < 2 and were excluded from the fitting. The fits to the model are shown in Figs. 3c (D estimated) and 3d (D fixed). When D was an estimated parameter the fit gave $R = 6.1$ μm, $f_i = 0.23$, $D = 1.40 \times 10^{-3}$ mm^2/s and $S_0 = 0.994$. When D was fixed at 1.36×10^{-3} mm^2/s the estimates were $R = 6.1$ μm, $f_i = 0.22$ and $S_0 = 0.993$. The fitted value of D was therefore only 3 % higher than that obtained from the independent measurement, and fixing D was observed to have little impact on the estimates of R, f_i, and S_0.

Figure 4 shows the histograms obtained from the bootstrap-style simulations used to investigate the precision of the microstructural estimates obtained from the phantom data. The confidence intervals that were used in these simulations (derived using (4)) ranged from 0.01 to 0.06. The top row shows the results when all four model parameters were estimated, and the bottom row shows the results obtained when D was fixed. Overall, fixing D was found to have little effect on the mean and SD of R, f_i, and S_0 estimates. When D was a fitted parameter, the mean ± SD over the 10000 fits were $R = (6.2 \pm 0.9)$ μm, $f_i = 0.24 \pm 0.03$, $D = (1.40 \pm 0.09) \times 10^{-3}$ mm^2/s, and $S_0 = 0.994 \pm 0.009$. When D was fixed, the values were $R = (6 \pm 1)$ μm, $f_i = 0.22 \pm 0.03$, and $S_0 = 0.993 \pm 0.008$. Taking the SD of these distributions as a measure of the precision of the parameter estimates, these results suggest that fixing D to the free fluid value has little impact on the

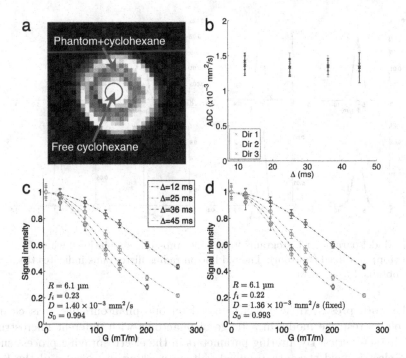

Fig. 3. (a) $G = 0\,\mathrm{mT/m}$, $\Delta = 12\,\mathrm{ms}$ image; the red circle defines the free cyclohexane ROI, and the lower-signal annulus corresponds to the phantom region. (b) Free cyclohexane ADC as a function of Δ. (c) Signals (circles) and model fitting (dashed lines) as a function of G and Δ; error bars correspond to the 95 % ci as described. (d) As in (c) but with D fixed.

precision of the cell size or volume fraction estimated from the phantom data. This also suggests that the diffusivity measured for the free cyclohexane provides a good estimate of the unhindered diffusivity in the phantom. The radius histograms in Fig. 4 also indicate the mean radius determined from SEM, 7.9 μm (red lines). The standard error on this estimate is ≈ 0.09 μm; an error bar showing this would be approximately the same width as the red line so has been omitted. The precision of the two size estimates suggests that R is lower than the outer sphere size measured using SEM. Qualitatively, this is expected given the non-zero thickness of the sphere wall, though measurements of this thickness are needed to see if this alone accounts for the difference. Modelling assumptions, sphere manufacturing imperfections and bias due to the use of LS fitting may also contribute to the difference. The estimated free diffusivity is consistent with the free cyclohexane ADC, and the volume fraction is plausible. Work to establish a ground truth volume fraction using high-resolution computed tomography is ongoing, which will allow the accuracy of the f_i estimate to be assessed. The close agreement between the model estimates and ground truth observations for R and D, combined with the very close agreement between theory and Monte Carlo simulations (Fig. 1), provides strong evidence in support of the use of the analytic model in (1)–(3) for assessing micron-scale spherical structures using DW-MRI.

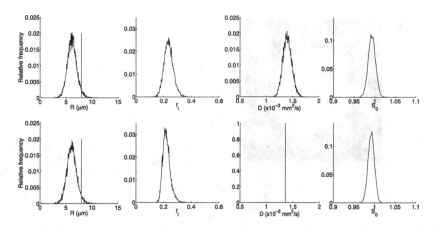

Fig. 4. Model parameter histograms from bootstrap-style simulations, when D is estimated (top) and fixed (bottom). The red line on radius histograms indicates the mean radius obtained from SEM.

The work presented here has focussed on one phantom, but it is clearly desirable to test the model in a range of phantoms with different microstructural characteristics. By altering parameters in the electrospraying process such as the electric field strength (applied voltage/working distance) and the flow rates of the polymer solutions, the inner radius of the resultant spheres, and the shell thickness, can be controlled. This approach has been used previously to generate electrospun fibre phantoms with different diameters [11,15]. Typically, the electrospraying technique is capable of producing spheres in the micron and sub-micron size range, and we envisage being able to produce spheres over a physiologically-relevant size range. For example, a previous electrospraying study generated spheres with diameters ranging from $0.6 - 36\,\mu\mathrm{m}$, although these were not hollow [24]. The bulk size of the phantom is mainly dependent on the sphere collecting efficiency and the length of time over which the electrospraying process is carried out. For example, the phantom used in this study had a length of $\sim 9\,\mathrm{mm}$ and an inner/outer annular radius of $\sim 0.7\,\mathrm{mm}/1.3\,\mathrm{mm}$, and was produced over a period of 1–2 h. While we do not currently have data regarding the reproducibility of the sphere phantom construction process, based on previous experience of generating fibre phantoms with co-electrospinning, we expect the reproducibility to be reasonably good.

Finally, it should be noted that the phantom investigated here is clearly a vast oversimplification of actual tumour tissue, lacking intra- and extra-cellular structures, such as cell nuclei and collagen, respectively, as well as lacking a vascular component. The simplicity of the phantom is intended to facilitate the validation of a simple mathematical model, which is not designed to capture all aspects of tumour microstructure. Future work will look at applying the model to progressively more complex systems, such as modified phantoms and in vitro and in vivo tumour models, with the aim of developing an understanding of which aspects of tumour microstructure the DW-MRI signal is sensitive to.

6 Conclusions

This work described in silico and experimental validation of a biophysical model of the DW-MRI signal. Good agreement was found between Monte Carlo simulations and the analytic model, which was then used to obtain microstructural estimates from a novel physical phantom. While further characterisation of the phantom is needed to fully assess the accuracy of the DW-MRI estimates, the difference between the MR and SEM radii is qualitatively consistent with the nonzero thickness of the sphere walls. The estimated free diffusivity is consistent with the free cyclohexane ADC, and the estimated volume fraction is plausible. These phantoms may prove useful for evaluating the accuracy and precision of estimates from models relevant to the characterisation of tumour tissue.

Acknowledgments. The authors thank Matt Hall for assistance with the simulations, and acknowledge the assistance given by IT Services and the use of the Computational Shared Facility at The University of Manchester. This work was supported by the MRC and AstraZeneca, and used facilities funded by the BBSRC. This work was supported by CRUK [C8742/A18097]. This is a contribution from the Cancer Imaging Centre in Cambridge and Manchester, which is funded by the EPSRC and Cancer Research UK.

References

1. Roberts, T.P.L., Rowley, H.A.: Diffusion weighted magnetic resonance imaging in stroke. Eur. J. Radiol. **45**, 185–194 (2003)
2. Padhani, A.R., Liu, G., Koh, D.M., Chenevert, T.L., Thoeny, H.C., Takahara, T., Dzik-Jurasz, A., Ross, B.D., Van Cauteren, M., Collins, D., Hammoud, D.A., Rustin, G.J.S., Taouli, B., Choyke, P.L.: Diffusion-weighted magnetic resonance imaging as a cancer biomarker: consensus and recommendations. Neoplasia **11**, 102–125 (2009)
3. Stanisz, G.J., Szafer, A., Wright, G.A., Henkelman, R.M.: An analytical model of restricted diffusion in bovine optic nerve. Magn. Reson. Med. **37**, 103–111 (1997)
4. Assaf, Y., Blumenfeld-Katzir, T., Yovel, Y., Basser, P.J.: AxCaliber: a method for measuring axon diameter distribution from diffusion MRI. Magn. Reson. Med. **59**, 1347–1354 (2008)
5. Barazany, D., Basser, P.J., Assaf, Y.: In vivo measurement of axon diameter distribution in the corpus callosum of rat brain. Brain **132**, 1210–1220 (2009)
6. Alexander, D.C., Hubbard, P.L., Hall, M.G., Moore, E.A., Ptito, M., Parker, G.J.M., Dyrby, T.B.: Orientationally invariant indices of axon diameter and density from diffusion MRI. NeuroImage **52**, 1374–1389 (2010)
7. Panagiotaki, E., Walker-Samuel, S., Siow, B., Johnson, S.P., Rajkumar, V., Pedley, R.B., Lythgoe, M.F., Alexander, D.C.: Noninvasive quantification of solid tumor microstructure using VERDICT MRI. Cancer Res. **74**, 1902–1912 (2014)
8. Hall, M.G., Alexander, D.C.: Convergence and parameter choice for Monte-Carlo simulations of diffusion MRI. IEEE Trans. Med. Imaging **28**, 1354–1364 (2009)
9. Yeh, C.H., Schmitt, B., Le Bihan, D., Li-Schlittgen, J.R., Lin, C.P., Poupon, C.: Diffusion microscopist simulator: a general Monte Carlo simulation system for diffusion magnetic resonance imaging. PLoS ONE **8**, e76626 (2013)

10. Fieremans, E., De Deene, Y., Delputte, S., Özdemir, M.S., Achten, E., Lemahieu, I.: The design of anisotropic diffusion phantoms for the validation of diffusion weighted magnetic resonance imaging. Phys. Med. Biol. **53**, 5405–5419 (2008)

11. Hubbard, P.L., Zhou, F.L., Eichhorn, S.J., Parker, G.J.M.: Biomimetic phantom for the validation of diffusion magnetic resonance imaging. Magn. Reson. Med. **73**, 299–305 (2015)

12. Siow, B., Drobnjak, I., Chatterjee, A., Lythgoe, M.F., Alexander, D.C.: Estimation of pore size in a microstructure phantom using the optimised gradient waveform diffusion weighted NMR sequence. J. Magn. Reson. **214**, 51–60 (2012)

13. Dietrich, O., Hubert, A., Heiland, S.: Imaging cell size and permeability in biological tissue using the diffusion-time dependence of the apparent diffusion coefficient. Phys. Med. Biol. **59**, 3081–3096 (2014)

14. Zhou, F.L., Hubbard, P.L., Eichhorn, S.J., Parker, G.J.M.: Jet deposition in near-field electrospinning of patterned polycaprolactone and sugar-polycaprolactone core-shell fibres. Polymer **52**, 3603–3610 (2011)

15. Zhou, F.L., Hubbard, P.L., Eichhorn, S.J., Parker, G.J.M.: Coaxially electrospun axon-mimicking fibers for diffusion magnetic resonance imaging. ACS Appl. Mater. Interfaces **4**, 6311–6316 (2012)

16. Malyarenko, D., Galbán, C.J., Londy, F.J., Meyer, C.R., Johnson, T.D., Rehemtulla, A., Ross, B.D., Chenevert, T.L.: Multi-system repeatability and reproducibility of apparent diffusion coefficient measurement using an ice-water phantom. J. Magn. Reson. Imaging **37**, 1238–1246 (2013)

17. Zhang, L., Huang, J., Si, T., Xu, R.X.: Coaxial electrospray of microparticles and nanoparticles for biomedical applications. Expert Rev. Med. Devices **9**, 595–612 (2012)

18. Murday, J.S., Cotts, R.M.: Self-diffusion coefficient of liquid lithium. J. Chem. Phys. **48**, 4938–4945 (1968)

19. Neuman, C.H.: Spin echo of spins diffusing in a bounded medium. J. Chem. Phys. **60**, 4508–4511 (1974)

20. Price, W.S., Barzykin, A.V., Hayamizu, K., Tachiya, M.: A model for diffusive transport through a spherical interface probed by pulsed-field gradient NMR. Biophys. J. **74**, 2259–2271 (1998)

21. Bland, J.M., Altman, D.G.: Measuring agreement in method comparison studies. Stat. Methods Med. Res. **8**, 135–160 (1999)

22. Walker-Samuel, S., Orton, M., McPhail, L.D., Robinson, S.P.: Robust estimation of the apparent diffusion coefficient (ADC) in heterogeneous solid tumors. Magn. Reson. Med. **62**, 420–429 (2009)

23. Kristoffersen, A.: Optimal estimation of the diffusion coefficient from non-averaged and averaged noisy magnitude data. J. Magn. Reson. **187**, 293–305 (2007)

24. Yao, J., Lim, L.K., Xie, J., Hua, J., Wang, C.H.: Characterization of electrospraying process for polymeric particle fabrication. J. Aerosol Sci. **39**, 987–1002 (2008)

Shape Analysis

Anisotropic Distributions on Manifolds: Template Estimation and Most Probable Paths

Stefan Sommer[(✉)]

DIKU, University of Copenhagen, Copenhagen, Denmark
`sommer@diku.dk`

Abstract. We use anisotropic diffusion processes to generalize normal distributions to manifolds and to construct a framework for likelihood estimation of template and covariance structure from manifold valued data. The procedure avoids the linearization that arise when first estimating a mean or template before performing PCA in the tangent space of the mean. We derive flow equations for the most probable paths reaching sampled data points, and we use the paths that are generally not geodesics for estimating the likelihood of the model. In contrast to existing template estimation approaches, accounting for anisotropy thus results in an algorithm that is not based on geodesic distances. To illustrate the effect of anisotropy and to point to further applications, we present experiments with anisotropic distributions on both the sphere and finite dimensional LDDMM manifolds arising in the landmark matching problem.

Keywords: Template estimation · Manifold · Diffusion · Geodesics · Frame bundle · Most probable paths · Anisotropy

1 Introduction

Among the most important tasks in medical imaging is building statistical models that best describe a set of observed data. For data in Euclidean space, a basic approach is finding the mean and performing PCA on the centered data, a procedure that can be considered fitting a normal distribution to observations [20]. This approach can be extended to non-Euclidean spaces, in particular to Riemannian manifolds, by finding a Fréchet mean on the manifold and performing PCA in the tangent space of the mean (PGA, [2]), or by formulating a latent variable model in a tangent space (Probabilistic PGA, [24]). The difference between the mean and the observed data is generally represented by tangent vectors that specify the initial velocity of geodesic paths with endpoints close to the observations. This approach effectively linearizes the curved manifold [18].

In this paper, we will advocate for a different approach: we will generalize the fit of normal distributions to data without linearizing to a tangent space. Euclidean normal distributions with anisotropic covariances can be generalized to manifolds by taking limits of stochastic paths starting at a source point and propagating with stochastic velocities sampled from normal distributions. Avoiding the linearization of the manifold, the proposed procedure uses this class of

© Springer International Publishing Switzerland 2015
S. Ourselin et al. (Eds.): IPMI 2015, LNCS 9123, pp. 193–204, 2015.
DOI: 10.1007/978-3-319-19992-4_15

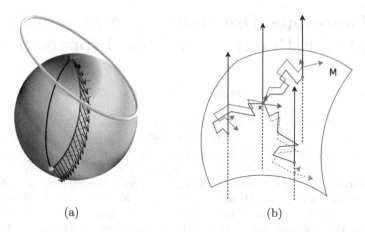

(a)   (b)

Fig. 1. (a) The sphere $\mathbb{S}^2$ and optimal paths for different costs: (black curve) a geodesic between the north pole and a point on the southern hemisphere; (blue curve) a most probable path (MPP) between the points for an anisotropic diffusion starting at the north pole with covariance diag$(2, .5)$ as indicated by the horizontal ellipsis at the north pole. The covariance is proportional to the squared length of the vectors that constitute a frame for $T_{(0,0,1)}\mathbb{S}^2$. The frame is parallel transported along the MPP (arrows). The MPP increases the movement in the direction of minor variance as it reaches the southern hemisphere. Compare with Fig. 2 (a,b). (b) Frame bundle diffusion: for each $x \in M$, the fibers (black arrows) contain frames X_α for $T_x M$. The stochastic paths from x (blue) transport the initial frame X_α (red vectors) horizontally in the frame bundle by parallel transport (green curves and vectors). The map $\pi : FM \to M$ sends a point and frame $(z, Z_\alpha) \in FM$ to the base point $z \in M$ (Color figure online).

distributions to find the most likely source point and covariance structure for explaining the data. The intrinsic definition of the statistical model has a significant side effect: while tangent vectors of geodesics are conventionally used as placeholders of data because geodesics are locally length minimizing, the *most probable paths* between source and data points under the anisotropic model are not geodesics. They are curves that depend on the covariance structure and the curvature of the manifold, and they provide a natural representation of data as the most probable ways of reaching observations given the statistical model.

1.1   Content and Outline

We construct an intrinsic statistical approach to modeling anisotropic data in manifolds using diffusions processes. We describe how the Eells-Elworthy-Malliavin construction of Brownian motion defines a space of probability distributions and how the non-linear template estimation problem can be recast using this construction. We argue for why the *most probable paths* are more natural than geodesics for representing data under the model and for approximating likelihood, and we derive analytical expressions for the flow equations by identifying the paths as projections of extremal curves on a sub-Riemannian manifold.

The paper ends with numerical experiments on the sphere for visualization and further on the LDDMM manifold of landmarks that is widely used in medical imaging and computational anatomy.

The paper thus presents an entirely new approach to one of the most import tasks in medical imaging: template and covariance estimation. The focus is on the theoretical insight behind the construction. The experiments presented indicate the effect of the new model without attempting to constitute a thorough evaluation on medical data. We will explore that further in future work.

While the paper necessarily uses differential geometry, we seek to only include technical details strictly needed for the exposition. Likewise, in order to clearly express the differential geometric ideas, analytical details of stochastic differential equations will be omitted.

2   Background

The data observed in a range of medical imaging applications can only be properly modeled in nonlinear spaces. Differentiable manifolds are therefore used for shape models from the Kendall shape spaces [8], to embedded curves [11] and m-reps and related models [15]. In computational anatomy, the LDDMM framework [23] provides a range of nonlinear geometries dependent on the data types to be matched: landmarks, curves, surfaces, images and tensors lead to different manifolds.

The goal of template estimation is to find a representative for a population of observations [6], for example as a Fréchet mean. Template estimation can be considered a non-linear generalization of the Euclidean space mean estimation. The Principal Geodesic Analysis (PGA, [2]) goes beyond the mean or template by modeling the covariance structure and linearizing data to the tangent space of the mean. Geodesic PCA (GPCA, [5]) and Horizontal Component Analysis (HCA, [16]) likewise provide low dimensional models of manifold valued data by seeking to generalize the Euclidean principal component analysis procedure. Probabilistic PGA [24] builds a latent variable model similar to [20] by the geodesic spray of linearly transformed latent variables. Generalizing Euclidean statistical tools to properly handling curved geometries [14] remain a challenging problem.

The frame bundle was used for dimensionality reduction with HCA [16] and later for Diffusion PCA (DPCA, [17]). While the current paper builds a statistical model similar to the DPCA construction, the focus is on the influence of anisotropy, in particular on the optimal curves, and on likelihood approximation.

For template estimation [6] and first order models such as [21], geodesic curves play a fundamental role. The Fréchet mean minimizes squared geodesic distances, and the momentum representation in the Lie algebra, the tangent space at identity, uses momenta or velocity vectors as representatives of the observed samples. Geodesics and geodesic distances take the role of difference vectors and norms in Euclidean space because differences between the template and the observed data cannot be represented by vectors in the nonlinear geometry. Geodesic paths are used because they are locally length minimizing. The fundamental argument in this paper is that in the case of anisotropy, a different family of curves and distance metrics can be used: the most probable paths for anisotropic distributions and log-likelihoods, respectively.

3   A Class of Anisotropic Distributions

In Euclidean space, the normal distribution $\mathcal{N}(\mu, \Sigma)$ can be defined as the transition probability of a driftless diffusion process with stationary generator Σ stopped at time $t = 1$, i.e. as the solution of the stochastic differential equation $dX_t = \Sigma^{1/2} \circ X_t$. Here, the probability density $p_{\mu,\Sigma}(y)$ is given by the marginal density of all sample paths ending at y. Formally, $p_{\mu,\Sigma}(y) = \int_{x_0=\mu, x_1=y} \tilde{p}_{\Sigma}(x_t) dx_t$ where the path density $\tilde{p}_{\Sigma}(x_t) = \int_0^1 f_{\Sigma}(\dot{x}_t) dt$ integrates the density of a normal distribution $\mathcal{N}(0, \Sigma)$ on the infinitesimal steps $\dot{x}_t$.[1]

In the Euclidean case, the distribution of $y \sim \mathcal{N}(\mu, \Sigma)$ can equivalently be specified both using the difference vector $y - \mu \sim \mathcal{N}(0, \Sigma)$ between observations and mean and using the density $p_{\mu,\Sigma}(y)$ that comes from the path density $\tilde{p}_{\Sigma}$ as above. The latter definition is however much more amenable to the nonlinear situation where a displacement vector $y - \mu$ does not have intrinsic meaning. In a differentiable manifold M, vector space structure is lost but infinitesimal displacements remain in the form of tangent vectors in the tangent spaces $T_x M$, $x \in M$. The path density $\tilde{p}_{\Sigma}$ therefore allows a more natural generalization to the nonlinear situation.

We here outline a construction of anisotropic normal distributions using diffusion processes. We present the discussion in the continuous limit omitting the stochastic analysis needed when the time steps of the stochastic paths goes to zero.

3.1   Stochastic Diffusion Processes on Manifolds

Let M be a manifold with affine connection ∇, and possibly Riemannian metric g. Isotropic diffusions can then be constructed as eigenfunctions of the Laplace-Beltrami operator. The Eells-Elworthy-Malliavin construction of Brownian motion (see e.g. [4]) provides an equivalent construction[2] that also extends to anisotropic diffusions. The starting point is the frame bundle FM that consists of pairs (x, X_α) of points $x \in M$ and frames X_α at x. A frame at x is a collection of $n = \dim M$ tangent vectors in $T_x M$ that together constitute a basis for the tangent space. The frame can thereby be considered an invertible linear map $\mathbb{R}^n \to T_x M$. If (x, X_α) is a point in FM, the frame X_α can be considered a representation of the square root covariance matrix $\Sigma^{1/2}$ that we used above and thus a representation for a diffusion process starting at x. The frame being invertible implies that the square root covariance has full rank.

---

[1] We use the notation $\tilde{p}(x_t)$ for path densities and $p(y)$ for point densities.

[2] If M has more structure, e.g. being a Lie group or a homogeneous space, additional equivalent ways of defining Brownian motion and heat semi-groups exist.

The difficulty in defining a diffusion process from (x, X_α) lies in the fact that the frame X_α cannot in general be defined globally on the manifold. A frame $X_{\alpha,t}$ can however be defined at a point x_t close to x by parallel transport along a curve from x to x_t. It is a fundamental property of curvature denoted holonomy [10] that this transport depends on the chosen curve, and the transport is therefore not unique. The Eells-Elworthy-Malliavin construction handles this by constructing the diffusion in FM directly so that each stochastic path carries with it the frame by parallel transport. If dU_t is a solution to such a diffusion in FM, U_t projects to a process X_t in M by the projection $\pi : FM \to M$ that maps (x, X_α) to the base point x. Different paths reaching x hit different elements of the fiber $\pi^{-1}(x)$ due to the holonomy, and the projection thus essentially integrates out the holonomy. The solutions at $t = 1$ which we will use are stochastic variables, and we write $\int_{\mathrm{Diff}}(x, X_\alpha)$ for the map from initial conditions to X_1. If M has a volume form, the stochastic variable X_1 has a density which generalizes the Euclidean density $p_{\mu,\Sigma}$ above.

3.2 Parallel Transport and Horizontallity

The parallel transport of a frame X_α from x to a frame $X_{\alpha,t}$ on x_t defines a map from curves x_t on M to curves $(x_t, X_{\alpha,t})$ in FM called a horizontal lift. The tangent vectors of lifted curves $(x_t, X_{\alpha,t})$ define a subspace of the frame bundle tangent space $T_{(x_t, X_{\alpha,t})}FM$ that is denoted the horizontal subspace $H_{(x_t, X_{\alpha,t})}FM$. This space of dimension n is naturally isomorphic to $T_{x_t}M$ by the map $\pi_* : (\dot{x}_t, \dot{X}_{\alpha,t}) \mapsto \dot{x}_t$ and it is spanned by n vector fields $H_i(x_t, X_{\alpha,t})$ called horizontal vector fields. Using the horizontal vector fields, the FM diffusion U_t is defined by the SDE

$$dU_t = \sum_{i=1}^{n} H_i(U_t) \circ W_t \tag{1}$$

where W_t is an $\mathbb{R}^n$ valued Wiener process. The diffusion thereby only flows in the horizontal part of the frame bundle, see Fig. 1 (b). Note that if M is Euclidean, the solution X_t is a stationary diffusion process.

This way of linking curves and transport of frames is also denoted "rolling without slipping" [4]. The procedure is defined only using the connection ∇ and its parallel transport. A Riemannian metric is therefore not needed at this point (though a Riemannian metric can be used to define a connection). A volume form on M, for example induced by a Riemannian metric, is however needed when we use densities for likelihoods later.

3.3 Why Parallel Transport?

In Euclidean space, the matrix $\Sigma^{1/2}$ being the square root of the covariance matrix specifies the diffusion process. In the manifold situation, the frame $X_{\alpha,0}$ takes the place of $\Sigma^{1/2}$ by specifying the covariance of infinitesimal steps.

The parallel transport provides a way of linking tangent spaces, and it therefore links the covariance at x_0 with the covariance at x_t. Since the acceleration $\nabla_{\dot{x}_t} X_{\alpha,t}$ vanishes when $X_{\alpha,t}$ is parallel transported, this can be interpreted as a transport of covariance between two tangent spaces with no change seen from the manifold, i.e. no change measured by the connection ∇. While $\Sigma^{1/2}$ can be defined globally in Euclidean space, each sample path will here carry its own transport of $X_{\alpha,0}$, and two paths ending at $y \in M$ will generally transport the covariance differently. The global effect of this stochastic holonomy can seem quite counterintuitive when related to the Euclidean situation but the infinitesimal effect is natural as a transport with no change seen from ∇.

4   Model and Estimation

The Euclidean procedure of mean estimation followed by PCA can be given a probabilistic interpretation [20] as a maximum likelihood estimate (MLE) of the matrix W in the latent variable model $y = Wx + \mu + \epsilon$. Here x are isotropically normally distributed $\mathcal{N}(0, I)$ latent variables, and ϵ is noise $\epsilon \sim \mathcal{N}(0, \sigma^2 I)$. The marginal distribution of y is with this model normal $\mathcal{N}(\mu, C_\sigma)$, $C_\sigma = WW^T + \sigma^2 I$. The MLE for μ is the sample mean, and finding the MLE for W is equivalent to performing PCA when $\sigma \to 0$. See also [24].

We here setup the equivalent model under the assumption that $y \in M$ has distribution $y \sim \tilde{X}_1$ resulting from a diffusion (1) in FM with $X_1 = \int_{\text{Diff}}(x, X_\alpha)$ for some $(x, X_\alpha) \in FM$ and with $\tilde{X}_1 = X_1 / \int_M X_1$ the probability distribution resulting from normalizing X_1. The source (x, X_α) of the diffusion is equivalent to the pair (μ, W) in the Euclidean situation. If M has a volume form, for example resulting from a Riemannian metric, we let $p_{(x, X_a)}$ denote the density of $\tilde{X}_1$. Then following [17], we define the log-likelihood

$$\ln \mathcal{L}(x, X_\alpha) = \sum_{i=1}^{N} \ln p_{(x, X_\alpha)}(y_i)$$

of a set of samples $\{y_1, \ldots, y_N\}$, $y \in M$. Maximum likelihood estimation is then a search for $\arg\max_{(x, X_\alpha) \in FM} \ln \mathcal{L}(x, X_\alpha)$. The situation is thus completely analogous to the Euclidean situation the only difference being that the diffusion is performed in FM and projected to M. If M is Euclidean, the PCA result is recovered.[3]

4.1   Likelihood Estimation

Computing the transition probabilities $p_{(x, X_\alpha)}(y_i)$ directly is computationally demanding as it amounts to evaluating the solution of a PDE in the frame

---

[3] In both cases, the representation is not unique because different matrices W/frames X_α can lead to the same diffusion. Instead, the MLE can be specified by the symmetric positive matrix $\Sigma = WW^T$ or, in the manifold situation, be considered an element of the bundle of symmetric positive covariant 2-tensors.

bundle FM. Instead, a simulation approach can be employed [13] or estimates of the mean path among the stochastic paths reaching y_i can be used [17]. Here, we will use the probability of the most probable stochastic paths reaching y_i as an approximation.

The template estimation algorithm is often considered a Fréchet mean estimation, i.e. a minimizer for the geodesic distances $d(x, y_i)^2$. With isotropic covariance, $d(x, y_i)^2$ corresponds the conditional path probability $\tilde{p}_{(x, X_\alpha)}(x_t | x_1 = y_i)$ defined below. We extend this to the situation when X_α defines an anisotropic distribution by making the approximation

$$p_{(x, X_\alpha)}(y_i) \approx \underset{c_t, c_0 = x, c_1 = y_i}{\arg\max} \tilde{p}_{(x, X_\alpha)}(c_t). \tag{2}$$

We will compute the extremizers, the most probable paths, in the next section.

4.2 Metric and Rank

The covariance X_α changes the transition probability and the energy of paths. It does not in general define a new Riemannian metric. As we will see below, it defines a sub-Riemannian metric on FM but this metric does not in general descend to M. The reason being that different paths transport X_α differently to the same point, and a whole distribution of covariances thus lies in the fiber $\pi^{-1}(x)$ of each $x \in M$. A notable exception is if M already has a Riemannian metric g and X_α is unitary in which case the metric does descend to g itself.

This fact also highlights the difference with metric estimation [22] in that the proposed frame estimation does not define a metric. Here, the emphasis is placed on probabilities of paths from a source point in contrast to the symmetric distances arising from a metric.

The model above is described for a full rank $n = \dim M$ frame X_α. The MLE optimization will take place over FM which is $n + n^2$ dimensional. The frame can be replaced by $k < n$ linearly independent vectors, and a full frame can be obtained by adding these to an orthogonal basis arising from a metric g. This corresponds to finding the first k eigenvectors in PCA. We use this computationally less demanding approach for the landmark matching examples.

5 Most Probable Paths

We will here derive flow equations for a formal notion of most probable paths between source and observations under the model. We start by defining the log-probability of observing a path.

In the Euclidean situation, for any finite number of time steps, the sample path increments $\Delta x_{t_i} = x_{t_{i+1}} - x_{t_i}$ of a Euclidean stationary driftless diffusion are normally distributed $\mathcal{N}(0, (\delta t)^{-1} \Sigma)$ with log-probability

$$\ln \tilde{p}_\Sigma(x_t) \propto -\frac{1}{\delta t} \sum_{i=1}^{N-1} \Delta x_{t_i}^T \Sigma^{-1} \Delta x_{t_i} - c_\Sigma.$$

Formally, the log-probability of a differentiable path can in the limit be written

$$\ln \tilde{p}_{\Sigma}(x_t) \propto - \int_0^1 \|\dot{x}_t\|_{\Sigma}^2 dt - c_{\Sigma} \tag{3}$$

with the norm $\| \cdot \|_{\Sigma}$ given by the inner product $\langle v, w \rangle_{\Sigma} = \langle \Sigma^{-1/2} v, \Sigma^{-1/2} w \rangle$. This definition transfers to paths for manifold valued diffusions. Let $(x_t, X_{\alpha,t})$ be a path in FM and recall that $X_{\alpha,t}$ represents $\Sigma^{1/2}$ at x_t. Since $X_{\alpha,t}$ defines an invertible map $\mathbb{R}^n \to T_{x_t} M$ by virtue of being a basis for $T_{x_t} M$, the norm $\| \cdot \|_{\Sigma}$ in (3) has an analogue in the norm $\| \cdot \|_{X_{\alpha,t}}$ defined by the inner product

$$\langle v, w \rangle_{X_{\alpha,t}} = \langle X_{\alpha,t}^{-1} v, X_{\alpha,t}^{-1} w \rangle_{\mathbb{R}^n} \tag{4}$$

for vectors $v, w \in T_{x_t} M$. The norm defines a corresponding path density $\tilde{p}_{(x,X_\alpha)}(x_t)$. The transport of the frame in effect defines a transport of inner product along the sample paths: the paths carry with them the inner product defined by the covariance $X_{\alpha,0}$ at x_0. Because $X_{\alpha,t}$ is parallel transported, the derivative of the inner product by means of the connection is zero. If M has a Riemannian metric g and $X_{\alpha,0}$ is an orthonormal basis, the new inner product will be exactly g. The difference arise when $X_{\alpha,0}$ is anisotropic.

The Onsager-Machlup functional [3] for most probable paths on manifolds differ from (4) in including a scalar curvature correction term. Defining the path density using (4) corresponds to defining the probability of a curve through its anti-development in $\mathbb{R}^n$. In [1], the relation between the two notions is made precise for heat diffusions. Taking the maximum of (3) gives a formal interpretation of geodesics as most probable paths for the pull-back path density of the stochastic development when Σ is unitary. We here proceed using (4) without the scalar correction term.

5.1   Flow Equations

Recall that geodesic paths for a Riemannian metric g are locally length and energy minimizing, and they satisfy the flow equation $\ddot{x}_t^k + \Gamma_{ij}^k \dot{x}_t^i \dot{x}_t^j = 0$. The super and subscripts indicate coordinates in a coordinate chart, and the Einstein summation convention implies a sum over repeated indices. We are interested in computing the most probable paths between points $x, y \in M$, i.e. the mode of the density $\tilde{p}_{(x,X_\alpha)}(x_t)$ where (x, X_α) is the starting point of a diffusion (1). By (3) and (4), this corresponds to finding minimal paths of the norm $\| \cdot \|_{X_{\alpha,t}}$, i.e. minimizers

$$x_t = \underset{c_t, c_0 = x, c_1 = y}{\arg \min} \int_0^1 \|\dot{c}_t\|_{X_{\alpha,t}}^2 dt. \tag{5}$$

This turns out to be an optimal control problem with nonholonomic constraints [19]. The problem can be approached by using the horizontal lift between tangent vectors in $T_{x_t} M$ and curves in $H_{(x_t, X_{\alpha,t})} FM$ coming from the map π_*: For vectors $\tilde{v}, \tilde{w} \in H_{(x_t, X_{\alpha,t})} FM$, the inner product $\langle v, w \rangle_{X_{\alpha,t}}$ lifts to the inner product

$$\langle \tilde{v}, \tilde{w} \rangle_{HFM} = \langle X_{\alpha,t}^{-1} \pi_*(\tilde{v}), X_{\alpha,t}^{-1} \pi_*(\tilde{w}) \rangle_{\mathbb{R}^n}$$

on $H_{(x_t, X_{\alpha,t})} FM$. This defines a (non bracket-generating) sub-Riemannian metric on TFM that we denote G, and (5) is equivalent to solving

$$(x_t, X_{\alpha,t}) = \underset{(c_t, C_{\alpha,t}), c_0 = x, c_1 = y}{\arg\min} \int_0^1 \|(\dot{c}_t, \dot{C}_{\alpha,t})\|_{HFM}^2 dt, \ (\dot{c}_t, \dot{C}_{\alpha,t}) \in H_{(c_t, C_{\alpha,t})} FM.$$
(6)

The requirement on the frame part $\dot{C}_{\alpha,t}$ to be horizontal is the nonholonomic constraint. Solutions of (6) are sub-Riemannian geodesics. Sub-Riemannian geodesics satisfy the Hamilton-Jacobi equations [19]

$$\dot{y}_t^k = G^{kj}(y_t)\xi_{t,j}, \quad \dot{\xi}_{t,k} = -\frac{1}{2}\frac{\partial G^{pq}}{\partial y^k}\xi_{t,p}\xi_{t,q}$$
(7)

similar to the geodesic equations for a Riemannian metric. In our case, y_t will be points in the frame bundle $y_t = (x_t, X_{\alpha,t})$ and $\xi_t \in T^*FM$ are covectors or momenta. Just as the geodesic equations can be written using a coordinate chart $(x^1, \ldots, x^n)$, the Hamilton-Jacobi equations have concrete expressions in coordinate charts. The first part of the system is in our case

$$\dot{x}^i = W^{ij}\xi_j - W^{ih}\Gamma_h^{j\beta}\xi_{j\beta}, \quad \dot{X}_\alpha^i = -\Gamma_h^{i\alpha}W^{hj}\xi_j + \Gamma_k^{i\alpha}W^{kh}\Gamma_h^{j\beta}\xi_{j\beta}$$
(8)

where (x^i) are coordinates on M, X_α^i are coordinates for the frame X_α, and $\Gamma_h^{i\alpha}$ are the Christoffel symbols following the notation of [12]. The matrix W encodes the inner product in coordinates by $W^{kl} = \delta^{\alpha\beta}X_\alpha^k X_\beta^l$. The corresponding equations for $(\xi_{i,t}, \xi_{i_\alpha,t})$ are

$$\dot{\xi}^i = W^{hl}\Gamma_{l,i}^{k\delta}\xi_h\xi_{k\delta} - \frac{1}{2}\left(\Gamma_{k,i}^{h\gamma}W^{kh}\Gamma_h^{k\delta} + \Gamma_k^{h\gamma}W^{kh}\Gamma_{h,i}^{k\delta}\right)\xi_{h\gamma}\xi_{k\delta}$$

$$\dot{\xi}^{i_\alpha} = \Gamma_{k,i_\alpha}^{h\gamma}W^{kh}\Gamma_h^{k\delta}\xi_{h\gamma}\xi_{k\delta} - \left(W^{hl}{}_{,i_\alpha}\Gamma_l^{k\delta} + W^{hl}\Gamma_{l,i_\alpha}^{k\delta}\right)\xi_h\xi_{k\delta}$$
(9)

$$\qquad - \frac{1}{2}\left(W^{hk}{}_{,i_\alpha}\xi_h\xi_k + \Gamma_k^{h\gamma}W^{kh}{}_{,i_\alpha}\Gamma_h^{k\delta}\xi_{h\gamma}\xi_{k\delta}\right)$$

where $\Gamma_{l,i}^{k\delta}$ denotes derivatives of the Christoffel symbols with respect to the ith component. We denote the concrete form (8), (9) of the Hamilton-Jacobi Equations (7) for MPP equations.

Note that while the geodesic equations depend on $2n$ initial conditions, the flow equations for the most probable paths dependent on $2(n+n^2)$ initial conditions. The first n encode the starting position on the manifold and the next n^2 the starting frame. The remaining $n + n^2$ coordinates for the momentum allows the paths to "twist" more freely than geodesics as we will see in the experiments section. Alternatively, a system of size $2(n + kn)$ can be obtained using the low-rank approach described above resulting in reduced computational cost.

6   Experiments

The aim of the following experiments is to both visualize the nature of the most probable paths and how they depend on the initial covariance of the diffusion

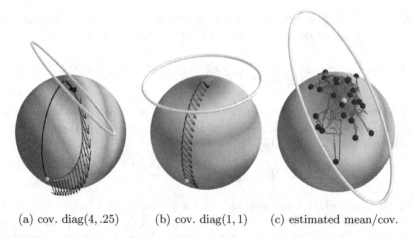

(a) cov. diag(4, .25)   (b) cov. diag(1, 1)   (c) estimated mean/cov.

Fig. 2. Diffusions on the sphere $\mathbb{S}^2$ with different covariances. Compare with Fig. 1 (a). (a,b) The MPPs are geodesics only with isotropic covariance, and they deviate from geodesics with increasing anisotropy. (c) Estimated mean (yellow dot) from samples (black) with stochastic paths (thin, gray) and MPPs (thick, lighter gray). Ellipsis shows the estimated covariance. Surfaces are colored by estimated densities (color figure online).

and to show that the framework can be applied on a manifold that is widely used in medical imaging. We perform experiments on the sphere to satisfy the first goal, and we implement the MPP equations for the finite dimensional manifold used for LDDMM landmark matching for the second goal. The code and scripts for producing the figures is available at http://github.com/stefansommer/dpca.

6.1   Sphere

In the Figs. 1 and 2, we visualize the difference between MPPs and geodesics on the 2-sphere $\mathbb{S}^2$. The computations are performed in coordinates using the stereographic projection, and the MPP equations (8), (9) are numerically integrated. Optimization for finding MPPs between points and for finding the MLE template and covariance below is performed using a standard `scipy` optimizer. The figures clearly show how the MPPs deviate from being geodesic as the covariance increases. In the isotropic case, the curve is geodesic as expected.

Figure 2 (c) shows 24 points sampled from a diffusion with anisotropic covariance. The samples arise as endpoints of stochastic paths. We perform MLE of the most likely mean x and covariance represented by a frame X_α at x. The figure shows the sample paths together with the MPPs under the model determined by the MLE. The difference between the estimated and true covariance is $< 5\%$.

6.2   Landmarks

The landmark matching problem [7] consists in finding paths ϕ_t of diffeomorphisms of a domain Ω that move finite sets of landmarks $(p_1, \ldots, p_m)$ to different

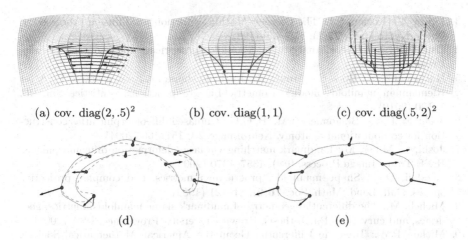

(a) cov. diag$(2, .5)^2$ (b) cov. diag$(1, 1)$ (c) cov. diag$(.5, 2)^2$

(d)   (e)

Fig. 3. Anisotropic matching and mean/covar. estimation on the LDDMM landmark manifold. The differences between the optimal paths (black curves) for the upper row matching problem is a result of anisotropy. Arrows show the covariance frame X_α. Subfigure (d) shows the MPP that move one of the ten corpora callosa into correspondence with the estimated mean (e). Arrows show the estimated major variance direction that corresponds to the Euclidean first PCA eigenvector.

sets of landmarks $(q_1, \ldots, q_m)$ through the action $\phi_t \cdot p = (\phi(p_1), \ldots, \phi(p_m))$. Given a metric on Diff$(\Omega)$, the problem reduces to finding geodesics on a finite dimensional manifold Q of point positions [23]. We will show examples of landmark geodesics and MPPs, and we will show how mean shape and covariance can be estimated on a dataset of outlines of corpora callosa.

Here, $Q = (x_1^1, x_1^2, \ldots, x_m^1, x_m^2)$ has metric $g(v, w) = \sum_{i,j=1}^m v K^{-1}(x_i, x_j) w$ where K^{-1} is the inverse of the matrix $K_j^i = K(x_i, x_j)$ of the Gaussian kernel The Christoffel symbols for this metric are derived in [9].

Figure 3, upper row, shows three examples of matching two landmarks with fixed anisotropic covariance (a,c) and the geodesic isotropic case (b). The frame X_α is displayed with arrows on (a,c). The anisotropy allows less costly movement in the horizontal direction (a) and vertical direction (c) resulting in different optimal paths. In Fig. 3, lower row, the result of template estimation on a set of ten outlines of corpora callosa represented by landmarks is shown. The landmarks are sampled along the outlines, and the MLE for the mean and major variance direction is found (e). Subfigure (d) shows the MPP that move one of the shapes towards the mean, and the major variance vector is displayed by arrows on the shapes.

References

1. Andersson, L., Driver, B.K.: Finite dimensional approximations to wiener measure and path integral formulas on manifolds. J. Funct. Anal. **165**(2), 430–498 (1999)
2. Fletcher, P., Lu, C., Pizer, S., Joshi, S.: Principal geodesic analysis for the study of nonlinear statistics of shape. IEEE Trans. Med. Imaging **23**(8), 995–1005 (2004)

3. Fujita, T., Kotani, S.I.: The Onsager-Machlup function for diffusion processes. J. Math. Kyoto Univ. **22**(1), 115–130 (1982)
4. Hsu, E.P.: Stochastic Analysis on Manifolds. American Mathematical Society, Providence (2002)
5. Huckemann, S., Hotz, T., Munk, A.: Intrinsic shape analysis: geodesic PCA for Riemannian manifolds modulo isometric Lie group actions. Statistica Sin. **20**, 1–100 (2010)
6. Joshi, S., Davis, B., Jomier, B.M., B, G.G.: Unbiased diffeomorphic atlas construction for computational anatomy. NeuroImage **23**, 151–160 (2004)
7. Joshi, S., Miller, M.: Landmark matching via large deformation diffeomorphisms. IEEE Trans. Image Process. **9**(8), 1357–1370 (2000)
8. Kendall, D.G.: Shape manifolds, procrustean metrics, and complex projective spaces. Bull. Lond. Math. Soc. **16**(2), 81–121 (1984)
9. Micheli, M.: The differential geometry of landmark shape manifolds: metrics, geodesics, and curvature. Ph.D. thesis, Brown University, Providence, USA (2008)
10. Michor, P.W.: Topics in Differential Geometry. American Mathematical Society, Providence (2008)
11. Michor, P.W., Mumford, D.: Riemannian geometries on spaces of plane curves. J. Eur. Math. Soc. **8**, 1–48 (2004)
12. Mok, K.P.: On the differential geometry of frame bundles of Riemannian manifolds. J. Fur Die Reine Angew. Math. **1978**(302), 16–31 (1978)
13. Nye, T.: Construction of distributions on Tree-Space via diffusion processes. Mathematisches Forschungsinstitut Oberwolfach (2014). http://www.mfo.de/document/1440a/preliminary_OWR_2014_44.pdf
14. Pennec, X.: Intrinsic statistics on Riemannian manifolds: basic tools for geometric measurements. J. Math. imaging Vis. **25**(1), 127–154 (2006)
15. Siddiqi, K., Pizer, S.: Medial Representations: Mathematics, Algorithms and Applications. Computational Imaging and Vision, 1st edn. Springer, Heidelberg (2008)
16. Sommer, S.: Horizontal dimensionality reduction and iterated frame bundle development. In: Nielsen, F., Barbaresco, F. (eds.) GSI 2013. LNCS, vol. 8085, pp. 76–83. Springer, Heidelberg (2013)
17. Sommer, S.: Diffusion processes and PCA on manifolds. Mathematisches Forschungsinstitut Oberwolfach (2014). http://www.mfo.de/document/1440a/preliminary_OWR_2014_44.pdf
18. Sommer, S., Lauze, F., Hauberg, S., Nielsen, M.: Manifold valued statistics, exact principal geodesic analysis and the effect of linear approximations. In: Daniilidis, K., Maragos, P., Paragios, N. (eds.) ECCV 2010, Part VI. LNCS, vol. 6316, pp. 43–56. Springer, Heidelberg (2010)
19. Strichartz, R.S.: Sub-Riemannian geometry. J. Differ. Geom. **24**(2), 221–263 (1986). http://projecteuclid.org/euclid.jdg/1214440436
20. Tipping, M.E., Bishop, C.M.: Probabilistic principal component analysis. J. Roy. Stat. Soc. B **61**(3), 611–622 (1999)
21. Vaillant, M., Miller, M., Younes, L., Trouv, A.: Statistics on diffeomorphisms via tangent space representations. NeuroImage **23**(Supplement 1), S161–S169 (2004)
22. Vialard, F.-X., Risser, L.: Spatially-varying metric learning for diffeomorphic image registration: a variational framework. In: Golland, P., Hata, N., Barillot, C., Hornegger, J., Howe, R. (eds.) MICCAI 2014, Part I. LNCS, vol. 8673, pp. 227–234. Springer, Heidelberg (2014)
23. Younes, L.: Shapes and Diffeomorphisms. Springer, Heidelberg (2010)
24. Zhang, M., Fletcher, P.: Probabilistic principal geodesic analysis. In: NIPS, pp. 1178–1186 (2013)

A Riemannian Framework for Intrinsic Comparison of Closed Genus-Zero Shapes

Boris A. Gutman[1,2](✉), P. Thomas Fletcher[3], M. Jorge Cardoso[2],
Greg M. Fleishman[1], Marco Lorenzi[2], Paul M. Thompson[1],
and Sebastien Ourselin[2]

[1] Imaging Genetics Center, INI,
University of Southern California, Los Angeles, USA
bgutman@gmail.com
[2] Center for Medical Image Computing,
University College London, London, UK
[3] School of Computing, University of Utah, Salt Lake City, USA

Abstract. We present a framework for intrinsic comparison of surface metric structures and curvatures. This work parallels the work of Kurtek et al. on parameterization-invariant comparison of genus zero shapes. Here, instead of comparing the embedding of spherically parameterized surfaces in space, we focus on the first fundamental form. To ensure that the distance on spherical metric tensor fields is invariant to parameterization, we apply the conjugation-invariant metric arising from the L^2 norm on symmetric positive definite matrices. As a reparameterization changes the metric tensor by a congruent Jacobian transform, this metric perfectly suits our purpose. The result is an intrinsic comparison of shape metric structure that does not depend on the specifics of a spherical mapping. Further, when restricted to tensors of fixed volume form, the manifold of metric tensor fields and its quotient of the group of unitary diffeomorphisms becomes a proper metric manifold that is geodesically complete. Exploiting this fact, and augmenting the metric with analogous metrics on curvatures, we derive a complete Riemannian framework for shape comparison and reconstruction. A by-product of our framework is a near-iso-metric and curvature-preserving mapping between surfaces. The correspondence is optimized using the fast spherical fluid algorithm. We validate our framework using several subcortical boundary surface models from the ADNI dataset.

Keywords: Shape analysis · Riemannian metric · Surface registration · Cortical surface

1 Introduction

Analysis of surfaces plays an important role in medical image processing. Surfaces representing boundaries of functionally and structurally distinct regions, such as the cortex and subcortical structures, can be locally analyzed and compared in lieu of full volumetric analysis. Succinct and easily visualized, such a representation offers tremendous power for morphometric analysis. However, the non-Euclidean nature of surface geometry significantly complicates this approach compared to volume-based methods.

© Springer International Publishing Switzerland 2015
S. Ourselin et al. (Eds.): IPMI 2015, LNCS 9123, pp. 205–218, 2015.
DOI: 10.1007/978-3-319-19992-4_16

A number of computational tools for surface analysis have been developed. Gu et al., developed a conformal mapping algorithm [1] for spherical mapping and formulated a landmark-matching energy as a Mobius transform. A relaxation of the conformal energy, the quasi-conformal mapping of Zeng et al. [2] simultaneously solves the Beltrami equations and minimizes curvature mismatch. Shi et al. [3] applies fluid registration to the flat 2D domain after conformally mapping a surface with prescribed boundaries. Spherical Demons [4], a less straightforward adaptation of a Euclidean registration algorithm, applies the diffeomorphic demons algorithm [5] to the sphere, matching curvature-derived intensity functions to match sulcal patterns of the cortex. A similar approach is taken [6], adapting fluid registration [7] to the sphere. Yet another family of algorithms computes high-dimensional embeddings of surfaces based on eigenfunctions of the Laplace-Beltrami operator [8]. This elegant approach locally adapts the metric tensor by scaling in order to more closely match the embeddings of two surfaces in the Euclidean sense.

Many of these methods produce reasonable and often quite good results for a wide range of problems. The "missing link" in much of the work above is the restriction of the problem to registration. Once the surfaces are registered it is not generally possible to know how one of the surfaces may develop to become the other, or how further deformation in the same direction may look. Comparison of surfaces is out of sync with the spatial alignment procedure, either using local setting-specific features, such as cortical thickness or radial distance, or applying deformation-based analysis after the registration step. An example the latter is surface Tensor-Based Morphometry (shape TBM) [9]. With this in mind, it is clear that a framework unifying surface registration, comparison, and reconstruction is ultimately desired.

In some sense, the "holy grail" of morphometric analysis of any kind that addresses the issue above is the development of a Riemannian manifold with non-vanishing geodesics. Developing the appropriate Riemannian metric for one's object of interest, such as curves, surfaces, or deformation fields, immediately allows the application of various tools from the Riemannian machinery. Examples of these tools include computing manifold statistics, geodesic shooting and parallel transport of velocities for predicting longitudinal change, etc. [10–12]. Well-known examples of Riemannian manifold structures in medical imaging have been developed for the space of diffeomorphisms (LDDMM) [13], curves in $\mathbb{R}^n$ [14], as well as surface embeddings [15, 16] and diffusion tensors [12]. Reference [17] applies the large deformation framework to compute distances between surfaces as the length of the path in the space of diffeomorphism resulting from morphing one boundary onto another. An improvement on this is suggested in [15], measuring distances on the deformation of the surface itself rather than in the ambient space as done in [17]. Closer still to our work here, Kurtek et al. [16] developed a Riemannian framework for surfaces of spherical topology, using "q-map" representation. The L^2 distance on q-maps, or simply the surface embedding locally weighted by the square root of the volume form, is shown to be invariant under spherical automorphisms. From this, a definition of a path length is developed, encapsulating the degree of spatial deformation between surfaces up to rotation and spherical remapping of one surface over the other. A path-straightening algorithm explicitly parameterized in time is then implemented, allowing both geodesic computation and interpolation. The beauty of this Riemannian approach lies in the ability to directly reconstruct the surface from the representation, which is not found in the surface-based methods discussed above. However, the representation is still of the surface *embedding*, with all the resulting nuisances. To overcome this, some standard heuristics are applied to the initial surfaces, namely centering each shape at the origin. Thus, a local change in the surface has a global effect on the representation. More importantly, the approach applies to the space S of smooth functions from the 2-sphere to $\mathbb{R}^n$, without any regard for the intrinsic metric structure of the surface. One undesirable effect of this is that the resulting geodesics may enter regions of S corresponding to surfaces with unrealistically severe metric distortion.

Hoping to avoid these confounds, we instead begin with the notion of intrinsic surface representation that is already invariant to nuisance parameters such as Euclidean motion, while capturing the metric structure. Our ultimate goal is a metric space on a complete surface representation. By "complete," we mean a representation from which a surface can be reconstructed uniquely up to initialization parameters. In general, the ability to reconstruct the object from the representation is not guaranteed, as some of the examples of Riemannian settings above show.

A basic result from surface geometry, the Fundamental Theorem of Surfaces states that a surface can be uniquely represented up to Euclidean motion with two smooth symmetric tensor fields satisfying certain integrability. With the additional constraint that the first of the tensor fields is positive definite, a surface can be reconstructed given an initial frame. The first of these fields is the Riemannian metric tensor on the surface g_{ij}, while the second is the Second Fundamental Form *II*, or "shape tensor." In this work, we mainly focus on the metric tensor. To develop a distance on metric tensors of surfaces, we turn to the work of Ebin [18] and others [19, 20] who have developed a Riemannian framework for the general manifold of metrics tensors. Applying the results to our case – pullback metrics on the 2-sphere induced from the mapped surfaces – we develop a parameterization-invariant comparison of surface metric structures. We show how this measure can be extended to be a metric, when the metric tensor space is restricted to a sub-manifold of fixed-form metrics. Augmenting this distance with metrics on curvatures, we develop a complete representation for surfaces of spherical topology. We apply our method to several brain structures. We show that our method leads to an equiareal mapping between surfaces that is as-conformal-as-possible.

2   A Riemannian Metric on the Space of Metric Tensors

Given an n-dimensional manifold M, the space of all smooth symmetric tensor fields $\Sigma(M) = \{h : TM \times TM \to \mathbb{R} | h \,\varepsilon\, Sym(n)\}$ and the subspace of Σ of positive definite tensors $\mathcal{M}(M) = \{h : TM \times TM \to \mathbb{R} | h \in SPD(n)\}$, our problem above can be restated generally as finding a suitable metric on $\mathcal{M}$, such that the group of diffeomorphisms on M acts on $\mathcal{M}$ by isometry. Ebin et al. [18] showed that the L^2 Riemannian metric on the tangent bundle of $\mathcal{M}$, each fiber of which is identified with Σ, indeed satisfies this criteria: given $g \in \mathcal{M}, h, k \in \Sigma \cong T_g \mathcal{M}$, the metric can be written as:

$$(h, k)_g = \int_M \langle h, k \rangle_g d\mu_g, \tag{1}$$

where $\langle h, k \rangle_g$ is the inner product induced by g, $\langle h, k \rangle_g = tr(g^{-1}hg^{-1}k)$, and μ_g is the volume form also induced by g. This metric produces geodesics on $\mathcal{M}$ whose length can be computed point-wise and in closed form. In other words, a geodesic on $\mathcal{M}$ is a one-parameter family of metrics g_t on M, with the tensor at a point $x \in M$, $g(x)$ depending only on $g_0(x)$ and $g_0'(x)$. Applying these results to our concrete case, we take M to be the 2-sphere $\mathbb{S}^2$, and consider the space of metrics pulled back from spherically parameterized surfaces $S = \{S : \mathbb{S}^2 \to \mathbb{R}^3 | S \in C^\infty\}$, expressed in canonical coordinates on $T\mathbb{S}^2$ as $g_{i,j} = S_i^T S_j$. We illustrate an example of this representation in Fig. 1. A reparameterization $\varphi \in \Phi = \{\phi : \mathbb{S}^2 \to \mathbb{S}^2 | \phi, \phi^{-1} \in C^2\}$ acts on g by conjugation with the pushforward (Jacobian) $D\varphi : T_x\mathbb{S}^2 \to T_{\varphi(x)}\mathbb{S}^2$, $\varphi \circ g = D\varphi^T g D\varphi$. Given two parameterized surfaces $A, B \in S$, a closed-form solution for the geodesic distance between g_A and g_B at a point x is [21]

$$D(g_A[x], g_B[x]) = \sqrt{\int_0^1 \langle g_t'(x), g_t'(x) \rangle_{g_{t(x)}} dt} = \left\| \mathrm{Log}\left[g_A^{-1/2} g_B g_A^{-1/2} \right] \right\|_F. \tag{2}$$

This metric is indeed invariant under simultaneous spherical re-mappings of A and B, since $D(g_A, g_B) = D(D\varphi^T g_A D\varphi, D\varphi^T g_B D\varphi)$. These results are derived in [21].

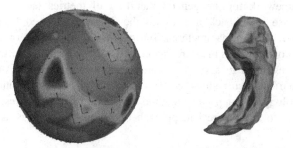

Fig. 1. Metric tensor fields and mean curvature – a nearly complete surface representation. Tensors are displayed as their eigenvectors in $T\mathbb{S}^2$ with magnitude corresponding to the eigenvalues. If Gaussian curvature (not shown) is also known, the information on the left is sufficient to reconstruct the hippocampal surface on the right.

3   Parameterization-Invariant Metric Tensor Comparison

While the measure above is pointwise-invariant to conjugation, integrating the expression following (1) does not in fact le to a measure that is invariant. This is due to the changing volume form in (1). As we will see, a trade-off must be made between three desirable properties of a shape comparison measure: **1.** Invariance under actions by Φ; **2.** Point-wise independence; **3.** Metric property. Only two of these three properties can be satisfied simultaneously on $\mathcal{M}$. The first of these is crucial for intrinsic shape comparison, for if it fails to hold, the measure is subject to the arbitrary nature of an initial spherical parameterization. The third property can be useful for all the reasons described in the introduction, such as computing intrinsic means and transporting trajectories. The second property is attractive for the ease of computation it implies: the problem reduces to minimizing the integral of the pointwise measures over M. For now, we choose to preserve the first two properties. This requires us to modify the volume form on $\mathbb{S}^2$ to be symmetric with respect to A and B, and independent of the spherical mapping. We define our measure as

$$P(A,B) = \int_{\mathbb{S}^2} \left\| \mathrm{Log}\left[g_A^{-1/2} g_B g_A^{-1/2} \right] \right\|_F^2 [det(g_A)det(g_B)]^{1/4} d\mathbb{S}^2 \qquad (3)$$

The volume form $[det(g_A)det(g_B)]^{1/4} d\mathbb{S}^2$ remains unchanged after a re-mapping $[det(g_A^{\varphi})det(g_B^{\varphi})]^{1/4} df(\mathbb{S}^2) = [det(g_A)det(g_B)]^{1/4} det(D\varphi)d\mathbb{S}^2 \det(D\varphi^{-1}) = [det(g_A) det(g_B)]^{1/4} d\mathbb{S}^2$. Together with the result from the previous section, this shows that $P(\varphi \circ A, \varphi \circ B) = P(A,B)$. Finding the global minimum of P by re-parameterizing one surface over the other, we obtain a comparison between the two surfaces' metric structures that is independent of parameterization and therefore intrinsic:

$$P^*(A,B) = \min_{\varphi \in \Phi} P(A, \varphi \circ B), A, B \in \mathcal{S}. \qquad (4)$$

The measure above is appealing: it leads to a mapping between two surfaces that minimizes metric distortion with a mixture of equiareal and conformal mapping between the surfaces. The minimization reduces to a standard registration problem over spherical automorphisms, with the cost function (3). Further, the mapping between the two surfaces retains its metric-preserving property regardless of the initial spherical mapping: here the sphere is a "dummy space," only needed as a standard canonical space for computational convenience. However, we cannot say that $P^*(A,B)$ is a metric.

4 Metrics on $M_\mu \backslash \Phi_U$ and on the Space of Surfaces

The change in the volume form due to reparameterization prevents a straightforward generalization of $(\cdot, \cdot)_g$. To the quotient space $\mathcal{M}\backslash\Phi$. This is the reason for the breakdown in the metric property of the measure $P^*(A,B)$. However, the submanifold $\mathcal{M}_\mu$ of metrics which correspond to a fixed measure μ admits this generalization. $\mathcal{M}_\mu$ is a metric space under $(\cdot, \cdot)_g$, with the geodesic distance defined as usual: $d(g_A, g_B) = \min_{g_0 = g_A, g_1 = g_B} \sqrt{\int_0^1 (g_t', g_t')_{g_t} dt}$. Taking its quotient by the appropriate restriction of Φ to maps with a unitary pushforward $\Phi_U = \{\phi \in \Phi | det(D\phi) = 1\}$, we see that $\mathcal{M}_\mu \backslash \Phi_U$ is also a metric space under the related metric

$$d^*(g_A, g_B) = \min_{\phi_t \in \{\varphi_t : [0,1] \to \Phi_U\}} d(g_A, \phi_t \circ g_B)$$

$$= \min_{\substack{g_0 = g_A, g_1 = g_B \\ \phi_t \in \{\varphi_t : [0,1] \to \Phi_U\}}} \sqrt{\int_0^1 \left(g_t'(\phi_t), g_t'(\phi_t) \right)_{g_t} dt} \quad (5)$$

Further, it is known that $\mathcal{M}_\mu \backslash \Phi_U$ is geodesically complete [19], i.e. the exponential map is defined on the entire tangent space. In particular, this means that geodesic shooting is possible following transport of any velocity between any pair of points on $\mathcal{M}_\mu \backslash \Phi_U$. The obvious choice for a concrete example of $\mathcal{M}_\mu$ is the set of metrics arising from area-preserving spherical maps, i.e. $\mathcal{S}_m = \{ S \in \mathcal{S} | det(g_S) = m \}$ for some constant m. Ensuring scale invariance, we further restrict $\mathcal{S}_m$ to $\mathcal{S}_1$ by rescaling surfaces to have area 4π.

Restricting the space of allowable parameterizations to $\mathcal{S}_1$ may seem like a high price to pay for the ability to use the Riemannian machinery. Yet, it is least restrictive among the three standard parameterizations: conformal, Tuette and equiareal. The genus-zero conformal mapping, for example, only has six degrees of freedom, while the Tuette energy has a unique minimum [1]. The registration arising from this restriction is an equiareal mapping that is as-conformal-as-possible. Thus, we can still expect the resulting registration to approximate near-isometric maps, though perhaps not as well as an unconstrained optimization of $P^*(A, B)$. A generic path between two points g_A, g_B on $\mathcal{M}(\mathcal{S}_1) \backslash \Phi_U$ may be parameterized at a point on $\mathbb{S}^2$ using a family of diffeomorphisms $\phi_t \in \{ \varphi_t : [0,1] \to \Phi_U \}$ as

$$g_t(\phi_t) = g_A^{1/2} e^{t \text{Log} \left[g_A^{-1/2} D\phi_t^T (\phi_t \circ g_B) D\phi_t g_A^{-1/2} \right]} g_A^{1/2}.$$

The velocity takes the form

$$g_t'(\phi_t) = g_A^{1/2} \left(\int_0^1 e^{\alpha t S(t)} [S(t) + t S'(t)] e^{(1-\alpha)t S(t)} d\alpha \right) g_A^{1/2},$$

$$S(t) = \text{Log} \left[g_A^{-1/2} D\phi_t^T (\phi_t \circ g_B) D\phi_t g_A^{-1/2} \right].$$

The geodesic path length can then be written as

$$\mathfrak{D}^*(A, B) = d^*(g_A, g_B), A, B \in \mathcal{S}_1$$

In general, the fact that Φ_U acts on $\mathcal{M}_\mu$ by isometry does not imply that ϕ_t is stationary, i.e. $\phi_t' \neq 0$ [19]. Nevertheless, this simplifying assumption leads to a far more tractable problem. Indeed, the authors in [16] implicitly make the same assumption. With this simplification at ha, we write our intrinsic metric on the metric structures of genus-zero shapes as

$$\mathfrak{D}(A, B) = \min_{\varphi \in \Phi_U} P(A, \varphi \circ B), A, B \in \mathcal{S}_1 \quad (6)$$

The metric $\mathfrak{D}(A, B)$ allows us to compute intrinsic distances between metric structures of surfaces of spherical topology. Yet, the metric structures alone do not represent surfaces uniquely. As a simple example, an inflated and a deflated tennis ball have zero distance between them on $\{\mathcal{M}(\mathcal{S}_1)\backslash\Phi_U, \mathfrak{D}(\cdot, \cdot)\}$. To achieve a unique representation, curvature information must be invoked. In principle, any surface can be reconstructed locally given an initial coordinate frame, if g and $II = n^T S_{ij}$ are known [22]. The last term is the shape tensor in local coordinates, where n is the surface normal. The reconstruction can be done following two integrations, so long as the Gauss-Codazzi equations are satisfied:

$$L_2 - M_1 = L\Gamma_{12}^1 + M(\Gamma_{12}^2 - \Gamma_{11}^1) - N\Gamma_{11}^2$$
$$-N_1 + M_2 = L\Gamma_{22}^1 + M(\Gamma_{22}^2 - \Gamma_{12}^1) - N\Gamma_{12}^2, \tag{7}$$

where the shape tensor is expressed explicitly as $II = \begin{pmatrix} L & M \\ M & N \end{pmatrix}$, and Γ_{ij}^k are the Christoffel symbols. Given a global parameterization with spherical boundary conditions, we can derive II using (7) from the mean and Gaussian curvature only, $H = tr(\vartheta)/2, K = det(\vartheta)$, where the shape operator $\vartheta = IIg^{-1}$. Several approaches are possible, including explicitly solving (7) numerically. A simpler approach [23] solves for the normal curvatures from H, K, and fits ϑ locally by solving a least squares problem; the shape tensor can then be computed as $II = \vartheta g$. The implication is that we only need to define a distance on two scalar quantities in addition to g. Because H, K are invariant to parameterization, L^2 distances on fields of curvatures on $\mathbb{S}^2$ are trivially invariant to action by Φ_U. We then define our genus-zero shape metric as the 1-product metric on $\mathfrak{S} = \{\mathcal{M}(\mathcal{S}_1) \times C^2(\mathbb{S}^2) \times C^2(\mathbb{S}^2)\}\backslash\Phi_U$,

$$\mathcal{L}(A, B) = \mathfrak{D}(A, B) + D_{L^2\backslash\Phi_U}(H_A, H_B) + D_{L^2\backslash\Phi_U}(K_A, K_B). \tag{8}$$

Here, $C^2(\mathbb{S}^2) = \{f : \mathbb{S}^2 \to \mathbb{R} | f \in C^2\}$, and the usual L^2 distance modified by Φ_U,

$D_{L^2\backslash\Phi_U}(a, b) = \min_{\phi_t \in \{\varphi_t : [0,1] \to \Phi_U\}} \sqrt{\int_0^1 \int_{\mathbb{S}^2} (a - \phi_t \circ b)^2 d\mathbb{S}^2 dt}$. Given two spherically parameterized surfaces A, B, the geodesic connecting them on $\mathfrak{S}$ can be parameterized explicitly at every point on $\mathbb{S}^2$ as

$$\{g_t, H_t, K_t\} = \{g_t(\phi_t), H_A + t(\phi_t \circ H_B - H_A), K_A + t(\phi_t \circ K_B - K_A)\}, \tag{9}$$

where $\phi_t \in \{\varphi_t : [0, 1] \to \Phi_U\}$ is solution of the optimization problem in (8). Here, as before, we make the simplifying assumption that ϕ_t is stationary.

5   Solving for ϕ with Fluid Registration on $\mathbb{S}^2$

We adapt an optimization approach similar to [6]. Briefly, spherical warps are parameterized by tangential vector fields $u : \mathbb{S}^2 \to T\mathbb{S}^2$, with $\varphi[u(x), x] = x\sqrt{1 - \|u(x)\|^2} - u(x)$, with u, x expressed in ambient $\mathbb{R}^3$ coordinates. The length of the geodesic on $\mathbb{S}^2$ connecting x and $\varphi[u(x), x]$ is the arcsine of $\|u(x)\|$. This parameterization was also used in [4]. The drawback is that warps transferring points more than 90 degrees cannot be modeled. This still allows for very large deformations, while simplifying the computation.

Fluid registration is based on modeling the simplified Navier-Stokes equation $\mu \Delta v(x, t) + (\lambda + \mu) \vec{\nabla} \left(\vec{\nabla} \cdot v(x, t) \right) = -F[\varphi[u(x, t), x]]$. The force field F represents the gradient of the objective function, and λ, μ are Lame coefficients [7]. The time-varying velocity v is integrated explicitly over time to obtain u. In [6], the authors use the material derivative to account for the effect of the Jacobian when updating u by the instantaneous velocity: $\frac{\partial u}{\partial t} = [D\varphi]v$, where $\frac{\partial u}{\partial t}$ is expressed in local coordinates in $T_{\varphi(x)}\mathbb{S}^2$. The pushforward $D\varphi$ connecting local frames at x and $\varphi(x)$ can be computed as $D\varphi = \left[\frac{\partial y}{\partial s}, \frac{\partial y}{\partial t} \right]^T_{y=\varphi(x)} \left[\frac{\partial \varphi}{\partial x} \right] \left[\frac{\partial y}{\partial s}, \frac{\partial y}{\partial t} \right]_{y=x}$, where s, t are local coordinates of tangent spaces, and

$$\frac{\partial \varphi}{\partial x} = I \left(1 - \|u\|^2 \right)^{1/2} - x \left[\left(\frac{\partial u}{\partial x} \right) u \right]^T \left(1 - \|u\|^2 \right)^{-1/2} - \left(\frac{\partial u}{\partial x} \right). \tag{10}$$

Accounting for the non-linearity in the parameterization of φ to update the field u in the Eulerian frame, we must find $u(x, t + \delta t)$ for a small time step δt, so that $\varphi[u(x, t + \delta t), x] = \varphi[u(x, t), x] \sqrt{1 - \left\| \delta t \frac{\partial u}{\partial t} \right\|^2} - \delta t \frac{\partial u}{\partial t}$. This can be done using the cross-product matrix $G(x)$, where $G(x)y = x \times y$, by $u(x, t + \delta t) = G^2 \varphi[u(x, t + \delta t), x]$.

We approximate the solution to the Navier-Stokes equation by filtering the force field with a Gaussian kernel, $v \approx - \mathbf{K}_\sigma * F$, which is a solution of the isotropic diffusion equation $\frac{\partial v}{\partial t} = -\Delta v$, $\sigma = \sqrt{2t}$, where Δ is the spherical *vector* Laplacian. This can be solved efficiently with vector spherical harmonics $\mathbf{B}_{lm}, \mathbf{C}_{lm}$, $\mathbf{K}_\sigma * \mathbf{v}(p) = \sum_{\substack{l=1 \\ |m| \le l}}^{\infty} e^{-l(l+1)\sigma} [\mathbf{B}_{lm} \langle \mathbf{B}_{lm}, \mathbf{v} \rangle + \mathbf{C}_{lm} \langle \mathbf{C}_{lm}, \mathbf{v} \rangle]$. See [6] for details.

The force field F coincides with the direction minimizing the cost function corresponding to the shape metric (8):

$$\mathcal{C}(A, B, u) = P(A, \varphi[u] \circ B) + \int_{\mathbb{S}^2} (H_A - \varphi[u] \circ H_B)^2 + (K_A - \varphi[u] \circ K_B)^2 d\mathbb{S}^2$$
$$+ R \int_{\mathbb{S}^2} (\log det[D\varphi[u]])^2 d\mathbb{S}^2 \tag{11}$$

The second term is simply an L^2 minimization problem, whose gradient is well-known. The last term, ensuring that the remapping φ remains in Φ_U, is similar to a regularization term used in 3D image registration [24]. The first term contains the most novelty; here, we derive its Euler-Lagrange equation. In detail,

$$P(A, \varphi[u] \circ B) = \int_{\mathbb{S}^2} L(\varphi[u, x], x) d\mathbb{S}^2, \quad L = \|LogX(\varphi[u, x], x)\|^2, \tag{12}$$

where $X(\varphi[u,x],x) = g_A^{-1/2}(x)D\phi^T(x)g_B(\varphi[u,x])D\phi(x)g_A^{-1/2}(x)$. Note that we have dropped the determinant terms, as they remain unchanged under Φ_U. For simplicity, we first derive the E-L equations at $u \equiv 0$. Since $\frac{\partial}{\partial t}\|\text{Log}X(t)^2\| = 2tr[\|\text{Log}XX^{-1}\frac{d}{dt}X\|]$, [21] the Lagrangian derivative with respect to u is

$$\frac{\partial L}{\partial u^i} = -2tr\left[\text{Log}X\,X^{-1}g_A^{-1/2}\frac{\partial}{\partial x^i}\{g_B(x)\}g_A^{-1/2}\right]. \qquad (13)$$

We show the second-order terms for the first coordinate only:

$$\frac{\partial L}{\partial\left(\frac{\partial u^1}{\partial x^1}\right)} = -2tr\left[\text{Log}X\,X^{-1}g_A^{-1/2}\begin{pmatrix}2g_{B,11} & g_{B,21}\\ g_{B,21} & 0\end{pmatrix}g_A^{-1/2}\right], \qquad (14)$$

$$\frac{\partial L}{\partial\left(\frac{\partial u^1}{\partial x^2}\right)} = -2tr\left[\text{Log}X\,X^{-1}g_A^{-1/2}\begin{pmatrix}0 & g_{B,11}\\ g_{B,11} & 2g_{B,21}\end{pmatrix}g_A^{-1/2}\right].$$

The expressions for the second coordinate are analogous. The descent direction minimizing $P(A, \varphi[u] \circ B)$ is then

$$F^j = \sum_{i=1}^2 \frac{d}{dx^i}\frac{\partial L}{\partial\left(\frac{\partial u^j}{\partial x^i}\right)} - \frac{\partial L}{\partial u^j}. \qquad (15)$$

In fact, estimates at $u \equiv 0$ are sufficient to perform the entire optimization: we only need to transport the metric fields by the current deformation to compute the gradient at an arbitrary u using (13–15).

6 Implementation Details

6.1 Initialization

We initially compute area-preserving spherical maps using Freidel's robust mapping [6]. We then perform all our computations on a regular spherical grid with direct reference to the original triangle meshing of both the parameterization and the original mesh. We maintain a harmonic bandwidth between 64 and 256, which corresponds to roughly between 16 K and 260 K control points. Due to the local nature of fluid registration, we must have a good initialization. We take an approach similar to [6], performing a coarse global search over the space of rotations to match the curvatures.

6.2 Tensor and Curvature Estimation

In order to compute the metric tensors in local spherical coordinates, we fit a quadratic surface at each regular grid point, but using the original meshing. The fitting is done with respect to all the vertices in the 1-ring of faces around the triangle containing the regular grid point. We then compute g and $\frac{\partial g}{\partial x}$ in local coordinates analytically from the fitted coefficients. At each iteration of the fluid algorithm, the original spherical parameterization of the moving mesh B is brought forward by $p \rightarrow \varphi^{-1}(p)$, and the transformed tensors are computed fresh over the new spherical mesh. We estimate curvatures directly on the original mesh following [23]. Curvature estimates on tri-angle meshes are notoriously noisy, and we apply mild Laplacian smoothing directly on the original mesh to H and K to obtain reasonable estimates. These are then interpolated onto the regular grid.

6.3 Surface Reconstruction

In Sect. 4, we proposed to reconstruct a surface by first solving for the shape tensor. In practice, we take a more direct approach, solving an auxiliary least squares problem based on discrete differential geometry operators [23]. Given a spherical mesh $m = \langle V, E \rangle$, $|x| = 1 \forall x \in V$, and g, H, K defined at each vertex, the mesh representing an embedding in space, $\langle S(V), E \rangle$ minimizes three least-squares problems:

$$E_g = \sum_{x \in V} A(x) \sum_{y \in N_1(x)} \left[(Sx - Sy)^2 - (x - y)^T g(x)(x - y) \right]^2,$$

$$E_H = \sum_{x \in V} A(x) \left(\left\langle \left[\sum_{y \in N_1(x)} \frac{(\cot a_{xy} + \cot b_{xy})(Sx - Sy)}{4A(x)} \right], n \right\rangle - H(x) \right)^2,$$

$$E_K = \sum_{x \in V} A(x) \left(\frac{2\pi - \left[\sum_{y,z \in N_1(x), yz \in E} \cos^{-1} \frac{\langle (Sy-Sx),(Sz-Sx) \rangle}{|(Sy-Sx)||(Sz-Sx)|} \right]}{A(x)} - K(x) \right)^2.$$

Here, n is the surface normal, $A(x)$ is the area element, and a_{xy}, b_{xy} are angles opposite edge xy. On a regular spherical grid, the area element is estimated as $A(x) = \frac{1}{2} det(g)^{\frac{1}{2}} \sin \theta(x) \left(\frac{\pi}{BW} \right)^2$, for bandwidth BW. The initial conditions are set using a single spherical triangle (x, y, z), so that $Sx = 0$, $Sy = \left(\|y - x\|_{g(x)}, 0, 0 \right)$. $Sz = \left(\|z - x\|_{g(x)} \cos \omega, \|z - x\|_{g(x)} \sin \omega, 0 \right)$, $\omega = \cos^{-1} \frac{\langle z-x, y-x \rangle_{g(x)}}{\|z-x\|_{g(x)} \|y-x\|_{g(x)}}$, $\langle p, q \rangle_g = p^T g q$.

7 Experiments

We applied our metric tensor registration to hippocampal and caudate surfaces of 100 Alzheimer's patients (AD) and 100 controls. In addition, we applied our method to a pair of cortical surfaces from different subjects from the same dataset. In all cases, the fluid registration was performed in 3 stages, with the kernel of the vector Gaussian set to $\sigma = 10^{-1}, \sigma = 10^{-2}, \sigma = 10^{-3}$. In general, we found that better overall results are achieved if an additional non-linear registration step is taken before this process, only minimizing curvature mismatch. Overall computation time at $BW = 128$ is on the order of 10 min, requiring 10–100 iterations at each stage.

In the first experiment, we tested the metric-preserving property of our method compared to curvature-only registration. We illustrate with a pair of caudate surfaces in Fig. 2. The angle distortion is far more widespread in the curvature-only case, indicating that the cost function in (11) preserves the metric structure between the two surfaces. Comparing distributions of distortion in hippocampal registration shows the same point. We compared the mean difference between distortion levels of the two registration approaches. Random pairs of subjects' hippocampi were registered, using the entire dataset. Unsurprisingly, the metric distance method lead to significantly lower distortion, t $= -19.9$.

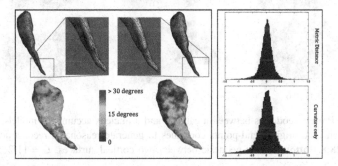

Fig. 2. Left Panel: Metric distortion using only curvature matching (left), and metric tensor registration (right). The top caudate surface is registered to the bottom one. Colors represent absolute angle distortion between the surfaces. **Right Panel:** Distributions of angle distortion in radians for hippocampal surface registration (Color figure online).

To test the reliability of our surface reconstruction method, we computed the geodesics between a surface model of the nucleus accumbens, and a caudate model. While this is certainly not representative of a real application, it is a good test of robustness of our method. Equally reasonable results hold for cortical metric registration. We illustrate the results in Fig. 3.

To examine the usefulness of the shape distance itself, we compared the annual rate of change in hippocampal and caudate shape between AD patients and controls. Shape change was computed as the geodesic length between corresponding surfaces over 1 year. We also made the same comparison using change in hippocampal and caudate volume. Results are displayed in Table 1. It is encouraging to see that shape change in our framework is somewhat more sensitive to disease effects.

Table 1. Rate of change difference between AD and controls: shape and volume.

	Left Hippocampus	Right Hippocampus	Left Caudate	Right Caudate
Shape	$\mathcal{L}_{AD} - \mathcal{L}_{CTL} = 0.81$ $P = 0.0002$	0.92 $P < 0.0001$	0.64 $P = 0.0014$	0.98 $P = 0.0007$
Volume (mm^3)	20.1 $P = 0.001$	23.2 $P < 0.0001$	12.4 $P = 0.027$	11.7 $P = 0.003$

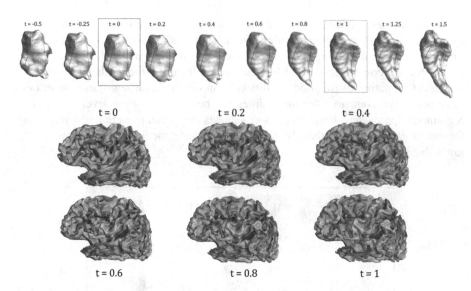

Fig. 3. Top Panel: geodesics between a caudate and a nucleus accumbens models. Extending the path beyond the original end-points continues to generate reasonable reconstructions. Path length $\mathcal{L} = 28.8$ **Bottom Panel:** geodesic between two cortical surfaces. $\mathcal{L} = 11.2$

8 Conclusion

We have presented a Riemannian framework for analyzing metric structures of shapes that are topologically equivalent to the sphere. Our "metric space of metrics" is defined by a conjugation-invariant distance on symmetric (0,2)-tensors. When augmented with metrics on curvature maps, the product space becomes a proper metric space of shapes. Due to computational constraints, we do not optimize our geodesics over the entire set of paths in this space, but restrict the search to paths up to a stationary diffeomorphism. Because our geodesic path lengths can then be computed in closed form, this results in a very efficient algorithm: no path-straightening is required. We show that the geodesic search in our space leads to robust near-isometric and curvature-preserving mapping, with the ability to reconstruct surfaces along the path. Our measure is able to detect disease-related shape change in subcortical structures with greater sensitivity than volume. While we do not consider size and rigid motion in our framework, metrics on affine transformations already exist [25]. These can be joined with the metric presented here for a more complete analysis of objects in space.

References

1. Gu, X., Wang, Y., Chan, T.F., Thompson, P.M., Yau, S.T.: Genus zero surface conformal mapping and its application to brain surface mapping. IEEE Trans. Med. Imaging **23**, 949–958 (2004)

2. Zeng, W., Lui, L.M., Luo, F., Chan, T.F.-C., Yau, S.-T., Gu, D.X.: Computing quasiconformal maps using an auxiliary metric and discrete curvature flow. Numer. Math. **121**, 671–703 (2012)
3. Shi, J., Thompson, P.M., Gutman, B., Wang, Y.: Surface fluid registration of conformal representation: application to detect disease burden and genetic influence on hippocampus. NeuroImage **78**, 111–134 (2013)
4. Yeo, B.T.T., Sabuncu, M.R., Vercauteren, T., Ayache, N., Fischl, B., Golland, P.: Spherical demons: fast diffeomorphic landmark-free surface registration. IEEE Trans. Med Imaging **29**, 650–668 (2010)
5. Vercauteren, T., Pennec, X., Perchant, A., Ayache, N.: Diffeomorphic demons: efficient non-parametric image registration. NeuroImage **45**, S61–S72 (2009)
6. Gutman, B.A., Madsen, S.K., Toga, A.W., Thompson, P.M.: A family of fast spherical registration algorithms for cortical shapes. In: Shen, L., Liu, T., Yap, P.-T., Huang, H., Shen, D., Westin, C-Fk (eds.) MBIA 2013. LNCS, vol. 8159, pp. 246–257. Springer, Heidelberg (2013)
7. Christensen, G.E., Rabbitt, R.D., Miller, M.I.: Deformable templates using large deformation kinematics. IEEE Trans. Med. Imaging **5**, 1435–1447 (1996)
8. Yonggang, S., Rongjie, L., Wang, D.J.J., Pelletier, D., Mohr, D., Sicotte, N., Toga, A.W.: Metric optimization for surface analysis in the Laplace-Beltrami embedding space. IEEE Trans. Med. Imaging **33**, 1447–1463 (2014)
9. Wang, Y., Yuan, L., Shi, J., Greve, A., Ye, J., Toga, A.W., Reiss, A.L., Thompson, P.M.: Applying tensor-based morphometry to parametric surfaces can improve MRI-based disease diagnosis. NeuroImage **74**, 209–230 (2013)
10. Fletcher, P.T., Venkatasubramanian, S., Joshi, S.: The geometric median on Riemannian manifolds with application to robust atlas estimation. NeuroImage **45**, S143–S152 (2009)
11. Joshi, S.H., Joshi, A.A., Gutman, B., Toga, A.W., McMahon, K., De Zubicaray, G., Martin, N., Wright, M.J., Thompson, P.M.: Genetic influences on sulcal patterns of the brain. In: 2012 9th IEEE International Symposium on Biomedical Imaging (ISBI), pp. 414–417 (2012)
12. Fletcher, P.T., Joshi, S.: Riemannian geometry for the statistical analysis of diffusion tensor data. Signal Process. **87**, 250–262 (2007)
13. Miller, M.I., Younes, L.: Group actions, homeomorphisms, and matching: a general framework. Int. J. Comput. Vision **41**, 61–84 (2001)
14. Joshi, S.H., Klassen, E., Srivastava, A., Jermyn, I.: An efficient representation for computing geodesics between n-dimensional elastic shapes. In: Proceedings of IEEE Conference on Computer Vision and Pattern Recognition (2007)
15. Bauer, M., Bruveris, M.: A new Riemannian setting for surface registration. In: 3rd MICCAI Workshop on Mathematical Foundations of Computational Anatomy, pp. 182–194 (2011)
16. Kurtek, S., Klassen, E., Zhaohua, D., Jacobson, S.W., Jacobson, J.B., Avison, M.J., Srivastava, A.: Parameterization-invariant shape comparisons of anatomical surfaces. IEEE Trans. Med. Imaging **30**, 849–858 (2011)
17. Qiu, A., Younes, L., Miller, M.I., Csernansky, J.G.: Parallel transport in diffeomorphisms distinguishes the time-dependent pattern of hippocampal surface deformation due to healthy aging and the dementia of the Alzheimer's type. NeuroImage **40**, 68–76 (2008)
18. Ebin, D.G.: On the space of Riemannian metrics. Bull. Am. Math. Soc. **74**(5), 1001–1003 (1968)
19. Clarke, B.: The metric geometry of the manifold of Riemannian metrics over a closed manifold. Calc. Var. **39**, 533–545 (2010)
20. Bauer, M., Bruveris, M., Michor, P.W.: Overview of the geometries of shape spaces and diffeomorphism groups. J. Math. Imaging Vision **50**, 60–97 (2014)

21. Moakher, M.: A differential geometric approach to the geometric mean of symmetric positive-definite matrices. SIAM J. Matrix Anal. Appl. **26**, 735–747 (2005)
22. Millman, R.S., Parker, G.D.: Elements of Differential Geometry. Prentice-Hall, Englewood Cliffs (1977)
23. Meyer, M., Desbrun, M., Schröder, P., Barr, A.: Discrete differential-geometry operators for triangulated 2-manifolds. In: Hege, H.-C., Polthier, K. (eds.) Visualization and Mathematics III, pp. 35–57. Springer, Heidelberg (2003)
24. Leow, A.D., Yanovsky, I., Chiang, M.C., Lee, A.D., Klunder, A.D., Lu, A., Becker, J.T., Davis, S.W., Toga, A.W., Thompson, P.M.: Statistical properties of Jacobian maps and the realization of unbiased large-deformation nonlinear image registration. IEEE Trans. Med. Imaging **26**, 822–832 (2007)
25. Woods, R.P.: Characterizing volume and surface deformations in an atlas framework: theory, applications, and implementation. NeuroImage **18**(3), 769–788 (2003)

Multi-atlas Fusion

Multi-atlas Segmentation as a Graph Labelling Problem: Application to Partially Annotated Atlas Data

Lisa M. Koch[1]([✉]), Martin Rajchl[1], Tong Tong[1], Jonathan Passerat-Palmbach[1], Paul Aljabar[1,2], and Daniel Rueckert[1]

[1] Biomedical Image Analysis Group, Imperial College London, London, UK
l.koch@imperial.ac.uk
[2] Division of Imaging Sciences and Biomedical Engineering, King's College London, London, UK

Abstract. Manually annotating images for multi-atlas segmentation is an expensive and often limiting factor in reliable automated segmentation of large databases. Segmentation methods requiring only a proportion of each atlas image to be labelled could potentially reduce the workload on expert raters tasked with labelling images. However, exploiting such a database of partially labelled atlases is not possible with state-of-the-art multi-atlas segmentation methods. In this paper we revisit the problem of multi-atlas segmentation and formulate its solution in terms of graph-labelling. Our graphical approach uses a Markov Random Field (MRF) formulation of the problem and constructs a graph connecting atlases and the target image. This provides a unifying framework for label propagation. More importantly, the proposed method can be used for segmentation using only partially labelled atlases. We furthermore provide an extension to an existing continuous MRF optimisation method to solve the proposed problem formulation. We show that the proposed method, applied to hippocampal segmentation of 202 subjects from the ADNI database, remains robust and accurate even when the proportion of manually labelled slices in the atlases is reduced to 20%.

1 Introduction

In recent years, major efforts have been undertaken towards building large medical image databases, e.g. in population studies. As the wealth of data increases, automated segmentation of images becomes crucial while manually annotating them becomes prohibitive. In particular, robust and accurate segmentation techniques relying on minimal manual input become increasingly desirable.

Atlas-based segmentation has proven to be a successful and robust tool for a number of applications. Many of these techniques [1,2,7] rely on label propagation from multiple suitable atlases after non-linear registration to a target image. The target segmentation can be formed by label fusion of the propagated labels, for example by applying a majority vote rule [1,7] or another combination strategy such as a weighted average based on global or local similarity measures

© Springer International Publishing Switzerland 2015
S. Ourselin et al. (Eds.): IPMI 2015, LNCS 9123, pp. 221–232, 2015.
DOI: 10.1007/978-3-319-19992-4_17

between the target and atlas images [2]. Other combination strategies include STAPLE [20], where label fusion weights are estimated with an Expectation-Minimisation algorithm, or Joint Label Fusion [19], where correlations among atlases are taken into account. To account for high local anatomical variability between images, patch-based segmentation [5,17] has been introduced, where the label fusion step employs a non-local weighted average of voxel labels in a small neighbourhood of the atlas images, with weights based on the similarities of patches centred on the compared voxels. Considerable improvements to results obtained with label propagation can be achieved by using the label propagation results as prior probabilities in subsequent refinement steps, combining them with regularisation terms and an intensity model in a Markov Random Field (MRF) formulation [11–13]. It has been shown that in general, segmentation accuracy decreases when fewer [7] or less suitable [1] atlases are used.

All of the above methods rely on the availability of fully annotated atlas data. However, segmentation methods requiring only a proportion of each atlas image to be labelled (while no knowledge is necessary about the remaining voxels) could reduce the workload of raters who manually label these atlases. [9] proposed an extension to STAPLE [20] which, to our knowledge, is the only existing multi-atlas segmentation method that uses partially annotated atlas data. However, partial annotations have been used in the context of interactive segmentation. In [4], regions of an image were manually labelled to enable automated segmentation of the remaining image. In particular, an MRF energy function [10] was formulated on a graph constructed on the regular image grid in which annotated voxels are connected to virtual terminal nodes with infinite weights. The MRF energy minimisation problem was efficiently solved by finding a min-cut/max-flow on the graph with graph-cuts [4]. An iterative graph-cuts approach [16] has been proposed to reduce user interaction compared to [4].

Some applications of graph-cuts employ MRF energy functions that have been formulated for labelling on graphs connecting more than one image. Recently, [6] applied graph-cuts for tumor segmentation based on PET and CT image pairs by minimising an MRF energy function which penalises segmentation differences between a PET and CT image of the same subject. [15] proposed a prostate segmentation algorithm in which multiple 2D slices were extracted from a 3D image at different angles. Exploiting axial symmetry, the 2D slices were simultaneously segmented using a max-flow algorithm which penalised segmentation differences between slices at similar angles. The max-flow algorithm they used is an extension of the recently proposed Continuous Max-Flow (CMF), which solves a continuous counterpart to the discrete min-cut/max-flow problem [21]. CMF can be computed using a reliable, highly parallelisable multiplier-based algorithm with guaranteed convergence, making it suitable for the optimisation of large labelling problems in parallel computing environments.

Combining aspects of multi-atlas segmentation with recent developments in min-cut/max-flow methods [15,21], and with the goal of successfully exploiting partially labelled images for segmentation, we propose a segmentation framework incorporating three novel contributions:

1. We revisit the labelling problem in existing multi-atlas segmentation methods and express the solution in terms of labelling a graph which connects the target and atlas images. We formulate an MRF energy function on this graph and show analytically that its solution is equivalent to existing multi-atlas segmentation methods [2,7]. We then show how spatial regularisation and intensity models [11] can be readily incorporated in the proposed formulation.
2. We provide a generalisation of the Continuous Max-Flow algorithm which can efficiently minimise energy functions on graphs connecting multiple images. The proposed generalised CMF is applied to the graph labelling problem formulated here. However, as it is highly parallelisable, its scalability to large graphs could make it useful for solving large-scale MRF frameworks beyond the scope of this work.
3. We show that the proposed method can provide automated segmentations using partially annotated atlas data. To evaluate the method, we apply it to hippocampal segmentation in 202 Magnetic Resonance (MR) images of the ADNI database and investigate its performance under varying proportions of labelled voxels per atlas image.

2   Method

In the following sections, we revisit multi-atlas segmentation (Sect. 2.1) and show how it can be viewed as a labelling problem on a graph connecting atlases and the target image (Sect. 2.2). In Sect. 2.3 we discuss extensions to the proposed MRF energy function to integrate label propagation, regularisation, as well as intensity models into a single comprehensive framework. Furthermore, we show how the proposed methodology can be applied to segmentation problems where only partially annotated atlas data are available (Sect. 2.4). The optimisation of the proposed energy function is discussed in Sect. 2.5.

2.1   Multi-atlas Label Propagation

For multi-atlas segmentation [2,7] using R images, all atlas images $j \in \{1, \ldots, R\}$ are registered to the target image i. For convenience we assume $i = R + 1$. The label maps l_j associated with the atlas images j are then propagated to the target. Figure 1a shows an example atlas set with corresponding label maps, and an unlabelled target image. Each voxel $x \in \Omega$ in the target image i is labelled using some combination strategy, e.g. a weighted average of atlas labels $l_j(x)$:

$$l_i(x) = \arg\max_L \sum_{j=1}^{R} \beta_{ij}(x) \delta(l_j(x) = L) \tag{1}$$

Here $\delta(.)$ is an indicator function. The weights $\beta_{ij}(x)$ can be uniform (which is equivalent to a majority vote rule) or based on global or local similarity measures between images i and j. Suitable measures were investigated in [2].

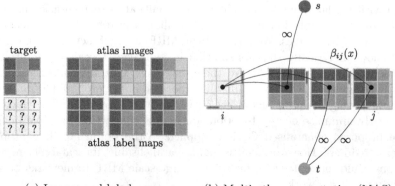

(a) Images and label maps   (b) Multi-atlas segmentation (MAS)

Fig. 1. (a) An example dataset with an unlabelled target image on the left, atlas images and corresponding manual annotations (blue and red depict different labels) on the right. (b) In MAS, each voxel x in target image i is labelled by label propagation from atlases $j \in \{1, \ldots, R\}$ with fusion weights $\beta_{ij}(x)$. This can also be interpreted as a graph labelling problem, where atlas voxels are connected to the terminal nodes with infinitely weighted edges (Color figure online).

2.2   Reformulation as a Graph Labelling Problem

As an alternative perspective, we can construct a graph to model the relationship of shared information between the atlases and the target. According to the above labelling scenario, this graph connects each voxel x in the target image i to the corresponding voxels in the atlas images j with an edge weighted by $\beta_{ij}(x)$. Figure 1b visualises this configuration. To find a labelling on the graph, we can formulate a potential function V that penalises conflicting labels in voxels connected by a high weight $\beta_{ij}(x)$, e.g.

$$V(l_i(x), l_j(x)) = \beta_{ij}(x)\delta(l_j(x) \neq l_i(x)) \tag{2}$$

This assigns a high penalty when the target and atlas labels differ and the atlas is considered similar to the target i, as defined by the similarity measure $\beta_{ij}(x)$. In the case of a majority vote, the weights are uniform, e.g. $\beta_{ij}(x) = 1$. The cost for labelling an individual voxel x in image i can then be calculated as follows:

$$E_{\text{propagation}}(l_i(x)) = \sum_{j=1}^{R} V(l_i(x), l_j(x)) \tag{3}$$

$$= \sum_{j=1}^{R} \beta_{ij}(x)\delta(l_j(x) \neq l_i(x)) \tag{4}$$

$$= \sum_{j=1}^{R} \beta_{ij}(x) - \sum_{j=1}^{R} \beta_{ij}(x)\delta(l_j(x) = l_i(x)) \tag{5}$$

In this formulation the labels in the atlases are fixed. This is achieved by assigning infinite unary potentials to the atlas voxels (visualised as infinitely weighted edges to the terminal nodes in Fig. 1b for the binary case). Voxels in the target image are assumed to be conditionally independent since spatially neighbouring voxels in the target image are not connected in the graph (in contrast to the setting for regularisation in many vision problems [10]). The optimal label can therefore be found by minimising $E_{\text{propagation}}\left(l_i(x)\right)$ independently for all voxels:

$$l_i(x) = \arg\min_L \quad E_{\text{propagation}}\left(l_i(x) = L\right) \tag{6}$$

$$= \arg\min_L \quad -\sum_{j=1}^{R}\beta_{ij}(x)\delta(l_j(x) = L) \tag{7}$$

$$= \arg\max_L \quad \sum_{j=1}^{R}\beta_{ij}(x)\delta(l_j(x) = L), \tag{8}$$

which leads to the same result as the vote rule in Eq. 1. This demonstrates that multi-atlas segmentation can be expressed in terms of a graph optimisation problem. It is important to note that patch-based segmentation (PBS [5,17]) can also be expressed in this framework. In this case we can use a slightly different graph structure as the label fusion step in PBS takes into account multiple voxels in a neighbourhood of x in each atlas instead of just one voxel at location x.

While this alternative problem formulation does not provide any immediate benefits over traditional multi-atlas segmentation in itself (because it is equivalent), it has two advantages: (1) it allows easy integration of additional components and therefore provides a unifying reformulation for existing multi-atlas segmentation methods, as shown in Sect. 2.3 and (2) the graphical approach extends to segmentation using partially annotated atlases (Sect. 2.4).

2.3 Unified Label Propagation Framework

As we are interpreting the whole dataset, comprising target and atlas images, as one graph satisfying Markov properties, we can assign unary potentials (data terms) to each voxel in all images, and pairwise potentials to each pair of voxels [10]. In the previous section, we proposed assigning pairwise potentials between target and atlas voxels for label propagation. In addition, we assigned infinite unary potentials to the atlas voxels since their labels are fixed. It is important to note that a data term can be specified for the target image as well, using prior probabilities, intensity models of the data, or a combination of both. Lastly, we can incorporate spatial regularisation with pairwise potentials between adjacent voxels within an image. The propagation, data, and regularisation terms can be combined to a comprehensive labelling energy function on the whole graph:

$$E(l) = E_{\text{data}}(l) + E_{\text{regularisation}}(l) + E_{\text{propagation}}(l) \tag{9}$$

As mentioned in the introduction, many existing multi-atlas segmentation methods (e.g. [11,13]) use an MRF formulation to improve label propagation results

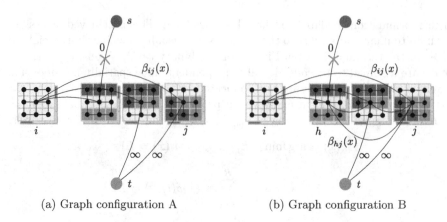

(a) Graph configuration A　　　　　　(b) Graph configuration B

Fig. 2. Graph connections with partially annotated atlas data (blue and red depict different labels), based on the example dataset of Fig. 1a. Voxels with missing labels (white) are disconnected from terminal nodes. Spatial regularisation is enabled in all images. (a) Voxels at each location x in the target image are connected to voxels in atlases j. (b) Additionally, atlas voxels are connected to voxels in other atlases (Color figure online).

with the benefits of regularisation and intensity data models. However, these approaches use probabilistic label propagation results as prior probabilities (i.e. unary potentials) in a *subsequent* refinement step, therefore adding the MRF optimisation as a separate post-processing step. The above comprehensive formulation treats label propagation as part of the optimisation process, and therefore unifies all the components within a single framework. Using the above general formulation, it is possible to open-up a new field of applications, namely segmentation using partially annotated atlas data.

2.4　Segmentation Using Partially Annotated Atlas Data

In the graph setting proposed in the previous sections, an atlas label is characterised by an infinitely weighted connection to a terminal node. For a partially annotated atlas image, unlabelled voxels may simply be disconnected from the terminal nodes. In a multi-atlas segmentation problem as described by Fig. 1b, this translates to a segmentation based only on the available labels. In this case, however, there is no guarantee that each location in the target image can be segmented (depending on the extent of missing labels in the atlases at specific voxel locations), and performance is degraded for low proportions of labelled voxels. We therefore propose the following two graph configurations (Fig. 2): **(A)** Labels are propagated from atlases to the target, i.e. label propagation edges $\beta_{ij}(x)$ are used as in the multi-atlas segmentation case. Additionally, spatial regularisation is used in all images so that labels may be shared between similar regions with labelled and unlabelled voxels, and which can then be propagated to the target image. **(B)** Instead of only propagating labels between target and atlases, atlas images are also interconnected. This serves to facilitate the propagation, especially when manual labels are very scarce.

2.5 Optimisation

It has been shown that MRF energy functions consisting of unary and pairwise terms can be minimised using min-cut/max-flow approaches if the pairwise terms are metric or semi-metric [3], yielding globally optimal results for binary labelling problems and approximately globally optimal results for multiple labels [3]. Recently, [21] proposed a continuous max-flow (CMF) algorithm in the 2D or 3D domain (i.e. a single image) which is highly parallelisable in contrast to discrete graph-based methods [21]. As the proposed energy function can be optimised for a large graph consisting of voxels in all images and their interactions, this approach was used and extended for graphs between multiple images.

Analogous to discrete max-flow approaches, the energy function on the graph can be minimised by maximising a source flow p^s through the network, subject to flow conservation and capacity constraints on the edges. In the original CMF algorithm [21], spatial flows $\mathbf{p} = [p_x, p_y, p_z]^T$ exist between adjacent voxels in the image domain Ω (for regularisation) and source and sink flows $p^{s,t}$ between voxels and terminal nodes. The optimisation is performed with a variational approach by introducing a Lagrange multiplier $u(x)$ to incorporate the constraints [21]. It has been shown that the resulting $u(x)$ corresponds to the globally optimal labelling [21]. While CMF has been extended to multi-label segmentation problems [22], we restrict the scope of this paper to binary labelling problems.

In the following, we propose a generalisation of CMF from a single image to an arbitrary configuration of interconnected images to account for any user-defined choice of inter-image relationships $\beta_{ij}(x)$. Figure 3 shows the capacity constraints and introduces the notation for inter-image flows $r_{ij}(x)$ (for label propagation), spatial flows $\mathbf{p}_i(x)$ (for regularisation) and terminal flows $p_i^{s,t}(x)$ (for unary priors). The notation is similar to [15], where inter-image constraints were used in a different context. To satisfy flow conservation, the sum of all in-

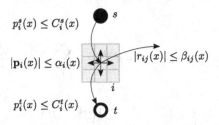

Fig. 3. Notation for flow constraints $\beta_{ij}(x), C_i^{s,t}(x), \alpha_i(x)$ for propagation, data term and regularisation, and corresponding inter-image flows $r_{ij}(x)$, source and sink flows $p_i^{s,t}(x)$ and spatial flows $\mathbf{p}_i(x)$ at location x in image i.

and outgoing flows $\rho_i(x)$ at each node must be zero, i.e.

$$\rho_i(x) = \text{div } \mathbf{p}_i(x) - p_i^s(x) + p_i^t(x) + \sum_{j=1, j \neq i}^{n} r_{ij}(x) = 0, \tag{10}$$

where $r_{ij}(x) = -r_{ji}(x)$ and n is the number of images in the graph. This leads to the Lagrangian function

$$L(u, p^s, p^t, \mathbf{p}, r) = \sum_{i=1}^{n} \left(\int_{\Omega} p_i^s dx + <u_i, \rho_i> - \frac{c}{2} \|\rho_i\|^2 \right), \tag{11}$$

which can be solved iteratively by optimising each variable $u, p^s, p^t, \mathbf{p}, r$ separately [15,21]. The novel component compared to [15,21] is the use of inter-image flows $r_{ij}(x)$ between any pair of images i, j. We therefore show in particular the optimisation step at iteration k for $r_{ij}(x)$ while fixing all other variables:

$$r_{ij}^{k+1} = \underset{|r_{ij}| \leq \beta_{ij}}{\arg\max} \quad L(u, p^s, p^t, \mathbf{p}, r) \tag{12}$$

$$= \underset{|r_{ij}| \leq \beta_{ij}}{\arg\max} \quad u_i^k r_{ij}^k + u_j^k r_{ji}^k \tag{13}$$

$$-\frac{c}{2} \left\| (\text{div } \mathbf{p}_i - p_i^s + p_i^t)^k + \sum_{l=1, l \neq i, j}^{n} r_{il}^k + r_{ij}^k \right\|^2$$

$$-\frac{c}{2} \left\| (\text{div } \mathbf{p}_j - p_j^s + p_j^t)^k + \sum_{l=1, l \neq j, i}^{n} r_{jl}^k + r_{ji}^k \right\|^2$$

$$= \underset{|r_{ij}| \leq \beta_{ij}}{\arg\max} \quad -\frac{c}{2} \left\| (\text{div } \mathbf{p}_i - p_i^s + p_i^t)^k + \sum_{l=1, l \neq i, j}^{n} r_{il}^k - \frac{u_i^k}{c} + r_{ij}^k \right\|^2 \tag{14}$$

$$-\frac{c}{2} \left\| (\text{div } \mathbf{p}_j - p_j^s + p_j^t)^k + \sum_{l=1, l \neq j, i}^{n} r_{jl}^k - \frac{u_j^k}{c} - r_{ij}^k \right\|^2$$

$$= \underset{|r_{ij}| \leq \beta_{ij}}{\arg\max} \quad -\frac{c}{2} \left\| J_i^k + r_{ij}^k \right\|^2 - \frac{c}{2} \left\| J_j^k - r_{ij}^k \right\|^2 \tag{15}$$

where

$$J_i^k = (\text{div } \mathbf{p}_i - p_i^s + p_i^t)^k + \sum_{l=1, l \neq i, j}^{n} r_{il}^k - \frac{u_i^k}{c} \tag{16}$$

This leads to

$$r_{ij}^{k+1} = \begin{cases} -\beta_{ij}, & \frac{1}{2}(J_j^k - J_i^k) \leq -\beta_{ij}, \\ \frac{1}{2}(J_j^k - J_i^k), & |\frac{1}{2}(J_j^k - J_i^k)| \leq \beta_{ij}, \\ \beta_{ij} & \text{otherwise.} \end{cases} \tag{17}$$

After convergence, a binary segmentation can be found by thresholding the resulting solution for u, e.g. at 0.5.

3   Application to Segmentation of Partially Labelled Hippocampus Data

Manually annotating medical images is very time consuming, placing a major burden on clinical experts tasked with labelling large datasets. The images are typically manually annotated slice-by-slice, therefore reducing the proportion of annotated slices while retaining robust and accurate segmentation is an important goal. With the following experiments we investigate the potential of the proposed method to provide accurate hippocampal segmentation using partially annotated atlas data. While demonstrating a scenario where a proportion of atlas *slices* are annotated, the framework proposed in this paper could be applied to different configurations of partial labels, for example to datasets where different regions are annotated in different images.

Data and Experiment Setup. The proposed method was applied to 202 images from the ADNI database [8] for which reference segmentations of the hippocampus were available through ADNI. All images were affinely aligned to the MNI152 template space and intensity-normalised [14]. A leave-one-out procedure was performed for evaluation where, for each target subject, the 10 most similar subjects were selected as atlases using normalised mutual information in a region of interest around the hippocampus. The selected atlases were non-rigidly registered to the target subject [18] with a control-point spacing of 5 mm.

Partially Annotated Atlases. Manual labels of a proportion q of slices in the atlas images were used for segmentation of the target image, while source and sink connections were removed in the remaining slices (as shown in Fig. 2). The selected slice positions were evenly distributed but varied in different atlases. For the spatial regularisation constraints (Fig. 3), we chose

$$\alpha_i(x) = c \exp\left(-\frac{\|\nabla I(x)\|^2}{2\sigma^2}\right), \qquad (18)$$

which is a continuous equivalent of the regularisation term used in [11]. The parameters $c = 0.1$ and $\sigma = 50$ were heuristically tuned for the comparison methods introduced below. We report results for two graph configurations proposed in Sect. 2.4: Graph labelling using (a) connections between target and atlases (GLa) and (b) connections between all pairs of images (GLb). The similarity measure $\beta_{ij}(x)$ was chosen as a function of the local mean squared distance (LMSD) as recommended by [2] for hippocampus segmentation. The LMSD was evaluated in a cubic neighbourhood of radius 5 around each location [2].

Fully Annotated Atlases. We compared the proposed method to locally weighted multi-atlas segmentation (MAS [2]) with different numbers of atlases. The propagated atlas labels were fused with a weighted average as in Eq. 1. The label fusion was implemented using the proposed framework (since we have shown in Eq. 8 that this formulation is equivalent to MAS). We also compared

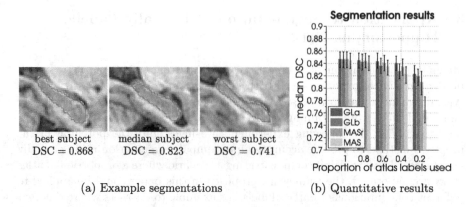

(a) Example segmentations   (b) Quantitative results

Fig. 4. (a) Best, median, and worst segmentation results (red) obtained with GLa using 20 % of available atlas slices, compared to the reference segmentation (yellow) (b) Median DSC and interquartile range for the proposed (blue) and comparison (green) methods using different proportions of atlas labels. The proposed methods use a proportion of slices, whereas the comparison methods use a proportion of images for segmentation (Color figure online).

against a variation of MAS using regularisation in the target image (MASr). Regularisation parameters (for MASr) and $\beta_{ij}(x)$ were chosen as in the proposed method to guarantee fair comparisons.

Results. Experiments were run for $q = \{1, 0.8, 0.6, 0.4, 0.2\}$, where $q = 1$ means that the 10 selected atlases were fully labelled. To measure the effect of partial annotations compared to full annotations, for proportion q, exactly the same number of labelled voxels were available to both the proposed methods and the comparison methods: either as a proportion of slices in each image (labelled voxels were distributed amongst all atlases), or as a proportion of the complete atlas set. This means that for the comparison methods MAS and MASr, fewer (but fully labelled) atlas images were used. Segmentation accuracy is reported with the median Dice Similarity Coefficient (DSC) and interquartile range. As the results were not normally distributed, statistical significance is measured using the two-sided Wilcoxon signed-rank test and is reported for $p < 10^{-4}$.

As expected, segmentation accuracy decreased when less atlases were used [7]. This was observed most strongly in MAS, while spatial regularisation (MASr) increased segmentation accuracy considerably, particularly when fewer atlases were used. The proposed methods GLa and GLb are identical to MASr for $q = 1$ where all atlas voxels are labelled. As the proportion of labelled voxels decreased, GLa was significantly more accurate than MASr for $q = 0.6$, $q = 0.4$ and $q = 0.2$. In GLb, where atlas images were densely interconnected, improvements over MAS and MASr could only be found for $q = 0.2$. The most distinct differences between the methods could be observed when only 20 % of the atlas voxels were labelled. Median DSC values are 0.823(0.03) and 0.819(0.03) for GLa and GLb compared to 0.764(0.04) and 0.810(0.04) for MAS and MASr. Figure 4a shows example segmentations for GLa, for which the runtime per subject on a single CPU was 5 min when computation was limited to the hippocampal region.

4   Discussion and Conclusion

The experiments show that with the proposed method and graph configuration A (Fig. 2a), segmentation accuracy remained stable when reducing the proportion of labelled atlas voxels down to 40 %. The segmentation results were still relatively accurate at 20 %, so the required user input could be reduced considerably. In particular, the proposed method significantly outperformed multi-atlas segmentation using fewer, but fully labelled atlases. This suggests that it could be worthwhile to allocate resources for partially annotating more images instead of fully annotating few images. More generally, we demonstrated that partially annotated images, a resource that is not usually exploited, can be utilised for multi-atlas segmentation.

In order to provide a framework for multi-atlas segmentation using partially annotated atlases, we make two key methodological contributions: We take a new perspective on the well-studied problem of multi-atlas segmentation and formulate it as a graph-labelling problem on a graph between target and atlas images. The proposed framework unifies a number of existing atlas-based segmentation methods (e.g. [2,7,11]) and can incorporate label propagation, regularisation, and intensity models in a single and comprehensive optimisation problem. In the scope of this paper, we have limited ourselves to label propagation and regularisation. In future work, these components will be further developed, and suitable intensity models will be investigated.

Furthermore, we have proposed a generalisation of the Continuous Max-Flow [21] algorithm for parallelisable optimisation of energy functions on graphs between interconnected images of any configuration. In this work, graphs were constructed between target and atlas images to establish an analogy to multi-atlas segmentation scenarios. However, the proposed method could be used for segmenting large-scale, partially labelled datasets.

References

1. Aljabar, P., Heckemann, R.A., Hammers, A., Hajnal, J.V., Rueckert, D.: Multi-atlas based segmentation of brain images: atlas selection and its effect on accuracy. NeuroImage **46**(3), 726–38 (2009)
2. Artaechevarria, X., Munoz-Barrutia, A., Ortiz-de Solórzano, C.: Combination strategies in multi-atlas image segmentation: application to brain MR data. IEEE Trans. Med. Imaging **28**(8), 1266–1277 (2009)
3. Boykov, Y., Veksler, O., Zabih, R.: Fast approximate energy minimization via graph cuts. IEEE Trans. PAMI **23**(11), 1222–1239 (2001)
4. Boykov, Y., Jolly, M.-P.: Interactive organ segmentation using graph cuts. In: Delp, S.L., DiGoia, A.M., Jaramaz, B. (eds.) MICCAI 2000. LNCS, vol. 1935, pp. 276–286. Springer, Heidelberg (2000)
5. Coupé, P., Manjón, J.V., Fonov, V., Pruessner, J., Robles, M., Collins, D.L.: Patch-based segmentation using expert priors: application to hippocampus and ventricle segmentation. NeuroImage **54**(2), 940–954 (2011)

6. Han, D., Bayouth, J., Song, Q., Taurani, A., Sonka, M., Buatti, J., Wu, X.: Globally optimal tumor segmentation in PET-CT Images: a graph-based co-segmentation method. In: Székely, G., Hahn, H.K. (eds.) IPMI 2011. LNCS, vol. 6801, pp. 245–256. Springer, Heidelberg (2011)

7. Heckemann, R.A., Hajnal, J.V., Aljabar, P., Rueckert, D., Hammers, A.: Automatic anatomical brain MRI segmentation combining label propagation and decision fusion. NeuroImage 33(1), 115–126 (2006)

8. Jack, C.R., Bernstein, M., Fox, N.C., Thompson, P., Alexander, G., Harvey, D., Borowski, B., Britson, P., Whitwell, J., Ward, C., Dale, A., Felmlee, J., Gunter, J., Hill, D., Killiany, R., Schuff, N., Fox-Bosetti, S., Lin, C., Studholme, C., DeCarli, C., Krueger, G., Ward, H., Metzger, G., Scott, K., Mallozzi, R., Blezek, D., Levy, J., Debbins, J., Fleisher, A., Albert, M., Green, R., Bartzokis, G., Glover, G., Mugler, J., Weiner, M.: The Alzheimer's disease neuroimaging initiative (ADNI): MRI methods. Magn. Reson. Imaging 27(4), 685–691 (2008)

9. Landman, B.A., Asman, A., Scoggins, A., Bogovic, J., Xing, F., Prince, J.: Robust statistical fusion of image labels. IEEE Trans. Med. Imaging 31(2), 512–522 (2012)

10. Li, S.: Markov random field models in computer vision. In: ECCV, pp. 361–370 (1994)

11. van der Lijn, F., den Heijer, T., Breteler, M., Niessen, W.J.: Hippocampus segmentation in MR images using atlas registration, voxel classification, and graph cuts. NeuroImage 43(4), 708–720 (2008)

12. Lötjönen, J.M., Wolz, R., Koikkalainen, J.R., Thurfjell, L., Waldemar, G., Soininen, H., Rueckert, D.: Fast and robust multi-atlas segmentation of brain magnetic resonance images. NeuroImage 49(3), 2352–2365 (2010)

13. Makropoulos, A., Gousias, I.S., Ledig, C., Aljabar, P., Serag, A., Hajnal, J.V., Edwards, D., Counsell, S.J., Rueckert, D.: Automatic whole brain MRI segmentation of the developing neonatal brain. IEEE Trans. Med. Imaging 33(9), 1818–1831 (2014)

14. Nyúl, L.G., Udupa, J.K.: On standardizing the MR image intensity scale. Magn. Reson. Med. 42(6), 1072–1081 (1999)

15. Qiu, W., Yuan, J., Ukwatta, E., Sun, Y., Rajchl, M., Fenster, A.: Prostate segmentation: an efficient convex optimization approach with axial symmetry using 3D TRUS and MR images. IEEE Trans. Med. Imaging 33(4), 947–960 (2014)

16. Rother, C., Kolmogorov, V., Blake, A.: Grabcut: Interactive foreground extraction using iterated graph cuts. ACM Trans. Graph. 23(3), 309–314 (2004)

17. Rousseau, F.: A supervised patch-based approach for human brain labeling. IEEE Trans. Med. Imaging 30(10), 1852–1862 (2011)

18. Rueckert, D., Sonoda, L.I., Hayes, C., Hill, D.L.G., Leach, M.O., Hawkes, D.J.: Nonrigid registration using free-form deformations: application to breast MR images. IEEE Trans. Med. Imaging 18(8), 712–721 (1999)

19. Wang, H., Suh, J., Das, S., Pluta, J., Craige, C., Yushkevich, P.: Multi-atlas segmentation with joint label fusion. IEEE Trans. PAMI 35(3), 611–623 (2012)

20. Warfield, S.K., Zou, K.H., Wells, W.M.: Simultaneous truth and performance level estimation (STAPLE): an algorithm for the validation of image segmentation. IEEE Trans. Med. Imaging 23(7), 903–921 (2004)

21. Yuan, J., Bae, E., Tai, X.: A study on continuous max-flow and min-cut approaches. In: CVPR, pp. 2217–2224 (2010)

22. Yuan, J., Bae, E., Tai, X.-C., Boykov, Y.: A continuous max-flow approach to potts model. In: Daniilidis, K., Maragos, P., Paragios, N. (eds.) ECCV 2010, Part VI. LNCS, vol. 6316, pp. 379–392. Springer, Heidelberg (2010)

Keypoint Transfer Segmentation

C. Wachinger[1,2]([✉]), M. Toews[3], G. Langs[1,4], W. Wells[1,3], and P. Golland[1]

[1] Computer Science and Artificial Intelligence Lab, MIT, Cambridge, USA
wachinger@csail.mit.edu
[2] MGH, Harvard Medical School, Boston, USA
[3] BWH, Harvard Medical School, Boston, USA
[4] CIR, Department of Biomedical Imaging and Image-Guided Therapy,
Medical University of Vienna, Vienna, Austria

Abstract. We present an image segmentation method that transfers label maps of entire organs from the training images to the novel image to be segmented. The transfer is based on sparse correspondences between keypoints that represent automatically identified distinctive image locations. Our segmentation algorithm consists of three steps: (i) keypoint matching, (ii) voting-based keypoint labeling, and (iii) keypoint-based probabilistic transfer of organ label maps. We introduce generative models for the inference of keypoint labels and for image segmentation, where keypoint matches are treated as a latent random variable and are marginalized out as part of the algorithm. We report segmentation results for abdominal organs in whole-body CT and in contrast-enhanced CT images. The accuracy of our method compares favorably to common multi-atlas segmentation while offering a speed-up of about three orders of magnitude. Furthermore, keypoint transfer requires no training phase or registration to an atlas. The algorithm's robustness enables the segmentation of scans with highly variable field-of-view.

1 Introduction

Is atlas-based segmentation without dense correspondences possible? Typical registration- and patch-based segmentation methods [3,7,15,16] compute correspondences for each location in the novel image to be segmented to the training images. These correspondences are either obtained from dense deformation fields or from the retrieval of similar patches. For scans with a large field-of-view, such approaches become computationally intense. We propose a segmentation method based on distinctive locations in the image - *keypoints*. In contrast to manually selected landmarks [14], keypoints are automatically extracted as local optima of a saliency function [12]. Matches between keypoints in test and training images provide correspondences for a sparse set of image locations, which we use to transfer entire organ segmentations. Working with sparse correspondences and transferring whole organ maps makes our method computationally efficient. The probabilistic fusion of organ maps yields a segmentation accuracy comparable to that of state-of-the-art methods, while offering orders of magnitude of speed-up.

© Springer International Publishing Switzerland 2015
S. Ourselin et al. (Eds.): IPMI 2015, LNCS 9123, pp. 233–245, 2015.
DOI: 10.1007/978-3-319-19992-4_18

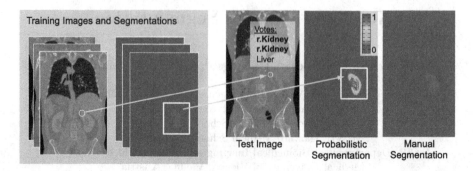

Fig. 1. Illustration of keypoint transfer segmentation. First, keypoints (white circles) in training and test images are matched (arrow). Second, voting assigns an organ label to the test keypoint (r.Kidney). Third, matches from the training images with r.Kidney as labels are transferred to the test image, creating a probabilistic segmentation. We show the manual segmentation for comparison.

Keypoint matching offers the additional advantage of robustness in establishing correspondences between images with varying field-of-view. This property is important when using manually annotated whole-body scans to segment clinical scans with a limited field-of-view. In clinical practice, the diagnostic focus is commonly on a specific anatomical region. To minimize radiation dose to the patient and scanning time, only the region of interest is scanned. The alignment of scans with a limited field-of-view to full abdominal scans is challenging with intensity-based registration, especially when the initial transformation does not roughly align anatomical structures. The efficient and robust segmentation through keypoint transfer offers a practical tool to handle the growing number of clinical scans.

Figure 1 illustrates the keypoint transfer segmentation. Keypoints are identified at salient image regions invariant to scale. Each keypoint is characterized by its geometry and a descriptor based on a local gradient histogram. After keypoint extraction, we obtain the segmentation in three steps. First, keypoints in the test image are matched to keypoints in the training images based on the geometry and the descriptor. Second, reliable matches vote on the organ label of the keypoint in the test image. In the example, two matches vote for right kidney and one for liver, resulting in a majority vote for right kidney. Third, we transfer the segmentation mask for the entire organ for each match that is consistent with the majority label vote; this potentially transfers the organ map from one training image multiple times if more than one match is identified for this training image. The algorithm also considers the confidence of the match in the keypoint label voting. Keypoint transfer does not require a training stage. Its ability to approximate the organ shape improves as the number of manually labeled images grows.

1.1 Related Work

Several methods have been previously demonstrated for segmenting large field-of-view scans. Entangled decision forests [13] and a combination of discriminative and generative models [8] have been proposed for the segmentation of CT scans. A combination of local and global context for simultaneous segmentation of multiple organs has been explored [11]. Organ detection based on marginal space learning was proposed in [20]. The application of regression forests for efficient anatomy detection and localization was described in [4]. In contrast to previously demonstrated methods, our algorithm does not require extensive training on a set of manually labeled images.

We evaluate our method on the publicly available Visceral dataset [10,19]. Multi-atlas segmentation on the Visceral data was proposed in [6,9], which we use as a baseline method in our experiments. Our work builds on the identification of keypoints, defined as a 3D extension [18] of the popular scale invariant feature transform (SIFT) [12]. In addition to image alignment, 3D SIFT features were also applied to study questions related to neuroimaging [17]. In contrast to previous uses of the 3D SIFT descriptor, we use it to transfer information across images.

2   Method

In atlas-based segmentation, the training set includes images $\mathcal{I} = \{I_1, \ldots, I_n\}$ and corresponding segmentations $\mathcal{S} = \{S_1, \ldots, S_n\}$, where $S_i(x) \in \{1, \ldots, \eta\}$ for η labels. The objective is to infer segmentation S for test image I. Instead of aligning training images to the test image with deformable registration, we automatically extract anatomical features from the images and use them to establish sparse correspondences. We identify keypoints that locally maximize a saliency function. In the case of SIFT, it is the difference-of-Gaussians [12]

$$\{(x_i, \sigma_i)\} = \text{local arg max}_{x, \sigma} |f(x, \kappa\sigma) - f(x, \sigma)|, \tag{1}$$

where x_i and σ_i are the location and scale of keypoint i, $f(\cdot, \sigma)$ is the convolution of the image I with a Gaussian kernel of variance σ^2, and κ is a multiplicative scale sampling rate. The identified local extrema in scale-space correspond to distinctive spherical image regions. We characterize the keypoint by a descriptor F^D computed in a local neighborhood whose size depends on the scale of the keypoint. We work with a 3D extension of the image gradient orientation histogram [18] with 8 orientation and 8 spatial bins. This description is scale and rotation invariant and further robust to small deformations. Constructing the descriptors from image gradients instead of intensity values facilitates comparisons across subjects.

We combine the 64-dimensional histogram F^D with the location $F^x \in \mathbb{R}^3$ and scale $F^\sigma \in \mathbb{R}$ to create a compact 68-dimensional representation F for each salient image region. We let F_I denote the set of keypoints extracted from the test image I and $\mathcal{F}_{\mathcal{I}} = \{\mathcal{F}_{I_1}, \ldots, \mathcal{F}_{I_n}\}$ denote the set of keypoints extracted from the training images $\mathcal{I}$. We assign a label to each keypoint in $\mathcal{F}_{I_i}$ according to the organ that contains it, $\mathcal{L} = S_i(\mathcal{F}^x)$ for $\mathcal{F} \in \mathcal{F}_{I_i}$. We only keep keypoints within the segmented organs and discard those in the background. The organ label L is unknown for the keypoints in the test image and is inferred with a voting algorithm as described later in this section.

2.1 Keypoint Matching

The first step in the keypoint-based segmentation is to match each keypoint in the test image with keypoints in the training images. Some of these initial matches might be incorrect. We employ a two-stage matching procedure with additional constraints to improve the reliability of the matches. First, we compute a match $\mathcal{M}(F)_i$ for a test keypoint $F \in F_I$ to keypoints in a training image $\mathcal{F}_{I_i}$ by identifying the nearest neighbor based on the descriptor and scale constraints

$$\mathcal{M}(F)_i = \arg\min_{\mathcal{F} \in \mathcal{F}_{I_i}} \|F^D - \mathcal{F}^D\|, \quad \text{s.t.} \quad \varepsilon_\sigma^{-1} \leq \frac{F^\sigma}{\mathcal{F}^\sigma} \leq \varepsilon_\sigma, \tag{2}$$

where we set a loose threshold on the scale allowing for variations up to a factor of $\varepsilon_\sigma = 2$. We use the distance ratio test to discard keypoint matches that are not reliable [12]. The distance ratio is computed between the descriptors of the closest and second-closest neighbor. We reject all matches with a distance ratio of greater than 0.9.

To further improve the matches, we impose loose spatial constraints on the matches, which requires a rough alignment. For our dataset, accounting for translation was sufficient at this stage; alternatively a keypoint-based pre-alignment could be performed [18]. We estimate the mode of the translations t_i proposed by the matches $\mathcal{M}_i$ from training image I_i with the Hough transform [2]. Mapping the training keypoints with t_i yields a rough alignment of the keypoints and enables an updated set of matches with an additional spatial constraint

$$\mathcal{M}(F)_i = \arg\min_{\mathcal{F} \in \mathcal{F}_{I_i}} \|F^D - \mathcal{F}^D\|, \quad \text{s.t.} \quad \varepsilon_\sigma^{-1} \leq \frac{F^\sigma}{\mathcal{F}^\sigma} \leq \varepsilon_\sigma, \quad \|F^x - \mathcal{F}^{x+t_i}\|_2 < \varepsilon_x,$$

where we set the spatial threshold ε_x to keep 10% of the closest matches. As before, we discard matches that do not fulfill the distance ratio test.

We define a distribution $p(m)$ over matches, where a match m associates keypoints in the test image I and training images I_i. We use kernel density estimation on translations proposed by all matches $\mathcal{M}_i$ between keypoints in the test image and those in the i-th training image. For a match $m \in \mathcal{M}_i$, the probability $p(m)$ expresses the translational consistency of the match m with respect to all other matches in $\mathcal{M}_i$. This non-parametric representation accepts multi-modal distributions, where the keypoints in the upper abdomen may suggest a different transformation than those in the lower abdomen.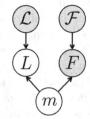

2.2 Keypoint Voting

After establishing matches for keypoints in the test image, we estimate an organ label L for each keypoint in the test image based on the generative model illustrated above. The latent variable m represents the keypoint matches found in the previous step. Keypoint labeling is helpful to obtain a coarse representation of the image, including rough location of organs. Additionally, we use the keypoint labels to guide the image segmentation as described in the next section. For inference of keypoint labels, we marginalize over the latent random variable m and use the factorization from the graphical model to obtain

$$p(L, F, \mathcal{L}, \mathcal{F}) = \sum_{m \in \mathcal{M}(F)} p(L, F, \mathcal{L}, \mathcal{F}, m) \tag{3}$$

$$= \sum_{m \in \mathcal{M}(F)} p(L|\mathcal{L}, m) \cdot p(F|\mathcal{F}, m) \cdot p(m), \tag{4}$$

where $\mathcal{M}(F)$ contains matches for keypoint F across all training images. The marginalization is computationally efficient, since we only compute and evaluate a sparse set of matches. We define the label likelihood

$$p(L = l|\mathcal{L}, m) = \begin{cases} 1 & \text{if } \mathcal{L}_{m(F)} = l, \\ 0 & \text{otherwise,} \end{cases} \tag{5}$$

where $\mathcal{L}_{m(F)}$ is the label of a training keypoint that the match m assigns to the test keypoint F. The keypoint likelihood is based on the descriptor of the keypoint

$$p(F|\mathcal{F}, m) = \frac{1}{\sqrt{2\pi\tau^2}} \exp\left(-\frac{\|F^D - \mathcal{F}^D_{m(F)}\|_2^2}{2\tau^2}\right), \tag{6}$$

where we set $\tau^2 = \max_m \|F^D - \mathcal{F}^D_{m(F)}\|_2^2$. We assign the most likely organ label to the keypoint

$$\hat{L} = \arg\max_{l \in \{1, \dots, \eta\}} p(L = l|F, \mathcal{L}, \mathcal{F}) = \arg\max_{l \in \{1, \dots, \eta\}} p(L = l, F, \mathcal{L}, \mathcal{F}). \tag{7}$$

2.3   Keypoint Segmentation

Here, we introduce a generative model for image segmentation based on keypoint matches and keypoint voting. The latent image segmentation S depends on the keypoint label L and the training segmentations $\mathcal{S}$. A further dependency exists between the test image I and the training images $\mathcal{I}$. All relations between test and training images or keypoints depend on the matches, which bring them into correspondence. We let $\mathcal{I}_m$ denote the training image identified with match m after the transformation implied by the match has been applied. $\mathcal{S}_m$ is similarly defined to be the selected and transformed segmentation map. We infer the segmentation S by marginalizing over the latent random variables and using the factorization from the graphical model

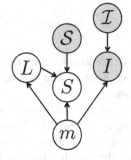

$$p(S, I, \mathcal{S}, \mathcal{I}, \mathcal{L}) = \sum_{m \in \mathcal{M}} \sum_{L} p(S, I, \mathcal{S}, \mathcal{I}, \mathcal{L}, L, m) \tag{8}$$

$$= \sum_{m \in \mathcal{M}} \sum_{L} p(S|L, \mathcal{S}, m) \cdot p(I|\mathcal{I}, m) \cdot p(L|m) \cdot p(m). \tag{9}$$

The likelihood of image segmentation causes keypoints to transfer entire organ label maps

$$p(S|L, \mathcal{S}, m) \propto \begin{cases} 1 & \text{if } S^L = \mathcal{S}_m^L, \\ 0 & \text{otherwise,} \end{cases} \tag{10}$$

where S^L and $\mathcal{S}_m^L$ are the regions with label L in the test and training segmentations, respectively. This likelihood further restricts keypoints to only transfer segmentations with the same label. We also investigate the transfer of organ segmentations that are different from the keypoint labels in our experimental evaluation.

For the label likelihood we consider $p(L|m) \propto p(L) \cdot \delta(\mathcal{L}_m, \hat{L})$. The Kronecker delta δ only allows training keypoints to transfer their votes that are consistent with the majority vote in Eq. (7). This improves the robustness of the method because even if single matches propose to assign the wrong label to the test keypoint, such matches are discarded for the segmentation, as long as they do not reach the majority. The probability $p(L)$ models the certainty of the label voting for the keypoint in Eq. (7).

The image likelihood assumes conditional independence of the locations x on the image grid Ω and models the local similarity between test and training image

$$p(I(x)|\mathcal{I}, m) = \frac{1}{\sqrt{2\pi\nu}} \exp\left(-\frac{(I(x) - \mathcal{I}_m(x))^2}{2\nu^2}\right), \tag{11}$$

where ν^2 is the intensity noise variance. We obtain the final segmentation $\hat{S}(x)$ by selecting the most likely label

$$\hat{S}(x) = \arg\max_{l \in \{1,\ldots,\eta\}} p(S(x) = l|I(x), \mathcal{S}, \mathcal{I}, \mathcal{L}) = \arg\max_{l \in \{1,\ldots,\eta\}} p(S(x) = l, I(x), \mathcal{S}, \mathcal{I}, \mathcal{L}).$$

We account for not transferring the background surrounding the organ by assigning $\hat{S}(x)$ to the background label if the maximal probability in the voting is below 15 %.

We illustrate the mechanism for computing the segmentation likelihood $p(S(x) = \text{liver})$ on an example of liver. We sum across all matches to all the training images. Only matches that involve training keypoints with the label of liver are considered, identified by $\delta(\mathcal{L}_m, \hat{L})$. Further, the label of liver must be assigned to the test keypoint L.

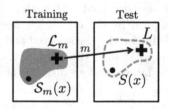

If the match satisfies these requirements, the entire liver label map is transferred with the transformation proposed by the match m; this step is modeled by $P(S|L, \mathcal{S}, m)$. The transfer affects the segmentation likelihood $p(S(x))$ only if location x is within the spatial extent of the transferred liver label map. To increase the robustness and accuracy of the segmentation, we weigh the transferred segmentation according to the certainty in the keypoint label voting $p(L)$, in the match $p(m)$, and in the local intensity similarity of the test and training image $p(I(x)|\mathcal{I}, m)$.

We also investigate the potential improvement of the segmentation by accounting for affine organ variations across subjects. If there are at least three matches for an organ between one training image and the test image, we estimate an organ-specific affine transformation. We apply the random sample consensus (RANSAC) algorithm [5] to determine the transformation parameters with the highest number of inliers. In our experimental evaluation, the organ-wide affine transformation did not achieve a robust improvement of segmentation accuracy and is therefore not reported in the results. The affine transformation may not improve results because we transfer organ labels multiple times per scan for different translations, which already accounts for organ variability in combination with the weighted voting across subjects.

Table 1. Keypoint voting statistics per organ for ceCT (top) and wbCT (bottom): the average number of keypoints per organ, the average fraction of keypoints that get labeled, and the average fraction of correct keypoints labels. Keypoints are not assigned labels if there exists no reliable match. We omit background keypoints from the training images. Only about one third of the background keypoints are labeled.

Organs	Liver	Spleen	Aorta	Trachea	R.Lung	l.Lung	r.Kid	l.Kid	r.PM	l.PM	Bckgrnd
# Keypts	13.6	4.0	7.6	3.0	29.7	24.7	12.1	12.2	2.5	3.0	526.0
% Labeled	0.73	0.89	0.98	1.00	0.95	0.92	0.98	0.99	0.94	0.92	0.33
% Correct	0.87	0.91	0.97	0.99	1.00	1.00	0.98	1.00	0.99	0.93	0.00
# Keypts	6.0	2.6	5.6	4.4	28.2	24.0	6.7	9.0	2.5	2.5	637.2
% Labeled	0.93	0.98	1.00	1.00	0.98	0.98	0.98	0.99	0.98	1.00	0.35
% Correct	0.82	0.87	0.92	1.00	0.99	0.99	0.98	0.96	1.00	0.93	0.00

3 Results

We perform experiments on 20 contrast-enhanced CT (ceCT) scans and on 20 whole-body CT (wbCT) scans from the Visceral dataset re-sampled to 2 mm isotropic voxels [10]. We segment 10 anatomical structures (liver, spleen, aorta, trachea, left/right lung, left/right kidney, left/right psoas major muscle (PM)). Image dimensions are roughly $217 \times 217 \times 695$ for wbCT and $200 \times 200 \times 349$ for ceCT. We set $\nu = 300$ for lungs and trachea and $\nu = 50$ for all other organs. We perform leave-one-out experiments by using one image as test and the remaining 19 images as training images. We compare our method to multi-atlas segmentation with majority voting (MV) [7,15] and locally-weighted label fusion (LW) [16] using ANTS [1] for deformable registration. We quantify the segmentation accuracy with the Dice volume overlap between manual and automatic segmentation.

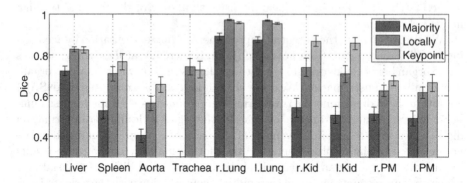

Fig. 2. Segmentation accuracy for ten organs on ceCT images for majority voting, locally-weighted voting, and keypoint transfer. Bars indicate the mean Dice and error bars correspond to standard error.

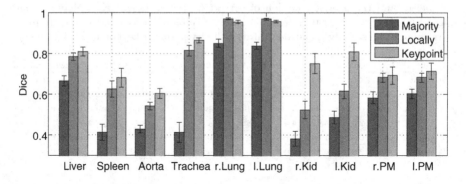

Fig. 3. Segmentation accuracy for ten organs on wbCT images for majority voting, locally-weighted voting, and keypoint transfer. Bars indicate the mean Dice and error bars correspond to standard error.

Table 1 reports statistics for the voting on keypoint labels. The average number of keypoints varies across organs. Keypoints are not labeled if they do not receive reliable matches that pass the spatial constraint and the distance ratio test. Focusing on reliable keypoints improves the performance of the algorithm because it is possible that certain keypoints in the test image do not appear in the training set. For the keypoints that are labeled, the voting accuracy is high. All of the votes on background keypoints in the test image are incorrect, since we do not include background keypoints in the training set. However, only about one third of the background keypoints receives labels. The remaining background keypoints have limited impact on the segmentation as long as there is no bias in transferring organ maps to a specific location.

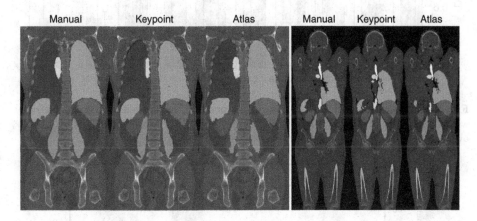

Fig. 4. Coronal views of example segmentation results for ceCT (left) and wbCT (right) overlaid on the intensity images. Each series reports segmentations in the following order: manual, keypoint transfer, locally-weighted multi-atlas.

Figures 2 and 3 report segmentation results for ceCT and wbCT scans, respectively, comparing keypoint transfer to multi-atlas segmentation. Locally-weighted voting outperforms majority voting for all anatomical structures. Keypoint transfer segmentation yields segmentation accuracy comparable to that of locally-weighted voting for most structures and better accuracy for the segmentation of kidneys; the increase in Dice for kidneys is about 0.15 on ceCT and about 0.2 on wbCT. In these experiments, the transfer of segmentations that are different from the keypoint label did not achieve a robust improvement and are therefore not reported. Figure 4 illustrates segmentation results for ceCT and wbCT.

Figure 5 reports the average segmentation result for ceCT scans when varying the number of training scans from 5 to 15; the evaluation is on the five images not included in the training set. The segmentation accuracy generally increases with the number of training scans. This result suggests that averaging over segmentations of a larger number of subjects helps in recovering the true shape of the organ. The availability of larger datasets in the future may therefore further improve the segmentation results. An atlas selection scheme that only transfers organs from overall similar subjects may be helpful, which could be efficiently implemented based on keypoints.

Figure 6 reports the runtime of keypoint transfer segmentation and multi-atlas label fusion. The segmentation with keypoint transfer is about three orders of magnitude faster. On ceCT scans, the extraction of keypoints takes about

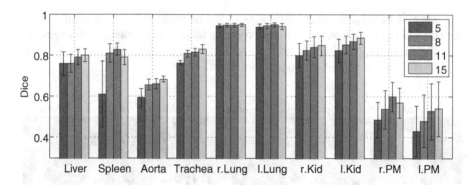

Fig. 5. Segmentation accuracy for ten organs on ceCT images with keypoint transfer with the number of training images ranging from 5 to 15. Bars indicate the mean Dice over five test images and error bars correspond to standard error.

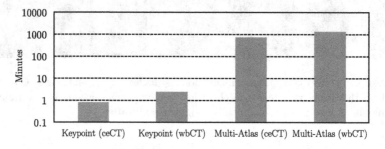

Fig. 6. Average runtimes (in minutes) of the segmentation of ten organs in one image with keypoint transfer and multi-atlas label fusion for ceCT and wbCT. The time is displayed on the logarithmic scale.

30 s and the segmentation transfer takes 16 s, yielding a segmentation time for ten organs that is below one minute. The segmentation transfer is implemented in Matlab without parallelization. For multi-atlas segmentation, the pairwise deformable registration consumes most of the runtime. We also experimented with creating a probabilistic atlas, which reduces computational costs. However, the iterative estimation of the atlas is also expensive and the high anatomical variability of the abdomen makes the summarization challenging.

In addition to the segmentation of abdominal and whole-body scans, we also evaluated the segmentation of scans with limited field-of-view. In clinical practice, such partial scans frequently occur because of a specific diagnostic focus. To test the performance of the algorithm, we crop ceCT and wbCT images around the kidneys and the spleen, as shown in Fig. 7. For spleen images, we found a substantial improvement by transferring organ segmentations that are different from the keypoint label. Figure 7 reports results for segmenting the spleen byonly using spleen keypoints and by also using lung and liver keypoints. In the partial scans, we notice a slight decrease in segmentation accuracy, compared to working on the full scans. However, the keypoint transfer is overall robust to variations in the field-of-view and enables segmentation without modifications of the algorithm. We do not report results for the multi-atlas segmentation in this experiment because the registration between the cropped images and the training images failed. Since the initial alignment does not lead to a rough overlap of the target regions, it is a very challenging registration problem. While it may be possible to develop initialization techniques that improve the alignment, we consider it a major advantage of the keypoint transfer that no modification is required to handle limited field-of-view scans.

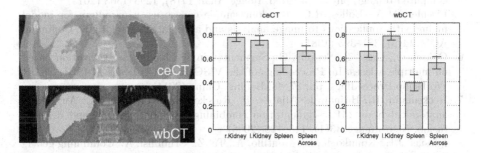

Fig. 7. Coronal views of scans with limited field-of-view showing the kidneys or the spleen, illustrated for ceCT and wbCT, respectively. Bars indicate the mean Dice and error bars correspond to standard error. 'Spleen Across' corresponds to using lung and liver keypoints to transfer spleen segmentations.

4 Conclusion

We introduced an image segmentation method based on keypoints that transfers label maps of entire organs. Relying on sparse correspondences between keypoints in the test and training images increases the efficiency of the method. Keypoint matches are further robust to variations in the field-of-view of the images, which enables segmentation of partial scans. Our algorithms for the keypoint voting and the segmentation transfer were derived from generative models, where latent random variables were marginalized out. The accuracy of our segmentation compares favorably to multi-atlas segmentation, while requiring about three orders of magnitude less computation time.

Acknowledgements. This work was supported in part by the Humboldt foundation, the National Alliance for Medical Image Computing (U54-EB005149), the NeuroImaging Analysis Center (P41-EB015902), the National Center for Image Guided Therapy (P41-EB015898), and the Wistron Corporation.

References

1. Avants, B.B., Epstein, C.L., Grossman, M., Gee, J.C.: Symmetric diffeomorphic image registration with cross-correlation: evaluating automated labeling of elderly and neurodegenerative brain. Med. Image Anal. **12**(1), 26–41 (2008)
2. Ballard, D.: Generalizing the hough transform to detect arbitrary shapes. Pattern Recogn. **13**(2), 111–122 (1981)
3. Coup, P., Manjn, J.V., Fonov, V., Pruessner, J., Robles, M., Collins, D.L.: Patch-based segmentation using expert priors: application to hippocampus and ventricle segmentation. NeuroImage **54**(2), 940–954 (2011)
4. Criminisi, A., Robertson, D., Konukoglu, E., Shotton, J., Pathak, S., White, S., Siddiqui, K.: Regression forests for efficient anatomy detection and localization in computed tomography scans. Med. Image Anal. **17**(8), 1293–1303 (2013)
5. Fischler, M.A., Bolles, R.C.: Random sample consensus: a paradigm for model fitting with applications to image analysis and automated cartography. Commun. ACM **24**(6), 381–395 (1981)
6. Goksel, O., Gass, T., Szekely, G.: Segmentation and landmark localization based on multiple atlases. In: Proceedings of the VISCERAL Challenge at ISBI, CEUR Workshop Proceedings, pp. 37–43, Beijing, China (2014)
7. Heckemann, R., Hajnal, J., Aljabar, P., Rueckert, D., Hammers, A.: Automatic anatomical brain MRI segmentation combining label propagation and decision fusion. NeuroImage **33**(1), 115–126 (2006)
8. Iglesias, J.E., Konukoglu, E., Montillo, A., Tu, Z., Criminisi, A.: Combining generative and discriminative models for semantic segmentation of CT scans via active learning. In: Székely, G., Hahn, H.K. (eds.) IPMI 2011. LNCS, vol. 6801, pp. 25–36. Springer, Heidelberg (2011)
9. Jiménezdel Toro, O., Müller, H.: Hierarchical multi-structure segmentation guided by anatomical correlations. In: Proceedings of the VISCERAL Challenge at ISBI, CEUR Workshop Proceedings, pp. 32–36, Beijing, China (2014)
10. Langs, G., Hanbury, A., Menze, B., Müller, H.: VISCERAL: towards large data in medical imaging — challenges and directions. In: Greenspan, H., Müller, H., Syeda-Mahmood, T. (eds.) MCBR-CDS 2012. LNCS, vol. 7723, pp. 92–98. Springer, Heidelberg (2013)
11. Lay, N., Birkbeck, N., Zhang, J., Zhou, S.K.: Rapid Multi-organ Segmentation Using Context Integration and Discriminative Models. In: Gee, J.C., Joshi, S., Pohl, K.M., Wells, W.M., Zöllei, L. (eds.) IPMI 2013. LNCS, vol. 7917, pp. 450–462. Springer, Heidelberg (2013)
12. Lowe, D.G.: Distinctive image features from scale-invariant keypoints. Int. J. Comput. Vis. **60**(2), 91–110 (2004)
13. Montillo, A., Shotton, J., Winn, J., Iglesias, J.E., Metaxas, D., Criminisi, A.: Entangled decision forests and their application for semantic segmentation of CT images. In: Székely, G., Hahn, H.K. (eds.) IPMI 2011. LNCS, vol. 6801, pp. 184–196. Springer, Heidelberg (2011)
14. Potesil, V., Kadir, T., Brady, S.: Learning new parts for landmark localization in whole-body CT scans. IEEE Trans. Med. Imaging **33**(4), 836–848 (2014)
15. Rohlfing, T., Brandt, R., Menzel, R., Maurer, C., et al.: Evaluation of atlas selection strategies for atlas-based image segmentation with application to confocal microscopy images of bee brains. NeuroImage **21**(4), 1428–1442 (2004)
16. Sabuncu, M., Yeo, B., Van Leemput, K., Fischl, B., Golland, P.: A generative model for image segmentation based on label fusion. IEEE Trans. Med. Imaging **29**, 1714–1729 (2010)

17. Toews, M., Wells III, W., Collins, D.L., Arbel, T.: Feature-based morphometry: discovering group-related anatomical patterns. NeuroImage **49**(3), 2318–2327 (2010)

18. Toews, M., Wells III, W.M.: Efficient and robust model-to-image alignment using 3D scale-invariant features. Med. Image Anal. **17**(3), 271–282 (2013)

19. Jiménez del Toro, O., et al.: VISCERAL - VISual Concept Extraction challenge in RAdioLogy. In: Goksel, O. (ed.) Proceedings of the VISCERAL Challenge at ISBI, No. 1194 in CEUR Workshop Proceedings, pp. 6–15 (2014)

20. Zheng, Y., Georgescu, B., Comaniciu, D.: Marginal space learning for efficient detection of 2D/3D anatomical structures in medical images. In: Prince, J.L., Pham, D.L., Myers, K.J. (eds.) IPMI 2009. LNCS, vol. 5636, pp. 411–422. Springer, Heidelberg (2009)

Fast Image Registration

Finite-Dimensional Lie Algebras for Fast Diffeomorphic Image Registration

Miaomiao Zhang[✉] and P. Thomas Fletcher

Scientific Computing and Imaging Institute, University of Utah,
Salt Lake City, UT, USA
miaomiao@sci.utah.edu

Abstract. This paper presents a fast geodesic shooting algorithm for diffeomorphic image registration. We first introduce a novel finite-dimensional Lie algebra structure on the space of bandlimited velocity fields. We then show that this space can effectively represent initial velocities for diffeomorphic image registration at much lower dimensions than typically used, with little to no loss in registration accuracy. We then leverage the fact that the geodesic evolution equations, as well as the adjoint Jacobi field equations needed for gradient descent methods, can be computed entirely in this finite-dimensional Lie algebra. The result is a geodesic shooting method for large deformation metric mapping (LDDMM) that is dramatically faster and less memory intensive than state-of-the-art methods. We demonstrate the effectiveness of our model to register 3D brain images and compare its registration accuracy, run-time, and memory consumption with leading LDDMM methods. We also show how our algorithm breaks through the prohibitive time and memory requirements of diffeomorphic atlas building.

1 Introduction

Deformable image registration is a fundamental tool in medical image analysis that is used for several tasks, including anatomical comparisons across individuals, alignment of functional data to a reference coordinate system, and atlas-based image segmentation. In many applications, it is desirable that image transformations be diffeomorphisms, i.e., differentiable, bijective mappings with differentiable inverses. Such diffeomorphic mappings ensure several properties of the transformed images: (1) topology of objects in the image remain intact; (2) no non-differentiable artifacts, such as creases or sharp corners, are created; and (3) the process can be inverted, for instance, to move back and forth between two individuals, or between an atlas and an individual. An elegant mathematical formulation for diffeomorphic image registration is that of Large Deformation Diffeomorphic Metric Mapping (LDDMM), first proposed by Beg et al. [5]. In this setting, the group of diffeomorphisms is equipped with a Riemannian metric, giving rise to a variational principle that expresses the optimal image registration as a geodesic flow. The result is a distance metric between images that quantifies their geometric similarity. Having a distance metric is a critical component in

S. Ourselin et al. (Eds.): IPMI 2015, LNCS 9123, pp. 249–260, 2015.
DOI: 10.1007/978-3-319-19992-4_19

statistical analysis of anatomical shape, including regression, longitudinal analysis, and group comparisons, as it provides a mathematical foundation for fitting a statistical model to image data via minimization of the sum-of-squared residual distances.

A major barrier to the widespread use of LDDMM, especially in large imaging studies, is its high computational cost and large memory footprint. The original algorithm by Beg et al. computes a geodesic path by gradient descent of a time-varying velocity field. This requires expensive numerical solutions to partial differential equations for the gradient evaluation, as well as time integration of the velocities to compute the diffeomorphic transformation, all of which must be done on dense spatial grids for numerical accuracy. Furthermore, convergence of the algorithm can be slow and prone to getting stuck in local minima, as is often the case with relaxation methods. Addressing some of these weaknesses, Vialard et al. [14] introduced a geodesic shooting algorithm for diffeomorphic image matching. This takes advantage of the fact that a geodesic is determined by its initial momentum at time zero via the geodesic evolution equations. Using a control theory formulation, Vialard et al. then derive the necessary adjoint equations to carry gradients of the image match at the endpoint of the geodesic back to a gradient in the initial momentum. They demonstrated that this led to better convergence and more reliable estimates of the initial momentum. It also avoids having to store the entire time-varying velocity field from one iteration to the next, as just the initial momentum is sufficient to encode the current geodesic. However, despite these advantages, the geodesic shooting and backward adjoint equations must also be solved numerically on a dense grid and are still prohibitively time consuming.

Another class of diffeomorphic registration methods are the "greedy" algorithms, that is, algorithms that iteratively apply gradient updates to a single deformation field, rather than update a full time-dependent flow each iteration. Algorithms in this class include the original diffeomorphic image registration algorithm of Christensen et al. [6] and the diffeomorphic demons algorithm of Vercauteren et al. [13]. Greedy methods are much faster and more memory efficient than LDDMM, but they do not minimize a global variational problem and do not provide a distance metric between images. They also lack the initial velocity parameterization that geodesic methods possess. Such a parameterization is important for statistical analysis because it represents deformations in a linear vector space, which is amenable to statistical models such as principal component analysis [12] and regression [10]. Arsigny et al. [2] introduced the concept of a stationary velocity field representation for diffeomorphisms and demonstrated that one-parameter subgroup flows of diffeomorphisms could be computed efficiently. A similar strategy is used by the DARTEL image registration method of Ashburner [3]. While stationary velocity fields again are more efficient in time and memory than LDDMM, they do not provide distance metrics on the space of diffeomorphisms.

In this paper, we show that it is possible to have a fast diffeomorphic image registration algorithm that retains the metric properties of LDDMM. To do this, we introduce a novel theoretical framework for diffeomorphic image registration based on representing discretized velocity fields as elements in a finite-dimensional Lie algebra. A somewhat surprising feature of our proposed framework is that not only is our algorithm faster than state-of-the-art LDDMM algorithms, it is actually able to converge to better solutions, i.e., lower values of the registration objective function.

2   Background on LDDMM and Geodesic Shooting

In this section we give a brief overview of LDDMM and set up the notation we will use. We consider images defined on a cyclical domain, i.e., a d-dimensional torus, $\Omega = \mathbb{R}^d/\mathbb{Z}^d$. An image will be a square-integrable function on Ω, that is, an element of $L^2(\Omega, \mathbb{R})$. Let $\mathrm{Diff}^\infty(\Omega)$ denote the Lie group of smooth diffeomorphisms on Ω. The Lie algebra for $\mathrm{Diff}^\infty(\Omega)$ is the space $V = \mathfrak{X}^\infty(T\Omega)$ of smooth vector fields on Ω, which is the tangent space at the identity transform. We equip V with the weak Sobolev metric:

$$\langle v, w \rangle_V = \int_\Omega (Lv(x), w(x))dx, \tag{1}$$

where $L = (I - \alpha\Delta)^s$ is a symmetric, positive-definite, differential operator for some scalar, $\alpha > 0$, and integer power, s. The dual to the tangent vector v is a momentum, $m = Lv \in V^*$. The notation (m, v) denotes the pairing of a momentum vector $m \in V^*$ with a tangent vector $v \in V$. The metric L is an invertible operator, and $K = L^{-1}$ maps the momentum vector $m \in V^*$ back to the tangent vector $v = Km \in V$.

LDDMM: In the LDDMM framework, we will consider diffeomorphisms that are generated by flows of time-varying velocity fields from V. More specifically, consider a time-varying velocity field, $v : [0,1] \to V$, then we may define the flow $t \mapsto \phi_t \in \mathrm{Diff}^s(\Omega)$ as a solution to the equation

$$\frac{d\phi_t}{dt}(x) = v_t \circ \phi_t(x).$$

The registration between two images, $I_0, I_1 \in L^2(\Omega, \mathbb{R})$, is the minimizer of the energy,

$$E(v_t) = \int_0^1 \|v_t\|_V^2 \, dt + \frac{1}{2\sigma^2}\|I_0 \circ \phi_1^{-1} - I_1\|_{L^2}^2. \tag{2}$$

Geodesic Shooting: Given an initial velocity, $v_0 \in V$, at $t = 0$, the geodesic path $t \mapsto \phi_t \in \mathrm{Diff}^\infty(\Omega)$ under the right-invariant Riemannian metric (1) is uniquely determined by the Euler-Poincaré equations (EPDiff) [1,9],

$$\frac{\partial v}{\partial t} = -\mathrm{ad}_v^\dagger v = -K\mathrm{ad}_v^* m$$

$$= -K\left[(Dv)^T m + Dm\,v + m\,\mathrm{div}\,v\right], \tag{3}$$

where D denotes the Jacobian matrix, and the operator ad^* is the dual of the negative Lie bracket of vector fields,

$$\mathrm{ad}_v w = -[v, w] = Dvw - Dwv. \tag{4}$$

By integrating Eq. (3) forward in time, we generate a time-varying velocity $v_t : [0, 1] \rightarrow V$, which itself is subsequently integrated in time by the rule $(d\phi_t(x)/dt) = v_t \circ \phi_t(x)$ to arrive at the geodesic path, $\phi_t(x) \in \mathrm{Diff}^s(\Omega)$. Details are found in [14, 15]. Noting that the geodesic ϕ_t is fully determined by the initial condition v_0, we can rewrite the LDDMM image matching objective function (2) in terms of the initial velocity v_0 as

$$E(v_0) = (Lv_0, v_0) + \frac{1}{2\sigma^2} \|I_0 \circ \phi_1^{-1} - I_1\|^2. \tag{5}$$

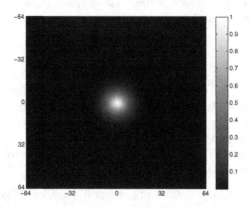

Fig. 1. Fourier coefficients of the discretized K operator on a 128×128 grid, with parameters $\alpha = 3$, $s = 3$.

3   Finite-Dimensional Lie Algebras of Diffeomorphism

While the Lie algebra $V = \mathfrak{X}^\infty(\Omega)$ is an infinite-dimensional vector space, we must of course approximate smooth vector fields in V with finite-dimensional discretizations in order to represent them on a computer. In this section, we show that careful choices for the discretization of vector fields and their corresponding Lie brackets leads to a representation that is itself a finite-dimensional Lie algebra. The key observation is that the K operator is a low-pass filter, and as such, suppresses high frequency components in the velocity fields (see, for example, Fig. 1). As the K operator appears as the last operation on the right-hand side of the EPDiff Eq. (3), we can see that the velocity fields in the geodesicevolution do not develop high frequency components. This suggests that a standard implementation of geodesic shooting, using high-resolution velocity fields, wastes a lot of effort computing the high frequency components, which just end up being forced to zero by K. Instead, we propose to use a low-dimensional discretization of velocity fields as bandlimited signals in the Fourier domain.

More specifically, let $\tilde{V}$ denote the space of bandlimited velocity fields on Ω, with frequency bounds $N_1, N_2, \ldots, N_d$ in each of the dimensions of Ω. It will be convenient to represent an element $\tilde{v} \in \tilde{V}$ in the Fourier domain. That is, let $\tilde{v} \in \tilde{V}$ be a multidimensional array: $\tilde{v}_{k_1,k_2,\ldots,k_d} \in \mathbb{C}^d$, where $k_i \in 0, \ldots, N_i - 1$ is the frequency index along the ith axis. Note that to ensure $\tilde{v}$ represents a real-valued vector field in the spatial domain, we have the constraint that $\tilde{v}_{k_1,\ldots,k_d} = \tilde{v}^*_{N_1-k_1,\ldots,N_d-k_d}$, where $*$ denotes the complex conjugate. There is a natural inclusion mapping, $\iota : \tilde{V} \to V$, of $\tilde{V}$ into the space V of smooth vector fields, given by the Fourier series expansion:

$$\iota(\tilde{v})(x_1,\ldots,x_d) = \sum_{k_1=0}^{N_1} \cdots \sum_{k_d=0}^{N_d} \tilde{v}_{k_1,\ldots,k_d} e^{2\pi k_1 x_1} \cdots e^{2\pi k_d x_d}. \tag{6}$$

Next, we define an operator that is a discrete analog of (4), the Lie bracket on continuous vector fields. First, we will denote by $\tilde{D}\tilde{v}$ the central difference Jacobian matrix of a discrete vector field, $\tilde{v} \in \tilde{V}$. This can be computed in the discrete Fourier domain as a tensor product $\tilde{D}\tilde{v} = \eta \otimes \tilde{v}$, where $\eta \in \tilde{V}$ is given by

$$\eta_{k_1,k_2,\ldots,k_d} = (i\sin(2\pi k_1), \ldots, i\sin(2\pi k_d)).$$

Second, we note that pointwise multiplication of matrix and vector field in the spatial domain corresponds to convolution in the Fourier domain. Because convolution between two bandlimited signals does not preserve the bandlimit, we must follow a convolution operation by truncation back to the bandlimits, N_j, in each dimension. We denote this truncated convolution operator between a matrix and a vector field as $\star$. Now we are ready to define our discrete bracket operator for any two vectors $\tilde{v}, \tilde{w} \in \tilde{V}$ as

$$[\tilde{v}, \tilde{w}] = (\tilde{D}\tilde{v}) \star \tilde{w} - (\tilde{D}\tilde{w}) \star \tilde{v}. \tag{7}$$

The next theorem proves that this operation satisfies the properties to be a Lie bracket on $\tilde{V}$.

Theorem 1. *The vector space $\tilde{V}$, when equipped with the bracket operation (7), is a finite-dimensional Lie algebra. That is to say, $\forall \tilde{x}, \tilde{y}, \tilde{z} \in \tilde{V}$ and $a, b \in \mathbb{R}$, the following properties are satisfied:*

(a) Linearity: $[a\tilde{x} + b\tilde{y}, \tilde{z}] = a[\tilde{x}, \tilde{z}] + b[\tilde{y}, \tilde{z}]$,
(b) Anticommutativity: $[\tilde{x}, \tilde{y}] = -[\tilde{y}, \tilde{x}]$,
(c) Jacobi identity: $[\tilde{x}, [\tilde{y}, \tilde{z}]] + [\tilde{z}, [\tilde{x}, \tilde{y}]] + [\tilde{y}, [\tilde{z}, \tilde{x}]] = 0$.

Proof. Linearity and anticommutativity are immediate. We have

(a) Linearity:

$$[a\tilde{x} + b\tilde{y}, \tilde{z}] = \tilde{D}(a\tilde{x} + b\tilde{y}) \star \tilde{z} - \tilde{D}\tilde{z} \star (a\tilde{x} + b\tilde{y})$$
$$= a(\tilde{D}\tilde{x} \star \tilde{z} - \tilde{D}\tilde{z} \star \tilde{x}) + b(\tilde{D}\tilde{y} \star \tilde{z} - \tilde{D}\tilde{z} \star \tilde{y})$$
$$= a[\tilde{x}, \tilde{z}] + b[\tilde{y}, \tilde{z}],$$

(b) Anticommutativity:

$$[\tilde{x}, \tilde{y}] = \tilde{D}\tilde{x} \star \tilde{y} - \tilde{D}\tilde{y} \star \tilde{x} = -\left(\tilde{D}\tilde{y} \star \tilde{x} - \tilde{D}\tilde{x} \star \tilde{y}\right) = -[\tilde{y}, \tilde{x}].$$

(c) Jacobi identity: The proof of the Jacobi identity follows closely that of the continuous case. First, note that the iterated central difference operator results in a third-order tensor:

$$\tilde{D}^2\tilde{x} = \tilde{D}\tilde{D}\tilde{x} = \eta \otimes \eta \otimes \tilde{x}.$$

Much like the Hessian tensor of a vector-valued function in the continuous case, the discrete Hessian is also symmetric with respect to contraction with a pair of vectors. That is,

$$(\tilde{D}^2\tilde{x} \star \tilde{y}) \star \tilde{z} = (\tilde{D}^2\tilde{x} \star \tilde{z}) \star \tilde{y},$$

where the convolution between $\tilde{D}^2\tilde{x}$ and $\tilde{y}$ is now analogous to the pointwise contraction of a third-order tensor field with a vector field in spatial domain.

Next, we note that the product rule of differentiation also carries over to the discrete Fourier representation, and we have the identity

$$\tilde{D}(\tilde{D}\tilde{x} \star \tilde{y}) = \tilde{D}^2\tilde{x} \star \tilde{y} + \tilde{D}\tilde{x} \star \tilde{D}\tilde{y},$$

where the second convolution operator is analogous to pointwise matrix field multiplication in the spatial domain. We then have

$$[\tilde{x}, [\tilde{y}, \tilde{z}]] = [\tilde{x}, \tilde{D}\tilde{y} \star \tilde{z} - \tilde{D}\tilde{z} \star \tilde{y}]$$
$$= \tilde{D}\tilde{x} \star (\tilde{D}\tilde{y} \star \tilde{z} - \tilde{D}\tilde{z} \star \tilde{y}) - \tilde{D}(\tilde{D}\tilde{y} \star \tilde{z} - \tilde{D}\tilde{z} \star \tilde{y}) \star \tilde{x}$$
$$= \tilde{D}\tilde{x} \star \tilde{D}\tilde{y} \star \tilde{z} - \tilde{D}\tilde{x} \star \tilde{D}\tilde{z} \star \tilde{y} - (\tilde{D}^2\tilde{y} \star \tilde{z}) \star \tilde{x} - \tilde{D}\tilde{y} \star \tilde{D}\tilde{z} \star \tilde{x}$$
$$+ (\tilde{D}^2\tilde{z} \star \tilde{y}) \star \tilde{x} + \tilde{D}\tilde{z} \star \tilde{D}\tilde{y} \star \tilde{x} \tag{8}$$

Similarly, we rewrite the other two terms as

$$[\tilde{z}, [\tilde{x}, \tilde{y}]] = \tilde{D}\tilde{z} \star \tilde{D}\tilde{x} \star \tilde{y} - \tilde{D}\tilde{z} \star \tilde{D}\tilde{y} \star \tilde{x} - (\tilde{D}^2\tilde{x} \star \tilde{y}) \star \tilde{z} - \tilde{D}\tilde{x} \star \tilde{D}\tilde{y} \star \tilde{z}$$
$$+ (\tilde{D}^2\tilde{y} \star \tilde{x}) \star \tilde{z} + \tilde{D}\tilde{y} \star \tilde{D}\tilde{x} \star \tilde{z} \tag{9}$$

$$[\tilde{y}, [\tilde{z}, \tilde{x}]] = \tilde{D}\tilde{y} \star \tilde{D}\tilde{z} \star \tilde{x} - \tilde{D}\tilde{y} \star \tilde{D}\tilde{x} \star \tilde{z} - (\tilde{D}^2\tilde{z} \star \tilde{x}) \star \tilde{y} - \tilde{D}\tilde{z} \star \tilde{D}\tilde{x} \star \tilde{y}$$
$$+ (\tilde{D}^2\tilde{x} \star \tilde{z}) \star \tilde{y} + \tilde{D}\tilde{x} \star \tilde{D}\tilde{z} \star \tilde{y} \tag{10}$$

Finally, by combining the Eqs. (8–10), and using the symmetric rule above, we obtain

$$[\tilde{x}, [\tilde{y}, \tilde{z}]] + [\tilde{z}, [\tilde{x}, \tilde{y}]] + [\tilde{y}, [\tilde{z}, \tilde{x}]] = 0.$$

4   Estimation of Diffeomorphic Image Registration

In this section, we present a geodesic shooting algorithm for diffeomorphic image registration using our finite-dimensional Lie algebra representation. This is a gradient descent algorithm on an initial velocity $\tilde{v}_0 \in \tilde{V}$. Geodesic shooting of $\tilde{v}_0$ proceeds entirely in the reduced finite-dimensional Lie algebra, producing a time-varying velocity, $t \mapsto \tilde{v}_t \in \tilde{V}$. Such a geodesic path in $\tilde{V}$ can consequently generate a flow of diffeomorphisms, $t \mapsto \phi_t \in \text{Diff}^\infty(\Omega)$, in the following way. Using the inclusion mapping $\iota : \tilde{V} \to V$ defined in (6), we can generate the diffeomorphic flow as

$$\frac{d\phi_t(x)}{dt} = \iota(\tilde{v}_t) \circ \phi_t(x), \qquad x \in \Omega.$$

This leads to a modification for the energy function (5) for LDDMM, where we now parameterize diffeomorphisms by the finite-dimensional velocity $\tilde{v}_0$:

$$E(\tilde{v}_0) = \|\tilde{v}_0\|_{\tilde{L}}^2 + \frac{1}{2\sigma^2}\|I_0 \circ \phi_1^{-1} - I_1\|^2. \tag{11}$$

Here the metric on $\tilde{V}$ is given by the discretized version of the $\tilde{L}$ operator. The Fourier transformation of $L = (-\alpha\Delta + I)^s$ is a diagonal operator. Discretizing this operator by only keeping the frequencies up to our bandlimits, N_j, we get a diagonal matrix $\tilde{L}$. Analogous to the L operator, this $\tilde{L} : \tilde{V} \to \tilde{V}^*$ maps a tangent vector in Fourier domain to its dual momentum vector $\tilde{m}$. For a 3D grid, the coefficients $\tilde{L}_{ijk}$ of this operator at coordinate (i, j, k) in the Fourier domain are

$$\tilde{L}_{ijk} = \left[-2\alpha\left(\cos\frac{2\pi i}{W} + \cos\frac{2\pi j}{H} + \cos\frac{2\pi k}{D}\right) + 7\right]^s,$$

where W, H, D are the dimension of each direction. Vice versa, the Fourier coefficients of the K operator are $\tilde{K}_{ijk} = \tilde{L}_{ijk}^{-1}$.

Before describing the details of our diffeomorphic image matching algorithm, we first provide an outline of the general steps. Beginning with the initialization $\tilde{v}_0 = 0$, the gradient descent algorithm to minimize the energy (11) proceeds by iterating the following:

1. **Forward shooting of $\tilde{v}_0$:** Forward integrate the geodesic evolution equations on $\tilde{V}$ to generate $\tilde{v}_{t_k}$ at discrete time points $t_1 = 0, t_2, \ldots, t_T = 1$.
2. **Compute the diffeomorphism ϕ_1^{-1}:** Compute the inverse diffeomorphism, ϕ_1^{-1}, by integrating the negative velocity field backward in time.
3. **Compute gradient at $t = 1$:** Compute the gradient, $\nabla_{\tilde{v}_1} E$, of the energy (11) at $t = 1$.
4. **Bring gradient to $t = 0$ by adjoint Jacobi field:** Integrate the reduced adjoint Jacobi field equations in $\tilde{V}$ to get the gradient update $\nabla_{\tilde{v}_0} E$.

We note that Steps 2 and 3 are computed at the full resolution of the input images in the spatial domain. However, Steps 1 and 4 to compute the geodesic and the adjoint Jacobi fields are computed entirely in the finite-dimensional space $\tilde{V}$, resulting in greatly reduced computation time and memory requirements. We now provide details for the computations in each of these steps.

4.1   Geodesic Shooting in the Finite-Dimensional Lie Algebra

In the previous section, we introduced a finite-dimensional Lie algebra. Analogous to the EPDiff Eq. (3), we define its geodesic evolution equation as

$$\frac{\partial \tilde{v}}{\partial t} = -\text{ad}_{\tilde{v}}^{\dagger}\tilde{v} = -\tilde{K}\text{ad}_{\tilde{v}}^{*}\tilde{m}, \tag{12}$$

where the operator $\text{ad}^{*} : \tilde{V}^{*} \to \tilde{V}^{*}$ is the dual of the negative finite-dimensional Lie bracket of vector fields in the Fourier space, and its discrete formulation is

$$\text{ad}_{\tilde{v}}^{*}\tilde{m} = (\tilde{D}\tilde{v})^{T} \star \tilde{m} + \tilde{D}\tilde{m} \star \tilde{v} + \tilde{m} \star (\tilde{\Gamma}\tilde{v}), \tag{13}$$

where $\tilde{\Gamma}\tilde{v}$ is divergence of the discrete vector field $\tilde{v}$. It is computed as sum of the point-wise multiplication $\tilde{\Gamma}\tilde{v} = \sum_{k_1=0}^{N_1} \cdots \sum_{k_d=0}^{N_d} \eta_i \tilde{v}_i$, where η_i is the Fourier coefficient of the central differential operator on each dimension.

Plugging (13) back into the geodesic evolution Eq. (12), we have

$$\frac{\partial \tilde{v}}{\partial t} = -\text{ad}_{\tilde{v}}^{\dagger}\tilde{v} = -\tilde{K}\left[(\tilde{D}\tilde{v})^{T} \star \tilde{m} + \tilde{D}\tilde{m} \star \tilde{v} + \tilde{m} \star (\tilde{\Gamma}\tilde{v})\right]. \tag{14}$$

4.2   Adjoint Jacobi Fields

The computation of the gradient term in our model requires the adjoint Jacobi fields, which are used to integrate the gradient term at $t = 1$ backward to the initial point $t = 0$. To derive this, consider a variation of geodesics $\gamma :$ $(-\epsilon, \epsilon) \times [0,1] \to \text{Diff}^{\infty}(\Omega)$, with $\gamma(0,t) = \phi_t$ and $\gamma(s,0) = \text{Id}$. Such a variation corresponds to a variation of the initial velocity $(d/dt)\gamma(s,0) = v_0 + s\delta v_0$. The variation $\gamma(s,t)$ produces a "fan" of geodesics, illustrated in Fig. 2. Taking the derivative of this variation results in a Jacobi field: $J_v(t) = d\gamma/ds(0,t)$.

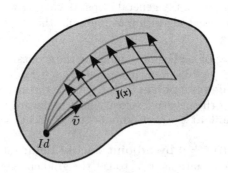

Fig. 2. Jacobi fields

In this paper, we use a simple version of reduced Jacobi field from Bullo [7], which is also used by [8]. Under the right invariant metric of diffeomorphisms, we define a vector $U(t) \in \tilde{V}$ as a right trivialized reduced Jacobi field $U(t) = J_{\tilde{v}}(t)\phi(t)^{-1}$, and a variation of the right trivialized reduced velocity $\tilde{v}$ is $\delta\tilde{v}$.

By introducing adjoint variables $\hat{U}, \delta\hat{v} \in \tilde{V}$, we have the adjoint Jacobi equations as

$$\frac{d\hat{U}}{dt} = -\mathrm{ad}_{\tilde{v}}^{\dagger}\hat{U}$$

$$\frac{d\delta\hat{v}}{dt} = -\hat{U} - \mathrm{sym}_{\tilde{v}}^{\dagger}\delta\hat{v}, \tag{15}$$

where $\mathrm{sym}_v^{\dagger}\delta\hat{v} = -\mathrm{ad}_v\delta\hat{v} + \mathrm{ad}_{\delta\hat{v}}^{\dagger}v$. For more details on the derivation of the adjoint Jacobi field equations, see [7].

5 Results

We demonstrate the effectiveness of our proposed model using real 3D OASIS MRI brain data. The MRI have resolution $128 \times 128 \times 128$ and are skull-stripped, intensity normalized, and co-registered with rigid transforms. We use $\alpha = 3.0, s = 3.0, \sigma = 0.03$ with $T = 10$ time-steps in geodesic shooting for all the experiments in this paper.

Image Registration. We tested our algorithm for geodesic shooting for pairwise image registration at different levels of truncated dimension $N =$

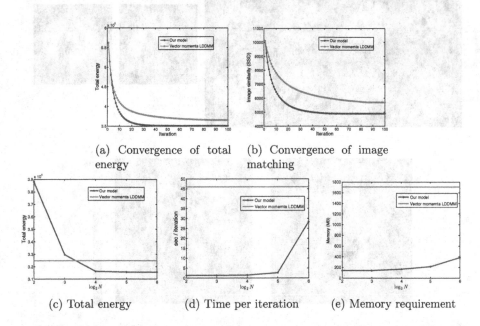

(a) Convergence of total energy

(b) Convergence of image matching

(c) Total energy

(d) Time per iteration

(e) Memory requirement

Fig. 3. Comparison between our model at different scale of truncated dimension and vector momenta LDDMM for (a) convergence of total energy with $N = 16$ truncated dimension; (b) convergence of image matching with $N = 16$ truncated dimension; (c) total energy; (d) time consumption per iteration; (e) memory requirement.

$4, 8, 16, 32, 64$. We compared the total energy formulated in (5), time consumption, and memory requirement of our model versus the open source implementation of vector momenta LDDMM [11] (https://bitbucket.org/scicompanat/vectormomentum). For comparison, we use the same integration method and (α, s, σ, T) parameters for both models.

Figure 3 displays the comparison of convergence, time, and memory at different levels of truncated dimensions. It indicates that our model gains better registration accuracy but with much less time and memory. We see that our method actually achieves a lower overall energy than vector momenta LDDMM for truncated dimension $N = 16$ and higher. Note that increasing the dimension beyond $N = 16$ does not improve the image registration energy, indicating that $N = 16$ is sufficient to capture the transformations between images. We emphasize that

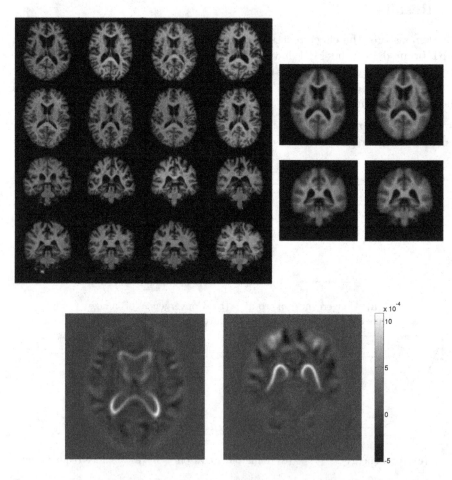

Fig. 4. Top left: axial and coronal slices from 8 of the input 3D MRIs. Middle to right: atlas estimated by our model and vector momenta LDDMM. Bottom: axial and coronal view of atlas intensity difference.

we used the same full-dimensional registration energy from (2) for all runs so that they would be comparable. In addition, our model arrives at the optimal solution for $N = 16$ in 1.59 s per iteration, and 168.4 MB memory. In comparison, vector momenta LDDMM requires 46 s per iteration, and 1708.1 MB memory.

Atlas Building. We also used our algorithm to build an atlas from a set of 3D brain MRIs from the OASIS database, consisting of 60 healthy subjects between the age of 60 to 95. We initialize the template I as the average of image intensities, and set the truncated dimension as $N = 16$ that was shown to be optimal in the previous section. We used a message passing interface (MPI) parallel programming implementation for both our model and vector momenta LDDMM, and scattered each image onto an individual processor. With 100 iterations for gradient descent, our model builds the atlas in 7.5 min, while the vector momenta LDDMM in [11] requires 2 h.

The left side of Fig. 4 shows the axial and coronal slices from 8 of the selected 3D MRI dataset. The right side shows the atlas image estimated by our algorithm, followed by the atlas estimated by vector momenta LDDMM. We see from the difference image between the two atlas results that our algorithm generated a very similar atlas to vector momenta LDDMM, but at a fraction of the time and memory cost.

6   Conclusion

We presented a fast geodesic shooting algorithm for diffeomorphic image registration. Our method is the first to introduce a finite-dimensional Lie algebra that can represent discretized velocity fields of diffeomorphisms in a lower-dimensional space. Another key contribution of this finite-dimensional Lie algebra is that we can compute the geodesic evolution equations, as well as the adjoint Jacobi field equations required for gradient descent methods entirely in a low-dimensional vector space. This leads to a dramatically fast diffeomorphic image registration algorithm without loss in accuracy. This work paves the way for efficient computations in large statistical studies using LDDMM. Other speed up strategies, for instance, a second-order Gauss-Newton step, similar to the one proposed in   [4], or a multi-resolution optimization scheme could be added on top of our algorithm for further speed improvement. Another interesting possibility is that our algorithm could make inference by Monte Carlo sampling of diffeomorphisms [16] more feasible.

Acknowledgments. This work was supported by NIH Grant 5R01EB007688 and NSF CAREER Grant 1054057.

References

1. Arnol'd, V.I.: Sur la géométrie différentielle des groupes de Lie de dimension infinie et ses applications à l'hydrodynamique des fluides parfaits. Ann. Inst. Fourier **16**, 319–361 (1966)

Fast Optimal Transport Averaging
of Neuroimaging Data

A. Gramfort[1,2]([⊠]), G. Peyré[3], and M. Cuturi[4]

[1] Institut Mines-Télécom, Telecom ParisTech, CNRS LTCI, Paris, France
alexandre.gramfort@telecom-paristech.fr
[2] NeuroSpin, CEA Saclay, Bat. 145, 91191 Gif-sur-Yvette, Cedex France
[3] CNRS and CEREMADE, Université Paris-Dauphine, Paris, France
[4] Graduate School of Informatics, Kyoto University, Kyoto, Japan

Abstract. Knowing how the Human brain is anatomically and functionally organized at the level of a group of healthy individuals or patients is
the primary goal of neuroimaging research. Yet computing an average of
brain imaging data defined over a voxel grid or a triangulation remains
a challenge. Data are large, the geometry of the brain is complex and
the between subjects variability leads to spatially or temporally non-
overlapping effects of interest. To address the problem of variability, data
are commonly smoothed before performing a linear group averaging. In
this work we build on ideas originally introduced by Kantorovich [18] to
propose a new algorithm that can average efficiently non-normalized data
defined over arbitrary discrete domains using transportation metrics. We
show how Kantorovich means can be linked to Wasserstein barycenters in
order to take advantage of the entropic smoothing approach used by [7].
It leads to a smooth convex optimization problem and an algorithm with
strong convergence guarantees. We illustrate the versatility of this tool
and its empirical behavior on functional neuroimaging data, functional
MRI and magnetoencephalography (MEG) source estimates, defined on
voxel grids and triangulations of the folded cortical surface.

1 Introduction

Computing the average of some observations may seem like a trivial problem, yet
it remains an active topic of research in mathematics, statistics and applications
such as medical imaging. The problem of atlas computation from images [17], or
meshes [11], or the problem of group analysis from functional imaging data [25]
are particularly relevant for this field. The challenge is that natural phenomena
are usually described in terms of physical and temporal event locations, along
with their intensity. While Euclidean averaging is standard and has some benefits
such as low computation time, this procedure ignores the geometry of the space
the observations belong to; the image of an average brain image obtained by
Euclidean averaging of individual voxels does not yield the image of the brain
of an average individual.

Starting from observations defined on a regular or irregular grid, our aim is to
provide a *model-free* approach to *average* them that only builds upon geometric

© Springer International Publishing Switzerland 2015
S. Ourselin et al. (Eds.): IPMI 2015, LNCS 9123, pp. 261–272, 2015.
DOI: 10.1007/978-3-319-19992-4_20

Fast Optimal Transport Averaging
of Neuroimaging Data

A. Gramfort[1,2]($\boxtimes$), G. Peyré[3], and M. Cuturi[4]

[1] Institut Mines-Télécom, Telecom ParisTech, CNRS LTCI, Paris, France
`alexandre.gramfort@telecom-paristech.fr`
[2] NeuroSpin, CEA Saclay, Bat. 145, 91191 Gif-sur-Yvette, Cedex France
[3] CNRS and CEREMADE, Université Paris-Dauphine, Paris, France
[4] Graduate School of Informatics, Kyoto University, Kyoto, Japan

Abstract. Knowing how the Human brain is anatomically and function-ally organized at the level of a group of healthy individuals or patients is the primary goal of neuroimaging research. Yet computing an average of brain imaging data defined over a voxel grid or a triangulation remains a challenge. Data are large, the geometry of the brain is complex and the between subjects variability leads to spatially or temporally non-overlapping effects of interest. To address the problem of variability, data are commonly smoothed before performing a linear group averaging. In this work we build on ideas originally introduced by Kantorovich [18] to propose a new algorithm that can average efficiently non-normalized data defined over arbitrary discrete domains using transportation metrics. We show how Kantorovich means can be linked to Wasserstein barycenters in order to take advantage of the entropic smoothing approach used by [7]. It leads to a smooth convex optimization problem and an algorithm with strong convergence guarantees. We illustrate the versatility of this tool and its empirical behavior on functional neuroimaging data, functional MRI and magnetoencephalography (MEG) source estimates, defined on voxel grids and triangulations of the folded cortical surface.

1 Introduction

Computing the average of some observations may seem like a trivial problem, yet it remains an active topic of research in mathematics, statistics and applications such as medical imaging. The problem of atlas computation from images [17], or meshes [11], or the problem of group analysis from functional imaging data [25] are particularly relevant for this field. The challenge is that natural phenomena are usually described in terms of physical and temporal event locations, along with their intensity. While Euclidean averaging is standard and has some benefits such as low computation time, this procedure ignores the geometry of the space the observations belong to; the image of an average brain image obtained by Euclidean averaging of individual voxels does not yield the image of the brain of an average individual.

Starting from observations defined on a regular or irregular grid, our aim is to provide a *model-free* approach to *average* them that only builds upon geometric

© Springer International Publishing Switzerland 2015
S. Ourselin et al. (Eds.): IPMI 2015, LNCS 9123, pp. 261–272, 2015.
DOI: 10.1007/978-3-319-19992-4_20

arguments. An example of such data are functional MRI (fMRI) data defined on a voxel grid or a triangulated cortical surface. The approach aims to be intrinsically geometric in the sense that it *only* requires the prior knowledge of a metric between the locations on the grid. The technique aims to be versatile in the sense that it can be applied to weighted samples taking values on a discretized space with no assumptions on the regularity of the metric.

The approach we propose is inspired by optimal transport theory [26] and can be seen as an extension of the Wasserstein barycenter problem [1,7,22], which aims at estimating a probability measure which bests approximates a family of probability measures in the Wasserstein metric sense. The challenge of using optimal transport in the setting we consider comes from the fact that Wasserstein distances (and their barycenters) are defined for *probability* measures only. While some data are normalized such the Orientation Diffusion Function (ODF) in diffusion MRI [10], a number of medical imaging data are non-normalized. Here we bypass this limitation using a generalization of optimal transport distances proposed by [18]. This extension comes at a price, since it introduces an additional parameter (the cost of adding or removing mass) which can be difficult to tune. We propose a simple way to mitigate this problem by introducing a natural constraint on the overall mass of the barycenter, which we set to be equal to the average of the masses of all samples. We provide an efficient method to compute Kantorovich means by building upon the first algorithm of [7]. We provide intuitions on the behavior of our method and demonstrate its relevance with simulations and experimental results obtained with fMRI and MEG data which are neuroimaging data defined on a voxel grid or a triangulation of the folded cortical mantle.

This paper is organized as follows. We start in Sect. 2 with a reminder on optimal transport and the Kantorovich metric for non-normalized measures. We introduce Kantorovich means in Sect. 3 and describe efficient algorithms to compute them. Section 4 contains simulations and results on publicly available fMRI data with 20 subjects and MEG data with 16 subjects.

2   Optimal Transport Between (Un)Normalized Measures

We introduce in this section Wasserstein distances for non-negative measures on a finite metric space (Ω, D). Simply put, we consider normalized histograms on a grid of locations, and assume the distance between any two locations is provided. Next, we extend Wasserstein distances to non-negative vectors of *bounded mass*.

Notations. Let d be the cardinal of Ω. Relabeling arbitrarily all the elements of Ω as $\{1, \cdots, d\}$ we represent the set of non-negative measures on Ω by the non-negative orthant $\mathbb{R}_+^d$. Let $\mathbf{1}_d$ be the d-dimensional vector of ones. For any vector $u \in \mathbb{R}^d$ we write $|u|_1$ for the l_1 norm of u, $\sum_{i=1}^d |u_i|$. When $u \in \mathbb{R}_+^d$ we also call $|u|_1$ the (total) *mass* of vector u. Let $M = [m_{ij}] \in \mathbb{R}_+^{d \times d}$ be the matrix that describes the metric between all locations in Ω, namely $m_{ij} = D(i,j), i, j \leq d$.

Wasserstein Distance for Normalized Histograms. Consider two vectors $a, b \in \mathbb{R}_+^d$ such that $|a|_1 = |b|_1$. Both can be interpreted as histograms on Ω of the same mass. A non-trivial example of such normalized data in medical imaging is the discretized ODF used for diffusion imaging data [10]. For $p \geq 1$, the p-Wasserstein distance $W_p(a, b)$ between a and b is the pth root of the optimum of a linear program, known as a *transportation problem* [4, §7.2]. A transport problem is a network flow problem on a bipartite graph with cost M^p (the pairwise distance matrix M raised element-wise to the power p), and feasible set of flows $U(a, b)$ (known as the transportation polytope of a and b), where $U(a, b)$ is the set of $d \times d$ nonnegative matrices such that their row and column marginals are equal to a and b respectively:

$$U(a, b) \stackrel{\text{def}}{=} \{T \in \mathbb{R}_+^{d \times d} \mid T\mathbf{1}_d = a, \, T^T\mathbf{1}_d = b\}. \tag{1}$$

Given the constraints induced by a and b, one naturally has that $U(a, b)$ is empty when $|a|_1 \neq |b|_1$ and non-empty when $|a|_1 = |b|_1$ (in which case one can easily check that the matrix $ab^T / |a|_1$ belongs to that set). The p-Wasserstein distance $W_p(a, b)$ raised to the power p (written $W_p^p(a, b)$ below) is equal to the optimum of a parametric Optimal Transport (**OT**) problem on d^2 variables,

$$W_p^p(a, b) = \mathbf{OT}(a, b, M^p) \stackrel{\text{def}}{=} \min_{T \in U(a,b)} \langle T, M^p \rangle, \tag{2}$$

parameterized by the marginals a, b and matrix M^p.

Optimal Transport for Unnormalized Measures. If the total masses of a and b differ, namely $|a|_1 \neq |b|_1$, the definition provided above is not useful because $U(a, b) = \emptyset$. Several extensions of the OT problem have been proposed in that setting; we recall them here for the sake of completeness. In the computer vision literature, [23] proposed to handle that case by: *(i) relaxing* the equality constraints of $U(a, b)$ to inequality constraints $T\mathbf{1}_d \leq a, T^T\mathbf{1}_d \leq b$ in Eq. (1); *(ii) adding an equality constraint* on the total mass of the solution $\mathbf{1}_d^T T\mathbf{1}_d = \min(|a|_1, |b|_1)$; *(iii) dividing* the minimum of $\langle T, M \rangle$ under constraints *(i,ii)* by $\min(|a|_1, |b|_1)$. This modification does not, however, result in a metric. [20] proposed later a variant of this approach called EMD-hat that incorporates constraints *(i,ii)* but *(iii')* adds to the optimal cost $\langle T^\star, M \rangle$ a constant times $\min(|a|_1, |b|_1)$. When that constant is large enough M, [20] claim that EMD-hat is a metric. We also note that [2] proposed a quadratic penalty between the differences of masses and made use of a dynamic formulation of the transportation problem.

Kantorovich Norms for Signed Measures. We propose to build on early contributions by Kantorovich to define a generalization of optimal transport distance for unnormalized measures, making optimal transport applicable to a wider class of problems, such as the averaging of functional imaging data. [18] proposed such a generalization as an intermediary result of a more general definition, the *Kantorovich norm* for signed measures on a compact metric space, which was itself extended to separable metric spaces by [15]. We summarize this idea here by simplifying it to the case of interest in this paper where Ω is a finite (of size d) probability space, in which case signed measures are equivalent to vectors in $\mathbb{R}^d$. [18] propose first a norm for vectors z in the orthogonal of 1_d (vectors z such that $z^T 1_d = 0$), by considering the 1-Wasserstein distance between the positive and negative parts of z, $\|z\|_K = W_1(z_+, z_-)$. A penalty vector $\Delta \in \mathbb{R}^d_+$ is then introduced to define the norm $\|x\|_K$ of any vector x as the minimal value of $\|z\|_K + \Delta^T |z - x|$ when z is taken in the space of all vectors z with zero sum, and $|z - x|$ is the element-wise absolute value of the difference of vectors z and x. For this to define a true norm in $\mathbb{R}^d$, Δ must be such that $\Delta_i \geq \max_j m_{ij}$ and $|\Delta_i - \Delta_j| \leq m_{ij}$. The distance between two arbitrary non-negative vectors a, b of different mass is then defined as $\|a - b\|_K$. As highlighted by [26, p.108], and if we write e_i for the ith vector of the canonical basis of $\mathbb{R}^d$, this norm is the maximal norm in $\mathbb{R}^d$ such that for any $i, j \leq d$, $\|e_i - e_j\|_K = m_{ij}$, namely the maximal norm in the space of signed measures on Ω such that the norm between two Dirac measures coincides with Ω's metric between these points.

Kantorovich Distances for Unnormalized Nonnegative Measures. Reference [14] noticed that Kantorovich's distance between unnormalized measures can be cast as a regular optimal transport problem. Indeed, one simply needs to: *(i)* add a *virtual point* ω to the set $\Omega = \{1, \cdots, d\}$ whose distance $D(i, \omega) = D(\omega, i)$ to any element i in Ω is set to Δ_i; *(ii)* use that point ω as a buffer when comparing two measures of different mass. The appeal of Kantorovich's formulation in the context of this work is that it boils down to a classic optimal transport problem, which can be approximated efficiently using the smoothing approach of [6] as discussed in Sect. 3. To simplify our analysis in the next section, we only consider non-negative vectors (histograms) $a \in \mathbb{R}^d_+$ such that their total mass is upper bounded by a known positive constant. This assumption alleviates the definition of our distance below, since it does not require to treat separately the cases where either $|a|_1 \geq |b|_1$ or $|a|_1 < |b|_1$ when comparing $a, b \in \mathbb{R}^d_+$. Note also that this assumption always holds when dealing with finite collections of data. Without loss of generality, this is equivalent to considering vectors a in $\mathbb{R}^d_+$ such that $|a|_1 \leq 1$ with a simple rescaling of all vectors by that constant. We define next the Kantorovich metric on S_d, where $S_d = \{u \in \mathbb{R}^d_+, |u|_1 \leq 1\}$.

Definition 1 (Kantorovich Distances on S_d). *Let $\Delta \in \mathbb{R}^d_+$ such that $\Delta_i \geq \max_j m_{ij}$ and $|\Delta_i - \Delta_j| \leq m_{ij}$. Let $p \geq 0$. For two elements a and b of S_d, we write $\alpha = 1 - |a|_1 \geq 0$ and $\beta = 1 - |b|_1 \geq 0$. Their p-Kantorovich distance raised to the power p is*

$$K^p_{p\Delta}(a, b) = \mathbf{OT}\left(\begin{bmatrix} a \\ \alpha \end{bmatrix}, \begin{bmatrix} b \\ \beta \end{bmatrix}, \hat{M}^p\right), \text{ where } \hat{M} = \begin{bmatrix} M & \Delta \\ \Delta^T & 0 \end{bmatrix} \in \mathbb{R}^{d+1 \times d+1}_+. \quad (3)$$

The Kantorovich distance inherits all metric properties of Wasserstein distances: the mapping which to a vector a associates a vector $[a; 1 - |a|_1] \in \Sigma_{d+1}$ can be regarded as a feature map, to which the standard Wasserstein distance using $\hat{M}$ (which is itself a metric matrix) is applied.

3 Kantorovich Mean of Unnormalized Measures

Consider now a collection $\{b^1, \cdots, b^N\}$ of N non-negative measures on (Ω, D) with mass upper-bounded by 1, namely N vectors in S_d. Let $\beta^j = 1 - |b^j|$ be the deficient mass of b^j. Our goal in this section is to find, given a vector of virtual costs Δ and an exponent p, a vector a in S_d which minimizes the sum of its p-Kantorovich distances $K^p_{p\Delta}$ to all the b^j,

$$a \in \operatorname*{argmin}_{u \in S_d} \frac{1}{N} \sum_{j=1}^{N} K^p_{p\Delta}(u, b^j) = \operatorname*{argmin}_{u \in S_d} \frac{1}{N} \sum_{j=1}^{N} \mathbf{OT}\left(\begin{bmatrix} u \\ 1-|u|_1 \end{bmatrix}, \begin{bmatrix} b^j \\ \beta^j \end{bmatrix}, \hat{M}^p\right). \quad \text{(P1)}$$

Because of the equivalence between Kantorovich distances for points in S_d and Wasserstein distances in the $d+1$ simplex, this problem can be naturally cast as a Wasserstein barycenter problem [1] with metric $\hat{M}$. Problem (P1) can be cast as a linear program with $N(d+1)^2$ variables. For the applications we have in mind, where d is of the order or larger than 10^4, solving that program is not tractable. We discuss next computational approaches to solve it efficiently.

Smooth Optimal Transport. References [22] and [5] have proposed efficient algorithms to solve the Wasserstein barycenter problem in low dimensional Euclidean spaces. These approaches are not, however, suitable when one considers observations on the cortex, for which *all pairs shortest path* metrics (inferred from a graph structure connecting all voxels) are preferred over Euclidean metrics. To solve Problem (P1) we turn instead to a recent series of algorithms proposed in [3,7] and [8] that all exploit the regularized OT approach suggested in [6]. Among these recent approaches, we propose to build in this work upon the first algorithm in [7], which can be easily modified to incorporate constraints on a. This flexibility will prove useful in the next section.

The strategy of [7] is to regularize directly the optimal transport problem by an entropic penalty, whose weight is parameterized by a parameter $\lambda > 0$,

$$\mathbf{OT}_\lambda(a, b, M^p) \stackrel{\text{def}}{=} \min_{T \in U(a,b)} \langle T, M^p \rangle - \frac{1}{\lambda} H(T),$$

where $H(T)$ stands for the entropy of the matrix T seen as an element of the simplex of size d^2, $H(T) \stackrel{\text{def}}{=} -\sum_{ij} t_{ij} \log(t_{ij})$. As shown by [7], the regularized transport problem $\mathbf{OT}_\lambda$ admits a unique optimal solution. As such, $\mathbf{OT}_\lambda(a, b, M^p)$ is a differentiable function of a whose gradient can be recovered through the solution of the corresponding smoothed dual optimal transport. Without elaborating further on this approach, we propose to simply replace all expressions that involve an optimal transport problem $\mathbf{OT}$ in our formulations by their smoothed counterpart $\mathbf{OT}_\lambda$.

Sensitivity of Kantorovich Means to the Parameter Δ. The magnitude of the solution a to Problem (P1) depends directly on the virtual distance Δ. Suppose, for instance, that $\Delta = \varepsilon 1_d$ with ε arbitrarily small. In that case a should converge to a unit mass on the last (virtual) bin and would therefore be equal to the null histogram $\mathbf{0}_d$ on the d other bins. If, on the contrary, $\Delta = \gamma \mathbf{1}_d$ and γ is large, we obtain that $K_{p\Delta}^p(a,b)/\gamma$ grows as $||a|_1 - |b|_1|$. Therefore a minimum of Problem (P1) would necessarily need to have a total mass that minimizes $\sum_j ||a|_1 - |b^j|_1|$, namely a total mass equal to the median mass of all b^j. This sensitivity of the solution a to the magnitude of Δ may be difficult to control. Choosing adequate values for Δ, namely setting the distance of the virtual point to the d other points, may also be a difficult parameter choice. To address this issue we propose to simplify our framework by introducing an equality constraint on the mass of the barycenter a in our definition, and let Δ be any non-negative vector, typically set to a large quantile of the distribution of all pairwise distances M_{ij}^p times the vector of ones $\mathbf{1}_d$. Under these assumptions, we can now propose p-Kantorovich means with a constraint on the total mass of a. Remaining parameters in our approach are therefore only p and λ. In practice we will fix $p = 1$, which corresponds to the Earth Mover's Distance [23], and use a high λ, namely a small entropic regularization of order $1/\lambda$, which has also the merit of making Problem (P1) strongly convex. λ is set in our experiments to $100/\mathrm{median}(M)$, where $\mathrm{median}(M)$ is the median of all pairwise distances $\{M_{ij}\}_{ij}$.

Definition 2 (p-Kantorovich Means with Constrained Mass). *Let $\Delta \in \mathbb{R}_+^d$ and $p \geq 0$. A Kantorovich mean with a target mass $\rho \leq 1$ of a set of N histograms $\{b^1, \cdots, b^N\}$ in S_d is the unique vector a in S_d such that:*

$$a \in \underset{\substack{a \in S_d \\ |a|_1 = \rho}}{\operatorname{argmin}} \frac{1}{N} \sum_j \mathbf{OT}_\lambda(a, b^j, \hat{M}^p).$$

We provide in Algorithm 1 an implementation of [7, Alg.1]. Unlike their version, we only consider a fixed step-length exponentiated gradient descent, and add a mass renormalization step. We set the default mass of the barycenter to be the mean of the masses of all histograms. We use the notation $\circ$ for the elementwise (Schur) product of vectors. Note that the computations of N dual optima in line 7 of Algorithm 1 below can be vectorized and computed using only matrix-matrix products. We use GPGPUs to carry out these computations.

4   Application to the Averaging of Neuroimaging Data

Neuromaging data are defined on a grid of voxels, eventually restricted to the brain volume, or on a triangulation of the cortical mantle obtained by segmentation of MRI data. Examples of data most commonly analyzed on a grid are fMRI data, while neural activity estimates derived from MEG/EEG data are often restricted to the cortical surface [9]. Anatomical data such as cortical thickness, which is a biomarker of certain neurodegenerative pathologies, is also defined on the surface. In all cases the data are defined on a discrete set of points (voxels or vertices) which have a natural distance given by the geometry of the brain. The data are also non-normalized as they represent physical or statistical quantities, such as thickness in millimeters or F statistics. Such data are therefore particularly well adapted to the algorithm proposed in this paper: they are defined on discrete space, are non-normalized and there exists a natural ground metric.

Algorithm 1. p-Kantorovich Barycenter with Constrained Mass

1: **Input**: $\{b^1, \cdots, b^N\} \subset S_d$, metric M, quantile q, $p \geq 0$, entropic regularizer $\lambda > 0$,
   step size c.
2: Compute mean mass $\rho = \frac{1}{N} \sum_i |b^j|_1$.
3: Form virtual cost vector $\Delta = \text{quantile}(M, q\%)\mathbf{1}_d$.
4: Form augmented $d+1 \times d+1$ ground metric $\hat{M}$ as in Equation (3)
5: Set $a = \mathbf{1}_{d+1}/(d+1)$.
6: **while** a changes **do**
7:   Compute all dual optima α^j of $\mathbf{OT}_\lambda(a, b^j, \hat{M})$ using [7, Alg.3]
8:   $a \leftarrow a \circ \exp(-c\frac{1}{N} \sum_{j=1}^N \alpha^j)$; (gradient update)
9:   $a_i \leftarrow \begin{cases} \rho a_i / \sum_{l=1}^d a_l & \text{if } i \leq d, \\ 1 - \rho & \text{if } i = d+1. \end{cases}$ (projection on the simplex/mass constraint)
10: **end while**
11: **Output** $a_{1:d} \in S_d$.

The difficulty when averaging neuroimaging data is the anatomo-functional variability: every brain is different. The standard approach to compensate for this variability across subjects is to smooth the data to favor the overlap of signal of interest after the individual data have been ported to a common space using anatomical landmarks (anatomical registration). Volume data are typically redefined in MNI space while surface data are transferred to an average cortical surface, using for instance the FreeSurfer software[1]. When working with fMRI the spatial variability is commonly compensated by smoothing the data with an isotropic Gaussian kernel of Full Width at Half Maximum (FWHM) between 6 and 8 mm. MEG and EEG suffer from the same spatial variability, but also from the temporal variability of neural responses which is compensated by low pass filtering the data. By employing a transportation metric informed by the geometry of the domain, this smoothing procedure as well as the setting of the kernel bandwidth are not needed.

In the following experiments we focus on spatial averaging, although extension to spatiotemporal data is straightforward provided the metric is defined along the time axis. When working with a voxel grid the distance is the Euclidian distance taking into account the voxel size in millimeters, and when working on a cortical triangulation, the distance used is the geodesic distance computed on the folded cortical mantle. We now present results of a simulation study where standard averaging with Gaussian smoothing is compared to Kantorovich means. Simulation results are followed by experimental results obtained with fMRI data from 20 subjects and MEG data on a population of 16 subjects.

Simulation Setup. In this experiment using on a triangulation of the cortex, we simulated signals of interest in two brain regions using the functional parcellation provided by the FreeSurfer software. We used regions Broadman area 45 (BA45) and the visual area MT. We simulated for a group of 100 subjects

---

[1] https://surfer.nmr.mgh.harvard.edu/.

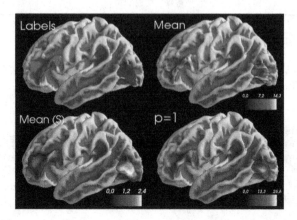

Fig. 1. Simulation results with focal random signals generated in areas/labels BA45 (yellow) and MT (red) in a group of 100 subjects. Data are defined on a surface with 10,024 vertices (FreeSurfer fsaverage 5). One shows the standard averaging referred to as *Mean*, the averaging after Gaussian smoothing is referred to as *Mean (S)* (mean after Gaussian smoothing with FWHM=8 mm), and the Kantorovich mean (p=1). The result *Mean* shows the focal signals with random positions in the labels delineated in green. The Kantorovich mean highlights clear foci of activations in the ROIs without smearing the activation as with Gaussian smoothing which furthermore significantly dampens the amplitudes (Color figure online).

random positive signals in these two regions. For each subject and each region, the signal is focal at a random location with a random amplitude generated with a truncated Gaussian distribution (mean 5, std. dev. 1.). We use here focal signals to exemplify the effect of optimal transport. Such signals could correspond to dipolar activations derived from MEG/EEG using dipole fitting methods [24] or sparse regression techniques [13,27].

Figure 1 presents the locations of the two regions (labels), the averages with and without Gaussian smoothing and the Kantorovich average. Gaussian smoothing leads to a highly blurred average which exceeds the extent of the regions of interest, while it also strongly reduces the amplitudes of the signals, potentially washing out the statistical effects. The peak amplitudes obtained with optimal transport are also higher and closer to the individual peak amplitudes. One can clearly observe the limitations of Gaussian smoothing, which furthermore requires to set the bandwidth of the kernel. The Kantorovich average nicely highlights two foci of signals at the group level.

Results on fMRI data. We used here fMRI data analyzed on a voxel grid. It corresponds to 20 subjects from the database described in [21]. We average here the standardized effect of interest induced by left hand button press. In Fig. 2-a we show the Euclidian average without smoothing. In Fig. 2-b we report results obtained by classical averaging following Gaussian smoothing with FWHM of 8 mm. Figure 2-c shows the Kantorovich mean with constrained mass. One can observe that this barycenter highlights a clear active region without requiring

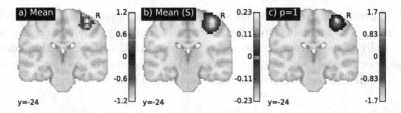

Fig. 2. Averaging of the standardized effect of interest on fMRI data. From left to right, a) the Euclidian mean without smoothing, b) the Euclidian mean with smoothing (FWHM=8 mm), c) the Kantorovich mean with Euclidian ground metric and p=1. The later result highlights a clear foci of activations in the ROI without smearing the activation nor damping the amplitudes as much as the kernel smoothing.

any kernel smoothing. It also leads to a amplitude in the average standardized effect around 1.7 which is much higher than the 0.23 obtained when smoothing.

Results on MEG data. We now evaluate the benefit of the proposed approach on experimental data. These data were acquired with a Neuromag VectorView system (Elekta Oy, Helsinki, Finland) with 306 sensors arranged in 102 triplets, each comprising two orthogonal planar gradiometers and one magnetometer. Subjects are presented with images containing faces of familiar (famous) or unfamiliar persons and so called "scrambled" faces. See [16] for more details. Dataset contains 16 subjects. For each one, event related fields (ERF) were obtained by averaging about 200 repetitions of recordings following stimuli presentations. Data were band pass filtered between 1 and 40 Hz. Following standard MEG source localization pipelines [12], a noise covariance was estimated from prestimulus time intervals and used for source reconstruction with the cortically constrained dSPM method [9]. The values obtained with dSPM can be considered as F statistics, where high values are located in active regions.

In Fig. 3, we present results at a single time point, 190 ms after stimulus onset, which corresponds to the time instant where the dSPM amplitudes are maximum. Data correspond the visual presentation of *famous faces*. In green, is the border of the primary visual cortex (V1) provided by the FreeSurfer functional atlas. One can observe that the Kantorovich barycenter yields a more focal average nicely positioned in the middle of the calcarine fissure where V1 is located. Such a strong activation in V1 is expected in such an experiment consisting of visual stimuli. To investigate more subtle cognitive effects, such as the response of the fusiform face area (FFA) reported about 170 ms after stimulation in the literature [16,19], we report results obtained on contrasts of ERFs measured after famous faces presentations *vs.* scrambled faces. As illustrated in Fig. 4, Kantorovich mean nicely delineates a focal source of activity in the ventral part of the cortex known as the fusiform gyrus.

These results show that Kantorovich means provides focal activation at the population level despite the challenging problem of inter-subject anatomo-functional variability. They avoid the smearing of the signal or statistical effects of interests which naturally occur when data are spatially smoothed before standard averaging. Note again that here no smoothing parameter with FWHM in millimeters is manually specified. Their solution only depends on the metric naturally derived from the geometry of the cortical surface. With a cortical triangulation containing 10,024 vertices and 16 subjects the computation on a Tesla K40 GPU of one barycenter takes less than 1 min.

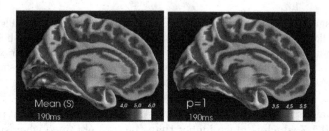

Fig. 3. Average of dSPM estimates derived from MEG ERF data on a group of 16 subjects stimulated with pictures of famous faces. From left to right: standard mean and Kantorovich mean. The left hemisphere is displayed in medial view. In green is the border of the primary visual cortex (V1) provided by FreeSurfer. One can observe that the Kantorovich mean has its peak amplitude within V1 (Color figure online).

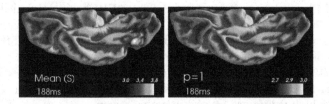

Fig. 4. Group averages (16 subjects) of dSPM estimates derived from MEG ERF data obtained by contrasting the famous faces stimulation with the scrambled faces. From left to right: standard mean and the Kantorovich mean. The right hemisphere is displayed in ventral view. Optimal transport results highlight a focal activity in the Fusiform gyrus known to be implicated in face processing [19].

5   Conclusion

The contributions of this work are two-fold. First, by considering non-normalized measures particularly relevant for medical imaging data we extend the current state of the art in barycenter estimation using transportation metrics. Following recent contributions on discrete optimal transport we propose a smoothed version of the transport problem that leads us to an efficient optimization algorithm. While many contributions on optimal transport work only in one or two dimensions on a regular grid, our approach can cope with the complex geometry of the brain (irregular grids and surfaces). Only the definition of a ground metric is here required. The algorithm proposed involves simple operations that are particularly adapted to modern GPU hardware and allows us to compute barycenters on full brain data in a few minutes.

Second, with simulations defined on the cortex triangulation, a publicly available fMRI dataset with 20 subjects and an MEG dataset processed with a standard analysis pipeline with 16 subjects we demonstrated the ability of the method to clearly highlight activation foci while avoiding the need to smooth the data. The fMRI data showed a clear activation in the right motor cortex and on the MEG data we showed that the proposed approach better identified activation foci in the primary visual cortex and the fusiform gyrus. Both findings, that are consistent with previous neuroscience literature, show that method proposed yields more accurate results than the current pipelines which furthermore requires to set a kernel bandwidth parameter. The removal of any free parameter in the pipeline is a way towards more reproducible neuroimaging results.

Due to the non-linearity of the approach the estimation of statistical threshold shall be performed with non-parametric permutation tests. When thresholding barycenters as presented in Sect. 4 it is expected that one will obtain clear clusters.

Acknowledgements. A. Gramfort was supported by the ANR grant THALAMEEG, ANR-14-NEUC-0002-01. M. Cuturi gratefully acknowledges the support of JSPS young researcher A grant 26700002, the gift of a K40 card from NVIDIA and fruitful discussions with K.R. Müller. The work of G. Peyré has been supported by the European Research Council (ERC project SIGMA-Vision).

References

1. Agueh, M., Carlier, G.: Barycenters in the Wasserstein space. SIAM J. Math. Anal. **43**(2), 904–924 (2011)
2. Benamou, J.D.: Numerical resolution of an unbalanced mass transport problem. ESAIM. Math. Model. Numer. Anal. **37**(5), 851–868 (2003)
3. Benamou, J.D., Carlier, G., Cuturi, M., Nenna, L., Peyré, G.: Iterative bregman projections for regularized transportation problems. arXiv preprint arXiv:1412.5154 (2014)
4. Bertsimas, D., Tsitsiklis, J.: Introduction to linear optimization. Athena Scientific Belmont, Boston (1997)
5. Bonneel, N., Rabin, J., Peyré, G., Pfister, H.: Sliced and radon wasserstein barycenters of measures. J. Math. Imaging Vis. **51**(1), 1–24 (2014)
6. Cuturi, M.: Sinkhorn distances: lightspeed computation of optimal transport. Adv. Neural Inf. Process. Sys. **26**, 2292–2300 (2013)
7. Cuturi, M., Doucet, A.: Fast computation of wasserstein barycenters. In: Proceedings of the 31st International Conference on Machine Learning (ICML-14) (2014)
8. Cuturi, M., Peyré, G., Rolet, A.: A smoothed dual approach for variational wasserstein problems. arXiv preprint arXiv:1503.02533 (2015)
9. Dale, A., Liu, A., Fischl, B., Buckner, R.: Dynamic statistical parametric neurotechnique mapping: combining fMRI and MEG for high-resolution imaging of cortical activity. Neuron **26**, 55–67 (2000)

10. Descoteaux, M., Deriche, R., Knosche, T., Anwander, A.: Deterministic and probabilistic tractography based on complex fibre orientation distributions. IEEE Trans. Med. Imaging **28**(2), 269–286 (2009)

11. Durrleman, S., Prastawa, M., Charon, N., Korenberg, J.R., Joshi, S., Gerig, G., Trouvé, A.: Morphometry of anatomical shape complexes with dense deformations and sparse parameters. NeuroImage **101**, 35–49 (2014)

12. Gramfort, A., Luessi, M., Larson, E., Engemann, D., Strohmeier, D., Brodbeck, C., Parkkonen, L., Hämäläinen, M.: MNE software for processing MEG and EEG data. NeuroImage **86**, 446–460 (2014)

13. Gramfort, A., Strohmeier, D., Haueisen, J., Hämäläinen, M., Kowalski, M.: Time-frequency mixed-norm estimates: Sparse M/EEG imaging with non-stationary source activations. NeuroImage **70**, 410–422 (2013)

14. Guittet, K.: Extended kantorovich norms: a tool for optimization. Technical repot 4402, INRIA (2002)

15. Hanin, L.: An extension of the kantorovich norm. Contemp. Math **226**, 113–130 (1999)

16. Henson, R.N., Wakeman, D.G., Litvak, V., Friston, K.J.: A parametric empirical bayesian framework for the EEG/MEG inverse problem: generative models for multisubject and multimodal integration. Front. Hum. Neuro. **5**(76), 141–153 (2011)

17. Joshi, S., Davis, B., Jomier, M., Gerig, G.: Unbiased diffeomorphic atlas construction for computational anatomy. NeuroImage **23**, 151–160 (2004)

18. Kantorovich, L., Rubinshtein, G.: On a space of totally additive functions, vestn. Vestn Lening. Univ. **13**, 52–59 (1958)

19. Kanwisher, N., Mcdermott, J., Chun, M.M.: The fusiform face area: a module in human extrastriate cortex specialized for face perception. J. Neurosci. **17**, 4302–4311 (1997)

20. Pele, O., Werman, M.: A linear time histogram metric for improved SIFT matching. In: Forsyth, D., Torr, P., Zisserman, A. (eds.) ECCV 2008, Part III. LNCS, vol. 5304, pp. 495–508. Springer, Heidelberg (2008)

21. Pinel, P., Thirion, B., Meriaux, S., Jobert, A., Serres, J., Le Bihan, D., Poline, J., Dehaene, S.: Fast reproducible identification and large-scale databasing of individual functional cognitive networks. BMC neuroscience **8**, 91 (2007)

22. Rabin, J., Peyré, G., Delon, J., Bernot, M.: Wasserstein barycenter and its application to texture mixing. In: Bruckstein, A.M., ter Haar Romeny, B.M., Bronstein, A.M., Bronstein, M.M. (eds.) SSVM 2011. LNCS, vol. 6667, pp. 435–446. Springer, Heidelberg (2012)

23. Rubner, Y., Guibas, L., Tomasi, C.: The earth movers distance, multi-dimensional scaling, and color-based image retrieval. In: Proceedings of the ARPA Image Understanding Workshop, pp. 661–668 (1997)

24. Scherg, M., Von Cramon, D.: Two bilateral sources of the late AEP as identified by a spatio-temporal dipole model. Electroencephalogr. Clin. Neurophysiol. **62**(1), 32–44 (1985)

25. Thirion, B., Pinel, P., Mériaux, S., Roche, A., Dehaene, S., Poline, J.B.: Analysis of a large fMRI cohort: statistical and methodological issues for group analyses. NeuroImage **35**(1), 105–120 (2007)

26. Villani, C.: Optimal transport: Old and New. Springer, Heidelberg (2009)

27. Wipf, D., Ramirez, R., Palmer, J., Makeig, S., Rao, B.: Analysis of empirical bayesian methods for neuroelectromagnetic source localization. In: Proceedings of the Neural Information Processing Systems (NIPS) (2007)

Deformation Models

Joint Morphometry of Fiber Tracts and Gray Matter Structures Using Double Diffeomorphisms

Pietro Gori[1]([✉]), Olivier Colliot[1,2], Linda Marrakchi-Kacem[1,3], Yulia Worbe[1],
Alexandre Routier[1], Cyril Poupon[3], Andreas Hartmann[1], Nicholas Ayache[4],
and Stanley Durrleman[1]

[1] Inria Paris-Rocquencourt, Sorbonne Universités,
UPMC Univ Paris 06 UMR S1127, Inserm U1127, CNRS UMR 7225,
CATI, ICM, 75013 Paris, France
pietro.gori@inria.fr
[2] Departments of Neurology and Neuroradiology,
AP-HP, Pitié-Salpêtrière Hospital, 75013 Paris, France
[3] Neurospin, CEA, Gif-sur-yvette, France
[4] Asclepios Project-team, Inria Sophia Antipolis, Sophia Antipolis, France

Abstract. This work proposes an atlas construction method to jointly
analyse the relative position and shape of fiber tracts and gray matter
structures. It is based on a *double diffeomorphism* which is a composition of two diffeomorphisms. The first diffeomorphism acts only on the
white matter keeping fixed the gray matter of the atlas. The resulting
white matter, together with the gray matter, are then deformed by the
second diffeomorphism. The two diffeomorphisms are related and jointly
optimised. In this way, the first diffeomorphisms explain the variability
in *structural connectivity* within the population, namely both changes in
the connected areas of the gray matter and in the geometry of the pathway of the tracts. The second diffeomorphisms put into correspondence
the homologous anatomical structures across subjects. Fiber bundles are
approximated with *weighted prototypes* using the metric of *weighted currents*. The atlas, the covariance matrix of deformation parameters and
the noise variance of each structure are automatically estimated using
a Bayesian approach. This method is applied to patients with Tourette
syndrome and controls showing a variability in the structural connectivity of the left cortico-putamen circuit.

1 Introduction

The brain could be seen as an interlinked multi-object anatomical complex.
Both gray and white matter consist of different structures (objects) which can
be segmented respectively as 3D surfaces (cortical surface and sub-cortical structures) or as sets of 3D tracts (fiber bundles resulting from tractography algorithms). The shape of these objects can then be analysed in order, for instance,
to find morphological characteristics of brain disorders. Most studies examine

© Springer International Publishing Switzerland 2015
S. Ourselin et al. (Eds.): IPMI 2015, LNCS 9123, pp. 275–287, 2015.
DOI: 10.1007/978-3-319-19992-4_21

these objects independently focusing on a single anatomical structure [9–13]. Others propose multi-object analysis considering only a particular kind of mesh, either only sub-cortical structures [5–8] or only fiber-bundles [14–16]. However, an abnormal brain development due to a neuropsychiatric disorder can influence not only the shape of individual structures but also their organization. An example is the syndrome of Gilles de la Tourette (GTS) which is thought to be associated with mis-connections of the cortico-striato-pallido-thalamic circuits [3]. These circuits need to be analysed as a whole, studying not only the shape of both white and gray matter components but also their relative position.

A technique to study this problematic is the atlas construction. It permits to estimate an average shape complex of the population under study called template complex and the 3D deformations of the embedding space which warp the template complex to the shape complexes of each subject. Previous works [2,5,8,9] have defined these 3D deformations as a diffeomorphism which prevents shape components to intersect, fold or shear during deformation. This allows the joint analysis of series of objects while guaranteeing preservation of the anatomical organization. However, such a global change of coordinates assumes that the relative position between structures *in contact with each other* does not change across subjects. This implies that a particular fiber bundle should link the same areas of the cortical surface and basal ganglia across the whole population. This assumption precludes the study of changes in structural connectivity which could be caused by an abnormal brain development as in GTS.

To overcome this problem we propose to replace a *single diffeomorphism* with a *double diffeomorphism* which is a composition of two diffeomorphisms. Given a template complex, the idea is to use the first diffeomorphism to deform only the white matter of the template while keeping fixed the gray matter and then to use the second diffeomorphism to deform the resulting white matter together with the gray matter. The first diffeomorphism makes the fiber bundles slide on the fixed cortical surface and basal ganglia. It can be seen as a relative motion with respect to the template gray matter considered as a fixed anatomical reference frame delineating the boundaries of the functional and anatomical territories. The second diffeomorphism puts in correspondence the structures of the template with the homologous ones of the subject. It is a global change of coordinates which brings all the structures in the coordinate system of the subject. The two diffeomorphisms are linked since they both deform the white matter and they are optimised together. This permits to find the composition of diffeomorphisms which allows to separate the variations due to a different structural connectivity (first diffeomorphism) to the ones related to a global shape difference (second diffeomorphism). An illustrative matching toy example in Fig. 1 clarifies in which situations double diffeomorphisms are necessary.

In order to deal with the considerable amount of fibers resulting from tractography algorithms, we rely on the approximation scheme introduced in [4]. Fiber bundles are approximated with weighted prototypes represented as "tubes". They are chosen among the fibers and their radius is related to the number of fibers approximated. This new representation is based on the metric of weighted currents [4], an extension of the framework of currents. As usual currents, it does not require point-correspondence between fibers or fiber-correspondence between

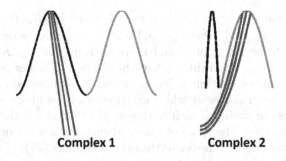

Fig. 1. Two shape complexes composed by a pseudo cortex, divided into a black and green area, and a red pseudo fiber bundle. A single diffeomorphism could not capture the differences in structural connectivity and put in correspondence both structures. A double diffeomorphism would first move the fiber bundle from the left to the right gyrus and then it would change the shape of the gyri, producing an accurate matching (Color figure online).

bundles. Two fibers modelled as weighted currents are considered similar if their pathways are alike and their endpoints are close to each other. This metric makes therefore possible to match correctly also the extremities of two fiber bundles and not only their central part as in usual currents. This is fundamental in order to retrieve the connectivity changes at the end of the first diffeomorphism.

The atlas is estimated using a generative statistical model similar to the one in [2] adapted to double diffeomorphisms. The proposed Bayesian model uses similar priors as in [1] which enables to automatically estimate the noise variance of each structure and the covariance matrix of the deformation parameters for both diffeomorphisms. The set of noise variances represent a trade-off between each data-term and the two deformation regularity terms.

In Sect. 2, we first introduce how we model the brain structures summarizing the framework of weighted currents and weighted prototypes. We then present the proposed framework of *double diffeomorphism* and include it into a Bayesian atlas construction method. In Sect. 3, we first apply our new scheme to a toy matching example comparing its performance with the one of a single diffeomorphism. Then, we build an atlas with the proposed technique using real data.

2   Bayesian Double Diffeomorphic Atlas Construction

2.1   Object Representation

Gray Matter. Gray matter objects are modelled as 3D surfaces, where we assume vertex correspondence across subjects. The norm of the difference between two meshes is defined as the sum of squared differences between pair of vertices.

White Matter. Fiber bundles are modelled as *weighted currents* [4]. Let X and Y be two fibers which can be modelled as polygonal lines of Q and Z segments respectively. We define $\{f^a, f^b\}$ for X and $\{t^a, t^b\}$ for Y as the vectors containing the coordinates of their extremities. The inner product between these two tracts in the framework of weighted currents is given by: $K_a(f^a, t^a) K_b(f^b, t^b)$ $\sum_{i=1}^{Q} \sum_{j=1}^{Z} \alpha_i^T K_g(x_i, y_j) \beta_j$ where $\{x_i, \alpha_i\}$ and $\{y_j, \beta_j\}$ are the centres and tangent vectors of the segments of X and Y respectively and K_a, K_b and K_g are Gaussian kernels whose bandwidth is fixed by the user. The last one defines the range of interaction between the points of X and Y, as in usual currents, while K_a and K_b set the distances at which extremities of the fibers are considered close. Two fibers are similar if their pathways are alike and if their extremities are close to each other. The space of weighted currents is a vector space, which implies that a fiber bundle B is seen as the sum of its fibers $\{F_i\}$: $B = \sum_i F_i$. This makes possible to easily compare two fiber bundles, which do not need to have the same number of fibers, by expanding the inner product $< \sum_i F_i, \sum_j F_j' >$.

Weighted Prototypes. A fiber bundle B is approximated with a set of weighted prototypes $\{\tau_i M_i\}$ chosen among the fibers [4]. The prototype M_i is modelled as a weighted current and its weight τ_i is linked to the number of fibers approximated. This approximation scheme is controlled by the residual error: $||B - \sum_{i=1}^{K} \tau_i M_i||_{W^*}^2$ in the space of weighted currents. It permits to reduce the number of fibers to analyse while preserving connectivity (location of the fiber endpoints on the gray matter) and geometry (pathway of the fibers).

2.2 Double Diffeomorphic Deformation

Let N be the number of subjects and M the number of objects. All structures of subject i can be seen as a shape complex $S_i = \{S_{ij}\}_{j=1...M} = S_i^W \cup S_i^G$ which is modelled as a *double deformation* of a common template complex $T = T^W \cup T^G$ plus a residual noise $\epsilon_i = \{\epsilon_i^W, \epsilon_i^G\}$ where $T = \{T_j\}_{j=1...M}$, $\epsilon_i = \{\epsilon_{ij}\}_{j=1...M}$ and the upper indices W and G refer to the White and Gray matter respectively:

$$S_i = \phi_i^{All}\left(\phi_i^W(T^W) \cup T^G\right) + \epsilon_i \tag{1}$$

The first deformation ϕ_i^W deforms the white matter keeping fixed the gray, thus modeling the changes in the relative position between white and gray matter objects. The second deformation ϕ_i^{All} matches both gray and white matter (the latter already deformed by ϕ_i^W). Both deformations depend on subject i and they are the last deformation of a flow of diffeomorphisms built by integrating a time-varying vector field $v_i(t, x) = v_{it}(x)$ ($t \in [0, 1]$, $x \in \mathbf{R}^3$) (see [5] for details). The two vector fields $v_{it}^{All}(x)$ and $v_{it}^W(x)$ are defined by two different sets of control points c^{All} and c^W shared among the whole population, and by two sets of 3D vectors, called momenta, α_i^{All} and α_i^W linked to the control points and specific to each subject i: $v_{it}^{All}(x(t)) = K(x(t), c^{All}(t))\alpha_i^{All}(t)$ and $v_{it}^W(x(t)) = K(x(t), c^W(t))\alpha_i^W(t)$, where $K(x(t), c(t))$ represents a block matrix of Gaussian kernels with equal fixed width for both deformations. Control points and momenta evolve in time according to the differential equations:

$$\dot{c}_i(t) = K(c_i(t), c_i(t))\alpha_i(t) = F^c(c_i(t), \alpha_i(t)) \qquad c_i(0) = c(0) = c_0$$
$$\dot{\alpha}_i(t) = -\alpha_i(t)^T \alpha_i(t) \nabla_1 K(c_i(t), c_i(t)) = F^\alpha(c_i(t), \alpha_i(t)) \quad \alpha_i(0) = \alpha_{i0} \tag{2}$$

This system of ODEs is valid for both diffeomorphisms: $L_i^{All/W}(t)=\{c_i^{All/W}(t),$ $\alpha_i^{All/W}(t)\}$ and it can be summarized as $\dot{L}_i^{All/W}(t) = F(L_i^{All/W}(t))$. The last diffeomorphisms $\phi_i^{All}(1)$ and $\phi_i^{W}(1)$ are completely parametrized by the initial conditions of the systems: $L_i^{All/W}(0) = L_{i0}^{All/W} = \{c_0^{All/W}, \alpha_{i0}^{All/W}\}$. Thus, in order to deform the template complex T, we first integrate forward in time $\dot{L}_i^{W}(t)$ starting from L_{i0}^{W} and we use these values to deform only the white objects of the template complex (T^W) integrating forward in time:

$$\dot{T}_i^{W}(t) = K(T_i^{W}(t), c_i^{W}(t))\alpha_i^{W}(t) \qquad T_i^{W}(0) = T_{i0}^{W} \qquad (3)$$

The deformed white matter template, together with the un-deformed gray matter template (T^G), are then used as starting point for the second deformation All: $T^{All}(0) = T^W(1) \cup T^G(0)$. $\dot{L}_i^{All}(t)$ is integrated forward in time starting from L_{i0}^{All} and the global template T^{All} is deformed using a similar equation as Eq. 3. Omitting the index i for clarity purpose, the composition is computed as:

$$\begin{bmatrix} L^W(0) \\ T^W(0) \end{bmatrix} \xrightarrow{\phi^W} \begin{bmatrix} L^W(1) \\ \boxed{T^W(1)} \end{bmatrix} \xrightarrow{} \boxed{T^W(1)} \cup T^G(0) = T^{All}(0) \begin{bmatrix} L^{All}(0) \\ T^{All}(0) \end{bmatrix} \xrightarrow{\phi^{All}} \begin{bmatrix} L^{All}(1) \\ T^{All}(1) \end{bmatrix}$$

2.3 Optimization Procedure

We show here how to estimate the template complex $T = T^W \cup T^G$ and the deformation parameters $L_{i0}^{All} = \{c_0^{All}, \alpha_{i0}^{All}\}$, $L_{i0}^{W} = \{c_0^{W}, \alpha_{i0}^{W}\}$ which characterize respectively the invariants and the variability of the set of anatomical configurations. This is performed using a Bayesian framework like in [1,2,17]. Assuming independence between the variables, we model α_{i0}^{All} and α_{i0}^{W} as multivariate Gaussian variables: $p(\alpha_{i0}^{W}|\Gamma_\alpha^W) \sim N(0, \Gamma_\alpha^W)$, $p(\alpha_{i0}^{All}|\Gamma_\alpha^{All}) \sim N(0, \Gamma_\alpha^{All})$ as well as the residual noise ϵ_i: $p(\epsilon_{ij}^G|\sigma_j^2) \sim N(0, \sigma_j^2 Id)$ and $p(\epsilon_{ij}^W|\sigma_j^2) \sim N(0, \sigma_j^2(K_j^W)^{-1}) \propto \frac{1}{|\sigma_j^2|^{\Lambda_j/2}} \exp\left[-\frac{1}{2\sigma_j^2}||\Pi(S_{ij}^W - \phi_i^{All}(\phi_i^W(T_j^W)))||_{W_{\Lambda_j}^*}^2\right]$ where Λ_j refers to the size of the j-th grid on which both the shapes and the template of the j-th white matter structure are projected in order to define probability density functions (space of weighted currents is infinite). Moreover we add priors on $\{\sigma_j^2\}$, Γ_α^{All} and Γ_α^W using Inverse Wishart distributions: $\sigma_j^2 \sim \mathcal{W}^{-1}(P_j, w_j)$, $\Gamma_\alpha^{All} \sim \mathcal{W}^{-1}(P_\alpha^{All}, w_\alpha^{All})$, $\Gamma_\alpha^W \sim \mathcal{W}^{-1}(P_\alpha^W, w_\alpha^W)$ where the matrices P_α^W, P_α^{All} and the scalars $w_\alpha^W, w_\alpha^{All}$, $\{P_j\}$, $\{w_j\}$ are hyper-parameters. Both the template complex T and the control points $\{c_0^W\}$ and $\{c_0^{All}\}$ have a uniform prior distribution. The parameters $\Theta = \{\{\sigma_j^2\}, \Gamma_\alpha^{All}, \Gamma_\alpha^W, \{c_0^{All}\}, \{c_0^W\}, T\}$ should be estimated considering $\{\alpha_{i0}^{All}\}$ and $\{\alpha_{i0}^{W}\}$ as latent variables and $\{S_i\}$ as observations using, for instance, Monte Carlo sampling procedures (as in [17]). This process would be very time-consuming and we have thus opted for a faster MAP estimation, where $\{\alpha_{i0}^{All}\}$ and $\{\alpha_{i0}^{W}\}$ are considered as parameters Θ. The (minus) log posterior distribution of Θ given the observations $\{S_i\}$ is equal to:

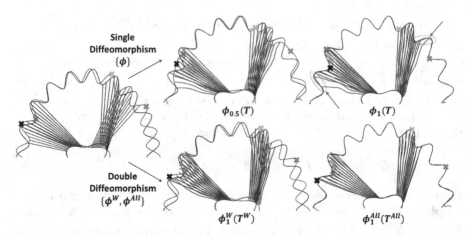

Fig. 2. Matching between the green structures towards the red ones. In the first row it is used one diffeomorphism (ϕ) whereas in the second row it is shown the proposed double diffeomorphic scheme $\phi^W \cup \phi^{All}$. These four structures represent the cortical surface, the basal ganglia and two fiber bundles connecting them. The first two are modelled as varifolds (see [5]) and the last two as weighted currents. We have used the same modeling and deformation parameters for the two settings. The four coloured X represent some peaks and valleys that are inverted in the first row and conserved in the second one. The red arrows highlight the matching errors using one diffeomorphism (Color figure online).

$$
\boxed{\sum_{j=1}^{M}\sum_{i=1}^{N}\frac{1}{2\sigma_j^2}\left(\|S_{ij}-T_{ij}^{All}(1)\|^2+\frac{P_jw_j}{N}\right)}+\boxed{\sum_{j=1}^{M}\frac{1}{2}(w_j+\Lambda_jN)\log(\sigma_j^2)}+
$$

$$
\boxed{\frac{1}{2}\sum_{i=1}^{N}(\alpha_{i0}^{All})^T(\Gamma_\alpha^{All})^{-1}\alpha_{i0}^{All}}+\frac{(w_\alpha^{All}+N)}{2}\log(|\Gamma_\alpha^{All}|)+\frac{w_\alpha^{All}}{2}tr((\Gamma_\alpha^{All})^{-1}P_\alpha^{All})+
$$

$$
\boxed{\frac{1}{2}\sum_{i=1}^{N}(\alpha_{i0}^{W})^T(\Gamma_\alpha^{W})^{-1}\alpha_{i0}^{W}}+\frac{(w_\alpha^{W}+N)}{2}\log(|\Gamma_\alpha^{W}|)+\frac{w_\alpha^{W}}{2}tr((\Gamma_\alpha^{W})^{-1}P_\alpha^{W})
$$

$$(4)$$

$\|\cdot\|$ refers to the norm of weighted currents for white matter objects ($\|\cdot\|_{W_{\Lambda_j}^*}$) and to the L^2 norm for gray matter objects where Λ_j is equal to the number of vertices. The framed terms refer respectively to the data-terms and to the regularity of both diffeomorphisms. The other terms are due to the use of priors.

Gradient descent. This cost function is minimized using a gradient descent scheme. $\{\sigma_j^2\}, \Gamma_\alpha^{All}, \Gamma_\alpha^{W}$ have a closed form solution which is equal to: $\hat{\Gamma}_\alpha = \frac{\sum_{i=1}^{N}[(\alpha_{i0})(\alpha_{i0})^T]+w_\alpha P_\alpha^T}{(w_\alpha+N)}$, which is the weighted sum between the sample covariance matrix of the deformation parameters and the prior, and to $\hat{\sigma}_j^2 =$

$\frac{\sum_{i=1}^{N}||S_{ij}-T_{ij}^{All}(1)||^2+w_j P_j}{(w_j+N\Lambda_j)}$, which is also a weighted sum between the data term of the j-th object and the prior. In order to compute the derivatives with respect to $\{c_0^{All}\}$, $\{c_0^{W}\}$, T^{W}, T^{G}, $\{\alpha_{i0}^{All}\}$ and $\{\alpha_{i0}^{W}\}$, we rewrite the cost function as:

$$E[T_0^{W}, T_0^{G}, \{c_0^{All}\}, \{\alpha_{i0}^{All}\}, \{c_0^{W}\}, \{\alpha_{i0}^{W}\}] = \sum_{i=1}^{N} D_i[T_i^{All}(1)] + R[L_{i0}^{All}] + R[L_{i0}^{W}]$$

subject to
$$\begin{cases} \dot{L}_i^{All}(t) = F[L_i^{All}(t)] & L_i^{All}(0) = L_{i0}^{All} = \{c_0^{All}, \alpha_{i0}^{All}\} \\ \dot{L}_i^{W}(t) = F[L_i^{W}(t)] & L_i^{W}(0) = L_{i0}^{W} = \{c_0^{W}, \alpha_{i0}^{W}\} \\ \dot{T}_i^{W}(t) = G[T_i^{W}(t), L_i^{W}(t)] & T^{W}(0) = T_0^{W} \\ \dot{T}_i^{All}(t) = G[T_i^{All}(t), L_i^{All}(t)] & T_i^{All}(0) = T_i^{W}(1) \cup T^{G}(0) \end{cases}$$

$$(5)$$

where $G[T_i(t), L_i(t)] = K(T_i(t), c_i(t))\alpha_i(t)$ and $D_i[T_i^{All}(1)]$, $R[L_{i0}^{All}]$ and $R[L_{i0}^{W}]$ are respectively the first, second and third framed terms of Eq. 4. Using the calculus of variations as in [5,18] (see Appendix) we obtain:

$$\begin{cases} \nabla_{c_0^{All}} E = \sum_{i=1}^{N} \xi_{ci}^{All}(0) + \nabla_{c_0^{All}} R[L_{i0}^{All}] & \nabla_{c_0^{W}} E = \sum_{i=1}^{N} \xi_{ci}^{W}(0) + \nabla_{c_0^{W}} R[L_{i0}^{W}] \\ \nabla_{\alpha_{i0}^{All}} E = \xi_{\alpha i}^{All}(0) + \nabla_{\alpha_{i0}^{All}} R[L_{i0}^{All}] & \nabla_{\alpha_{i0}^{W}} E = \xi_{\alpha i}^{W}(0) + \nabla_{\alpha_{i0}^{W}} R[L_{i0}^{W}] \\ \nabla_{T_0^{G}} E = \sum_{i=1}^{N} \theta_i^{All,G}(0) & \nabla_{T_0^{W}} E = \sum_{i=1}^{N} \theta_i^{W}(0) \end{cases}$$

$$(6)$$

where $\xi_i^{All} = \{\xi_{\alpha i}^{All}, \xi_{ci}^{All}\}$, $\xi_i^{W} = \{\xi_{\alpha i}^{W}, \xi_{ci}^{W}\}$, $\theta_i^{All} = \{\theta_i^{All,G}, \theta_i^{All,W}\}$, $\{\theta_i^{W}\}$ satisfy:

$$\begin{cases} \dot{\theta}_i^{All}(t) = -(\partial_{T_i^{All}} G_i^{All}(t))^T \theta_i^{All}(t) & \theta_i^{All}(1) = \nabla_{T_i^{All}(1)} D_i \\ \dot{\theta}_i^{W}(t) = -(\partial_{T_i^{W}} G_i^{W}(t))^T \theta_i^{W}(t) & \theta_i^{W}(1) = \theta_i^{All,W}(0) \\ \dot{\xi}_i^{All}(t) = -(\partial_{L_i^{All}} G_i^{All}(t))^T \theta_i^{All}(t) + (d_{L_i^{All}} F_i^{All}(t))^T \xi_i^{All}(t) & \xi_i^{All}(1) = 0 \\ \dot{\xi}_i^{W}(t) = -(\partial_{L_i^{W}} G_i^{W}(t))^T \theta_i^{W}(t) + (d_{L_i^{W}} F_i^{W}(t))^T \xi_i^{W}(t) & \xi_i^{W}(1) = 0 \end{cases}$$

$$(7)$$

where $G_i^{All}(t) = G[T_i^{All}(t), L_i^{All}(t)]$, $G_i^{W}(t) = G[T_i^{W}(t), L_i^{W}(t)]$, $F_i^{All}(t) = F[L_i^{All}(t)]$ and $F_i^{W}(t) = F[L_i^{W}(t)]$. Once obtained T_1^{All} from current values of control points and momenta, it is used to compute the gradient of the data terms $\nabla_{T_i^{All}(1)} D_i$. This information is brought back at time 0 by integrating backward the ODEs of the *All* auxiliary variables in Eq. 7. These results are used to update $c_0^{All}, \{\alpha_{i0}^{All}\}, T_0^{G}$ whereas the values concerning the white matter objects $(\theta_i^{All,W}(0))$ are used as final values of the variable θ_i^{W}. This is the key element that connects the two diffeomorphisms. The ODEs of the W auxiliary variables in Eq. 7 are then integrated backward and these values are used to update $c_0^{W}, \{\alpha_{i0}^{W}\}, T_0^{W}$. ODEs are integrated with the Euler's method using 10 steps. Here, the flow of information goes from *All* to W, contrary to Sect. 2.2, and it can be summed up as:

$$\begin{bmatrix} \theta^{All,W}(1) \\ \theta^{All,G}(1) \\ \xi_\alpha^{All}(1) \\ \xi_c^{All}(1) \end{bmatrix} \int_1^0 \begin{bmatrix} \left[\theta^{All,W}(0) = \theta^W(1)\right] \int_1^0 \begin{bmatrix} \xi_c^W(1) \\ \xi_\alpha^W(1) \end{bmatrix} \begin{bmatrix} \xi_c^W(0) \longrightarrow \nabla_{c_0^W} E \\ \xi_\alpha^W(0) \longrightarrow \nabla_{\alpha_0^W} E \\ \theta^W(0) \longrightarrow \nabla_{T_0^W} E \end{bmatrix} \\ \theta^{All,G}(0) \longrightarrow \nabla_{T_0^G} E \\ \xi_\alpha^{All}(0) \longrightarrow \nabla_{\alpha_0^{All}} E \\ \xi_c^{All}(0) \longrightarrow \nabla_{c_0^{All}} E \end{bmatrix}$$

3   Experiments

Figure 2 shows a comparison between a single and a double diffeomorphic matching applied to a toy example. The structural connectivity is different since the fiber bundles end in different folds of the cortex. Using a single diffeomorphism the cortical surface changes its folding since a peak becomes a valley and vice-versa (see the four coloured X), and at the same time the fiber bundles are not

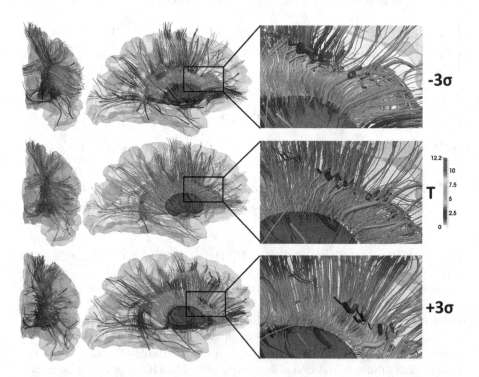

Fig. 3. Displacement of the fiber bundle template deformed with the first mode of PCA based on the covariance matrix of the deformation parameters of the first diffeomorphism at $\pm 3\sigma$, keeping fixed the gray matter templates. Colors refer to the magnitude of the displacement from the template, shown in gray in the middle row (Color figure online).

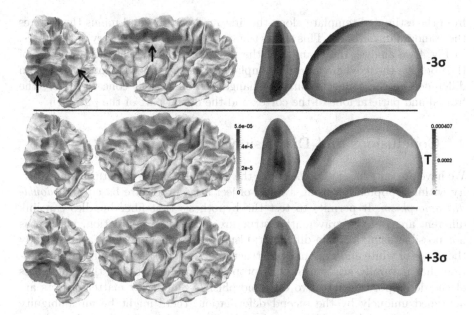

Fig. 4. Fiber bundle template deformed with the first mode of PCA based on the covariance matrix of the deformation parameters of the first diffeomorphism at $\pm 3\sigma$, keeping fixed the gray matter templates. Colors refer to the probability densities of the endpoints of the fibers onto the gray matter templates (Color figure online).

well matched. Instead, using a double diffeomorphism we can first see the relative motion of the fiber bundles with respect to the fixed cortex and basal ganglia which highlights the differences in structural connectivity. Then, all structures are well matched via the second global diffeomorphism. In this case the cortex is simply shifted without modifying its folding structure, which is more sensible since the two cortical surfaces have the same number of folds.

We have also built an atlas with 2 controls and 3 patients subject to GTS using left cortex, putamen and the fiber bundle connecting them. The cortex is segmented using FreeSurfer and the putamen with FSL, in both cases there is a vertex-correspondence between subjects. The fiber bundle comes from a deterministic tractography [3]. The templates of cortex and putamen have been initialised as the average of the vertices. For the fiber bundle template, we have first gathered the fibers of all subjects in a single bundle which has then been approximated as a set of weighted prototypes [4]. Both Figs. 3 and 4 show the first mode of PCA based on the estimated covariance matrix of the deformation parameters of the first diffeomorphism W applied to the fiber bundle template keeping fixed the templates of cortex and putamen. Given the important structural changes that are likely to occur in GTS patients [3], we may assume that controls and patients create separate clusters, so that the first mode of PCA on the pooled data mostly highlights the effects of the pathology on the anatomy and structural connectivity. Figure 3 highlights the displacement of the points from the estimated template along the first mode at plus and minus three times the standard deviation σ. This shows the variability of the geometry of the fibers. In Fig. 4 we analyse the changes of the probability density of the endpoints of the fibers on the fixed gray matter templates. This permits to point out the main differences in the connected areas. Changes in connections concern mainly the frontal and parietal lobe of the cortex and the dorsal part of the putamen.

4   Conclusions and Discussion

We have presented a method to study the variability of the structural connectivity within a population using a multi-object atlas procedure based on a *double diffeomorphism*. It permits to test the hypothesis that fiber bundles can link different areas of the gray matter structures across the population, which was not possible using a single diffeomorphism. This scheme permits also to study the shape of white and gray matter structures typical of the population. A question that naturally arises using the proposed method is about the uniqueness of the decomposition into two diffeomorphisms. Since gray matter objects are deformed uniquely by the second deformation, there might be an ambiguity concerning the regions which contain only white matter structures. In order to obtain a unique decomposition, we have chosen a scale of deformation so that white matter objects are deformed by the second diffeomorphism in a correlated way with respect to at least one gray matter structure. Furthermore, our algorithm is limited for now to cases in which we can assume that there is a point-correspondence among the cortical surfaces in the population. In future works, we will try to adapt our technique for considering also subjects showing different cortical gyrifications. We have applied this technique to a population of 3 patients with GTS and 2 controls using left cortex, putamen and the fiber bundle connecting them. We have shown that the main variation in structural connectivity within the population is in the frontal and parietal lobe of the cortex and in the dorsal part of the putamen. This could indicate the principal variability between patients and controls. Future works will extend this technique to a larger population considering all the cortico-striato-pallido-thalamic circuits. This will permit to verify our preliminary results about atypical structural connections in the cortico-putamen circuit which likely result from abnormal brain development due to GTS [3].

Acknowledgements. The research leading to these results has received funding from the program "Investissements d'avenir" ANR-10-IAIHU-06.

Appendix

We compute here the gradient of the criterion for atlas construction. A variation in the white system δL_{i0}^{W} produces a variation in the path of control points and momenta $\delta L_{i}^{W}(t)$ and consequently $\delta T_{i}^{W}(t)$. In parallel, δL_{i0}^{All} produces a variation in $\delta \boldsymbol{L}_i^{All}(t)$ which , together with $\delta \boldsymbol{T}_{i1}^W$, induces a variation in the global template $\delta \boldsymbol{T}_i^{All}(t)$ and then in the criterion δE:

$$\delta E = \sum_{i=1}^{N} \nabla_{\boldsymbol{T}_{i1}^{All}}(D_i[\boldsymbol{T}_{i1}^{All}])^T \delta \boldsymbol{T}_{i1}^{All} + \nabla_{\boldsymbol{L}_{i0}^{All}}(R[\boldsymbol{L}_{i0}^{All}])^T \delta \boldsymbol{L}_{i0}^{All} + \nabla_{\boldsymbol{L}_{i0}^{W}}(R[\boldsymbol{L}_{i0}^{W}])^T \delta \boldsymbol{L}_{i0}^{W}$$

$$\delta \dot{\boldsymbol{L}}_i^{All}(t) = (d_{\boldsymbol{L}_{it}^{All}} F_i^{All}(t))^T \delta \boldsymbol{L}_{it}^{All} \qquad\qquad \delta \boldsymbol{L}_i^{All}(0) = \delta \boldsymbol{L}_{i0}^{All}$$

$$\delta \dot{\boldsymbol{L}}_i^{W}(t) = (d_{\boldsymbol{L}_{it}^{W}} F_i^{W}(t))^T \delta \boldsymbol{L}_{it}^{W} \qquad\qquad \delta \boldsymbol{L}_i^{W}(0) = \delta \boldsymbol{L}_{i0}^{W}$$

$$\delta \dot{\boldsymbol{T}}_i^{W}(t) = (\partial_{\boldsymbol{T}_{it}^{W}} G_i^{W}(t))^T \delta \boldsymbol{T}_{it}^{W} + (\partial_{\boldsymbol{L}_{it}^{W}} G_i^{W}(t))^T \delta \boldsymbol{L}_{it}^{W} \qquad \delta \boldsymbol{T}^W(0) = \delta \boldsymbol{T}_0^{W}$$

$$\delta \dot{\boldsymbol{T}}_i^{All}(t) = (\partial_{\boldsymbol{T}_{it}^{All}} G_i^{All}(t))^T \delta \boldsymbol{T}_{it}^{All} + (\partial_{\boldsymbol{L}_{it}^{All}} G_i^{All}(t)])^T \delta \boldsymbol{L}_{it}^{All} \quad \delta \boldsymbol{T}_i^{All}(0) = \delta \boldsymbol{T}_{i1}^{W} \cup \delta \boldsymbol{T}_0^{G}$$

As in [5] we denote: $R_{st} = \exp(\int_s^t d_{\boldsymbol{L}_u} F(u) du)$ and $V_{st} = \exp(\int_s^t \partial_{\boldsymbol{T}_u} G(u) du)$ which are valid for both frameworks W and All and where we have omitted the index i for clarity purpose. The two first ODEs are linear whereas the last two are linear with source term: $\delta \boldsymbol{L}(t) = R_{0t} \delta \boldsymbol{L}_0$, $\delta \boldsymbol{T}(t) = \int_0^t V_{ut} \partial_{\boldsymbol{L}_u} G(u) \delta \boldsymbol{L}(u) du + V_{0t} \delta \boldsymbol{T}_0$. Calling $\boldsymbol{Y}^W$ and $\boldsymbol{Y}^G$ the white and gray matter objects of $\boldsymbol{T}^{All}$:

$$\delta \boldsymbol{Y}^W(t) = \left(\int_0^t V_{ut}^{All} \partial_{\boldsymbol{L}^{All}} G^{All}(u) R_{0u}^{All} du \right) \delta \boldsymbol{L}_0^{All} + V_{0t}^{All} \delta \boldsymbol{T}_0^{W} +$$

$$V_{0t}^{All} \int_0^1 \partial_{\boldsymbol{T}^W} G^W(s) \delta \boldsymbol{T}^W(s) ds + V_{0t}^{All} \int_0^1 \partial_{\boldsymbol{L}^W} G^W(s) \delta \boldsymbol{L}^W(s) ds$$

Using the Fubini's theorem, the 3rd term is equal to: $\left(V_{0t}^{All} \int_0^1 V_{u1}^{W} \partial_{\boldsymbol{L}^W} G^W(u) \right.$ $\left. R_{0u}^W du \right) \delta \boldsymbol{L}_0^{W} - \left(V_{0t}^{All} \int_0^1 \partial_{\boldsymbol{L}^W} G^W(u) R_{0u}^W du \right) \delta \boldsymbol{L}_0^{W} + (V_{0t}^{All} V_{01}^{W}) \delta \boldsymbol{T}_0^{W} - V_{0t}^{All} \delta \boldsymbol{T}_0^{W}$. The 4th term becomes: $\left(V_{0t}^{All} \int_0^1 \partial_{\boldsymbol{L}^W} G^W(s) R_{0s}^W ds \right) \delta \boldsymbol{L}_0^{W}$. Plugging them into δE:

$$\nabla_{\boldsymbol{L}_0^{All}} E = \left(\int_0^1 (R_{0u}^{All})^T (\partial_{\boldsymbol{L}^{All}} G^{All}(u))^T (V_{u1}^{All})^T du \right) \nabla_{\boldsymbol{T}_1^{All}} D + \nabla_{\boldsymbol{L}_0^{All}} R^{All}$$

$$\nabla_{\boldsymbol{L}_0^{W}} E = \left(\int_0^1 (R_{0u}^{W})^T (\partial_{\boldsymbol{L}^W} G^{W}(u))^T (V_{u1}^{W})^T du \right) (V_{01}^{All})^T \nabla_{\boldsymbol{Y}_1^{W}} D + \nabla_{\boldsymbol{L}_0^{W}} R^{W}$$

$$\nabla_{\boldsymbol{T}_0^{W}} E = (V_{01}^{W})^T (V_{01}^{All})^T \nabla_{\boldsymbol{Y}_1^{W}} D$$

$$\nabla_{\boldsymbol{T}_0^{G}} E = (V_{01}^{All})^T \nabla_{\boldsymbol{Y}_1^{G}} D$$

Calling $\theta^{All,G}(t) = (V_{t1}^{All})^T \nabla_{\boldsymbol{Y}_1^{G}} D$, $\theta_t^{All,W} = (V_{t1}^{All})^T \nabla_{\boldsymbol{Y}_1^{W}} D$, $\theta^{All}(t) = \{\theta^{All,G}(t), \theta^{All,W}(t)\}$, $\theta^{W}(t) = (V_{t1}^{W})^T \theta_0^{All,W}$, $\xi^{All}(t) = \int_t^1 (R_{tu}^{All})^T (\partial_{\boldsymbol{L}^{All}} G^{All}$ $(u))^T \theta^{All}(u) du$ and $\xi^{W}(t) = \int_t^1 (R_{tu}^{W})^T (\partial_{\boldsymbol{L}^W} G^{W}(u))^T \theta^{W}(u) du$ we obtain the results in Eq. 6.

References

1. Allassonnière, S., Amit, Y., Trouvé, A.: Toward a coherent statistical framework for dense deformable template estimation. J. Roy. Statist. Soc. B **69**(1), 3–29 (2007)
2. Gori, P., Colliot, O., Worbe, Y., Marrakchi-Kacem, L., Lecomte, S., Poupon, C., Hartmann, A., Ayache, N., Durrleman, S.: Bayesian atlas estimation for the variability analysis of shape complexes. In: Mori, K., Sakuma, I., Sato, Y., Barillot, C., Navab, N. (eds.) MICCAI 2013, Part I. LNCS, vol. 8149, pp. 267–274. Springer, Heidelberg (2013)
3. Worbe, Y., Marrakchi-Kacem, L., Lecomte, S., Valabregue, R., Poupon, F., Guevara, P., Tucholka, A., Mangin, J.F., Vidailhet, M., Lehericy, S., Hartmann, A., Poupon, C.: Altered structural connectivity of cortico-striato-pallido-thalamic networks in Gilles de la Tourette syndrome. Brain **138**, 472–482 (2014). doi:10.1093/brain/awu311
4. Gori, P., Colliot, O., Marrakchi-Kacem, L., Worbe, Y., De Vico Fallani, F., Chavez, M., Lecomte, S., Poupon, C., Hartmann, A., Ayache, N., Durrleman, S.: A prototype representation to approximate white matter bundles with weighted currents. In: Golland, P., Hata, N., Barillot, C., Hornegger, J., Howe, R. (eds.) MICCAI 2014, Part III. LNCS, vol. 8675, pp. 289–296. Springer, Heidelberg (2014)
5. Durrleman, S., Prastawa, M., Charon, N., Korenberg, J.R., Joshi, S., Gerig, G., Trouvé, A.: Morphometry of anatomical shape complexes with dense deformations and sparse parameters. NeuroImage **101**, 35–49 (2014). doi:10.1016/j.neuroimage.2014.06.043
6. Chen, T., Rangarajan, A., Eisenschenk, S.J., Vemuri, B.C.: Construction of a neuroanatomical shape complex atlas from 3D MRI brain structures. NeuroImage **60**(3), 1778–1787 (2012)
7. Gorczowski, K., Styner, M., Jeong, J.Y., Marron, J.S., Piven, J., Hazlett, H.C., Pizer, S.M., Gerig, G.: Multi-object analysis of volume, pose, and shape using statistical discrimination. IEEE Trans. Pattern Anal. Mach. Intell. **32**(4), 652–661 (2010)
8. Qiu, A., Miller, M.I.: Multi-structure network shape analysis via normal surface momentum maps. NeuroImage **42**(4), 1430–1438 (2008)
9. Ma, J., Miller, M.I., Younes, L.: A bayesian generative model for surface template estimation. Int. J. Biomed. Imaging **16**, 1–14 (2010). doi:10.1155/2010/974957
10. Davies, R.H., Twining, C.J., Cootes, T.F., Taylor, C.J.: Building 3-D statistical shape models by direct optimization. IEEE. Trans. Med. Imag. **29**(4), 961–981 (2010)
11. Hufnagel, H., Pennec, X., Ehrhardt, J., Ayache, N., Handels, H.: Computation of a probabilistic statistical shape model in a Maximum-a-posteriori framework. Methods. Inf. Med. **48**(4), 314–319 (2009)
12. Niethammer, M., Reuter, M., Wolter, F.-E., Bouix, S., Peinecke, N., Koo, M.-S., Shenton, M.E.: Global medical shape analysis using the laplace-beltrami spectrum. In: Ayache, N., Ourselin, S., Maeder, A. (eds.) MICCAI 2007, Part I. LNCS, vol. 4791, pp. 850–857. Springer, Heidelberg (2007)
13. Joshi, S.H., Cabeen, R.P., Joshi, A.A., Sun, B., Dinov, I., Narr, K.L., Toga, A.W., Woods, R.P.: Diffeomorphic sulcal shape analysis on the cortex. IEEE Trans. Med. Imaging **31**(6), 1195–1212 (2012)
14. Durrleman, S., Fillard, P., Pennec, X., Trouvé, A., Ayache, N.: Registration, atlas estimation and variability analysis of white matter fiber bundles modeled as currents. Neuroimage **55**(3), 1073–1090 (2011)

15. O'Donnell, L.J., Westin, C.F., Golby, A.J.: Tract-based morphometry for white matter group analysis. Neuroimage **45**(3), 832–844 (2009)
16. Wassermann, D., Rathi, Y., Bouix, S., Kubicki, M., Kikinis, R., Shenton, M., Westin, C.-F.: White matter bundle registration and population analysis based on gaussian processes. In: Székely, G., Hahn, H.K. (eds.) IPMI 2011. LNCS, vol. 6801, pp. 320–332. Springer, Heidelberg (2011)
17. Zhang, M., Singh, N., Fletcher, P.T.: Bayesian estimation of regularization and atlas building in diffeomorphic image registration. In: Gee, J.C., Joshi, S., Pohl, K.M., Wells, W.M., Zöllei, L. (eds.) IPMI 2013. LNCS, vol. 7917, pp. 37–48. Springer, Heidelberg (2013)
18. Marsland, S., McLachlan, R.: A hamiltonian particle method for diffeomorphic image registration. In: Karssemeijer, N., Lelieveldt, B. (eds.) IPMI 2007. LNCS, vol. 4584, pp. 396–407. Springer, Heidelberg (2007)

A Robust Probabilistic Model for Motion Layer Separation in X-ray Fluoroscopy

Peter Fischer[1]([✉]), Thomas Pohl[2], Thomas Köhler[1], Andreas Maier[1],
and Joachim Hornegger[1]

[1] Pattern Recognition Lab and Erlangen Graduate School in Advanced Optical
Technologies (SAOT), FAU Erlangen-Nürnberg, Erlangen, Germany
peter.fischer@fau.de
[2] Siemens Healthcare, Forchheim, Germany

Abstract. Fluoroscopic images are characterized by a transparent projection of 3-D structures from all depths to 2-D. Differently moving structures, for example due to breathing and heartbeat, can be described approximately using independently moving 2-D layers. Separating the fluoroscopic images into the motion layers is desirable to facilitate interpretation and diagnosis. Given the motion of each layer, it is state of the art to compute the layer separation by minimizing a least-squares objective function. However, due to high noise levels and inaccurate motion estimates, the results are not satisfactory in X-ray images.

In this work, we propose a probabilistic model for motion layer separation. In this model, we analyze various data terms and regularization terms theoretically and experimentally. We show that a robust penalty function is required in the data term to deal with noise and shortcomings of the image formation model. For the regularization term, we propose to enforce smoothness of the layers using bilateral total variation. On synthetic data, the mean squared error between the estimated layers and the ground truth is improved by 18 % compared to the state of the art. In addition, we show qualitative improvements on real X-ray data.

1 Introduction

Minimally-invasive interventions are often guided by fluoroscopic X-ray imaging. X-ray imaging offers good temporal and spatial resolution and high contrast of interventional devices and bones. However, the soft-tissue contrast is low and the patient and the physician are exposed to ionizing radiation. In addition to the low soft-tissue contrast, the loss of 3-D information due to the transparent projection to 2-D complicates interpretation of the fluoroscopic images. To simplify the analysis, fluoroscopic images can be decomposed into independently moving layers. Each layer contains similarly moving structures, leading to the separation of background structures like bones from moving soft-tissue like the heart or the liver. In addition, other post-processing algorithms like segmentation or frame interpolation can benefit from the motion layer separation. Another clinically relevant post-processing application is digital subtraction angiography (DSA). DSA is performed by subtracting a reference frame. However, if there is too

© Springer International Publishing Switzerland 2015
S. Ourselin et al. (Eds.): IPMI 2015, LNCS 9123, pp. 288–299, 2015.
DOI: 10.1007/978-3-319-19992-4_22

much motion, the selection of an appropriate reference frame is difficult. In particular for coronary arteries, complex respiratory and cardiac motion complicate traditional DSA and make motion layer separation a good alternative [17].

In the literature, multiple approaches to layer separation have been investigated. Layer separation is sometimes combined with motion estimation, but we limit ourselves to layer separation in this work. Close et al. estimate rigid motion of each layer in a region of interest [3]. The layers are computed by stabilizing the sequence w.r.t. the layer motion and subsequent averaging. Preston et al. jointly estimate motions and layers using a coarse-to-fine variational framework [10], but the results are not physically meaningful motions or layers. In [14], an iterative scheme for motion and layer estimation is used. For layer separation, a constrained least-squares optimization problem is solved. Weiss estimates a static layer from a transparent image sequence exploiting the sparsity of images in the gradient domain [16]. Zhang et al. assume the motions as given and solve a constrained least-squares problem for estimating the layers [17].

So far, regularization has rarely been applied to aid layer separation. Exception are [10], where a layer gradient penalty is introduced, and [16], where the objective function implicitly favors smooth layers. In other areas of image processing, regularization is widely used. Inverse problems in image processing, often formulated to minimize an energy function, benefit from regularization, for example denoising [11], image registration [7], and super-resolution [4]. Total variation is a popular, edge-preserving regularization that was originally introduced for denoising [11]. Super resolution is conceptually similar to layer separation and is often formulated as a probabilistic model with robust regularization, e.g., bilateral total variation [4].

In this paper, we introduce a novel probabilistic model for layer separation in transparent image sequences. As likelihood and prior in the Bayesian model, we propose to use a robust data term and edge-preserving regularization. In particular, a non-convex data term is used that is robust w.r.t. noise, errors in the image formation model, and errors in the motion estimates. Furthermore, we theoretically analyze different spatial regularization terms for layer separation. Inference in the Bayesian model leads to maximum a posteriori estimation of the layers, as opposed to the previously used maximum likelihood. In the experiments, we extensively compare possible data and regularization terms. We show that layer separation can benefit from our robust approach.

2   Materials and Methods

2.1   Image Formation Model

In this paper, we are interested in separating X-ray images $I^t \in \mathbb{R}^{W \times H}$, $t \in \{1, \ldots, T\}$ into different motion layers L_l, where each layer may undergo independent non-rigid 2-D motion v_l^t. A motion layer can roughly be assigned to each source of motion, e.g., breathing, heartbeat, and background.

In our spatially discrete formulation, the images and layers are vectorized to $\boldsymbol{I}^t, \boldsymbol{L}_l \in \mathbb{R}^{WH}$. The transformation of a layer by its motion and subsequent interpolation is modeled in the system matrix $\boldsymbol{W}_l^t \in \mathbb{R}^{WH \times WH}$ [14]

$$I^t = \sum_{l=1}^{N} W_l^t L_l + \epsilon^t, \tag{1}$$

where we introduce ϵ^t to account for model errors and observation noise. N is the number of layers in the image sequence. This model is justified by the log-linearity of Lambert-Beer's law applied to X-ray attenuation. In W_l^t, we use bilinear interpolation, but the method generalizes to other interpolation or point spread functions. Boundary treatment for image pixels moving outside of the spatial support of the layers is to take the nearest layer pixel. Alternatively, the layer support can be increased to cover all motions in the current sequence [15]. For all images and layers, the joint forward model is used

$$I = WL + \epsilon, \tag{2}$$

where $I = \left(I^{1\mathsf{T}}, \ldots, I^{T\mathsf{T}}\right)^{\mathsf{T}}$, $L = \left(L_1^{\mathsf{T}}, \ldots, L_N^{\mathsf{T}}\right)^{\mathsf{T}}$, and $\epsilon = \left(\epsilon^{1\mathsf{T}}, \ldots, \epsilon^{T\mathsf{T}}\right)^{\mathsf{T}}$. The system matrix $W = \left(W^{1\mathsf{T}}, \ldots, W^{T\mathsf{T}}\right)^{\mathsf{T}}$ is composed of matrices $W^t = \left(W_1^t, \ldots, W_N^t\right)$ to transform all layers to a certain point in time.

2.2   Probabilistic Approach to Layer Separation

The goal of layer separation is to find the layers L given the images I and the motions encoded in W. From a Bayesian point of view, the observed images I, the noise ϵ, and the layers L are random variables. Assuming conditionally independent observed images, the posterior probability of the layers given the images $p(L|I)$ is given by

$$p(L|I) = \frac{p(L)\,p(I|L)}{p(I)} = \frac{p(L)\prod_{t=1}^{T} p(I_t|L)}{p(I)}, \tag{3}$$

with the prior probability for the layers $p(L)$ and the likelihood $p(I_t|L)$ for each image given the layers. Common priors in image processing are defined on local neighborhoods, such that Eq. (3) corresponds to a Markov random field. The maximum a posterior (MAP) estimate

$$\hat{L} = \underset{L}{\operatorname{argmax}}\, p(L) \prod_{t=1}^{T} p(I_t|L) \tag{4}$$

yields the statistically optimal layers for the given model and input images. In previous work, no probabilistic motivation [3] or maximum likelihood (ML) estimation was often used [14,17], implicitly assuming a uniform prior $p(L)$.

By applying the logarithm and negating, the probabilistic formulation can be equivalently regarded as an energy. Assuming positive values, it is possible to write prior $p(L)$ and likelihood $p(I_t|L)$ as $p(L) = \frac{1}{Z_R}\exp(-\lambda R(L))$ and $p(I_t|L) = \frac{1}{Z_D}\exp(-D(I_t,L))$, where Z_R, Z_D are partition functions to normalize the probabilities. Consequently, MAP inference as in Eq. (4) turns into energy minimization

$$\hat{L} = \underset{L}{\operatorname{argmin}} \, \lambda R\left(L\right) + \sum_{t=1}^{T} D\left(I_t, L\right),\tag{5}$$

where $D\left(I_t, L\right)$ is the data term, $R\left(L\right)$ the regularization, and $\lambda \in \mathbb{R}_0^+$ the regularization weight. In the following sections, we concretize $D\left(I_t, L\right)$ and $R\left(L\right)$.

2.3 Data Term

The data term describes how deviations from the image formation model are penalized. From a probabilistic point of view, it corresponds to an assumption on the observation noise ϵ^t. The classic choice of a least-squares data term

$$D_{L_2}\left(I_t, L\right) = \left\| I^t - W^t L \right\|_2^2 \tag{6}$$

corresponds to a Gaussian noise model, which has been used in most of the prior work [10,14,17] and is a fitting model for images with good photon statistics [9]. This model is easy to optimize by solving a sparse linear system of equations. Its major drawback is the sensitivity to outliers, i.e., a few erroneous measurements lead to artifacts in the estimated layers. However, outliers are very common in X-ray layer separation, for example due to errors in motion estimation, which is challenging in X-ray without knowing the layers (Sect. 2.6). Another important source of outliers is the simplified image formation model (Sect. 2.1). Many effects occurring in X-ray images are not captured by this model, e.g., foreshortening and out-of-plane motion.

The least absolute deviation corresponds to a Laplacian noise model

$$D_{L_1}\left(I_t, L\right) = \left\| I^t - W^t L \right\|_1, \tag{7}$$

which is more robust to outliers and still a convex function. In contrast to Eq. (6), it is not smooth due to the non-differentiability at 0. Therefore, a smooth approximation to the L_1-norm is helpful for gradient-based optimization schemes, e.g., the Charbonnier function $\|z\|_1 \approx \phi(z) = \sqrt{z^2 + \tau^2} - \tau$, for $\tau > 0$ [13].

A non-convex data term can be derived using a generalization of the Charbonnier function $\phi_\alpha(z) = \left(z^2 + \tau^2\right)^\alpha - \tau^{2\alpha}$ [13]. $\phi(z)$ is equivalent to $\phi_{0.5}(z)$ and z^2, as used in D_{L_2}, is equivalent to $\phi_1(z)$. Then, the general data term is

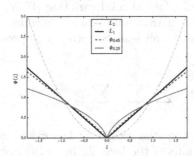

Fig. 1. Behavior of different penalty functions (best viewed in color) (Color figure online).

$$D_{\text{Charb.}}\left(\boldsymbol{I}_t, \boldsymbol{L}\right) = \sum_{k=1}^{WH} \phi_\alpha\left(\left[\boldsymbol{I}^t - \boldsymbol{W}^t\boldsymbol{L}\right]_k\right). \tag{8}$$

$[\boldsymbol{x}]_k$ extracts the k-th component of $\boldsymbol{x}$. Using the generalized Charbonnier function, the value of α can be tuned to fit the statistics of the observation noise. τ is only required for numerical reasons and set to 0.01. The penalty functions are visualized in Fig. 1. It is evident that L_1 and L_2 are convex penalties, and that large deviations are penalized less by $\phi_\alpha(z)$ with smaller values of α.

2.4   Regularization Term

Common priors in image processing favor smoothness of the images. The most basic prior is based on Tikhonov regularization and penalizes high gradients

$$R_{L_2}\left(\boldsymbol{L}\right) = \sum_{l=1}^{N} \|\boldsymbol{\nabla}\boldsymbol{L}_l\|_2^2, \tag{9}$$

where $\boldsymbol{\nabla}$ is a matrix computing the spatial derivatives for each layer. As image gradients in natural images are heavy-tailed, Eq. (9) leads to oversmoothed images. For layer separation, the L_2 regularization term is particularly counterproductive. Assume a certain gradient at an image location has to be represented somehow by the layers. The L_2-norm gives the lowest penalty if all layers contribute equally to the image gradient. However, this corresponds to a separation into two equal layers.

To better preserve edges in the layers, the total variation (TV) regularization

$$R_{\text{TV}}\left(\boldsymbol{L}\right) = \sum_{l=1}^{N} \|\boldsymbol{\nabla}\boldsymbol{L}_l\|_1 \tag{10}$$

is useful [11], which again leads to a convex optimization problem. In contrast to the L_2-norm, the L_1-norm does neither hinder nor enforce layer separation. Sparse solutions, i.e., an image gradient is represented by a single layer, have the same energy as equal gradients in all layers.

In super-resolution, bilateral total variation (BTV) is a popular regularizer [4]. It generalizes TV regularization to include a wider spatial support of $2P+1$ pixels in each dimension, can lead to better edge preservation, and is convex. BTV is defined as

$$R_{\text{BTV}}\left(\boldsymbol{L}\right) = \sum_{l=1}^{N} \sum_{m=-P}^{P} \sum_{n=-P}^{P} \beta^{|m|+|n|} \|\boldsymbol{L}_l - \boldsymbol{S}_v^m \boldsymbol{S}_h^n \boldsymbol{L}_l\|_1, \tag{11}$$

where $0 \le \beta \le 1$ is a spatial weighting factor and $\boldsymbol{S}_v^m$ ($\boldsymbol{S}_h^n$) corresponds to vertical (horizontal) shifts of the layer $\boldsymbol{L}_l$ by m (n) pixels.

All the aforementioned regularization terms are spatially independent. Additional information for layer regularization can be gained from the images, i.e., the regularization term can be generalized to $R(\boldsymbol{I}, \boldsymbol{L})$. For example, the image gradient offers information about the desired position and direction of the layer gradients. Preston et al. use this to define the regularization term

$$R_{\text{Pres.}}(\boldsymbol{I}, \boldsymbol{L}) = \sum_{t=1}^{T}\sum_{l=1}^{N}\sum_{k=1}^{WH}\left(\left\|\nabla\left[\boldsymbol{W}_l^t\boldsymbol{L}_l\right]_k\right\|_2 - \left(\nabla\left[\boldsymbol{W}_l^t\boldsymbol{L}_l\right]_k\right)^{\mathsf{T}}\boldsymbol{n}_k^t\right) \qquad (12)$$

to remove the penalty if the layer gradient is in the same direction as the image gradient [10], which is computed using ∇. The image gradient is thresholded

$$\boldsymbol{n}_k^t = \begin{cases} \dfrac{\nabla[\boldsymbol{I}^t]_k}{\left\|\nabla[\boldsymbol{I}^t]_k\right\|_2} & \text{if } \left\|\nabla[\boldsymbol{I}^t]_k\right\|_2 > \delta \\ 0 & \text{else} \end{cases}, \qquad (13)$$

such that small gradients caused by noise do not influence the regularization. Other than that, the magnitude of the image gradient is not important. Consequently, at a single position the gradients of multiple layers can point in the same direction without increasing the energy. An advantage of this regularization term is that layer gradients with magnitude 0 always lead to 0 energy. In this sense, it is a TV regularization that is switched off if the layer gradient points in the same direction as the image gradient.

Inspired by [16], we define another regularization term that uses image gradient information. Assuming sparsity of layer gradients, it is likely that an observed image gradient comes from a single layer. Therefore, the magnitude of the layer gradient should be the same as the image gradient, as in the regularization term

$$R_{\text{Weiss}}(\boldsymbol{I}, \boldsymbol{L}) = \sum_{t=1}^{T}\sum_{l=1}^{N}\left\|\nabla\boldsymbol{W}_l^t\boldsymbol{L}_l - \nabla\boldsymbol{I}^t\right\|_1. \qquad (14)$$

For the layer that explains the corresponding image gradient, 0 energy is incurred. However, the remaining layers all create an energy of $\|\nabla\boldsymbol{I}\|_1$. The minimum value of this regularization term is not attained for a layer without gradients, as in TV or L_2-regularization. Instead, it is attained when the layer gradient is equal to the median of the image gradients over time [16], where the layer motion is compensated in the image. As the image gradient is sparse and the layer motions are independent, the median is often close to 0. For the previously described regularization terms, the L_1-norm can be replaced by the generalized Charbonnier penalty ϕ_α to enforce sparsity even more.

Figure 2 shows the effects of the different regularizers. R_{L_2} focuses on large gradients in the layer, leading to oversmoothing. R_{TV} is more robust, i.e., the relative penalty on large gradients is reduced compared to R_{L_2}. R_{BTV} is a smoothed version of R_{TV}, because the spatial shifts cover a wider area. R_{Weiss} has no penalty for the gradients of Fig. 2a. However, a penalty must be paid for image gradients that are not explained by this layer, which could lead to worse separation. $R_{\text{Pres.}}$ is identical to R_{TV}, except that the TV penalty is switched off if there is an image gradient. Due to their dependence on the layer motions, $R_{\text{Pres.}}$ and R_{Weiss} have artifacts for inexact motion estimates.

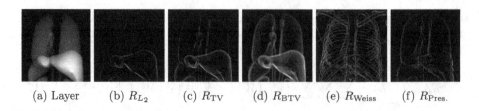

(a) Layer   (b) R_{L_2} (c) R_{TV} (d) R_{BTV} (e) R_{Weiss} (f) $R_{Pres.}$

Fig. 2. Penalty of the ground truth layer (a) for different regularization terms. Dark corresponds to low and bright to high penalty (best viewed in color) (Color figure online).

2.5   Numerical Optimization

The layer estimation problem is processed in a coarse-to-fine pyramid. This ensures that an approximate solution is found quickly on low-resolution images and greatly reduces computation time. In contrast to [17], we estimate all layers on all resolutions. Thus, the coarse-to-fine pyramid is mainly used for speeding up the convergence. In addition, it helps to avoid local minima for the non-convex energy terms involving the generalized Charbonnier penalty.

The optimization method on each level is limited-memory Broyden-Fletcher-Goldfarb-Shanno with bound constraints (L-BFGS-B). This method requires smooth gradients, so all L_1-norms are approximated by the Charbonnier function. For some combinations of data terms and regularization terms, specialized solvers exist that are much faster. For example, a L_2 data term with L_2 regularization can be solved in closed form using the pseudo-inverse, and L_2 data term with TV regularization can be optimized using a split-Bregman solver [5]. However, as we prefer generality over runtime in this work, we always use L-BFGS-B. Optimization is run until convergence on each level of the pyramid. Boundary conditions are enforced for the layers that can be derived from the additive image formation model, e.g., non-negativity [14].

2.6   Sources of Layer Motions

An important prerequisite for our approach to layer extraction from fluoroscopic images is the motion of each layer. By itself, this is a challenging problem. However, there are several applications where this is feasible.

The first application is joint layer and motion estimation. The layers and their motions are assumed to be unknown and jointly estimated from a fluoroscopic sequence. This can be optimized using an alternation scheme, with the two subtasks of motion estimation given the layers and layer estimation given the motions. For the latter, the proposed method of this paper is applicable. In particular for this application, it can not be presupposed that the given layer motions are accurate. Consequently, robust methods are mandatory.

The second application is post-processing of fluoroscopic sequences. Separated motion layers are useful for improved interpretation of the image content. Dense motion of the background can be computed using robust parametric registration methods [1]. More complex motion patterns require more effort. A possibility is tracking of control points, devices [6] or anatomical curves [2]. To get a dense motion field from the tracking results, interpolation methods like thin-plate splines (TPS) can be used. In post-processing, there is enough time to accurately perform these tasks.

2.7 Experiments

Synthetic data is used for quantitative analysis and real X-ray data for qualitative results. The synthetic data is created by independently projecting different organs of the XCAT phantom to 2-D [8,12]. The resulting layers are transformed using 2-D motion fields. The 2-D motion is created by TPS interpolation of manual control point motions. In total, we use two datasets, each with $N = 2$ layers and $T = 10$ images of size $W = H = 250$ and with a dynamic range of $[0, 1]$. On the synthetic data, we simulate different types of errors. First, we add measurement noise in the form of Gaussian and Laplacian noise to the image intensities ($\sigma_{Gauss} = \sigma_{Laplace} = 0.01$). Second, we simulate registration and model errors by smoothing the ground truth motion field and randomly disturbing it by adding Gaussian noise to the motion vectors ($\sigma_{motion} = 1.5$ px). In addition, two images of the sequence are translated randomly ($\sigma_{trans} = 4.0$ px). For each of the datasets, 10 instances with random errors are created. As the error measure for ground truth comparison, we use a modified version of the mean squared error (MSE). As a uniform intensity offset can not be determined using layer separation, the means of the layers are subtracted before computing the MSE.

The real X-ray data consists of a sequence of 10 images of $W = 670$, $H = 1000$. The required layer motions are extracted from the images manually. In each image, the motion of ~25 control points is annotated. The motion of these control points is converted to a dense motion field using TPS interpolation.

To find the parameters for each method, we perform grid search. For $D_{Cha.}$, α is searched in $\{0.25, 0.3, 0.35, 0.4, 0.45, 0.5\}$. For the regularizers, λ is searched in $\{0.0001, 0.0005, 0.001, 0.005, 0.01, 0.05, 0.1, 0.5, 1.0, 5\}$ while α is fixed. The threshold for the gradient magnitude δ in $R_{Pres.}$ is set to 0.01 [10]. The parameters of R_{BTV} are searched in $\beta = \{0.5, 0.7, 0.9\}$ and $P = \{3, 5\}$. For each experiment, 10 different random instances with the same error and noise type are used as training data. We use forward differences to approximate spatial derivatives ∇. The coarse-to-fine pyramid is implemented with a downsampling factor of 0.5 and 6 levels.

3 Results

3.1 Analysis of Data Terms

To analyze the behavior of different data terms, we apply ML estimation without regularization for each of them. For $D_{Cha.}$, the grid search yields $\alpha = 0.25$, $\beta = 0.5$, and $P = 5$. The MSE decreases with increasing robustness of the data term, see Table 1. Qualitatively, the errors in D_{L_2} correspond to artifacts at positions of wrong motion. Note that D_{L_2} is the common data term in the state of the art [10,14,17]. Using robust data terms, these artifacts in the layers are removed.

Table 1. MSE ($\cdot 10^{-3}$) for different data terms on synthetic test data (mean $\pm$ std). Grid search determined $\alpha = 0.25, \beta = 0.5, P = 5$ for $D_{\text{Cha.}}$.

	D_{L_2}	D_{L_1}	$D_{\text{Cha.}}$
MSE	8.9 ± 5.6	8.5 ± 5.5	8.3 ± 5.4

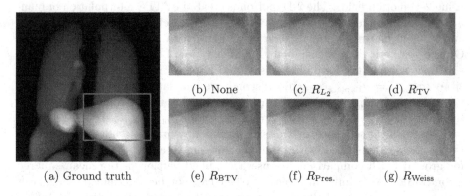

(a) Ground truth   (b) None   (c) R_{L_2} (d) R_{TV}

(e) R_{BTV} (f) $R_{\text{Pres.}}$ (g) R_{Weiss}

Fig. 3. View of a region of interest (red) of a layer extracted using different regularization terms. $D_{\text{Cha.}}$ is used in all cases (Colour figure online).

3.2   Analysis of Regularization Terms

We investigate all combinations of $D_{\text{Cha.}}$ with $\alpha = 0.25$ and the introduced regularization terms. The respective regularization weights are listed in Table 2, together with the experimental results. All regularization methods improve the MSE compared to ML estimation. The image-driven regularizers $R_{\text{Pres.}}$ and R_{Weiss} have only a small effect, as training assigned low weights. This means that using higher weights for these regularizers deteriorates the results. With an MSE of $7.3 \cdot 10^{-3}$, R_{BTV} is the best regularizer in our experiments. R_{TV} is second, as it also preserves edges. Since R_{BTV} is a generalization of R_{TV}, it is more flexible. R_{BTV} has the highest runtime as multiple finite differences are evaluated. R_{Weiss} and $R_{Pres.}$ are slow as well, since they must be computed for each point in time.

A qualitative impression of the effect of the regularization is given in Fig. 3 for a region of interest. The robust data term already removed most of the outliers. The main difference between the regularization terms the denoising performance, including edge preservation. In Fig. 4, we highlight the the difference between the state of the art and the proposed robust probabilistic model. D_{L_2} has blurred edges and a high-noise level, while our method is closer to the ground truth.

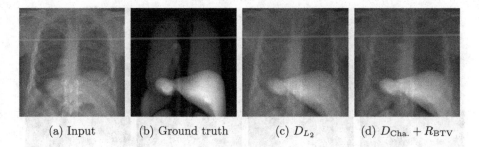

| (a) Input | (b) Ground truth | (c) D_{L_2} | (d) $D_{\text{Cha.}} + R_{\text{BTV}}$ |

Fig. 4. An image of the input sequence (a), a ground truth layer (b), and the corresponding layer extracted with the state of the art (c) and our method (d).

Table 2. Value of regularization weight λ found using grid search on training data, MSE ($\cdot 10^{-3}$), and runtime [s] on test data (mean $\pm$ std).

	-	R_{L_2}	R_{TV}	R_{BTV}	$R_{\text{Pres.}}$	R_{Weiss}
λ	-	1.0	0.5	0.1	0.05	0.0001
MSE	8.3 ± 5.4	8.1 ± 5.5	7.8 ± 5.3	7.3 ± 5.7	8.1 ± 5.0	8.3 ± 5.4
Runtime	55.8 ± 9.2	50.0 ± 8.1	42.5 ± 9.6	203 ± 114	116 ± 18.4	117 ± 25.5

3.3 Real X-ray Data

For the real X-ray data, the same parameters as in Table 2 are used. The experiments on real data have to deal with many sources of error. The manual labeled motion is inaccurate, because it is only based on a few sparse control points. In addition, the layered image formation model is not fulfilled here. A reconstructed layer from an X-ray sequence containing soft tissue motion of the heart, lung and diaphragm is shown in Fig. 5. Ribs, spine, and skin markers are static and should be removed from the shown layer. The state-of-the-art D_{L_2} data term without regularization creates artifacts and smooths edges (bottom left). D_{L_1} and $D_{\text{Cha.}}$ are able to suppress most of the artifacts. High noise levels are visible for all data terms (top left).

All regularizers help to reduce this noise. As $R_{\text{Pres.}}$ and R_{Weiss} have similar results, only the former is shown. Both do not sufficiently suppress noise. R_{TV} and R_{BTV} smooth the noise and preserve the edges, for example near the diaphragm and the heart shadow. In contrast, R_{L_2} slightly blurs edges and does not suppress noise. R_{BTV} is best at reducing streak artifacts (bottom middle).

4   Conclusions and Outlook

In this paper, a Bayesian probabilistic model for layer separation in transparency was presented. As this model is only a rough approximation of the real X-ray image generation process, it has to tolerate many outliers. To this end, we introduce robust data terms and robust regularization for motion layer separation in

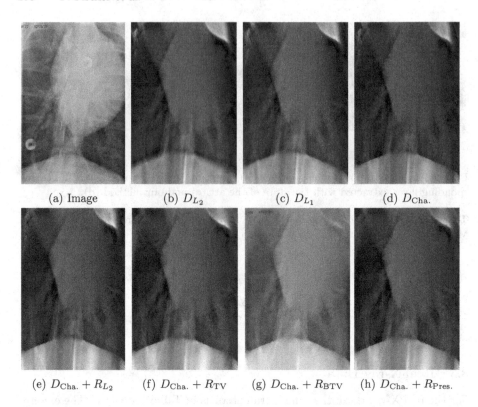

(a) Image   (b) D_{L_2} (c) D_{L_1} (d) $D_{Cha.}$

(e) $D_{Cha.} + R_{L_2}$ (f) $D_{Cha.} + R_{TV}$ (g) $D_{Cha.} + R_{BTV}$ (h) $D_{Cha.} + R_{Pres.}$

Fig. 5. Layer extracted from a real X-ray sequence using different combinations of data and regularization term (contrast enhanced for display).

fluoroscopy. A slowly increasing penalty function like the generalized Charbonnier is crucial in the data term. Furthermore, we showed that robust regularization like BTV yields semantically better separation. Image-driven regularization did not improve upon BTV, but might help in joint motion and layer estimation [10].

For the future, there are several areas for possible improvements. The image formation model can be extended to better model true X-ray physics, e.g., scattering. Joint motion and layer estimation with anatomically plausible layers would greatly enhance the practical usefulness. Another issue is runtime. Although the coarse-to-fine approach considerably reduces runtime, the current configuration of the optimizer requires up to a minute for computing the layers. The runtime can be improved using preconditioning or specialized solvers [5].

Acknowledgments. The authors gratefully acknowledge funding by Siemens Healthcare and of the Erlangen Graduate School in Advanced Optical Technologies (SAOT) by the German Research Foundation (DFG) in the framework of the German excellence initiative. The concepts and information presented in this paper are based on research and are not commercially available.

References

1. Black, M.J., Anandan, P.: The robust estimation of multiple motions: parametric and piecewise-smooth flow fields. Comput. Vis. Image Underst. **63**(1), 75–104 (1996)
2. Cao, Y., Wang, P.: An adaptive method of tracking anatomical curves in X-ray sequences. In: Ayache, N., Delingette, H., Golland, P., Mori, K. (eds.) MICCAI 2012, Part I. LNCS, vol. 7510, pp. 173–180. Springer, Heidelberg (2012)
3. Close, R.A., Abbey, C.K., Morioka, C.A., Whiting, J.S.: Accuracy assessment of layer decomposition using simulated angiographic image sequences. IEEE Trans. Med. Imaging **20**(10), 990–998 (2001)
4. Farsiu, S., Robinson, M.D., Elad, M., Milanfar, P.: Fast and robust multiframe super resolution. IEEE Trans. Image Process. **13**(10), 1327–1344 (2004)
5. Goldstein, T., Osher, S.: The split Bregman method for L1-regularized problems. SIAM J. Imaging Sci. **2**(2), 323–343 (2009)
6. Heibel, H., Glocker, B., Groher, M., Pfister, M., Navab, N.: Interventional tool tracking using discrete optimization. IEEE Trans. Med. Imaging **32**(3), 544–555 (2013)
7. Hermosillo, G., Chefd'Hotel, C., Faugeras, O.: Variational methods for multimodal image matching. Int. J. Comput. Vision **50**(3), 329–343 (2002)
8. Maier, A., Hofmann, H., Berger, M., Fischer, P., Schwemmer, C., Wu, H., Müller, K., Hornegger, J., Choi, J.H., Riess, C., Keil, A., Fahrig, R.: CONRAD-a software framework for cone- beam imaging in radiology. Med. Phys. **40**(11) (2013)
9. Manhart, M., Kowarschik, M., Fieselmann, A., Deuerling-Zheng, Y., Royalty, K., Maier, A., Hornegger, J.: Dynamic iterative reconstruction for interventional 4-D c-arm CT perfusion imaging. IEEE Trans. Med. Imaging **32**(7), 1336–1348 (2013)
10. Preston, J.S., Rottman, C., Cheryauka, A., Anderton, L., Whitaker, R.T., Joshi, S.: Multi-layer deformation estimation for fluoroscopic imaging. In: Gee, J.C., Joshi, S., Pohl, K.M., Wells, W.M., Zöllei, L. (eds.) IPMI 2013. LNCS, vol. 7917, pp. 123–134. Springer, Heidelberg (2013)
11. Rudin, L.I., Osher, S., Fatemi, E.: Nonlinear total variation based noise removal algorithms. Phys. D **60**(14), 259–268 (1992)
12. Segars, W., Mahesh, M., Beck, T., Frey, E., Tsui, B.: Realistic CT simulation using the 4D XCAT phantom. Med. Phys. **35**(8), 3800–3808 (2008)
13. Sun, D., Roth, S., Black, M.J.: A quantitative analysis of current practices in optical flow estimation and the principles behind them. Int. J. Comput. Vision **106**(2), 115–137 (2014)
14. Szeliski, R., Avidan, S., Anandan, P.: Layer extraction from multiple images containing reflections and transparency. In: CVPR, vol. 1, pp. 246–253. IEEE (2000)
15. Tipping, M.E., Bishop, C.M.: Bayesian image super-resolution. In: Becker, S., Thrun, S., Obermayer, K. (eds.) Advances in Neural Information Processing Systems, vol. 15, pp. 1303–1310. MIT Press, Cambridge (2003)
16. Weiss, Y.: Deriving intrinsic images from image sequences. In: ICCV, vol. 2, pp. 68–75. IEEE (2001)
17. Zhang, W., Ling, H., Prummer, S., Zhou, K.S., Ostermeier, M., Comaniciu, D.: Coronary tree extraction using motion layer separation. In: Yang, G.-Z., Hawkes, D., Rueckert, D., Noble, A., Taylor, C. (eds.) MICCAI 2009, Part I. LNCS, vol. 5761, pp. 116–123. Springer, Heidelberg (2009)

Poster Papers

Weighted Hashing with Multiple Cues for Cell-Level Analysis of Histopathological Images

Xiaofan Zhang[1], Hai Su[2], Lin Yang[2], and Shaoting Zhang[1]([✉])

[1] Department of Computer Science, UNC Charlotte, Charlotte, NC 28223, USA
shaoting@cs.rutgers.edu
[2] J. Crayton Pruitt Family Department of Biomedical Engineering,
University of Florida, Gainesville, FL 32611, USA

Abstract. Recently, content-based image retrieval has been investigated for histopathological image analysis, focusing on improving the accuracy and scalability. The main motivation is to interpret a new image (i.e., query image) by searching among a potentially large-scale database of training images in real-time. Hashing methods have been employed because of their promising performance. However, most previous works apply hashing algorithms on the whole images, while the important information of histopathological images usually lies in individual cells. In addition, they usually only hash one type of features, even though it is often necessary to inspect multiple cues of cells. Therefore, we propose a probabilistic-based hashing framework to model multiple cues of cells for accurate analysis of histopathological images. Specifically, each cue of a cell is compressed as binary codes by kernelized and supervised hashing, and the importance of each hash entry is determined adaptively according to its discriminativity, which can be represented as probability scores. Given these scores, we also propose several feature fusion and selection schemes to integrate their strengths. The classification of the whole image is conducted by aggregating the results from multiple cues of all cells. We apply our algorithm on differentiating adenocarcinoma and squamous carcinoma, i.e., two types of lung cancers, using a large dataset containing thousands of lung microscopic tissue images. It achieves 90.3 % accuracy by hashing and retrieving multiple cues of half-million cells.

1 Introduction

Content-based image retrieval (CBIR) has been an effective approach in analyzing medical images [1–3]. It aims to retrieve and visualize relevant medical images with diagnosis information, which assist doctors to make consistent clinical decisions. Successful use cases include clinical pathology, mammogram analysis, and categorization of X-ray images [1,4–7]. Recently, the research focus of CBIR for medical images has been on the efficient and large-scale methods, and several benchmarks have been designed, such as Image CLEF and VISCERAL [2,8].

© Springer International Publishing Switzerland 2015
S. Ourselin et al. (Eds.): IPMI 2015, LNCS 9123, pp. 303–314, 2015.
DOI: 10.1007/978-3-319-19992-4_23

The motivation of leveraging large databases of training images is that they have the potential to offer abundant information to precisely interpret the new data. However, the scalability or efficiency of these algorithms is usually an issue. In this paper, we design a scalable CBIR algorithm to tackle a challenging problem, differentiating lung cancers using histopathological images. Lung cancer is one of the most common cancers [9]. There are four typical histologic types of lung cancers, including adenocarcinoma, squamous carcinoma, small cell carcinoma, and large cell carcinoma, each of which needs a different treatment [10]. Therefore, early diagnosis and differentiation of these four types is clinically important. Bronchial biopsy is one of the most effective diagnosis methods to differentiate them, with the aid of Computer Aided Diagnosis (CAD) systems [11–13]. Many previous methods emphasize the diagnosis of small cell vs. non-small cell (i.e., adenocarcinoma, squamous carcinoma, and large cell carcinoma) types of lung cancers, achieving promising accuracy. On the other hand, differentiation of the adenocarcinoma and squamous carcinoma, both of which are non-small cells, is much more difficult, while it is also clinically significant, since management protocols of these two types of cancers are different [14]. This is challenging because the difference between the adenocarcinoma and squamous carcinoma highly depends on the cell-level information, e.g., its morphology, texture and appearance, requiring to analyze multiple cues of all cells for accurate diagnosis. In fact, thoroughly examining cell-level information is necessary for many use cases of biopsy or histopathological image analysis. To this end, a potential solution proposed recently is to extract high-dimensional local texture features (e.g., SIFT [15]) that align with the cell-level information, and then compress them as binary codes via hashing-based CBIR algorithms [16] to improve the computational efficiency. Hashing methods [17–20] have been intensively investigated in machine learning communities, which enable fast approximated nearest neighbors (ANN) search for scalability. However, information loss is inevitable in such holistic approximation of cell-level information. Segmenting and hashing each cell offers a potential solution [21], and our framework also follows this strategy. Nonetheless, it only utilizes one type of features, while multiple cues should be examined for accurate classification.

Different from these previous methods, our proposed framework is able to (1) hash multiple cues of all cells with weights, and (2) accommodate new training data on-the-fly. Specifically, each cue of a cell is represented as binary codes through supervised hashing with kernels [20]. Then, the importance of such hash entry is determined adaptively according to its discriminativity for differentiating different classes, based on several measures such as probability scores. Given these probability scores, we integrate multiple features by considering importance. An additional benefit of this design is that the hashing results of multiple cues can be updated on-the-fly when handling new training samples. The classification of the whole image is conducted by aggregating the results of multiple cues of all cells. We evaluate our algorithm on this specific problem of differentiating lung cancers, using a large dataset containing 1120 lung microscopic tissue images acquired from hundreds of patients, achieving an accuracy of 90.3 % within several seconds by searching among half-million cells.

The rest of the paper is organized as follows. Section 2 presents our framework for real-time cell examination by hashing multiple cues of cells, including details of the hashing method, probabilistic-based weighting schemes, and aggregation of multiple cues. Section 3 shows the experimental results and comparisons. Section 4 draws the concluding remarks and shows future directions.

2   Methodology

2.1   Overview

The overview of our proposed framework is illustrated in Fig. 1. It includes automatic cell detection and segmentation, supervised hashing that generates binary codes from multiple types of image features, and the probabilistic-based weighting scheme that decides the importance of the hash entry for each cell. Specifically, the segmentation is based on the off-the-shelf method [22], while many other methods and systems are also applicable for this task [23, 24].

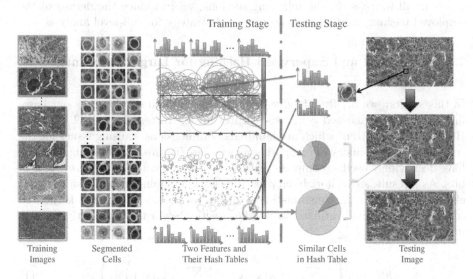

| Training Images | Segmented Cells | Two Features and Their Hash Tables | Similar Cells in Hash Table | Testing Image |

Fig. 1. Overview of our framework. In the training stage, the input is histopathological images representing two types of lung cancers. Green stands for adenocarcinoma, and yellow stands for squamous carcinoma. First, all cells are detected and segmented from these images. Second, two types of texture features are extracted and compressed as binary codes by hashing methods. These hash codes are visualized in two hash tables, representing two features, according to their ability to differentiate two categories (details in Sect. 2.3). In the testing stage, all cells are segmented from the query image, from which feature and binary codes are obtained using the same preprocess. Each cell is mapped into hash tables to search for the most similar cases, which are used to interpret the category of this unknown cell. The hash entries of two features are then integrated to enhance the accuracy. Finally, the results of all cells are aggregated to classify the testing image (Color figure online).

After segmenting all cells from the training images, a large-scale database of half-million cell patches is created. Then, two types of texture features [25, 26] are extracted for each cell, within the segmented region. After that, kernelized and supervised hashing (KSH) [20] is employed as a baseline to compress these features as binary code, since it can bridge the semantic gap of image appearances and their labels, which is essential for medical image retrieval. However, different from hashing the whole image, hashing cells (i.e., sub-regions of the whole image) is more challenging, due to cells' high intra-class but low inter-class variations. Therefore, traditional hashing methods result in low-discriminative hash entries. In addition, it is necessary to integrate multiple features from each cell, so the information can be largely explored. Our solution is the probabilistic-based weighting schemes that stress discriminative hash entries, and the integration of multiple cues of cells through the probability scores. Given a testing image, the same framework is utilized to segment cells, extract their features, and hash them for real-time comparison with the training database. Each cell is assigned with multiple weights or probability scores after this matching process. Finally, the classification of the testing image is achieved by aggregating the probability scores of all its cells. In the following sections, we introduce the details of the employed hashing method and our proposed strategy for cell-level analysis.

2.2 Kernelized and Supervised Hashing for Large-Scale Image Retrieval

In this section, we briefly introduce the hashing method employed as our baseline. For each segmented cell, two features are extracted, i.e., GIST [25] and HOG [26], and both of which are hundreds of dimensions, causing issues for the computational efficiency of comparing all samples. To this end, hashing methods have been widely used to compress features into binary codes with merely tens of bits. As a result, such short binary features allow mapping into a hash table for efficient retrieval, e.g., constant-time. To improve the accuracy, the kernelized scheme [18] is usually utilized to handle practical data that is mostly linearly inseparable:

$$h = sgn\left(\sum_{j \in anchors}\left(\kappa(\mathbf{x}_j, \mathbf{y}) - \frac{1}{n}\sum_{i=1}^{n}\kappa(\mathbf{x}_j, \mathbf{x}_i)\right)a_j\right), \tag{1}$$

where $\mathbf{y}$ is the feature (e.g., GIST or HOG) to be compressed as binary code, $\mathbf{x}_i$ with i from 1 to n means all training samples, i.e., cell patches, $\mathbf{x}_j$ denotes the anchors, i.e., random samples selected from the data, h is the kernelized hashing method taking the sign value of a kernel function with kernel κ, and a_j is the coefficient determining hash functions. The resulting binary codes can be used for indexing and differentiating different categories. Although kernelized scheme well solves the linear inseparability problem of features, it is still not able to provide accurate retrieval or classification of cell images, because of their large variations. Therefore, supervised information [20] can be leveraged to bridge the semantic gap by designing more discriminative hash functions:

$$\min_{A \in \mathbb{R}^{m \times r}} \mathcal{Q}(A) = \left\| \frac{1}{r} sgn(\bar{K}_l A)(sgn(\bar{K}_l A))^T - S \right\|_F^2 \tag{2}$$

where S is a matrix encoding the supervised information (e.g., 1 for same category and -1 for different categories, which is applicable to multi-class problems) and A is the model parameter to compute hashing code, and $\bar{K}_l = [\bar{\mathbf{k}}(\mathbf{x}_1), \cdots, \bar{\mathbf{k}}(\mathbf{x}_l)]^T \in \mathbb{R}^{l \times m}$ is the matrix form of the kernel function, in which $\bar{\mathbf{k}}(\mathbf{x}_i)$ is a kernelized vectorial map $\mathbb{R}^d \mapsto \mathbb{R}^m$, $A = [\mathbf{a}_1, \cdots, \mathbf{a}_r] \in \mathbb{R}^{m \times r}$. The optimization of $\mathcal{Q}$ is based on Spectral Relaxation [27] for convexification, which is used as a warm start, and Sigmoid Smoothing that applies standard gradient descent technique for accurate hashing.

Indexing these compressed features in a hash table, our framework can match each cell of the testing image with all cells in the training database in constant-time. The category of each cell is decided straightforwardly with the majority logic of retrieved cells, and the whole image is hence classified by aggregating results of all cells from the testing image. The whole process is very efficient and takes 1–2 s.

2.3 Weighted Hashing with Multiple Cues

Despite its efficacy in large-scale image retrieval, KSH still has several limitations when dealing with our use case, which requires to hash a large number of cell images. First of all, it builds hash functions for one type of feature, while it is preferred to model multiple cues of cells for accurate classification. Second, multiple cells can be mapped into the same hash entry using KSH, i.e., the hamming distances among them are zero. In this case, one may use majority voting to decide the label of a testing cell image having the same hash entry. However, cell images from different categories can be easily mapped into the same hash entry, due to image noise, erroneous segmentation results, and the low inter-class variations. In other words, not all hash entries are reliable for classification. Figure 2 visualizes the hash tables of two features, GIST [25] and HOG [26], representing the texture characteristics of cells. The entries in each hash table are illustrated according to the distribution of cells mapped into them, such as the ratio between two categories and the number of cells mapped into that entry. The indecisive hash entries are usually around the 0.5 ratio, indicating equal opportunity for either category. The small circles in Fig. 2 are also not reliable, since only few cells are mapped there, which can be easily affected by the image noise or erroneous segmentation. A potential solution is to identify reliable hash entries and omit indecisive one, by heuristically select or prune them via feature selection. However, this may involve tuning parameters and have difficulties in modeling multiple cues of cells because of lacking the consistent measures. Furthermore, it is hard to guarantee that the selected hash entry is sufficiently discriminative for classification. Therefore, we introduce a unified formulation to solve these problems in a principled way. First, probability scores

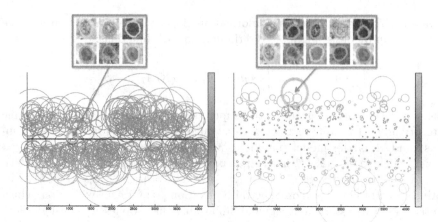

Fig. 2. We visualize hash tables and their entries according to cells mapped into them, and each circle represents one entry. The left hash table corresponds to HOG feature, and the right is GIST. The x-axis represents different hash entries corresponding to 12 bits, indicating 4096 different entries. The y-axis means the ratio between the adenocarcinoma and squamous carcinoma, ranging from 0 to 1, which is also visualized as different colors. The size of each circle denotes the number of cells mapped into that entry. As shown in the figures, different features may result in diverse cell distributions in the hash table, making it essential to explore consistent measures for feature fusion.

are assigned to each hash entry, based on its ability to differentiate different categories. Then, such probability scores can be integrated from different types of features, by emphasizing reliable hash entries of certain features. In this section, we introduce the details of our method.

Probabilistic-Based Weights for Hashing: We define three types of weights to emphasize discriminative hash entries. These weights can be consistently compared among different hash tables, representing multiple features.

- The first weight is defined as the conditional probability of a cell belonging to the ith category when its hash entry is H: $P(L_i|H) = P(L_i, H)/P(H) = |\{\text{cell} : l(\text{cell}) = L_i, \text{cell} \in S_H\}|/|S_H|$, where $S_H = \{\text{cell} : h(\text{cell}) = H\}$ is the set of cells mapped into a specific hash entry H, $|S|$ is the number of element in set S, $h(\text{cell})$ is the hash entry of this cell, $l(\text{cell})$ is the label of a cell image and L_i means the ith label or category. This represents the confidence of assigning a label to this hash entry. Instead of giving hash entry a hard label by majority voting and ignoring the minority categories, this soft assignment from probability distribution on all categories can fully utilize training data's information in the hash entry.
- The second weight is based on the information entropy E_H that is calculated from the probability distribution of each category in a hash entry: $E_H = -\sum_{i \in \text{labels}} P(L_i|H) \log(P(L_i|H))$. The entropy measures uncertainty

of a hash entry. High entropy means that it is not discriminative enough, e.g., cells mapped into the same hash entry H are evenly distributed in all categories. To reduce the importance of these non-discriminative entries, we define $W_H^E = 1 - E_H$.

- The third weight is decided according to the number of cells mapped into this entry. Entries with fewer cells are assigned lower weights, since they may be easily affected by image noise and erroneous segmentation results, i.e., less reliable compared to entries with more cells. The third weight W_H^S is defined as: $W_H^S = |S_H|/\sum_{k=0}^{2^r-1} |S_k|$, where r is the number of hash bits, representing 2^r hash values.

Combining these three weights together, we can get a probability-based score $W_{i,H} = W_H^S W_H^E P(L_i|H)$ for hash value H in the ith category. With these weights, we can utilize all training samples and reduce the influence of hash entries that are not discriminative. During the training process, $P(L_i|H)$, W_H^E and W_H^S can be computed for all hash entries. The category of a whole testing image is decided by arg $\max_{\{i\}} \sum_{\text{cell} \in \text{query}} W_{i,H_{\text{cell}}}$, where H_{cell} is the hash value of the cell belonging to the query or testing image.

Feature Fusion and Selection for Hashing Entries: Since these weights are based on probabilities, they are comparable among multiple features. For example, hash entries that are able to differentiate different categories should be advocated in different features. Therefore, feature fusion and selection can also be designed based on the proposed framework. When there are multiple types of features, hash tables are built for each of them and the weights of every hash entries in these hash tables are calculated during the training stage. To search cells for the query image, we first extract those types of features, denoted as F_j, $j \in \{1, 2, ..., N\}$, where N is the number of features, map them into hash entries H_{F_j} in these hash tables, and calculate their weights $W_{i,H_{F_j}}$. For feature fusion, the weights can be accumulated as $W_{i,H} = \sum_{j=1}^{N} W_{i,H_{F_j}}$, indicating that all these features contribute equally to the classification. For feature selection, the maximum of the weights can be chosen, $W_{i,H} = max(W_{i,H_{F_1}}, ..., W_{i,H_{F_N}})$, meaning that the most reliable one (e.g., discriminative feature) is selected and the others are ignored. Both feature fusion and selection methods are conducted in a cell-specific fashion, instead of on the whole image. Therefore, the strengths of multiple features can be fully explored on the cell-level.

This framework is also able to accommodate new samples efficiently. This online updating scheme can be achieved by storing not only the weights but also the number of cells in each category. Given new samples, we can update the cell number in their mapped hash entries, re-calculate and update the weights based on such information. The computational overhead is negligible. To summarize, the whole framework includes cell segmentation, hashing, and retrieval. The probability scores are assigned to each hash entry, and they are aggregated within the whole image for the final classification. This process is computationally efficient, with small overhead in the aggregation of probabilities. Benefited from the thorough analysis of multiple cues from each individual cell, this framework can achieve promising accuracy without sacrificing the efficiency.

3 Experiments

In this section, we conduct extensive experiments to evaluate our weighted hashing with multiple features for cell-level analysis. Our dataset is collected from the Cancer Genome Atlas (TCGA) [28], including 57 adenocarcinoma and 55 squamous carcinoma. 10 patches with 1712×952 resolution, i.e., region-of-interests (ROIs), are cropped from each whole slide scanned pathology specimens, by consulting with certified pathologists. Generally, the ROIs mainly consist of cancer cells. The lymphocytes regions which have different visual patterns than the representative tumor regions are avoided. All the data are prepared and labeled based on the independent confirmation of the pathologists. There are around half-million cells segmented for large-scale image retrieval, including nearly 20 K adenocarcinoma cells and 30 K squamous carcinoma cells. We evaluate the efficacy of our proposed framework in terms of the classification accuracy and computational efficiency. The evaluations are conducted on a 3.40 GHz CPU with 4 cores and 16 G RAM, in MATLAB and C++ implementation.

Table 1. We report the quantitative comparisons of the classification accuracy and efficiency, based on the mean value, standard deviation and running time. We compare with several methods which have been used for histopathological image analysis, including kNN [29], SVM [30] and KSH [20,31], using GIST [25] and HOG [26] features to represent cells' texture.

	Adeno	Squamous	Mean	Variance	Time(s)
kNN-GIST	0.567	0.933	0.750	0.076	~2600
kNN-HOG	0.354	0.820	0.587	0.063	~2600
SVM-GIST	0.925	0.533	0.729	0.072	~50
SVM-HOG	0.775	0.583	0.679	0.094	~50
KSH-GIST	0.925	0.658	0.792	0.081	1.22
KSH-HOG	0.757	0.748	0.753	0.082	1.22
Weight-GIST	0.833	0.875	0.854	0.052	1.70
Weight-HOG	0.818	0.793	0.806	0.065	1.70
Feature fusion	0.895	0.903	**0.899**	0.064	3.45
Feature selection	0.903	0.903	**0.903**	0.062	3.45

During the evaluation, 25 % patients are randomly selected as the testing data, and the remaining cases are used as the training. This procedure is repeated tens of times to get the mean and standard deviation. As shown in Table 1, we compare our algorithm with several methods that have been employed for histopathological image classification, including k-nearest neighbor (kNN) method [29] which is usually chosen as the baseline for comparison, Support Vector Machine (SVM) [30] that uses supervised information to improve the accuracy, and KSH [20,31] that is used as our baseline to generate binary codes.

For fair comparison, same features (GIST [25] and HOG [26]) are used for all compared methods, and their parameters and kernel selections are optimized by cross-validation. In general, these compared methods do not achieve very accurate results, with 75.0 % and 58.7 % for kNN using two features, 72.9 % and 67.9 % for SVM and 79.2 % and 75.3 % for KSH, even though they thoroughly analyze all segmented cells, same as our algorithm. The main reason is twofold. First, the cell images have high intra-class but low inter-class variations, and the number of two classes is not balanced. Second, same as most segmentation methods, ours is not perfectly accurate, especially for cell images with noise. These inaccurate segmentation results can adversely affect the classification accuracy. Supervised information used in SVM and KSH can alleviate this problem and improve the accuracy, while the results are still not promising.

Using our probabilistic-based weighting scheme, the accuracy is improved to 85.4 % for GIST and 80.6 % for HOG, around 6 % better than the baseline hashing method. The reason is that these weights emphasize certain hash entries that are more discriminative and have more "evidence" than others (i.e., more cells are mapped into that entry), alleviating the issue of high intra-class but low inter-class variations. Furthermore, our weighting scheme reduces the importance of unreliable features, most of which are extracted from inaccurate segmentations. Therefore, it ensures the robustness of the classification module, making it less sensitive to the segmentation accuracy or image

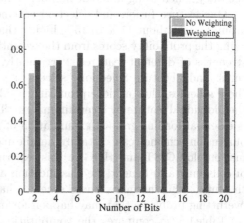

Fig. 3. Classification accuracy of KSH [20] (no weighting) and the weighted hashing applied for five rounds, with different number of hashing bits (2 to 20).

noise. In fact, this not only benefits the classification accuracy, but also is compatible with the paradigm of cell-level analysis, given the fact that most existing cell segmentation methods are still not perfect.

This weighted hashing framework has one important parameter, i.e., the number of hash bits. In our experiments, we have used 12 bits for classification, indicating 4096 hash entries. Theoretically, using one bit is already sufficient for binary classification, i.e., differentiation of two types of cells. However, as shown in Fig. 2, some hash entries may not be reliable and have to be pruned, due to image noise and inaccurate segmentations. Therefore, it is necessary to use many hash entries, which also enable multi-label classification. On the other hand, it is also preferred to have enough samples mapped into each hash entry, so the weight W_H^S can be effective and benefit the classification accuracy. Therefore, the number of hash bits should not be very large either. For example, using

20 hash bits can result in one million hash entries, sufficiently representing half million cells in our dataset. In addition, using a large number of hash bits (e.g., 64 bits) may reduce the computational and memory efficiency, since hash table is no longer an option owing to the memory constraint. Therefore, we have chosen 12 bits for this task, mapping half million cells to 4096 hash values and hence ensuring sound accuracy of classification without sacrificing the efficiency. This is also demonstrated by our experiments shown in Fig. 3. Note that this parameter is not that sensitive to different values, i.e., good accuracy in a certain range of values. This is critical to an automatic framework for histopathological image analysis, since tuning sensitive parameters is infeasible when conducting this large-scale and cell-level analysis. Furthermore, Fig. 3 also shows that our weighting scheme consistently improves the hashing method for classification accuracy, when using different number of hash bits.

Our feature fusion and selection schemes further improve the accuracy to around 90 %, about 11 % to 15 % higher than the KSH with single feature. Utilizing the probability scores from the weighting stage, we can naturally integrate strengths of different features. Particularly, "Feature Fusion" combines all features, and "Feature Selection" selects the best one. Despite the simplicity of these schemes, they achieve promising results, i.e., both strategies can improve the individual feature by a certain margin. Therefore, using multiple cues of cells is essential for fine-grained examination of histopathological images. Note that our fusion schemes can certainly handle more than two features, although we just employ GIST and HOG in this experiment. Other morphological features of cells may also benefit the classification accuracy, and will be investigated in the future. Furthermore, these schemes have no parameter to tune, avoiding overfitting problems that may happen for many learning-based fusion methods.

Table 1 also compares the computational efficiency of these methods, i.e., testing time. Hashing methods are always efficient, since they compress each feature into 12 bits, allowing constant time access using a hash table. Therefore, KSH achieves 1–2 s classification time, much faster than kNN and SVM. Both weighting and fusion schemes have computational overhead (i.e., 0.5 s), while it is negligible in practice. In general, the classification stage is very efficient, and can be used for large-scale and cell-level analysis. However, the segmentation and preprocessing can take tens of seconds, which are the bottleneck for real-time analysis. Currently, we have around one thousand images with half million cells. We expect to apply it on much larger databases (e.g., hundreds of millions of cells) or whole slide images in the future. In this case, parallel computing may be necessary to ensure the computational efficiency for both preprocessing and classification. Fortunately, our framework for cell-level analysis can be parallelled straightforwardly. For example, the whole slide image can be divided as multiple patches, and each patch can be processed by one node of the cluster for cell segmentation and classification independently. In general, the computational efficiency of our framework is very promising and has the potential to handle large-scale databases.

4   Conclusions

In this paper, we proposed an efficient framework for cell-level analysis of histopathological images, by conducting CBIR in a large amount of cell images. This large-scale retrieval is based on weighted hashing with multiple features, which is able to analyze multiple cues of cells and model them in hash entries. We applied this framework on the differentiation of two types of lung cancers, the adenocarcinoma and squamous carcinoma, and achieved promising accuracy and efficiency. In the future, we plan to apply our framework on larger databases and whole slides images, and investigate the correlation of database sizes and the classification accuracy. We also plan to evaluate our method on other use cases of histopathological image analysis.

References

1. Comaniciu, D., Meer, P., Foran, D.J.: Image-guided decision support system for pathology. Mach. Vis. Appl. **11**(4), 213–224 (1999)
2. Müller, H., Geissbühler, A., Ruch, P.: ImageCLEF 2004: combining image and multi-lingual search for medical image retrieval. In: Peters, C., Clough, P., Gonzalo, J., Jones, G.J.F., Kluck, M., Magnini, B. (eds.) CLEF 2004. LNCS, vol. 3491, pp. 718–727. Springer, Heidelberg (2005)
3. Syeda-Mahmood, T., Turaga, P., Beymer, D., Wang, F., Amir, A., Greenspan, H., Pohl, K.: Shape-based similarity retrieval of doppler images for clinical decision support. In: CVPR, pp. 855–862. IEEE (2010)
4. Foran, D.J., Yang, L., et al.: Imageminer: a software system for comparative analysis of tissue microarrays using content-based image retrieval, high-performance computing, and grid technology. JAMIA **18**(4), 403–415 (2011)
5. Dy, J.G., Brodley, C.E., Kak, A., Broderick, L.S., Aisen, A.M.: Unsupervised feature selection applied to content-based retrieval of lung images. TPAMI **25**(3), 373–378 (2003)
6. El-Naqa, I., Yang, Y., Galatsanos, N.P., Nishikawa, R.M., Wernick, M.N.: A similarity learning approach to content-based image retrieval: application to digital mammography. TMI **23**(10), 1233–1244 (2004)
7. Greenspan, H., Pinhas, A.T.: Medical image categorization and retrieval for PACS using the GMM-KL framework. TITB **11**(2), 190–202 (2007)
8. Langs, G., Hanbury, A., Menze, B., Müller, H.: VISCERAL: towards large data in medical imaging — challenges and directions. In: Greenspan, H., Müller, H., Syeda-Mahmood, T. (eds.) MCBR-CDS 2012. LNCS, vol. 7723, pp. 92–98. Springer, Heidelberg (2013)
9. Siegel, R., Naishadham, D., Jemal, A.: Cancer statistics, 2013. CAJC **63**(1), 11–30 (2013)
10. Freeman, D.L.: Harrison's principles of internal medicine. JAMA **286**(8), 506 (2001)
11. Kayser, G., Riede, U., Werner, M., Hufnagl, P., Kayser, K.: Towards an automated morphological classification of histological images of common lung carcinomas. Elec. J. Pathol. Histol. **8**, 022–03 (2002)

12. Thunnissen, F., Diegenbach, P., Van Hattum, A., Tolboom, J., van der Sluis, D., Schaafsma, W., Houthoff, H., Baak, J.R.: Further evaluation of quantitative nuclear image features for classification of lung carcinomas. Pathol. Res. Pract. **188**(4), 531–535 (1992)

13. Mijović, Ž., Mihailović, D., Kostov, M.: Discriminant analysis of nuclear image variables in lung carcinoma. Facta Univ. Ser. Med. Biol. **15**(1), 28–32 (2008)

14. Edwards, S., Roberts, C., McKean, M., Cockburn, J., Jeffrey, R., Kerr, K.: Preoperative histological classification of primary lung cancer: accuracy of diagnosis and use of the non-small cell category. Am. J. Clin. Path. **53**(7), 537–540 (2000)

15. Lowe, D.G.: Distinctive image features from scale-invariant keypoints. IJCV **60**(2), 91–110 (2004)

16. Zhang, X., Yang, L., Liu, W., Su, H., Zhang, S.: Mining histopathological images via composite hashing and online learning. In: Golland, P., Hata, N., Barillot, C., Hornegger, J., Howe, R. (eds.) MICCAI 2014, Part II. LNCS, vol. 8674, pp. 479–486. Springer, Heidelberg (2014)

17. Datar, M., Immorlica, N., Indyk, P., Mirrokni, V.S.: Locality-sensitive hashing scheme based on p-stable distributions. In: SoCG, pp. 253–262. ACM (2004)

18. Kulis, B., Grauman, K.: Kernelized locality-sensitive hashing for scalable image search. In: CVPR (2009)

19. Andoni, A., Indyk, P.: Near-optimal hashing algorithms for approximate nearest neighbor in high dimensions. In: FOCS, Berkeley, CA, 21–24 October 2006

20. Liu, W., Wang, J., Ji, R., Jiang, Y.G., Chang, S.F.: Supervised hashing with kernels. In: CVPR, pp. 2074–2081 (2012)

21. Zhang, X., Su, H., Yang, L., Zhang, S.: Fine-grained histopathological image analysis via robust segmentation and large-scale retrieval. In: CVPR. IEEE (2015)

22. Xing, F., Su, H., Neltner, J., Yang, L.: Automatic ki-67 counting using robust cell detection and online dictionary learning. TBME **61**(3), 859–870 (2014)

23. Carpenter, A.E., Jones, T.R., Lamprecht, M.R., Clarke, C., Kang, I.H., Friman, O., Guertin, D.A., Chang, J.H., Lindquist, R.A., Moffat, J., et al.: Cellprofiler: image analysis software for identifying and quantifying cell phenotypes. Genome Biol. **7**(10), R100 (2006)

24. Arteta, C., Lempitsky, V., Noble, J.A., Zisserman, A.: Learning to detect cells using non-overlapping extremal regions. In: Ayache, N., Delingette, H., Golland, P., Mori, K. (eds.) MICCAI 2012, Part I. LNCS, vol. 7510, pp. 348–356. Springer, Heidelberg (2012)

25. Oliva, A., Torralba, A.: Modeling the shape of the scene: a holistic representation of the spatial envelope. IJCV **42**(3), 145–175 (2001)

26. Dalal, N., Triggs, B.: Histograms of oriented gradients for human detection. In: CVPR, vol. 1, pp. 886–893 (2005)

27. Weiss, Y., Torralba, A., Fergus, R.: Spectral hashing. In: NIPS (2008)

28. National Cancer Institute: The cancer genome atlas retrieved from https://tcga-data.nci.nih.gov (2013)

29. Tabesh, A., Teverovskiy, M., Pang, H.Y., Kumar, V.P., Verbel, D., Kotsianti, A., Saidi, O.: Multifeature prostate cancer diagnosis and gleason grading of histological images. TMI **26**(10), 1366–1378 (2007)

30. Doyle, S., Agner, S., Madabhushi, A., Feldman, M., Tomaszewski, J.: Automated grading of breast cancer histopathology using spectral clustering with textural and architectural image features. In: ISBI, pp. 496–499 (2008)

31. Zhang, X., Liu, W., Dundar, M., Badve, S., Zhang, S.: Towards large-scale histopathological image analysis: hashing-based image retrieval. TMI **34**(2), 496–506 (2015)

Multiresolution Diffeomorphic Mapping
for Cortical Surfaces

Mingzhen Tan[1,4] and Anqi Qiu[1,2,3,4]([✉])

[1] Department of Biomedical Engineering,
National University of Singapore, Singapore, Singapore
biequa@nus.edu.sg
[2] Clinical Imaging Research Center,
National University of Singapore, Singapore, Singapore
[3] Singapore Institute for Clinical Sciences, Singapore, Singapore
[4] NUS Graduate School for Integrative Sciences and Engineering,
Singapore, Singapore

Abstract. Due to the convoluted folding pattern of the cerebral cortex, accurate alignment of cortical surfaces remains challenging. In this paper, we present a multiresolution diffeomorphic surface mapping algorithm under the framework of large deformation diffeomorphic metric mapping (LDDMM). Our algorithm takes advantage of multiresolution analysis (MRA) for surfaces and constructs cortical surfaces at multiresolution. This family of multiresolution surfaces are used as natural sparse priors of the cortical anatomy and provide the anchor points where the parametrization of deformation vector fields is supported. This naturally constructs tangent bundles of diffeomorphisms at different resolution levels and hence generates multiresolution diffeomorphic transformation. We show that our construction of multiresolution LDDMM surface mapping can potentially reduce computational cost and improves the mapping accuracy of cortical surfaces.

1 Introduction

The human cortex is a convoluted sheet that forms folding patterns. Because of this, functionally distinct regions are close to each other in a volume space but geometrically distant in terms of distance measured along the cortex. Such geometric property of the cortex has been well preserved in the cortical surface model [4,7,9,13,20]. Thus, surface-based analysis, in particular, surface-based registration for optimizing the alignment of anatomical and functional data across individuals, has received great attention in both anatomical and functional studies [8,10,17,20,21].

Most of the advanced cortical surface registration approaches have been implemented in the spherical coordinates based on either folding patterns [10,15] or landmarks (sulcal or gyral curves) [8,17]. In particular, landmark-based spherical mappings provide flexibility to choose sulcal or gyral curves in functional activation areas for the improvement of the alignment in regions of interest

© Springer International Publishing Switzerland 2015
S. Ourselin et al. (Eds.): IPMI 2015, LNCS 9123, pp. 315–326, 2015.
DOI: 10.1007/978-3-319-19992-4_24

(ROIs) [1] even though the gyral or sulcal curves are the coarse representation of the cortex. Nevertheless, the landmark or folding pattern based spherical mappings require the spherical reparametrization of the cortical surface in which adjacent gyri with distinct functions are well separated. This surface reparametrization process introduces large distance and area distortion that potentially affects the quality of the surface alignment. To avoid such distortion, one would expect to directly align the cortical surfaces in their own coordinates. Vaillant and Glaunès [18] first introduced a vector-valued measure acting on vector fields as geometric representation of surfaces in their own space and then imposed a Hilbert space structure on it, whose norm was used to quantify the geometric similarity between two surfaces in their own coordinates. Since then, the vector-valued measure has been incorporated as a matching functional in the variational problems of large deformation diffeomorphic metric surface and curve mapping (LDDMM) [18,19,22]. It has been shown that first aligning gyral/sulcal curves and then cortical surfaces have great improvement in mapping cortical surfaces when compared to directly mapping cortical surfaces alone [21]. This gives an idea of multiresolution mapping for reducing computational cost and improving cortical surface alignment.

Multiresolution diffeomorphic mapping has been proposed for images. LDDMM with a mixture of kernels was introduced for aligning images [3], providing the mathematical foundation of a multiresolution diffeomorphic image mapping. However, the weights associated with kernels were not straightforward to determined and its computation remained the same as that of the image mapping algorithm in [2]. Rather than a simple weighted mixture of kernels, large deformation diffeomorphic kernel bundle mapping (LDDKBM) was proposed to allow multiple kernels at multiple scales incorporated in the registration of images [16]. It combines sparsity priors with the kernel bundle resulting in compact representations across scales. The results demonstrated tremendous improvement on image mapping.

Paper Contributions. This paper presents a multiresolution surface mapping algorithm under the LDDMM framework. We take advantage of a multiresolution analysis of surfaces, constructing coarse-to-fine surfaces that become natural sparse priors of the cortical anatomy. The vertices on the surface at individual resolutions provide the anchor points where the parametrization of deformation vector fields is supported. This naturally constructs tangent bundles of diffeomorphisms at different resolution levels, similar to LDDKBM [16], and hence generates multiresolution diffeomorphic transformation. We show that our construction of multiresolution LDDMM surface mapping can potentially reduce computational cost and improves the mapping accuracy of cortical surfaces.

2   Methods

2.1   Multiresolution Analysis for Surfaces

In this study, we adopt multiresolution analysis (MRA) for arbitrary surfaces from Lounsbery et al. [12] to construct coarse-to-fine surface meshes. The method, which is related to the mathematical foundations of wavelets, decomposes a poly-hedral surface into 2 separate components, namely a low-resolution surface and a corresponding collection of coefficients containing the removed "details". This process, when performed iteratively, produces a family of surfaces, wherein each successive surface is of a lower resolution than its predecessor. A recovery process, known as "synthesis", reverses the decomposition such that the original high-resolution surface could be progressively reproduced from any member of the family. We can thus define a chain of nested function spaces $\mathbf{V}^{(0)} \subset \mathbf{V}^{(1)} \subset \cdots$, such that $f \in \mathbf{V}^{(r)}$ is a function at resolution r, $r \in [0, R]$, with the level of detail increasing as r increases.

Let $T = (\{x_i\}, \{\Sigma_{ijk}\})$ be a triangular surface mesh, where $\{x_i\}, i = 1, \ldots, N$ is a set of vertices and $\{\Sigma_{ijk}\}$ a set of simplices, with each simplex Σ_{ijk} as a three tuple of points x_i, x_j, x_k. Given a mesh $T^{(r)}$ at level r, with coordinates $X^{(r)} = [x_1, \ldots, x_i, \ldots, x_{N^{(r)}}]$, where $x_i \in \mathbb{R}^3$ and $N^{(r)}$ is the number of vertices on $T^{(r)}$. The new vertices on $T^{(r+1)}$, denoted as $\hat{X}^{(r+1)}$, can be given as

$$\hat{X}^{(r+1)} = X^{(r)} A_{N^{(r)} \times M}, \tag{1}$$

where A is an $N^{(r)} \times M$ matrix for a simple subdivision scheme (where all elements of $A_j = 0$ except for $A_{ij} = A_{kj} = 0.5$) and M is the number of the new vertices on $T^{(r+1)}$, $X^{(r+1)} = [X^{(r)}, \hat{X}^{(r+1)}]$. Given an "averaging matrix" $B_{N^{(r+1)} \times N^{(r+1)}}$, a general subdivision scheme can be rewritten as

$$X^{(r+1)} = X^{(r)} [I_{N^{(r)} \times N^{(r)}} \quad A] B = \tilde{X}^{(r+1)} B = X^{(r)} P^{(r)}, \tag{2}$$

where $\tilde{X}^{(r+1)} = X^{(r)} [I_{N^{(r)} \times N^{(r)}} \quad A]$, $P^{(r)} = [I_{N^{(r)} \times N^{(r)}} \quad A] B$.

As explained in [12], surfaces can be parametrized with a function $S(y)$, where y is defined on a base (coarsest) mesh $T^{(0)}$, i.e. y is a point on one of the simplices in $\Sigma_{ijk}^{(0)}$ and can be tracked through a predefined subdivision process to a limit surface. We begin by first defining $S^{(0)}(y) := y$. Let $S^{(r-1)}(y)$ be found in a simplex $\Sigma_{abc}^{(r)}$ with vertices $(\tilde{x}_a, \tilde{x}_b, \tilde{x}_c)$, $\tilde{x}$ found in $\hat{X}^{(r)}$. Using the barycentric coordinates $(\lambda_a, \lambda_b, \lambda_c)$ such that $S^{(r-1)}(y) = \lambda_a \tilde{x}_a + \lambda_b \tilde{x}_b + \lambda_c \tilde{x}_c$, we can induce a bijective map $S^{(r-1)}(y) \to S^{(r)}(y)$ where

$$S^{(r)}(y) = \lambda_a x_a + \lambda_b x_b + \lambda_c x_c, \qquad x \in X^{(r)} \tag{3}$$

and (x_a, x_b, x_c) corresponds to $(\tilde{x}_a, \tilde{x}_b, \tilde{x}_c)$ of the simplex $\Sigma_{abc}^{(r)}$. Then, $S(y) := \lim_{r \to \infty} S^{(r)}(y)$. In matrix form,

$$S^{(r)}(y) = \boldsymbol{\lambda}^{(r)}(y)(X^{(r)})^T. \tag{4}$$

It follows that

$$S^{(r)}(y) = \boldsymbol{\lambda}^{(r)}(y)(X^{(r-1)} P^{(r-1)})^T \tag{5}$$

$$= \boldsymbol{\lambda}^{(r)}(y)(P^{(r-1)})^T \cdots (P^{(0)})^T (X^{(0)})^T. \tag{6}$$

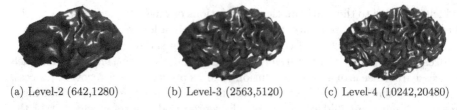

(a) Level-2 (642,1280)   (b) Level-3 (2563,5120)   (c) Level-4 (10242,20480)

Fig. 1. Increasing levels of $X^{(r)}$ from left to right. Subcaptions indicates the corresponding levels, number of vertices, and number of faces - "Level-r (no. of vertices, no. of faces)".

In other words, surfaces when parameterized into meshes, can be henceforth understood as functions from a small collection of triangles into $\mathbb{R}^3$. The subdivision of triangles allows us to move from one resolution to another, providing a family of surfaces for registration. We show three resolutions of the brain cortex in Fig. 1.

2.2 Multiresolution Large Deformation Diffeomorphic Metric Mapping for Surfaces

Now, we state a variational problem for mapping two surfaces under the framework of LDDMM. LDDMM assumes that transformation can be generated from one to another via flows of diffeomorphisms φ_t, which are solutions of ordinary differential equations $\dot{\varphi}_t = v_t(\varphi_t), t \in [0,1]$, starting from the identity map $\varphi_0 = \text{Id}$. They are therefore characterized by time-dependent velocity vector fields $v_t, t \in [0,1]$. We define a metric distance between a target surface S_{targ} and an atlas surface S_{atlas} as the minimal length of curves $\varphi_t \cdot S_{atlas}, t \in [0,1]$, in a shape space such that, at time $t = 1$, $\varphi_1 \cdot S_{atlas} = S_{targ}$. Lengths of such curves are computed as the integrated norm $\|v_t\|_V$ of the vector field, where $v_t \in V$ and V is a reproducing kernel Hilbert space with kernel k_V and norm $\|\cdot\|_V$. To ensure solutions are diffeomorphisms, V must be a space of smooth vector fields. The duality isometry in Hilbert spaces allows us to express the lengths in terms of $m_t \in V^*$, interpreted as momentum such that $\forall u \in V, \langle m_t, u \circ \varphi_t \rangle_2 = \langle k_V^{-1} v_t, u \rangle_2$, and $\langle m, u \rangle_2$ denotes the $\mathbb{L}^2$ inner product between m and u, With a slight abuse of symbols, it is the result of the natural pairing between m and v in cases where m is singular (e.g., a measure). This identity is classically written as $\varphi_t^* m_t = k_V^{-1} v_t$, where φ_t^* is referred to as the pullback operation on a vector measure, m_t. Using the identity $\|v_t\|_V^2 = \langle k_V^{-1} v_t, v_t \rangle_2 = \langle m_t, k_V m_t \rangle_2$ and the fact that energy-minimizing curves coincide with constant-speed length-minimizing curves, we obtain the metric distance between the atlas and target, $\rho(S_{atlas}, S_{targ})$, by minimizing $\|v_t\|_V^2$, such that $\varphi_1 \cdot S_{atlas} = S_{targ}$ at time $t = 1$ [5]. We associate this with the variational problem in the form of

$$J(m_t) = \inf_{m_t : \dot{\varphi}_t = k_V m_t(\varphi_t), \varphi_0 = \text{Id}} \rho(S_{atlas}, S_{targ})^2$$
$$+ \gamma E(\varphi_1 \cdot S_{atlas}, S_{targ}), \tag{7}$$

where E is defined based vector-valued measure as introduced in [18]. For any two surfaces S_1 and S_2, $E(S_1, S_2)$ is defined as

$$E(S_1, S_2) = \sum_{f,g} N_f^t k_W(c_g, c_f) N_g - 2\sum_{f,q} N_f^t k_W(c_f, c_q) Nq \\ + \sum_{q,p} N_q^t k_W(c_q, c_p) N_r, \tag{8}$$

where f, g are simplices from S_1 while q, p are simplices from S_2. N_g is then the normal vector pointing out of the centre, c_g, of simplex g. k_W is a Gaussian kernel with bandwidth σ_W. The metric distance $\rho(S_{atlas}, S_{targ})^2$ could be easily computed as $\int_0^1 \|v_t\|_V^2 dt$.

We now construct the multiresolution diffeomorphic mapping for surfaces under the framework of LDDMM. In the previous section, we show that a surface, S, may be sequentially subsampled into meshes of decreasing resolution $T^{(r)} \ldots T^{(1)}$. With a slight abuse of notation, let us define these meshes as the discretization of the surface, rewriting $T^{(r)}$ as $S^{(r)}$, such that $\lim_{r \to \infty} S^{(r)} \to S$. The duality isometry of m_t with v_t allows defining the smooth vector field, v_t through m_t, where m_t can sparsely anchor at the vertices on $S^{(r)}$. Therefore, it is natural to seek $m_t^{(r)}$ defined at the vertices on $S^{(r)}$ and then construct the smooth vector field, $w_t^{(r)} = k_V^{(r)} m_t^{(r)}$, where the size of $k_V^{(r)}$ can be adapted to the sparse level of the vertices on $S^{(r)}$. From this construction, $w_t^{(r)}, r = 0, 1, \ldots, R$ can be defined via momentum $m_t^{(r)} \otimes \delta_x, x \in S^{(r)}, r = 0, 1, \ldots, R$ and construct independent tangent spaces of diffeomorphisms, $w^{(r)} \in W^{(r)}$. The family of vector fields forms reproducing kernel Hilbert spaces, which could be summed across multiple resolutions, i.e., $\vartheta_t(w_t) = \sum_{r=0}^R w_t^{(r)}$, to form one single vector field for the flow equation $\dot{\varphi}_t^\vartheta = \vartheta_t(\varphi_t^\vartheta)$. Through this family of vector fields, we redefine $\rho^{MRA}(S_{atlas}, S_{targ})$ by minimizing $\int_0^1 \sum_{r=0}^R \|w_t^{(r)}\|_{W^{(r)}}^2 dt$ such that $\varphi_1^\vartheta \cdot S_{atlas} = S_{targ}$ at time $t = 1$, where $\|w_t^{(r)}\|_{W^{(r)}}^2 = \langle (k_V^{(r)})^{-1} w_t^{(r)}, w_t^{(r)} \rangle_2 = \langle m_t^{(r)}, k_V^{(r)} m_t^{(r)} \rangle_2$. This construction of $\rho^{MRA}(S_{atlas}, S_{targ})$ is in turn similar to that proposed for the large deformation diffeomorphic kernel bundle mapping (LDDKBM) for the registration of images [16].

We now modify Eq. (7) to the variational problem for the multiresolution LDDMM surface mapping in the form of

$$J(m_t) = \inf_{m_t^{(r)} : \dot{\varphi}_t^\vartheta = \sum_{r=0}^R k_V^{(r)} m_t^r(\varphi_t^\vartheta), \varphi_0^\vartheta \doteq \mathrm{Id}} \rho^{MRA}(S_{atlas}, S_{targ})^2 \\ + \gamma E(\varphi_1 \cdot S_{atlas}^{(R)}, S_{targ}^{(R)}), \tag{9}$$

where $m_t = \{m_t^{(r)}\}$. We can rewrite this variational problem as

$$J(m_t) = \inf_{m_t^{(r)} : \dot{\varphi}_t^\vartheta = \sum_{r=0}^R k_V^{(r)} m_t^r(\varphi_t^\vartheta), \varphi_0^\vartheta \doteq \mathrm{Id}} \int_0^1 \sum_{r=0}^R \|w_t^{(r)}\|_{W^{(r)}}^2 dt \\ + \gamma E(\varphi_1 \cdot S_{atlas}^{(R)}, S_{targ}^{(R)}), \tag{10}$$

where $w_t^{(r)}(\cdot) = \sum_{i=1}^{N^{(r)}} k_V^{(r)}(\cdot, x_i) m_t^{(r)}(x_i)$ and $x_i \in S^{(r)}$.

2.3 Gradient Computation and Implementation

To reduce the computational cost, we minimize Eq. (10) at *each* resolution level when R gradually increases from $0, 1, 2, \cdots$. We use the gradient descent method to solve Eq. (10) when R is fixed and the method presented in [14] to speed up the computation of the Gaussian transform.

We now compute the gradient of J in Eq. (10) with respect to $\boldsymbol{m}_t = \{m_t^{(r)}\}$. We begin by considering a variation in the vector field $w_{t,\varepsilon}^{(r)} = w_t^{(r)} + \varepsilon \tilde{w}_t^{(r)}$. The corresponding variation of $x_{j,1} = \varphi_1^\vartheta(x_j)$ is

$$\tilde{x}_{j,1} = \partial_\varepsilon x_{j,1}|_{\varepsilon=0} = \int_0^1 d_{x_{j,t}} \varphi_{t1}^\vartheta \tilde{w}_t^{(r)}(x_{j,t}) dt, \tag{11}$$

where $\varphi_{t1} := \varphi_1 \circ \varphi_t^{-1}$. Based on the derivation from [18], the variation of E is

$$\partial_\varepsilon E|_{\varepsilon=0} = \int_0^1 \langle k_V^{(r)}(x_{j,t}, \cdot)(d_{x_{j,t}} \varphi_{t1}^\vartheta)^* \nabla_{x_{j,t}} E, \tilde{w}_t^{(r)} \rangle dt.$$

This implies that the gradient of E in the space $\mathbb{L}^2([0,1], W^{(r)})$ of vector fields, at a particular level r is of the form

$$\nabla E(t, \cdot) = \sum_j k_V^{(r)}(x_{j,t}, \cdot)(d_{x_{j,t}} \varphi_{t1}^\vartheta)^* \nabla_{x_{j,t}} E. \tag{12}$$

In this way, we have reduced the gradient computations to $\nabla_{x_{j,t}} E$, (the derivative of the data attachment term, E, with respect to the vertices in $x_{j,t}$). When the surface is represented using vector-valued measure, $\nabla_{x_{j,t1}} E$ is given in [18]. The Jacobian of the transformation, $d_{x_{j,t}} \varphi_{t1}^\vartheta$, is given by the following relationship (refer to [11] for further details)

$$\frac{d}{dt}(d_{x_{j,t}} \varphi_{t1}^\vartheta) = -d_{x_{j,t}} \varphi_{t1}^\vartheta d_{x_{j,t}} \vartheta. \tag{13}$$

Finally, using Eq. (13), we can directly compute

$$\frac{d}{dt} \nabla_{x_{j,t}} E = -(d_{x_{j,t}} \vartheta(w_t))^* \nabla_{x_{j,t}} E, \tag{14}$$

which can be integrated backwards from $t = 1$ to 0. For a given resolution, the gradient of $\int_0^1 \sum_{r=0}^R \|w_t^{(r)}\|_{W^{(r)}}^2 dt$ is $2w_t^{(r)}$. The gradient of the cost functional J with respect to $w_t^{(r)}$ is then

$$\nabla_{w_t^{(r)}} J(x) = 2 \sum_j k_V^{(r)}(x_{j,t}, x) \left[\gamma(d_{x_{j,t}} \varphi_{t1}^\vartheta)^* \nabla_{x_{j,t}} E + m_{j,t}^{(r)} \right]. \tag{15}$$

We can hence write the gradient of J with respect to $m_t^{(r)}$ as

$$\nabla_{m_t^{(r)}} J(x) = 2\gamma(d_{x_{j,t}} \varphi_{t1}^\vartheta)^* \nabla_{x_{j,t}} E + 2m_t^{(r)}. \tag{16}$$

We now summarize the optimization with the following algorithm:

Algorithm 1

Given S_{atlas}, S_{targ}, use Eq. (5) and obtain $\{S_{atlas}^{(r)}\}, \{S_{targ}^{(r)}\}, r \in \{0, 1, \cdots, R\}$.

for $R = 0, 1, 2, \cdots$ **do**

   Step 1: Compute the gradient $\nabla_{m_t^{(R)}} J_t(x)$ using Eqs. (13), (14) and (16).

   Step 2: Update $m_t^{(R)}$ using $m_t^{(R)} = m_t^{(R),old} - \epsilon \nabla_{m_t^{(R)}} J(x)$,

   where ϵ is an adaptive gradient descent step size. Evaluate J.

   Step 3: Repeat steps 1,2 until J is optimized at level R.

   Step 4: Initialize $m_t^{(R+1)}$. Assume $X^{(R)}$ and $X^{(R+1)}$ to be sets respectively containing vertices of $S^{(R)}$ and $S^{(R+1)}$.

   if $x \in X^{(R+1)} \cap X^{(R)}$ **then**
   $$m_t^{(R+1)}(x) = m_t^{(R)}(x).$$
   else if $x \in X^{(R+1)}/X^{(R)}$ **then**
   $$m_t^{(R+1)}(x) = m_t^{(R)}(x)P^{(R)}$$
   end if

end for

3 Experiments

In this section, we will first show experiments on real datasets using the proposed registration algorithm and the LDDMM surface mapping in [18]. We will then show the computation time and evaluate the mapping accuracy of the two mapping algorithms. For all experiments, we use a Gaussian kernel, i.e. $k_V(x, y) := \exp(-\|x - y\|_2/\sigma_V)$.

Figure 2 illustrates one example of the mapping results using the proposed method. Both atlas and target surfaces have 10242 vertices and 20480 faces. The final deformed atlas showed on panel (d) was obtained using the proposed mapping algorithm with four resolution levels respectively associated with the diffeomorphic kernels of $\sigma_V = \{25, 10, 5, 1\}$. In panel (f), we visually examine the deformed atlas by plotting the minimum distance (mm) from every vertex of the target surface to every other vertex on the deformed source. The mean and standard deviation of the minimum distance is 0.8238 ± 0.565.

We visually compared this mapping result with that obtained using the LDDMM surface mapping in [18]. To make the two mapping algorithms comparable, the mapping procedure was the same except that the LDDMM surface mapping was only applied to the finest level of the surfaces and $\sigma_V = 1$. From Fig. 3(c), we can see that the LDDMM surface mapping method tends to have the undesirable behaviour of 'inwards folding' (regions with in-folding indicated with tiny black arrows) along the precentral gyrus, while this is not observed using the proposed coarse-to-fine method.

Next, we aligned the atlas to 5 cortical surfaces using the same mapping procedures as those introduced above for both the proposed method and the LDDMM surface mapping. Table 1 lists the parameter setting and the computational cost averaged across the 5 cortical surfaces. In general, the computational time is much less for the all four levels in the proposed method. This is due to

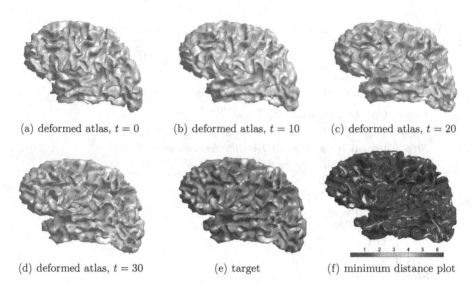

(a) deformed atlas, $t = 0$ (b) deformed atlas, $t = 10$ (c) deformed atlas, $t = 20$

(d) deformed atlas, $t = 30$ (e) target   (f) minimum distance plot

Fig. 2. An example of cortical surface mapping using the proposed algorithm with time for the diffeomorphic flow was discretized into 30 steps. Panels (a, e) respectively show the atlas and target surfaces, while panels (b,c) show the intermediate mapping results (deformed atlas at time steps of 10 and 20) and panel (d) illustrates the deformed atlas. Panel (f) shows the minimum distance from a point on the target to every other point on the deformed atlas.

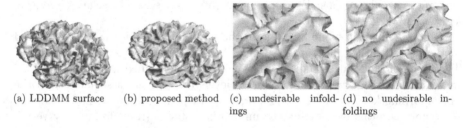

(a) LDDMM surface   (b) proposed method   (c) undesirable infold-ings   (d) no undesirable in-foldings

Fig. 3. This figure shows the comparison between the LDDMM surface mapping and the proposed method for cortical surface registration. Panels (a) and (b) are the deformed atlases obtained using LDDMM surface mapping and the proposed method, respectively. The second row shows a closer view of the region around the central sulcus. Panels (c,d) respectively correspond to those from the LDDMM algorithm and the proposed method. Black arrows on panel (c) point out the locations with undesired infolding features.

the initialization provided by the low resolution surfaces, which allows the gradient optimization at high resolutions, (where the computation is more costly), to converge quickly.

We also evaluated the mapping accuracy of the two methods using surface alignment consistency (SAC) that was initially introduced by Van Essen [6]. The SAC quantifies the anatomical variability of a sulcal region among a group

Table 1. Average computational parameters and time for both methods, using the `Matlab` software. For the MRA-LDDMM, the average time taken is the runtime for the entire set of σ_V for that particular level, at a specific σ_W (bandwidth of the data-attachment term). The LDDMM runtime records the entire time taken to go through the same set of decreasing σ_W used by the MRA-LDDMM.

Method	Level	# of faces	# of points	σ_V	Time taken
MRA-LDDMM	1	320	162	25	49.4s
MRA-LDDMM	2	1280	642	25,10	541.3s
MRA-LDDMM	3	5120	2563	25,10,5	1986.7s
MRA-LDDMM	4	20480	10242	25,10,5,1	3903.0s
LDDMM	-	20480	10242	1	96341s

of subjects that can be characterized by the cortical mapping. A larger value indicates better mapping. With prior information such as delineated surface regions, the SAC is given as $\sum_{i=1}^{N}(i-1)n(i)/(N-1)(N_{\text{total}})$, where N is the total number of subjects used, $n(i)$ is the number of points that were mapped correctly for i number of times and N_{total} is the total number of nodes associated with a particular region.

In our experiment, we manually delineated seventeen sulcal regions on all the cortical surfaces (see details in [21]). The delineated regions are shown in Fig. 4. Figure 5 shows the comparison of SAC values for the LDDMM surface mapping and the proposed method at the last 2 levels. As expected, the SAC values of the proposed method increases as the surface resolution becomes finer. The SAC was also higher for the larger and more prominent sulci such as the Central Sulcus, Cingulate Sulcus, Sylvian Fissure, Superior Precentral Sulcus and Superior Temporal Sulcus. At level 3 (or 4) of the proposed mapping method, the SAC values were uniformly greater than those obtained using the LDDMM surface mapping for all seventeen sulcal regions.

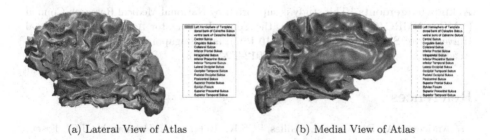

(a) Lateral View of Atlas   (b) Medial View of Atlas

Fig. 4. Seventeen sulcal regions are illustrated on the atlas surface.

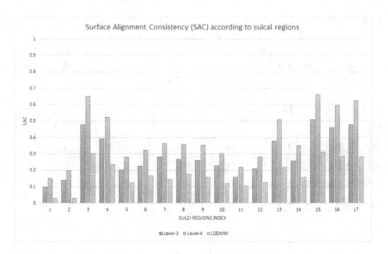

Fig. 5. Surface alignment consistency (SAC) for the LDDMM surface mapping and the proposed method. Indexed sulci regions 1-17 are respectively: Dorsal bank of Calcarine Sulcus(1), Ventral bank of Calcarine Sulcus(2), Central Sulcus(3), Cingulate Sulcus(4), Collateral Sulcus(5), Inferior Frontal Sulcus(6), Intraparietal Sulcus(7), Inferior Precentral Sulcus(8), Inferior Temporal Sulcus(9), Lateral Occipital Sulcus(10), Occipital Temporal Sulcus(11), Parietal Occipital Sulcus(12), Postcentral Sulcus(13), Superior Frontal Sulcus(14), Sylvian Fissure(15), Superior Precentral Sulcus(16), Superior Temporal Sulcus(17).

4   Conclusion

This paper introduced the multiresolution diffeomorphic mapping for cortical surfaces. We showed that this algorithm improves alignment as compared to the LDDMM-surface algorithm [18]. It has potential to reduce the computational time.

Acknowledgements. This study is supported by National Medical Research Council (NMRC; NMRC/CBRG/0039/2013), the Young Investigator Award at the National University of Singapore (NUSYIA FY10 P07), and Singapore Ministry of Education Academic Research Fund Tier 2 (MOE2012-T2-2-130).

References

1. Anticevic, A., Dierker, D.L., Gillespie, S.K., Repovs, G., Csernansky, J.G., Essen, D.C.V., Barch, D.M.: Comparing surface-based and volume-based analyses of functional neuroimaging data in patients with schizophrenia. Neuroimage **41**(3), 835–848 (2008)
2. Beg, M.F., Miller, M.I., Trouvé, A., Younes, L.: Computing large deformation metric mappings via geodesic flows of diffeomorphisms. Int. J. Comput. Vision **61**(2), 139–157 (2005)

3. Bruveris, M., Risser, L., Vialard, F.X.: Mixture of kernels and iterated semidirect product of diffeomorphisms groups. Multiscale Model. Simul. **10**(4), 1344–1368 (2012)
4. Clouchoux, C., Coulon, O., Rivière, D., Cachia, A., Mangin, J.-F., Régis, J.: Anatomically constrained surface parameterization for cortical localization. In: Duncan, J.S., Gerig, G. (eds.) MICCAI 2005. LNCS, vol. 3750, pp. 344–351. Springer, Heidelberg (2005)
5. Du, J., Younes, L., Qiu, A.: Whole brain diffeomorphic metric mapping via integration of sulcal and gyral curves, cortical surfaces, and images. NeuroImage **56**(1), 162–173 (2011)
6. Essen, D.C.V.: A population-average, landmark- and surface-based (pals-b12) atlas of human cerebral cortex. Neuroimage **28**, 635–662 (2005)
7. van Essen, D.: Surface-based approaches to spatial localization and registration in primate cerebral cortex. NeuroImage **23**, s97–s107 (2004)
8. van Essen, D.: A population-average, landmark- and surface-based (PALS) atlas of human cerebral cortex. NeuroImage **28**, 635–662 (2005)
9. Fischl, B., Sereno, M.I., Dale, A.M.: Cortical surface-based analysis II: inflation, flattening, and a surface-based coordinate system. NeuroImage **9**, 195–207 (1999)
10. Fischl, B., Sereno, M.I., Tootell, R.B.H., Dale, A.M.: High-resolution intersubject averaging and a coordinate system for the cortical surface. Hum. Brain Mapp. **8**, 272–284 (1999)
11. Glaunès, J., Trouvé, A., Younes, L.: Diffeomorphic matching of distributions: a new approach for unlabelled point-sets and sub-manifolds matching. In: CVPR, pp. 712–718. IEEE Computer Society (2004)
12. Lounsbery, M., DeRose, T.D., Warren, J.: Multiresolution analysis for surfaces of arbitrary topological type. ACM Trans. Graph. (TOG) **16**(1), 34–73 (1997)
13. Lyttelton, O., Boucher, M., Robbins, S., Evans, A.: An unbiased iterative group registration template for cortical surface analysis. NeuroImage **34**, 1535–1544 (2007)
14. Morariu, V.I., Srinivasan, B.V., Raykar, V.C., Duraiswami, R., Davis, L.S.: Automatic online tuning for fast gaussian summation. In: Advances in Neural Information Processing Systems, pp. 1113–1120 (2009)
15. Robbins, S., Evans, A., Collins, D., Whitesides, S.: Tuning and comparing spatial normalization methods. Med. Image Anal. **8**(3), 311–323 (2004)
16. Sommer, S., Lauze, F., Nielsen, M., Pennec, X.: Sparse multi-scale diffeomorphic registration: the kernel bundle framework. J. Math. Imaging Vis. **46**, 292–308 (2013)
17. Thompson, P.M., Schwartz, C., Lin, R.T., Khan, A.A., Toga, A.W.: Three-dimensional statistical analysis of sulcal variability in the human brain. J. Neurosci. **16**(13), 4261–4274 (1996)
18. Vaillant, M., Glaunès, J.: Surface matching via currents. In: Christensen, G.E., Sonka, M. (eds.) IPMI 2005. LNCS, vol. 3565, pp. 381–392. Springer, Heidelberg (2005)
19. Vaillant, M., Qiu, A., Glaunès, J., Miller, M.I.: Diffeomorphic metric surface mapping in subregion of the superior temporal gyrus. NeuroImage **34**, 1149–1159 (2007)
20. van Essen, D.C., Drury, H.A., Joshi, S., Miller, M.I.: Functional and structural mapping of human cerebral cortex: solutions are in the surfaces. Proc. Natl. Acad. Sci. **95**, 788–795 (1998)

21. Zhong, J., Phua, D.Y.L., Qiu, A.: Quantitative evaluation of lddmm, freesurfer, and caret for cortical surface mapping. NeuroImage **52**(1), 131–141 (2010). http://www.sciencedirect.com/science/article/B6WNP-4YT6D56-2/2/9c94d7bf0 b64e4c1c4c639d412997bb7
22. Zhong, J., Qiu, A.: Multi-manifold diffeomorphic metric mapping for aligning cortical hemispheric surfaces. Neuroimage **49**, 355–365 (2010)

A Comprehensive Computer-Aided Polyp Detection System for Colonoscopy Videos

Nima Tajbakhsh[1]([⊠]), Suryakanth R. Gurudu[2], and Jianming Liang[1]

[1] Department of Biomedical Informatics, Arizona State University,
Scottsdale, AZ, USA
{Nima.Tajbakhsh,Jianming.Liang}@asu.edu
[2] Division of Gastroenterology and Hepatology, Mayo Clinic, Scottsdale, AZ, USA
Gurudu.Suryakanth@mayo.edu

Abstract. Computer-aided detection (CAD) can help colonoscopists reduce their polyp miss-rate, but existing CAD systems are handicapped by using either shape, texture, or temporal information for detecting polyps, achieving limited sensitivity and specificity. To overcome this limitation, our key contribution of this paper is to fuse all possible polyp features by exploiting the strengths of each feature while minimizing its weaknesses. Our new CAD system has two stages, where the first stage builds on the robustness of shape features to reliably generate a set of candidates with a high sensitivity, while the second stage utilizes the high discriminative power of the computationally expensive features to effectively reduce false positives. Specifically, we employ a unique edge classifier and an original voting scheme to capture geometric features of polyps in context and then harness the power of convolutional neural networks in a novel score fusion approach to extract and combine shape, color, texture, and temporal information of the candidates. Our experimental results based on FROC curves and a new analysis of polyp detection latency demonstrate a superiority over the state-of-the-art where our system yields a lower polyp detection latency and achieves a significantly higher sensitivity while generating dramatically fewer false positives. This performance improvement is attributed to our reliable candidate generation and effective false positive reduction methods.

1 Introduction

Colon cancer most often develop from colonic polyps. However, polyp grow slowly and it typically take years for polyps to develop into cancer, making colon cancer amenable to prevention. Colonoscopy is the preferred procedure for preventing colon cancer. The goal of colonoscopy is to find and remove polyps before turning into cancer. Despite its demonstrated utility, colonoscopy is not a perfect procedure. A recent clinical study [5] reports that a quarter of polyps are missed during colonoscopy. Computer-aided polyp detection can help colonoscopists reduce their polyp miss-rate, in particular, during long and back-to-back procedures where fatigue and inattentiveness may result in miss detection of polyps.

© Springer International Publishing Switzerland 2015
S. Ourselin et al. (Eds.): IPMI 2015, LNCS 9123, pp. 327–338, 2015.
DOI: 10.1007/978-3-319-19992-4_25

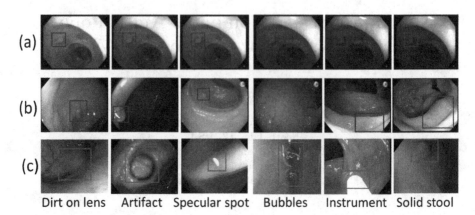

Fig. 1. Significant variation in visual characteristics of polyps. (a) Color and appearance variation of the same polyp due to varying lighting conditions. (b) Texture and shape variation among polyps. Note how the distance between the polyps and colonoscopy camera determines the availability of polyp texture. (c) Other polyp-like structures in the colonoscopic view (Color figure online).

However, designing a high-performance system for computer-aided polyp detection is challenging: (1) Polyps appear differently in color, and even the same polyp, as shown in Fig. 1(a), may look differently due to varying lighting conditions. (2) Polyps have large inter- and intra-morphological variations. As shown in Fig. 1(b), the shapes of polyps vary considerably from one to another. The intra-shape variation of polyps is caused by various factors, including the viewing angle of the camera and the spontaneous spasms of the colon. (3) Visibility of the texture on the surface of polyps is also varying due to biological factors and distance between the polyps and the colonoscopy camera. This can be seen in Fig. 1(b) where texture visibility decrease as the polyps distance from the capturing camera. The significant variations among polyps suggest that there is no single feature that performs the best for detecting all the polyps.

As a result, to achieve a reliable polyp detection system, it is critical to fuse all possible features of polyps, including shapes, color, and texture. Each of these features has strengths and weaknesses. Among these features, geometric shapes are most robust because polyps, irrespective of their morphology and varying levels of protrusion, have at least one curvilinear head at their boundaries. However, this property is not highly specific to polyps. This is shown in Fig. 1(c) where non-polyp structures exhibit similar geometric characteristics to polyps. Texture features have the weakness of limited availability; however, when visible, they can distinguish polyps from some non-polyp structures such as specular spots, dirt, and fecal matter. In addition, temporal information is available in colonoscopy and may be utilized to distinguish polyps from bubbles or other artifacts that only briefly appear in colonoscopy videos.

Our key contribution of this paper is an idea to exploit the strengths of each feature and minimize its weaknesses. To realize this idea, we have developed a new system for polyp detection with two stages. The first stage builds on the robustness of shape features of polyps to reliably generate a set of candidate detections with a high sensitivity, while the second stage utilizes the high discriminative power of the computationally expensive features to effectively reduce false positive detections. More specifically, we employ a unique edge classifier coupled with a voting scheme to capture geometric features of polyps in context and then harness the power of convolutional deep networks in a novel score fusion approach to capture shape, color, texture, and temporal information of the candidates. Our experimental results based on the largest annotated polyp database demonstrate that our system achieves high sensitivity to polyps and generates significantly less number of false positives compared to state-of-the-art. This performance improvement is attributed to our reliable candidate generation and effective false positive reduction methods.

2   Related Works

Automatic polyp detection in colonoscopy videos has been the subject of research for over a decade. Early methods, e.g., [1,3] for detecting colonic polyps utilized hand-crafted texture and color descriptors such as LBP and wavelet transform. However, given large color variation among polyps and limited texture availability on the surface of polyps (See Fig. 1), such methods could offer only a partial solution. To avoid such limitations, more recent techniques have considered temporal information [6] and shape features [2,7,9–11], reporting superior performance over the early polyp detection systems. Despite significant advancements, state-of-the-art polyp detection methods fail to achieve a clinically acceptable performance. For instance, to achieve the polyp sensitivity of 50 %, the system suggested by Wang et al. [11] generates 0.15 false positives per frame or approximately 4 false positive per second. Similarly, the system proposed in [10], which is evaluated on a significantly larger dataset, generates 0.10 false positives per frame. Clearly, such systems that rely on a subset of polyp characteristics are not clinically viable—a limitation that this paper aims to overcome.

3   Proposed Method

Our computer-aided polyp detection system is designed based on our algorithms [7,8,10], consisting of 2 stages where the first stage utilizes geometric features to reliably generate polyp candidates and the second stage employs a comprehensive set of deep features to effectively remove false positives. Figure 2 shows a schematic overview of the suggested method.

3.1   Stage 1: Candidate Generation

Our unique polyp candidate generation method exploits the following two properties: (1) polyps have distinct appearance across their boundaries, (2) polyps,

Stage 1: candidate generation **Stage 2: candidate classification**

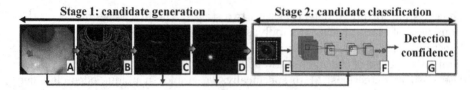

Fig. 2. Our system consists of 2 stages: candidate generation and classification. Given a colonoscopy frame (A), we first obtain a crude set of edge pixels (B). We then refine this edge map using a classification scheme where the goal is to remove as many non-polyp boundary pixels as possible (C). The geometric features of the retained edges are then captured through a voting scheme, generating a voting map whose maximum indicates the location of a polyp candidate (D). In the second stage, a bounding box is estimated for each generated candidate (E) and then a set of convolution neural networks—each specialized in one type of features—are applied in the vicinity of the candidate (F). Finally, the CNNs are aggregated to generate a confidence value (G) for the given polyp candidate.

irrespective of their morphology and varying levels of protrusion, feature at least one curvilinear head at their boundaries. We capture the first property with our image characterization and edge classification schemes, and capture the second property with our voting scheme.

Constructing Edge Maps. Given a colonoscopy image, we use Canny's method to extract edges from each input channel. The extracted edges are then put together in one edge map. Next, for each edge in the constructed edge map, we determine edge orientation. The estimated orientations are later used for extracting oriented patches around the edge pixels.

Image Characterization. Our patch descriptor begins with extracting an oriented patch around each edge pixel. The patch is extracted so that the containing boundary is placed vertically in the middle of the patch. This representation allows us to capture desired information across the edges independent of their orientations. Our method then proceeds with forming 8×16 sub-patches all over the extracted patch. Each sub-patch has 50% overlap with the neighboring sub-patches. For a compact representation, we compress each sub-patch into a 1D signal S by averaging intensity values along each column. We then apply a 1D discrete cosine transform (DCT) to the resulting signal:

$$C_k = \frac{2}{n}w(k)\sum_{i=0}^{n-1} S[i]\cos(\frac{2i+1}{2n}\pi k) \tag{1}$$

where

$$w(k) = 1/\sqrt{2}, k = 0 \text{ and } w(k) = 1, 1 \leq k \leq n - 1.$$

With the DCT, the essential information of the intensity signal can be summarized in a few coefficients. We discard the DC component C_0 because the average patch intensity is not a robust feature—it is affected by a constant change in patch intensities. However, the next 3 DCT coefficients $C_1 - C_3$ are more reliable and provide interesting insight about the intensity signal. C_1 measures whether the average patch intensity along the horizontal axis is monotonically decreasing (increasing) or not, C_2 measures the similarity of the intensity signal against a valley (ridge), and finally C_3 checks for the existence of both a valley and a ridge in the signal. The higher order coefficients $C_4 - C_{15}$ may not be reliable for feature extraction because of their susceptibility to noise and other degradation factors in the images.

The selected DCT coefficients $C_1 - C_3$ are still undesirably proportional to linear illumination scaling. We therefore apply a normalization treatment. Mathematically,

$$C_i = \frac{C_i}{\sqrt{C_1^2 + C_2^2 + C_3^2}}, i = 1, 2, 3.$$

Note that we use the norm of the selected coefficients for normalization rather than the norm of entire DCT coefficients. By doing so, we can avoid the expensive computation of all the DCT components. The final descriptor for a given patch is obtained by concatenating the normalized coefficients selected from each sub-patch.

The suggested patch descriptor has 4 advantages. First, our descriptor is fast because compressing each sub-patch into a 1D signal eliminates the need for expensive 2D DCT and that only a few DCT coefficients are computed from each intensity signal. Second, due to the normalization treatment applied to the DCT coefficients, our descriptor achieves invariance to linear illumination changes, which is essential to deal with varying lighting conditions (see Fig. 1). Third, our descriptor is rotation invariant because the patches are extracted along the dominant orientation of the containing boundary. Fourth, our descriptor handles small positional changes by selecting and averaging overlapping sub-patches in both horizontal and vertical directions.

Edge Classification. Our classification scheme has 2 layers. In the first layer, we learn a discriminative model to distinguish between the boundaries of the structures of interest and the boundaries of other structures in colonoscopy images. The structures of interest consists of polyps, vessels, lumen areas, and specular reflections. Specifically, we collect a stratified set of $N_1 = 100,000$ oriented patches around the boundaries of structures of interest and r andom structures in the training images, $S^1 = \{(p_i, y_i) | y_i \in \{p, v, l, s, r\}, i = 1, 2, ..., N_1\}$. Once patches are extracted, we train a five-class random forest classifier with 100 fully grown trees. The resulting probabilistic outputs can be viewed as the similarities between the input patches and the predefined structures of interest. Basically, the first layer receives low-level image features from our patch descriptor and then produces mid-level semantic features.

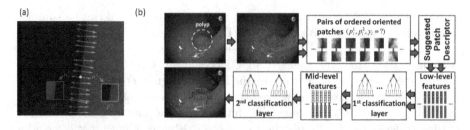

Fig. 3. (a) A pair of image patches $\{p_i^1, p_i^2\}$ extracted from an edge pixel. The green and red arrows show the two possible normal directions $\{n_i^1, n_i^2\}$ for a number of selected edges on the displayed boundary. The normal directions are used for patch alignment. (b) The suggested edge classification scheme given a test image. The edges that have passed the classification stage are shown in green. The inferred normal directions are visualized with the blue arrows for a subset of the retained edges (Color figure online).

In the second layer, we train a 3-class random forest classifier with 100 fully grown trees. Specifically, we collect $N_2 = 100,000$ pairs of oriented patches, of which half are randomly selected from the polyp boundaries and the rest are selected from random non-polyp edge segments. For an edge pixel at angle θ, one can obtain two oriented image patches $\{p_i^1, p_i^2\}$ by interpolating the image along the two possible normal directions $\{n_i^1, n_i^2\}$. As shown in Fig. 3(a), for an edge pixel on the boundary of a polyp, only one of the normal directions points to the polyp region. Our classification scheme operates on each pair of patches with two objectives: (1) to classify the underlying edge into polyp and non-polyp categories, and (2) to determine the desired normal direction among n_i^1 and n_i^2 such that it points towards the polyp location. Henceforth, we refer to the desired normal direction as "voting direction".

Once image pairs are collected, we order the patches $\{p_i^1, p_i^2\}$ within each pair according to the angles of their corresponding normal vectors, $\angle n_i^1 < \angle n_i^2$. In this way, the patches are represented in a consistent order. Each pair of ordered patches is then assigned a label $y_i \in \{0, 1, 2\}$, where "0" indicates that the underlying edge does not lie on a polyp boundary, "1" indicates that the edge lies on a polyp boundary and that n_i^1 is the voting direction, and "2" indicates that the edge lies on a polyp boundary but n_i^2 shows the voting direction. Mathematically, $S^2 = \{(p_i^1, p_i^2, y_i) | y_i \in \{0, 1, 2\}, i = 1, 2, ..., N_2\}$. To generate semantic features, each pair of ordered patches undergoes the image characterization followed by the first classification layer. The resulting mid-level features are then concatenated to form a feature vector f_i. This process is repeated for N_2 pairs of ordered patches, resulting in a labeled feature set, $\{(f_i, y_i) | y_i \in \{0, 1, 2\}, i = 1, 2, ..., N_2\}$, which is needed to train the second classifier. We train a 3-class classifier to learn both edge labels and the voting directions (embedded in y_i). Figure 3(b) illustrates how the suggested edge classification scheme operates given a test image.

Candidate Localization. Our voting scheme is designed to generate polyp candidates in regions surrounded by curvy boundaries. The rationale is such boundaries can represent the heads of polyps. In our voting scheme, each edge that has passed the classification stage, casts a vote along its voting direction (inferred by the edge classifier). The vote cast by the voter v at a receiver pixel $r = [x, y]$ is computed as

$$M_v(x, y) = \begin{cases} C_v \exp(\frac{-\|\vec{vr}\|^2}{\sigma_F}) \cos(\angle \vec{n^*vr}), & \text{if } \angle \vec{n^*vr} < \pi/2 \\ 0, & \text{if } \angle \vec{n^*vr} \geq \pi/2 \end{cases} \qquad (2)$$

where the exponential and cosinusoidal functions enable smooth vote propagation, which we will later use to estimate a bounding box around each generated candidate. In Eq. 2, C_{v_i} is the classification confidence, $\vec{vr}$ is the vector connecting the voter and receiver, σ_F controls the size of the voting field, and $\angle \vec{n^*vr}$ is the angle between the voting direction n^* and $\vec{vr}$. Figure 4(a) shows the voting field for an edge pixel lying at 135 degree. As seen, due to the condition set on $\angle \vec{n^*vr}$, the votes are cast only in the region pointed by the voting direction.

It is essential for our voting scheme to prevent vote accumulation in the regions that are surrounded by low curvature boundaries. For this purpose, our voting scheme first groups the voters into 4 categories according to their voting directions, $V^k = \{v_i | \frac{k\pi}{4} < mod(\angle n_i^*, \pi) < \frac{(k+1)\pi}{4}\}$, $k = 0...3$. Our voting scheme then proceeds by accumulating votes of each category in a separate voting map. To produce the final voting map, we multiply the accumulated votes generated in each category. A polyp candidate is then generated where the final voting map has the maximum vote accumulation (MVA). Mathematically,

$$MVA = \arg\max_{x,y} \prod_{k=0}^{3} \sum_{v \in V^k} M_v(x, y). \qquad (3)$$

Comparing Fig. 4(b) and (c) clarifies how the suggested edge grouping mitigates vote accumulation between parallel lines, assigning higher temperature to only regions surrounded by curvy boundaries. Another important characteristic of our voting scheme is the utilization of voting directions. As shown in Fig. 4(d), casting votes along both possible normal directions can result in mislocalized candidates; however, incorporating voting directions allows for more accurate candidate localization (Fig. 4(e)).

3.2   Stage 2: Candidate Classification

Our candidate classification method begins with estimating a bounding box around each polyp candidate followed by a novel score fusion framework based on convolutional neural networks (CNNs) [4] to assign a confidence value to each generated candidate.

Bounding Box Estimation. To measure the extent of the polyp region, we estimate a narrow band around each candidate, so that it contains the voters that have contributed to vote accumulation at the candidate location. In other

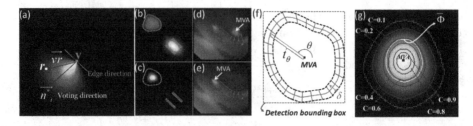

Fig. 4. (a) The generated voting map for an edge pixel lying at 135 degree. (b) Without edge grouping, all the votes are accumulated in one voting map, which results in undesirable vote accumulation between the parallel lines. (c) With the suggested edge grouping, higher temperature is assigned to only within the curvy boundaries. (d) Casting votes along both possible normal directions can result in a candidate placed outside the polyp region. (e) Casting votes only along the inferred voting directions results in a successful candidate localization. (f) A narrow band is used for estimating a bounding box around candidates. (g) A synthetic shape and its corresponding voting map. The isocontours and the corresponding representative isocontour are shown in blue and white, respectively (Color figure online).

words, the desired narrow band will enclose the polyp boundary and thus can be used to estimate a bounding box around the candidate location. As shown in Fig. 4(f), the narrow band B consists of a set of radial lines ℓ_θ parameterized as $\ell_\theta : MVA + t[\cos(\theta), \sin(\theta)]^T, t \in [t_\theta - \frac{\delta}{2}, t_\theta + \frac{\delta}{2}]$, where δ is the bandwidth, and t_θ is the distance between the candidate location and the corresponding point on the band skeleton at angle θ. Once the band is formed, the bounding box is localized so that it fully contains the narrow band around the candidate location (see Fig. 4(f)). The bounding box will be later used for data augmentation where we extract patches in multiple scales around the polyp candidates.

To estimate the unknown δ and t_θ for a given candidate, we use the isocontours of the corresponding voting map. The isocontour Φ_c of the voting map V is defined as $\Phi_c = \{(x, y) | V(x, y) = c \times M\}$ where M denotes the maximum of the voting map and c is a constant between 0 and 1. As shown in Fig. 4(g), the isocontours of the voting map, particularly those located farther away from the candidate, have the desirable feature of following the shape of the actual boundary from which the votes have been cast at the candidate location. Therefore, one can estimate the narrow band's parameters from the isocontours such that the band encloses the object's boundary. However, in practice, the shape of far isocontours are undesirably influenced by other nearby voters in the scene. We therefore obtain the representative isocontour $\bar{\Phi}$ by computing the median shape of the isocontours of the voting map (see Fig. 4(g)). We have experimented with different sets of isocontours and found out that as long as their parameter c is uniformly selected between 0 and 1, the resulting representative isocontour serves the desired purpose.

Let d_{iso}^i denotes the distance between the ith point on the representative iso-countour $\bar{\Phi}$ and the candidate location. We use d_{iso}^i to predict d_{obj}^i, the distance between the corresponding point on the object boundary and the candidate location. For this purpose, we employ a second order polynomial regression model

$$d_{obj}^i = b_0 + b_1(d_{iso}^i) + b_2(d_{iso}^i)^2,$$

(4)

where b_0, b_1, and b_2 are the regression coefficients that are estimated using a least square approach. Once the model is constructed, we take the output of the model d_{obj} at angle θ with respect to MVA as t_θ and the corresponding prediction interval as the bandwidth δ.

Probability Assignment. We propose a score fusion framework based on convolutional neural networks (CNNs) that can learn and integrate color, texture, shape, and temporal information of polyps in multiple scales for more accurate candidate classification. We choose to use CNNs because of their superior performance in major object detection challenges. The attractive feature of CNNs is that they jointly learn a multi-scale set of image features and a discriminative classifier during a supervised training process. While CNNs are known to learn discriminate patterns from raw pixel values, it turns out that preprocessing and careful selection of the input patches can have a significant impact on the performance of the subsequent CNNs. Specifically, we have found out that partial illumination invariance achieved by histogram equalizing the input patches significantly improves the performance of the subsequent CNNs and that curse of dimensionality caused by patches with more than 3 channels results in CNNs with inferior performance.

Considering these observations, we propose a 3-way image presentation that is motivated by the three major types of polyp features suggested in the literature: (1) for color and texture features, we collect histogram-equalized color patches P_C around each polyp candidate; (2) for temporal features, we form 3-channel patches P_T by stacking histogram-equalized gray channel of the current frame and that of the previous 2 frames; (3) for shape in context, we form 3-channel patches P_S by stacking the gray channel of the current frame and the corresponding refined edge channel and voting channel produced in the candidate generation stage (see Fig. 2).

We collect the three sets of patches P_C, P_T, and P_S from candidate locations in the training videos, label each individual patch depending on whether the underlying candidate is a true or false positive, and then train a CNN for each set of the patches. Figure 5(a) shows the test stage of the suggested score fusion framework. Given a new polyp candidate, we collect the three sets of patches in multiple scales and orientations around the candidate location, apply each of the trained CNNs on the corresponding patches, and take the maximum response for each CNN, resulting in three probabilistic scores. The final classification confidence is computed by averaging the resulting three scores.

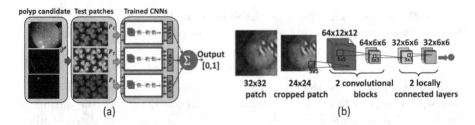

Fig. 5. (a) The test stage of the suggested score fusion framework. (b) Network layout used for training the deep convolution networks.

4   Experiments

For evaluation, we have used 40 short colonoscopy videos. We have randomly halved the database at video level into the training set containing 3800 frames with polyps and 15100 frames without polyps, and the test set containing 5700 frames with polyps and 13200 frames without polyps. Each colonoscopy frame in our database comes with a binary ground truth image. For performance evaluation, we consider a detection as a true (false) positive if it falls inside (outside) the white region of the ground truth image.

Our candidate generation stage yielded a sensitivity of 73.6 % and 0.8 false positives/frame. For candidate classification, we used Krizhevsky's GPU implementation [4] of CNNs. With data augmentation, we collected 400,000 32×32 patches for P_C, P_T, and P_S where half of the patches were extracted around false positive candidates and the rest around true positive candidates. Specifically, for a candidate with an $N \times N$ bounding box, we extracted patches at three scales $sN \times sN$ with $s \in \{1, 1.2, 1.4\}$ and then resized them to 32×32 patches. Furthermore, we performed data augmentation [4] by extracting patches at multiple orientations and translation in each given scale. We have used the layout shown in Fig. 5(b) for all the CNNs used in this paper.

Figure 6(a) shows FROC analysis of the suggested system. As seen, our system based on the suggested score fusion approach shows a relatively stable performance over a wide range of voting fields. For comparison, we have also reported the performance of our system based on individual CNNs trained using color patches (P_C), temporal patches (P_T), and shape in context patches (P_S). We have also experimented with the channel fusion approach where color, shape, and temporal patches are stacked for each polyp candidate followed by training one CNN for the resulting 9-channel training patches. To avoid clutter in the figure, only their best performance curves obtained by $\sigma_F = 70$ are shown. As seen in Fig. 6(a), the proposed score fusion framework yields the highest performance, achieving 50 % sensitivity at 0.002 FPs/frame, outperforming [10] with 0.10 FPs/frame at the same sensitivity.

FROC analysis is widely used for evaluating computer-aided detection systems designed for static datasets such as CT scans and mammograms. However, for temporal or sequence-based datasets such as colonoscopy videos, it has the

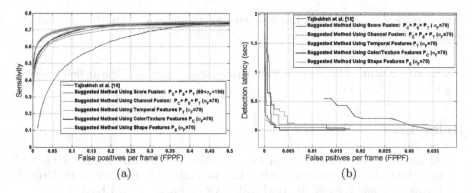

Fig. 6. (a) Analysis of FROC. (b) Analysis of polyp detection latency.

drawback of excluding the factor of time. While it is desirable for a polyp detection system to detect as many polyp instances as possible, it is also important to measure how quickly a polyp is detected after it appears in the video. We therefore employ a new performance curve [8] that measures the polyp detection latency with respect to the number of false positives. Briefly, if t_1 denotes the arrival frame of the polyp, t_2 denotes the frame in which the polyp is detected, and fps is the frame rate of the video, the detection latency is then computed as $\Delta T = (t_2 - t_1)/fps$. As with FROC, we change a threshold on the detection confidences and then at each operating point measure the median polyp detection latency of the test positive shots and the number of false positives in the entire test set. As seen in Fig. 6(b), different variations of our system yield significantly less number of false positives than our previous work [10] at nearly all operating points.

On a desktop computer with a 2.4 GHz quad core Intel and an Nvidia GeForce GTX 760 video card, our system processes each image at 2.65 s, which is significantly faster than [11] with run-time of 7.1 s and [2] with run-time of 19 s. We should note that a very large fraction of the computation time (2.6 s) is caused by the candidate generation stage and that the candidate classification based on CNNs is extremely fast because CNNs are only applied to the candidate location in each frame. We expect a significant speedup of our system using parallel computing optimization.

5   Conclusion

We proposed a new computer-aided polyp detection system for colonoscopy videos. Our system was based on context-aware shape features to generate a set of candidates and convoluational neural networks to reduce the generated false positives. We evaluated our system using the widely-used FROC analysis, achieving 50 % sensitivity at 0.002 FPs/frame, outperforming state-of-the-art systems [10,11], which generate 0.15 FPs/frame and 0.10 FPs/frame at 50 % sensitivity, respectively. We also evaluated our system using a latency analysis, demonstrating a significantly lower polyp detection latency than [10] particularly in low false positive rates.

Acknowledgment. This research has been supported by an ASU-Mayo Clinic research grant.

References

1. Alexandre, L.A., Nobre, N., Casteleiro, J.: Color and position versus texture features for endoscopic polyp detection. In: International Conference on BioMedical Engineering and Informatics, BMEI 2008, vol. 2, pp. 38–42. IEEE (2008)
2. Bernal, J., Snchez, J., Vilario, F.: Towards automatic polyp detection with a polyp appearance model. Pattern Recogn. **45**(9), 3166–3182 (2012)
3. Karkanis, S.A., Iakovidis, D.K., Maroulis, D.E., Karras, D.A., Tzivras, M.: Computer-aided tumor detection in endoscopic video using color wavelet features. IEEE Trans. Inform. Technol. Biomed. **7**(3), 141–152 (2003)
4. Krizhevsky, A., Sutskever, I., Hinton, G.E.: Imagenet classification with deep convolutional neural networks. In: Advances in Neural Information Processing Systems, pp. 1097–1105 (2012), https://code.google.com/p/cuda-convnet/
5. Leufkens, A., van Oijen, M., Vleggaar, F., Siersema, P.: Factors influencing the miss rate of polyps in a back-to-back colonoscopy study. Endoscopy **44**(05), 470–475 (2012)
6. Park, S.Y., Sargent, D., Spofford, I., Vosburgh, K.: A-Rahim, Y.: A colon video analysis framework for polyp detection. IEEE Trans. Biomed. Eng. **59**(5), 1408–1418 (2012)
7. Tajbakhsh, N., Chi, C., Gurudu, S.R., Liang, J.: Automatic polyp detection from learned boundaries. In: 2014 IEEE 11th International Symposium on Biomedical Imaging (ISBI), pp. 97–100. IEEE (2014)
8. Tajbakhsh, N., Gurudu, S.R., Liang, J.: Automatic polyp detection in colonoscopy videos using an ensemble of convolutional neural networks. In: Biomedical Imaging (ISBI), 2015 IEEE 12th International Symposium on. pp. 79–83. IEEE (2015)
9. Tajbakhsh, N., Gurudu, S.R., Liang, J.: A classification-enhanced vote accumulation scheme for detecting colonic polyps. In: Yoshida, H., Warfield, S., Vannier, M.W. (eds.) Abdominal Imaging 2013. LNCS, vol. 8198, pp. 53–62. Springer, Heidelberg (2013)
10. Tajbakhsh, N., Gurudu, S.R., Liang, J.: Automatic polyp detection using global geometric constraints and local intensity variation patterns. In: Golland, P., Hata, N., Barillot, C., Hornegger, J., Howe, R. (eds.) MICCAI 2014, Part II. LNCS, vol. 8674, pp. 179–187. Springer, Heidelberg (2014). http://dx.doi.org/10.1007/978-3-319-10470-6_23
11. Wang, Y., Tavanapong, W., Wong, J., Oh, J., de Groen, P.: Part-based multi-derivative edge cross-section profiles for polyp detection in colonoscopy. IEEE J. Biomed. Health Inform. **PP**(99), 1–1 (2013)

A Feature-Based Approach to Big Data Analysis of Medical Images

Matthew Toews[1](✉), Christian Wachinger[2], Raul San Jose Estepar[1],
and William M. Wells III[1]

[1] Brigham and Women's Hospital, Harvard Medical School, Boston, USA
{mt,rjosest,sw}@bwh.harvard.edu
[2] Computer Science and Artificial Intelligence Laboratory,
Massachussetts Institute of Technology, Cambridge, USA
wachinger@csail.mit.edu

Abstract. This paper proposes an inference method well-suited to large sets of medical images. The method is based upon a framework where distinctive 3D scale-invariant features are indexed efficiently to identify approximate nearest-neighbor (NN) feature matches in $O(log\ N)$ computational complexity in the number of images N. It thus scales well to large data sets, in contrast to methods based on pair-wise image registration or feature matching requiring $O(N)$ complexity. Our theoretical contribution is a density estimator based on a generative model that generalizes kernel density estimation and K-nearest neighbor (KNN) methods. The estimator can be used for on-the-fly queries, without requiring explicit parametric models or an off-line training phase. The method is validated on a large multi-site data set of 95,000,000 features extracted from 19,000 lung CT scans. Subject-level classification identifies all images of the same subjects across the entire data set despite deformation due to breathing state, including unintentional duplicate scans. State-of-the-art performance is achieved in predicting chronic pulmonary obstructive disorder (COPD) severity across the 5-category GOLD clinical rating, with an accuracy of 89 % if exact and one-off predictions are considered correct.

1 Introduction

Systems for storing and transmitting digital data are increasing rapidly in size and bandwidth capacity. Data collection projects such as COPDGene (19,000 lung CT scans of 10,000 subjects) [1] offer unprecedented opportunities to learn from large medical image sets, for example to discover subtle aspects of anatomy or pathology only observable in subsets of the population. For this, image processing algorithms must scale with the quantities of available data.

Consider an algorithm designed to discover and characterize unknown clinical phenotypes or disease subclasses from a large set of N images. Two major challenges that must be addressed are computational complexity and robust statistical inference. The fundamental operation required is often image-to-image

© Springer International Publishing Switzerland 2015
S. Ourselin et al. (Eds.): IPMI 2015, LNCS 9123, pp. 339–350, 2015.
DOI: 10.1007/978-3-319-19992-4_26

similarity evaluation, which incurs a prohibitive computational complexity cost of $O(N)$ when performed via traditional pair-wise methods such as registration [2,3] or feature matching [4,5]. For example, computing the pairwise affinity matrix between 416 low resolution brain scans via efficient deformable registration requires about one week on a 50 GHz cluster computer [2]. Furthermore, robustly estimating variables of interest requires coping with myriad confounds, including arbitrarily misaligned data, missing data due to resection or variable scan cropping (e.g. in order to reduce ionizing radiation exposure), inter-subject anatomical variability including abnormality, intra-subject variability due to growth and deformation (e.g. lung breathing state), inter-scanner variability in multi-site data, to name a few.

The technical contribution of this paper is a computational framework that provides a solution to both of these challenges. The framework is closely linked to large-scale data search methods where data are stored and indexed via nearest neighbor (NN) queries [6,10]. Images are represented as collections of distinctive 3D scale-invariant features [7,8], information-rich observations of salient image content. Robust, local image-to-image similarity is computed efficiently in $O(log\ N)$ computational complexity via approximate nearest neighbor search.

The theoretical contribution is a novel estimator for class-conditional densities in a Naive Bayes classification formulation, representing a hybrid of kernel density [11] and KNN [12] methods. A mixture density is estimated for each input feature of a new image as the weighted sum of (1) a variable bandwidth kernel density computed from a set of nearest neighbors and (2) a background distribution over unrelated features. This estimator achieves state-of-the-art performance in automatically predicting the 5-class GOLD severity label from a large multi-site data set, improving upon previous results based on lung-specific image processing pipelines and single-site data [13,28,29]. Furthermore, subject-level classification is used to identify all instances duplicate subjects in a large set of 19,000 subjects, despite deformation due to breathing state.

2   Related Work

Our work derives from two main bodies of research, local invariant image feature methods and density estimation. Here, a local feature refers to a salient image patch or region identified via an interest operator, e.g. extrema of the difference-of-Gaussian operator in the popular scale-invariant feature transform (SIFT) [7]. Local features effectively serve as a reduced set of information-rich image content that enable highly efficient image processing algorithms, for example feature correspondence in $O(log\ N)$ computational complexity via fast approximate NN search methods [9,10]. Early feature detection methods identified salient image locations [14], scale-space theory [15] lead to the development of so-called scale-invariant [7] and affine-invariant [16] feature detection methods capable of repeatedly detecting the same image pattern despite global similarity and affine image transforms, in addition to intensity variations.

Once detected, salient image regions are cropped and spatially normalized to patches of size D voxels, then encoded as compact, highly distinctive descriptors for efficient indexing, e.g. the gradient orientation histogram (GoH) representation [7]. Note that there is a tradeoff between the patch dimension D and the number of unique samples available to populate the space of image patches $\mathbb{R}^D$. At one extreme, voxel-size patches lead to a densely sampled but relatively uninformative R^1 space, while at the other extreme, entire images provide an information-rich but severely under-sampled R^N space. Intermediately-sized observations have been shown to be most effective for tasks such as classification [17]. Note also that many patches are rarely observed in natural medical images, and the typical set of patches is concentrated within a subspace or manifold $\mathcal{M} \in \mathbb{R}^D$. Furthermore, local saliency operators further restrict the manifold to a subset of highly informative patches $\mathcal{M} \bullet \in \mathcal{M}$, as common, uninformative image patterns are not detected, e.g. non-localizable boundary structures or regions of homogenous image intensity.

Salient image content can thus be modeled as a set of local features, e.g. within a spatial configuration or as an unordered bag-of-features representation when inter-feature spatial relationships are difficult to model. Probabilistic models for inference typically require estimating densities from feature data. Nonparametric density estimators such as KDE or KNN estimators are particularly useful as an explicit model of the joint distribution is not required. They can be computed on-the-fly without requiring computationally expensive training, e.g. via instance-based or lazy-learning methods [13,18,19]. KDE seeks to quantify density from kernel functions centered around training samples [11,20], whereas KNN estimators seek to quantify the density at a point from a set of K nearest neighbor samples [12,13,18,19]. An interesting property of KNN estimators is that when used in classification, their prediction error is asymptotically upper bounded by no more than twice the optimal Bayes error rate as the number of data grow [12]. This property is particularly relevant given the increasing size of medical image data sets.

In the context of medical image analysis, scale-invariant features have been used to align and classify 3D medical image data [8,21,22], however they have not yet been adapted to large-scale indexing and inference. Although our work here focuses on inference, the feature-based correspondence framework is generally related to medical image analysis methods using nearest neighbors or proximity graphs across image data, including subject-level recognition [5], manifold learning [2,3,23], in particular methods based on local image characteristics [24,25] and multi-atlas labeling [26].

The experimental portion of this paper investigates chronic pulmonary obstructive disorder (COPD) in a large set of multi-site lung CT images. A primary focus of COPD imaging research has been to characterize and classify disease phenotypes. Song et al. investigate various 2D feature descriptors for classifying lung tissues including local binary patterns and gradient orientation histograms [27]. Several authors propose subject-level COPD prediction as an avenue of exploratory research. Sorensen et al. [13] use texture patches in a binary classification COPD = (0,1) scenario on single-site data to achieve an area-under-the-curve (AUC) classification of 0.71. Mets et al. [28] use densitometric measures computed from single-site data of 1100 male subjects, to achieve an AUC value of 0.83 for binary COPD classification. Gu et al. [29] use automatic lung segmentation and densitometric measures to classify single-site data according to the GOLD range, achieving an exact classification rate of 0.37, or 0.83 if classification into neighboring categories is considered correct. A major challenge is classifying multi-site data acquired across different sites and scanners. On a large multi-site data set, our method achieves exact and one-off classification rates of 0.48 and 0.89, respectively, which to our knowledge are the highest rates reported for GOLD classification.

3   Method

3.1   Estimating Class Probabilities

Let $f_i \in \mathbb{R}^D$ be a D-dimensional vector encoding the appearance of a scale-normalized image patch, e.g. a scale-invariant feature descriptor, and let $F = \{f_i\}$ be a set of such features extracted in an image. Let C be a clinical variable of interest, e.g. a discrete measure of disease severity, defined over a set of M values $[1, \ldots, m]$. Finally let C_i represent the value of C associated with feature f_i.

We seek the posterior probability $p(C|F)$ of clinical variable C conditioned on feature data F extracted in a query image, which can be expressed as

$$p(C|F) \propto p(C)p(F|C) = p(C) \prod_i p(f_i|C). \qquad (1)$$

In Eq. (1), the first equality follows from Bayes' rule, and the second from the so-called Naive Bayes assumption of conditional feature independence. This strong assumption is often made for computational convenience when modeling the true joint distribution over all features F is intractable. Nevertheless, it often leads to robust, effective modeling even in contexts where conditional independence does not strictly hold. Conditional independence is reasonable in the case of local image observations f_i, as patches separated in scale and space do not typically exhibit direct correlations. On the RHS of Eq. (1), $p(C)$ is a prior distribution over the clinical variable of interest C, and $p(f_i|C)$ is the likelihood function of C associated with observed image feature f_i.

We use a robust variant of kernel density estimation for calculating the class conditional likelihood densities:

$$p(f_i|C) \propto \left[\sum_{j:C_j=C} \frac{N}{N_C} \exp\left(-\frac{d^2(f_i, f_j)}{\alpha^2 + 1} \right) \right] + \beta \frac{N_C}{N}. \qquad (2)$$

Here N_C is the number of features of class C in the training data, and $N = \sum_C N_C$ is the total feature count. $d(f_i, f_j)$ is the distance between f_i and neighboring descriptor f_j, here the Euclidean distance between descriptors. α is an adaptive kernel bandwidth parameter that is empirically set to d_{NN_i} for each input feature f_i, i.e. the distance between f_i and the nearest neighboring descriptor f_j in a data base of training data:

$$d_{NN_i} = min_j \{ \, d(f_i, f_j) \, \}. \tag{3}$$

Finally, β is a weighting parameter empirically set to $\beta = 1$ in experiments for best performance. Note that the overall scale of the likelihood is unimportant, as normalization can be performed after the product in Eq. (1) is computed.

In practice, Eq. 2 is computed for each f_i from a set of $KNN_i = \{ \, (f_j, C_j) \, \}$ of K feature/label pairs (f_j, C_j) identified via an efficient approximate KNN search over a set of training feature data. Because the adaptive exponential kernel falls off quickly, it is not crucial to determine an optimal K as in some KNN methods [18], but rather to set K large enough include all features contributing to the kernel sum. Inuitively, the two terms in Eq. 2 are designed as a mixture model that is aimed at increasing the robustness of estimates when some of the features are "uninformative". The first term is a density estimator that accounts for informative features in the data. It is a variant that combines aspects of kernel density estimation and KNN density estimation, using a kernel where the bandwidth is scaled by the distance to the first nearest neighbor as in Breiman et al. [20]. The second term $\beta \frac{N_C}{N}$ provides a default estimate for the case of uninformative features, curiously this class-specific value results in noticeably superior classification performance than a value that is uniform across classes.

3.2 Computational Framework

To scale to large data sets of medical images, our inference method focuses on rapidly indexing a large set of image features. A variety of local feature detectors exist, we adopt a 3D generalization of the SIFT algorithm [8], where the location and scale of distinctive image patches are detected as extrema of a difference-of-Gaussian operator. Once detected, patches are reoriented, rescaled to a fixed size (11^3 voxels) and transformed into a GoH representation over 8 spatial bins and 8 orientation bins, resulting in a 64-element feature descriptor. Finally, rank-ordering [30] transforms descriptor elements into an ordinal representation, where elements take on their rank in an array sorted according to GoH value. Once extracted, descriptors can be stored in tree data structures for efficient NN indexing. Again, $d(f_i, f_j)$ can be defined according to a variety of measures such as geodesic distance, here we adopt the Euclidean distance between descriptor elements. Exact NN search is difficult for high dimensional descriptors, however approximate KNN methods can be used to identify NNs with high probability in $O(log \, N)$ search time, for example via randomized K-D search tree [9].

4   Experiments

Experiments focus on analyzing Chronic Obstructive Pulmonary Disorder (COPD), an important health problem and a leading cause of death. We test our method on lung CT images from the COPDGene data set [1] acquired for the purpose of characterizing COPD phenotypes and associated genetic links. The COPDGene dataset consists of 19,000 lung CT images of 10,300 subjects with clinical and demographic labels, where expiration and inspiration images are acquired for most subjects. Data are acquired at 21 clinical centers with CT scanners from a variety of different vendors, making the dataset a diverse multi-site test bed for practical big data algorithms. The clinical COPD measurement of interest is the GOLD score, which quantifies COPD severity on a scale of 0–4 based on spirometry measurements.

The only data preprocessing step in our pipeline is 3D scale-invariant feature extraction from images using the implementation described in [8]. Note that feature extraction is robust to variations in image geometry and intensity, and domain-specific pre-processing steps such as lung segmentation are unnecessary. Feature extraction is a one-time processing step, requiring on the order of 20 s for an image of size 256^3 voxels (0.6 mm isotropic resolution), after which features can be efficiently indexed. All feature extraction was performed on a commodity cluster computing system over the course of several hours. Each lung CT image results in approximately 5000 features, and the set of 19,000 images results in a total of 95,000,000 features. While the original image data occupies 3.8 TB when gzip-compressed, the feature data requires only 8.6 GB, representing a data reduction of 440X. Feature extraction can thus be viewed as a form of lossy compression, where the goal is to retain as much salient information as possible while significantly reducing the memory footprint. Given the relatively small size and usefulness of feature data, it may be useful to include it as part of a standard markup for efficiently indexing future image formats, e.g. DICOM extensions.

4.1   Computer-Assisted COPD Prediction

A primary goal of the COPDGene project is to identify disease phenotypes in order to better understand and characterize COPD. To this end, we investigate computer-assisted prediction of COPD, based on the five GOLD categories ranging from 0 to 4 in increasing order of severity. For clarity we experiment with a balanced set of data with 523 images per GOLD category, for a total of 2615 images and 13,000,000 features. We use only expiratory images in order to evaluate algorithm performance in isolation from confounds such as shape change during breathing. Maximum a-posterior (MAP) estimation is used to predict the most probable GOLD score C_{MAP} for each new feature set F in a leave-one-out manner:

$$C_{MAP} = \underset{C}{\mathrm{argmax}} \left\{ p(C|F) \right\}. \qquad (4)$$

Note that for experiments, the prior $p(C)$ from Eq. (1) is taken to be uniform. The leave-one-out methodology is implemented efficiently using the K-D search tree method of Muja and Lowe [9] to compute NN correspondences. In this method, features are indexed in a set of independent search trees, whose data splits are chosen randomly amongst the subset of feature descriptor elements exhibiting the highest variability. As a figure of merit we consider both the accuracy of exact prediction and one-off prediction, i.e. where C_{MAP} predicts a GOLD score one off from the true label. Prediction is also tested on various training set sizes, in order to investigate the effect on prediction accuracy. Graphs of prediction results are shown in Fig. 1, and Table 1 lists the confusion matrix for prediction on 2615 training subjects.

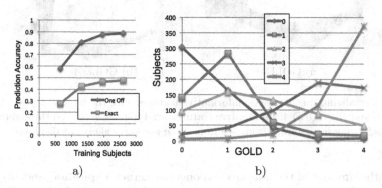

a)   b)

Fig. 1. (a) GOLD prediction accuracy (one-off and exact) as a function of the number of training subjects. (b) Curves for predicted vs. actual GOLD values for all 2615 training subjects. State-of-the art classification is achieved, with an accuracy of 48 % for exact prediction and 89 % for one-off prediction. Note the gradual transitions across predicted GOLD labels in (b), as expected in the case of a COPD severity continuum.

Table 1. Confusion matrix for COPD GOLD category prediction, 523 subjects per category using K = 100. Bold values indicate exact prediction.

GOLD	Predicted GOLD				
	0	1	2	3	4
0	**303**	164	43	5	8
1	141	**283**	60	21	18
2	95	160	**132**	87	49
3	21	43	98	**188**	173
4	5	9	21	114	**374**

In our method, feature-wise densities $p(f_i|C)$ quantify the informativeness of individual features f_i with respect to labels C_i, e.g. as in feature-based morphometry [21]. These densities may be useful in investigating and characterizing COPD phenotypes, this is a topic of ongoing investigation in our group. Figure 2 shows the 20 features with the highest $p(f_i|C)$ for images from either extreme of the GOLD severity rating.

Parameter K is typically important in KNN estimation methods, however our method does not vary significantly with changes in K above a certain value

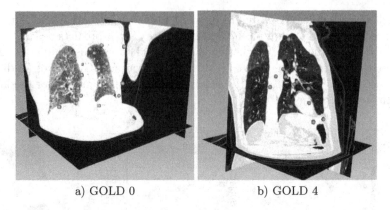

a) GOLD 0   b) GOLD 4

Fig. 2. Visualizing the 20 disease-informative features with the highest $p(f_i|C)$ for (a) GOLD 0 and (b) GOLD 4. Informative features are typically scattered throughout the lungs and range in size from from 2–5 mm. Note feature scale is not displayed.

due to the drop-off of the adaptive exponential kernel. Figure 3(a) and (b) illustrate inter-feature distances and their weighted kernel values for several typical features across K = 100 neighbors. The result of prediction tends to stabilize for $K \geq 100$. We attempted KNN density estimation for various values of K via standard counting as in [13], however classification performance was relatively poor and varied noticeably with values of K. We found the best means of improving performance was to adopt the kernel weighting scheme in Eq. (2).

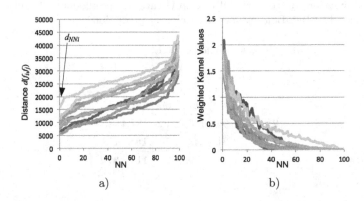

a)   b)

Fig. 3. (a) NN feature distance $d(f_i, f_j)$ for 10 typical features f_i and K = 100 neighbors f_j, sorted by increasing distance right-to-left. (b) Weighted kernel values of Eq. (2) for the same features and neighbors, note kernel values become negligible by K = 100.

Although the training sets used here for prediction here are balanced in terms of the number of subjects, individual images produce different numbers of features. Figure 4(a) shows the feature counts N_C for GOLD categories. Figure 4(b)

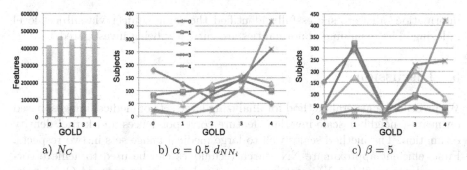

Fig. 4. Graph (a) illustrates feature counts N_C over GOLD categories. Graphs (b) and (c) illustrate skewed prediction from unoptimal kernel parameters in Eq. (2), (b) $\alpha = 0.5 \, d_{NN_i}$ and (c) from $\beta = 5$.

and (c) show how changes in either α or β result in prediction that is noticeably skewed towards or away from GOLD categories (e.g. here GOLD 1, 3 or 4) with higher feature counts.

4.2 Subject-Level Indexing

Large, multi-site image data sets can quickly become difficult to manage. Image labeling errors may be introduced in DICOM headers [31], and images of subjects may be inadvertently duplicated, removed or modified, compromising the data integrity and usefulness. We propose subject-level indexing to identify all instances of the same subject within a data set, in a manner similar to recent work in brain imaging [5], in order to inspect and verify data integrity. Subject ID is used as the clinical label of interest C, and inference seeks to identify highly probable labels $p(C|F)$ given feature data F from a test subject. Note that inference must be robust to large deformations due to inhale and exhale state, our method accomplishes this purely from local feature appearance information, parameters of feature geometry are not used (i.e. image location, scale, orientation).

Subject-level indexing effectively computes the image-to-image affinity matrix between all 19,000 image feature sets. The processing time is $\approx 6\,h$ on a laptop (MacBook Pro) using a single core, with a breakdown of $\approx 1\,h$ for data read-in and $\approx 5\,h$ for KNN feature correspondence ($\approx 1\,s$ per subject). This is effectively equivalent to $\approx 180,000,000$ pair-wise image registrations (assuming a symmetric registration technique). Note that here, correspondences are established across significant lung shape variation due to breathing state, as both expiration and inspiration are used. To our knowledge, all images are correctly grouped according to subject labels, using an empirically determined threshold on the posterior probability. A set of 65 images are flagged as abnormal, either duplicate images (unusually high posterior probability indicating identical feature sets) or different images of the same subject (high posterior probability). A partial list 20 unintentional duplicate subject scans was compiled from genetic information, all were successfully identified the same subject via subject-level indexing. The remaining abnormalities are currently being investigated.

5   Discussion

We presented a general method for analyzing large sets of medical images, based on nearest neighbor scale-invariant feature correspondences and kernel density estimation. The method scales well to large medical image sets in two respects. First, efficient approximate NN search techniques can be used to achieve correspondence in $O(log\ N)$ computational complexity, as to opposed $O(N)$ pairwise image or feature matching algorithms which quickly become intractable for large data sets. Second, probabilistic inference can be performed on-the-fly from feature data, without parametric models or potentially expensive training procedures. A hybrid KDE-KNN kernel density estimator with an adaptive bandwidth parameter is used to robustly estimate likelihood factors from nearest neighbor features.

Our method is demonstrated on 19,000 lung CT images of 10,300 subjects from the multi-site COPDGene data set. Subject-level indexing demonstrates that images of the same subject can be robustly identified across deformation due to breathing, and erroneous instances of subject duplication can be flagged. State-of-the-art results are obtained for multi-site multi-class prediction of clinical GOLD scores, improving on methods involving special purpose lung segmentation and densitometric measures. The prediction result is important, because it suggests the existence of disease-related anatomical patterns that could help to better understand COPD. It may be that the 3D SIFT representation is particularly well-tuned to anatomical structure of lung parenchyma related to COPD. Future work will focus on analysis of disease-informative features, identifying disease phenotypes. One avenue will be to incorporate feature geometry (e.g. location, scale) within modeling. Finally, our method is general and could be used to organize large sets of general medical image data, e.g. brain or full-body scans. Software described in this paper will be provided for to the public for research use.

We believe there is a good deal of potential for studying large sets of medical images via the local feature framework, e.g. 3D SIFT features or other suitable data-driven extractors. While they may be a coarse approximation to the original image, local features often contain enough salient information to robustly and efficiently perform tasks such registration or classification. This is particularly true where the quantity of data an algorithm is capable of exploiting begins to compensate for the coarseness of its representation, i.e. via efficient search methods. The general framework can be used to efficiently generate proximity graphs between large sets of medical image data, and may thus be useful in the context of other computational approaches such as manifold learning [2,32].

Acknowledgements. This research was supported by NIH grants P41EB015902, P41EB015898 5K25HL104085, 5R01HL116931 and 5R01HL116473.

References

1. Regan, E.A., Hokanson, J.E., Murphy, J.R., Make, B., Lynch, D.A., Beaty, T.H., Curran-Everett, D., Silverman, E.K., Crapo, J.D.: Genetic epidemiology of COPD (COPDGene) study design. COPD: J. Chronic Obstr. Pulm. Dis. **7**(1), 32–43 (2011)
2. Gerber, S., Tasdizen, T., Thomas Fletcher, P., Joshi, S., Whitaker, R.: Manifold modeling for brain population analysis. Med. Image Anal. **14**(5), 643–653 (2010)
3. Hamm, J., Ye, D.H., Verma, R., Davatzikos, C.: Gram: a framework for geodesic registration on anatomical manifolds. Med. Image Anal. **14**(5), 633–642 (2010)
4. Toews, M., Zöllei, L., Wells, W.M.: Feature-based alignment of volumetric multi-modal images. In: Gee, J.C., Joshi, S., Pohl, K.M., Wells, W.M., Zöllei, L. (eds.) IPMI 2013. LNCS, vol. 7917, pp. 25–36. Springer, Heidelberg (2013)
5. Wachinger, C., Golland, P., Reuter, M.: *BrainPrint*: identifying subjects by their brain. In: Golland, P., Hata, N., Barillot, C., Hornegger, J., Howe, R. (eds.) MICCAI 2014, Part III. LNCS, vol. 8675, pp. 41–48. Springer, Heidelberg (2014)
6. Brin, S.: Near neighbor search in large metric spaces. In: VLDB, pp. 574–584 (1995)
7. Lowe, D.G.: Distinctive image features from scale-invariant keypoints. IJCV **60**(2), 91–110 (2004)
8. Toews, M., Wells III, W.M.: Efficient and robust model-to-image alignment using 3D scale-invariant features. Med. Image Anal. **17**(3), 271–282 (2013)
9. Muja, M., Lowe, D.: Scalable nearest neighbour algorithms for high dimensional data. IEEE Trans. Pattern Anal. Mach. Intell. **36**(11), 2227–2240 (2014)
10. Kleinberg, J.M.: Two algorithms for nearest-neighbor search in high dimensions. In: ACM symposium on Theory of computing, pp. 599–608 (1997)
11. Terrell, G.R., Scott, D.W.: Variable kernel density estimation. Ann. Stat. **20**, 1236–1265 (1992)
12. Cover, T., Hart, P.: Nearest neighbor pattern classification. IEEE Trans. Inf. Theory **13**(1), 21–27 (1967)
13. Sorensen, L., Nielsen, M., Lo, P., Ashraf, H., Pedersen, J.H., De Bruijne, M.: Texture-based analysis of COPD: a data-driven approach. IEEE Trans. Med. Imaging **31**(1), 70–78 (2012)
14. Moravec, H.P.: Visual mapping by a robot rover. In: Proceedings of the 6th International Joint Conference on Artificial Intelligence, pp. 598–600 (1979)
15. Lindeberg, T.: Feature detection with automatic scale selection. IJCV **30**(2), 79–116 (1998)
16. Mikolajczyk, K., Schmid, C.: Scale and affine invariant interest point detectors. IJCV **60**(1), 63–86 (2004)
17. Ullman, S., Vidal-Naquet, M., Sali, E.: Visual features of intermediate complexity and their use in classification. Nat. Neurosci. **5**(7), 682–687 (2002)
18. Toussaint, G.T.: Proximity graphs for nearest neighbor decision rules: recent progress. In: Interface 34 (2002)
19. Yu, A., Grauman, K.: Predicting useful neighborhoods for lazy local learning. In: Advances in Neural Information Processing Systems, pp. 1916–1924 (2014)
20. Breiman, L., Meisel, W., Purcell, E.: Variable kernel estimates of multivariate densities. Technometrics **19**(2), 135–144 (1977)
21. Toews, M., Wells III, W.M., Collins, D.L., Arbel, T.: Feature-based morphometry: discovering group-related anatomical patterns. NeuroImage **49**(3), 2318–2327 (2010)

22. Gill, G., Toews, M., Beichel, R.R.: Robust initialization of active shape models for lung segmentation in CT scans: a feature-based atlas approach. Int. J. Biomed. Imaging **2014**, Article ID 479154, 7p (2014)

23. Singh, N., Thomas Fletcher, P., Samuel Preston, J., King, R.D., Marron, J., Weiner, M.W., Joshi, S.: Quantifying anatomical shape variations in neurological disorders. Med. Image Anal. **18**(3), 616–633 (2014)

24. Aljabar, P., Wolz, R., Srinivasan, L., Counsell, S.J., Rutherford, M.A., Edwards, A.D., Hajnal, J.V., Rueckert, D.: A combined manifold learning analysis of shape and appearance to characterize neonatal brain development. IEEE Trans. Med. Imaging **30**(12), 2072–2086 (2011)

25. Ye, D.H., Hamm, J., Kwon, D., Davatzikos, C., Pohl, K.M.: Regional manifold learning for deformable registration of brain MR images. In: Ayache, N., Delingette, H., Golland, P., Mori, K. (eds.) MICCAI 2012, Part III. LNCS, vol. 7512, pp. 131–138. Springer, Heidelberg (2012)

26. Aljabar, P., Heckemann, R.A., Hammers, A., Hajnal, J.V., Rueckert, D.: Multi-atlas based segmentation of brain images: atlas selection and its effect on accuracy. Neuroimage **46**(3), 726–738 (2009)

27. Song, Y., Cai, W., Zhou, Y., Feng, D.D.: Feature-based image patch approximation for lung tissue classification. IEEE TMI **32**(4), 797–808 (2013)

28. Mets, O.M., Buckens, C.F., Zanen, P., Isgum, I., van Ginneken, B., Prokop, M., Gietema, H.A., Lammers, J.W.J., Vliegenthart, R., Oudkerk, M., et al.: Identification of chronic obstructive pulmonary disease in lung cancer screening computed tomographic scans. JAMA **306**(16), 1775–1781 (2011)

29. Gu, S., Leader, J., Zheng, B., Chen, Q., Sciurba, F., Kminski, N., Gur, D., Pu, J.: Direct assessment of lung function in COPD using CT densitometric measures. Physiol. Meas. **35**(5), 833 (2014)

30. Toews, M., Wells III, W.M.: SIFT-RANK: ordinal description for invariant feature correspondence. In: 2009 IEEE Conference on Computer Vision and Pattern Recognition (CVPR), pp. 172–177. IEEE (2009)

31. Guld, M.O., Kohnen, M., Keysers, D., Schubert, H., Wein, B., Bredno, J., Lehmann, T.M.: Quality of DICOM header information for image categorization. In: International Symposium on Medical Imaging, vol. 4685, pp. 280–287. SPIE (2002)

32. Torki, M., Elgammal, A.: Putting local features on a manifold. In: 2010 IEEE Conference on Computer Vision and Pattern Recognition (CVPR), pp. 1743–1750. IEEE (2010)

Joint Segmentation and Registration Through the Duality of Congealing and Maximum Likelihood Estimate

Boris Flach[(⊠)] and Archibald Pontier

Czech Technical University in Prague, Prague, Czech Republic
`flachbor@cmp.felk.cvut.cz`

Abstract. In this paper we consider the task of joint registration and segmentation. A popular method which aligns images and simultaneously estimates a simple statistical shape model was proposed by E. Learned-Miller and is known as congealing. It considers the entropy of a simple, pixel-wise independent distribution as the objective function for searching the unknown transformations. Besides being intuitive and appealing, this idea raises several theoretical and practical questions, which we try to answer in this paper. First, we analyse the approach theoretically and show that the original congealing is in fact the DC-dual task (difference of convex functions) for a properly formulated Maximum Likelihood estimation task. This interpretation immediately leads to a different choice for the algorithm which is substantially simpler than the known congealing algorithm. The second contribution is to show, how to generalise the task for models in which the shape prior is formulated in terms of segmentation labellings and is related to the signal domain via a parametric appearance model. We call this generalisation *unsupervised congealing*. The new approach is applied to the task of aligning and segmenting imaginal discs of Drosophila melanogaster larvae.

Keywords: Congealing · MLE · DC-duality · Joint segmentation and registration

1 Introduction

The main goal of this paper is to consider models and methods for joint registration and segmentation. Many applications in medical and biological imaging require to solve these two tasks simultaneously because any attempt to solve them sequentially leads to suboptimal results [11]. Consider for example the task of analysing spatial gene expression patterns for hundreds (if not thousands) genes in imaginal discs of *Drosophila melanogaster* larvae (see Fig. 1). For this purpose, it is obviously necessary to co-register (align) all images into a common reference frame. A group-wise alignment based solely on their intensities (colours) is, however, impossible, simply because the spatial distribution of intensities in the discs varies strongly for different genes. On the other hand,

© Springer International Publishing Switzerland 2015
S. Ourselin et al. (Eds.): IPMI 2015, LNCS 9123, pp. 351–362, 2015.
DOI: 10.1007/978-3-319-19992-4_27

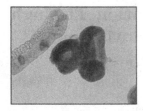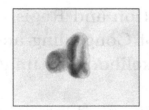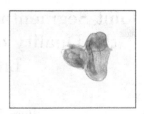

Fig. 1. Microscope images of Drosophila melanogaster imaginal discs with gene expression patterns (Color figure online).

it is also not possible to segment the images first by using intensity statistics for foreground and background only, simply because these statistics may vary substantially from image to image and because the images quite often contain parts of other objects as well.

A popular method which aligns images and simultaneously estimates a simple statistical shape model was proposed by E. Learned-Miller in [9] and is known as *congealing*. It considers the entropy of a simple, pixel-wise independent distribution as the objective function for searching the unknown transformations. This idea is indeed intuitive and appealing. Quite a few works were following it and have proposed different variants and generalisations of this approach [1,5,7,10].

Besides from being intuitive and appealing, this idea raises several theoretical and practical questions. Firstly, entropy minimisation is not a commonly accepted estimator in mathematical statistics. Secondly, from the algorithmic point of view, one has to minimise a non convex function depending on many variables. Almost all methods that apply congealing solve the optimisation task by block-wise local coordinate descent without a guarantee to converge to a local minimum. And finally, from the conceptual view, we may wish to decouple the shape model from the signal domain and to formulate it in terms of segmentation labellings. This will require unsupervised estimation (learning).

In this paper we try to answer at least some of the raised questions. First, we show that the original congealing is in fact the DC-dual task (difference of convex functions) for a properly formulated Maximum Likelihood estimation task. This interpretation immediately leads to a different choice for the algorithm which is substantially simpler and faster than the known congealing algorithm.

The second contribution is to show how to generalise the task for models in which the shape is formulated in terms of segmentation labellings and is related to the signal domain via a parametric appearance model. We show how to estimate the parameters of the shape model together with the parameters of the appearance model and the collection of transformations given a set of object images. We call this generalisation *unsupervised congealing*.

In the experimental section we first apply the new, unsupervised congealing to artificially generated images. This allows to compare the results with the known ground truth. In the second, and main part of this section we apply the newly proposed method to the task of aligning and segmenting imaginal discs and compare it with a previously published approach [6].

2 Theory

In the first part of this section we will show that supervised congealing, as introduced in [9], is indeed the DC-dual of a Maximum Likelihood estimation task. To avoid overloading with technicalities like boundary effects, infinite dimensional function spaces etc., we consider a simple probabilistic model for binary images defined on a two dimensional discrete torus $\mathbb{T}_n^2$.

2.1 Notations and Model

Let $\mathcal{S}(\mathbb{T}_n^2)$ denote the set of all binary images $\mathbf{s}\colon \mathbb{T}_n^2 \to \{0,1\}$ defined on the two dimensional discrete torus $\mathbb{T}_n^2$. We will denote the value of the image $\mathbf{s}$ in a particular node $i \in \mathbb{T}_n^2$ of the torus by s_i.

Let us consider the following family of pixelwise independent probability distributions on $\mathcal{S}(\mathbb{T}_n^2)$

$$p_{\mathbf{u},T}(\mathbf{s}) = \frac{1}{Z}\exp\langle \mathbf{u}, T\mathbf{s}\rangle , \qquad (1)$$

where $\mathbf{u}$ is a real valued field of parameters defined on $\mathbb{T}_n^2$ and $T \in \mathcal{T}$ denotes an orthogonal linear transformation $T\colon \mathcal{S}(\mathbb{T}_n^2) \to \mathcal{S}(\mathbb{T}_n^2)$, for example rigid body transformations. Notice that the normalising factor Z is independent of T as a consequence. For the sake of simplicity we assume here that $\mathcal{T}$ is the set of all discrete translations of the torus.

Suppose now, that we are given a set of binary images $\mathbf{s}^\ell$, $\ell \in L$, each of them independently generated by one of the distributions $p_{\mathbf{u},T^\ell}$. All of them share the parameter vector $\mathbf{u}$, but each of them has a different $T^\ell \in \mathcal{T}$. Both, the vector $\mathbf{u}$ and the collection of transformations $\mathbf{T} = (T^1,\ldots,T^L)$ are unknown and should be estimated from the given sample of (binary) images.

2.2 DC-duality of MLE and Congealing

Applying the Maximum Likelihood Estimator (MLE) for this task, means to solve the following optimisation problem

$$\frac{1}{L}\sum_\ell \langle \mathbf{u}, T^\ell \mathbf{s}^\ell\rangle - \log Z(\mathbf{u}) \to \max_{\mathbf{u},\mathbf{T}}. \qquad (2)$$

The normalisations factor (considered as a function of $\mathbf{u}$) is easy to compute

$$\log Z(\mathbf{u}) = \sum_{i\in\mathbb{T}_n^2} \log(1+e^{u_i}). \qquad (3)$$

We may rewrite the optimisation task equivalently by

$$\underbrace{\log Z(\mathbf{u})}_{g(\mathbf{u})} - \underbrace{\frac{1}{L}\sum_\ell \max_{T\in\mathcal{T}}\langle \mathbf{u}, T\mathbf{s}^\ell\rangle}_{h(\mathbf{u})} \to \min_{\mathbf{u}}. \qquad (4)$$

This is a DC program, because we have to minimise a difference of convex functions. Every DC program has a related DC dual program which has the same optimal value as the primal one

$$g(\mathbf{u}) - h(\mathbf{u}) \to \min_{\mathbf{u}} \tag{5}$$

$$h^*(\mathbf{v}) - g^*(\mathbf{v}) \to \min_{\mathbf{v}}, \tag{6}$$

where for a given function g, g^* is its Fenchel conjugate defined by

$$g^*(\mathbf{v}) = \sup_{\mathbf{u}} \{ \langle \mathbf{v}, \mathbf{u} \rangle - g(\mathbf{u}) \} \tag{7}$$

See e.g. [2,3] for the theory of DC programs, duality and related algorithms.

Let us have a closer look at the DC-dual program (6). It is easy to prove, that the Fenchel conjugate of $g(\mathbf{u}) = \log Z(\mathbf{u})$ is the (negative) entropy

$$g^*(\mathbf{v}) = \sum_{i \in \mathbb{T}_n^2} v_i \log v_i + (1 - v_i) \log(1 - v_i), \tag{8}$$

where we use the convention that $x \log x$ is zero if $x = 0$ and is $+\infty$ if x is negative. Let us compute the Fenchel conjugate of the function $h(\mathbf{u})$

$$h^*(\mathbf{v}) = \max_{\mathbf{u}} \left\{ \langle \mathbf{v}, \mathbf{u} \rangle - \max_{\mathbf{T}} \frac{1}{L} \sum_{\ell} \langle \mathbf{u}, T^\ell \mathbf{s}^\ell \rangle \right\} \tag{9}$$

$$= \max_{\mathbf{u}} \min_{\mathbf{T}} \left\langle \mathbf{v} - \frac{1}{L} \sum_{\ell} T^\ell \mathbf{s}^\ell, \mathbf{u} \right\rangle. \tag{10}$$

This problem has the form $\max_{\mathbf{u}} \min_{i \in I} \langle \mathbf{a}^i, \mathbf{u} \rangle$. Its value is either infinity if the origin does not lie in the convex hull of the vectors $\mathbf{a}^i$, $i \in I$ or zero in the opposite case. It follows from Gordan's lemma (see e.g. [4]). Hence, we obtain $h^*(\mathbf{v}) = \delta_C(\mathbf{v})$, where the indicator function $\delta_C(\mathbf{v})$ is 0 for $\mathbf{v}$ in C and $+\infty$ otherwise. The set C is the convex hull of all possible average images, i.e.

$$C = \text{conv} \left\{ \frac{1}{L} \sum_{\ell} T^\ell \mathbf{s}^\ell \,\middle|\, \forall T^1, \dots, T^L \in \mathcal{T} \right\}. \tag{11}$$

From all that we see that (6) requires to minimise the entropy (8) on the convex polytope C. Since the entropy is a concave function, the minimum is attained at an extremal point (vertex) of C. This in turn is precisely the task which congealing aims to solve. Hence, we proved the following theorem.

Theorem 1. *For the model family* (1) *and any (finite) set $\mathcal{T}$ of orthogonal transformations $T \colon \mathcal{S}(\mathbb{T}_n^2) \to \mathcal{S}(\mathbb{T}_n^2)$, congealing and MLE are DC-duals of each other. In particular, their optimal values are equal.*

2.3   A DC-algorithm

Congealing aims at solving the dual task (6) directly, i.e. to minimise the entropy (8) as a function of $\mathbf{v} = \frac{1}{L} \sum_\ell T^\ell \mathbf{s}^\ell$ w.r.t. to all possible collections of transformations $\mathbf{T} = (T^1, \ldots, T^L)$. This is usually done by block-wise local coordinate descent. Given the current $\mathbf{T}^{(k)}$, the algorithm tries to improve the entropy by sequentially probing local changes for each T^ℓ. Such an approach lacks a guarantee to converge to a local minimum.

Another option is to apply a DC algorithm. This type of algorithm aims at solving the primal and the dual task simultaneously, by constructing a pair of sequences $\mathbf{u}^{(k)}$, $\mathbf{v}^{(k)}$ in an alternating way

$$(a) \quad \mathbf{v}^{(k)} \in \partial h(\mathbf{u}^{(k)}) \tag{12}$$

$$(b) \quad \mathbf{u}^{(k+1)} \in \partial g^*(\mathbf{v}^{(k)}), \tag{13}$$

where $\partial h(\mathbf{u})$ denotes the sub-differential of a convex function h at point $\mathbf{u}$. In the case being considered, the algorithm reads as follows. Choose an initial $\mathbf{u}^{(0)}$ and repeat applying the following two steps until convergence

(a) Find $T^\ell \in \arg\max_T \langle \mathbf{u}^{(k)}, T\mathbf{s}^\ell \rangle$ for each image $\mathbf{s}^\ell$ independently. Set

$$\mathbf{v}^{(k)} = \frac{1}{L} \sum_\ell T^\ell \mathbf{s}^\ell. \tag{14}$$

(b) Since g^* is differentiable in the interior of its domain, its unique subgradient is given by the derivative, i.e., we have

$$u_i^{(k+1)} = \log v_i^{(k)} - \log(1 - v_i^{(k)}). \tag{15}$$

Remark 1. The DC algorithm solves the same task as the congealing algorithm but is substantially simpler and faster than the latter. The main reason is that step (a) decomposes into independent minimisation tasks for each image $\mathbf{s}^\ell$ and, moreover, the objective is a simple scalar product. Notice that these alignment tasks are similar but simpler than the corresponding tasks in approaches, where the entropy similarity measure is replaced with a least-squares similarity measure [5]. The function h being polyhedral guarantees that the DC-algorithm will almost surely converge to a local minimum of the primal task (see [3]). Finally we would like to mention here that all results given above are valid also for multivalued images.

2.4   Unsupervised Congealing

Let us consider the following generalisation of the congealing task. We will assume that the shape model (1) is formulated in terms of binary valued segmentation labellings $\mathbf{s}$. We assume furthermore, that the segmentations are (statistically) related to the images $\mathbf{x} \colon \mathbb{T}_n^2 \to F$ (where F is a feature space) by a parametric, pixel-wise conditionally independent appearance model. The joint model is therefore given by

$$p(\mathbf{x}, \mathbf{s}) = \frac{1}{Z(\mathbf{u})} \exp \langle \mathbf{u}, T\mathbf{s} \rangle \, p_\theta(\mathbf{x} \mid \mathbf{s}), \tag{16}$$

where θ denotes the parameters of the appearance model. In contrast with [12], θ is a parameter to be estimated, thus there is no need to marginalize it.

We consider the following unsupervised learning task. We are given a set of images $\mathbf{x}^\ell$, $\ell \in L$, each of them independently generated by one of the distributions $p_{\mathbf{u}, T^\ell}(\mathbf{s}) \cdot p_{\theta_\ell}(\mathbf{x} \mid \mathbf{s})$. All of them share the parameter vector $\mathbf{u}$, but each of them has a different $T^\ell \in T$ and a different parameter θ_ℓ. All parameter values are unknown. Moreover, the generated segmentations are also unknown. Given the sample of images $\mathbf{x}^\ell$, $\ell \in L$, we want to estimate the vector $\mathbf{u}$, the collection of transformations $\mathbf{T} = (T^1, \ldots, T^L)$ and the collection of parameters $\theta = (\theta_1, \ldots, \theta_L)$. The corresponding MLE task reads

$$\log Z(\mathbf{u}) - \frac{1}{L} \sum_{\ell \in L} \max_{T, \theta} \log \sum_{\mathbf{s}} \exp \langle \mathbf{u}, T\mathbf{s} \rangle \, p_\theta(\mathbf{x}^\ell \mid \mathbf{s}) \to \min_{\mathbf{u}}. \tag{17}$$

This is again a DC program and the corresponding DC algorithm reads as follows. Choose an initial $\mathbf{u}^{(0)}$ and repeat applying the following two steps until convergence

(a) Given $\mathbf{u}^{(k)}$, solve the task

$$(\theta^\ell, T^\ell) \in \arg \max_{\theta, T} \sum_{\mathbf{s}} \exp \left\langle \mathbf{u}^{(k)}, T\mathbf{s} \right\rangle p_\theta(\mathbf{x}^\ell \mid \mathbf{s}) \tag{18}$$

for each image $\mathbf{x}^\ell$, $\ell \in L$ independently. Given the solutions, compute the gradient

$$\mathbf{v}^{(k)} = \nabla_{\mathbf{u}} \frac{1}{L} \sum_{\ell \in L} \log \sum_{\mathbf{s}} \exp \langle \mathbf{u}, T^\ell \mathbf{s} \rangle \, p_{\theta_\ell}(\mathbf{x}^\ell \mid \mathbf{s}) \Big|_{\mathbf{u}^{(k)}} \tag{19}$$

(b) Compute the improved estimate of $\mathbf{u}$

$$u_i^{(k+1)} = \log v_i^{(k)} - \log(1 - v_i^{(k)}). \tag{20}$$

The computation of the gradient in (19) is rather straightforward, because all parts of the model probability (16) factorise pixel-wise. Summation over $\mathbf{s}$ in (19) is therefore tractable and can be performed in closed form. It results in

$$\mathbf{v}^{(k)} = \nabla_{\mathbf{u}} \ldots = \frac{1}{L} \sum_{\ell \in L} T^\ell \mathbf{b}^\ell, \tag{21}$$

where $\mathbf{b}^\ell$ denotes the posterior foreground probability for pixels of image $\mathbf{x}^\ell$ in its frame. Denoting by $\tilde{\mathbf{u}} = (T^\ell)^{-1} \mathbf{u}^{(k)}$ the current shape model $\mathbf{u}^{(k)}$ transformed into the image frame of $\mathbf{x}^\ell$, these probabilities are given by

$$b_i^\ell = p(s_i = 1 \mid x_i^\ell) = \frac{e^{\tilde{u}_i} \, p_{\theta_\ell}(x_i^\ell \mid s_i = 1)}{p_{\theta_\ell}(x_i^\ell \mid s_i = 0) + e^{\tilde{u}_i} \, p_{\theta_\ell}(x_i^\ell \mid s_i = 1)} \tag{22}$$

It remains to discuss the task (18), which has to be solved for each image given the current estimate $\mathbf{u}^{(k)}$ of the shape model. It requires to estimate the translation T^ℓ and the parameters θ_ℓ of the appearance model. This can be done by a standard Expectation Maximisation algorithm which is tractable due to same reasons as discussed for the computation of the gradient in the second sub-step of the DCA iteration.

The EM algorithm reads here as follows. Start with an initial estimate of the translation T^ℓ and the parameters θ_ℓ for the image $\mathbf{x}^\ell$. For instance, this could be those estimated for the image $\mathbf{x}^\ell$ in the previous cycle of the DCA algorithm. Iterate the following steps until convergence.

- **E-step.** Given the current estimate of T^ℓ and θ_ℓ, compute the posterior foreground probabilities $\mathbf{b}^\ell$ for all pixels in the image frame as in (22).
- **M-step.** The M-step consists in solving two subtasks. The first one re-estimates the translation by solving

$$T^\ell \in \arg\max_T \left\langle \mathbf{u}^{(k)}, T\mathbf{b}^\ell \right\rangle. \tag{23}$$

It is precisely the same subtask as in the DCA algorithm for standard congealing. The second subtask re-estimates the parameters of the appearance model for the given image $\mathbf{x}^\ell$

$$\theta_\ell \in \arg\max_\theta \sum_{i \in \mathbb{T}_n^2} \left[b_i^\ell \log p_\theta(x_i^\ell \mid s_i = 1) + (1 - b_i^\ell) \log p_\theta(x_i^\ell \mid s_i = 0) \right]. \tag{24}$$

Altogether this results in a double loop algorithm. Within each iteration of the outer DCA loop, which re-estimates the shape model $\mathbf{u}$, we have to run an inner EM algorithm loop for each image $\mathbf{x}^\ell$ in order to re-estimate the translation T^ℓ and the parameters of the appearance model θ_ℓ. All the sub-steps of this double loop algorithm are tractable and easy to implement.

3   Experiments

3.1   Artificial Images

In the first experiment we tested the method for artificially generated colour images $\mathbf{x}^\ell$, $\ell \in L$. For this we have fixed a pixel-wise independent shape model for binary valued segmentations of size 200×231. The (grey coded) foreground probabilities are shown in Fig. 2. We also fix a basic appearance model by choosing two multivariate normal distributions in the colour space, one per segment. Then 50 images of size given above were generated as follows. We randomly generate a binary segmentation $\mathbf{s}^\ell$ and translate it by a vector randomly chosen in the range ± 15 pixels in each dimension. We also randomly perturb the parameters of the normal distributions of the appearance model and use it to generate the colour image $\mathbf{x}^\ell$ from the segmentation $T^\ell \mathbf{s}^\ell$. Two such pairs are shown in Fig. 2.

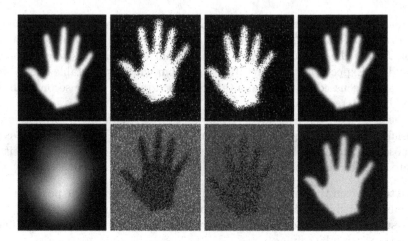

Fig. 2. Artificial images, top row: true shape model, two translated segmentations, true model (repeated). Bottom row: initial shape model, images generated for the segmentations above, final model found by the DCA algorithm.

The 50 images $\mathbf{x}^\ell$ are the input for the unsupervised congealing. The initial model parameters for the algorithm were chosen as follows. The initial shape model $\mathbf{u}^{(0)}$ favours (a-priori) foreground in the centre of the reference frame and background at the borders (see Fig. 2). The initial parameters for the two normal distributions were set to be equal for background and foreground centred at the midpoint of the colour space.

The DCA algorithms estimates all the parameters of the model, i.e., $\mathbf{u}$, and T^ℓ, θ_ℓ, $\ell \in L$, where we have restricted the search space for the translations to ± 20 pixels in each dimension. It runs until convergence of the log likelihood (17). The EM algorithms within each step of the outer loop of the DCA algorithm are run for each of the images $\mathbf{x}^\ell$ until convergence w.r.t. T and θ. We have implemented the algorithm both in Matlab and Python. The only "regularisation" we use, is to require all foreground and background probabilities of the shape model to be strictly positive (forcing them to stay above some prespecified value, e.g. 0.01). Optionally, the current estimate of the shape model can be averaged locally after each cycle of the DCA algorithm. The runtime for a standard Intel i7 processor is less than 10 min. Figure 3 shows the convergence of the log likelihood. It can be seen that not much more than ten cycles of the DCA algorithm were needed to converge. The average number of EM cycles (per image) spent in the inner loops is shown in the same figure.

The final estimated shape model is shown in Fig. 2. The per pixel Kullback Leibler divergence from the true model is 0.055. The translations T^ℓ found for the images $\mathbf{x}^\ell$ differ from the true ones by at most ± 1 pixel in each dimension.

3.2 Aligning and Segmenting Eye Disc Images

In the second experiment we test the proposed method for microscope images of Drosophila melanogaster larvae imaginal discs with stained mRNA for the

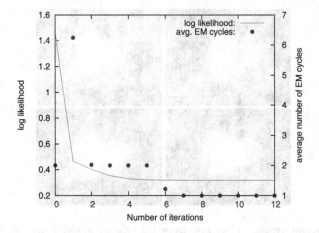

Fig. 3. Convergence of the DCA algorithm. Red: negative log likelihood per pixel, blue: average number of EM cycles per image in the DCA cycle (Color figure online).

expression of different genes. We have randomly chosen 194 images of eye discs and roughly pre-registered them (based on intensities only) by using Elastix [8].

The unsupervised congealing as described in Sect. 2.4 was run on the pre-registered colour images $(200 \times 150 \, \text{px})$ with initialisation similar to the one described in Sect. 3.1 for artificial images. However, instead of an exhaustive search over translations in each DCA cycle, we incrementally improve the result by restricting the search range by ± 10 pixels centered on the current estimate. Choosing a larger range has no influence on the final results. The following additional "regularisation" (compare with Sect. 2.4) was used in this experiment. To prevent the covariance matrices of the multivariate normal distributions from degeneration, we require their determinants to be larger than a pre-specified value. If the determinant falls under this value we add a scaled identity matrix to the covariance matrix.

The convergence of the algorithm observed in this experiment is similar to the convergence reported for the artificial images. Usually less that 20 DCA cycles were needed to converge with similar numbers of EM cycles per image in the inner loop. The runtime of an experiment never exceeded 20 min.

For comparison we use the approach proposed in [6] as a baseline. It is rather a pipeline – segmentation and registration are applied consecutively. First, each image is segmented by thresholding a local Laplacian filter. It is then improved by applying some morphological operations. The last sub-step is to apply a distance transform. The resulting (multi-level) images are then aligned by using the standard congealing approach as proposed in [9]. We have re-implemented the method and applied it to our images. Unfortunately we were not able to get satisfactory results, because the method depends on several parameters (domain of the Laplace filter, thresholds, size of the structure element, etc.) the values of which are not reported. We were able to find a parameter combination leading to reasonable results provided that the distance transform was not applied before congealing.

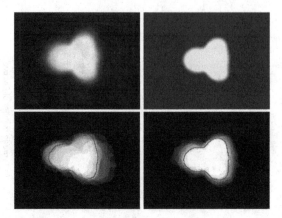

Fig. 4. Alignment results. First row from left: shape model found by the baseline method and by our method (grey-coded foreground probabilities). Second row from left: averaged aligned true segmentations for the baseline method and for our method. The red curves show the outline of the shape model (thresholded at 0.5 foreground probability (Color figure online).

For a fair comparison we use only the alignment results. The reason is the following. In contrast to our method, the shape model obtained by the baseline method has no influence on the segmentations. Therefore we have chosen a subset of 15 images, segmented them by hand and consider these segmentations as ground truth. The translations found for these images, when running the respective methods for the whole sample, were used to align the segmentations into the reference frame of the obtained shape model. We report the entropy of the averaged segmentation (in the reference frame). We also compute the Jaccard similarity coefficient[1] for each of the segmentations and the shape model (thresholded at foreground probability 0.5) and report the average over all 15 images.

The shape models found by the algorithms when applied to the 194 pre-registered images are shown in the first row of Fig. 4. The averages of the aligned true segmentations are shown in the second row of the same figure. Our method achieves per pixel entropy 0.0685 and average Jaccard index 0.764. This is substantially better than 0.1002 and 0.6500 respectively as obtained by the baseline method. This clearly shows that models and resulting algorithms for joint segmentation and alignment improve not only the segmentations but also the alignment.

Finally, we show some segmentations obtained by our method (Fig. 5). Notice that they are obtained from the posterior probabilities for foreground computed for each image in the last DCA cycle (see (21)). If the learned model is used to align and segment new images, then we run the EM algorithm for the image as described in Sect. 2.4 without changing the shape model. As can be seen,

---

[1] $|A \cap B|/|A \cup B|$.

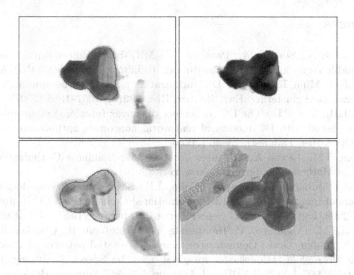

Fig. 5. Eye disc images overlaid with the outline of all connected components of the segmentations found by our method.

the prior shape model successfully aligns the disc objects and interprets foreign objects as background in most cases. However, the segmentations themselves are not yet satisfactory. The reason for this is the so far simple shape model and the limited class of transformations. This restricts the expressive power of the joint model.

4   Conclusions

We have shown how to generalise an entropy based alignment approach from signal based models to more complex models with latent segment variables keeping at the same time the corresponding algorithm for joint alignment and segmentation simple and fast. This was achieved by a thorough theoretical analysis of the task.

By applying the new algorithm to artificial images and microscope images of Drosophila melanogaster larvae imaginal disc, we have demonstrated that methods for joint alignment and segmentation outperform sequential approaches even considering alignment only. The segmentation results obtained in experiments are not completely satisfactory yet. We believe that the reason for this is the simple shape model and the limited class of transformations we have used so far. Therefore we plan to enrich the model by more complex shape model components as Markov Random Fields and to generalise the corresponding algorithm for the use with a richer class of transformations.

References

1. Komodakis, N., Sotiras, A., Paragios, N.: MRF-based diffeomorphic population deformable registration and segmentation. Technical Report 6837, INRIA (2009)
2. An, L.T.H., Minh, L.H., Tao, P.D.: Optimization based DC programming and DCA for hierarchical clustering. Eur. J. Oper. Res. **183**(3), 1067–1085 (2007)
3. An, L.T.H., Tao, P.D.: The DC (difference of convex functions) programming and DCA revisited with DC models of real world nonconvex optimization problems. Ann. Oper. Res. **133**(1–4), 23–46 (2005)
4. Borwein, J.M., Lewis, A.S.: Convex Analysis and Nonlinear Optimization. CMS Books in Mathematics. Springer, New York (2000)
5. Cox, M., Sridharan, S., Lucey, S., Cohn, J.F.: Least-squares congealing for large numbers of images. In: IEEE 12th International Conference on Computer Vision, ICCV 2009, Kyoto, Japan, 27 September–4 October, pp. 1949–1956 (2009)
6. Harmon, C.L., Ahammad, P., Hammonds, A., Weiszmann, R., Celniker, S.E., Sastry, S.S., Rubin, G.M.: Comparative analysis of spatial patterns of gene expression in *Drosophila melanogaster* imaginal discs. In: Speed, T., Huang, H. (eds.) RECOMB 2007. LNCS (LNBI), vol. 4453, pp. 533–547. Springer, Heidelberg (2007)
7. Huang, G., Mattar, M., Lee, H., Learned-Miller, E.G.: Learning to align from scratch. In: Pereira, F., Burges, C.J.C., Bottou, L., Weinberger, K.Q. (eds.) Advances in Neural Information Processing Systems 25, pp. 764–772. Currant Associates Inc. (2012)
8. Klein, S., Staring, M., Murphy, K., Viergever, M.A., Pluim, J.P.W.: Elastix: a toolbox for intensity-based medical image registration. IEEE Trans. Med. Imaging **29**(1), 196–205 (2010)
9. Learned-Miller, E.G.: Data driven image models through continuous joint alignment. IEEE Trans. Pattern Anal. Mach. Intell. **28**(2), 236–250 (2006)
10. Liu, X., Tong, Y., Wheeler, F.W.: Simultaneous alignment and clustering for an image ensemble. In: IEEE 12th International Conference on Computer Vision, ICCV 2009, Kyoto, Japan, 27 September–4 October, pp. 1327–1334 (2009)
11. Pohl, K.M., Fisher, J., Grimson, W.E.L., Kikinis, R., Wells, W.M.: A bayesian model for joint segmentation and registration. NeuroImage **31**(1), 228–239 (2006)
12. Zöllei, L., Jenkinson, M., Timoner, S.J., Wells, W.M.: A Marginalized MAP approach and EM optimization for pair-wise registration. In: Karssemeijer, N., Lelieveldt, B. (eds.) IPMI 2007. LNCS, vol. 4584, pp. 662–674. Springer, Heidelberg (2007)

Self-Aligning Manifolds for Matching Disparate Medical Image Datasets

Christian F. Baumgartner[1]([envelope]), Alberto Gomez[1], Lisa M. Koch[2],
James R. Housden[1], Christoph Kolbitsch[1], Jamie R. McClelland[3],
Daniel Rueckert[2], and Andy P. King[1]

[1] Division of Imaging Sciences, King's College London, London, UK
christian.baumgartner@kcl.ac.uk
[2] Biomedical Image Analysis Group, Department of Computing,
Imperial College London, London, UK
[3] Centre for Medical Image Computing, University College London, London, UK

Abstract. Manifold alignment can be used to reduce the dimensionality of multiple medical image datasets into a single globally consistent low-dimensional space. This may be desirable in a wide variety of problems, from fusion of different imaging modalities for Alzheimer's disease classification to 4DMR reconstruction from 2D MR slices. Unfortunately, most existing manifold alignment techniques require either a set of prior correspondences or comparability between the datasets in high-dimensional space, which is often not possible. We propose a novel technique for the 'self-alignment' of manifolds (SAM) from multiple dissimilar imaging datasets without prior correspondences or inter-dataset image comparisons. We quantitatively evaluate the method on 4DMR reconstruction from realistic, synthetic sagittal 2D MR slices from 6 volunteers and real data from 4 volunteers. Additionally, we demonstrate the technique for the compounding of two free breathing 3D ultrasound views from one volunteer. The proposed method performs significantly better for 4DMR reconstruction than state-of-the-art image-based techniques.

1 Introduction

Relating individual images of multiple image datasets is a frequent problem in the analysis of medical images. This may, for example, be the matching of images of a population acquired with different imaging protocols [5], matching respiratory motion states in different modalities [12] or matching motion states in dynamic images of the same modality acquired from different views [1,2,13]. In this work we will focus on the latter problem.

An example of this problem is navigator-less 4D magnetic resonance (MR) reconstruction from 2D sagittal MR slices acquired over a period of time at different slice positions [1,2,13]. Such images have applications in motion corrected reconstruction of PET/MR images [1,2], or as input for motion models for radiotherapy guidance [13]. Another example of relating disparate datasets is the compounding of free breathing 3D ultrasound (US) images from different

© Springer International Publishing Switzerland 2015
S. Ourselin et al. (Eds.): IPMI 2015, LNCS 9123, pp. 363–374, 2015.
DOI: 10.1007/978-3-319-19992-4_28

views for the purpose of reducing artefacts and increasing the effective field of view [16]. Even though such data is acquired with the same modality, it may appear very dissimilar as the different views either visualise different anatomical regions (MR slices) or a similar region from a different view point (US views).

Dimensionality reduction techniques (i.e. manifold learning) have been used to map a single dataset into a low-dimensional embedding, e.g. for deriving navigators for MR gating [14] or for respiratory motion modelling [6]. Manifold Alignment (MA) is a class of techniques which transforms manifold embeddings from two or more datasets into a single, globally consistent space. MA techniques can be performed either semi-supervised, i.e. using a set of prior correspondences between some data points known beforehand, or unsupervised by deriving correspondences from similarities between the data in high-dimensional space.

For example, [14] reduced the dimensionality of US images acquired using a wobbler probe at different angles to 1 and adjusted the resulting curves for flipping and scaling based on information about the acquisition order. This is a simple form of semi-supervised MA. Another example of a semi-supervised technique is [5], where embeddings in higher dimensions were aligned. Lombaert et al. [7] proposed an unsupervised MA technique for matching cortical surfaces based on spectral matching. The authors aligned embeddings obtained using Laplacian Eigenmaps by employing a point set registration algorithm, which took into account features derived from the high-dimensional data such as e.g. cortical thickness. Later, the authors extended this work to obtain diffeomorphic transformations between cortical surfaces [8]. Another unsupervised technique was proposed by [1]. The authors embedded the manifolds of dynamic MR data acquired from different coronal slice positions in groups of two for the purpose of 4DMR reconstruction. In this work the correspondences between the different datasets were based on similarities in image space of neighbouring slice positions.

In some MA applications, prior correspondences may be unavailable and comparison in the high-dimensional space may not be possible due to the different appearance of the data or potentially due to the datasets being of a different type altogether. To the best of our knowledge the only MA technique which requires neither prior correspondences nor comparability of the high-dimensional data was proposed by [15]. The authors proposed to establish correspondences between the datasets by considering similarities of the local neighbourhood within each of the datasets to be aligned. Unfortunately, the approach requires iterating through all of the permutations of the local neighbourhood of each point, which is only computationally tractable for very small neighbourhoods.

In this work, we propose a method for the 'self-alignment of manifolds' (SAM) of medical images. This means that the manifolds of multiple datasets are mapped into a globally consistent space without prior correspondences or inter-dataset comparisons in the high-dimensional space. The method can be used to align manifolds from medical imaging datasets which depict different anatomy or the same anatomy from different views, and that are hence not directly comparable. The method is inspired by work from the graph matching literature, and establishes correspondences between multiple datasets based on their internal graph structure. This allows to avoid inter-dataset comparisons in the original high-dimensional space.

We apply the method to two problems in medical imaging which require matching of respiratory positions of different views which are hard to compare in image space: the 4D reconstruction of MR volumes from sagittal slices acquired at different slice positions and the compounding of free breathing 3D US sequences acquired from two different views.

2 Theory

In this section we describe the theoretical basis for our approach. We first present theory relating to manifold learning and alignment, introduce our notation, and show how locally linear embeddings (LLE) [11], a commonly used manifold learning technique, can be extended to align arbitrary numbers of manifolds. We then describe how an arbitrary number of manifolds can be aligned without prior correspondences or inter-dataset comparisons in the high-dimensional space.

2.1 Manifold Learning

In non-linear dimensionality reduction the underlying assumption is that a dataset X consisting of N high-dimensional points $X = [\mathbf{x_1}, \ldots, \mathbf{x_N}] \in \mathbb{R}^{D \times N}$ (e.g. a time series of N images with D pixels each) lies on a manifold $\mathcal{M}$ which can be described by much fewer dimensions. Manifold learning techniques map each point $\mathbf{x_i}$ in the high-dimensional dataset to a low-dimensional point $\mathbf{y_i} \in \mathbb{R}^d$, where $d \ll D$, while preserving the local neighbourhood structure of the high-dimensional points on $\mathcal{M}$. The low-dimensional points form a new low-dimensional dataset $Y \in \mathbb{R}^{d \times N}$.

LLE models the locality of the high-dimensional space by first constructing a graph of the data points and then calculating the weights which reconstruct each high-dimensional point as a linear combination of its k-nearest neighbours. The optimal contribution of each point j to the reconstruction of i is given by the weights W_{ij} and can be calculated as described in [11]. The embedding preserving this structure is given by the Y minimising the cost function

$$\phi(Y) = \sum_i ||\mathbf{y}_i - \sum_{j \in \eta(i)} W_{ij}\mathbf{y}_j||^2 = Tr(YMY^T). \tag{1}$$

Here, $\eta(i)$ is the neighbourhood of each point i and $Tr(\cdot)$ is the trace operator. This optimisation problem can be solved by calculating the eigendecomposition of the centred reconstruction weight matrix $M = (I - W)^T(I - W)$. The embedding Y is given by the eigenvectors corresponding to the second smallest to $d+1$ smallest eigenvalues of M [11].

It is well known that when manifold learning is applied to time series of medical images under free breathing, the low dimensional coordinates $\mathbf{y}_i$ contain useful information about the motion. In particular, when reducing the data to a one dimensional space ($d = 1$) the embedding strongly correlates with a respiratory navigator obtained by traditional means [14]. Baumgartner et al. [1] showed that embeddings in higher dimensions can give additional information on respiratory variation such as hysteresis or respiratory drift over time.

2.2 Manifold Alignment by Simultaneous Embedding

Medical image datasets which have the same source of motion often lie on similar low-dimensional manifolds. Within the context of this work the different datasets are free breathing images acquired from different views, i.e. different slice positions (MR) or different probe locations (US). Bringing the manifolds into a globally consistent coordinate system allows the matching of images at similar respiratory positions between the different views.

Unfortunately, the embeddings obtained using manifold learning techniques are arbitrary with respect to the sign of the eigenvectors (i.e. arbitrary flipping). In addition, the manifolds obtained from different datasets often feature small but significant differences in shape such as small rotations or scaling differences, which further complicate their alignment. In order to relate the respiratory positions of L different datasets $X_1, \ldots, X_L : X_\ell = [\mathbf{x}_1^{(\ell)}, \ldots, \mathbf{x}_N^{(\ell)}]$ (e.g. free breathing images obtained from L different views) in the low-dimensional space, first the underlying manifold embeddings $Y_1, \ldots, Y_L$ must be aligned.

Our solution to the alignment problem is to formulate a joint cost function and then compute an embedding for all datasets simultaneously in one embedding step. This approach is the general case for L datasets of the formulation proposed in [1] for two datasets. However, to the best of our knowledge, LLE has not been extended to embed $L > 2$ datasets simultaneously. This can be done by augmenting the cost function from Eq. (1) as follows:

$$\phi_{tot}(Y_1, ..., Y_L) = \sum_{\ell=1}^{L} \phi_\ell(Y_\ell) + \frac{\mu}{2} \sum_{\substack{n=1,m=1 \\ m \neq n}}^{L} \sum_{i,j}^{N} U_{ij}^{(nm)} ||\mathbf{y}_i^{(n)} - \mathbf{y}_j^{(m)}||^2, \quad (2)$$

where ϕ_ℓ is given by Eq. (1). The second term of Eq. (2) is the cost function relating all datasets to each other. $U^{(nm)}$ is a similarity kernel relating points from dataset n to dataset m. Large values in $U^{(nm)}$ force corresponding points to be close together in the resulting embedding. μ is a weighting parameter which governs the influence of the inter-dataset terms. ϕ_{tot} can be rewritten in matrix form as $\phi_{tot} = Tr(VHV^T)$, where V is a $d \times (N \cdot L)$ matrix containing the concatenated embeddings, $V = [Y_1, \ldots, Y_L]$, and

$$H = \begin{bmatrix} M^{(1)} + \mu\sum_p D^{(1p)} & -\mu U^{(12)} & \cdots & -\mu U^{(1L)} \\ -\mu U^{(21)} & M^{(2)} + \mu\sum_p D^{(2p)} & \cdots & -\mu U^{(2L)} \\ \vdots & & \ddots & \vdots \\ -\mu U^{(L1)} & -\mu U^{(L2)} & \cdots & M^{(L)} + \mu\sum_p D^{(Lp)} \end{bmatrix} \quad (3)$$

Here, the diagonal degree matrices $D^{(nm)}$ are given by $D_{ii}^{(nm)} = \sum_j U_{ij}^{(nm)}$. Under the scaling constraint $\sum_{\ell=1}^{L} Y_\ell^T Y_\ell = 1$, the embeddings V are given by the second smallest to $d + 1$ smallest eigenvectors of H.

2.3 Similarity Without Correspondences

All previous work on simultaneous embeddings has either used known prior correspondences to define the similarity kernels $U^{(nm)}$ [5], or has used similarity measures between the high-dimensional data to define it [1,8]. The notable exception is [15] which we discussed in the introduction. For many applications, however, it is desirable to simultaneously embed medical image datasets which are not comparable in image space and for which prior correspondences are not easily obtainable. This problem is effectively one of finding a suitable inter-dataset similarity kernel $U^{(nm)}$ that connects datasets X_n, X_m but which is *not* based on comparisons between datasets in the high-dimensional space.

In this paper we propose a novel, robust method for deriving an inter-dataset similarity kernel. Instead of directly comparing the data from different datasets in the high-dimensional space we first analyse the internal graph structure of each dataset and derive a characteristic feature vector for each node. In the next step we compare these feature vectors across datasets. This approach is an extension of the method proposed in [3] for graph matching.

Deriving a Characteristic Feature Vector for Each Node. For each dataset X we form a fully connected, weighted graph $\mathcal{G} = \{V, E, C\}$, connecting each node in V to every other with edges E. The edge weights C_{ij} connecting node V_i to V_j are given by a Gaussian kernel

$$C_{ij} = e^{\frac{-||\mathbf{x}_i - \mathbf{x}_j||^2}{2\sigma_1^2}},$$

where $\mathbf{x}_i, \mathbf{x}_j$ are the high-dimensional data points of X, and σ_1 is a shape parameter. Note that C_{ij} is formed by intra-dataset comparisons only.

As noted in [3], the steady-state distribution of a (lazy) random walk, i.e. the probability $\mathbf{p}_i$ of ending up at a particular node V_i after $t \to \infty$ time steps, can provide information about each node's location in the graph. In a lazy random walk the walker remains at their current node V_i with probability 0.5 at each time step and walks to a random neighbour V_j with a probability given by the edge weights C_{ij} the other half of the time. The state of the random walk in a weighted graph after $t + 1$ time steps is given by $\mathbf{p}^{(t+1)} = \frac{1}{2}(I + CB^{-1})\mathbf{p}^{(t)}$, where B is the diagonal degree matrix given by $B_{ii} = \sum_j C_{ij}$. The steady state distribution is stationary and is given by

$$\mathbf{p}^* = \frac{B\mathbf{1}}{\mathbf{1}^T B\mathbf{1}}. \tag{4}$$

In [3], $\mathbf{p}^*$ was used to perform graph matching. In our experiments, $\mathbf{p}^*$ alone was not sufficiently robust to align our datasets. Therefore, to increase the robustness of this measure we propose to additionally analyse the neighbourhood of each node. For each V_i we select the r-nearest neighbours and evaluate their $\mathbf{p}^*$ as well, by forming an average over the neighbourhood:

$$\pi_i^{(r)} = \frac{1}{|\eta(i)|} \sum_{j \in \eta(i)} \mathbf{p}_j^*. \tag{5}$$

A single value of r does not produce a rich enough descriptor of local graph structure. Therefore, we systematically increase the value of r from 1 to a maximum neighbourhood R, resulting in a feature vector $\mathbf{r_i} = [\mathbf{p}_i^*, \pi_i^{(1)}, \ldots, \pi_i^{(R)}]$ for each node V_i. This feature is highly characteristic for each node in the graph.

Matching Graph Nodes Across Datasets. The feature vectors $\mathbf{r_i}^{(\ell)}$ are derived for each dataset ℓ as described above. Next, a similarity kernel $\tilde{U}^{(nm)}$, connecting two datasets n and m, is formed as

$$\tilde{U}_{ij}^{(nm)} = e^{\frac{-||\mathbf{r_i}^{(n)} - \mathbf{r_j}^{(m)}||^2}{2\sigma_2^2}}, \tag{6}$$

where σ_2 is another shape parameter. A one-to-one matching between the two datasets maximising the similarity is found using the Hungarian algorithm as in [3]. This forms the final similarity kernel $U_{ij}^{(nm)}$, that can be substituted into Eq. (2).

3   Materials and Applications

In the following we show how to apply our novel self-aligning manifolds algorithm to the reconstruction of accurate 4DMR sequences of the liver from sagittal 2D slices, and the simultaneous gating and compounding of 3D liver US images.

3.1   Application to 4DMR Reconstruction

We acquired high-resolution 2D MR slices from L anatomical slice positions such that the whole liver was covered. In contrast to [1] we used sagittal slices because most respiratory motion occurs in the sagittal plane. The acquisitions were carried out on a Phillips Achieva 3T MR scanner using a T1-weighted gradient echo sequence with an acquired in-plane image resolution of $1.4 \times 1.4\,\text{mm}^2$ and a slice thickness of $8\,\text{mm}$. To cover the liver, typically around 30 slice positions were needed and each slice position was sampled 100 times. No gating was applied and the acquisition of one slice took $\sim 270\,\text{ms}$, resulting in a typical total acquisition time of $\sim 14\,\text{min}$. For the synthetic experiments we generated such data in a realistic manner from other scans as will be described in the following section.

The image data from the L slice positions form L high-dimensional datasets $X_1, \cdots, X_L$, where each X_ℓ contains all slices acquired at slice position ℓ. For each of the acquired slices we aim to reconstruct a 3D volume by stacking appropriate images from all other slice positions such that the respiratory position is consistent in the whole volume. The sequence of reconstructed 3D volumes from each slice results in the 4DMR sequence. To achieve this we first applied our novel technique to reduce the dimensionality of these datasets and embed them in an aligned, globally consistent way, such that any two low dimensional points $\mathbf{y}_i^{(n)}, \mathbf{y}_j^{(m)}$ from slice positions n and m, which are embedded close to each other, correspond to the high-dimensional images $\mathbf{x}_i^{(n)}, \mathbf{x}_j^{(m)}$, which have similar respiratory positions. Thus, for the 4DMR reconstruction it suffices to look up the nearest neighbour of each slice in the low-dimensional space for each other slice position and stack the corresponding 2D images into a volume.

Generation of Synthetic 2D MR Slice-by-Slice Data. Baumgartner et al. [1] generated synthetic data by deriving motion fields from low-resolution 3D MR volumes and then transforming a breathhold scan using these motion fields. The drawback of this approach is that every slice position has exactly the same sampling of motion states, which is unrealistic and makes the MA problem artificially easy. We solve this problem by first forming a motion model [10] to derive a large number of synthetic volumes and then randomly sampling each slice position.

We acquired 50 low-resolution 3D MR dynamic scans using the same sequence as described in [1]. Next, we derived 50 3D transformations from these volumes by registering them to a manually selected exhale volume using B-spline registration [9] to obtain a set of grid displacements $\mathbf{b}^{(t)}(\mathbf{c})$ for each image t at grid location $\mathbf{c}$. Additionally, we acquired a single breathhold volume consisting of all sagittal slice positions covering the liver using the same acquisition protocol as was used for the real acquisitions. In the next step we derived two 1D signals $s_1^{(t)}, s_2^{(t)}$ from the 3D image data by analysing the image intensities within small boxes on the diaphragm and chest [10]. We chose two signals to increase the amount of respiratory variabilities captured in the resulting model. Next, we formed a motion model [10] by fitting a linear function of the time series of signal values to the displacements of each B-spline grid point, i.e.

$$\mathbf{b}(\mathbf{c}) = \alpha_1(\mathbf{c}) + \alpha_2(\mathbf{c})s_1 + \alpha_3(\mathbf{c})s_2, \tag{7}$$

where $\alpha_1, \alpha_2, \alpha_3$ are the parameters of the motion model.

Next, we fitted a 2D distribution to the signal values using kernel density estimation. From this distribution we sampled 200 synthetic signal pairs $\tilde{s}_1, \tilde{s}_2$. By substituting these values into Eq. (7) we obtained 200 synthetic B-spline transformations. These transformations were then applied to the slice-by-slice breathhold volume to obtain 200 synthetic slice-by-slice volumes. Lastly, we randomly sampled 100 different time points from each slice position without replacement, generating the final synthetic dataset. This approach has two main advantages: (1) more realistic sampling of respiratory positions, (2) the ability to generate datasets of arbitrary size from a 50 s scan.

3.2 Application to 3D Ultrasound Gating and Compounding

For this application we acquired freehand 3D US images of the liver from two overlapping views for 22 s at 14 frames/second (i.e. ~ 300 frames per view). We used a Phillips iE33 US system with a X3-1 matrix array transducer. The data from the two views make up two datasets X_1, X_2. The first 2 s of the acquisition from each view were performed at an end-exhale breathhold.

The compounding of the two views will lead to an extended field of view and reduced noise artefacts. The objective is to obtain a number of such compounded volumes, each of which has a consistent respiratory position. For this purpose we binned the imaging data from both views in the low-dimensional space such that all images in one bin originated from approximately the same respiratory state, and then for each bin reconstructed a compounded volume.

To achieve the binning, we reduced the dimensionality of the two US sequences, X_1, X_2, using SAM such that their embeddings Y_1, Y_2 lay in a globally consistent space. We restricted ourselves to $d = 2$ in this experiment to simplify the binning. We defined 5×5 bins in the embedded space as shown in Fig. 3a, and selected only the ones which contain 5 or more images from each view. We then rigidly registered the breathhold of view 2 to the one of view 1 to obtain a transformation correcting for the different probe location [4]. After adjusting each image from view 2 using this transformation, we applied the compounding algorithm proposed in [16] to combine the images from each bin.

4   Experiments and Results

4.1   4DMR Reconstruction

We evaluated this method on synthetic data derived from 6 healthy volunteer scans and real data from 4 healthy volunteers.

Experiment 1: Synthetic 4DMR Reconstruction. We generated synthetic data as described in Sect. 3.1 from 6 volunteer scans. In order to evaluate the reconstruction accuracy of our method we reconstructed a volume $\tilde{V}_s$ from each slice s in the dataset, and measured its L2-distance to the ground truth volume V_s from which the slice was originally sampled, i.e. $E_s = ||\tilde{V}_s - V_s||$. Since the distribution of E_s was skewed we report the median reconstruction errors.

In addition to the proposed SAM technique we computed this error for two other image based image reconstruction techniques: simultaneous groupwise manifold alignment (SGA) [1] and a method based purely on direct comparisons between images which we will refer to as PIM [2]. Both SGA and PIM compare only neighbouring slice positions and were initially proposed for coronal slices which have smaller changes in appearance between adjacent slice positions. For SGA we used the optimal parameters proposed in [1]. For SAM we chose the following parameters by manual tuning: $\mu = 10^{-5}$, $\sigma_1 = 1, \sigma_2 = 0.15, k = 30$, $d = 4, R = 99$. PIM does not have parameters which require tuning.

The reconstruction errors for each subject using the different methods are shown in Fig. 1a. SAM performed significantly better ($p < 0.001$) than the two other techniques for all volunteers expect for volunteer 5 where SGA performed similarly. Significance was assessed using a Wilcoxon signed rank test. SGA and PIM regularly failed to propagate respiratory information across the medial slices. SAM, which embeds all slice positions simultaneously without image comparisons did not suffer from this problem. Coronal views of a single time point of the 4D reconstructions formed from the sagittal input slices for volunteers 2 and 4 are shown in Fig. 1b.

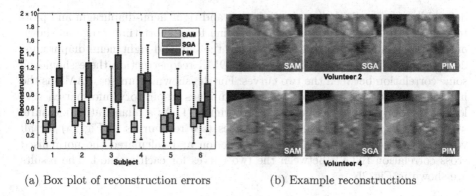

(a) Box plot of reconstruction errors   (b) Example reconstructions

Fig. 1. Results of synthetic 4DMR reconstruction experiment. (a) Box plot of reconstruction errors. (b) Coronal slices through a single time-point of the 4DMR reconstructions obtained using the three methods for two volunteers. The green and purple areas denote positive and negative differences to the ground truth (Color figure online).

Experiment 2: 4DMR Reconstruction from Real Data. We acquired real slice-by-slice data from 4 volunteers and formed 4DMR reconstructions as explained in Sect. 3.1. We again evaluated against SGA and PIM, and used the same parameters as above for all methods. On the left-hand side of Fig. 2a we show examples of coronal slices through single time-frames of the 4DMR reconstruction of volunteer 2. All three methods show reasonable looking reconstructions. However, as in Experiment 1, the respiratory information does not always propagate through medial slices for SGA and PIM. To illustrate this we

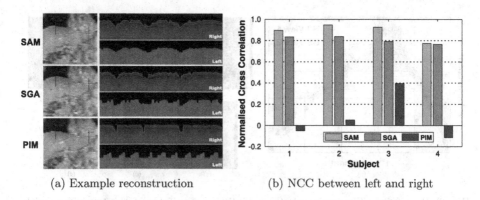

(a) Example reconstruction   (b) NCC between left and right

Fig. 2. Results of the real 4DMR reconstruction. (a) Coronal slice through a single time point of the 4DMR sequence obtained using the three compared methods and line profiles extracted from the left and right hemi-diaphragm from sagittal slices indicated by the blue lines (the right line is at a more posterior position on this slice). (b) NCC between the left and right line profiles over the entire duration of the 4DMR sequence (Color figure online).

defined lines on sagittal slices from the left and right hemi-diaphragm and plotted the 4DMR reconstruction along this line for a short time range as shown on the right-hand side of Fig. 2a. Because the left and right hemi-diaphragms do not move independently, in a correct 4DMR reconstruction there should be some correlation between the two curves. For the shown volunteer, SAM has the highest correlation. For the other two techniques respiratory information gets lost in the body middle as before in Experiment 1. As a quantitative measure, we extracted curves from such line profiles (see red curves in Fig. 2a) for all volunteers for the entire 4DMR reconstruction and calculated the normalised cross correlation (NCC) between the two curves for each method. The results are shown in Fig. 2b.

4.2   Experiment 3: 3D Ultrasound Compounding

We acquired and gated US data from two views from one healthy volunteer as described in Sect. 3.2. We used the following parameter values for SAM: $\mu = 10^{-4}$, $\sigma_1 = 1, \sigma_2 = 0.2, k = 20$, $R = 200$. Two single frames of the two views are shown in Fig. 3c. The gating resulted in 8 bins with more than 5 volumes from each view. These are highlighted in green in Fig. 3a. In Fig. 3b we show the reconstructions from these 8 gates. We did not compare against SGA or PIM because the views are not similar enough in image space to apply those methods. By observing the liver boundary indicated by the arrow in the first frame, it can be verified that the gates order the data from exhale to inhale. For comparison a compounded volume of all acquired images without gating is shown in Fig. 3d in which the same structure appears blurred. In Fig. 3e a 3D rendering of gate 1 is shown.

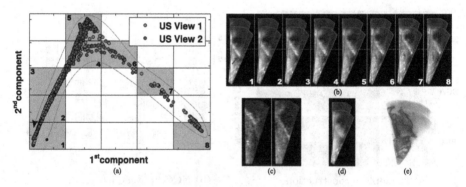

Fig. 3. Results of US experiment. (a) Self-aligned manifolds of the two views, with gates for binning. The arrow indicates the path around the manifold during one full breath. (b) Reconstructed gates, (c) Single frames from the two views, (d) Compounded volume without gating, (e) 3D rendering of compounded gate 1.

5   Discussion and Conclusion

We have proposed a novel method for self-aligning manifold embeddings which can reduce the dimensionality of multiple datasets into a single globally consistent space. The method is completely unsupervised and requires neither prior correspondences nor comparability of the datasets in high-dimensional space. We applied the method to two problems from the domain of free breathing 4D image reconstruction: 4D US view compounding and 4DMR reconstruction.

In our 4DMR experiments we were able to obtain significantly better reconstructions from sagittal slices than two state-of-the-art image based techniques. We restricted the 3D US demonstration to two views for simplicity. However, in principle an arbitrary number of views can be combined in this manner, e.g. to obtain motion images of the entire liver. This would have potential application in radiotherapy planning or motion modelling.

We believe that the idea of self-aligning manifolds will find application in a wide range of problems. Since the method does not require the images to be comparable in high-dimensional space, it could also be applied to matching the motion in multi-modal image pairs, such as PET and MR for motion corrected PET reconstruction [1,2,6], or the alignment of pre-treatment MR or CT images to intra-treatment imaging such as real-time US images for image-guided interventions [10]. Lastly, the potential of this technique is not limited to analysing motion. The globally consistent embedded space of multiple datasets could also be used as input features for further statistical analysis such as classification of Alzheimer's disease from images acquired with different modalities [5].

The proposed method relies on a simultaneous dimensionality reduction of all datasets in one embedding step. An alternative approach to MA without correspondences is to embed each dataset separately and then perform a point cloud registration based solely on the shape of the manifold. We investigated such an approach, but found the SAM approach to be preferable for two reasons. First, the problem of the arbitrary orientation of the eigenvectors (i.e. the flipping) is not trivial to solve if the high-dimensional image data are not directly comparable. Secondly, the shape of the embeddings may vary significantly from dataset to dataset impeding shape-based registration techniques. The simultaneous embedding neatly solves both of these problems.

In order to formulate the similarity kernel we build on work proposed in the graph matching literature, in particular the work by [3]. Graph matching and MA are, in fact, strongly related techniques. The key difference is that in graph matching one is typically interested in a one-to-one correspondence between graph nodes. In MA, on the other hand, we obtain a continuous low-dimensional space in which we can form more complex relations between all the data points.

One limitation of our technique is that it requires the graph structure to be in some way characteristic of the way data was generated. This is true for dynamic images during free breathing, however we believe that most real datasets in medical imaging will have such a structure.

Acknowledgements. This work was funded by EPSRC programme grant EP/H0464 10/1. This research was supported by the National Institute for Health Research (NIHR) Biomedical Research Centre at Guy's and St. Thomas' NHS Foundation Trust and King's College London. The views expressed are those of the authors and not necessarily those of the NHS, the NIHR or the Department of Health.

References

1. Baumgartner, C.F., Kolbitsch, C., Balfour, D.R., Marsden, P.K., McClelland, J.R., Rueckert, D., King, A.P.: High-resolution dynamic MR imaging of the thorax for respiratory motion correction of PET using groupwise manifold alignment. Med. Image Anal. **18**(7), 939–952 (2014)
2. Dikaios, N., Izquierdo-Garcia, D., Graves, M.J., Mani, V., Fayad, Z.A., Fryer, T.D.: MRI-based motion correction of thoracic PET: initial comparison of acquisition protocols and correction strategies suitable for simultaneous PET/MRI systems. Eur. Radiol. **22**(2), 439–446 (2012)
3. Gori, M., Maggini, M., Sarti, L.: Exact and approximate graph matching using random walks. IEEE T. Pattern Anal. **27**(7), 1100–1111 (2005)
4. Grau, V., Becher, H., Noble, J.A.: Registration of multiview real-time 3-D echocardiographic sequences. IEEE T. Med. Imaging **26**(9), 1154–1165 (2007)
5. Guerrero, R., Ledig, C., Rueckert, D.: Manifold alignment and transfer learning for classification of Alzheimer's disease. In: Wu, G., Zhang, D., Zhou, L. (eds.) MLMI 2014. LNCS, vol. 8679, pp. 77–84. Springer, Heidelberg (2014)
6. King, A.P., Buerger, C., Tsoumpas, C., Marsden, P.K., Schaeffter, T.: Thoracic respiratory motion estimation from MRI using a statistical model and a 2-D image navigator. Med. Image Anal. **16**(1), 252–264 (2012)
7. Lombaert, H., Grady, L., Polimeni, J.R., Cheriet, F.: Fast brain matching with spectral correspondence. In: Székely, G., Hahn, H.K. (eds.) IPMI 2011. LNCS, vol. 6801, pp. 660–673. Springer, Heidelberg (2011)
8. Lombaert, H., Sporring, J., Siddiqi, K.: Diffeomorphic spectral matching of cortical surfaces. In: Gee, J.C., Joshi, S., Pohl, K.M., Wells, W.M., Zöllei, L. (eds.) IPMI 2013. LNCS, vol. 7917, pp. 376–389. Springer, Heidelberg (2013)
9. Modat, M., Ridgway, G.R., Zeike, A.T., Lehmann, M., Barnes, J., Hawkes, D.J., Fox, N.C., Ourselin, S.: Fast free-form deformation using graphics processing units. Comput. Meth. Prog. Bio. **98**(3), 278–284 (2010)
10. McClelland, J.R., Hawkes, D.J., Schaeffter, T., King, A.P.: Respiratory motion models: a review. Med. Image Anal. **17**(1), 19–42 (2013)
11. Roweis, S.T., Saul, L.K.: Nonlinear dimensionality reduction by locally linear embedding. Science **290**(5500), 2323–2326 (2000)
12. Thielemans, K., Rathore, S., Engbrant, F., Razifar, P.: Device-less gating for PET/CT using PCA. In: Proceedings of the IEEE NSS/MIC, pp. 3904–3910. IEEE (2011)
13. von Siebenthal, M., Székely, G., Lomax, A.J., Cattin, P.C.: Systematic errors in respiratory gating due to intrafraction deformations of the liver. Med. Phys. **34**, 3620–3629 (2007)
14. Wachinger, C., Yigitsoy, M., Rijkhorst, E., Navab, N.: Manifold learning for image-based breathing gating in ultrasound and MRI. Med. Image Anal. **16**(4), 806–818 (2011)
15. Wang, C., Mahadevan, S.: Manifold alignment without correspondence. In: Proceedings of the IJCAI, pp. 1273–1278 (2009)
16. Yao, C., Simpson, J., Schaeffter, T., Penney, G.: Multi-view 3D echocardiography compounding based on feature consistency. Phys. Med. Biol. **56**(18), 6109 (2011)

Leveraging EAP-Sparsity for Compressed Sensing of MS-HARDI in (k, q)-Space

Jiaqi Sun, Elham Sakhaee, Alireza Entezari, and Baba C. Vemuri$^{(\boxtimes)}$

CISE Department, University of Florida, Gainesville, FL 32611, USA
vemuri@cise.ufl.edu

Abstract. Compressed Sensing (CS) for the acceleration of MR scans has been widely investigated in the past decade. Lately, considerable progress has been made in achieving similar speed ups in acquiring multi-shell high angular resolution diffusion imaging (MS-HARDI) scans. Existing approaches in this context were primarily concerned with sparse reconstruction of the diffusion MR signal $S(\mathbf{q})$ in the $\mathbf{q}$-space. More recently, methods have been developed to apply the compressed sensing framework to the 6-dimensional joint $(\mathbf{k}, \mathbf{q})$-space, thereby exploiting the redundancy in this 6D space. To guarantee accurate reconstruction from partial MS-HARDI data, the key ingredients of compressed sensing that need to be brought together are: (1) the function to be reconstructed needs to have a sparse representation, and (2) the data for reconstruction ought to be acquired in the dual domain (i.e., incoherent sensing) and (3) the reconstruction process involves a (convex) optimization.

In this paper, we present a novel approach that uses partial Fourier sensing in the 6D space of $(\mathbf{k}, \mathbf{q})$ for the reconstruction of $P(\mathbf{x}, \mathbf{r})$. The distinct feature of our approach is a sparsity model that leverages surfacelets in conjunction with total variation for the joint sparse representation of $P(\mathbf{x}, \mathbf{r})$. Thus, our method stands to benefit from the practical guarantees for accurate reconstruction from partial $(\mathbf{k}, \mathbf{q})$-space data. Further, we demonstrate significant savings in acquisition time over diffusion spectral imaging (DSI) which is commonly used as the benchmark for comparisons in reported literature. To demonstrate the benefits of this approach, we present several synthetic and real data examples.

1 Introduction

Diffusion weighted MRI is a non-invasive way to probe the axonal fiber connectivity in the body by making the MR signal sensitive to water diffusion through tissue. In diffusion weighted MRI, the water diffusion is fully characterized by the diffusion Probability Density Function (PDF) called the ensemble average propagator (EAP) [1]. Under the narrow pulse assumption, the EAP denoted by $P(\mathbf{r})$ and the diffusion signal attenuation $E(\mathbf{q})$ are related through the Fourier transform [1]:

This research was funded in part by the AFOSR FA9550-12-1-0304 and NSF CCF-1018149 grants to Alireza Entezari and the NIH grant NS066340 to Baba C. Vemuri.

© Springer International Publishing Switzerland 2015
S. Ourselin et al. (Eds.): IPMI 2015, LNCS 9123, pp. 375–386, 2015.
DOI: 10.1007/978-3-319-19992-4_29

$$P(\mathbf{r}) = \int E(\mathbf{q}) \exp(-2\pi j \mathbf{q} \cdot \mathbf{r}) d\mathbf{q} \qquad (1)$$

where, $E(\mathbf{q}) = S(\mathbf{q})/S_0$, S_0 is the diffusion signal with zero diffusion gradient, $\mathbf{q}$ is the vector along which the diffusion gradient is applied and $\mathbf{r}$ is the radial vector in the dual space defined through the Fourier relationship above. $P(\mathbf{r})$ at each voxel, captures all the information needed to perform tractography since it is well known that the peaks of this distribution correspond to the local fiber orientations.

In order to estimate the $P(\mathbf{r})$, one normally acquires the diffusion-weighted MR data by sampling $E(\mathbf{q})$ in the $\mathbf{q}$-space along different diffusion sensitizing gradient directions, $\mathbf{q}_k$ (with $1 \leq k \leq N$), spanning a unit hemisphere either over a single shell or multiple shells [2]. For every gradient direction $\mathbf{q}_k$, a full 3-D acquisition in the $\mathbf{k}$-space follows. In order to reconstruct $P(\mathbf{r})$ with a reasonable angular accuracy, a substantial number of sensitizing gradient directions, on multiple shells, are necessary (e.g., $N = 180$). The time incurred in this extensive data acquisition is the key problem making high angular resolution diffusion imaging impractical for clinical use. Very recently however, novel techniques such as multi-band imaging have been implemented, in connection with the well known connectome project, to speed up the acquisition of MS-HARDI [3]. However, these techniques do not exploit the redundancy present in the $(\mathbf{k}, \mathbf{q})$-space which is the main theme of our work in this paper. Thus, the methods presented in this paper maybe applied in addition to the multi-banding techniques to achieve further gains in acquisition time.

Compressed sensing has been applied to magnetic resonance image (MRI) acquisition quite successfully by under sampling in the $\mathbf{k}$-space (frequency space) and still achieving accurate signal reconstruction from this sparse sampling [4]. In the context of diffusion MRI acquisition, there have been some attempts at applying compressed sensing concepts to diffusion spectral imaging (DSI) [5–7]. These techniques reported to use approximately 200 gradient directions to achieve accurate diffusion MR signal reconstruction and this amounts to over forty minutes of scan time which is not practical in many situations such as for movement disorder and Autism patients. As an alternative, there has been some ground breaking work reported in literature on reducing the number of directions along which the magnetic field gradients that are applied to acquire the data in order to achieve sparse reconstruction of the signal and the EAP [8–10]. They however did not apply the compressed sensing jointly to $(\mathbf{k}, \mathbf{q})$-space.

More recently, Mani et al. [11] proposed compressed sensing in $(\mathbf{k}, \mathbf{q})$-space by jointly under-sampling $\mathbf{k}$ and $\mathbf{q}$ spaces. This was achieved by under-sampling the $\mathbf{k}$-space randomly for each direction q. Another recent development in the same vein was reported in [12], where joint $(\mathbf{k}, \mathbf{q})$-space compressed sensing is proposed while the sparsity is enforced in the $\mathbf{q}$-space. Naturally their reconstruction is again geared to recovering the $S(\mathbf{k}, \mathbf{q})$ signal, first. To achieve the EAP reconstruction their method employs the typical Fourier transform relationship between $S(\mathbf{k}, \mathbf{q})$ and $P(\mathbf{x}, \mathbf{r})$ post reconstruction of $S(\mathbf{k}, \mathbf{q})$ (using the dual spherical polar Fourier basis) and thus fails to exploit the incoherence between $P(\mathbf{x}, \mathbf{r})$ and $S(\mathbf{k}, \mathbf{q})$.

In this paper, we present a novel technique based on advances in sampling theory to alleviate this time and cost expensive acquisition process that will make MS-HARDI a more viable imaging technique in the clinic. We pose the diffusion-weighted imaging problem as a six-dimensional sampling problem in the 6-dimensional $(\mathbf{k}, \mathbf{q})$-space (i.e., (k_x, k_y, k_z) and (q_x, q_y, q_z)). The diffusion sensitized MR signal and the EAP are related through the 6-dimensional Fourier transform given by,

$$S(\mathbf{k}, \mathbf{q}) = \int_{\mathbb{R}^3} \int_{\mathbb{R}^3} P(\mathbf{x}, \mathbf{r}) \exp(-2\pi j (\mathbf{x}^t \mathbf{k} + \mathbf{q}^t \mathbf{r})) \, d\mathbf{r} \, d\mathbf{x} \qquad (2)$$

For simplicity, we omitted the scaling factor $S(\mathbf{x}, \mathbf{0})$ from the Fourier transform in the equation above.

In order to utilize the compressed sensing principles to achieve accurate reconstruction from partial data, the sparsity constraint is often enforced in the space domain while the sensing occurs in the (dual) frequency space. The notion of incoherent sensing formalizes the idea that sensing basis (e.g., Fourier) and representational basis (e.g., Dirac) are dual to each other; thus yielding full incoherence. Since $(\mathbf{k}, \mathbf{q})$ and $(\mathbf{x}, \mathbf{r})$ spaces are Fourier duals of each other and the acquisition occurs in $(\mathbf{k}, \mathbf{q})$-space, we seek to reconstruct with sparsity constraints in $(\mathbf{x}, \mathbf{r})$-space. The key distinction between our approach and existing approaches is that, enforcing sparsity in $P(\mathbf{x}, \mathbf{r})$ entitles us to leverage incoherent sensing, not only in $\mathbf{k}$, but also in the q-space simultaneously. Therefore, our approach presented here stands to benefit from practical guarantees for accurate reconstruction from partial $(\mathbf{k}, \mathbf{q})$ data. We then combine the $(\mathbf{k}, \mathbf{q})$ sampling with sparse reconstruction to exploit the principle of compressed sensing for reconstruction of $P(\mathbf{x}, \mathbf{r})$. The key ingredient enabling sparse representation for $P(\mathbf{x}, \mathbf{r})$ is accomplished using surfacelet basis. The most attractive feature of surfacelet basis is the inherent directional selectivity that leads to a sparse representation in the $\mathbf{r}$-space. For further details, see Sect. 2.2.

The rest of the paper is organized as follows, in Sect. 2, we present the theoretical formulation of the sampling and reconstruction problem. Section 3 contains several synthetic and real data experiments demonstrating the performance of our method. Finally, we wrap up in Sect. 4 with conclusions.

2   Formulation

In this section, we present the theoretical formulation for our full 6D Compressed Sensing (CS) and sparse reconstruction of the field of EAPs, $P(\mathbf{x}, \mathbf{r})$.

2.1   Compressed Sensing

The significant achievement of the CS theory [13,14] is the ability to reconstruct a function from partial data given the function has a sparse representation. The three ingredients of the CS framework necessary to guarantee accurate reconstruction are:

- **Sparsity:** The function to be reconstructed needs to be sparsely representable, possibly in some transform domain.
- **Incoherent Sensing:** The data for reconstruction must be acquired in a domain incoherent (e.g., dual) to the domain in which the function is sparsely representable.
- **Nonlinear Reconstruction:** The reconstruction problem involves an (convex) optimization process.

In the case of diffusion MR imaging, with the presence of the Fourier dual relationship between $(\mathbf{k}, \mathbf{q})$ and $(\mathbf{x}, \mathbf{r})$ space, as illustrated in Eq. (2), the above conditions will be met when a proper sparsifying transform is applied to $P(\mathbf{x}, \mathbf{r})$. In this work, we propose to use surfacelets as a choice of sparsifying basis for representation of EAPs.

2.2   The Surfacelet Transform

Measuring the diffusion of water molecules along several directions in HARDI acquisitions is an attempt to capture diffusion anisotropy. It is well known that EAPs capture this local information quite adequately. The key question then is, how best to represent the EAPs that are to be reconstructed from patially sensed data in $(\mathbf{k}, \mathbf{q})$-space? Thus, the primary goal here (in accordance with the principles of CS described above) is to find a basis in which EAPs with their inherent directional information are sparsely representable.

Wavelets, as a common choice of sparsifying transforms, lack directional sensitivity and exhibit inadequacy in efficiently capturing orientational features. As geometric generalizations to wavelets, directional decomposition methods, e.g., ridgelets [15], have been proposed to detect the orientational structures in a signal. Although these transforms can be generalized to higher dimensions, they are only optimal for 2D signals such as images. The three dimensional curvelet (3D-Curvelet) was suggested in [16] for detecting/representing directional information and geometry of the object; however, its high redundancy factor (i.e., ratio of the number of transformed coefficients to the number of signal elements) makes the problem size excessively large, hence, limits its application in diffusion MR image analysis.

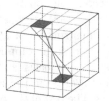

Fig. 1. Frequency partitioning of surfacelet transform

Surfacelets [17], on the other hand, are real three-dimensional transforms and were shown to be particularly efficient for sparse approximation of volumetric data [18]. They have a low redundancy factor (~ 4) and are able to capture directional information which is predominant in the $\mathbf{q}$-space diffusion sensitized MR signal.

The surfacelet transform is implemented as a combination of a multi-scale pyramid with 3D directional filter banks (3D-DFB) [17]. The basis functions are a spatial domain representation of symmetric pyramids partitioning the frequency space. Figure 1 depicts the support of one surfacelet basis in the frequency domain.

Let Ω denote the rectangular 3-D volume within which we desire to reconstruct the EAPs. Let the total number of voxels in Ω be N_s. In this work, we propose to reconstruct the EAP at each voxel in Ω on a grid within the voxel. In order to fully exploit the power of surfacelet transform, we further restrict this grid to be a cube and denote the length of the side of this cube by N_r. Let P_i ($i = 1, \ldots, N_s$) be the EAP at the ith voxel, thus, $P_i \in \mathbb{R}^{N_r \times N_r \times N_r}$. P_i can then be expressed in surfacelet basis $\varphi_m^{(l)}(.)$, corresponding to different scales (l) and spectral directions (m) as:

$$P_i(\mathbf{r}) = \sum_{m,l} c_{m,l} \varphi_m^{(l)}(\mathbf{r}) \tag{3}$$

Let $\mathbf{c}_i := [c_{m,l}]$ be the vector formed by surfacelet coefficients of the ith voxel and denote the surfacelet transform with $\mathcal{S}$. We can then write $\mathbf{c}_i = \mathcal{S}(P_i)$ and seek for a sparse coefficient vector by minimizing ℓ_1 norm of $\mathbf{c}_i$ for each voxel, as described in Sect. 2.3. When we represent the voxel location by $\mathbf{x}$, surfacelet transform of $P(\mathbf{x}, \mathbf{r})$ is essentially $\mathcal{S}(P_i)$ applied on all N_s voxels separately and simultaneously.

The low redundancy factor along with tree-structured (fast) implementation makes the surfacelets practically suitable in dMRI applications, while directional decomposition makes it well-suited for recovering the geometry of EAPs.

2.3 Problem Formulation

Equipped with the sparsifying ability of the surfacelet transform upon EAPs, we are now able to apply the CS theory to achieve direct reconstruction of EAPs from a set of partial samples of $S(\mathbf{k}, \mathbf{q})$. Denote the measured $(\mathbf{k}, \mathbf{q})$-space data over Ω by S and let $\mathscr{F}_u$ be the undersampled 6-D Fourier Transform. We formulate the EAP reconstruction problem as the following optimization problem:

$$\hat{P} = \arg\min_{P} \left\{ \frac{1}{2} \|\mathscr{F}_u(P) - S\|_F^2 + \mu \sum_{i=1}^{N_s} \|\mathcal{S}(P_i)\|_1 + \gamma \|P\|_{TV_s} \right\} \tag{4}$$

where, μ and γ control the balance between the sparsity regularization and the spatial smoothness regularization. $\mathcal{S}(P_i)$ denotes the coefficients obtained by applying the surfacelet transform to the EAP at the ith voxel in Ω.

In the above objective function, the l_1 norm of the surfacelet coefficients is minimized which promotes sparsity [13,14] in the surfacelet representation. In addition, we leverage the sparsity of the gradients in the field of EAPs via a total variation (TV) penalty term. The TV norm over the field of EAPs, where each EAP is represented by a volume of size N_s, is denoted by $\|\cdot\|_{TV_s}$ and is defined as follows. First, let us define the total variation of the kth component of an EAP, $k = 1, \ldots, N_r^3$, over Ω. In this context, we adopt the anisotropic TV norm in our formulation. Represent the kth component of an EAP in the voxel (r, s, t) of Ω by $P_{(r,s,t)}^k$, and represent the 3D volume formed by all of $P_{(r,s,t)}^k$ by P^k.

P^k can be regarded as a discrete scalar valued function defined on a 3-D rectangular grid Ω, $P^k : \Omega \to \mathbb{R}$. Therefore, the anisotropic total variation of P^k can be defined as:

$$TV_{aniso_{3,1}}(P^k) = \sum_{r,s,t} \left\{ \left| P^k_{(r+1,s,t)} - P^k_{(r,s,t)} \right| + \left| P^k_{(r,s+1,t)} - P^k_{(r,s,t)} \right| + \left| P^k_{(r,s,t+1)} - P^k_{(r,s,t)} \right| \right\}$$

(5)

Then, the total variation of P over the spatial domain can be defined as follows:
$$\|P\|_{TV_s} = \left\{ \sum_{k=1}^{N_r^3} \left[TV_{aniso_{3,1}}(P^k) \right]^\alpha \right\}^{\frac{1}{\alpha}} . \text{ In this work, we use } \alpha = 1.$$

2.4 Solution Using the Split Bregman Algorithm

We solve the optimization problem in Eq. (4) by employing the well known Split Bregman method [19]. The problem in Eq. (4) can now be reformulated as:

$$\hat{P} = \arg\min_P \left\{ \frac{1}{2} \|\mathscr{F}_u(P) - S\|_F^2 + \mu \sum_{i=1}^{N_s} \|\mathbf{c}_i\|_1 + \gamma \|P\|_{TV_s} \right\}$$

$$s.\,t.\ P_i = \mathcal{S}^\star(\mathbf{c}_i),\ \ i = 1,\ldots,N_s$$

(6)

where, $\mathcal{S}^\star$ denotes the inverse surfacelet transform and P_i is defined as in Sect. 2.3. We can now convert this problem into an unconstrained one by introducing the Lagrange multipliers λ_i:

$$\hat{P} = \arg\min_P \left\{ \frac{1}{2} \|\mathscr{F}_u(P) - S\|_F^2 + \mu \sum_{i=1}^{N_s} \|\mathbf{c}_i\|_1 + \gamma \|P\|_{TV_s} + \sum_{i=1}^{N_s} \frac{\lambda_i}{2} \|P_i - \mathcal{S}^\star(\mathbf{c}_i)\|_F^2 \right\}.$$

(7)

In this work we choose to assign $\lambda_1 = \lambda_2 = \cdots = \lambda_{N_s} = \lambda$, then, Eq. (7) is simplified to:

$$\hat{P} = \arg\min_P \left\{ \frac{1}{2} \|\mathscr{F}_u(P) - S\|_F^2 + \mu \sum_{i=1}^{N_s} \|\mathbf{c}_i\|_1 + \gamma \|P\|_{TV_s} + \frac{\lambda}{2} \sum_{i=1}^{N_s} \|P_i - \mathcal{S}^\star(\mathbf{c}_i)\|_F^2 \right\}.$$

(8)

The Split Bregman algorithm is used to find the optimal solution to the above problem through the following iterations, where t denotes the iteration index:

$$(P^{(t+1)}, \mathbf{c}_i^{(t+1)}) = \arg\min_{P,\mathbf{c}_i} \left\{ \frac{1}{2} \|\mathscr{F}_u(P) - S\|_F^2 + \mu \sum_{i=1}^{N_s} \|\mathbf{c}_i\|_1 + \gamma \|P\|_{TV_s} \right.$$

$$\left. + \frac{\lambda}{2} \sum_{i=1}^{N_s} \|P_i - \mathcal{S}^\star(\mathbf{c}_i) - \mathbf{b}_i^{(t)}\|_F^2 \right\}$$

(9)

$$\mathbf{b}_i^{(t+1)} = \mathbf{b}_i^{(t)} + (\mathcal{S}^\star(\mathbf{c}_i^{(t+1)}) - P_i^{(t+1)})$$

$$\text{for each } i = 1,\ldots,N_s$$

(10)

The minimization in (9) can be performed by iteratively minimizing with respect to P and c_i separately. The entire algorithm is summarized below.

Algorithm.
Split Bregman for EAP reconstruction from partial $(\mathbf{k}, \mathbf{q})$ data

---

Input: Partial $(\mathbf{k}, \mathbf{q})$-space data S
Output: Reconstructed EAP
  Initialization: $P^{(0)} = \mathscr{F}^{-1}(S^0)$
  while $\|\mathscr{F}_u(P^{(t)}) - S\|_F^2 < tol$ **do**
    for $n = 1$ **to** N **do**
      $P^{(t+1)} =$
        $\arg\min_P \left\{ \frac{1}{2} \|\mathscr{F}_u(P) - S\|_F^2 + \gamma \|P\|_{TV_s} + \frac{\lambda}{2} \sum_{i=1}^{N_s} \|P_i - S^\star(c_i^{(t)}) - b_i^{(t)}\|_F^2 \right\}$
      for $i = 1$ **to** N_s **do**
        $c_i^{(t+1)} = \arg\min_{c_i} \left\{ \mu \|c_i\|_1 + \frac{\lambda}{2} \|P_i^{(t+1)} - S^\star(c_i) - b_i^{(t)}\|_F^2 \right\}$
      end for
    end for
    for $i = 1$ **to** N_s **do**
      $b_i^{(t+1)} = b_i^{(t)} + (S^\star(c_i^{(t+1)}) - P_i^{(t+1)})$
    end for
    $t = t + 1$
  end while

As illustrated above, we initialize P to be the inverse Fourier Transform of the zero-filled partial data S (by filling the unkown value to be 0), denoted by S^0. The number of inner iterations in the above algorithm N is set to be 1 as suggested in [19].

3   Experimental Results

To demonstrate the performance of our approach, we present experimental results on several synthetic and real datasets in this section.

We use conventional diffusion spectral imaging (DSI) data as the ground truth for comparisons of the reconstruction performance. The $(\mathbf{k}, \mathbf{q})$-space data, acquired for the connectome project, that is composed of 515 diffusion weighted images was considered as fully sampled data. We perform the undersampling of the DSI data with a radial line sampling scheme. It is one of the most widely used schemes for partial Fourier sensing [4], and the theoretical justification for it from a CS perspective was presented in [20].

The undersampling of the entire $(\mathbf{k}, \mathbf{q})$-space is achieved by applying 3-D radial line sampling in $\mathbf{k}$ and $\mathbf{q}$ spaces respectively. We conducted experiments at various rates of undersampling in the joint $(\mathbf{k}, \mathbf{q})$-space. In addition to that, $\mathbf{q}$-space-only and $\mathbf{k}$-space-only undersampling were also performed, respectively, for comparisons.

3.1 Synthetic Data Experiments

We synthesized a fully sampled DSI dataset, $\hat{S}(\mathbf{x}, \mathbf{q})$, over a grid of size $12 \times 12 \times 12$. Each slice consisted of two straight "fiber" bundles crossing each other in the center and a circular "fiber" bundle crossing with the two straight ones at the corners. To fully demonstrate the performance of our method on data sets with complex local geometry, we further increased the complexity of the data set by making the two straight "fiber" bundles gradually rotate throughout the 12 slices. The diffusion signals were generated using a mixture of Gaussian functions, each being a rotated version of a Gaussian distribution function with zero mean and diagonal covariance matrix Cov = diag{20, 20, 400}. The $(\mathbf{k}, \mathbf{q})$-space data was generated from the $(\mathbf{x}, \mathbf{q})$-space data through a 3-D Fourier Transform (relating $\mathbf{x}$ to $\mathbf{k}$) for each gradient direction $\mathbf{q}$.

We applied conventional DSI reconstruction on the fully sampled synthetic data, to obtain the ground truth field of EAPs. The performance of the reconstruction was quantitatively evaluated by the normalized sum-of-squares error (NSSE) between the reconstructed EAP ($P_{REC}(\mathbf{x}, \mathbf{r})$) and the ground truth EAP ($P_{GT}(\mathbf{x}, \mathbf{r})$), defined as NSSE $= \frac{\sum_{\mathbf{x}, \mathbf{r}} \|P_{GT}(\mathbf{x}, \mathbf{r}) - P_{REC}(\mathbf{x}, \mathbf{r})\|_2^2}{\sum_{\mathbf{x}, \mathbf{r}} \|P_{GT}(\mathbf{x}, \mathbf{r})\|_2^2}$. We tested our method at various undersampling levels (i.e., partial Fourier sensing rates). At each level, three different undersampling schemes were performed on fully sampled data, namely joint $(\mathbf{k}, \mathbf{q})$-space undersampling, $\mathbf{q}$-space only undersmapling and $\mathbf{k}$-space only undersampling. The reconstruction accuracy for each combination of undersampling level and scheme is computed as the average of 15 repetitions. To demonstrate the advantages of partial sensing in the joint 6-D $(\mathbf{k}, \mathbf{q})$-space compared to partial $\mathbf{k}$ or partial $\mathbf{q}$ sensing, we compared the reconstruction accuracy of these three undersampling schemes at identical sampling rates.

To assess the performance of the proposed method in the presence of noise, we carried out another experiment where various levels of Rician noise was added to the synthetic $(\mathbf{x}, \mathbf{q})$-space data. The noise level is measured by SNR, defined as SNR $= E/\sigma$, E being the mean magnitude of the noise-free signal and σ the standard deviation of the noise. We analyzed the accuracy of reconstruction measured by NSSE, with various undersampling rates and undersampling schemes.

Quantitative results of the reconstruction on partial data (noise-free) with various undersampling rates for different undersampling schemes are presented in Fig. 2(a) and the effects of noise on reconstruction accuracy are shown in Fig. 2(b). As shown in the plots, in both noise-free and noisy case, the proposed compressed sensing in joint $(\mathbf{k}, \mathbf{q})$-space has a better EAP reconstruction accuracy than when undersampling is performed in $\mathbf{k}$-space or $\mathbf{q}$-space only. And with as little as 10–15 % of the original data, our method is able to reconstruct the EAPs with very high accuracy even in the presence of noise. As evident from Fig. 2(b), at a moderate level of noise, there is little degradation in the reconstruction accuracy compared to the noise-free case, and at a high level of noise, our method still maintains satisfactory performance. Since NSSE is depicted using a log scale, the reader is cautioned about larger values of NSSE being compressed.

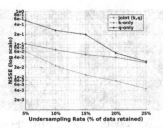

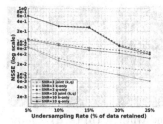

(a) Reconstruction accuracy on noise-free data

(b) Reconstruction accuracy in presence of various levels of noise

Fig. 2. Quantitative EAP reconstruction results for synthetic data.

To further assess the results visually, we plotted the reconstructed EAPs as well as the ground truth EAPs at $\mathbf{r} = 4.5$ for each voxel and showcase selected slices below. In Fig. 3, for slice #12, we show the ground truth EAP field and reconstructed EAP fields with various undersampling schemes from 15 % of the full noise-free DSI data. Considering the complexity of the data and the low undersampling rate, our method with joint $(\mathbf{k}, \mathbf{q})$-space undersampling obtained a reconstruction fairly close to the ground truth. While in the $\mathbf{k}$-only undersampling case, false crossings appear at voxels with no crossings (as highlighted in green boxes). In the $\mathbf{q}$-only case, however, the recovered EAP profiles appear to be of poor quality as depicted in the region marked with a red box. In Fig. 4, we present a visualization of the EAP reconstruction from slice #7 of the noisy data with $SNR = 10$, reconstructed with 15 % of the full DSI data. Compared to $\mathbf{k}$-only and $\mathbf{q}$-only cases, the joint $(\mathbf{k}, \mathbf{q})$-space undersampling yields more accurate reconstructions with respect to the lobe orientations as well as the presence of crossings (representative regions are highlighted in colored boxes).

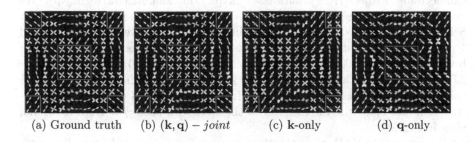

(a) Ground truth   (b) $(\mathbf{k}, \mathbf{q}) - joint$ (c) k-only   (d) q-only

Fig. 3. Visualization of EAP reconstruction for synthetic noise-free data. Ground truth EAP field and reconstructed EAP fields with different undersampling schemes at a rate of 15 % for slice #12 of the noise-free data (Color figure online).

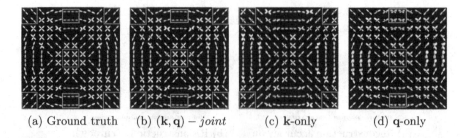

(a) Ground truth   (b) $(\mathbf{k}, \mathbf{q}) - joint$ (c) **k**-only   (d) **q**-only

Fig. 4. Visualization of EAP reconstruction for noise contaminated synthetic data. Ground truth EAP field and reconstructed EAP fields with different undersampling schemes at a rate of 15 % for slice #7 of the noisy data with SNR=10 (Color figure online).

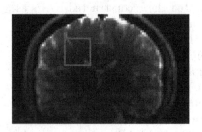

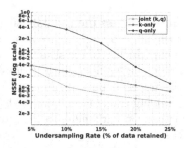

Fig. 5. Coronal view of slice #57 of the real dataset with ROI presented in the red box (Color figure online).

Fig. 6. Quantatitive EAP reconstruction results for real data.

3.2   Real Data Experiments

Real datasets used in the experiments were obtained from the MGH-USC Human Connectome Project(HCP) database (https://ida.loni.usc.edu/login.jsp). We evaluated the proposed method on data acquired using the DSI scheme on a Seimens 3T Connectom scanner, including 514 diffusion weighted images and 1 non-diffusion weighted image. The scan parameters are as follows: maximum b-value $b_{max} = 10,000\,s/mm^2$, TR $= 5900.0$ ms, TE $= 77.0$ ms, pixel size X $= 2.0$ mm, Y $= 2.0$ mm and slice thickness 2.0 mm, resulting in a $104 \times 104 \times 55$ volume. We picked a $12 \times 12 \times 12$ region from the dataset as our ROI for reconstruction and show the intersection of the ROI with slice #57 from a coronal view in Fig. 5.

We present the EAP reconstruction accuracy for various undersampling rates in Fig. 6 and visualization of the EAP fields for the coronal slice #57 (slice #11 in ROI) in Fig. 7. From Fig. 6 it is evident that the joint $(\mathbf{k}, \mathbf{q})$-space undersampling leads to higher accuracy in terms of NSSE over the **k**-only and **q**-only undersampling. The graph depicts that with 10–15 % of the fully sampled data our method yields high fidelity reconstruction of the EAPs. This leads to an acceleration by a factor of 6.7–10 over the standard DSI acquisition. From a comparison of the three reconstructed EAP fields with ground truth in Fig. 7, it is evident that the joint $(\mathbf{k}, \mathbf{q})$-space undersamping method correctly recovered most of the crossings and fiber orientations. However, with $\mathbf{k}$-only undersampling, false crossings and incorrect recovery of EAP lobe orientations are evident in several regions (highlighted in colored boxes). Further, with $\mathbf{q}$-only undersampling, spurious lobes are introduced leading to erroneous orientation information.

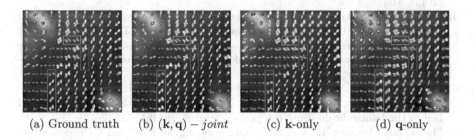

(a) Ground truth   (b) $(\mathbf{k}, \mathbf{q}) - joint$ (c) $\mathbf{k}$-only   (d) $\mathbf{q}$-only

Fig. 7. Visualization of EAP reconstruction for real data. Ground truth EAP field and reconstructed EAP fields with different undersampling schemes at rate 15 % for slice #11 in the ROI of real data (Color figure online)

In summary, through synthetic and real data experiments we have demonstrated that our method of direct reconstruction of EAPs from CS in joint $(\mathbf{k}, \mathbf{q})$-space yields superior results in comparison to CS applied to either $\mathbf{q}$-space or $\mathbf{k}$-space in isolation.

4   Conclusion

In this paper we presented a novel technique for direct reconstruction of the field of EAPs, $P(\mathbf{x}, \mathbf{r})$, from partial sampling in the 6D joint $(\mathbf{k}, \mathbf{q})$-space. The key distinguishing feature of our method from earlier reported works in literature is that we exploit the principle of Compressed Sensing which states that sensing and reconstruction ought to occur in mutually dual spaces. Consequently, since the data acquisition in diffusion MRI occurs in $(\mathbf{k}, \mathbf{q})$-space, the reconstruction ought to be performed in the $(\mathbf{x}, \mathbf{r})$-space. Moreover, using the Fourier transform relationship between $P(\mathbf{x}, \mathbf{r})$ and $S(\mathbf{k}, \mathbf{q})$, it is natural to exploit the aforementioned duality condition and seek a sparse representation of $P(\mathbf{x}, \mathbf{r})$. We achieved this sparsity through a surfacelet basis which are well known for their directional selectivity in signal/image processing literature. We presented reconstruction results for synthetic and real data demonstrating the performance of our algorithm. Our results show that we can achieve high fidelity of reconstruction of $P(\mathbf{x}, \mathbf{r})$ using just 10–15 % of the samples used in a full DSI acquisition. This leads to an acceleration rate of 6.7–10 in acquisition time thus making MS-HARDI a clinically viable diagnostic imaging tool. Our future work will focus on exploring benefits to be acrrued from different sampling schemes in the joint $(\mathbf{k}, \mathbf{q})$-space.

References

1. Callaghan, P.T.: Principles of Nuclear Magnetic Resonance Microscopy. Oxford University Press, Oxford (1991)
2. Tuch, D.S.: Q-ball imaging. Mag. Res. Med. (MRM) **52**, 1358–1372 (2004)
3. Ugurbil, K., Xu, J., et al.: Pushing spatial and temporal resolution for functional and diffusion MRI in the human connectome project. NeuroImage **80**, 80–104 (2013). Mapping the Connectome
4. Lustig, M., Donoho, D., Pauly, J.: Sparse MRI: the application of compressed sensing for rapid MR imaging. Mag. Res. Med. (MRM) **58**, 1182–1195 (2007)
5. Landman, B.A., Wan, H., Bogovic, J., van Zijl, P., Bazin, P.L., Prince, J.: Accelerated compressed sensing of diffusion-inferred intra-voxel structure through adaptive refinement. In: ISMRM (2010)
6. Lee, N., Singh, M.: Compressed sensing based DSI. In: ISMRM (2010)
7. Menzel, M., Khare, K., King, K.F., Tao, X., Hardy, C.J., Marinelli, L.: Accelerated DSI in the human brain using compressed sensing. In: ISMRM (2010)
8. Merlet, S.L., Deriche, R.: Continuous diffusion signal, EAP and ODF estimation via compressive sensing in diffusion MRI. Med. Image Anal. **17**, 556–572 (2013)
9. Merlet, S., Caruyer, E., Deriche, R.: Parametric dictionary learning for modeling EAP and ODF in diffusion MRI. In: Ayache, N., Delingette, H., Golland, P., Mori, K. (eds.) MICCAI 2012, Part III. LNCS, vol. 7512, pp. 10–17. Springer, Heidelberg (2012)
10. Michailovich, O.V., Rathi, Y., Dolui, S.: Spatially regularized compressed sensing for high angular resolution diffusion imaging. IEEE Trans. Med. Imaging **30**, 1100–1115 (2011)
11. Mani, M., Jacob, M., Guidon, A., Magnotta, V., Zhong, J.: Acceleration of high angular and spatial resolution diffusion imaging using compressed sensing with multichannel spiral data. Mag. Res. Med. (MRM) **73**, 126–138 (2015)
12. Cheng, J., Shen, D., Yap, P.T.: Joint k-q space compressed sensing for accelerated multi-shell acquisition and reconstruction of the diffusion signal and ensemble average propagator. In: ISMRM, p. 664 (2014)
13. Donoho, D.: Compressed sensing. IEEE Trans. Inf. Theory **52**, 1289–1306 (2006)
14. Candès, E., Tao, T.: Near-optimal signal recovery from random projections: universal encoding strategies? IEEE Trans. Inf. Theory **52**, 5406–5425 (2006)
15. Do, M.N., Vetterli, M.: Image denoising using orthonormal finite ridgelet transform. In: International Symposium on Optical Science and Technology, pp. 831–842. International Society of Optics and Photonics (2000)
16. Ying, L., Demanet, L., Candes, E.: 3D discrete curvelet transform. In: Optics & Photonics 2005, pp. 591413–591413. International Society of Optics and Photonics (2005)
17. Lu, Y.M., Do, M.N.: Multidimensional directional filter banks and surfacelets. IEEE Trans. Image Process. **16**, 918–931 (2007)
18. Xu, X., Sakhaee, E., Entezari, A.: Volumetric data reduction in a compressed sensing framework. Comput. Graph. Forum (CGF) **33**, 111–120 (2014). Special Issue on EuroVIS
19. Goldstein, T., Osher, S.: The split bregman method for l1-regularized problems. SIAM J. Imaging Sci. **2**, 323–343 (2009)
20. Willett, R.M.: Smooth sampling trajectories for sparse recovery in MRI. In: Proceedings of the 8th International Symposium on Biomedical Imaging, ISBI 2011, Chicago, Illinois, USA, pp. 1044–1047, 30 March – 2 April 2011

Multi-stage Biomarker Models for Progression Estimation in Alzheimer's Disease

Alexander Schmidt-Richberg[1]([✉]), Ricardo Guerrero[1], Christian Ledig[1], Helena Molina-Abril[2], Alejandro F. Frangi[2], Daniel Rueckert[1], and on behalf of the Alzheimers Disease Neuroimaging Initiative

[1] Biomedical Image Analysis Group, Imperial College London, London, UK
a.schmidt-richberg@imperial.ac.uk
[2] Center for Computational Imaging and Simulation Technologies (CISTIB), University of Sheffield, Sheffield, UK

Abstract. The estimation of disease progression in Alzheimer's disease (AD) based on a vector of quantitative biomarkers is of high interest to clinicians, patients, and biomedical researchers alike. In this work, quantile regression is employed to learn statistical models describing the evolution of such biomarkers. Two separate models are constructed using (1) subjects that progress from a cognitively normal (CN) stage to mild cognitive impairment (MCI) and (2) subjects that progress from MCI to AD during the observation window of a longitudinal study. These models are then automatically combined to develop a multi-stage disease progression model for the whole disease course. A probabilistic approach is derived to estimate the current disease progress (DP) and the disease progression rate (DPR) of a given individual by fitting any acquired biomarkers to these models. A particular strength of this method is that it is applicable even if individual biomarker measurements are missing for the subject. Employing cognitive scores and image-based biomarkers, the presented method is used to estimate DP and DPR for subjects from the Alzheimer's Disease Neuroimaging Initiative (ADNI). Further, the potential use of these values as features for different classification tasks is demonstrated. For example, accuracy of 64 % is reached for CN vs. MCI vs. AD classification.

1 Introduction

Alzheimer's disease (AD) is a progressive neurodegenerative condition and the most common form of dementia. Patients that show first symptoms like general memory loss are usually diagnosed as suffering from Mild Cognitive Impairment (MCI), an early stage of dementia. Later, throughout the disease, these symptoms are followed by behavioural changes and further cognitive and functional decline. Patients become less able to perform simple tasks and increasingly depend on carers' support. However, an objective staging of the disease is non-trivial due to the considerable variability in the patient's age at disease onset and the individual rate of progression [3]. Estimating the current disease severity

© Springer International Publishing Switzerland 2015
S. Ourselin et al. (Eds.): IPMI 2015, LNCS 9123, pp. 387–398, 2015.
DOI: 10.1007/978-3-319-19992-4_30

and the future rate of progression is of interest for patients and caregivers but also has potential to improve clinical trials as more homogeneous study groups can be recruited.

Most existing approaches with this aim employ the results of cognitive tests like the Clinical Dementia Rating – Sum of Boxes (CDR-SB) as biomarkers to characterise disease progression. Many of those methods (see e.g. [5] for a detailed overview) use Markov transition models and Cox proportional hazard models to estimate disease progression. However, as detailed in [5], the main limitations of these methods are "the use of a limited number of health states to capture events related to disease progression over time", and the fact that "a single symptom, such as cognition, is not able to characterise AD progression". Therefore, additional meaningful biomarkers that better describe anatomical changes can be quantified from imaging data. For example, [4,12] use an event-based model to determine the order in which CSF-, image- and cognition-based biomarkers become abnormal and then employ this information to assign a subject to one of several discrete disease stages.

As modelling disease progression by a number of discrete stages is a strong simplification, some approaches have been developed that acknowledge the course of disease as a continuous process. For example, Yang et al. [10] assume an exponential-shaped trajectory of the ADAS score. The authors then estimate a *time shift* γ indicating the disease progress of a subject by fitting its ADAS scores to this curve. Similarly, Delor et al. [2] compute a *disease onset time* by adjusting subjects according to their CDR-SB score.

The approach presented in this work builds upon these methods. Here, quantile regression is used to estimate typical trajectories of clinical biomarkers (see Sect. 2). In detail, two models are trained, one for the transition from CN to MCI and one for the MCI-to-AD conversion. These models are then combined to a multi-stage model for the whole course of the disease. Thereafter, a probabilistic model is derived that allows the estimation of a subjects current disease progress and rate of progression based on measured biomarker values. The approach is flexible with regard to the considered biomarkers, which can be based, for example, on cognitive scores, neuroimaging, or both. Moreover, missing measurements are handled in a natural way, this means, the approach can be employed even if the set of observed biomarkers is incomplete. The proposed disease progress estimation is evaluated in Sect. 3 using clinical data. Its applicability for different classification tasks is demonstrated at the end of this section.

2   Methods

To model disease progression, the existence of a set of biomarker values y_{sv}^b acquired from multiple subjects $s \in S = \{1, \dots, n_S\}$ during multiple visits $v \in V_s$ is assumed. Here, $b \in B_{sv}$ denotes the index of the biomarker. Each biomarker vector is associated with the time $t_{sv} \in T$ of acquisition, measured in days after the first (baseline) visit, as well as the diagnosis d_{sv} that was given during each visit. The number of visits can vary for each subject, $V_s \subseteq V = \{1, \dots, n_V\}$. Also, the biomarkers acquired at each visit might differ, such that $B_{sv} \subseteq B = \{1, \dots, n_B\}$.

In the training phase of the presented method, characteristic trajectories of biomarkers in the course of disease progression are learned based on a number of training subjects (Sect. 2.1). These models are then employed in the test phase to estimate how far and how fast test subjects have progressed along the disease trajectory (Sect. 2.2).

2.1   Model Learning

Aim of the model training phase is to learn the temporal trajectory of biomarker evolution throughout the disease by determining the probability that a certain biomarker b has a value y^b at a specified time point. More technically, each measured biomarker value y^b_{sv} is understood as an observation of a response variable Y^b at a *disease progress (DP)* $p_{sv} \in \mathbb{R}$ (the explanatory variable or covariate). The conditional distribution of Y^b given p is then denoted by $f_{Y^b}(y|p)$.

A *disease progression model* $\mathcal{M}(p)$ comprises the distributions of all biomarkers in B on a domain $P \subset \mathbb{R}$, such that $\mathcal{M}(p) = \{\mathcal{M}^1(p), \ldots, \mathcal{M}^{n_B}(p)\}$ with $\mathcal{M}^b(p) := f_{Y^b}(y|p)$ for $p \in P$. Another way of representing the model is by its q-quantile functions $y^b_q(p)$, which can be derived directly from $f_{Y^b}(y|p)$ (for example, the median trajectory is denoted by $y^b_{0.5}(p)$).

The learning of a model consists of three main steps. First, the training subjects have to be temporally aligned to establish correspondences between the time points of observation. Progression models are then estimated using quantile regression to learn the probability distributions $f_{Y^b}(y|p)$. Since temporal alignment is based on the point of conversion from either CN to MCI or MCI to AD, two separate models are learned. These two models are then combined to a multi-stage progression model.

Temporal Alignment of the Training Data. Temporal alignment aims at associating the time points t_{sv} of biomarker acquisition to the corresponding DP p_{sv}. In detail, the goal is to find a strictly monotonically increasing *time warp* function $\tau(t)$ that maps the subject-specific acquisition time $t_{sv} \in T$ to the population-based disease progress $p_{sv} \in P$, such that $p_{sv} = \tau(t_{sv})$. During model training, the time point t^0_s at which the clinical diagnosis changes and thus indicates transition to a more severe disease state is set to $p = 0$, that means

$$p_{sv} = \tau(t^0_s; t_{sv}) := t_{sv} - t^0_s. \tag{1}$$

For this reason, a specific model is trained for each transition phase (here, CN-to-MCI and MCI-to-AD). To identify t^0_s, the visits v^* and v^{**} with the last CN (MCI) and the first MCI (AD) diagnosis are determined. The time point of conversion is then assumed to be the average of these two visits, i.e. $t^0_s := 0.5 \cdot (t_{sv^*} + t_{sv^{**}})$.

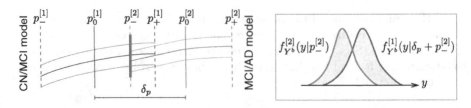

Fig. 1. Approach for automatically determining the optimal model offset δ_p.

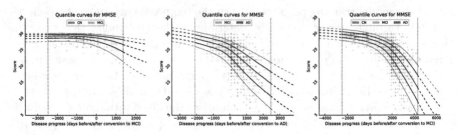

Fig. 2. Example of the model composition. First, separate models are trained for CN-to-MCI and MCI-to-AD converters. An optimal offset between these models is then automatically determined and model training is repeated with the whole set of samples (Colour figure online).

Learning Disease Progression Model. The conditional distributions f_{Y^b} are learned independently for each biomarker using quantile regression via *vector generalised additive models* (VGAMs) [11]. In contrast to logistic or exponential regression [10], VGAMs do not depend on prior assumptions on the functional form for each predictor variable other than their smoothness. However, the domain P of $\mathcal{M}^b(p)$ is limited to the progress interval contained in the sample set. This means P is given by $P = [p_-, p_+]$, with $p_- := \min_{s,v}(p_{sv})$ and $p_+ := \max_{s,v}(p_{sv})$ being the earliest and latest observed DP, respectively. Therefore, the models are extrapolated by a linear extension of the underlying predictor functions (see [11] for details) and $P = \mathbb{R}$ is assumed in the following.

Model Composition. To combine the CN/MCI and MCI/AD models, an optimal offset δ_p is determined by optimising the similarity of the models in the overlapping region. Given δ_p, the end point $p_+^{[1]}$ of the CN/MCI model $\mathcal{M}^{[1]}$ corresponds to $p_+^{[1]} - \delta_p$ in the MCI/AD model $\mathcal{M}^{[2]}$. Similarly, $\mathcal{M}^{[2]}(p_-^{[2]})$ corresponds to $\mathcal{M}^{[1]}(\delta_p + p_-^{[2]})$ (cf. Fig. 1). The quality of the fit is quantified by

$$\hat{\delta}_p := \operatorname*{argmax}_{\delta_p} \frac{1}{2}\left[\left(\mathcal{M}^{[1]}(p_+^{[1]}) - \mathcal{M}^{[2]}(p_+^{[1]} - \delta_p)\right) + \left(\mathcal{M}^{[1]}(\delta_p + p_-^{[2]}) - \mathcal{M}^{[2]}(p_-^{[2]})\right)\right]$$

with $\mathcal{M}^{[1]}(p) - \mathcal{M}^{[2]}(q) = \frac{1}{|B|}\sum_{b\in B}\int f_{Y^b}^{[1]}(y|p) - f_{Y^b}^{[2]}(y|q)\ dy$ being the area between the corresponding density functions (averaged over all biomarkers).

After determining $\hat{\delta}_p$, the multi-stage model is retrained using the full set of samples with $p = 0$ defined as the point of conversion from CN to MCI (see Fig. 2).

2.2 Progress Estimation

Once the disease progression model is built, the aim is to estimate the progress of any given subject. However, the point of conversion t_s^0 is usually unknown and thus Eq. (1) cannot be employed. Progress estimation is accomplished by finding the most likely time warp $\tau(t)$ that optimally fits the evolution of the biomarkers, as measured from the patient, into the progression model $\mathcal{M}$.

Let $\boldsymbol{t}_s = (t_{s1}, \ldots, t_{snv})^T$ be the vector containing the time points of all visits of subject s and $\tau(\boldsymbol{t}_s) = (\tau(t_{s1}), \ldots, \tau(t_{snv}))^T$. Let further $\boldsymbol{y}_s = (\boldsymbol{y}_{sv})_{v \in V_s}$ be the biomarker vector measured for s, with $\boldsymbol{y}_{sv} = (y_{sv}^b)_{b \in B_{sv}}$ denoting the values acquired at visit v. Based on $\boldsymbol{t}_s$, the most probable time warp $\hat{\tau}_s$ given $\boldsymbol{y}_s$ is determined by maximising the logarithm of the likelihood function $\mathcal{L}(\tau(\boldsymbol{t}_s) \mid \boldsymbol{y}_s)$. This means

$$\hat{\tau}_s := \underset{\tau}{\operatorname{argmax}} \ \log \mathcal{L}(\tau(\boldsymbol{t}_s) \mid \boldsymbol{y}_s) = \underset{\tau}{\operatorname{argmax}} \ \log f_{\boldsymbol{Y}}(\boldsymbol{y}_s \mid \tau(\boldsymbol{t}_s)) \tag{2}$$

with $\boldsymbol{Y} = (Y^1, \ldots, Y^{n_B})$. The joint probability of all observations y_{sv}^b is then

$$f_{\boldsymbol{Y}}(\boldsymbol{y}_s \mid \tau(\boldsymbol{t}_s)) = \prod_{v \in V_s} f_{\boldsymbol{Y}}(\boldsymbol{y}_{sv} \mid \tau(t_{sv})) = \prod_{v \in V_s} \prod_{b \in B_{sv}} f_{Y^b}(y_{sv}^b \mid \tau(t_{sv})) .$$

whereat all biomarker observations are assumed to be independent of each other.

A simple *translational time warp* parameterisation is given by

$$\tau(p^0; t) := p^0 + t. \tag{3}$$

Here, the *disease progress* (DP) $p^0 \in \mathbb{R}$ is an offset that indicates how far the subject has progressed in the course of disease at the time point of the first visit. However, this simple model cannot accommodate for different rates of progression, which are known to exist between subjects [3]. If $|V_s| > 1$, the extended *affine time warp* definition

$$\tau(p^0, r; t) := p^0 + rt \tag{4}$$

can be employed, where $r \in \mathbb{R}^+$ is a scaling factor indicating the *disease progression rate* (DPR). The optimal values $\hat{p}_s^0$ and $\hat{r}_s$ for DP and DPR are determined by maximising Eq. (2) over all p^0 and r, i.e. $\hat{\tau}_s(\cdot) \hat{=} \tau(\hat{p}_s^0, \hat{r}; \cdot)$. In general, more complex time warps definitions are possible.

3 Experiments and Results

This section evaluates the presented approach using data from the Alzheimer's Disease Neuroimaging Initiative (ADNI, Sect. 3.1). First, in Sect. 3.2, progression models are trained for all available biomarkers. These models are then employed to estimate DP and DPR. The applicability of these values for different classification tasks is shown in Sect. 3.3.

3.1   Materials

For this study, all subjects enrolled in either ADNI1, ADNIGO or ADNI2 (up to an acquisition date of 30/01/2014) were considered. For model training, all subjects were selected that converted either from CN to MCI (60 subjects) or from MCI to AD (248 subjects). The number of available biomarkers can vary between the training subjects (see below). To obtain consistent results in all experiments, the test set consists of the subjects with a stable diagnosis for which all biomarkers are present at baseline (bl), month 12 (m12) and month 24 (m24) visit. In total, these are 158 (88 male, 70 female) subjects classified as cognitive normal (CN), 90 (50 male, 40 female) patients with early MCI (EMCI), 94 (63 male, 31 female) with late MCI (LMCI), and 88 (45 male, 43 female) patients diagnosed with AD.

The set B of biomarkers considered in this work consists of cognitive scores and image-based features as detailed in the following. Biomarker values are corrected for age using a linear regression on the baseline samples of all control subjects.

Cognitive Scores B^{cog}: A number of cognitive tests are performed by subjects participating in the ADNI study at each visit. The achieved scores are used as biomarkers. These tests include the Minimental State Examination (MMSE), the Alzheimer's Disease Assessment Scale (ADAS 11 and ADAS 13), the Functional Activities Questionnaire (FAQ), the Clinical Dementia Rating – Sum of Boxes (CDR-SB) and the Rey Auditory Verbal Learning Test (RAVLT). Not every test score is available for each subject and visit, such that the absolute number of available training samples varies between 393 to 399 samples from 60 subjects for $\mathcal{M}^{[1]}$, and 1452 to 1480 samples from 248 subjects for $\mathcal{M}^{[2]}$.

Volumes of Brain Structures B^{vol}: Further, the volumes of 35 distinct brain structures are used as biomarkers. For this, MR scans are first automatically segmented into 134 regions using the whole brain segmentation proposed by [8], which is based on multi-atlas label propagation with expectation-maximisation based refinement (MALPEM). Here, brain atlases from the MICCAI 2012 Grand Challenge on Multi-Atlas Labeling[1] are employed. Corresponding manual expert segmentations are provided by Neuromorphometrics, Inc.[2] under academic subscription. The 30 atlas segmentations are transformed to an unsegmented scan and fused into a consensus probabilistic segmentation estimate using a local weighting approach. Subsequently, all 134 probabilistic label estimates are further refined using image intensity information.

To reduce the total number of models, left and right cortex are fused to single structures, resulting in 35 distinct anatomical regions. For procedural reasons, only segmentations for images acquired before 20/11/2013 were available, such that the total number of training samples for each structure is 219 (59 subjects) and 955 (247 subjects) for the two models.

---

[1] https://masi.vuse.vanderbilt.edu/workshop2012.

[2] http://Neuromorphometrics.com.

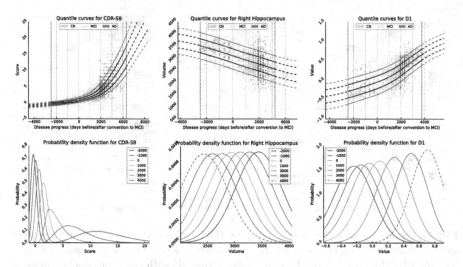

Fig. 3. Examples for the learned multi-stage disease progression models (Colour figure online).

Biomarkers Derived from Manifold Learning B^{ml}: Features obtained from MR images using manifold learning (ML) have been shown to contain valuable information about disease severity and progression [6]. The main idea of ML is to find a meaningful, low-dimensional representation of a high-dimensional feature space, such that similar scans also have similar coordinates in the low-dimensional manifold. This is achieved in three steps. First, the image regions that are most relevant with regard to information about disease state are automatically learned using sparse regression as in [6]. To compensate for varying intensity values in the images caused by different scanners and acquisition protocols, local binary patterns (LBP) are computed in a 26-connected neighbourhood for voxels within these regions and used as features in the high-dimensional space. The manifold is then learned using Laplacian eigenmaps. The local geometry is determined via a sparse similarity graph, built using the sum of squared differences (SSD) as similarity measure. Connections in the graph are made between the k nearest neighbours, with the additional constraint that an instance can only be connected to one instance per subject.

The manifold coordinates are computed for all training subjects with at least 5 visits, which results in 185 samples from 41 subjects available to train the CN/MCI model and 859 samples (155 subjects) for the MCI/AD model. The manifold dimension is chosen to be $d = 20$, that means 20 features are obtained per subject per visit and denoted as D1 to D20.

3.2   Model Learning and Progress Estimation

Progression models are trained for all 60 biomarkers. CDRSB and FAQ models could not be built for the CN-to-MCI transition because the majority of samples is clustered at $y = 0$. These biomarkers were therefore omitted for determining

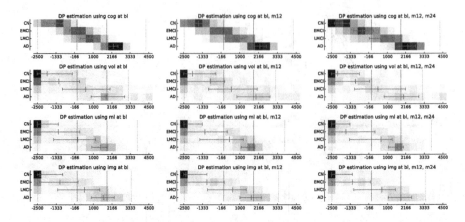

Fig. 4. Visualisation of the disease progress (DP) estimated with different biomarker settings (columns: number of visits; rows: biomarker sets). The distribution of DPs is indicated by the grey values. The x-axis gives the DP with solid and dashed lines at the points of conversion at $p = 0$ and $p = \delta_p$, and the mean model range p_- and p_+. The red bars show the median and 25th/75th percentile of the estimated DPs (Color figure online).

the model offset. Based on the remaining biomarkers, an $\hat{\delta}_p = 1860$ days is determined. Composed models are then retrained based on all samples and example results visualised in Fig. 3. Using the composed models, disease progression of all test subjects is estimated as proposed in Sect. 2.2. Plausibility of the estimated DPs is evaluated with regard to their ability do differentiate between the different diagnoses, that means to what extent an ordering of CN < EMCI < LMCI < AD is achieved. To this end, the disease progress $\hat{p}_s^0$ is estimated on the search space $[-2500, 4500]$ for all CN, EMCI, LMCI and AD subjects in the test set using several biomarker configurations. On the one hand, different sets of biomarkers B^{est} are considered for estimation: B^{cog}, B^{vol}, B^{ml}, as well as all imaging-based biomarkers $B^{\text{img}} := B^{\text{vol}} \cup B^{\text{ml}}$. On the other hand, biomarkers from one (baseline), two (baseline and m12) and three (baseline, m12 and m24) visits V^{est} are employed. The distribution of the estimated DPs depending on the diagnosis is visualised in Fig. 4.

3.3   Application: Classification

Image-Based Classification of Disease Stage. One of the main research topics of image-based analysis of Alzheimer's disease is the classification of subjects according to their diagnosis based on structural MR images. The high interest is highlighted by a classification challenge held in the course of MICCAI 2014[3]. The estimated DPs are therefore employed as single features to distinguish between CN and AD, CN and MCI, MCI and AD, and all three classes simultaneously. Support Vector Machines (SVMs) are used as classifiers. Corresponding to Sect. 3.2, DPs are estimated using the translational time warp

---

[3] http://caddementia.grand-challenge.org.

Table 1. Results for the image-based classification of subjects according to their diagnosis. Different imaging biomarkers acquired at a different number of visits are compared. For each test, the accuracies (ACC) of a 10-fold cross validation are given.

Biomarkers B^{est}	Visits V^{est}	CN/AD ACC	CN/MCI ACC	MCI/AD ACC	CN/MCI/AD ACC
B^{ml}	$\{bl\}$	0.89	0.71	0.82	0.63
	$\{bl, m12\}$	0.91	0.71	0.82	0.63
	$\{bl, m12, m24\}$	0.91	0.69	0.82	0.61
B^{vol}	$\{bl\}$	0.83	0.68	0.80	0.59
	$\{bl, m12\}$	0.86	0.68	0.78	0.58
	$\{bl, m12, m24\}$	0.85	0.69	0.78	0.58
B^{img}	$\{bl\}$	0.88	0.72	0.81	0.63
	$\{bl, m12\}$	0.90	0.71	0.83	0.64
	$\{bl, m12, m24\}$	0.90	0.71	0.83	0.64

definition (3) based on different biomarker settings and compared to each other. The cognitive scores are excluded because the diagnosis is made largely based on the CDR, such that including them biases the classification (e.g., classification accuracy reaches 1.0 for CN vs. AD and 0.96 for MCI vs. AD using B^{cog} at baseline). The results of a 10-fold cross validation are shown in Table 1.

Classification of Stable and Progressive MCI. Of high clinical interest is the task of identifying subjects with memory complaints that will develop Alzheimer's disease within a given period of time [9]. For example, this information is valuable to select subjects for clinical trials. Therefore, classification between MCI/AD converters and non-converters is performed using different features: A) DPs estimated with the time warp definition Eq. (3) using m12 measurements, B) DPs using baseline and m12 measurements (translational time warp Eq. (3)) and C) DPs and DPRs computed with the affine time warp Eq. (4) based on baseline and m12 visits. The set of converters (progressive MCI, pMCI) consists of all subjects that convert from MCI to AD between m12 and m36 visit. It is to be noted that these subjects are part of the training set used for learning the progression models, which introduces a bias in the test. However, adding one subject to a set of more than 1500 samples for the quantile regression barely changes the models, such that this effect can be neglected. Non-converters are test subjects with a stable MCI diagnosis (sMCI). In total, the data consists of 231 sMCI and 106 pMCI subjects. Weighted SVMs are used for classification to compensate for the unbalanced sets. Classification results are given in Table 2.

Classification of Subjects with Rapid Cognitive Decline (RCD). The rate of cognitive decline is known to vary considerably between subjects. It is therefore of interest for family and researchers alike to predict if a subject will suffer a rapid cognitive decline (RCD). Following [1], RCD is defined as a decrease of 8 or more MMSE points in the course of 2 years (28 subjects in the test set of 633 subjects). All remaining 605 test subjects are labeled as non-RCD. Classification results are given in Table 2.

Table 2. Results for the classification between subjects with stable and progressive MCI (sMCI vs. pMCI), and the identification of subjects with rapid cognitive decline (RCD). For all test, accuracy (ACC), sensitivity (SENS) and specificity (SPEC) of a 10-fold cross validation are given.

Biomarkers B^{est}	Visits V^{est}	Time warp $\tau(t)$	sMCI vs. pMCI ACC	SENS	SPEC	RCD vs. non-RCD ACC	SENS	SPEC
B^{cog}	{m12}	DP	0.78	0.82	0.76	0.89	0.90	0.89
	{bl, m12}	DP	0.77	0.82	0.75	0.84	0.83	0.84
	{bl, m12}	DP/DPR	0.79	0.82	0.78	0.92	0.97	0.92
B^{ml}	{m12}	DP	0.73	0.82	0.68	0.65	1.00	0.63
	{bl, m12}	DP	0.72	0.77	0.69	0.64	1.00	0.63
	{bl, m12}	DP/DPR	0.72	0.88	0.64	0.69	0.87	0.68
B^{vol}	{m12}	DP	0.68	0.59	0.71	0.73	0.83	0.73
	{bl, m12}	DP	0.68	0.54	0.74	0.74	0.87	0.73
	{bl, m12}	DP/DPR	0.66	0.68	0.66	0.75	0.83	0.74
B^{img}	{m12}	DP	0.68	0.71	0.67	0.70	0.90	0.69
	{bl, m12}	DP	0.70	0.65	0.72	0.72	0.87	0.71
	{bl, m12}	DP/DPR	0.71	0.84	0.64	0.73	0.83	0.73

4   Discussion

Visually assessed, the trained multi-stage models appear plausible for all biomarkers (cf. Figs. 2 and 3). In particular, the automatically determined offset of $\hat{\delta}_p = 1860$ days entails a smooth transition between CN/MCI and MCI/AD models and is in the same range as a manual fit would be. This indicates the validity of the presented approach for model composition.

While classic machine learning methods would be restricted to the set of training subjects for which all considered biomarkers are present, all available samples are used for model learning in the presented approach. For example, a subject's CDR-SB score is considered even though no MMSE was acquired.

The estimated DPs visualised in Fig. 4 show a good class separation. Naturally, the cognitive scores perform best for distinguishing between the four classes, while image-based measurements suffer from a larger inter-subject variability. Neither volumetric nor manifold features seem to be clearly superior. Adding measurements from multiple visits slightly reduces noise and increases class separability. A particular advantage of the presented approach for progress estimation is that all available data can be used without retraining the model. It is, for example, possible to estimate the DP if only cognitive scores are available for one visit and only image-based biomarkers for another visit. In this way, all available information can be employed in an optimal way.

The experiments show that DP and DPR are powerful features for different classification tasks. The results of the three-class classification of the disease stage are, for example, on par with [7] (even though not on exactly the same data and therefore not directly comparable). Interestingly, CN/MCI classification is worse and MCI/AD classification considerably better than in [7]. A possible explanation for this observation is the fact that fewer training samples were available from CN/MCI converters and the model is therefore less precise in this region. DP and DPR are also successfully employed to distinguish between stable and progressive MCI subjects and to identify patients with rapid cognitive decline. While not directly comparable (due to a different set of subjects), the results for sMCI vs. pMCI classification are on par with the literature (e.g., ACC = 0.67 is reported for MRI-based biomarkers in [9]). No results for an automatic RCD prediction have been published so far (to the best of our knowledge), however, classification accuracy is in the same range as for predicting conversion to AD and therefore appears reasonable. In all tests, cognitive scores excel as biomarkers. Interestingly, manifold coordinates perform better then volumetric features for separating stable from progressive MCI, but worse for RCD detection. The combination of the image-based features enhances robustness and performs best on average. Further, joint DP and DPR estimation considerably enhances classification of subjects with RCD.

In summary, classification results highlight the validity of the estimated DP and DPR values. However, the method still relies on the definition of meaningful biomarkers, as the superiority of B^{cog} in all experiments shows. In future work, it would therefore be interesting to employ biomarkers based on brain atrophy, tensor-based morphometry or PET imaging. Given enough training data, it would further be highly interesting to generate personalised models for certain groups, e.g. male and female patients or APoE ϵ4 positive and negative subjects.

5   Conclusion

In this work, a biomarker-based method for modelling disease progression from a cognitively normal stage to Alzheimer's disease was proposed. This was achieved by learning two separate models for the CN/MCI and MCI/AD transition phases using quantile regression and then combining these to a multi-stage model. Further, a probabilistic approach for estimating the disease progress and the rate of progression for any given subject was presented.

Model training and progression estimation were then evaluated on the ADNI database. The estimated DPs showed good class separability on the whole domain from CN to AD. DP and DPR were further successfully employed as features to classify subjects according to their disease stage, to differentiate between stable and progressive MCI and to identify subjects with rapid cognitive decline, highlighting the versatile applicability of the presented approach.

Acknowledgements. The research leading to these results has received funding from the European Union Seventh Framework Programme (FP7/2007 2013) under grant agreement no. 601055, VPH-DARE@IT.

References

1. Atchison, T.B., Bradshaw, M., Massman, P.J.: Investigation of profile difference between Alzheimer's disease patients declining at different rates: examination of baseline neuropsychological data. Arch. Clin. Neuropsychol. **19**(8), 1007–1015 (2004)
2. Delor, I., Charoin, J.E., Gieschke, R., Retout, S., Jacqmin, P.: Modeling Alzheimer's disease progression using disease onset time and disease trajectory concepts applied to CDR-SOB scores from ADNI. CPT Pharmacomet. Syst. Pharmacol. **2**(10), e78 (2013)
3. Doody, R.S., Pavlik, V., Massman, P., Rountree, S., Darby, E., Chan, W.: Predicting progression of Alzheimer's disease. Alzheimers Res. Ther. **2**(1), 2 (2010)
4. Fonteijn, H.M., Modat, M., Clarkson, M.J., Barnes, J., Lehmann, M., Hobbs, N.Z., Scahill, R.I., Tabrizi, S.J., Ourselin, S., Fox, N.C., Alexander, D.C.: An event-based model for disease progression and its application in familial Alzheimer's disease and Huntington's disease. NeuroImage **60**(3), 1880–1889 (2012)
5. Green, C., Shearer, J., Ritchie, C.W., Zajicek, J.P.: Model-based economic evaluation in Alzheimer's disease: a review of the methods available to model Alzheimer's disease progression. Value Health **14**(5), 621–630 (2011)
6. Guerrero, R., Ledig, C., Rueckert, D.: Manifold alignment and transfer learning for classification of Alzheimer's disease. In: Wu, G., Zhang, D., Zhou, L. (eds.) MLMI 2014. LNCS, vol. 8679, pp. 77–84. Springer, Heidelberg (2014)
7. Ledig, C., Guerrero, R., Tong, T., Gray, K., Schmidt-Richberg, A., Makropoulos, A., Heckemann, R., Rueckert, D.: Alzheimer's disease state classification using structural volumetry, cortical thickness and intensity features. In: MICCAI Workshop Challenge on Computer-Aided Diagnosis of Dementia Based on Structural MRI Data, pp. 55–64 (2014)
8. Ledig, C., Heckemann, R.A., Makropoulos, A., Hammers, A., Lötjönen, J., Menon, D., Rueckert, D.: Robust whole-brain segmentation: application to traumatic brain injury. Med. Image Anal. **21**(1), 40–58 (2015)
9. Trzepacz, P.T., Yu, P., Sun, J., Schuh, K., Case, M., Witte, M.M., Hochstetler, H., Hake, A.: Alzheimer's disease neuroimaging initiative: comparison of neuroimaging modalities for the prediction of conversion from mild cognitive impairment to Alzheimer's dementia. Neurobiol. Aging **35**(1), 143–151 (2014)
10. Yang, E., Farnum, M., Lobanov, V., Schultz, T., Verbeeck, R., Raghavan, N., Samtani, M.N., Novak, G., Narayan, V., DiBernardo, A.: Alzheimer's disease neuroimaging initiative: quantifying the pathophysiological timeline of Alzheimer's disease. J Alzheimers Dis. **26**(4), 745–753 (2011)
11. Yee, T.W.: Quantile regression via vector generalized additive models. Stat. Med. **23**(14), 2295–2315 (2004)
12. Young, A.L., Oxtoby, N.P., Daga, P., Cash, D.M., Fox, N.C., Ourselin, S., Schott, J.M., Alexander, D.C.: Alzheimer's disease neuroimaging initiative: a data-driven model of biomarker changes in sporadic Alzheimer's disease. Brain **137**(Pt 9), 2564–2577 (2014)

Measuring Asymmetric Interactions in Resting State Brain Networks

Anand A. Joshi[1,2]([✉]), Ronald Salloum[1], Chitresh Bhushan[1],
and Richard M. Leahy[1,2]

[1] Signal and Image Processing Institute,
University of Southern California, Los Angeles, CA, USA
ajoshi@sipi.usc.edu
[2] Brain and Creativity Institute,
University of Southern California, Los Angeles, CA, USA

Abstract. Directed graph representations of brain networks are increasingly being used to indicate the direction and level of influence among brain regions. Most of the existing techniques for directed graph representations are based on time series analysis and the concept of causality, and use time lag information in the brain signals. These time lag-based techniques can be inadequate for functional magnetic resonance imaging (fMRI) signal analysis due to the limited time resolution of fMRI as well as the low frequency hemodynamic response. The aim of this paper is to present a novel measure of necessity that uses asymmetry in the joint distribution of brain activations to infer the direction and level of interaction among brain regions. We present a mathematical formula for computing necessity and extend this measure to partial necessity, which can potentially distinguish between direct and indirect interactions. These measures do not depend on time lag for directed modeling of brain interactions and therefore are more suitable for fMRI signal analysis. The necessity measures were used to analyze resting state fMRI data to determine the presence of hierarchy and asymmetry of brain interactions during resting state. We performed ROI-wise analysis using the proposed necessity measures to study the default mode network. The empirical joint distribution of the fMRI signals was determined using kernel density estimation, and was used for computation of the necessity and partial necessity measures. The significance of these measures was determined using a one-sided Wilcoxon rank-sum test. Our results are consistent with the hypothesis that the posterior cingulate cortex plays a central role in the default mode network.

1 Introduction

Brain networks are primarily described in terms of functional connectivity and effective connectivity. Functional connectivity is defined as the temporal correlation between spatially remote neurophysiological events and effective connectivity is defined as the influence one neuronal system exerts over another [4].

This work is supported by the following grants: R01 EB009048, R01 NS074980, and R01 NS089212.

S. Ourselin et al. (Eds.): IPMI 2015, LNCS 9123, pp. 399–410, 2015.
DOI: 10.1007/978-3-319-19992-4_31

Functional connectivity refers only to an undirected relationship between two distinct brain regions. Effective connectivity, on the other hand, can be used to describe the brain network as a directed graph. Two popular model-driven approaches for measuring effective connectivity from fMRI data are structural equation modeling (SEM) [11] and dynamic causal modeling (DCM) [5]. In SEM, the covariances of activity between brain regions are used to calculate path coefficients representing the magnitudes of influences corresponding to directional paths. On the other hand, DCM models the brain as a nonlinear dynamic system in which external stimuli produce changes in brain activity. Responses to the stimuli are measured and used to estimate model parameters representing the effective connectivity between brain regions. Recently, DCM has been extended to resting state fMRI data [6]. Note that DCM models interactions at the neuronal rather than the hemodynamic level. Since changes in effective connectivity occur at a neuronal level, DCM is frequently the preferred method for making inferences about effective connectivity from fMRI data. However, a limitation of DCM is that it requires a priori knowledge and the estimation of a large number of parameters, which can be difficult in the context of resting state fMRI data analysis. Moreover, the parameters are affected by the sampling rate, and the neuronal parameters are often confounded by hemodynamic effects [18].

Several causality measures which incorporate time lag information have been used to analyze effective connectivity. One popular model-driven approach is Granger causality, which makes use of the notion of temporal prediction. In Granger causality, if the prediction of a time series Y could be improved by incorporating the knowledge of a second time series X, then X is said to have a causal influence on Y [16]. While Granger's method can be effective with electrophysiological recordings, the poor temporal resolution of fMRI ($\sim$1 s) makes it difficult to perform causal inference based on the past. Consequently, lag-based methods for computing directed interactions are not suitable for fMRI data analysis.

Instead of relying on time lag information, an alternative approach is to compute directed measures based on the joint distribution of time series measured in two or more regions of interest (ROIs). For example, Patel et al. [14] have used a pairwise conditional probability approach (referred to as the Patel tau measure) to study the relative difference between $P(Y|X)$ and $P(Y)$, and conversely, the relative difference between $P(X|Y)$ and $P(X)$, where X and Y denote the activation of two voxels or ROIs in a brain volume. Large differences indicate strong effective connectivity between the two voxels. Given strong effective connectivity between the two voxels, this metric is a measure of ascendancy between X and Y as determined by the ratio of their respective marginal activation probabilities. Specifically, for two connected voxels X and Y, X is said to be ascendant over Y whenever the marginal activation probability of X is larger than that of Y. Another non lag-based technique is the use of Bayesian networks, which rely on multivariate conditional probability distributions to measure effective connectivity [13,20]. A comprehensive review and comparison of effective connectivity techniques for fMRI data analysis is presented in [18], where it has been noted that non lag-based methods such as the Patel tau measure and Bayesian networks are best suited for effective connectivity analysis of fMRI data [2]. A limitation of Bayesian networks is that most techniques restrict the network topology by assuming the directed graph to be acyclic. Also, the Patel tau measure is limited in the sense that it is a bivariate measure and there are no known extensions to multivariate data. Another limitation of the Patel tau measure is that it cannot be applied directly to continuous-valued random variables.

In this paper, we present a method for directed graphical modeling of brain networks based on a notion of necessity. The ideas of logical necessity and suffi-ciency were emphasized by Mill [12] in his "method of difference" and "method of agreement" to explain the relationship between random events. These ideas have recently been extended to fuzzy sets by Ragin [15]. In contrast to these works, our method is based on the classical theory of random variables. Our necessity measure is independent of time lag and has some similarity to the Patel tau measure, but can work directly with continuous-valued random variables.

First, we present our model of necessity using an illustrative example. We then extend the definition of necessity to partial necessity, which can deal with multivariate data and is able to distinguish between direct and indirect rela-tionships in a brain network. The proposed necessity measures were applied to resting state fMRI data from the Human Connectome Project (HCP) database.

2   Materials and Methods

2.1   Mathematical Formulation of the Necessity Measure

In this section, we present the mathematical formulation of the proposed neces-sity measure. Let us denote two Bernoulli random variables by X and Y. We define the necessity of X to Y by

$$N(X \to Y) = \log_2 \frac{P(Y = 1|X = 1)}{P(Y = 1|X = 0)}.$$

This necessity measure determines the change in the odds of Y being active based on the activation or inactivation of X. The necessity measure takes val-ues on $[-\infty, \infty]$. Positive (negative) val-ues indicate that activation of X causes an increase (decrease) in the probability of activation of Y. The magnitude of the necessity value indicates the extent of the increase or decrease in this probability. For example, a necessity value of 1 means

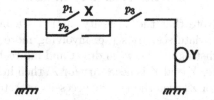

Fig. 1. An illustrative example of three switches and a lamp motivating the definition of the proposed necessity measure.

that activation of X causes the probability of activation of Y to double. The motivating example for this definition of necessity is a configuration of switches and lamps as shown in Fig. 1. The positions of the switches are modeled as Bernoulli random variables, with p_1, p_2, p_3 indicating the probabilities of these switches being on. The necessity of switch X for activation of lamp Y is given by

$$N(X \rightarrow Y) = \log_2 \frac{P(Y = 1|X = 1)}{P(Y = 1|X = 0)} = \log_2 \left(\frac{p_3}{p_3 p_2} \right) = -\log_2(p_2).$$

This value is consistent with the intuition: when $p_2 = 0$ (i.e. the switch in parallel to switch X is always off), the switch X becomes totally necessary for activation of the lamp Y as indicated by $N(X \rightarrow Y) = \infty$, while when $p_2 = 1$ (i.e. the switch in parallel to switch X is always on), the switch X becomes unnecessary for activation of Y as indicated by $N(X \rightarrow Y) = 0$. Note that in this example, the necessity value cannot be negative since p_2 takes values on $[0, 1]$.

Next, we extend this definition to continuous-valued random variables taking values in the $[0, 1]$ interval. For this purpose, we perform the following algebraic manipulation in the discrete-valued case:

$$N(X \rightarrow Y) = \log_2 P(Y = 1|X = 1) - \log_2 P(Y = 1|X = 0)$$

$$= \sum_{y=0}^{1} \sum_{x=0}^{1} y(2x - 1) \log_2 P(Y = y|X = x).$$

Extending this to continuous-valued random variables with range $[0, 1]$, we get

$$N(X \rightarrow Y) = \int_0^1 \int_0^1 y(2x - 1) \log_2 \left(\frac{P_{X,Y}(x, y)}{P_X(x)} \right) dx dy. \tag{1}$$

2.2 Partial Necessity Measure

Note that the necessity metric is a bivariate measure, and therefore in multivariate scenarios (i.e. involving more than two random variables) it does not distinguish between direct and indirect necessity. For example, if X is necessary for Y and Y is necessary for Z, then in this bivariate measure X is also necessary for Z, even though the necessity of X to Z is only indirect (or inherited). In order to study the necessity relationships of two random variables after conditioning on the remaining variables in a multivariate scenario, we introduce the following notion of partial necessity, analogous to the partial correlation measures used in undirected networks. Let S be a set of random variables. The partial necessity of X to Y is denoted as $N(X \to Y \,|\, \boldsymbol{W})$ where $\boldsymbol{W} = \boldsymbol{S} \backslash \{X, Y\}$ represents the remainder of the random variables, and is given by:

$$N(X \to Y \,|\, \boldsymbol{W}) = \int_{x,y,w} y(2x-1) \log_2 \left(\frac{p_{XY|\boldsymbol{W}}(x,y|\boldsymbol{w})}{p_{X|\boldsymbol{W}}(x|\boldsymbol{w})} \right) p(\boldsymbol{w}) \, d\boldsymbol{w}\,dx\,dy$$

$$= E_{\boldsymbol{W}} \left(\int_{x,y} y(2x-1) \log_2 \left(\frac{p_{XY|\boldsymbol{W}}(x,y|\boldsymbol{w})}{p_{X|\boldsymbol{W}}(x|\boldsymbol{w})} \right) dx\,dy \right).$$

Note that in this formulation, numerical implementation of the partial necessity measure involves computation of the multivariate integration over $\boldsymbol{w}$. This can be computationally expensive if the number of variables involved is large. In order to simplify the computation, we approximate the expectation by the sample mean as follows:

$$N(X \to Y \,|\, \boldsymbol{W}) \approx \frac{1}{T} \sum_{i=1}^{T} \int_{x,y} y(2x-1) \log_2 \left(\frac{p_{XY|\boldsymbol{W}}(x,y|\boldsymbol{w}(i))}{p_{X|\boldsymbol{W}}(x|\boldsymbol{w}(i))} \right) dx\,dy \quad (2)$$

where $\boldsymbol{w}(i)$ indicates the ith sample of $\boldsymbol{w}$, and T represents the number of samples. Note that we first perform kernel density estimation to compute the multivariate distribution of $X, Y, \boldsymbol{W}$ using all of the samples and then compute the conditional distributions at $\boldsymbol{W} = \boldsymbol{w}(i)$ (i.e. at each sample value). This formula is more computationally tractable because it eliminates the $p(\boldsymbol{w})$ term, and as a result, avoids the high-dimensional multivariate integration over $\boldsymbol{w}$. Note that in multivariate kernel density estimation, there is an exponential increase in the number of samples as the number of dimensions increases (referred to as the "curse of dimensionality") [9]. However, in this paper, we are dealing with two-dimensional conditional distributions, which may reduce the sensitivity of our measures to increases in the number of variables (or nodes in a network) relative to the full multivariate distribution, an issue we plan to explore further.

2.3   Interpretation and Properties of the Necessity Measures

In the previous section, a mathematical formulation of the necessity measures was presented. The purpose of this section is to provide an intuitive interpretation and discuss several interesting properties of these measures.

Let X and Y be two binary random variables. In terms of Boolean logic, when X is necessary for Y, Y must be zero whenever X is zero. This condition limits the support of the joint distribution of the two random variables, as illustrated in Fig. 2(a). The black squares represent the support of the joint distribution in the binary-valued case. We can see that the condition that X is necessary for Y requires cases to exist at the bottom-left corner and that no cases may exist at the upper-left corner. Note that when X is one, Y may either be zero or one, as indicated by the presence of black squares in the lower-right and upper-right corners, respectively. Generalizing these statements from binary to continuous-valued random variables results in the joint distribution denoted by the shaded triangle in Fig. 2(a).

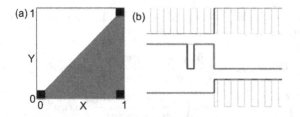

Fig. 2. (a) Asymmetry in the joint distribution of two random variables X and Y in the binary-valued case (denoted by black squares) and the continuous-valued case (denoted by the shaded triangle); (b) Hypothetical cases illustrating different cases of correlation and necessity between X (blue) and Y (orange) (Color figure online).

The proposed necessity measure can be used to indicate the presence of such asymmetry in the joint distribution of two random variables. A less restrictive form of asymmetry can be observed in the joint distribution of fMRI signals from two different ROIs. A scatter plot of activation of the posterior cingulate gyrus and inferior parietal lobule during resting state fMRI is shown in Fig. 3(a). This example illustrates that there are asymmetric relationships in the activation of these two ROIs, as indicated by the approximately lower-triangular joint distribution in Fig. 3(b).

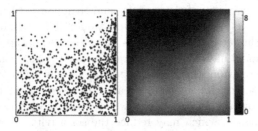

Fig. 3. (a) A scatter plot of activation of left posterior cingulate gyrus - dorsal (x-axis) and left inferior parietal lobule - angular gyrus (y-axis) from one of the resting-state fMRI data sets mentioned in Sect. 2.5; (b) Kernel density estimate of the joint distribution.

In order to highlight the difference between correlation and necessity measures, we consider the hypothetical cases shown in Fig. 2(b). The top row shows an example where X (blue) is not necessary for Y (orange) and there is no correlation between X and Y. The middle row shows a case where there is high correlation between X and Y but X is not necessary for Y. Finally, the bottom row shows a case where X is necessary for Y but there is low correlation between X and Y. These examples highlight the differences between necessity and correlation-based network representations. It is also important to point out that the correlation measure is undirected, while our necessity measure can indicate directed relationships. Although the above examples are not realistic representations of fMRI data, similar relationships can exist in the context of fMRI.

Also of interest is the relationship between statistical independence and necessity. When two events A and B are statistically independent, there is no necessity between A and B. Moreover, it can be verified that when A and B are conditionally independent given another event W, there is zero partial necessity between the two. These properties are desirable and are consistent with the intuitive requirement from such a measure.

2.4   Implementation of the Necessity Measures

The numerical implementation of the proposed necessity and partial necessity measures (as given by Eqs. 1 and 2) was performed in MATLAB. The integrations involved in the formulas were discretized using $\delta x = \delta y = .01$ and were computed over $[0, 1] \times [0, 1]$. Accurate estimation of the joint and conditional probability distributions is critical for computation of the necessity measures. We used the Kernel Density Estimation Toolbox for MATLAB (provided by http://www.ics.uci.edu/~ihler/code/kde.html) for the purpose of multivariate joint and conditional probability density estimation. This implementation uses "kd-trees," a hierarchical representation for point sets which caches sufficient statistics about point locations in order to achieve potential speedups in computation [8].

2.5   Application to fMRI Data

We applied the necessity and partial necessity measures to resting state fMRI data. The dataset used for this paper was provided by the Human Connectome Project (HCP), supported by the WU–Minn Consortium and McDonnell Center for Systems Neuroscience at Washington University [19]. The dataset consisted of 68 healthy participants in the HCP quarter 1 (released online: March 2013) [17]. For each participant, one resting state fMRI session (with left-to-right direction phase encoding) was analyzed. The scan parameters of the resting state fMRI data were: TR, 720 ms; TE, 33.1 ms; flip angle, 52°; field of view, 208 × 180 mm; slice thickness, 2.0 mm; 72 slices; voxels isotropic, 2.0 mm; multiband factor, 8; echo spacing, 0.58 ms; bandwidth (BW), 2290 Hz/Px; time points, 1200 [17].

This data was processed using the HCP preprocessing pipeline, which involves the use of a denoising process that combines independent component analysis (ICA) with an automated component classifier referred to as FIX (FMRIB's ICA-based X-noisifier) [7,17]. ICA is run using FSL's Multivariate Exploratory Linear Optimized Decomposition (MELODIC) with automatic dimensionality estimation. These components are fed into FIX, which determines which components need to be removed from the data. The HCP pipeline uses a grayordinate spatial coordinate system, which allows for combined cortical surface and subcortical volume analyses. Additionally, it reduces the storage and processing requirements for high spatial and temporal resolution data.

Note that our necessity measure requires an input in the range $[0, 1]$. ROI-wise time series were computed by averaging the fMRI signal over each ROI. The fMRI time series for each ROI was normalized by subtracting the mean, taking the absolute value, and then dividing by the standard deviation of the signals from all ROIs in a given network. Using the error function, the resulting signal was transformed to the $[0, 1]$ interval. Using this process, we computed the necessity measures between each pair of ROIs in a given network. For the analysis presented in this paper, we focused on the default mode network, in particular the following ROIs: (1) Posterior Cingulate Gyrus - Dorsal, (2) Posterior Cingulate Gyrus - Ventral, (3) Inferior Parietal Gyrus - Angular, (4) Inferior Parietal Gyrus - Supramarginal, and (5) Superior Frontal Gyrus. ROIs were defined by the HCP preprocessing pipeline, which uses FreeSurfer.

We also performed significance testing, explained as follows. In these studies, we are interested in comparing the necessity of X to Y with the necessity of Y to X, where X and Y represent the activations of two ROIs. In order to determine significance, we performed a one-sided Wilcoxon rank-sum test. The null hypothesis for this test is that necessity of X to Y is equal to that from Y to X in the study population. Rejection of the null hypothesis indicates that necessity of X to Y is greater than the necessity of Y to X, which suggests ascendancy of X over Y in the network. Note that this one-sided test does not consider the possibility that the necessity of Y to X is greater than the necessity of X to Y. To account for this possibility, we also performed hypothesis testing in the opposite direction (i.e. by exchanging X and Y). In the case of multiple ROIs, all pairwise necessity measures were computed and significance testing was performed in both directions for each pair. Multiple hypothesis correction was performed using false discovery rate (FDR = 0.05) with the Benjamin Hochberg procedure [1].

3   Results

We used the proposed necessity measures to determine the presence of hierarchy and asymmetry of brain interactions during resting state. First, we validated our measures using a simulation based on a model of directed interaction. The simulation demonstrates how partial necessity can distinguish between direct and indirect interactions. We then performed ROI-wise analysis on resting state fMRI data to study connectivity and directed interactions in the default mode network.

3.1   Simulation Based on a Model of Directed Interaction

In this section, we present a simulation to validate the proposed necessity and partial necessity measures. First, consider the following motivating example. Let C be the central hub in a network consisting of two other regions A and B, where we restrict the three variables to be binary-valued (1 indicating activation and 0 indicating inactivation). Suppose we model C as the maximum of A and B. In this case, if C is inactive, then both A and B must be inactive, indicating that activation of C is necessary for activation of A and B. Although this example restricts the variables to be binary-valued, we can extend this concept to the continuous-valued case, as illustrated by the following simulation. We selected three fMRI time series signals, each from a different ROI, and converted them to signals with range [0,1], as explained in Sect. 2.5. These signals are represented by X, W_1, and W_2. We then computed $Y = max(X, W_1)$ and $Z = max(Y, W_2)$, where we took the maximum at each time instant. We then analyzed the connectivity between X, Y, and Z. Intuitively, one would expect activation of Z to be necessary for activation of Y, and activation of Y to be necessary for activation of X. The Venn diagram in Fig. 4(a) depicts this subset/superset relationship, with Z being a superset of Y, and Y being a superset of X.

We studied the connectivity using the necessity and partial necessity measures, with a one-sided Wilcoxon rank-sum test as a test of significance, as explained in Sect. 2.5. Note that for a given pair of ROIs, say X and Y, we compared the values of $N(X \rightarrow Y)$ and $N(Y \rightarrow X)$, and reported the difference when there is significance. Figures 4(b) and (c) show block diagrams that illustrate the network connectivity, analyzed using the

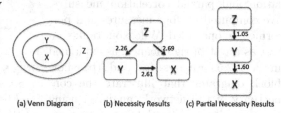

(a) Venn Diagram   (b) Necessity Results   (c) Partial Necessity Results

Fig. 4. Simulation of directed interaction. (a) Venn diagram illustrating the set relationship between random variables X, Y, and Z. Figures (b) and (c) are block diagrams illustrating the connectivity between X, Y, and Z, using the necessity and partial necessity measures, respectively.

necessity and partial necessity measures, respectively. The arrows indicate necessity (e.g. Y is necessary for X), with the number next to the arrow indicating the difference between the two necessity values. As expected, we can see that Z is necessary for Y, and Y is necessary for X. However, the necessity measure also shows a connection between Z and X, which is misleading because this is an indirect interaction. When we compute the partial necessity measure, only the direct interactions are found. Thus, when we are only interested in direct interactions, partial necessity may be the preferred analytical measure.

3.2 Analyzing Connectivity and Directed Interactions in the Default Mode Network

We used the proposed necessity measures to study connectivity and directed interactions in the default mode network for both the left and right hemispheres. We restricted our analysis to the following ROIs: (1) Posterior Cingulate Gyrus - Dorsal (PCG-D), (2) Posterior Cingulate Gyrus - Ventral (PCG-V), (3) Inferior Parietal Gyrus - Angular (IP-AG), (4) Inferior Parietal Gyrus - Supramarginal (IP-SMG), and (5) Superior Frontal Gyrus (SFG). Studies have shown that the posterior cingulate cortex forms a central node in the default mode network [3,10]. Figure 5 shows a plot of the difference between the necessity of PCG-D to IP-AG and the necessity of IP-AG to PCG-D across the study population. Results are shown for the necessity and partial necessity measures.

In both cases, the difference is consistently greater than zero across the subjects, indicating that there is asymmetry in the interaction of these two ROIs. In the following study, we compared our proposed necessity and partial necessity measures to the popularly used correlation and partial correlation measures. We computed all four measures and performed a one-sided Wilcoxon rank-sum test as a test of significance, as explained in Sect. 2.5. Figures 6(a) and (b) show block diagrams that illustrate the connectivity of the network, analyzed using the necessity and partial necessity measures, respectively. Each block represents an ROI in the network and each arrow indicates a necessity relationship between a pair of ROIs with the number next to the arrow representing the difference between the two necessity values (averaged over the subjects). Similar block diagrams were generated for the correlation and partial correlation measures, shown in Figs. 6(c) and (d), respectively. In the case of the necessity measures, we can see that the majority of the arrows are originating from the PCG. This indicates that activation of the PCG is necessary for activation of the other ROIs in the network, thus supporting the notion that the PCG is a central hub in the default mode network. However, this is not evident from the undirected correlation and partial correlation measures. Also, since the partial necessity measure shows the same connectivity as the necessity measure, this suggests that all of the necessity relationships are direct.

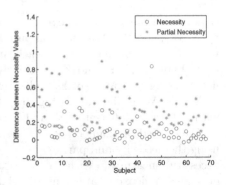

Fig. 5. Plot of the differences between the two necessity values (i.e. necessity of PCG-D to IP-AG minus necessity of IP-AG to PCG-D) across the study population. Corresponding results for partial necessity are also shown.

4   Discussion and Conclusion

We presented a measure of necessity and partial necessity for exploring asymmetric brain interactions during resting state. These measures are particularly useful in the context of fMRI data analysis because they do not depend on time lag information. We validated our measures using a simulation based on a model of directed interaction. Also, we used our measures to study connectivity in the default mode network. Fransson and Marrelec [3], and others, have conjectured that the posterior cingulate gyrus plays a central role in the default mode network [3,10]. Preliminary results from the necessity measures indicate that activation of the posterior cingulate gyrus is necessary for activation of other ROIs in the network, thus supporting the notion that this region acts as a central hub. While the proposed necessity measures depict subset relationships indicative of a hierarchy of brain activations, it is important to point out that the necessity measures do not indicate a cause-effect relationship. However, ascendancy has

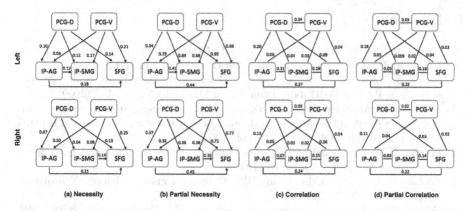

Fig. 6. Study of connectivity and directed interactions in the default mode network. We studied connectivity in the default mode network using four measures: (a) Necessity, (b) Partial necessity, (c) Correlation, and (d) Partial correlation. The ROIs we studied are as follows: PCG-D = Posterior Cingulate Gyrus - Dorsal; PCG-V = Posterior Cingulate Gyrus - Ventral; IP-AG = Inferior Parietal Lobule - Angular Gyrus; IP-SMG = Inferior Parietal Lobule - Supramarginal Gyrus; SFG = Superior Frontal Gyrus. The top and bottom rows illustrate connectivity in the left and right hemispheres, respectively. The results indicate that the posterior cingulate gyrus plays a central role in the default mode network, which is consistent with the literature.

been effectively used as a surrogate for causality in previous studies [14,18]. One limitation of the necessity measures is that they use fMRI signal intensities scaled to the [0, 1] interval as a measure of activation. As a result, the necessity measures can be sensitive to the preprocessing pipeline. We will explore the impact of preprocessing on the necessity measures in future studies. Another limitation is that the necessity measures do not take into consideration neurophysiological properties, such as the characteristics of the hemodynamic response and neuromuscular coupling. Also, the partial necessity measure requires computation of multivariate joint distributions and may become increasingly unstable with increasing dimension. We did however investigate the stability of the partial measure using bootstrapping. While within-subject variance increased relative to the non-partial measure, there was still sufficient consistency across subjects, as illustrated in Fig. 5, to detect statistically significant directed interactions.

Acknowledgement. Datasets were provided [in part] by the Human Connectome Project, WU-Minn Consortium (Principal Investigators: David Van Essen and Kamil Ugurbil; 1U54MH091657) funded by the 16 NIH Institutes and Centers that support the NIH Blueprint for Neuroscience Research; and by the McDonnell Center for Systems Neuroscience at Washington University.

References

1. Benjamini, Y., Yekutieli, D.: The control of the false discovery rate in multiple testing under dependency. Ann. Stat. **29**(4), 1165–1188 (2001)
2. Burge, J., Lane, T., Link, H., Qiu, S., Clark, V.P.: Discrete dynamic Bayesian network analysis of fMRI data. Hum. Brain Mapp. **30**(1), 122–137 (2009)
3. Fransson, P., Marrelec, G.: The precuneus/posterior cingulate cortex plays a pivotal role in the default mode network: evidence from a partial correlation network analysis. NeuroImage **42**(3), 1178–1184 (2008)
4. Friston, K.J.: Functional and effective connectivity in neuroimaging: a synthesis. Hum. Brain Mapp. **2**(1–2), 56–78 (1994)
5. Friston, K.J., Harrison, L., Penny, W.: Dynamic causal modelling. NeuroImage **19**(4), 1273–1302 (2003)
6. Friston, K.J., Kahan, J., Biswal, B., Razi, A.: A DCM for resting state fMRI. NeuroImage **94**, 396–407 (2014)
7. Glasser, M.F., Sotiropoulos, S.N., Wilson, J.A., Coalson, T.S., Fischl, B., Andersson, J.L., Xu, J., Jbabdi, S., Webster, M., Polimeni, J.R., et al.: The minimal preprocessing pipelines for the Human Connectome Project. NeuroImage **80**, 105–124 (2013)
8. Gray, A.G., Moore, A.W.: Very fast multivariate kernel density estimation via computational geometry. In: Proceedings of the Joint Statistical Meeting (2003)
9. Hwang, J.N., Lay, S.R., Lippman, A.: Nonparametric multivariate density estimation: a comparative study. IEEE Trans. Signal Process. **42**(10), 2795–2810 (1994)
10. Leech, R., Braga, R., Sharp, D.J.: Echoes of the brain within the posterior cingulate cortex. J. Neurosci. **32**(1), 215–222 (2012)
11. McIntosh, A., Gonzalez-Lima, F.: Structural equation modeling and its application to network analysis in functional brain imaging. Hum. Brain Mapp. **2**(1–2), 2–22 (1994)
12. Mill, J.S.: A system of logic: ratiocinative and Inductive. Green and Company, Longmans (1956)
13. Mumford, J.A., Ramsey, J.D.: Bayesian networks for fMRI: a primer. NeuroImage **86**, 573–582 (2014)
14. Patel, R.S., Bowman, F.D., Rilling, J.K.: A Bayesian approach to determining connectivity of the human brain. Hum. Brain Mapp. **27**(3), 267–276 (2006)
15. Ragin, C.C.: Fuzzy-Set Social Science. University of Chicago Press, Chicago (2000)
16. Roebroeck, A., Formisano, E., Goebel, R.: Mapping directed influence over the brain using Granger causality and fMRI. NeuroImage **25**(1), 230–242 (2005)
17. Smith, S.M., Beckmann, C.F., Andersson, J., Auerbach, E.J., Bijsterbosch, J., Douaud, G., Duff, E., Feinberg, D.A., Griffanti, L., Harms, M.P., et al.: Resting-state fMRI in the Human Connectome Project. NeuroImage **80**, 144–168 (2013)
18. Smith, S.M., Miller, K.L., Salimi-Khorshidi, G., Webster, M., Beckmann, C.F., Nichols, T.E., Ramsey, J.D., Woolrich, M.W.: Network modelling methods for fMRI. NeuroImage **54**(2), 875–891 (2011)
19. Van Essen, D.C., Smith, S.M., Barch, D.M., Behrens, T.E., Yacoub, E., Ugurbil, K.: The Wu-Minn Human Connectome Project: an overview. NeuroImage **80**, 62–79 (2013)
20. Wu, X., Li, J., Yao, L.: Determining effective connectivity from fMRI data using a gaussian dynamic Bayesian network. In: Huang, T., Zeng, Z., Li, C., Leung, C.S. (eds.) ICONIP 2012, Part I. LNCS, vol. 7663, pp. 33–39. Springer, Heidelberg (2012)

Shape Classification Using Wasserstein Distance for Brain Morphometry Analysis

Zhengyu Su[1]([⊠]), Wei Zeng[2], Yalin Wang[3], Zhong-Lin Lu[4], and Xianfeng Gu[1]

[1] Department of Computer Science, Stony Brook University, Brookhaven, USA
{zhsu,gu}@cs.stonybrook.edu
[2] School of Computing and Information Sciences, Florida International University,
Miami, USA
wzeng@cis.fiu.edu
[3] School of Computing, Informatics, and Decision Systems Engineering,
Arizona State University, Arizona, USA
Yalin.Wang@asu.edu
[4] Department of Psychology, Ohio State University, Ohio, USA
lu.535@osu.edu

Abstract. Brain morphometry study plays a fundamental role in medical imaging analysis and diagnosis. This work proposes a novel framework for brain cortical surface classification using Wasserstein distance, based on uniformization theory and Riemannian optimal mass transport theory.

By Poincare uniformization theorem, all shapes can be conformally deformed to one of the three canonical spaces: the unit sphere, the Euclidean plane or the hyperbolic plane. The uniformization map will distort the surface area elements. The area-distortion factor gives a probability measure on the canonical uniformization space. All the probability measures on a Riemannian manifold form the Wasserstein space. Given any 2 probability measures, there is a unique optimal mass transport map between them, the transportation cost defines the Wasserstein distance between them. Wasserstein distance gives a Riemannian metric for the Wasserstein space. It intrinsically measures the dissimilarities between shapes and thus has the potential for shape classification.

To the best of our knowledge, this is the first work to introduce the optimal mass transport map to general Riemannian manifolds. The method is based on geodesic power Voronoi diagram. Comparing to the conventional methods, our approach solely depends on Riemannian metrics and is invariant under rigid motions and scalings, thus it intrinsically measures shape distance. Experimental results on classifying brain cortical surfaces with different intelligence quotients demonstrated the efficiency and efficacy of our method.

Keywords: Brain morphometry · Wasserstein distance · Optimal mass transport

© Springer International Publishing Switzerland 2015
S. Ourselin et al. (Eds.): IPMI 2015, LNCS 9123, pp. 411–423, 2015.
DOI: 10.1007/978-3-319-19992-4_32

1 Introduction

Wasserstein distance has been widely studied and applied for shape analysis, due to its significant power to intrinsically compare similarities between shapes. Wang et al. [29] proposed a linear optimal transportation framework for comparing images. Schmitzer et al. [23] proposed Wasserstein based method for joint variational object segmentation and shape matching. Hong et al. [11] introduced a shape feature that characterizes local shape geometry for shape matching based on Wasserstein distance. However, these methods for shape analysis only work for 2D images. With the fast development of 3D scanning technologies, 3D shapes become more and more popular and analyzing 3D surfaces becomes important in medical imaging field.

3D surface based brain morphometry analysis usually takes brain thickness morphometry features [25]. Recent work [31,32] showed that surface area feature may be independent of cortical thickness and itself provides a unique and important morphometry feature to study brain structural MRI images. With the clinical questions of interest moving towards identifying very early signs of brain functional and diseases, the corresponding statistical differences at the group level become weaker and harder to identify. An efficient and effective framework with a rigorous theoretical guarantee to classify brain cortical surfaces into different categories would be highly desired for preclinical imaging study.

Due to the difficult boundary parameterization and high dimension, conventional 2D shape classification methods can not be easily extended to 3D shape classification problems. Many methods have been proposed in order to describe shapes. Statistical based method [4,22] represent objects with feature vectors in a multidimensional space, but they are not discriminating enough to make subtle distinctions between shapes. Topology based method [10] computes 3D shape similarity by comparing Multiresolutional Reeb Graphs, yet they can not describe the geometric differences. Geometry based method [17,20] compare 3D shapes by embedding them to into canonical space, but the classifications are too restrictive. Shape space models have been proposed to provide suitable mathematical and computational descriptions for both shape representation and comparisons [16,24,33].

Therefore, in this work we first generalized the optimal mass transport map from Euclidean metrics to Riemannian metrics, such that our proposed framework is applicable to any general Riemannian manifolds. The computation is based on geodesic power Voronoi diagram which is an extension of the work [30].

According to Poincare uniformization theorem [21], all shapes can be conformally mapped to one of three canonical spaces: the unit sphere, the Euclidean plane or the hyperbolic plane. The area-distortion factor by the uniformization map gives a probability measure on the canonical uniformization space. All the probability measures on a Riemannian manifold form the Wasserstein space. Given 2 probability measures, there exists a unique optimal mass transport map between them. The transportation cost induced by the optimal mass transport map defines the Wasserstein distance between the two probability measures. Wassertein distance gives a Riemannian metric for the Wasssertein space.

Figure 1 shows the computation of the proposed Riemannian optimal mass transport map between two brain cortical surfaces.

With the tools of uniformization mapping and our Riemannian optimal mass transport map, we proposed a novel framework for shape classification by Wasserstein distance. We applied our method for brain morphology study to classify human brain cortical surfaces with different intelligence quotient. The experimental results and comparisons with previous methods demonstrated the efficiency and efficacy of our method.

In summary, the main contributions of this work are as follows:

1. Introduced the optimal mass transport map to general Riemannian manifolds, which greatly improves the applicability of optimal mass transport map for shape analysis.
2. Presented a novel 3D shape classification framework for brain morphometry analysis using Wasserstein distance, based on uniformization theory and our Riemannian optimal mass transport map.

2 Previous Work

Brain morphometry study plays a fundamental role in medical imaging [14,18,19]. Chaplota et al. [7] introduced a method using wavelets as input to neural network self-organizing maps and support vector machine for brain MR images classification. Singh et al. [27] presented an approach to classify an autistic group from controls using structural image. Zacharaki et al. [34] proposed brain tumor classification method combining conventional MRI and perfusion MRI. Im et al. [12] studied the brain complexity by interpreting the variation of Fractal dimension in the cortical surface of normal controls through multiple regression analysis with cortical thickness, sulcal depth, and folding area.

Various surface based shape analysis and classification methods were also proposed to solve real 3D shape problems. Unnikrishnan et al. [26] presented a multi-scale operators on point clouds that captures variation in shapes. Mahmoudi et al. [20] represented shapes by computing the histogram of pairwise diffusion distances between all points. Kurtek et al. [16] provided a Riemannian framework for computing geodesic paths which are important for comparing and matching 3D shapes. Jermyn et al. [13] defined a general elastic metric on the space of parameter domains for shape comparisons and analysis.

Compared with the elastic shape metric methods [13,16], our metric is intrinsic yet theirs is extrinsic. The elastic shape (extrinsic) metric methods need to embed the surfaces into $\mathbb{R}^3$, which is not necessary in our method. The elastic shape metric assumes two shapes are isotopic. However, the proposed intrinsic method is applicable for general Riemannian manifolds. Our approach solely depends on Riemannian metrics and is invariant under rigid motions and scalings such that it intrinsically measures shape distance, and thus more effective and efficient for shape classification and brain morphology analysis.

3   Theory

This section briefly introduces the theoretic foundation, for thorough treatments, we refer readers to [9] for conformal geometry, and [6,15] for optimal mass transport theory.

3.1   Conformal Mapping

Suppose S is a topological surface, a *Riemannian metric* $\mathbf{g}$ on S is a family of inner products on the tangent planes. Locally, a metric tensor is represented as a positive definite matrix (g_{ij}). Let $\varphi : (S_1, \mathbf{g}_1) \to (S_2, \mathbf{g}_2)$ be a diffeomorphic map between two Riemannian surfaces, the *pull back metric* on the source induced by φ is $\varphi^* \mathbf{g}_2 = J^T \mathbf{g}_2 J$, where J is the Jacobian matrix of φ. The mapping is *conformal* or *angle-preserving*, if the pull back metric and the original metric differ by a scalar function, $\varphi^* \mathbf{g}_2 = e^{2\lambda} \mathbf{g}_1$, where $\lambda : S_1 \to \mathbb{R}$ is called the *conformal factor*.

Hamilton's surface Ricci flow conformably deforms the Riemannian metric proprotional to the curvature, such that the curvature evolves according to a non-linear heat diffusion process, and becomes constant everywhere.

Definition 1 (Surface Ricci Flow). *The normalized surface Ricci flow is defined as*

$$\frac{dg_{ij}(p,t)}{dt} = \left(\frac{4\pi\chi(S)}{A(0)} - 2K(p,t) \right) g_{ij}(p,t),$$

where $\chi(S)$ is the Euler characteristic number of the surface, $A(0)$ is the total area at the initial time.

Theorem 1 (Uniformization). *Suppose $(S, \mathbf{g})$ is a closed compact Riemannian surface with genus g, then there is a conformal factor function $\lambda : S \to \mathbb{R}$, such that the conformal metric $e^{2\lambda}\mathbf{g}$ induces constant Gaussian curvature. Depending on the $\chi(S)$ is positive, zero or negative, the const is $+1$, 0 or -1.*

In the current work, we apply surface Ricci flow to deform the human cortical surface to the unit sphere.

3.2   Optimal Mass Transport

The *Optimal mass transportation problem* was first raised by Monge [5] in the 18th century. Suppose $(S, \mathbf{g})$ is a Riemannian manifold with a metric $\mathbf{g}$. Let μ and ν be two probability measures on S with the same total mass $\int_S d\mu = \int_S d\nu$, $\varphi : S \to S$ be a diffeomorphism, the *pull back* measure induced by ν is $\varphi^* \nu = det(J)\nu \circ \varphi$. The mapping is called *measure preserving*, if the pull back measure equals to the initial measure, $\varphi^* \nu = \mu$. The *transportation cost* of φ is defined as

$$\mathcal{C}(\varphi) := \int_S d_{\mathbf{g}}^2(p, \varphi(p)) d\mu(p). \tag{1}$$

The optimal mass transportation problem is to find the measure preserving mapping, which minimizes the transportation cost,

$$\min_\varphi \mathcal{C}(\varphi)$$
$$s.t. \ \varphi : S \to S, \ \varphi^*\nu = \mu$$

In the 1940s, Kantorovich introduced the relaxation of Monge's problem and solved it using linear programming method [15].

Theorem 2 (Kantorovich). *Suppose $(M, \mathbf{g})$ is a Riemannian manifold, probability measures μ and ν have the same total mass, μ is absolutely continuous, ν has finite second moment, the cost function is the squared geodesic distance, then the optimal mass transportation map exists and is unique.*

If $S \subset \mathbb{R}^n$ is a convex domain in the Euclidean space, then Brenier proved the following theorem.

Theorem 3 (Brenier). *There is a convex function $u : S \to \mathbb{R}$, the optimal map is given by the gradient map $p \to \nabla u(p)$.*

Solving the optimal transportation problem is equivalent to solve the following Monge-Ampéré equation,

$$det\left(\frac{\partial^2 u}{\partial x_i \partial x_j}\right) \nu \circ \nabla u(\mathbf{x}) = \mu(\mathbf{x}).$$

3.3 Wasserstein Metric Space

Suppose $(S, \mathbf{g})$ is a Riemannian manifold with a Riemannian metric $\mathbf{g}$.

Definition 2 (Wasserstein Space). *For $p \geq 1$, let $\mathcal{P}_p(S)$ denote the space of all probability measures μ on M with finite p^{th} moment, for some $x_0 \in S$, $\int_S d(x, x_0)^p d\mu(x) < +\infty$, where d is the geodesic distance induced by $\mathbf{g}$.*

Given two probability μ and ν in $\mathcal{P}_p$, the Wasserstein distance between them is defined as the transportation cost induced by the optimal transportation map $\varphi : S \to S$,

$$W_p(\mu, \nu) := \inf_{\varphi^*\nu=\mu} \left(\int_M d_{\mathbf{g}}^p(x, \varphi(x)) d\mu(x)\right)^{\frac{1}{p}}.$$

The following theorem plays a fundamental role for the current work

Theorem 4. *The Wasserstein distance W_p is a Riemannian metric of the Wasserstein space $\mathcal{P}_p(S)$.*

Detailed proof can be found in [28].

3.4   Discrete Optimal Mass Transport

Let $P = \{p_1, p_2, \ldots, p_k\}$ be a discrete point set on S, $\mathbf{h} = \{h_1, h_2, \ldots, h_k\}$ be the *weight* vector.

Definition 3 (Geodesic Power Voronoi Diagram). *Given the point set P and the weight $\mathbf{h}$, the geodesic power voronoi diagram induced by $(P, \mathbf{h})$ is a cell decomposition of the manifold $(S, \mathbf{g})$, such that the cell associated with p_i is given by*

$$W_i := \{q \in S | d_{\mathbf{g}}^2(p_i, q) - h_i \le d_{\mathbf{g}}^2(p_j, q) - h_j\}.$$

Theorem 5 (Discrete Optimal Mass Transportation Map). *Given a Riemannian manifold $(S, \mathbf{g})$, two probability measures μ and ν are of the same total mass. ν is a Dirac measure, with discrete point set support $P = \{p_1, p_2, \cdots, p_k\}$, $\nu(p_i) = \nu_i$. There exists a weight $\mathbf{h} = \{h_1, h_2, \cdots, h_k\}$, unique up to a constant, the geodesic power Voronoi diagram induced by $(P, \mathbf{h})$ gives the optimal mass transportation map,*

$$\varphi : W_i \to p_i, i = 1, 2, \cdots, k,$$

furthermore

$$\int_{W_i} d\mu = \nu_i, \forall i.$$

Proof. Suppose $S = \cup_{i=1}^k \tilde{W}_i$ is another partition of the manifold, such that $\int_{\tilde{W}_i} d\mu = \nu_i$. The mapping $\tilde{\varphi} : \tilde{W}_i \to p_i$ is another measure-preserving mapping. By the definition of geodesic Voronoi diagram, given any point $p \in W_i$, suppose it belongs to $\tilde{W}_j$, then

$$d_{\mathbf{g}}^2(p, p_i) - h_i \le d_{\mathbf{g}}^2(p, p_j) - h_j,$$

this induces

$$\sum_{i=1}^k \int_{W_i} (d_{\mathbf{g}}^2(p, p_i) - h_i) d\mu(p) \le \sum_{j=1}^k \int_{\tilde{W}_j} (d_{\mathbf{g}}^2(q, p_i) - h_j) d\mu(q)$$

Then

$$\mathcal{C}(\varphi) - \sum \nu_i h_i \le \mathcal{C}(\tilde{\varphi}) - \sum \nu_j h_j$$

This shows for any measure preserving mapping, $\mathcal{C}(\tilde{\varphi}) \ge \mathcal{C}(\varphi)$.

The optimal weight for the geodesic power Voronoi diagram that induces the optimal transportation map can be found by

$$\frac{dh_i}{dt} = \nu_i - \int_{W_i(\mathbf{h})} d\mu. \tag{2}$$

4   Algorithm

4.1   Riemannian Optimal Mass Transport Map

This section gives the algorithmic implementation details for Riemannian optimal mass transport map (OMT-Map) generation using geodesic power Voronoi diagram.

Smooth metric surfaces can be approximated by piecewise linear triangle mesh. There are many ways to discretize a smooth surface, such that the piecewise linear metrics converge to the smooth metric, e.g., the sampling is uniform and the triangulation is geodesic Delaunay. The geodesics on the triangle meshes can be efficiently computed using the algorithms in [30].

First, we repeat subdividing the triangle mesh until the size of each triangle is small enough to ensure the accuracy. Then from each point p_i in the point set P, we compute the geodesics to reach every other vertex on the subdivided mesh, this gives the geodesic distance from every vertex to p_i. Repeat this for all vertices in P.

Third, we find the optimal weight. We initialize all the weights to be zeros, then update the weight using the formula

$$\frac{dh_i}{dt} = \nu_i - \int_{W_i(\mathbf{h})} \mu(p)dp.$$

Details of the algorithm can be found in Algorithm 1.

4.2   Wasserstein Distance

The OMT-Map algorithm can also be generalized to compute the Wasserstein distance between surfaces. Given two topological spherical surfaces $(S_1, \mathbf{g}_1)$, $(S_2, \mathbf{g}_2)$ with total area 4π. We first compute the conformal maps by [21] $\phi_1 : S_1 \to \mathbb{S}^2$ and $\phi_2 : S_2 \to \mathbb{S}^2$, where $\mathbb{S}^2$ is the unit sphere. The conformal factors $e^{2\lambda_1}$ and $e^{2\lambda_2}$ define two probability measures on the sphere, which can be computed by [21].

Then we discretize $\mathbb{S}^2$ into a discrete point set with measure (P, ν), where ν is computed as follows: first we compute geodesic voronoi diagram induced by P, suppose the Voronoi cell associated with p_i is W_i, then

$$\nu_i := \int_{W_i} e^{2\lambda(p)} dA(p),. \tag{3}$$

where dA is the spherical area element. Denote the measure $e^{2\lambda_1}dA$ as μ, use $(\mathbb{S}^2, \mu)$ and (P, ν) as inputs of Algorithm 1, we compute the Optimal Mass Transport map $T : \mathbb{S}^2 \to P$, $W_i(\mathbf{h}) \to p_i$, where $p_i \in P, i = 1, 2, \cdots, k$. Therefore, the Wasserstein distance between S_1 and S_2 can be computed by

$$Wasserstein(\mu, \nu) = \sum_{i=1}^{k} \int_{W_i} d_{\mathbf{g}}^2(x, T(x))^2 \mu(x)dx \tag{4}$$

Algorithm 2 gives the implementation details.

Algorithm 1. Riemannian Optimal Mass Transport Map

Input: A triangle mesh M, measure μ and Dirac measure $\{(p_1, \nu_1), (p_2, \nu_2), \cdots,$ $(p_k, \nu_k)\}$, $\int_M u(p)dp = \sum_{i=1}^{k} \nu_i$; a threshold ϵ.
Output: The unique discrete Optimal Mass Transport Map $\varphi : (M, \mu) \to (P, \nu)$.

Subdivide M for several levels, until each triangle size is small enough.
for all $p_i \in P$ **do**
    Compute the geodesic from p_i to every other vertex on M,
end for
$\mathbf{h} \leftarrow (0, 0, \cdots, 0)$.
repeat
    for all vertex v_j on M **do**
        Find the minimum weighted squared geodesic distance, decide which Voronoi
        cell v_i belongs to, $v_i \in W_t(\mathbf{h})$

$$t = argmin_k d_{\mathbf{g}}^2(v_j, p_k) + h_k$$

    end for
    for all $p_i \in P$ **do**
        Compute the current cell area $w_i = \int_{W_i(\mathbf{h})} d\mu$,
    end for
    for all $h_i \in \mathbf{h}$ **do**
        Update h_i, $h_i = h_i + \delta(\nu_i - w_i)$
    end for
until $|\nu_i - w_i| < \epsilon, \forall i$.
return Power geodesic Voronoi diagram.

Algorithm 2. Computing Wasserstein Distance

Input: Two topological spherical surfaces $(S_1, \mathbf{g}_1)$, $(S_2, \mathbf{g}_2)$.
Output: The Wasserstein distance between S_1 and S_2.

1. Scale and normalize S_1 and S_2 such that the total area of each surface is 4π.
2. Compute the conformal maps by [21] $\phi_1 : S_1 \to \mathbb{S}^2$ and $\phi_2 : S_2 \to \mathbb{S}^2$, where $\mathbb{S}^2$ is the unit sphere, and ϕ_1 and ϕ_2 are with normalization conditions: the mass center of the image points are at the sphere center.
3. Compute the conformal factors λ_1 and λ_2 by [8]. Construct the measure $\mu \leftarrow e^{2\lambda_1} dA$.
4. Discretize $\mathbb{S}^2$ into a discrete point set with measure (P, ν), where ν is computed by Eq. 3.
5. With $(\mathbb{S}^2, \mu)$ and (P, ν) as inputs of Algorithm 1, we compute the Riemannian Optimal Mass Transport map.
6. Wasserstein distance between S_1 and S_2 can be computed by Eq. 4.

---

5   Brain Cortical Surface Classification

There have been much research into the relation between human intelligence and human brain. Earlier works have studied some significant factors such as cortical surface area, cortical thickness and cortical convolution [12,18,19]. To validate the correctness of our framework in real applications, we applied our method for the classification problem of brain cortical surfaces with different intelligence quotient (IQ), and compared with some existing works.

The biological properties of interest by our method are as follows: The brain cortical surface is conformally mapped to the unit sphere, the conformal factor represents the area distortion. In fact, the area distortion factor encodes the complete information of the original Riemannian metric of the brain: due to the conformality of the mapping, the metric on brain equals to the product of the conformal factor and spherical metric. Therefore, Wasserstein distance between the conformal factors gives the distance between the Riemannian metrics of the cortical surfaces. The Gaussian curvatures on the brains are induced by their metrics. This method is stronger than solely comparing curvatures.

Data Preparation: The brain data is from the Center for Cognitive and Behavioral Brain Imaging at the Ohio State University. MRI recording was performed using a standard 12-channel head coil on a Siemens 3T Trio Magnetic Resonance Imaging System with TIM. The brain cortical surfaces are reconstructed from MRI images by FreeSurfer [2]. Our experimental dataset includes 50 males and 50 females, with ages ranging from 18 to 30 years uniformly distributed. Among all the brain data, we used the left hemisphere of the brain surface for experiments.

The intelligence quotient (IQ) was evaluated by an online version of Ravens Advanced Progressive Matrices (APM) [3]. The test consists of 36 questions and the IQ score is calculated by $N_{correctAnswers}/N_{total} * 100$. The IQ among the data ranges from 0 to 100, which are uniformly distributed. Figure 1 shows the computation of Wasserstein distance between two brain cortical surfaces. (a) shows an example of a 20-year-old female, with IQ score 88.89; (b) shows an example of a 21-year-old male, with IQ score 33.33.

Instead of claiming whether one human brain is intelligent or not, in our experimental settings we divided the IQ into three classes: A, B, and C, ranging from $A : [0, 33)$, $B : [33, 67)$ and $C : [67, 100]$. The data uniformly distributed in the three classes. For each gender, we randomly chose 12 examples from each class. Therefore, we created a training set of 72 examples, which is uniformly distributed with respect to gender and IQ. And the remaining examples are used as testing data.

For the classification experiments, we first computed the full pair-wise Wasserstein distance matrix based on our method. We indexed all the data of class A into $i = 1, 2, ..., 33$, data of class B into $i = 34, 35, ..., 66$ and data of class C into $i = 67, 68, ...100$. Figure 2(a) shows the visualization of the Wasserstein distance matrix encoded in a gray image. The distance is normalized from 0 to 1, where 0 indicates black and 1 indicates white. The entry of the matrix $M_{i,j}$ is the Wasserstein distance between brain data i and brain data j. Then we can clearly see that, mostly, two surfaces in the same class induce smaller Wasserstein distance, yet two surfaces in different classes induce larger Wasserstein distance. The results further demonstrated the power of Wasserstein distance for measuring shape similarities.

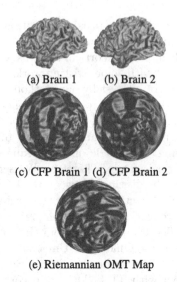

(a) Brain 1   (b) Brain 2

(c) CFP Brain 1 (d) CFP Brain 2

(e) Riemannian OMT Map

Fig. 1. The computation of Wasserstein distance between the left hemisphere brain cortical surfaces. (a) shows an example of a 20-year-old female, with IQ score 88.89; (b) shows an example of a 21-year-old male, with IQ score 33.33. (c) and (d) are the spherical conformal parameterization (CFP) of (a) and (b), respectively. (e) shows the Riemannian optimal mass transport (OMT) map result from (c) to (d), which induces the Wasserstein distance between (a) and (b).

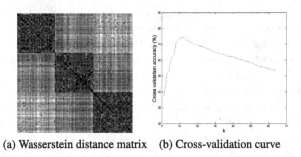

(a) Wasserstein distance matrix   (b) Cross-validation curve

Fig. 2. (a) Wasserstein distance matrix encoded in a gray image. The distance is normalized from 0 to 1, where 0 indicates black and 1 indicates white. The results show that, mostly, two surfaces in the same class induce smaller Wasserstein distance, yet two surfaces in different classes induce larger Wasserstein distance. (b) Cross-validation curve.

With the distance matrix, we classified the testing set by k-Nearest Neighbors (k-NN) classifier, where k is chosen to be 11 by running 9-fold cross-validation. The cross-validation curve is shown in Fig. 2 (b). Table 1 shows the classification rate of our method is 78.57 %.

To demonstrate the efficiency and advantages of our method, we compared our method with existing popular method. Previous work [14] shows that cortical surface area and cortical surface mean curvature have significant correlations to human intelligence, since they quantify the complexity of cortical foldings. Thus we computed the two cortical measurements and used surface area, mean curvature, and the combination of the two measurements as three types of features for classification, respectively. We used LIBSVM [1] as the classifier. Linear kernel and regularization parameter $C = 4.5$ were chosen by cross validation. Table 1 reports the classification rate of all the three comparison methods. The results indicated that our method outperforms previous methods.

Table 1. Classification rate (CR) of our method and previous methods based on cortical surface area, cortical surface mean curvature and combination of previous two cortical measurements. The results demonstrated the accuracy of our method.

Method	CR
Our method	78.57%
Surface Area	53.57%
Surface Mean Curvature	57.14%
Combination of Area and Curvature	67.85%

6 Conclusion and Future Work

This work introduces a novel 3D shape classification framework for brain morphology study using Wasserstein distance, based on uniformization theory and Riemannian optimal mass transport theory. We generalized the existing optimal mass transport map from Euclidean metrics to Riemannian metrics. The theoretical foundation is rigorous, and the computation is based on geodesic power Voronoi diagram.

Comparing to the existing methods, our algorithm solely depends on Riemannian metrics and is invariant under rigid motions and scalings, thus it intrinsically measures distance between shapes. We applied the proposed framework for classification of brain cortical surfaces with different intelligent quotient. The experimental results show that our method outperforms previous methods based on surface area and surface mean curvature. In the future, we will explore and validate broader applications in other medical imaging field by our framework.

References

1. http://www.csie.ntu.edu.tw/~cjlin/libsvm/
2. http://www.freesurfer.net/
3. Raven, J.C., et al.: Raven Manual: Section 4, Advanced Progressive Matrices. Oxford Psychologists Press Ltd., Oxford (1998)

4. Ankerst, M., Kastenmüller, G., Kriegel, H.-P., Seidl, T.: 3D shape histograms for similarity search and classification in spatial databases. In: Güting, R.H., Papadias, D., Lochovsky, F.H. (eds.) SSD 1999. LNCS, vol. 1651, pp. 207–226. Springer, Heidelberg (1999)
5. Bonnotte, N.: From Knothe's rearrangement to Brenier's optimal transport map, pp. 1–29 (2012). arXiv:1205.1099
6. Brenier, Y.: Polar factorization and monotone rearrangement of vector-valued functions. Com. Pure Appl. Math. 64, 375–417 (1991)
7. Chaplota, S., Patnaika, L., Jagannathanb, N.: Classification of magnetic resonance brain images using wavelets as input to support vector machine and neural network. Biomed. Signal Process. Control 1, 86–92 (2006)
8. Gu, X., Wang, Y., Yau, S.-T.: Geometric compression using riemann surface structure. Commun. Inf. Syst. 3(3), 171–182 (2003)
9. Gu, X., Yau, S.-T.: Computational Conformal Geometry. International Press, Boston (2008)
10. Hilaga, M., Shinagawa, Y., Kohmura, T., Kunii, T.: Topology matching for fully automatic similarity estimation of 3D shapes. In: SIGGRAPH 2001, vol. 21, pp. 203–212 (2001)
11. Hong, B.-W., Soatto, S.: Shape matching using multiscale integral invariants. IEEE TPAMI 37, 151–160 (2014)
12. Im, K., Lee, J., Yoon, U., Shin, Y., Hong, S., Kim, I., Kwon, J., Kim, S.: Fractal dimension in human cortical surface: multiple regression analysis with cortical thickness, sulcal depth and folding area. Hum. Brain Mapp. 27, 994–1003 (2006)
13. Jermyn, I.H., Kurtek, S., Klassen, E., Srivastava, A.: Elastic shape matching of parameterized surfaces using square root normal fields. In: Fitzgibbon, A., Lazebnik, S., Perona, P., Sato, Y., Schmid, C. (eds.) ECCV 2012, Part V. LNCS, vol. 7576, pp. 804–817. Springer, Heidelberg (2012)
14. Yang, J.J., Yoon, U., Yun, H., Im, K., Choi, Y.Y., Kim, S.I., Lee, K.H., Lee, J.-M.: Prediction for human intelligence using morphometric characteristics of cortical surface: partial least square analysis. Neuroscience 246, 351–361 (2013)
15. Kantorovich, L.V.: On a problem of monge. Uspekhi Mat. Nauk. 3, 225–226 (1948)
16. Kurtek, S., Klassen, E., Gore, J.C., Ding, Z., Srivastava, A.: Elastic geodesic paths in shape space of parameterized surfaces. TPAMI 34, 1717–1730 (2012)
17. Laga, H., Takahashi, H., Nakajima, M.: Three-dimensional point cloud recognition via distributions of geometric distances. In: Shape Modeling and Applications, pp. 15–23 (2006)
18. Luders, E., Narr, K., Bilder, R., Szeszko, P., Gurbani, M., Hamilton, L., Toga, A., Gaser, C.: Mapping the relationship between cortical convolution and intelligence: effects of gender. Cereb. Cortex 18, 2019–2026 (2008)
19. Luders, E., Narr, K., Bilder, R., Thompson, P., Szeszko, P., Hamilton, L., Toga, A.: Positive correlations between corpus callosum thickness and intelligence. Neuroimage 37, 1457–1464 (2007)
20. Mahmoudi, M., Sapiro, G.: Three-dimensional point cloud recognition via distributions of geometric distances. J. Graph. Models 71, 22–32 (2009)
21. Jin, M., Kim, J., Luo, F., Gu, X.: Discrete surface ricci flow. TVCG 14, 1030–1043 (2008)
22. Osada, R., Funkhouser, T., Chazelle, B., Dobkin, D.: Shape distributions. In: Symposium on Large Spatial Databases, vol. 21, pp. 807–832 (2002)
23. Schmitzer, B., Schnörr, C.: Object segmentation by shape matching with wasserstein modes. In: Heyden, A., Kahl, F., Olsson, C., Oskarsson, M., Tai, X.-C. (eds.) EMMCVPR 2013. LNCS, vol. 8081, pp. 123–136. Springer, Heidelberg (2013)

24. Srivastava, A., Klassen, E., Joshi, S.H., Jermyn, I.H.: Shape analysis of elastic curves in euclidean spaces. TPAMI **33**(7), 1415–1428 (2011)
25. Thompson, P.M., Hayashi, K.M., Doddrell, D.M., Toga, A.W.: Dynamics of gray matter loss in Alzheimer's disease. J. Neurosci. **23**, 994–1005 (2003)
26. Unnikrishnan, R., Hebert, M.: Multi-scale interest regions from unorganized point clouds. In: CVPR Workshop (2008)
27. Singh, V., Mukherjee, L., Chung, M.K.: Cortical surface thickness as a classifier. Med. Image Comput. Comput. Assist. Interv. **11**, 999–1007 (2008)
28. Villani, C.: Topics in Optimal Transportation. American Mathematical Society, Providence (2003)
29. Wang, W., Slepev, D., Basu, S., Ozolek, J.A., Rohde, G.K.: A linear optimal transportation framework for quantifying and visualizing variations in sets of images. IJCV **101**(2), 254–269 (2013)
30. Wang, X., Ying, X., Liub, Y.-J., Xin, S.-Q., Wang, W., Gu, X., Mueller-Wittig, W., He, Y.: Intrinsic computation of centroidal voronoi tessellation (CVT) on meshes. Comput. Aided Des. **58**, 51–61 (2015)
31. Winkler, A.M., Glahn, D.C.: Cortical thickness or grey matter volume? the importance of selecting the phenotype for imaging genetics studies. Neuroimage **53**(3), 1135–1146 (2010)
32. Winkler, A.M., Glahn, D.C.: Measuring and comparing brain cortical surface area and other areal quantities. Neuroimage **61**(4), 1428–1443 (2012)
33. Younes, L.: Spaces and manifolds of shapes in computer vision: an overview. Image Vis. Comput. **30**(6–7), 389–397 (2012)
34. Zacharaki, E.I., Wang, S., Chawla, S., Yoo, D.S., Wolf, R., Melhem, E.R., Davatzikosa, C.: Classification of brain tumor type and grade using mri texture and shape in a machine learning scheme. Magn. Reson. Med. **62**, 1609–1618 (2009)

Temporal Trajectory and Progression Score Estimation from Voxelwise Longitudinal Imaging Measures: Application to Amyloid Imaging

Murat Bilgel[1,2]($\boxtimes$), Bruno Jedynak[3], Dean F. Wong[4],
Susan M. Resnick[2], and Jerry L. Prince[1,3,4,5]

[1] Department of Biomedical Engineering, School of Engineering,
Johns Hopkins University, Baltimore, MD, USA
mbilgel1@jhu.edu
[2] Laboratory of Behavioral Neuroscience,
National Institute on Aging, NIH, Baltimore, MD, USA
[3] Department of Applied Mathematics and Statistics, School of Engineering,
Johns Hopkins University, Baltimore, MD, USA
[4] Department of Radiology, School of Medicine,
Johns Hopkins University, Baltimore, MD, USA
[5] Department of Electrical and Computer Engineering, School of Engineering,
Johns Hopkins University, Baltimore, MD, USA

Abstract. Cortical β-amyloid deposition begins in Alzheimer's disease (AD) years before the onset of any clinical symptoms. It is therefore important to determine the temporal trajectories of amyloid deposition in these earliest stages in order to better understand their associations with progression to AD. A method for estimating the temporal trajectories of voxelwise amyloid as measured using longitudinal positron emission tomography (PET) imaging is presented. The method involves the estimation of a score for each subject visit based on the PET data that reflects their amyloid progression. This amyloid progression score allows subjects with similar progressions to be aligned and analyzed together. The estimation of the progression scores and the amyloid trajectory parameters are performed using an expectation-maximization algorithm. The correlations among the voxel measures of amyloid are modeled to reflect the spatial nature of PET images. Simulation results show that model parameters are captured well at a variety of noise and spatial correlation levels. The method is applied to longitudinal amyloid imaging data considering each cerebral hemisphere separately. The results are consistent across the hemispheres and agree with a global index of brain amyloid known as mean cortical DVR. Unlike mean cortical DVR, which depends on *a priori* defined regions, the progression score extracted by the method is data-driven and does not make assumptions about regional longitudinal changes. Compared to regressing on age at each voxel, the longitudinal trajectory slopes estimated using the proposed method show better localized longitudinal changes.

Keywords: Progression score · Amyloid · Pittsburgh compound B · PiB · Longitudinal image analysis

© Springer International Publishing Switzerland 2015
S. Ourselin et al. (Eds.): IPMI 2015, LNCS 9123, pp. 424–436, 2015.
DOI: 10.1007/978-3-319-19992-4_33

1 Introduction

Cortical β-amyloid deposition is a neuropathological hallmark associated with Alzheimer's disease (AD), and begins years before any cognitive symptoms of AD are evident [8]. Studying within-subject longitudinal changes is limited by the number of follow-up visits. The relatively short span of longitudinal positron emission tomograpy (PET) studies of amyloid deposition compared to its hypothesized timeline makes it difficult to extensively study the longitudinal brain amyloid changes that occur in the preclinical stages of AD.

It is possible to "stitch" data across subjects in order to obtain temporal biomarker trajectories that fit an underlying model. This is the premise of the Disease Progression Score method, which has been applied to studying changes in cognitive and biological markers related to Alzheimer's disease [3,9]. It is assumed that there is an underlying progression score (PS) for each subject visit that is a linear transform of the subject's age, and given this PS, it is possible to place biomarker measurements across a group of subjects onto a common timeline. The linear transformation of age removes across-subject variability in baseline biomarker measures as well as in their rates of longitudinal progression. Each biomarker is associated with a parametric trajectory as a function of PS, whose parameters are estimated along with the PS for each subject.

Other methods for analyzing trajectories of biomarkers have been proposed. One approach involves fitting a piecewise linear model to longitudinal data assuming that each biomarker becomes abnormal a certain number of years before clinical diagnosis, and this duration is estimated for each biomarker to yield the longitudinal trajectories as a function of time to diagnosis [13]. In another approach, an event-based probabilistic framework is used to determine the ordering of changes in longitudinal biomarker measures as well as the appropriate thresholds for separating normal from abnormal measures [14]. The second method is agnostic to clinical diagnosis, but does not allow for the characterization of longitudinal biomarker trajectories except for determining the ordering of the change points. The first method does delineate the longitudinal trajectories for each biomarker, but requires knowledge of clinical diagnosis and therefore is not suitable for studying the earliest changes in healthy individuals.

Here, we adopt the disease progression score principle, but make two substantial innovations. First, the voxelwise PET measures constitute the biomarkers in the model. Since voxelwise PET measures have an underlying spatial correlation, we incorporate the modeling of the spatial correlations among the biomarker error terms and estimate the spatial correlations along with the subject and trajectory parameters. Modeling spatial correlations makes the inference of the subject-specific progression scores less susceptible to the inherent correlations among the voxels. Second, instead of using an alternating least-squares approach for parameter estimation, we formulate the model fitting as an expectation-maximization (EM) algorithm, which guarantees optimality and convergence. In experiments using this approach, we first show using simulated data that the model parameters are estimated accurately, then apply the method to each cerebral hemisphere separately using distribution volume ratio (DVR) images derived from Pittsburgh compound B (PiB) PET imaging, which show the distribution of amyloid. Models fitted using data for 75 participants with a total of 271 visits reveal that the precuneus and frontal lobes show the greatest longitudinal increases in amyloid, with smaller increases in lateral temporal and temporoparietal regions, and minimal increases in the occipital lobe and the sensorimotor strip. Results are consistent across the two hemispheres, and the estimated PS agrees with a widely used global index of brain amyloid known as mean cortical DVR.

2   Method

2.1   Model

The progression score s_{ij} for subject i at visit j is assumed to be a linear transformation of age t_{ij}:

$$s_{ij} = \alpha_i t_{ij} + \beta_i, \tag{1}$$

where (α_i, β_i) are assumed to be uniformly distributed random variables on a fixed and large domain $\Omega \subset \mathbb{R}^2$. The collection of K biomarker measurements (the intensities at each PiB-PET DVR voxel reflecting amyloid levels) make up the $K \times 1$ vector $\mathbf{y}_{ij}$. The longitudinal trajectories associated with these biomarkers are assumed have a linear form parameterized by $K \times 1$ vectors $\mathbf{a} = [a_1, a_2, \ldots, a_K]^T$ and $\mathbf{b} = [b_1, \ldots, b_K]^T$:

$$\mathbf{y}_{ij} = \mathbf{a}\, s_{ij} + \mathbf{b} + \boldsymbol{\varepsilon}_{ij}. \tag{2}$$

Here, $\boldsymbol{\varepsilon}_{ij} \sim \mathcal{N}_K(\mathbf{0}, R)$ is the observation noise. The covariance matrix R is assumed to be of the form $R = \lambda^2 C(\rho)$, where λ is a positive scalar and C is a correlation matrix parameterized by ρ. The parameters $(\mathbf{a}, \mathbf{b}, \lambda, \rho)$ make up $\boldsymbol{\theta}$.

2.2   Log-Likelihood Function

Let $\mathbf{y}_i$ be the vector consisting of all biomarker measurements stacked across all visits of subject i and let $\mathbf{u}_i = [\alpha_i, \beta_i]^T$. We then define $\mathbf{y} = \left[\mathbf{y}_1^T, \mathbf{y}_2^T, \ldots, \mathbf{y}_n^T\right]^T$ and $\mathbf{u} = \left[\mathbf{u}_1^T, \mathbf{u}_2^T, \ldots, \mathbf{u}_n^T\right]^T$, where n is the number of subjects. The pair $(\mathbf{y}, \mathbf{u})$ is the complete data. The complete log-likelihood for the model, ignoring the constants, is given by

$$\ell(\mathbf{y}, \mathbf{u} \mid \boldsymbol{\theta}) = -\sum_{i,j} \left[\log(\det R) + (\mathbf{y}_{ij} - Z_{ij}\mathbf{u}_i - \mathbf{b})^T R^{-1} (\mathbf{y}_{ij} - Z_{ij}\mathbf{u}_i - \mathbf{b}) \right], \tag{3}$$

where $Z_{ij} = \mathbf{a}\begin{bmatrix} t_{ij} & 1 \end{bmatrix}$ and $R = \lambda^2 C(\rho)$.

2.3   EM Algorithm Derivation

The observations $\mathbf{y}$ include biomarker measurements $\{\mathbf{y}_{ij}\}$ at each visit. The hidden variables $\mathbf{u}$ are the subject-specific parameters $\{\alpha_i\}$ and $\{\beta_i\}$. The unknown parameters are $\boldsymbol{\theta} = (\mathbf{a}, \mathbf{b}, \lambda, \rho)$.

E-Step: Let θ' be the previous estimate of the parameters. The expectation step involves evaluating an expression for

$$E\left[\ell\left(\mathbf{y},\mathbf{u}\mid\boldsymbol{\theta}\right)\mid\mathbf{y},\boldsymbol{\theta}'\right] = \sum_i \int f(\tilde{\mathbf{u}}_i\mid\mathbf{y}_i,\boldsymbol{\theta}')\ell\left(\mathbf{y}_i,\tilde{\mathbf{u}}_i\mid\boldsymbol{\theta}\right)d\tilde{\mathbf{u}}_i. \tag{4}$$

Note that

$$f(\mathbf{y}_i\mid\tilde{\mathbf{u}}_i,\boldsymbol{\theta}') = \phi(\mathbf{y}_i; Z_i'\tilde{\mathbf{u}}_i + \mathbf{b}_i', R_i') \tag{5}$$
$$= \phi(\hat{\mathbf{u}}_i'; \tilde{\mathbf{u}}_i, S_i'), \tag{6}$$

where

$$\hat{\mathbf{u}}_i' = \left(\sum_j Z_{ij}'^T R'^{-1} Z_{ij}'\right)^{-1} \sum_j Z_{ij}'^T R'^{-1}(\mathbf{y}_{ij} - \mathbf{b}'), \tag{7}$$

$S_i' = \left(\sum_j Z_{ij}'^T R'^{-1} Z_{ij}'\right)^{-1}$, and $\phi(\cdot; \boldsymbol{\mu}, \boldsymbol{\Sigma})$ is a multivariate Gaussian density with mean $\boldsymbol{\mu}$ and covariance $\boldsymbol{\Sigma}$. For ease of notation, we have used $\mathbf{b}_i'$ to denote $\mathbf{b}'$ stacked across the visits of subject i and R_i' to denote diagonally stacked R' matrices across the visits of subject i. Z_i' is obtained by diagonally stacking $Z_{ij}' = \mathbf{a}'\left[t_{ij}\ 1\right]$ across the visits of subject i.

The uniform prior assumption on $\mathbf{u}_i$ allows us to write $f(\tilde{\mathbf{u}}_i,\boldsymbol{\theta}') = 1/c$, where c is a constant. Rewriting the expectation using Bayes' rule and plugging in the result from (6) yields

$$E\left[\ell\left(\mathbf{y},\mathbf{u}\mid\boldsymbol{\theta}\right)\mid\mathbf{y},\boldsymbol{\theta}'\right] \propto \sum_i \int_\Omega \frac{\phi(\hat{\mathbf{u}}_i'; \tilde{\mathbf{u}}_i, S_i')}{f(\mathbf{y}_i,\boldsymbol{\theta}')}\ell\left(\mathbf{y}_i,\tilde{\mathbf{u}}_i\mid\boldsymbol{\theta}\right)d\tilde{\mathbf{u}}_i. \tag{8}$$

If Ω is large enough, we can approximate the expectation as an infinite domain integration over $\mathbf{u}_i$ to obtain

$$E\left[\ell\left(\mathbf{y},\mathbf{u}\mid\boldsymbol{\theta}\right)\mid\mathbf{y},\boldsymbol{\theta}'\right] \propto \sum_i \int \phi(\hat{\mathbf{u}}_i'; \tilde{\mathbf{u}}_i, S_i')\ell\left(\mathbf{y}_i,\tilde{\mathbf{u}}_i\mid\boldsymbol{\theta}\right)d\tilde{\mathbf{u}}_i \tag{9}$$

$$\propto -\sum_{i,j} \log[\det R] - \sum_{i,j}(\mathbf{y}_{ij} - \mathbf{b})^T R^{-1}(\mathbf{y}_{ij} - \mathbf{b})$$

$$+ 2\left(\sum_{i,j} s_{ij}'\mathbf{y}_{ij} - \mathbf{b}\sum_{i,j} s_{ij}'\right)^T R^{-1}\mathbf{a}$$

$$- \mathbf{a}^T R^{-1}\mathbf{a}\left(\frac{n}{\mathbf{a}'^T R'^{-1}\mathbf{a}'} + \sum_{i,j} s_{ij}'^2\right), \tag{10}$$

where $s_{ij}' = \left[t_{ij}\ 1\right]\hat{\mathbf{u}}_i'$.

M-Step: Let $g\left(\boldsymbol{\theta},\boldsymbol{\theta}'\right)$ be the function obtained at the end of the E-step. We set the derivatives $\frac{\partial g}{\partial \mathbf{a}}$ and $\frac{\partial g}{\partial \mathbf{b}}$ equal to 0 and solve for the parameters to obtain

$$\mathbf{a} = \frac{\sum_{i,j} s'_{ij}(\mathbf{y}_{ij} - \bar{\mathbf{y}})}{\frac{2n}{\mathbf{a}'^T R'^{-1} \mathbf{a}'} + \sum_{i,j} s'^2_{ij} - \frac{1}{\sum_i v_i}\left(\sum_{i,j} s'_{ij}\right)^2}, \tag{11}$$

$$\mathbf{b} = \frac{\left(\frac{2n}{\mathbf{a}'^T R'^{-1} \mathbf{a}'} + \sum_{i,j} s'^2_{ij}\right)\left(\sum_{i,j} \mathbf{y}_{ij}\right) - \left(\sum_{i,j} s'_{ij}\right)\left(\sum_{i,j} s'_{ij}\mathbf{y}_{ij}\right)}{\left(\sum_i v_i\right)\left(\frac{2n}{\mathbf{a}'^T R'^{-1} \mathbf{a}'} + \sum_{i,j} s'^2_{ij}\right) - \left(\sum_{i,j} s'_{ij}\right)^2}, \tag{12}$$

where v_i is the number of visits for subject i, and $\bar{\mathbf{y}} = \frac{1}{\sum_i v_i} \sum_{i,j} \mathbf{y}_{ij}$.

We must use numerical optimization to solve for the covariance parameters λ and ρ as a closed form solution does not exist. Instead of performing this optimization over the two parameters simultaneously, we perform coordinate descent: we first fix ρ at its previous estimate and optimize over λ, and then we fix λ and optimize over ρ. This process increases the value of the expectation instead of maximizing it, but the convergence property of the EM algorithm is not violated. This simplification allows us to write down a closed form solution for λ. When ρ is fixed, meaning that the covariance matrix C is fixed, we have that

$$\lambda = \sqrt{\frac{1}{K \sum_i v_i}\left[\frac{2n\mathbf{a}^T C^{-1}\mathbf{a}}{\mathbf{a}'^T R'^{-1}\mathbf{a}'} + \sum_{i,j}\left(\mathbf{y}_{ij} - \mathbf{a}s'_{ij} - \mathbf{b}\right)^T C^{-1}\left(\mathbf{y}_{ij} - \mathbf{a}s'_{ij} - \mathbf{b}\right)\right]}, \tag{13}$$

where $\mathbf{a}$ and $\mathbf{b}$ are as given in (11) and (12). We then optimize over ρ using a numerical method, fixing $\mathbf{a}, \mathbf{b}$ and λ at their current estimates as given in (11), (12) and (13):

$$\rho = \arg\max_{\rho} g\left(\boldsymbol{\theta}, \boldsymbol{\theta}'\right). \tag{14}$$

The EM steps are iterated until the relative change in the function $g(\boldsymbol{\theta}, \boldsymbol{\theta}')$ is less than a small tolerance. Upon convergence, the subject-specific parameters $\mathbf{u}_i = [\alpha_i, \beta_i]^T$ are estimated using (7).

2.4   Selection and Initialization of the Spatial Correlation Function

We obtain an initial fit assuming that $C = I_{K \times K}$ and calculate the empirical semivariogram using the robust estimator [5]

$$\hat{\gamma}(s) = \left(\frac{1}{2N(s)}\sum_{i,j}\sum_{d(k,k')=s}|r_{ijk} - r_{ijk'}|^{0.5}\right)^4 /(0.457 + 0.494/N(s)), \tag{15}$$

where $\mathbf{r}_{ij}$ is obtained by standardizing the residual $\mathbf{y}_{ij} - \mathbf{a}s_{ij} - \mathbf{b}$, $d(k, k')$ is the Euclidean distance between voxels k and k', and $N(s)$ is the number of voxel pairs that are separated by a distance s.

We consider the spatial correlation functions described in Table 1. Note that all of these spatial correlation functions yield valid correlation matrices C for $\rho > 0$, ensuring the positive semi-definiteness of the covariance matrix R. These functions are selected based on their similarity with the correlation pattern observed in our data, and we limit our consideration to functions described by a single parameter to simplify calculations. Using the identity that $\gamma(s) = 1 - h(s)$, where $\gamma(s)$ is the semivariogram calculated using observations with zero mean and unit variance and $h(s)$ is a correlation function, we convert the spatial correlation functions in Table 1 into semivariogram functions, and fit them to the empirical semivariogram. The function with the smallest sum of squared error is selected as the spatial correlation function for the data. We initialize ρ at the value obtained from the semivariogram fitting. The entries of the correlation matrix $C(\rho)$ are given by $C_{kk'} = h(d(k, k'); \rho)$. We perform the EM algorithm again, this time also estimating ρ along with the rest of the model parameters.

Table 1. Spatial correlation functions.

Exponential	$h(s; \rho) = e^{-s/\rho}$
Gaussian	$h(s; \rho) = e^{-(s/\rho)^2}$
Rational quadratic	$h(s; \rho) = \frac{1}{1+(s/\rho)^2}$
Spherical	$h(s; \rho) = \left(1 - \frac{3}{2}\frac{s}{\rho} + \frac{1}{2}\left(\frac{s}{\rho}\right)^3\right)\mathbb{1}(s < \rho)$

2.5 Implementation Details

The units of the estimated PS are arbitrarily defined. After fitting, we scale the PS values so that at baseline their mean is 0 and variance is 1. We also ensure that the median value of the subject-specific parameter α is positive so that increasing PS corresponds to increasing age. Given these scalings, the PS model is identifiable, as shown in [9].

The correlation parameter ρ must be positive, meaning that constrained optimization must be used to perform the maximization given in (14). Instead of using constraints, we reparametrize such that $\rho = e^{\log \rho} := e^{\rho_0}$. This enables unconstrained optimization over ρ_0, and ρ is set to e^{ρ_0} after this optimization.

C and R are sparse matrices. Limiting the optimization range to $[\rho_{\min}, \rho_{\max}]$ allows us to avoid computing the elements $C_{kk'}$ where the distance between voxels k and k' is larger than a threshold δ; we simply assign the value 0 to these elements of the correlation matrix. This distance threshold δ is picked such that the correlation matrix is numerically positive semi-definite when $\rho = \rho_{\max}$.

2.6 Image Acquisition and Preprocessing

We used longitudinal positron emission tomography (PET) data for participants with at least two visits from the Baltimore Longitudinal Study of Aging (BLSA) [12] neuroimaging substudy [11]. PET scans were acquired on a GE Advance scanner immediately following an intravenous bolus injection of Pittsburgh compound B (PiB), which binds to fibrillar β-amyloid. Dynamic PET data were acquired over 70 min, yielding 33 time frames each with $128 \times 128 \times 35$ voxels. Voxel size is $2 \times 2 \times 4.25\,\text{mm}^3$. Data for 75 participants, ages 55.7–92.4 at baseline, with a total of 271 visits were used.

The frames of each dynamic PET scan were aligned to the average of the first two minutes to remove motion [10]. For registration purposes, we obtained static images by averaging the first 20 min of the dynamic PET scan. Follow-up PET scans were rigidly registered onto the baseline PET within each participant using the 20-minute average images. Baseline magnetic resonance images (MRIs) were rigidly registered onto their corresponding 20-minute averages, and their FreeSurfer segmentations [6,7] were transformed accordingly. Distribution volume ratio (DVR) images were calculated in the native space of each PET image using the simplified reference tissue model with the cerebellar gray matter as reference tissue [15]. The MRIs coregistered with the PET were deformably registered [1] onto a study-specific template [2,4] and transformed to MNI space using a pre-calculated affine transformation. The resulting mappings were applied to the DVR images to bring them into the MNI space. The spatially normalized DVR images in MNI space were downsampled to have 4 mm isotropic voxels. The PS model was fitted separately to the left and right cerebral hemispheres. This served two purposes: first, to reduce the computational burden by using a smaller number of voxels in the fitting, and second, to enable the comparison of the estimated parameters and progression scores across the hemispheres for assessing model stability. We refer to the progression score calculated using the DVR images as PiB-PS.

3   Results

3.1   Simulation Experiments

We generated α_i, β_i, and a_k from independent uniform distributions in the range $[-1, 1]$, and b_k in the range $[-10, 10]$ for 100 subjects and 125 biomarkers that were arranged in a $5 \times 5 \times 5$ image with 4 mm isotropic voxels. Each subject was randomly assigned to have 2 to 5 visits, with 2 being more probable than 5. Age at baseline was generated independently for each subject from a uniform distribution in the range $[20, 80]$. The intervals between consecutive visits were randomly assigned to be 1, 2, or 3. PS was calculated as $s_{ij}^{(\text{truth})} = \alpha_i t_{ij} + \beta_i$ and standardized such that at baseline it had zero mean and unit variance. The subject-specific parameters α_i and β_i were normalized accordingly. Biomarker values (voxel values in the images) were calculated using the current values of the model parameters as $y_{ijk}^{(\text{truth})} = a_k s_{ij}^{(\text{truth})} + b_k$ and standardized to have zero mean and unit variance across all visits and subjects. The trajectory parameters a_k and b_k were normalized accordingly. Noise was generated from a multivariate normal distribution with covariance matrix $R = \lambda^2 C(\rho)$ for given λ and ρ, and added to the biomarker values to yield the observations y_{ijk}. The model fitting was then performed to recapture the model parameters $a_k, b_k, \alpha_i, \beta_i, \lambda$, and ρ.

We performed 100 simulation experiments for each combination of the following values of λ^2 and ρ: $\lambda^2 = 0.01, 0.05, 0.10, 0.15, 0.20$ and $\rho = 0, 2, 4, 6, 8$. For each experiment, we calculated the mean squared error for y and PS as

$$\text{MSE}_y = \frac{1}{K \sum_i v_i} \sum_{i,j,k} \left(\hat{y}_{ijk} - y_{ijk}^{(\text{truth})} \right)^2 \text{ and } \text{MSE}_{\text{PS}} = \frac{1}{\sum_i v_i} \sum_{i,j} \left(\hat{s}_{ij} - s_{ij}^{(\text{truth})} \right)^2,$$

(16)

where $\hat{y}_{ijk}$ and $\hat{s}_{ij}$ are the values obtained using the estimated parameters. These mean squared error values, averaged across the 100 simulations for each combination of λ^2 and ρ, are presented in Fig. 1. Since the biomarker values and baseline PS were scaled to have zero mean and unit variance, the mean squared error values are directly interpretable. The mean squared error is much lower than the unit variance associated with the biomarker values and baseline PS at all noise variances λ^2 and correlation parameters ρ, indicating that model fitting is accurate.

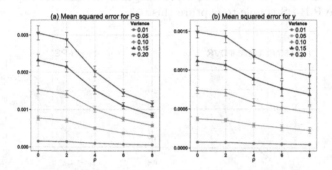

Fig. 1. The mean squared error for (a) the progression scores (PS) and (b) the biomarker values y, averaged across 100 simulations for each combination of the noise variance λ^2 and correlation parameter ρ. The error bars correspond to ± 1 standard deviation of the mean squared error across the 100 simulations.

3.2   DVR Images

Based on the sum of squared error of the fitted semivariograms over a 100 mm distance calculated using 20 equidistant points, the algorithm selected the exponential correlation function for both hemispheres. The correlation parameter ρ was using the value were obtained from the semivariogram fitting, as described in §2.4. At convergence, ρ was 14.2 for the left hemisphere and 14.8 for the right.

The estimates for the subject-specific variables α and β, as well as the PiB-PS across the cerebral hemispheres are presented in Fig. 2. The Pearson correlation coefficients across the hemispheres for α, β, and PiB-PS at baseline are $0.90, 0.89$, and 0.98, respectively.

PiB-PS, which reflects the progression of fibrillar amyloid-β deposition as measured by PiB-PET, reveals a pattern similar to that of mean cortical DVR,

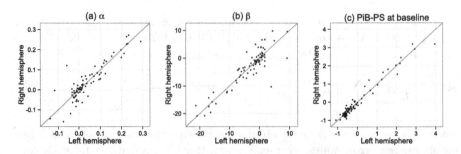

Fig. 2. Comparison of the subject-specific parameters (a) α, (b) β and (c) progression scores (PS) at baseline across the cerebral hemispheres. PiB = Pittsburgh compound B.

which is an average of DVR values across cortical regions that are early accumulators of amyloid (Pearson correlation coefficient at baseline = 0.93) (Fig. 3). The progression as measured using DVR images is not linearly associated with age, and the PiB-PS is able to capture this.

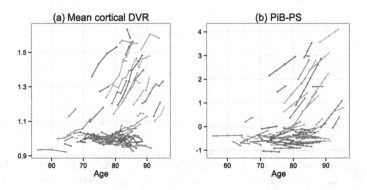

Fig. 3. (a) Mean cortical DVR and (b) PiB-PS averaged across left and right cerebral hemispheres plotted against age. The longitudinal data points are connected by lines within each subject. Different colors are used across subjects for visualization. DVR = Distribution volume ratio, PS = progression score, PiB = Pittsburgh compound B (Color figure online).

The trajectory slope parameters **a** estimated for the left and right cerebral hemispheres reveal largely symmetric patterns (Fig. 4), with the precuneus and frontal lobe showing the greatest increases in DVR with PiB-PS, smaller increases in lateral temporal and temporoparietal regions, and minimal increases in the occipital lobe and the sensorimotor strip.

The linear mixed effects model is commonly used to analyze the longitudinal trajectories of voxelwise imaging values. We compared the image of the trajectory slope parameter **a** to the image of the slope associated with the age term in a linear mixed effects model (Fig. 5). For visualization, the histogram of the slope

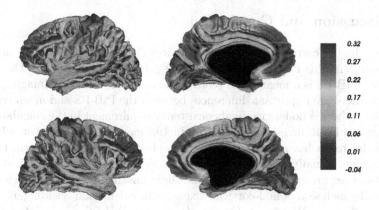

Fig. 4. Trajectory slope parameter **a** projected onto the inner cortical surface associated with the template space. Left hemisphere (*top*) and right hemisphere (*bottom*) lateral and medial cerebral surfaces. For each unit increase in PiB-PS, the DVR value increases by a_k at voxel k. DVR = Distribution volume ratio, PS = progression score, PiB = Pittsburgh compound B.

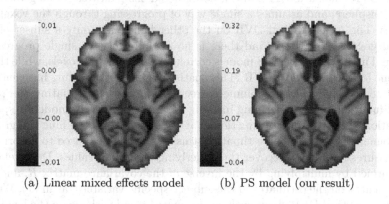

(a) Linear mixed effects model   (b) PS model (our result)

Fig. 5. Comparison of the image of the trajectory parameter **a** in (a) the progression score (PS) model to the image of the slope associated with the age term in (b) the linear mixed effects model. Longitudinal changes in the anterior frontal lobe are better contained within the cortical gray matter and lateral frontal lobe changes are more pronounced in the PS result.

image associated with the age term in the linear mixed effects model was matched to the histogram of the image of trajectory slope parameter **a** from the PS model. Overall, there are strong similarities in the two results. However, in the result from the PS model, longitudinal changes in the anterior frontal lobe are better contained within the cortical gray matter, and also lateral frontal lobe changes are more pronounced.

4   Discussion and Conclusion

PiB-PS is highly correlated with mean cortical DVR, the widely used measure for quantifying PiB-PET scans and assessing longitudinal change. This indicates that PiB-PS is a meaningful score extracted from voxelwise imaging data. However, there are important differences between the PiB-PS and mean cortical DVR. Since there is no longitudinal consistency requirement in the calculation of mean cortical DVR, its estimates exhibit fluctuations from visit to visit, whereas PiB-PS, due to the linear relationship assumed between age and PS in the model, exhibits longitudinally smoother trajectories. Furthermore, mean cortical DVR calculations require anatomical labels, and slight misalignment of the labels could result in the inclusion of non-cortical voxels in the calculation, yielding an incorrect mean cortical DVR value. On the other hand, PiB-PS is calculated on the whole hemisphere and does not use anatomical labels. Slight misregistration of boundary voxels has much less influence on the PiB-PS estimates since voxels with high registration errors are likely to have trajectory slope estimates close to 0 due to the lack of a clear relationship between voxel intensity and time.

There are several methodological differences between the PiB-PS and mean cortical DVR calculations. PiB-PS is constructed using all voxels in a given cerebral hemisphere, and assumes a single way of progressing through the voxelwise changes. The mean cortical DVR on the other hand, uses only a subset of the cortical gray matter voxels and there is no assumption of a single progression pattern. Furthermore, PiB-PS models correlations among the voxels, while this is not done for mean cortical DVR. This spatial correlation modeling has elements similar to voxelwise partial volume correction: instead of estimating the point spread function of the underlying imaging data, the purpose of modeling spatial correlations is to estimate a function that acts analogously to blur the ground truth biomarker values. The estimate of this function is then used to decorrelate the measures in order to recover the underlying biomarker values. Decorrelation is performed by multiplying by the inverse of the covariance matrix R, and has a direct effect on the estimates of the subject-specific variables, as in (7). We see that mean cortical DVR shows a slight downward trend with age in the low DVR group, most likely due to atrophy and the lack of partial volume correction. In contrast, this effect has flattened out for PiB-PS, possibly due to the modeling of the spatial correlation being similar to partial volume correction.

Deposition of cerebral amyloid is thought to affect both hemispheres in a symmetric fashion. The similarity of the subject-specific variables and the trajectory slopes estimated for the cerebral hemispheres indicates that the spatial PS model is not sensitive to slight changes in the data.

The PS model relies on the estimated progression scores rather than age for staging the subjects and assessing longitudinal change. This allows for alignment of subjects according to their amyloid burden and progression, yielding slope images that show better localized longitudinal changes compared to regressing on age using a linear mixed effects model. Certain longitudinal changes that could not be detected when regressing on age can be detected with the PS model due to this alignment of subjects. For example, the longitudinal amyloid increases in the frontal lobe did not extend to the lateral frontal regions in our linear mixed effects model analysis, whereas the PS model showed that these regions do exhibit longitudinal increases (Fig. 5).

The presented method is applicable to other types of medical imaging and biomarker data, and can be used to extract progression scores that reveal how each individual compares to the rest of the sample. For different types of medical images where a summary score such as the mean cortical DVR is not available, the progression score estimates provided by our method can be greatly informative for disease staging and potentially an early diagnosis. Calculation of PS using voxelwise imaging data not only yields a staging variable for the individuals, but also enables the comparison of voxelwise trajectories to determine the temporal ordering of changes. The model is amenable to a hypothesis testing framework to evaluate whether certain regions of the brain show the earliest or fastest changes.

Acknowledgment. This research was supported in part by the Intramural Research Program of the National Institutes of Health.

References

1. Avants, B.B., Epstein, C.L., Grossman, M., Gee, J.C.: Symmetric diffeomorphic image registration with cross-correlation: evaluating automated labeling of elderly and neurodegenerative brain. Med. Image Anal. **12**(1), 26–41 (2008)
2. Avants, B.B., Yushkevich, P., Pluta, J., Minkoff, D., Korczykowski, M., Detre, J., Gee, J.C.: The optimal template effect in hippocampus studies of diseased populations. NeuroImage **49**(3), 2457–2466 (2010)
3. Bilgel, M., An, Y., Lang, A., Prince, J., Ferrucci, L., Jedynak, B., Resnick, S.M.: Trajectories of Alzheimer disease-related cognitive measures in a longitudinal sample. Alzheimer's Dement. **10**(6), 735–742 (2014)
4. Bilgel, M., Carass, A., Resnick, S.M., Wong, D.F., Prince, J.L.: Deformation field correction for spatial normalization of PET images using a population-derived partial least squares model. In: Wu, G., Zhang, D., Zhou, L. (eds.) MLMI 2014. LNCS, vol. 8679, pp. 198–206. Springer, Heidelberg (2014)
5. Cressie, N., Hawkins, D.M.: Robust estimation of the variogram. J. Int. Assoc. Math. Geol. **12**(2), 115–125 (1980)
6. Dale, A., Fischl, B., Sereno, M.: Cortical surface-based analysis: I. segmentation and surface reconstruction. NeuroImage **194**, 179–194 (1999)
7. Desikan, R.S., Ségonne, F., Fischl, B., Quinn, B.T., Dickerson, B.C., Blacker, D., Buckner, R.L., Dale, A.M., Maguire, R.P., Hyman, B.T., Albert, M.S., Killiany, R.J.: An automated labeling system for subdividing the human cerebral cortex on MRI scans into gyral based regions of interest. NeuroImage **31**(3), 968–980 (2006)
8. Jack, C.R., Knopman, D.S., Jagust, W.J., Petersen, R.C., Weiner, M.W., Aisen, P.S., Shaw, L.M., Vemuri, P., Wiste, H.J., Weigand, S.D., Lesnick, T.G., Pankratz, V.S., Donohue, M.C., Trojanowski, J.Q.: Tracking pathophysiological processes in Alzheimer's disease: an updated hypothetical model of dynamic biomarkers. Lancet Neurol. **12**(2), 207–216 (2013)

9. Jedynak, B.M., Lang, A., Liu, B., Katz, E., Zhang, Y., Wyman, B.T., Raunig, D., Jedynak, C.P., Caffo, B., Prince, J.L.: A computational neurodegenerative disease progression score: method and results with the Alzheimer's disease neuroimaging initiative cohort. NeuroImage **63**(3), 1478–1486 (2012)

10. Jenkinson, M., Bannister, P., Brady, M., Smith, S.: Improved optimization for the robust and accurate linear registration and motion correction of brain images. NeuroImage **17**(2), 825–841 (2002)

11. Resnick, S.M., Goldszal, A.F., Davatzikos, C., Golski, S., Kraut, M.A., Metter, E.J., Bryan, R.N., Zonderman, A.B.: One-year age changes in MRI brain volumes in older adults. Cereb. Cortex **10**(5), 464–472 (2000)

12. Shock, N.W., Greulich, R.C., Andres, R., Arenberg, D., Costa Jr., P.T., Lakatta, E.G., Tobin, J.D.: Normal human aging: The Baltimore Longitudinal Study of Aging. Technical report, U.S. Government Printing Office, Washington, DC (1984)

13. Younes, L., Albert, M., Miller, M.I.: Inferring changepoint times of medial temporal lobe morphometric change in preclinical Alzheimer's disease. NeuroImage Clin. **5**, 178–187 (2014)

14. Young, A.L., Oxtoby, N.P., Daga, P., Cash, D.M., Fox, N.C., Ourselin, S., Schott, J.M., Alexander, D.C.: A data-driven model of biomarker changes in sporadic Alzheimer's disease. Brain **137**, 2564–2577 (2014)

15. Zhou, Y., Endres, C.J., Brašić, J.R., Huang, S.C., Wong, D.F.: Linear regression with spatial constraint to generate parametric images of ligand-receptor dynamic PET studies with a simplified reference tissue model. NeuroImage **18**(4), 975–989 (2003)

Predicting Semantic Descriptions from Medical Images with Convolutional Neural Networks

Thomas Schlegl[1]([✉]), Sebastian M. Waldstein[2], Wolf-Dieter Vogl[1,2],
Ursula Schmidt-Erfurth[2], and Georg Langs[1]

[1] Computational Imaging Research Lab, Department of Biomedical Imaging
and Image-guided Therapy, Medical University, Vienna, Austria
{thomas.schlegl,georg.langs}@meduniwien.ac.at
[2] Christian Doppler Laboratory for Ophthalmic Image Analysis,
Vienna Reading Center, Department of Ophthalmology and Optometry,
Medical University Vienna, Vienna, Austria

Abstract. Learning representative computational models from medical imaging data requires large training data sets. Often, voxel-level annotation is unfeasible for sufficient amounts of data. An alternative to manual annotation, is to use the enormous amount of knowledge encoded in imaging data and corresponding reports generated during clinical routine. Weakly supervised learning approaches can link volume-level labels to image content but suffer from the typical label distributions in medical imaging data where only a small part consists of clinically relevant abnormal structures. In this paper we propose to use a semantic representation of clinical reports as a learning target that is predicted from imaging data by a convolutional neural network. We demonstrate how we can learn accurate voxel-level classifiers based on weak volume-level semantic descriptions on a set of 157 optical coherence tomography (OCT) volumes. We specifically show how semantic information increases classification accuracy for intraretinal cystoid fluid (IRC), subretinal fluid (SRF) and normal retinal tissue, and how the learning algorithm links semantic concepts to image content and geometry.

1 Introduction

Medical image analysis extracts diagnostically relevant information such as position and segmentations of abnormalities, or the quantitative characteristics of appearance markers from imaging data. To this end, algorithms are typically trained on annotated data. While the detection of subtle disease characteristics requires large training data sets, annotation does not scale well, since it is costly, time consuming and error-prone. An alternative for learning classifiers or predictors from very large data sets is to rely on existing data generated during clinical routine, such as imaging data, and corresponding reports. We propose

---

T. Schlegl—This work has received funding from the European Union FP7 (KHRES-MOI FP7-257528, VISCERAL FP7-318068) and the Austrian Federal Ministry of Science, Research and Economy.

S. Ourselin et al. (Eds.): IPMI 2015, LNCS 9123, pp. 437–448, 2015.
DOI: 10.1007/978-3-319-19992-4_34

to learn the link between semantic information in textual clinical reports and imaging data, by training convolutional neural networks that predict semantic descriptions from images without additional annotation. Experiments show that the inclusion of semantic representations has advantages over standard multiple-instance learning with independent labels. It increases the classification accuracy of pathologies, and learns semantic concepts such as spatial position.

Learning from Medical Imaging Data. Typical clinical imaging departments generate hundreds of thousands of image volumes per year that are assessed by clinical experts. The image and textual information comprise a rich source of knowledge about epidemiology and imaging markers that are a crucial reference during clinical routine and treatment guidance. They promise to serve as basis for the detection of imaging biomarkers, co-morbidities, and subtle signatures that are relevant for treatment decisions. Training reliable classifiers or segmentation algorithms is crucial in their processing, but requires annotated training data. While supervised learning based on annotated imaging data yields accurate classification results, annotation becomes unfeasible for large data. At the same time, expert reports created during clinical routine offer detailed descriptions of observations in the imaging data, and could fill this gap. They are currently largely unexploited.

Contribution. In this paper we propose a method to use the semantic content of textual reports linked to the image data instead of voxel-wise annotations for the training of an image classifier. We evaluate if the semantic information in medical reports can improve weakly supervised learning of abnormality detectors over standard multiple-instance learning with independent labels. Since medical reports not only list observations (pathologies) but also semantic concepts of their locations, we learn the relationship between these semantic terms and specific local entities in the imaging data, together with their location. The algorithm has to learn a mapping from image location to semantic location information encoded in a semantic target vector. The benefits of this algorithm are two-fold. First, we can estimate semantic descriptions from imaging data, second, we learn an accurate voxel-wise classifier without the need for voxel-wise classification in the training data.

Related Work. Weakly supervised learning approaches use binary class labels that indicate the presence or absence of an object of the corresponding class in an image or volume. Multiple-instance learning [1] is a form of weakly supervised learning to solve this problem, and views images as labeled bags of instances. A positive class label is assigned to the bag of examples if at least one example belongs to the class. The negative class label is assigned to all examples of the bag if no example belongs to the class. The corresponding situation in medical imaging consists of information that *somewhere* in the image there is a certain abnormality. Weakly supervised approaches learn from these weak or noisy labels. Examples are the *Diverse Density* Framework by Maron and Lozano-Pérez [2], mappings among images and captions [3] using algorithms, such as

Random Forests [4] or Support Vector Machines [5]. A recently published work [6] presents a multi-fold multiple-instance learning approach for weakly supervised object category localization. The work of Verbeek et al. [7] is another weakly supervised learning example, wherein semantic segmentation models are learned using image-wide class labels. While these methods yield lower classification accuracy compared to voxel-wise training set labels, they have proven useful in computer vision on natural images. Unfortunately, this does not translate directly to medical imaging data. For example, a large part of data such as retinal spectral-domain optical coherence tomography (SD-OCT) images show normal tissue. While abnormalities typically cover only a tiny fraction of the volume, they are the focus of diagnostic attention and observations encoded in the textual report. Furthermore, abnormality appearance can be modulated by location. This puts standard multiple-instance learning at a disadvantage. Our work differs from these weakly supervised learning approaches in two aspects: (i) We do not extract local or global image descriptors but the visual input representation is learned by our network and adapts to imaging and tissue characteristics. (ii) We do not only use class labels depicting the global presence or absence of objects in the entire image but use semantic information from clinical reports.

We use convolutional neural networks (CNN) to learn representations and classifiers. They were introduced in 1980 by Fukushima [8], and have been used to solve various classification problems (cf. [9–11]). They can automatically learn translation invariant visual input representations, enabling the adaptation of visual feature extractors to data, instead of manual feature engineering. The application of CNN in the domain of medical image analysis ranges from manifold learning in the frequency domain of 3D brain *magnetic resonance* (*MR*) imaging data [12] to domain adaptation via unsupervised pre-training of CNN to improve lung tissue classification accuracy on *computed tomography* (*CT*) imaging data [13]. A weakly supervised approach using CNN performed on natural images was presented in [14]. Our work differs from the aforementioned approaches as: (i) we do not perform supervised (pre-) training, (ii) we use medical images and (iii) our classifier does not only predict global image labels indicating the presence or absence of object classes in an image but also corresponding location information.

2   Weakly Supervised Learning of Semantic Descriptions

A CNN is a hierarchically structured feed-forward neural network comprising one or more pairs of *convolution layers* and succeeding *max-pooling layers* (cf. [10,11,13]). The stack of convolution and max-pooling layer pairs is typically followed by one or more fully-connected layers and a terminal classification layer. We can train more than one stack of pairs of convolution and max-pooling layers feeding into the first fully-connected layer. This enables training CNNs based on multiple scales. We use a CNN to perform voxel-wise classification on visual inputs and corresponding quantitative spatial location information.

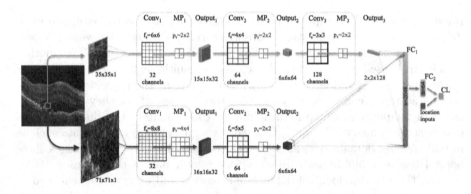

Fig. 1. Multi-scale CNN architecture used in our experiments. One stack of three pairs of convolution (*Conv*) and max-pooling layers (*MP*) uses input image patches of size 35×35. The second stack comprises two pairs of convolution and max-pooling layers and uses input image patches of size 71×71 (centered at the same position). The resulting outputs $Output_k$ of the k pairs of convolution $Conv_k$ and max-pooling MP_k layers are the inputs for the succeeding layers, with corresponding convolution filter sizes f_s and sizes of the pooling regions p_s. Our CNN also comprises two fully connected layers (*FC*) and a terminal classification layer (*CL*). The outputs of both stacks are connected densely with all neurons of the first fully-connected layer. The location parameters are fed jointly with the activations of the second fully-connected layer into the classification layer.

Figure 1 shows the architecture of the CNN. In the following we explain the specific representation of visual inputs and semantic targets.

2.1 Representing Inputs and Targets

The overall data comprises M tuples of medical imaging data, corresponding clinical reports and voxel-wise ground-truth class labels $\langle \mathbf{I}^m, \mathbf{T}^m, \mathbf{L}^m \rangle$, with $m = 1, 2, \ldots, M$, where $\mathbf{I}^m \in \mathbb{R}^{n \times n}$ is an intensity image (e.g., a slice of an SD-OCT volume scan of the retina) of size $n \times n$, $\mathbf{L}^m \in \{1, \ldots, K+1\}^{n \times n}$ is an array of the same size containing the corresponding ground-truth class labels and $\mathbf{T}^m$ is the corresponding textual report. During training we are only given $\langle \mathbf{I}^m, \mathbf{T}^m \rangle$ and train a classifier to predict $\mathbf{L}^m$ from $\mathbf{I}^m$ on new testing data. In this paper we propose a weakly supervised learning approach using semantic descriptions, where the voxel-level ground-truth class labels $\mathbf{L}^m$ are not used for training but only for evaluation of the voxel-wise prediction accuracy.

Visual and Coordinate Input Information. To capture visual information at different levels of detail we extract small square-shaped image patches $\dot{\mathbf{x}}_i^m \in \mathbb{R}^{\alpha \times \alpha}$ of size α and larger square-shaped image patches $\ddot{\mathbf{x}}_i^m \in \mathbb{R}^{\beta \times \beta}$ of size β with $\alpha < \beta < n$ centered at the same spatial position $\mathbf{c}_i^m$ in volume $\mathbf{I}^m$, where i is the index of the centroid of the image patch. For each image patch, we provide two additional quantitative location parameters to the network: *(i)* the 3D spatial coordinates $\mathbf{c}_i^m \in \Omega \subset \mathbb{R}^3$ of the centroid i of the image patches and *(ii)* the Euclidean distance $d_i^m \in \Omega \subset \mathbb{R}$ of the patch center i to a given reference structure (in our case: fovea) within the volume. We do not need to integrate these location parameters in the deep feature representation computation but inject them below the classification layer by concatenating the location parameters and activations of the fully-connected layer representing visual information (see Fig. 1). The same input information is provided for all experiments.

Semantic Target Labels. We assume that objects (e.g. pathology) are reported together with a textual description of their approximate spatial location. Thus a report $\mathbf{T}^m$ consists of K pairs of text snippets $\langle t_P^{m,k}, t_{Loc}^{m,k} \rangle$, with $k = 1, 2, \ldots, K$, where $t_P^{m,k} \in \mathcal{P}$ describes the occurrence of a specific object class term and $t_{Loc}^{m,k} \in \mathcal{L}$ represents the semantic description of its spatial locations. These spatial locations can be both abstract subregions (e.g., centrally located) of the volume or concrete anatomical structures. Note that $t_{Loc}^{m,k}$ does not contain quantitative values, and we do not know the link between these descriptions and image coordinate information. This semantic information can come in Γ orthogonal semantic groups (e.g., in (1) the lowest layer and (2) close to the fovea). That is, different groups represent different location concepts found in clinical reports. The extraction of these pairs from the textual document is based on semantic parsing [15] and is not subject of this paper. We decompose the textual report $\mathbf{T}^m$ into the corresponding **semantic target label** $\mathbf{s}^m \in \{0,1\}^{K \cdot \Sigma_\gamma n_\gamma}$, with $\gamma = 1, 2, \ldots, \Gamma$, where K is the number of different object classes which should be classified (e.g. cyst), and n_γ is the number of nominal region classes in one semantic group γ of descriptions (e.g., $n_\gamma = 3$ for upper vs. central vs. lower layer, $n_\gamma = 2$ for close vs. far from reference structure). I.e., lets assume we have two groups, then $\mathbf{s}^m$ is a K-fold concatenation of pairs of a binary *layer group* $g_1^k \in \{0,1\}^{n_1}$ with n_1 bits representing different layer classes and a binary *reference location group* $g_2^k \in \{0,1\}^{n_2}$ with n_2 bits representing relative locations to a reference structure. For all object classes, all bits of the layer group, and all bits of the reference location group are set to 1, if they are mentioned mutually with the respective object class in the textual report. All bits of the corresponding layer group and all bits of the corresponding reference location group are set to 0, where the respective object class is not mentioned in the report. The vector $\mathbf{s}^m$ of semantic target labels is assigned to all input tuples $\langle \dot{\mathbf{x}}_i^m, \ddot{\mathbf{x}}_i^m, \mathbf{c}_i^m, d_i^m \rangle$ extracted from the corresponding volume $\mathbf{I}^m$. Figure 2a shows an example of a semantic target label representation comprising two object classes. According to this binary representation the first object is mentioned mutually with layer classes 1, 2 and 3 and with reference location class 1 in the textual report. Figure 2c shows the corresponding volume information.

Voxel-wise Ground Truth Labels. To evaluate the algorithm, we use the ground-truth class label $l_i \in \{1, ..., K+1\}$ from $\mathbf{L}^m$ at the center position $\mathbf{c}_i^m$ of the patches for every multi-scale image patch pair $\langle \dot{\mathbf{x}}_i^m, \ddot{\mathbf{x}}_i^m \rangle$. Labels include the

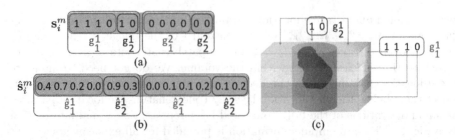

Fig. 2. (a) Example of a semantic target label comprising two object classes ($K = 2$). Each of which comprises a *layer group* g_1^k with 4 bits (layer 1,2,3, or 4) and a *reference location group* g_2^k with 2 bits (close or distant). (b) Prediction of a semantic description $\hat{s}_i^m$ that would lead to a corresponding object class label prediction $\hat{l}_i = 1$. (c) Visualization of the volume information which could lead to the given semantic target label shown in (a). (Best viewed in color) (Colour figure online)

reported observations $t_P^{m,k}$ and a healthy background label. l_i is assigned to the whole multi-scale image patch pair $\langle \dot{\mathbf{x}}_i^m, \ddot{\mathbf{x}}_i^m \rangle$ centered at voxel position i.

2.2   Training to Predict Semantic Descriptors

We train a CNN to predict the semantic description from the imaging data and the corresponding location information provided for the patch center voxels. We use tuples $\langle \dot{\mathbf{x}}_i^m, \ddot{\mathbf{x}}_i^m, \mathbf{c}_i^m, d_i^m, \mathbf{s}_i^m \rangle$ for weakly supervised training of our model. The training objective is to learn the mapping

$$f : \langle \dot{\mathbf{x}}_i^m, \ddot{\mathbf{x}}_i^m, \mathbf{c}_i^m, d_i^m \rangle \longmapsto \mathbf{s}_i^m \tag{1}$$

from multi-scale image patch pairs $\langle \dot{\mathbf{x}}_i^m, \ddot{\mathbf{x}}_i^m \rangle$, 3D spatial coordinates $\mathbf{c}_i^m$ and a distance value d_i^m to corresponding location specific noisy semantic targets $\mathbf{s}_i^m$ in a weakly supervised fashion. During testing we apply the mapping to new image patches in the test set. During classification, an unseen tuple $\langle \dot{\mathbf{x}}_i^m, \ddot{\mathbf{x}}_i^m, \mathbf{c}_i^m, d_i^m \rangle$ of multi-scale image patch pairs $\langle \dot{\mathbf{x}}_i^m, \ddot{\mathbf{x}}_i^m \rangle$ centered at voxel position i and corresponding location parameters $\mathbf{c}_i^m$ and d_i^m causes activations of the classification layer, which are the predictions of the semantic descriptions $\hat{\mathbf{s}}_i^m$. During training, all model parameters θ (weights and bias terms) of the whole model are optimized by minimizing the *mean squared error* between the actual volume-level semantic target labels $\mathbf{s}_i^m$ and the voxel-level probabilities of semantic descriptions $\hat{\mathbf{s}}_i^m$ predicted by the model.

2.3   Evaluation of Local Image Content Classification

We want to know if the proposed approach learns a link between semantic concepts and image content and location. To this end, we perform weakly supervised learning as described above. During testing, we apply the trained CNN to new data. We transform the voxel-wise predictions of semantic descriptions into voxel-level class labels and compare these labels with ground-truth labels on the testing data. Specifically we are interested in the increase of accuracy caused by the inclusion of semantic information into the training procedure. An object class may occur simultaneously in a number of layer classes within the layer group and in a number of reference location classes within the reference location group. But if an object class is present in an image, then this occurrence has to be reflected by the predictions of both groups. So, based on the predictions of the semantic descriptions $\hat{s}_i^m$ we compute the mean activation $\bar{a}_i^k$ of class k over the maximum activation within each semantic location group $\hat{g}_\gamma^k$:

$$\bar{a}_i^k = \frac{1}{\Gamma} \sum_{\gamma=1}^{\Gamma} max(\hat{g}_\gamma^k) \qquad (2)$$

Now we can compute location-adjusted predictions $\hat{l}_i$ for the class k having the highest mean activation:

$$\hat{l}_i = \begin{cases} 0, & \text{if } \bar{a}_i^k < 0.5, \forall \bar{a}_i^k, k = 1, 2, \ldots, K \\ \underset{k}{\text{argmax}}\,(\bar{a}_i^k), & \text{otherwise} \end{cases} \qquad (3)$$

If the mean activations of all classes are less than 0.5, the label 0 (*background class*) is assigned to the corresponding patch center. The resulting class label predictions $\hat{l}_i$ are assigned to the voxels in the center of the image patches. Based on these class label predictions $\hat{l}_i$ we now can measure the performance of our model in terms of misclassification errors on object class labels. Figure 2b shows an example of a prediction $\hat{s}_i^m$ of a semantic description comprising two object classes and two semantic groups. The corresponding object class-wise mean activations would evaluate to $\bar{a}_i^1 = 0.8$ and $\bar{a}_i^2 = 0.2$. According to equation (3) that would lead to the object class label prediction $\hat{l}_i = 1$.

3   Experiments

Data, Data Selection and Preprocessing. We evaluate the method on 157 clinical high resolution SD-OCT volumes of the retina with resolutions of $512 \times 128 \times 1024$ voxels (voxel dimensions $12 \times 47 \times 2\,\mu m$). The OCT data we use is not generated instantly but single slices (in the z/x-plane) are acquired sequentially to form the volume. Due to relatively strong anisotropy of the imaging data, we work with 2D in-plane (z/x) patches. From these volumes we extract pairs of 2D image patches (see Fig. 3a and b) with scales 35×35 and 71×71 for 300,000 positions. The positions of the patch centers within an image slice as well as the slice number within a volume are sampled randomly. A fast patch based image denoising related to non-local-means is applied as preprocessing step. Additionally, the intensity values of the image patches are normalized by transforming the data to zero-mean and unit variance. The human retina can be subdivided into different layers. We use an implementation of an automatic layer segmentation algorithm following [16] and based on the top and bottom layer we compute a retina mask. The voxel positions within this mask are normalized into the range [0, 1], where the voxels at the top and bottom layer (z-axis), the voxels in the first and last column of the image (x-axis) and the voxels in the first and last slice of the volume (y-axis) are assigned to the marginals 0 and 1 respectively (see Fig. 3c). These normalized 3D coordinates are used as location specific inputs. In every SD-OCT volume the position of the fovea is also annotated. We use the annotated position of the fovea as reference structure and provide the Euclidean distance of every image patch center as additional location specific input.

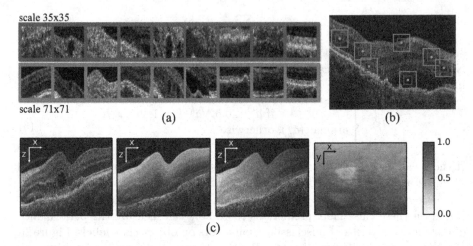

Fig. 3. (a) Visual inputs with two different scales. Patches in the same column share the centroid position. (b) Patch extraction at random positions from an SD-OCT intensity image: patches of size 35 × 35 (red), patches of size 71 × 71 (green) and corresponding patch centers (yellow). (c) Normalized coordinates of voxels within the retina. (Best viewed in color) (Colour figure online)

Evaluation. For the purposes of evaluation of voxel-wise classification performance we extract ground-truth class labels at the patch center positions from the corresponding volume with voxel-wise annotations. These labels are assigned to the whole corresponding image patches. In our data, 73.43 % of the patches are labeled as healthy tissue, 8.63 % are labeled as IRC and 17.94 % are labeled as SRF. Pairs of patches sampled at different positions within the same volume may partially overlap. We split the image patches on a patient basis into training and test set to perform 4-fold cross-validation, so that there is no patient both in the training, and the test set.

We train a classifier to perform 3-class classification between IRC, SRF and normal retinal tissue. Normal retinal tissue is handled as background class. We compare three approaches:

(1) **Naïve Weakly Supervised Learning:** We perform weakly supervised learning that links volume-level class labels to image content. We only use

the information which object class (pathology) is present in the volume. This results in a 3-class multiple-instance classification problem. The volume-level target label is assigned to all image patches of the corresponding volume.

(2) **Learning Semantic Descriptions:** We evaluate the performance of our proposed learning strategy. We use the volume-level semantic representation of the reported pathologies. We use semantic target labels encoding two pathologies (IRC and SRF) each of which comprises four bits for the layer group and two bits for the reference structure group resulting in a 12 bit semantic target vector (see Fig. 2). The semantic equivalent in a textual report for the four classes in the layer group would be *"ganglion cell complex"* (top layer of the retina), *"inner nuclear and plexiform layers"*, *"outer nuclear and plexiform layers"* and *"photoreceptor layers"* (bottom layers of the retina). The semantic equivalent for the two classes in the reference location group are *"foveal"* (in the vicinity of the fovea) and *"extrafoveal"* (at a distance from the fovea). This volume-level semantic representation is assigned to all image patches of the corresponding volume.

(3) **Supervised Learning:** We perform fully supervised learning using the voxel-level annotations of class labels. We evaluate what classification accuracy can be obtained when the maximum information at every single voxel-position - namely voxel-wise class labels - is available.

All experiments are performed using Python 2.6 with the Theano [17] library and run on a graphics processing unit (GPU) using CUDA 5.5.

3.1   Model Parameters

For every approach training of the CNN is performed for 200 epochs. We choose a multi-scale CNN architecture with two parallel stacks of pairs of convolution and max-pooling layers. These stacks take as input image patches of size 35×35 and 71×71 and comprise 3 and 2 pairs of convolution and max-pooling layers respectively (see Fig. 1). The outputs of the max-pooling layers on top of both stacks are concatenated and fed into a fully-connected layer with 2048 neurons. This layer is followed by a second fully-connected layer with 64 neurons. The activations of this layer are concatenated with the spatial location parameters of the patch centers and fed into the terminal classification layer. All layer parameters are learned during classifier training. The architecture of our multi-scale CNN and the detailed model parameters are shown in Fig. 1. The model parameters were found empirically due to preceding experiments using OCT data that differs in visual appearance from the data used in our presented experiments. The model parameters were tuned in these preceding experiments solely on the supervised training task to be a good trade-off between attainable classification accuracy and runtime efficiency. Thereafter they were fixed and used in all of our presented experiments to ensure comparability between the results of the different experiments.

Table 1. Confusion matrix of classification results and corresponding class-wise accuracies on (a) the naïve weakly supervised learning approach, (b) the weakly supervised learning approach using semantic descriptions and (c) the supervised learning approach.

		Prediction			
		Healthy	IRC	SRF	Accuracy
(a)	Healthy	**144329**	4587	70994	0.6563
	IRC	10391	**5653**	9718	0.2194
	SRF	4978	231	**48511**	0.9030
(b)	healthy	**173121**	10603	36186	0.7872
	IRC	2230	**22102**	1430	0.8579
	SRF	2963	1285	**49472**	**0.9209**
(c)	healthy	**214848**	2303	2759	**0.9770**
	IRC	2222	**23086**	454	**0.8961**
	SRF	3670	638	**49412**	0.9198

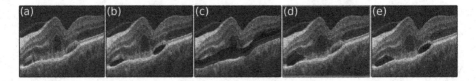

Fig. 4. (a) Intensity image of a single slice (zx-view) of a clinical SD-OCT scan of the retina. (b) Voxel-wise ground-truth annotations of IRC (red) and SRF (blue). Automatic segmentation results corresponding to voxel-wise class label predictions obtained with (c) the naïve weakly supervised learning approach, (d) our weakly supervised learning approach using semantic descriptions and (e) the supervised learning approach. On the class label predictions (c-e) no post-processing was performed. (Best viewed in color) (Colour figure online)

3.2   Classification Results

Experiment (1). The naïve weakly supervised learning approach represents the most restricted learning approach and serves as reference scenario. Classification results are shown in Table 1a. This approach yields a classification accuracy over all three classes of 66.30 %. Only 21.94 % of samples showing IRC are classified correctly, while the SRF class is classified relatively accurately (90.30 % of all patches showing SRF are correctly classified).

Experiment (2). The classification results of our proposed weakly supervised learning approach using semantic descriptions are shown in Table 1b. This approach yields a classification accuracy over all three classes of 81.73 % with lower accuracy for the healthy class (78.72 %) compared to SRF (92.09 % accuracy) which is also the best performance on SRF over all three approaches.

Experiment (3). As expected, the supervised learning approach performs best. This approach yields a overall classification accuracy over all three classes of 95.98 %. Classification results are shown in Table 1c. While it has most difficulties with IRC (89.61 % accuracy) it still obtains the highest accuracy for IRC over all three approaches. This approach also performs best for the healthy class (97.70 % accuracy). Figure 4 shows a comparison of voxel-wise classification results obtained by the different approaches. For each of the three training approaches the computation of the voxel-wise map took below 10 s.

4   Discussion

We propose a weakly supervised learning method using semantic descriptions to improve classification performance when no voxel-wise annotations but only textual descriptions linked to image data are available. A CNN learns optimal multi-scale visual representations and integrates them with location specific inputs to perform multi-class classification. We evaluated the accuracy of the proposed approach on clinical SD-OCT data of the retina and compared its performance on class label prediction accuracy with naïve weakly supervised learning and with fully supervised learning. Experiments demonstrate that based on volume-level semantic target labels the model learns voxel-level predictions of object classes. Including semantic information substantially improves classification performance. In addition to capturing the structure in intensity image patches and building a pathology specific model, the algorithm learns a mapping from 3D spatial coordinates and Euclidean distances to the fovea to semantic description classes found in reports. That is, the CNN learns diverse abstract concepts of "location". The learning approach can be applied to automatic classification and segmentation on medical imaging data for which corresponding report holds semantic descriptions in the form of pathology - anatomical location pairs.

Exploiting semantics over naïve weakly supervised learning has several benefits. The latter performs poorly for classes occurring only in few volumes or in a vanishingly low amount of voxels. While this is a characteristic of many diagnostically relevant structures in medical imaging, weakly supervised learning performed particularly poorly on them (e.g., IRC), while exhibiting the strongest bias towards the SRF class in our experiments. This can be explained by the fact that many volumes show SRF resulting in a large amount of patches having the (false) noisy SRF class label. Our approach achieves higher classification accuracy on class labels over all three classes by approximately 15 %. Results indicate that semantic descriptions which provide class occurrences and corresponding abstract location information provide a rich source to improve classification tasks in medical image analysis where no voxel-wise annotations are available. This is important, because in many cases medical images have associated textual descriptions generated and used during clinical routine. The proposed approach enables the use of these data on a scale for which annotation would not be possible.

References

1. Dietterich, T.G., Lathrop, R.H., Lozano-Pérez, T.: Solving the multiple instance problem with axis-parallel rectangles. Artif. Intell. **89**(1), 31–71 (1997)
2. Maron, O., Lozano-Pérez, T.: A framework for multiple-instance learning. In: NIPS '97 Proceedings of the 1997 Conference on Advances in Neural Information Processing Systems 10, pp. 570–576. MIT press, Cambridge (1998)
3. Srivastava, N., Salakhutdinov, R.: Multimodal learning with deep Boltzmann machines. In: Advances in Neural Information Processing Systems 25 (NIPS 2012), vol. 25, pp. 2231–2239 (2012)
4. Leistner, C., Saffari, A., Santner, J., Bischof, H.: Semi-supervised random forests. In: 12th International Conference on Computer Vision, pp. 506–513, IEEE (2009)
5. Zhou, Z.H., Zhang, M.L.: Multi-instance multi-label learning with application to scene classification. In: Proceedings of Neural Information Processing Systems (NIPS), vol. 19, pp. 1609–1616 (2007)
6. Cinbis, R.G., Verbeek, J., Schmid, C.: Multi-fold MIL training for weakly supervised object localization. In: Conference on Computer Vision and Pattern Recognition, IEEE (2014)
7. Verbeek, J., Triggs, B.: Region classification with markov field aspect models. In: Conference on Computer Vision and Pattern Recognition, pp. 1–8, IEEE (2007)
8. Fukushima, K.: Neocognitron: a self-organizing neural network model for a mechanism of pattern recognition unaffected by shift in position. Biol. Cybern. **36**(4), 193–202 (1980)
9. Lee, H., Grosse, R., Ranganath, R., Ng, A.Y.: Unsupervised learning of hierarchical representations with convolutional deep belief networks. Commun. ACM **54**(10), 95–103 (2011)
10. Ciresan, D., Meier, U., Schmidhuber, J.: Multi-column deep neural networks for image classification. In: Conference on Computer Vision and Pattern Recognition, pp. 3642–3649, IEEE (2012)
11. Krizhevsky, A., Sutskever, I., Hinton, G.E.: Imagenet classification with deep convolutional neural networks. In: Advances in Neural Information Processing Systems 25 (NIPS 2012), vol. 25, pp. 1097–1105 (2012)
12. Brosch, T., Tam, R.: Manifold learning of brain MRIs by deep learning. Medical Image Computing and Computer-Assisted Intervention, pp. 633–640 (2013)
13. Schlegl, T., Ofner, J., Langs, G.: Unsupervised pre-training across image domains improves lung tissue classification. In: Menze, B., Langs, G., Montillo, A., Kelm, M., Müller, H., Zhang, S., Cai, W.T., Metaxas, D. (eds.) MCV 2014. LNCS, vol. 8848, pp. 82–94. Springer, Heidelberg (2014)
14. Oquab, M., Bottou, L., Laptev, I., Sivic, J.: Weakly supervised object recognition with convolutional neural networks. Technical Report HAL-01015140, INRIA (2014)
15. Pradhan, S., Ward, W., Hacioglu, K., Martin, J., Jurafsky, D.: Shallow semantic parsing using support vector machines. In: Proceedings of HLT/NAACL, pp. 233–240 (2004)
16. Garvin, M.K., Abràmoff, M.D., Wu, X., Russell, S.R., Burns, T.L., Sonka, M.: Automated 3-D intraretinal layer segmentation of macular spectral-domain optical coherence tomography images. IEEE Trans. Med. Imaging **28**(9), 1436–1447 (2009)
17. Bergstra, J., Breuleux, O., Bastien, F., Lamblin, P., Pascanu, R., Desjardins, G., Turian, J., Warde-Farley, D., Bengio, Y.: Theano: A CPU and GPU math expression compiler. In: Proceedings of the Python for Scientific Computing Conference (SciPy), vol. 4 (2010)

Bodypart Recognition Using Multi-stage Deep Learning

Zhennan Yan[1,2], Yiqiang Zhan[1(✉)], Zhigang Peng[1], Shu Liao[1],
Yoshihisa Shinagawa[1], Dimitris N. Metaxas[2], and Xiang Sean Zhou[1]

[1] Siemens Healthcare, Malvern, PA, USA
zhennany@cs.rutgers.edu, yiqiang.zhan@siemens.com
[2] CBIM, Rutgers University, Piscataway, NJ, USA

Abstract. Automatic medical image analysis systems often start from
identifying the human body part contained in the image. Specifically,
given a transversal slice, it is important to know which body part it
comes from, namely "slice-based bodypart recognition". This problem
has its unique characteristic - the body part of a slice is usually identified by local discriminative regions instead of global image context, e.g.,
a cardiac slice is differentiated from an aorta arch slice by the mediastinum region. To leverage this characteristic, we design a multi-stage
deep learning framework that aims at: (1) discover the local regions that
are discriminative to the bodypart recognition, and (2) learn a bodypart
identifier based on these local regions. These two tasks are achieved by
the two stages of our learning scheme, respectively. In the pre-train stage,
a convolutional neural network (CNN) is learned in a multi-instance
learning fashion to extract the most discriminative local patches from the
training slices. In the boosting stage, the learned CNN is further boosted
by these local patches for bodypart recognition. By exploiting the discriminative local appearances, the learned CNN becomes more accurate
than global image context-based approaches. As a key hallmark, our
method does not require manual annotations of the discriminative local
patches. Instead, it automatically discovers them through multi-instance
deep learning. We validate our method on a synthetic dataset and a large
scale CT dataset (7000+ slices from wholebody CT scans). Our method
achieves better performances than state-of-the-art approaches, including
the standard CNN.

1 Introduction

In recent decades, various automatic image analysis algorithms have emerged to
assist clinicians in the interpretation and assessment of medical images. These
algorithms range from fundamental image analysis tasks, e.g., anatomical landmark detection, organ segmentation to comprehensive computer-aided-diagnosis
(CAD) systems. Due to the highly diverse characteristics of different organ systems, medical image analysis algorithms are often designed/trained for specific

---

Z. Yan— This research work was mainly conducted during Zhennan's internship in
Siemens.

S. Ourselin et al. (Eds.): IPMI 2015, LNCS 9123, pp. 449–461, 2015.
DOI: 10.1007/978-3-319-19992-4_35

anatomies with priors (e.g. organ shape [16]). In order to invoke these algorithms properly in a real-world clinical system, it is important to automatically identify the human bodypart contained in the medical image in the first place. A correct identification of human bodypart not only improves the efficiency of the system - it is unnecessary to invoke a lung CAD algorithm on an abdominal scan, but also reduces the possible errors - applying a liver segmentation algorithm on a head scan may produce unexpected results. In addition, besides working as a pre-processing module of an automatic image analysis system, an efficient and robust body identification algorithm is also the key component of some use cases, e.g., medical image retrieval, CT dose estimation, etc.

A common form of medical imaging scans, especially CT and MR, is a 3D volume image consisted of a series of 2D slices. In this study, we focus on the bodypart identification in a 2D transversal slice, namely "slice-based bodypart recognition". Specifically, as shown in Fig. 1, human body is divided into continuous sections according to anatomical context. Given a 2D transversal slice, a slice-based bodypart recognition algorithm should be able to identify which section it belongs to. It is worth noting that slice-based bodypart recognition is the key of 3D bodypart identification because of two reasons. First, in some real-world systems, 3D volume is not always accessible. For example, in a client-server application, the server end might only receive the 3D volume data slice-by-slice due to the limited network speed. Second, 2D slice-based bodypart recognition provides the foundation of 3D bodypart identification. Given the bodypart identities of the starting and ending slices of a 3D volume, the 3D bodypart can be straightforwardly derived.

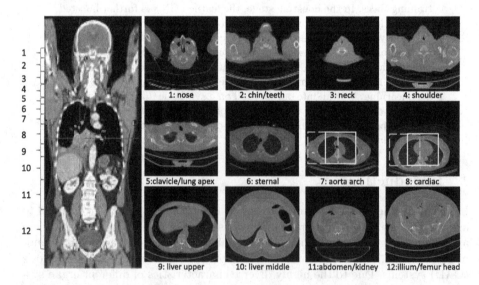

Fig. 1. Definition of body sections. Human body is divided into 12 continuous parts. Each parts may cover different ranges due to the variability of anatomies (Color figure online).

In slice-based bodypart recognition, since different body sections have diverse appearance characteristics and even same section may have large variability, it is almost impossible to "design" features that work commonly well for different body parts. Thus, deep learning technology, which can learn features and classifiers simultaneously, becomes a promising solution. However, slice-based bodypart recognition has its unique challenge which might not be solved by standard deep learning. As shown in Fig. 1, although image 7 and 8 belong to aorta arch and cardiac sections, respectively, their global appearance characteristics are quite similar. For these two slices, the only clues to differentiate them come from the local mediastinum region (indicated by the yellow boxes). While the standard deep learning framework is able to learn features, it cannot learn the local patches that are most discriminative for bodypart recognition. Hence, the classification power of the learned deep network may be limited. In fact, in face recognition community, Taigman et al. [12] also shows that only after the face (the local region of interest) is properly localized, can deep learning show its power in face recognition. However, while face is a well defined object and can be detected by mature algorithms, the discriminative local regions for bodypart recognition are not easy to define, not to mention that the effort to build these local detectors might be quite large.

In summary, in order to tackle the challenge of the slice-based bodypart recognition, two key questions need to be answered. First, which local regions are discriminative for bodypart recognition? Second, how to learn the local bodypart identifiers on them without time-consuming manual annotations? We answer these questions using a multi-stage deep learning scheme. In the pre-train stage, a convolutional neural network (CNN) is learned in a multi-instance learning fashion to "discover" the most discriminative local patches. Specifically, each slice is divided into multiple local patches. The deep network thus receives a set of labeled slices (bags), each containing multiple local patches (instances). The loss function of the CNN is adapted in a way that as long as one local patch (instance) is correctly labeled, the corresponding slice (bag) is considered as correct. In this way, the pre-trained CNN will be more sensitive to the discriminative local patches than others. Based on the responses of the pre-trained CNNs, discriminative and non-informative local patches are selected to further boost the pre-trained CNN. This is the second stage of our training scheme, namely "boosting stage". At run-time, a sliding window approach is employed to apply the boosted CNN to the subject image. As the CNN only has peaky responses on discriminative local patches, it essentially identifies bodypart by focusing on the most distinctive local information. Compared to global image context-based approaches, this local approach is expected to be more accurate and robust.

The major contributions of this work include: 1. We propose a multi-stage deep learning strategy to identify anatomy body parts by using discriminative local information; 2. Our method does not require annotations of the discriminative local patches. Instead, it automatically *discovers* these local patches through multi-instance deep learning. Thus our solution becomes highly scalable. 3. Our method is validated on a large scale of CT slices and shows superior performance than state-of-the-art methods.

2 Related Work

There are several bodypart recognition systems introduced in this decade. Park et al. [10] proposed an algorithm using energy information from Wavelet Transform to determine the body parts within a certain imaging modality. They used look-up tables to classify the imaging modality and body parts. Hong et al. [5] designed a framework to identify different body parts from a full-body input image. The method begins from establishing global reference frame and the head location. After determining the bounding box of the head, other body parts, i.e., neck, thorax cage, abdomen and pelvis, are localized one by one via different algorithms. These approaches use ad-hoc designed features and algorithms to identify major body parts with globally variant appearances. Some other studies use organ or landmark detection techniques [2,3,15]. These methods require large efforts to manually annotate organs or landmarks in the training stage.

The slice-based bodypart recognition is essentially an image classification problem, which has been extensively studied in computer vision and machine learning communities. Generally speaking, image classification methods can be categorized into two groups, global information-based and local information-based. Global information-based approaches extract features from the whole image. Conventional approaches rely on carefully hand-crafted features, e.g., GIST, SIFT, HOG and their variants. These features are extracted on dense grids or a few interested points and organized as bag of words to provide statistical summary of the spatial scene layouts without any object segmentation [7]. Such global representations followed by classical classifiers have been widely used in scene recognition or image classification [14]. Recently, deep learning based algorithms [1,6] have shown their superior in these tasks due to the ability of learning expressive nonlinear features and classifier simultaneously.

Although the global information-based approaches achieved good performances in some image classification problems, it is not sufficient or appropriate to recognize images whose characteristics are exhibited by local objects, e.g., jumbled image recognition [9] and multi-label image classification [13]. Local information-based approaches can achieve better performance here. For example, Szegedy et al. [11] utilized CNN for local object detection and recognition and achieved state-of-the-art performance on Pascal VOC database. However, in the training stage, they require manually annotated object bounding boxes, which is often time consuming. In another pioneer work, Felzenszwalb et al. [4] proposed a part-based deformable model using local information of object parts for object recognition and detection. The object's part locations are modeled as latent variables during training of a star-structured part-based model. In a more recent work, Wei et al. [13] applied objectness detection techniques followed by a CNN to provide multiple labels for an image. Based on the characteristics of slices from different body sections (see Fig. 1), a local information-based approach should be used in our study. Different from existing works, we aim to design an algorithm that is able to discover the most discriminative local regions without annotations or explicit object detection. Hence, the solution will become highly scalable.

3   Methodology

3.1   Problem Statement

Definitions: Slice-based bodypart recognition is a typical multi-class image classification problem that can be addressed by convolutional neural network (CNN). Denote $\mathbf{X}$ as the input slice/image, $\mathbf{W}$ as the CNN coefficients, and K as the number of body sections (classes). Standard CNN outputs a K dimension vector. Its kth component, $\mathbf{P}(k|\mathbf{X};\mathbf{W})$, indicates the probability of $\mathbf{X}$ belonging to class k given $\mathbf{W}$.

Given a training set $\mathcal{T} = \{\mathbf{X}_m, m = 1, ..., M\}$, with corresponding discrete labels $l_m \in \{1, ..., K\}$, the training algorithm of CNN aims to minimize the loss function:

$$L_1(\mathbf{W}) = \sum_{\mathbf{X}_m \in \mathcal{T}} - \log(\mathbf{P}(l_m|\mathbf{X}_m;\mathbf{W})). \tag{1}$$

Here, $\mathbf{P}(l_m|\mathbf{X}_m;\mathbf{W})$ indicates the probability of $\mathbf{X}_m$ being correctly classified as l_m.

CNN has shown impressive performance in image classification [6,13] due to its capability of modeling complex nonlinear functions and leveraging the context information of neighboring pixels. In these applications, standard CNN often takes the entire image as input, which is essentially a *global* learning scheme. In slice-based bodypart recognition, however, the distinctive information often comes from *local* patches (as shown in Fig. 1) and these local patches are distributed at different locations of the slices. The intrinsic conflicts between "global" and "local" may limit CNN's performance in our application. (One may argue that CNN can still learn local features through its convolutional layers. However, this situation only holds while local features always appear at the similar location of the image, which is not the case of bodypart recognition.) A toy example is presented to illustrate this problem. As shown in Fig. 2(a), two classes of binary images are synthesized by randomly positioning and combining 4 types of geometry elements, square, circle, triangle and diamond. While circle and diamond appear in both classes, triangle and square are exclusively owned by

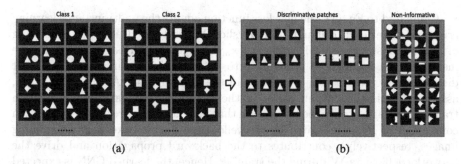

Fig. 2. A synthetic toy example. (a) Synthetic images of two classes. (b) The discriminative and non-informative local patches selected by the pre-trained CNN model.

Class1 and Class2, respectively (ref Sect. 4.1 for more details). Using standard CNN that takes the whole image as input, the classification accuracy is ~85 % (row "SCNN" of Table 1(a)), which implies it does not discover and learn the discriminative local patches: "triangle" and "square". Apparently, this problem will become trivial if we have the prior knowledge of the discriminative local patches and build local classifiers on them. However, in bodypart recognition, it is difficult to figure out the most discriminative local patches for different body sections. In addition, even with *adhoc* knowledge, it will take large efforts to annotate local patches and train local classifiers, which makes the solution non-scalable when body-sections are re-defined or the imaging modalities are changed.

In order to leverage the local information, more important, to "discover" the discriminative local patches for body-part identification, we propose a two-stage CNN learning framework that consists of pre-train and boosting stages, which will be detailed next.

3.2   Learning Stage I: Multi-instance CNN Pre-train

To exploit the local information, CNN needs to take some *discriminative* local patches of the slice as its input. The key problem here is how to *discover* these local patches through learning. This is the major task of the first stage of our CNN learning framework. A multi-instance learning strategy is employed to achieve this goal.

Given a training set $T = \{\mathbf{X}_m, m = 1, ..., M\}$ with corresponding labels l_m. Each training slice, $\mathbf{X}_m$, is divided into a set of local patches defined as $\mathcal{L}(X_m) = \{\mathbf{x}_{mn}, n = 1, ..., N\}$. These local patches become the basic training samples of the CNN and their labels are inherited from the original slices, i.e., all $\mathbf{x}_{mn} \in \mathcal{L}(X_m)$ share the same label l_m. While the structure of CNN is still the same as the standard one, the loss function is adapted as Eq. 2, where $\mathbf{P}(l_m|\mathbf{x}_{mn}; \mathbf{W})$ is the probability that the local patch $\mathbf{x}_{mn}$ is correctly classified as l_m.

$$L_2(\mathbf{W}) = \sum_{X_m \in T} - \log(\max_{\mathbf{x}_{mn} \in \mathcal{L}(\mathbf{X}_m)} \mathbf{P}(l_m|\mathbf{x}_{mn}; \mathbf{W})) \qquad (2)$$

Compared to Eq. (1), the new loss function adopts the multi-instance learning criterion. Here, each original training slice $\mathbf{X}_m$ is treated as a bag consisting of multiple instances (local patches), $\{\mathbf{x}_{mn}\}$. Within each bag (slice), only the instance with the highest probability to be correctly classified, i.e., the most discriminative local patch, is counted in the loss function. As shown in Fig. 3, assume R_{mn} is the output vector of the CNN on local patch $\mathbf{x}_{mn}$, for each training image $\mathbf{X}_m$, only the local patch that has the highest response at the l_mth component of R_{mn} (indicated by the yellow and purple boxes for two training images, respectively), contributes to the backward propagation and drive the network coefficients $\mathbf{W}$ during the training. Hence, the learned CNN is expected to have high responses on discriminative local patches.

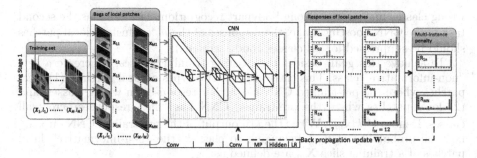

Fig. 3. Illustration of pre-train learning stage (Color figure online).

To ensure the learned CNN having stable high responses on descriminative local patches, we further incorporate the spatial continuity factor into the loss function as:

$$L_3(\mathbf{W}) = \sum_{X_m \in \mathcal{T}} -\log(\max_{\mathbf{x}_{mn} \in \mathcal{L}(\mathbf{X}_m)} \sum_{\mathbf{x} \in \mathfrak{N}(\mathbf{x}_{mn})} \mathbf{P}(l_m|\mathbf{x}; \mathbf{W})), \qquad (3)$$

where $\mathfrak{N}(\mathbf{x}_{mn})$ denotes the local patches in the neighborhood of $\mathbf{x}_{mn}$. According to Eq. (3), for each training slice, the local patch to be counted in the loss function is not the most *individually* discriminative one (i.e., with the highest probability of being correctly classified), but the one whose neighboring patches and itself are *overall* most discriminative. In this way, the selected discriminative local patches will be robust to image translation and artifacts.

3.3 Learning Stage II: CNN Boosting

The second stage of our learning framework aims to boost the pre-trained CNN using selected local patches.

The first type of selected local patches are the discriminative ones, i.e., these local patches on which the pre-trained CNN have high responses at the corresponding classs. For each slice $\mathbf{X}_m$, we select D discriminative local patches as:

$$\mathbf{A}_m = \underset{\mathbf{x}_{mn} \in \mathcal{L}(\mathbf{X}_m)}{\operatorname{argmax}_D} \mathbf{P}(l_m|\mathbf{x}_{mn}; \hat{\mathbf{W}}). \qquad (4)$$

Here, $\hat{\mathbf{W}}$ is the coefficients of the pre-trained CNN. $\operatorname{argmax}_D(.)$ is the operator that returns the arguments of the largest D elements.

Apart from the discriminative local patches, the remaining ones cannot be completely ignored in the boosting stage. For example, as shown in Fig. 1, the local patches containing lung regions (green dashed boxes) appear in both aortic arch and cardiac sections. For these "confusing" patches, CNN may generate similarly high responses for both aortic arch and cardiac classes. (Note that since the pre-trained CNN is only ensured to correctly classify one local patch per slice, the responses of the remaining patches are not guaranteed.) At runtime, when CNN is applied to the confusing patches, the high responses on other wrong classes may induce wrong bodypart recognition. Therefore, as the second task of the CNN boosting stage, the responses of these "confusing" local patches should be suppressed for *all* classes (body sections).

To achieve this goal, besides the existing training classes, we create a new "non-informative" class. This class includes two types of local patches: (1) local patches where the pre-trained CNN has higher responses on wrong classes, and (2) local patches where the pre-trained CNN has "flat" responses across all classes. Denote $\mathbf{P}(k|\mathbf{x}_{mn};\hat{\mathbf{W}})$ as the kth output of the pre-trained CNN on $\mathbf{x}_{mn}$, i.e., the probability of $\mathbf{x}_{mn}$ belonging to class k, the "non-informative" local patches of a training slice $\mathbf{X}_m$ are defined as:

$$\mathbf{B}_m = \{\mathbf{x}_{mn}|\ \underset{k\in\{1,\ldots,K\}}{\mathrm{argmax}}\ \mathbf{P}(k|\mathbf{x}_{mn};\hat{\mathbf{W}}) \neq l_m\}\cup\{\mathbf{x}_{mn}|\ \underset{k\in\{1,\ldots,K\}}{\mathrm{entropy}}\ \mathbf{P}(k|\mathbf{x}_{mn};\hat{\mathbf{W}}) > \theta\} \quad (5)$$

Recall the toy example, the selected discriminative and non-informative local patches are shown in Fig. 2(b). When the discriminative patches from Class1 and Class2 only contain "triangle" or "square", respectively, the non-informative patches may include circle, diamond or background. This is exactly in accordance to the fact that these two classes are only distinguishable by "triangle" and "square". It proves that our method is able to "discover" the key local patches without manually annotating them.

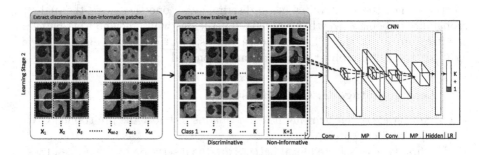

Fig. 4. Illustration of boosting learning stage.

After introducing the additional "non-informative" class, the LR layer of the CNN needs to have an additional output (see shadowed box in the rightmost diagram of Fig. 4). Other than that, the structure of the CNN keeps the same as the pre-trained CNN. Since the pre-trained CNN already captured some discriminative local appearance characteristics, all network layers except the last one inherit their coefficients from the pre-trained CNN as initial values. The coefficients are further adapted by minimizing:

$$L_4(\mathbf{W}) = \sum_{\mathbf{x}\in\mathbf{A}\bigcup\mathbf{B}} -\log(\mathbf{P}(l|\mathbf{x};\mathbf{W})), \quad (6)$$

where $\mathbf{A} = \bigcup_{\{m=1,\ldots,M\}}\mathbf{A}_m$ and $\mathbf{B} = \bigcup_{\{m=1,\ldots,M\}}\mathbf{B}_m$ denote the discriminative and non-informative local patches extracted from all training slices, respectively.

It is worth noting that since the "non-informative" local patches are not belonging to any body section class now, their responses on any body section class can be effectively suppressed during the CNN boost stage.

3.4   Run-Time Classification

The two-stage CNN learning algorithm is summarized in Algorithm 1. At runtime, the boosted CNN is applied for bodypart recognition in a large step sliding window way. Given a testing image $\mathbf{X}$, we first partition it into N overlapping local patches $\mathcal{L}(\mathbf{X}) = \{\mathbf{x}_n, n = 1, ..., N\}$. For each local patch $\mathbf{x}_n$, the boosted CNN outputs a vector with $K+1$ components $\{\mathbf{P}(k|\mathbf{x}_n; \mathbf{W}^{opt})|k = 1, ..., K+1\}$, where $\mathbf{W}^{opt}$ denotes the optimal coefficients of Eq. (6). Since the class $K+1$ is an artificially constructed "non-informative" one, local patches belong to this class should be ignored in determining the body section of the slice. Consequently, the class (body section) of the testing slice $\mathbf{X}$ is determined as:

$$C(\mathbf{X}) = c(\mathbf{x}_{n^*}), \quad \mathbf{x}_{n^*} = \underset{\mathbf{x}_n \in \mathcal{L}(\mathbf{X}); c(\mathbf{x}_n) \neq K+1}{\operatorname{argmax}} \mathbf{P}(c(\mathbf{x}_n)|\mathbf{x}_n; \mathbf{W}^{opt}), \qquad (7)$$

where $c(\mathbf{x}_n) = \operatorname{argmax}_{k \in \{1,...,K+1\}} \mathbf{P}(k|\mathbf{x}_n; \mathbf{W}^{opt})$.

Algorithm 1. Multi-stage deep learning

Input:
  Scalars M, N, K, dataset $(\mathbf{X}_m, l_m), \forall m \in \{1, \cdots, M\}$, CNN architecture
Output:
  Boosted CNN coefficients $\mathbf{W}^{opt}$
 1: Partition $\mathbf{X}_m$ into N overlapping local regions $\mathbf{x}_{mn}$
 2: Pre-train CNN on $(\mathbf{x}_{mn}, l_m)$ using multi-instance loss function (3), and obtain optimized $\hat{\mathbf{W}}$
 3: Extract $\mathbf{A}_m$ and $\mathbf{B}_m$ according to Eq. (4) and (5)
 4: Assign label l_m to each instance of $\mathbf{A}_m$, and label $K+1$ to each of $\mathbf{B}_m$
 5: Modify pre-trained CNN by adding one unit to LR, layers except LR inherit coefficients
 6: Boost CNN on set $\mathbf{A} \bigcup \mathbf{B}$ using loss function (6), and obtain optimized $\mathbf{W}^{opt}$

---

4   Experiments

4.1   Image Classification on Synthetic Data

We first demonstrate our method on a synthetic data set, which is constructed by 4 types of geometry elements: triangle, square, circle and diamond. Specifically, the size of all synthetic images are 60×60 with black background (intensity value 0). The basic geometry elements are created within a bounding-box 15×15 and random intensity values in $[1, 180]$. These elements are then transformed with random scales $[1, 1.4]$ in height and width, and randomly positioned on the image background. In constructing the two image classes, we ensure that the triangle and square only appear in Class1 and Class2, respectively. Circle and diamond can randomly appear in both classes. (Some examples of the synthetic images are shown in Fig. 2(a)). Overall, we create 400 training, 400 validation and 400 for testing samples (200 for each class).

If we applies standard CNN algorithm on the synthetic dataset, as shown in the "SCNN" row in Table 1(a), the classification accuracy is 85.6 %. This inferior performance results from the fact that the global CNN learning scheme may not learn the most discriminative local patches. On the contrary, by using our two-stage learning framework, as shown in Fig. 2(b), the most discriminative local patches are effectively extracted. All of them include either "triangle" (Class1) or "square"(Class2), which is exactly in accordance to the rule of generating these two classes. By leveraging the discriminative information of these local patches, our classification accuracy can reach 99.3 % ("BCNN2" row in Table 1(a)).

A comparison study is conducted using: (1) logistic regression (LR); (2) SVM; (3) standard CNN trained on whole image (SCNN); (4) local patch-based CNN without boost, i.e., the CNN trained by pre-train stage only (PCNN); (5) local patch-based CNN boosted without additional non-informative class (BCNN1); (6) local patch-based CNN boosted with both discriminative and non-informative patches (BCNN2). Methods (1)-(3) represent traditional learning (using image intensities as features) and deep learning approaches. Methods (4)-(5) are different variants of our proposed one (6), which are presented to verify the effects of each component of our method. The parameters of these comparison methods are optimized using the validation set.

Table 1. Classification accuracies by F1 score $= 2\frac{precision \cdot recall}{precision + recall}$ (%).

Class	(a) Synthetic Data			(b) CT Data												
	1	2	Total	1	2	3	4	5	6	7	8	9	10	11	12	Total
LR	60.6	65.6	63.4	35.3	50.9	33.0	57.3	33.2	34.4	52.5	58.7	40.1	26.1	40.4	71.4	56.1
SVM	86.0	86.0	86.0	54.9	48.9	52.4	58.0	41.8	40.2	58.6	60.3	41.4	38.0	39.0	71.4	57.7
SCNN	86.0	85.0	85.6	93.2	95.5	77.4	83.1	83.9	82.6	89.6	90.3	70.5	51.5	70.8	94.4	84.8
PCNN	96.3	96.2	96.3	95.8	94.1	71.0	83.8	73.8	82.5	95.9	94.7	72.0	60.6	78.2	95.8	88.2
BCNN1	90.4	90.1	90.3	95.5	94.2	68.8	82.5	80.8	85.2	96.1	94.2	69.4	60.3	76.0	95.0	87.3
BCNN2	99.2	99.3	99.3	91.9	96.7	78.8	87.5	82.1	85.0	95.7	95.1	72.0	64.8	82.6	97.9	89.8

As shown in Table 1(a), standard deep learning method (SCNN) is better than LR, which indicates deep learning can learn good features from raw data. By leveraging the local discriminative information, the CNN performance can be further improved (~11 % improvement from SCNN to PCNN). Among our local patch-based CNNs (PCNN, BCNN1 and BCNN2), BCNN1 shows the worst performance. It proves the importance of including an non-informative class in the boosting stage. BCNN2, which includes all designed components, achieves the best performance.

4.2   Bodypart Recognition of CT Slices

In this experiment, we applied our method to recognize the body section of transversal CT slices. As shown in Fig. 1, transversal CT slices are categorized into 12 classes corresponding to different body sections. Our experiment data includes 7489 transversal CT slices that were acquired from 675 patients with very different ages (1–90 years) using various imaging protocols (31 different kernels, pixel resolution $0.281\,mm - 1.953\,mm$). The appearances of this dataset thus become very diverse. The whole dataset is separated into 2340 training, 588 validation and 4561 testing subsets.

As a preprocessing step, all images are re-sampled to have $4\,mm \times 4\,mm$ pixel resolution and 90×90 in size. For each image, 50×50 local patches are extracted with step size 10 pixels. Thus, 25 local patches are extracted per image. Our CNN has two convolutional layers (with 9×9 filters) each followed by a 2×2 max-pooling layer. Its final two layers are a 600-node hidden layer and a LR layer with 12 (pre-train stage) or 13 (boosting stage) output nodes.

As shown in the "BCNN2" row of Table 1(b), our method can achieve the classification accuracy at 89.8 %. More detailed classification performance is shown by the confusion matrix in Fig. 5. In general, most errors appear close to the diagonal line, i.e., most mis-classifications

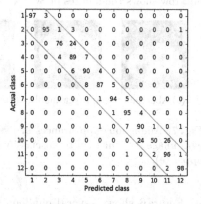

Fig. 5. Confusion matrix of BCNN2 on CT data. Values are normalized to $0 - 100$ in each row (Color figure online).

happen in the neighboring body sections. Qualitatively, **99.1 %** of the testing cases have "less-than-one neighboring class error" (within the red corridor in Fig. 5). In practice, this is an encouraging behavior, since this kind of errors are already acceptable for some use cases and they may be further fixed by post-processing algorithms. The computation time is $\sim 10\,ms$ per image, on a 64-bit desktop with i7–2600 (3.4 GHz) CPU, 16 GB RAM and NVIDIA GTX-660 3 GB GPU.

For comparison, we also tested other image classification methods, including (1) LR, (2) SVM, (3) SCNN, (4) PCNN, (5) BCNN1. In LR and SVM methods, we use dense SIFT [8] features followed by logistic regression and SVM classifiers, respectively. SCNN method is the standard CNN that takes the whole slice as input. Method (4)-(5) are the variants of our method as described in Sect. 4.1. Same network structure is used in all CNN-based methods. As shown in Table 1(b), although SCNN shows better performance than LR and SVM, its performance can be further improved by using local discriminative information. Compared to its variants, our method BCNN2 achieves the best performance, which proves the necessity of using all designed strategies.

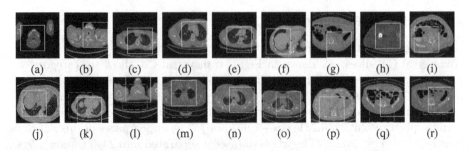

Fig. 6. Challenging examples on which other methods fail and BCNN2 succeeds. The first row shows the failures of SCNN. The second row shows the failures of PCNN.

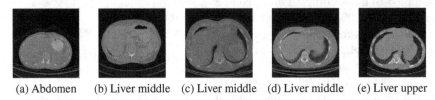

(a) Abdomen   (b) Liver middle   (c) Liver middle   (d) Liver middle   (e) Liver upper

Fig. 7. Ambiguous appearances of liver middle section. Methods may correctly deal with image (c), but tend to misclassify (b) to abdomen (a); and misclassify (d) to liver upper (e).

Figure 6 shows several challenging cases, on which other methods fail and our method succeeds. Since SCNN rely on global features, it fails because of mis-alignment (Fig. 6 (a)), partial field of view (Fig. 6 (f)) and local artifacts (Fig. 6 (h)), etc. The failure of PCNN is due to higher response on confusing local patches (indicated by green dashed boxes). For example, PCNN is misled by the local confusing patch and misclassifies Fig. 6 (j) (a "liver upper" slice) as "cardiac". On the contrary, our method can correctly classify all of them thanks to its capability of capturing the local characteristics (yellow boxes in Fig. 6) and suppressing the responses of the confusing local patches on any body section classes.

In Table 1(b), we also noticed that class 10 (liver middle section) has larger errors than others across *all* comparison algorithms, which may be contributed to the ambiguous appearances of this section. As shown in Fig. 7, "liver middle" slices (b) and (d) are misclassified as "abdomen" (a) or "liver upper" (e), respectively. However, due to the similar appearances, even a well trained professional may have very difficulty to distinguish them.

5   Conclusions

In this paper, we presented a novel multi-stage deep learning framework to tackle the bodypart recognition problem. The key idea is to automatically learn the discriminative local patches and exploit the local information for bodypart recognition. Importantly, since no manual annotations are required to label these local patches, our method do not need extensive annotations, hence, becomes very scalable. We evaluated our method on a synthetic dataset and a large scale CT dataset with 7000+ slices. The experimental results show clear improvements compared with state-of-the-art methods. The proposed framework is also easily extendable to other image classification tasks where local information is more important than global one.

References

1. Ciresan, D., Meier, U., Schmidhuber, J.: Multi-column deep neural networks for image classification. In: CVPR, pp. 3642–3649. IEEE (2012)
2. Criminisi, A., Shotton, J., Robertson, D., Konukoglu, E.: Regression forests for efficient anatomy detection and localization in CT studies. In: Menze, B., Langs, G., Tu, Z., Criminisi, A. (eds.) MICCAI 2010. LNCS, vol. 6533, pp. 106–117. Springer, Heidelberg (2011)
3. Donner, R., Menze, B.H., Bischof, H., Langs, G.: Global localization of 3D anatomical structures by pre-filtered Hough Forests and discrete optimization. Med. Image Anal. **17**(8), 1304–1314 (2013)
4. Felzenszwalb, P.F., Girshick, R.B., McAllester, D., Ramanan, D.: Object detection with discriminatively trained part-based models. TPAMI **32**(9), 1627–1645 (2010)
5. Hong, L., Hong, S.: Methods and apparatus for automatic body part identification and localization. US Patent App. 11/933,518, (15 May 2008)
6. Krizhevsky, A., Sutskever, I., Hinton, G.E.: Imagenet classification with deep convolutional neural networks. In: NIPS, pp. 1097–1105 (2012)
7. Lazebnik, S., Schmid, C., Ponce, J.: Beyond bags of features: Spatial pyramid matching for recognizing natural scene categories. In: CVPR, vol. 2, pp. 2169–2178. IEEE (2006)
8. Lowe, D.G.: Distinctive image features from scale-invariant keypoints. Int. J. Comput. Vis. (IJCV) **60**(2), 91–110 (2004)
9. Parikh, D.: Recognizing jumbled images: the role of local and global information in image classification. In: ICCV, pp. 519–526. IEEE (2011)
10. Park, J., Kang, G., Pan, S.B., Kim, P.: A novel algorithm for identification of body parts in medical images. In: Wang, L., Jiao, L., Shi, G., Li, X., Liu, J. (eds.) FSKD 2006. LNCS (LNAI), vol. 4223, pp. 1148–1158. Springer, Heidelberg (2006)
11. Szegedy, C., Toshev, A., Erhan, D.: Deep neural networks for object detection. In: NIPS, pp. 2553–2561 (2013)
12. Taigman, Y., Yang, M., Ranzato, M., Wolf, L.: Deepface: Closing the gap to human-level performance in face verification. In: CVPR, pp. 1701–1708. IEEE (2014)
13. Wei, Y., Xia, W., Huang, J., Ni, B., Dong, J., Zhao, Y., Yan, S.: CNN: Single-label to multi-label (2014). arXiv preprint arXiv:1406.5726
14. Yang, J., Yu, K., Gong, Y., Huang, T.: Linear spatial pyramid matching using sparse coding for image classification. In: CVPR, pp. 1794–1801. IEEE (2009)
15. Zhan, Y., Zhou, X.S., Peng, Z., Krishnan, A.: Active scheduling of organ detection and segmentation in whole-body medical images. In: Metaxas, D., Axel, L., Fichtinger, G., Székely, G. (eds.) MICCAI 2008, Part I. LNCS, vol. 5241, pp. 313–321. Springer, Heidelberg (2008)
16. Zhang, S., Zhan, Y., Dewan, M., Huang, J., Metaxas, D.N., Zhou, X.S.: Towards robust and effective shape modeling: Sparse shape composition. Med. Image Anal. **16**(1), 265–277 (2012)

Multi-subject Manifold Alignment of Functional Network Structures via Joint Diagonalization

Karl-Heinz Nenning[1]([✉]), Kathrin Kollndorfer[2], Veronika Schöpf[2], Daniela Prayer[2], and Georg Langs[1]

[1] Computational Imaging Research Lab, Medical University of Vienna, Vienna, Austria
karl-heinz.nenning@meduniwien.ac.at
[2] Department of Biomedical Imaging and Image-guided Therapy, Medical University of Vienna, Vienna, Austria

Abstract. Functional magnetic resonance imaging group studies rely on the ability to establish correspondence across individuals. This enables location specific comparison of functional brain characteristics. Registration is often based on morphology and does not take variability of functional localization into account. This can lead to a loss of specificity, or confounds when studying diseases. In this paper we propose multi-subject functional registration by manifold alignment via coupled joint diagonalization. The functional network structure of each subject is encoded in a diffusion map, where functional relationships are decoupled from spatial position. Two-step manifold alignment estimates initial correspondences between functionally equivalent regions. Then, coupled joint diagonalization establishes common eigenbases across all individuals, and refines the functional correspondences. We evaluate our approach on fMRI data acquired during a language paradigm. Experiments demonstrate the benefits in matching accuracy achieved by coupled joint diagonalization compared to previously proposed functional alignment approaches, or alignment based on structural correspondences.

1 Introduction

Functional magnetic resonance imaging (fMRI) is a valuable neuroscientific tool for deepening the understanding of the functional architecture of the brain, its relationship to cognition, or effects of disease and treatment. fMRI introduces numerous analytical challenges when seeking reliable answers to scientific or clinical questions. A particularly difficult issue is the link between function and anatomy. Relying on anatomical registration to establish correspondence before comparing function across individuals can introduce noise or confounds, if the location of functional regions varies or is correlated with disease. In this paper we propose a functional registration approach based on joint diagonalization of the functional connectivity relationship structure observed in multiple individuals.

K.-H. Nenning—This work was supported by the EU (FP7-ICT-2009-5/318068), and OeNB (15929).

S. Ourselin et al. (Eds.): IPMI 2015, LNCS 9123, pp. 462–473, 2015.
DOI: 10.1007/978-3-319-19992-4_36

A large body of research is focused on addressing fundamental challenges in analysing fMRI data such as low temporal resolution, noise, or motion artifacts. However, the potential disconnect between structure and function is only addressed in a small number of studies. It is relevant, because the brains anatomical structure can differ substantially across subjects , and the functional structure can even vary within the same subject [22]. Typical fMRI group studies assume functional correspondence after normalization to a common template space. However, since the localization and extent of functional areas varies across subjects within a certain spatial region, standard group analysis, such as the General Linear Model (GLM) [9] is degraded. Specifically, when studying the impact of damage to the brains functional architecture, the decoupling of changes in position and function is necessary. For instance, a brain tumor alters the anatomical structure, and might lead to functional reorganization, where other regions, possibly even on the opposite hemisphere, compensate for the function of the affected region [7].

In this work we propose a functional registration approach which overcomes the problem of structural and functional variability across individuals or pathologies, by uncoupling function from structure and aligning datasets based on their functional architecture. We propose to use coupled joint diagonalization [6] to learn correspondences, and mutually regularize the embedding representation of individual connectivity structures without using specific functional responses or localizers.

1.1 Related Work

Frist, we briefly review relevant related work on functional alignment, and previous work on manifold alignment related to the method proposed in this paper.

Incorporating functional information into anatomical registration has been shown to account for functional variability between subjects, and improve the inter-subject registration. For example, in [4] spatial patterns of functional response are used to guide anatomical registration, [12] uses progressive matching of multi-range functional connectivity patterns for spatial normalization, and [21] performs fine-tuning of anatomical alignment via a nonrigid registration that maximizes inter-subject correlation. Decoupling function from structure can be achieved via manifold learning. It captures the underlying structure of the relationships within a dataset (e.g. of functional signals) by embedding it into a new space where the Euclidean distance represents these relationships. Manifold alignment then allows to align the embeddings of multiple datasets based on similar intrinsic characteristics. Two general approaches to manifold alignment have been proposed in the literature: one-step and two-step approaches. In one-step approaches, multiple datasets are aligned simultaneously, whereas in two-step approaches, alignment is performed on individually created embeddings. Extensions to the basic concept of one-step alignment [10,25], have successfully been applied to align image datasets of different objects [23], textual datasets [27], or lung images of respiratory motion [1]. In [24], the authors proposed a basic two-step approach consisting of procrustes analysis of embedding maps with application for transfer learning. Two-step manifold alignment approaches were successfully used to map functionally coherent regions across a healthy population [14], to brain tumor patients [15], and for shape matching [16–18].

The benefit of two-step alignment is computational feasibility, whereas one-step manifold alignment techniques can only be applied on a small number of datasets with few sampling points, or with a sparsity constraint. Moreover, one-step alignment is particularly sensitive to subtle differences in the intrinsic structure of each dataset, affecting their applicability on many real-world problems. However, they have the favorable property to mutually regularize the individual embedding representations. The drawbacks of one-step alignment can be overcome with manifold alignment based on joint diagonalization of Laplacians [6,13]. The joint diagonalization approach finds the eigenbases of multiple Laplacian matrices of different datasets simultaneously. These eigenbases can be approximated by a small number of eigenvectors of the dataset specific Laplacians, reducing computational complexity of aligning multiple datasets with a large number of sampling points.

Most recent manifold alignment techniques require at least a small subset of correspondences between the datasets to be known. However, in the neurological context at the center of this paper, this information is generally not available, or not reliable. In this case, unsupervised manifold alignment, i.e. alignment without known correspondences, establishes a similarity measure between the datasets. As proposed in [26], correspondence weights are established based on a local pattern matching technique, and successfully applied to aligned protein data. An unsupervised two-step alignment approach was introduced in [20], where distances between sample points in the embedding space are used to establish parameterized distances curves and subsequently similarities are calculated between those. However, such correspondence estimation techniques are only reliable when there are distinct comparable intrinsic structures present, e.g. image datasets of different objects with comparable rotations.

1.2 Contribution

We propose a manifold alignment approach to build an atlas of functional network characteristics establishing functional correspondences between individuals. Diffusion maps [3] encode the functional architecture of each individual and initial correspondences are established via a two-step manifold alignment approach [15]. A subset of correspondence estimates between dense areas in this intial alignment is used to initiate coupled joint diagonalization that simultaneously finds common eigenbases of the functional connectivity structures and refined correspondences across all subjects [6].

2 Method

Diffusion maps [3] are used to encode the functional connectivity structure of each individual. Based on these subject-specific embeddings initial correspondences between fMRI datasets are established by a two-step manifold alignment approach [15]. It rearranges the spectral components based on spatial constraints, resulting in a population atlas of functional structure. Initial correspondence estimate pairs between datasets are drawn randomly from dense areas in this joint atlas. They initiate coupled joint diagonalization [6]. This results in refined correspondences, and a common eigenbasis, which represent the aligned underlying connectivity structure of a study group.

2.1 Spectral Representation of Functional Connectivity

We embed the whole-brain functional connectivity structure of each individual by diffusion maps [3], resulting in a functional geometry reflecting the functional organization of the brain. The fMRI data $\mathbf{I} \in \mathbb{R}^{T \times N}$ consists of N voxels $\mathbf{v}_i$ observed at T time points. The functional architecture of a brain state can be modeled as a connectivity graph G with vertices V representing the voxels, and edges E between these vertices. Let W denote the affinity matrix assigning weights to the egdes, where W_{ij} is the Pearson correlation coefficient between the time-series of vertex i and j. The spectral representation of the functional connectivity structure can be established via eigendecomposition of the normalized Laplacian matrix L, defined as $L = D^{-1/2}WD^{-1/2}$, where D is the diagonal matrix of node degrees, i.e. $d_i = \sum_j W(i,j)$. The normalized Laplacian is a symmetric version of the random walk matrix $L = D^{-1}W$, which is scaling invariant, and can be viewed as a diffusion process, where the transition probabilities for a diffusion time t between nodes can be expressed by L^t. Eigendecompostion of L results in eigenvalues Λ and corresponding eigenvectors Φ, where $\lambda_1 = 1 > \lambda_2 > \cdots > \lambda_n$. The dataset can be represented by a diffusion map with new embedding coordinates Ψ, where each vertex i in the original graph is represented by

$$\Psi_i^t = (\lambda_1^t \psi_1(x), \lambda_2^t \psi_2(x), \ldots, \lambda_d^t \psi_d(x)), \tag{1}$$

for every data point x in d dimensions of the embedding space. This translates the functional organization of a brain to a functional geometry Ψ, where the functional relations of the fMRI signals are captured by the diffusion distance D_t [15]. The diffusion distance $D_t(i,j)$ is defined as the probability of traveling from node i to node j in t steps, by considering all possible paths between these two nodes. The Euclidean distance in this new embedding space approximates the diffusion distance

$$D_t(x_i, x_j) = \| \psi_t(x_i) - \psi_t(x_j) \|^2. \tag{2}$$

Thus, the functional relationship between voxels of a brain is translated to Euclidean distances in a new embedding space, capturing the functional geometry of the dataset. This uncouples function from anatomy, and is the basis for functional registration of corresponding functional structures across individuals [15].

2.2   Initial Correspondence Estimates Across Individuals

We aim at aligning functionally equivalent areas across individuals. Assuming that for a majority of functional areas the spatial difference is small we use spatial correspondence for initialization. We perform an initial two-step manifold alignment following the initialization procedure in [15]. First, we align brain morphology to a common template [8]. Then, we orthonormally align individual embedding maps representing each subject based on correspondence defined by spatial position in the common template. For every subject specific embedding Ψ_s and template embedding Ψ_t, an orthonormal transformation matrix Q_{st} is calculated, accounting for rotations, sign flips and reordering of the spectral dimensions. Q_{st} is defined as

$$ Q_{st} = \underset{Q}{\mathrm{argmin}}(\sum_{c=1}^{C} w_c \parallel Q\Psi_{sc} - \Psi_{tc} \parallel^2), \tag{3} $$

where Ψ are the embeddings of s and t and w is the Euclidean distance between a pair c of corresponding voxels. After this initial alignment of embeddings, we perform nonrigid point cloud registration to refine the alignment and close potential gaps between the embedded sampling point distributions by Coherent Point Drift [19].

While preserving the functional relationship between brain regions, diffusion maps typically encode a distinct functionally coherent cluster of brain regions along a specific dimension, far from the origin in the leading dimensions of the embedding space. We use this property to obtain initial pairwise point-to-point correspondence estimates between two orthonormally aligned diffusion maps Ψ_s' and Ψ_t, resulting in n correspondence pairs $C = \{\langle i, j(i)\rangle\}_{i=1,\dots,n}$ with $j(i) = argmin_j \parallel \Psi_t(i) - \Psi_s'(j) \parallel^2$. For each pair of embeddings, a subset of q correspondence pairs C is selected based on their distance from the origin and used as initial coupling for joint diagonalization, described in the following section. Note that the purpose of this initial alignment is only to determine a subset of initial correspondence esimates. Sub-sequent joint diagonalization is based on the individual Laplacians and the correspondence pairs.

2.3   Joint Diagonalization

Joint diagonalization simultaneously finds the common eigenbases of the Laplacians of multiple datasets [2,6,13]. In theory, if multiple datasets share similar intrinsic structures, their Laplacians have similar eigenbases with variations in rotations, coefficient sign or ordering of spectral components. Joint diagonalization results in coupled eigenbases, which make the eigenbases of each individual dataset consistent. The basic joint diagonalization problem with full coupling can be formulated as an optimization problem of minimizing off-diagonal elements:

$$ \min_{V} \sum_{i=1}^{M} \mathbf{off}(V^T L_i V) \text{ with } V^T V = I, \tag{4} $$

where M is the number of different datasets, V is their common eigenbases, L_i are the dataset specific Laplacians. The off-diagonal penalty $\mathbf{off}(X)$ is typically defined as the sum of squared off diagonal elements $\mathbf{off}(X) = \parallel X - diag(X) \parallel_F^2$. This problem can be solved with the generalized Jacobi method (JADE method) [2]. It assumes full coupling with an equal amount of samples for every dataset, i.e. every sampling point in a dataset has a corresponding point in all other datasets. In our case we cannot assume identical numbers of sampling points or complete given correspondences between datasets. Instead we only use a sub-set of paired vertices to guide the joint diagonalization.

Coupled diagonalization allows to overcome these limitations [6, 13]. Only a subset of sparse point-wise correspondences is used to establish a coupling relation F. F_i is a $n_i \times q$ coupling matrix, where n_i is the number of data points and q is the number of correspondences. Based on this sparse subset, eigenbases V_i are established, such that $V_i^T L_i V_i$ is approximately diagonal and the eigenbases correspond for corresponding samples $F_i V_i \approx F_j V_j$. This results in multiple dataset specific eigenbases, contrary to the original joint diagonalization approach [2].

To incorporate the coupling between datasets, the formulation in Eq. 4 can be rewritten as

$$\min_{V_i} \sum_{i=1}^{M} \mathbf{off}(V_i^T L_i V_i) + \mu \sum_{i,j=1}^{M} \parallel F_i^T V_i - F_j^T V_j \parallel_F^2 \quad \text{with } V_i^T V_i = I, \quad (5)$$

where V_i are the dataset specific eigenbases, L_i the data specific Laplacians and μ is a coupling weight [6]. The sparse coupling between two datasets i and j is defined by corresponding points k_i and k_j and encoded as $F_i(k_i, q) = 1$ and $F_j(k_j, q) = 1$, with zeros elsewhere in the qth column. However, the coupling is not restricted to such point-wise coupling, and can contain any correspondence weighting. We use the leading k dimensions of the embedding, since they hold the majority of information. This reduces the computational complexity to an optimization problem with $k^2 M$ variables, instead of $\sum^{M} n_i^2$ variables for full eigenbases. Then, the formulation in Eq. 5 can be rewritten as

$$\min_{A_i} \sum_{i=1}^{M} \parallel A_i^T \bar{\Lambda}_i A_i \parallel_F^2 + \mu \sum_{i,j=1}^{M} \parallel F_i^T \bar{U}_i A_i - F_j^T \bar{U}_j A_j \parallel_F^2 \quad \text{with } A_i^T A_i = I, \quad (6)$$

where $\bar{U}_i$ are the first k eigenvectors of L_i and A_i is a $k \times k$ matrix with linear combination coefficients to be estimated [6, 13]. The specific eigenbases can be reconstructed with $\bar{V}_i = \bar{U}_i A_i$.

To solve Eq. 6, we employ an optimization on a Stiefel manifold with orthogonality constraints, introduced in [28]. Hereby, an unconstrained problem is solved by building the orthogonality constraint into the optimization method in the form of a projected descend. Following [6, 13], the cost function is rewritten to

$$\min_{A_i} \parallel A_i^T \bar{\Lambda}_i A_i \parallel_F^2 + \mu \sum_{j=1}^{M} \parallel F_i^T \bar{U}_i A_i - F_j^T \bar{U}_j A_j \parallel_F^2, \quad (7)$$

and solved for all A_i alternatingly, with the gradients for the off diagonal penalty given by

$$\nabla_{A_i} \parallel A_i^T \bar{\Lambda}_i A_i \parallel_F^2 = 4(\bar{\Lambda}_i A_i A_i^T \bar{\Lambda}_i A_i - \bar{\Lambda}_i A_i \bar{\Lambda}_i), \tag{8}$$

and the gradient for the coupling term given by

$$\nabla_{A_i} \parallel F_i^T \bar{U}_i A_i - F_j^T \bar{U}_j A_j \parallel_F^2 = 2\bar{U}_i^T F_i (F_i^T \bar{U}_i A_i - F_j^T \bar{U}_j A_j). \tag{9}$$

Coupled joint diagonalization can be viewed as a mixture between a one-step and a two-step manifold alignment approach. First, like in two-step alignment techniques, Laplacians are computed for each dataset. The eigenvectors and eigenvalues of each individual Laplacian are then used to find common eigenbases, following the principle of one-step manifold alignment approaches.

After coupled joint alignment every voxel in every individual is represented by a point in the joint embedding space. The final correspondences are determined by nearest neighbor search. For every voxel i in a dataset X, a corresponding voxel $\hat{j}$ in a dataset Y can be found by the minimal Euclidean distance between the aligned embedding maps Ψ_X and Ψ_Y: $\hat{j} = argmin_j \parallel \Psi_X(i) - \Psi_Y(j) \parallel^2$.

3   Evaluation

3.1   Data

We evaluate the alignment algorithm on fMRI data collected in study with a language related block design paradigm, comprising 12 healthy individuals. During the activation blocks, subjects are instructed to read nouns and mentally generate associated verbs. During the baseline block hash signs are presented. The fMRI was acquired on a 3 T unit (Philips Medical Systems, Best, The Netherlands) equipped with a 12 channel head coil, using a single shot echo planar imaging (EPI) sequence with TR/TE 3000/35 ms, $128 \times 128 \times 32\,mm$ Matrix, voxel size $1.8 \times 1.8 \times 4\,mm^3$, 100 volumes and a duration of 5 m comprising 5 task - rest alterations. Standard fMRI preprocessing is performed with FSL [11] and Freesurfer [8], including co-registration, motion-correction and removal of timepoints with extensive motion. The fMRI data is normalized to a common space via registration to the Freesurfer average cortical surface template in MNI space [5]. The time-series are projected onto this cortical surface and are normalized to have zero mean and unit variance. The preprocessing results in a total of 4718 cortical brain regions used for further analysis.

3.2   Evaluation

We evaluate if the alignment accurately matches areas that exhibit the same language task response activation. A standard GLM [9] activation analysis is performed on the fMRI data of each individual, and the obtained β parameters are transformed to z-scores. Since manifold alignment is performed without any direct activation information, we use the activation analysis as reference for validation of matching accuracy. In a leave-one-out cross validation, we label the

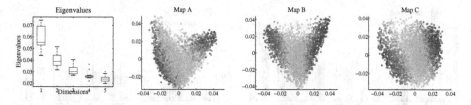

Fig. 1. The encoded information is reflected by the eigenvalues of the Laplacians. They indicate a dominance of the task structure, and the relation between task-negative (blue) and task-positive (red) networks can be observed as a smooth transition in the diffusion maps (Color figure online).

brain regions of a target subject with the z-scores of the closest region in the manifold atlas of the remaining subjects after alignment ('prediction'). We compare the z-scores of the subject specific GLM analysis on the target subject with the predicted z-scores by applying a cut-off and calculating the Dice-coefficient between predicted and measured z-scores. To illustrate the relationship between accuracy and z-score, we report results over a range of z-score values. We compare the alignment of two variants of the proposed approach and 2 alternative approaches. (1) Coupled joint diagonalization using initial correspondences in high density regions of the embedding space (**DG**), (2) coupled joint diagonalization using initial correspondences randomly distributed across the space (**DGrand**), (3) the orthonormal Procrustes alignment of functional connectivity manifolds based on spatial correspondences as used for initialization in [15] (**MA ortho**), and we establish correspondence based on the MNI coordinates of cortical vertices, i.e., relying entirely on the anatomical registration (**MNI**). We perform embedding of the fMRI data of each individual with a correlation threshold of zero, retaining only positive correlation values between brain regions.

3.3   Results: Alignment of Language Networks

Examples of embedded functional network structures are shown in Fig. 1 with the first two dimensions of the diffusion maps. The activation z-score is visualized by the color. Note that z-score information does not enter embedding or alignment. While the overall structure varies, the functional architecture is comparable: a common smooth transition between task-positive regions (red) and task-negative regions (blue). This can be explained by the fact that the intrinsic functional structure of each individual, modeled via correlation between time-series, is dominated by the task paradigm. This is supported by the eigenvalues of the Laplacians (Fig. 1 left), which reveal a rapid decrease in information encoded along each additional dimension, consistent across the study group. Therefore, we limit our further analysis only to the first 5 dimensions of the diffusion map embeddings.

Figure 2a shows the alignment accuracy of *MA ortho* using 1, 3 and 5 eigenvectors, analogously Fig. 2b shows the results for *DG*. A more liberal threshold

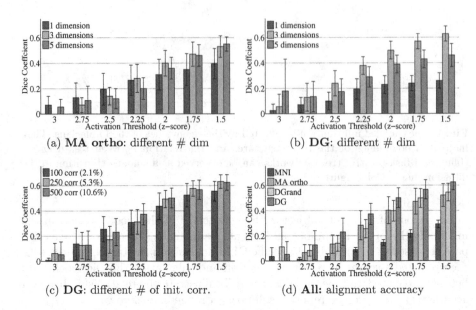

Fig. 2. Alignment accuracy: **(a)** Two step orthonormal manifold alignment for different z-score cut-offs and numbers of eigenvectors. **(b)** Alignment results for DG and 500 correspondences, shows highest alignment accuracy with the first 3 eigenvectors, although the first 5 eigenvectors are more sensitive at higher z-score thresholds. **(c)** As expected, DG with 500 correspondences (10.5%) yields overall best results, however comparable performance can be achieved with only 100 couplings (2.1%). **(d)** The overall comparison shows that our application of joint diagonalization yields better results compared to the two-step manifold alignment ($MA\ ortho$). The utilization of weighted correspondences (DG), yields better results compared to joint diagonalization with random pairs of correspondences ($DGrand$). As expected, performing transfer learning with the closest region on the cortex (MNI) performs underwhelming (Color figure online).

results in more voxels labeled as activated, which implicates a trend towards a higher dice score. A strict univariate GLM analysis might miss some voxels involved in a task, which can be found via network matching. Overall, diffusion maps with 3 dimensions achieve the best alignment results, which can be explained by the basic task-driven intrinsic functional connectivity structure of the language dataset. This is especially noticeable for DG, indicating that 3 common eigenbases are shared across the dataset. The impact on the number of initial correspondences during coupled joint diagonalization is shown in Fig. 2c. While 500 correspondences, 10.6% of points in the datasets, yield better results, even with 100 correspondences, which correspond to only 2.1% of sampling points, matching accuracy is comparable. Finally Fig. 2d compares all 4 alignment approaches. The coupled diagonalization approach (DG) is more accurate than the orthonormal two-step manifold alignment ($MA\ ortho$). Moreover, we observe the benefit of drawing initial correspondences during coupled

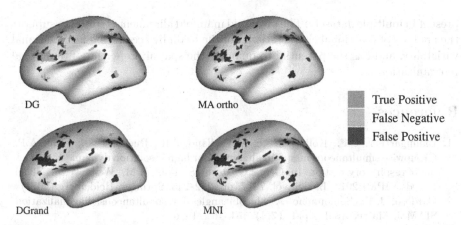

DG

MA ortho

DGrand

MNI

True Positive
False Negative
False Positive

Fig. 3. A single subject example of mapped activation with a z-score threshold of 2.5 on the left hemisphere. Our application of coupled diagonalization (DG) maps core regions related to language function successfully, with false positive and false negative mappings on the border areas (Color figure online).

joint diagonalization from dense regions in the atlas. When drawing random correspondences between closest points ($DGrand$), the joint diagonalization approach performs similar to the two-step manifold alignment method with spatial constraints. An example of matched activation maps is illustrated in Fig. 3. For one subject and a z-score threshold of 2.5 we compare the actual activation with the predicted activation. The core regions of the language related networks are mapped successfully, with false positive and false negative mappings located on the edges of these regions, which is analogous to the typical gaussian structure of GLM activation analysis in fMRI studies. Analogous to the quantitative results the coupled joint diagonalization (DG) most accurately predicts the language regions.

4   Conclusion

We propose coupled joint diagonalization to perform alignment of embedding representations of functional network structures. Sparse coupling reduces the computational complexity of the problem and facilitates manifold alignment for multiple datasets with a large amount of sampling points. In contrast to two-step approaches, joint alignment allows to draw upon multiple subject data simultaneously to learn a robust joint embedding. Estimating a subset of initial correspondences between functional datasets is challenging, and sub-sequent refinement and reestimation of correspondences after joint diagonalization exploits shared functional connectivity architecture, in order to establish correspondence despite spatial variability of functionally active regions. Manifold alignment allows for spectral embedding and clustering, or corresponding transfer learning on a group level, by taking advantage of common intrinsic structure present in multiple datasets. The proposed manifold alignment is suited to support the analysis of functional characteristics of the brain by accounting for functional variability, and has the potential to quantify the spatial properties of functional reorganization.

References

1. Baumgartner, C.F., Kolbitsch, C., McClelland, J.R., Rueckert, D., King, A.P.: Groupwise simultaneous manifold alignment for high-resolution dynamic MR imaging of respiratory motion. In: Gee, J.C., Joshi, S., Pohl, K.M., Wells, W.M., Zöllei, L. (eds.) IPMI 2013. LNCS, vol. 7917, pp. 232–243. Springer, Heidelberg (2013)
2. Cardoso, J.-F., Souloumiac, A.: Jacobi angles for simultaneous diagonalization. SIAM J. Matrix Anal. Appl. **17**(1), 161–164 (1996)
3. Coifman, R.R., Lafon, S.: Diffusion maps. Appl. Comput. Harmonic Anal. **21**(1), 5–30 (2006). Special Issue: Diffusion Maps and Wavelets
4. Conroy, B.R., Singer, B.D., Swaroop Guntupalli, J., Ramadge, P.J., Haxby, J.V.: Inter-subject alignment of human cortical anatomy using functional connectivity. NeuroImage **81**, 400–411 (2013)
5. Evans, A.C., Collins, D.L., Mills, S.R., Brown, E.D., Kelly, R.L., Peters, T.M.: 3D statistical neuroanatomical models from 305 mri volumes. In: 1993 IEEE Conference Record on Nuclear Science Symposium and Medical Imaging Conference, vol. 3, pp. 1813–1817, October 1993
6. Eynard, D., Kovnatsky, A., Bronstein, M.M., Glashoff, K., Bronstein, A.M.: Multimodal manifold analysis by simultaneous diagonalization of laplacians. IEEE Trans. Pattern Anal. Mach. Intell., PP(99), 1 (2015)
7. Fandino, J., Kollias, S.S., Wieser, H.G., Valavanis, A., Yonekawa, Y.: Intraoperative validation of functional magnetic resonance imaging and cortical reorganization patterns in patients with brain tumors involving the primary motor cortex. J. Neurosurg. **91**(2), 238–250 (1999)
8. Fischl, B.: Freesurfer. NeuroImage **62**(2), 774–781 (2012). 20 Years of fMRI
9. Friston, K.J., Holmes, A.P., Worsley, K.J., Poline, J.-P., Frith, C.D., Frackowiak, R.S.J.: Statistical parametric maps in functional imaging: A general linear approach. Hum. Brain Mapp. **2**(4), 189–210 (1994)
10. Ham, J., Lee, D., Saul, L.: Semisupervised alignment of manifolds. In: Proceedings of the Tenth International Workshop on Artificial Intelligence and Statistics (2005)
11. Jenkinson, M., Beckmann, C.F., Behrens, T.E.J., Woolrich, M.W., Smith, S.M.: Fsl. NeuroImage **62**(2), 782–790 (2012). 20 YEARS OF fMRI 20 YEARS OF fMRI
12. Jiang, D., Yuhui, D., Cheng, H., Jiang, T., Fan, Y.: Groupwise spatial normalization of fmri data based on multi-range functional connectivity patterns. NeuroImage **82**, 355–372 (2013)
13. Kovnatsky, A., Bronstein, M.M., Bronstein, A.M., Glashoff, K., Kimmel, R.: Coupled quasi-harmonic bases. Comput. Graph. Forum **32**(2(pt. 4)), 439–448 (2013)
14. Langs, G., Lashkari, D., Sweet, A., Tie, Y., Rigolo, L., Golby, A.J., Golland, P.: Learning an Atlas of a cognitive process in its functional geometry. In: Székely, G., Hahn, H.K. (eds.) IPMI 2011. LNCS, vol. 6801, pp. 135–146. Springer, Heidelberg (2011)
15. Langs, G., Sweet, A., Lashkari, D., Tie, Y., Rigolo, L., Golby, A.J., Golland, P.: Decoupling function and anatomy in atlases of functional connectivity patterns: Language mapping in tumor patients. NeuroImage **103**, 462–475 (2014)

16. Lombaert, H., Grady, L., Polimeni, J.R., Cheriet, F.: Focusr: Feature oriented correspondence using spectral regularization-a method for precise surface matching. IEEE Trans. Pattern Anal. Mach. Intell. **35**(9), 2143–2160 (2013)
17. Lombaert, H., Grady, L., Polimeni, J.R., Cheriet, F.: Fast brain matching with spectral correspondence. In: Székely, G., Hahn, H.K. (eds.) IPMI 2011. LNCS, vol. 6801, pp. 660–673. Springer, Heidelberg (2011)
18. Mateus, D., Horaud, R., Knossow, D., Cuzzolin, F., Boyer, E.: Articulated shape matching using laplacian eigenfunctions and unsupervised point registration. In: IEEE Conference on Computer Vision and Pattern Recognition, CVPR 2008, pp. 1–8, June 2008
19. Myronenko, A., Song, X.: Point set registration: Coherent point drift. IEEE Trans. Pattern Anal. Mach. Intell. **32**(12), 2262–2275 (2010)
20. Pei, Y., Huang, F., Shi, F., Zha, H.: Unsupervised image matching based on manifold alignment. IEEE Trans. Pattern Anal. Mach. Intell. **34**(8), 1658–1664 (2012)
21. Sabuncu, M.R., Singer, B.D., Conroy, B., Bryan, R.E., Ramadge, P.J., Haxby, J.V.: Function-based intersubject alignment of human cortical anatomy. Cereb. Cortex **20**(1), 130–140 (2010)
22. Smith, S.M., Beckmann, C.F., Ramnani, N., Woolrich, M.W., Bannister, P.R., Jenkinson, M., Matthews, P.M., McGonigle, D.J.: Variability in fmri: A reexamination of inter-session differences. Hum. Brain Mapp. **24**(3), 248–257 (2005)
23. Torki, M., Elgammal, A., Lee, C.S.: Learning a joint manifold representation from multiple data sets. In: 2010 20th International Conference on Pattern Recognition (ICPR), pp. 1068–1071, August 2010
24. Wang, C., Mahadevan, S.: Manifold alignment using procrustes analysis. In: Proceedings of the 25th International Conference on Machine Learning, ICML 2008, pp. 1120–1127 (2008)
25. Wang, C., Mahadevan, S.: A general framework for manifold alignment. In: AAAI Fall Symposium Series (2009)
26. Wang, C., Mahadevan, S.: Manifold alignment without correspondence. In: Proceedings of the 21st International Jont Conference on Artifical Intelligence, IJCAI 2009, pp. 1273–1278 (2009)
27. Wang, C., Mahadevan, S.: Multiscale manifold learning. In: Proceedings of the 27th AAAI Conference on Artificial Intelligence (2013)
28. Wen, Z., Yin, W.: A feasible method for optimization with orthogonality constraints. Math. Program. **142**(1–2), 397–434 (2013)

Brain Transfer: Spectral Analysis of Cortical Surfaces and Functional Maps

Herve Lombaert[1]([✉]), Michael Arcaro[2], and Nicholas Ayache[1]

[1] INRIA Sophia-Antipolis, Asclepios Team, Valbonne, France
herve.lombaert@inria.fr
[2] Princeton Neuroscience Institute, Princeton University, Princeton, USA

Abstract. The study of brain functions using fMRI often requires an accurate alignment of cortical data across a population. Particular challenges are surface inflation for cortical visualizations and measurements, and surface matching or alignment of functional data on surfaces for group-level analyses. Present methods typically treat each step separately and can be computationally expensive. For instance, smoothing and matching of cortices often require several hours. Conventional methods also rely on anatomical features to drive the alignment of functional data between cortices, whereas anatomy and function can vary across individuals. To address these issues, we propose *BrainTransfer*, a spectral framework that unifies cortical smoothing, point matching with confidence regions, and transfer of functional maps, all within minutes of computation. Spectral methods decompose shapes into intrinsic geometrical harmonics, but suffer from the inherent instability of eigenbasis. This limits their accuracy when matching eigenbasis, and prevents the *spectral transfer* of functions. Our contributions consist of, first, the optimization of a spectral transformation matrix, which combines both, point correspondence and change of eigenbasis, and second, *focused harmonics*, which localize the spectral decomposition of functional data. *BrainTransfer* enables the transfer of surface functions across interchangeable cortical spaces, accounts for localized confidence, and gives a new way to perform statistics directly on surfaces. Benefits of spectral transfers are illustrated with a variability study on shape and functional data. Matching accuracy on retinotopy is increased over conventional methods.

1 Introduction

Major brain activities occur on the cerebral cortex. The analysis of this thin, highly convoluted surface is therefore of particular interest to neuroscience, for instance, in studying vision and perception. The geometry of the cortex can be extracted from anatomical MRI, while neural activity can be measured via changes of blood flow in functional MRI. In order to establish shape and functional relationships across a population, fast and accurate algorithms are often sought for matching surfaces and functions on surfaces. Early approaches based on volumetric warping [1] ignore the complex geometry of the cortical folds, and consequently, produce misaligned cortical areas [2]. Recent surface-based

© Springer International Publishing Switzerland 2015
S. Ourselin et al. (Eds.): IPMI 2015, LNCS 9123, pp. 474–487, 2015.
DOI: 10.1007/978-3-319-19992-4_37

Shape Spectrum – Surface Functions can be written as composition of shape harmonics

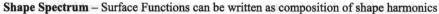
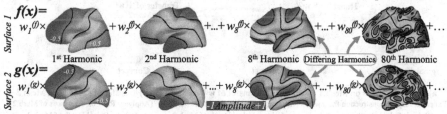

Fig. 1. Spectral Decomposition on Shapes – Any function $f(x)$ on surface 1 *(top row)*, or $g(x)$ on surface 2 *(bottom row)* can be written as a sum of weighted harmonics (coloring is harmonic amplitude). Spectral weights, $\mathbf{w}^{(f)}$ and $\mathbf{w}^{(g)}$, are not directly transferable between surfaces since harmonics may change sign (bases 8), and not correspond (differences in black isolines, incompatible bases 80) (Color figure online).

approaches, either slowly deform surfaces until matching [3,4], or inflate cortical surfaces to a spherical template [5–7]. Methods that flow surfaces into one another, such as LDDMM [8] and Currents [9,10], provide an elegant mathematical framework, with guarantees on diffeomorphism, but remain computationally expensive, and typically take several hours to match meshes with a few thousand vertices. On the other hand, spherical methods, such as FreeSurfer [5] and Spherical Demons [7], find correspondences on simplified spherical models of the cortex. These methods subsequently exploit extrinsic shape features, such as sulcal depth and mean curvature, to drive the alignment of the spherical models. Unfortunately, these approaches rely on an expensive inflation of cortical surfaces into spheres [11], which also requires a few hours to process high-resolution meshes. Moreover, current methods typically rely on anatomical features to drive the alignment of functional data across individuals, whereas their relation to function can vary across a population [12].

Spectral graph theory [13] recently offers a fast alternative for matching high-resolution cortical surfaces within minutes on a conventional laptop computer [14,15]. Spectral methods facilitate the correspondence problem by matching shapes in a spectral domain, rather than in the Euclidean space. Complex geometries, such as cortical surfaces, become reduced embeddings that are isometry-invariant, i.e., two shapes having the same intrinsic geometry, with identical geodesic distances between points, yield identical spectral embeddings, even if they have different extrinsic geometries. This is equivalent to comparing intrinsic vibration properties of shapes rather than their external configurations. However, a perturbation in shape isometry, such as expansion and compression of surfaces, changes the Laplacian eigenvectors in the spectral embeddings. This limited the use of spectral methods to coarse alignment [16] or global analysis [17,18]. Attempts were made to correct the perturbed embeddings with rigid [19] and nonrigid transformations [14,20], but all assume that Laplacian eigenvectors are *compatible* between shapes. These methods are in fact inherently flawed by the instability of the eigendecomposition. Eigenvectors can indeed change sign, orientation and shape, due to possible multiplicities of eigenvalues,

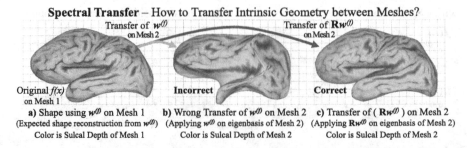

Spectral Transfer – How to Transfer Intrinsic Geometry between Meshes?

a) Shape using $w^{(f)}$ on Mesh 1
(Expected shape reconstruction from $w^{(f)}$)
Color is Sulcal Depth of Mesh 1

b) Wrong Transfer of $w^{(f)}$ on Mesh 2
(Applying $w^{(f)}$ on eigenbasis of Mesh 2)
Color is Sulcal Depth of Mesh 2

c) Transfer of ($Rw^{(f)}$) on Mesh 2
(Applying $Rw^{(f)}$ on eigenbasis of Mesh 2)
Color is Sulcal Depth of Mesh 2

Fig. 2. Spectral Transfer between Shapes – **(a)** Reconstruction of a function (here the point coordinates of mesh 1, $f(x) = (x, y, z)$), is correct when using the right eigenbasis of mesh 1. **(b)** Direct transfer of spectral weights, $w^{(f)}$, onto mesh 2 yields a wrong reconstruction. **(c)** Transfer must account for an optimal spectral transformation R. Color represents sulcal depth on respective meshes. Transfer of $w^{(f)}$ onto mesh 2 enables a direct comparison between depth maps **(a,c)** (Color figure online).

to ambiguities in shape symmetry, and to numerical instabilities. For instance, the Laplacian eigenvectors of a sphere have ambiguous orientations. This makes spectral embeddings hardly comparable for near spherical shapes. The underlying graph metric may also be adapted by an expensive conformal metric correction [21]. Laplacian eigenvectors provide nonetheless a set of basis functions on complex geometries [22–24], and enable, therefore, any surface function to be represented as a linear combination of harmonics. This is for instance exploited in Laplacian smoothing [25,26], where meshes are reconstructed with the coarser harmonics. The weights associated with each harmonic, capture intrinsic geometrical properties of the represented shape or function. These weights remain, however, incompatible between surfaces.

This paper proposes to ameliorate spectral approaches by enabling a *Spectral Transfer* of such weights across interchangeable harmonic bases. Surface functions, such as point coordinates or activation maps, become transferable from one surface onto another via a *spectral transformation* of the harmonic weights. We indeed assume that if any function can be expressed using a surface basis, there exist a transformation allowing the harmonic weights on one surface to be transferred on another surface [23,24]. In other words, a set of harmonic weights from one surface must be translated to the same language as on another surface. This requires the optimization of a spectral transformation matrix that combines both, a surface correspondence and a change of harmonic basis. Such spectral transfer provides a more robust formulation for spectral methods and handles naturally the sign changes as well as differences across Laplacian eigenvectors, including the *mixing* of eigenvectors in higher frequencies. In addition, this paper proposes *Focused Harmonics* in order to better capture geometrical properties within a region of interest. This is achieved by building a confidence map with a graph node weighting, which guides the spectral decomposition within regions of higher confidence. Localized functional maps, such as the visual area in the occipital lobe, can therefore be expressed with dedicated harmonics.

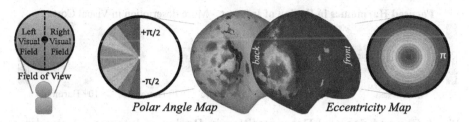

Fig. 3. Retinotopy – fMRI activation maps of visual inputs over the visual field: *(Left)* Polar angle map, varying with $[-\pi/2, +\pi/2]$ (lower/upper field), *(Right)* Eccentricity map, varying with $[0, \pi]$ (center/peripheral). Brain shows occipital lobe.

Our framework, *Brain Transfer*, enables the transfer of harmonic weights representing cortical shape and functional data across individuals. These harmonic weights capture intrinsic geometrical properties at multiscales, and can be linearly composed in order to reconstruct shapes and functions between subjects. We explore the parameter space of these harmonic weights via a principal component analysis over a dataset on retinotopy. Our results shows that our framework achieves similar accuracy in a fraction of the time as compared with conventional methods when matching cortical surfaces, and outperforms the state-of-the-art when matching functional data within the visual cortex.

2   Spectral Decomposition on Shapes

We begin by reviewing the fundamentals of spectral decomposition on shapes.

Surface Function Decomposition. Let us consider a compact manifold $\mathcal{M}$, and $f(x)$ a smooth function on $\mathcal{M}$. The Laplace-Beltrami operator on f is defined as the divergence of the function gradient, $\Delta f = -\text{div}\nabla f$, and admits an eigendecomposition $\Delta\phi = \lambda\phi$. This can be interpreted as finding the natural vibration amplitudes ϕ, at harmonic frequencies λ, of a membrane with shape $\mathcal{M}$. Since ϕ forms a basis on $\mathcal{M}$, any smooth function f can be represented as a linear combination $f = \sum_{i=0}^{\infty} w_i \phi_i$, where w_i's are harmonic weights. On a discrete representation, e.g., a triangulated mesh of $\mathcal{M}$, the general Graph Laplacian is often used. Let us build the graph $\mathcal{G} = \{\mathcal{V}, \mathcal{E}\}$ from the set of vertices, with positions $\mathbf{x} = (x, y, z)$, and the set of edges. We define the $|\mathcal{V}| \times |\mathcal{V}|$ weighted adjacency matrix W in terms of node affinities, e.g., $W_{ij} = \|\mathbf{x}_i - \mathbf{x}_j\|^{-2}$, and the diagonal degree matrix D as the sum $D_i = \sum_j W_{ij}$. The General Graph Laplacian is formulated as $\mathcal{L} = G^{-1}(D - W)$ [27], where G is a general node weighting matrix, typically diagonal with $G = D$. The decomposition, $\mathcal{L} = \mathbf{U}\Lambda\mathbf{U}^{-1}$, provides the eigenvalues $\Lambda = \text{diag}\left(\lambda_0, \lambda_1, ..., \lambda_{|\mathcal{V}|}\right)$ and its associated eigenfunctions $\mathbf{U} = (U_0, U_1, ..., U_{|\mathcal{V}|})$, that correspond respectively to the shape harmonic frequencies and bases on $\mathcal{M}$. Figure 1 shows how harmonics describe increasingly more complex geometrical properties as frequency augments. A surface function f is represented with:

Focused Harmonics in Region of Interest – More description in Visual Cortex

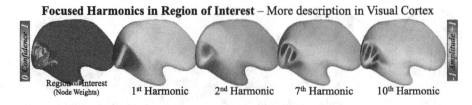

| Region of Interest (Node Weights) | 1st Harmonic | 2nd Harmonic | 7th Harmonic | 10th Harmonic |

Fig. 4. Focused Spectral Decomposition in Region of Interest – A confidence map indicates regions of confidence of a surface function. *(Left)* Higher confidence is given to the visual cortex, *(Right)* 1st to 10th harmonics. Stronger graph node weights produce focused harmonics, with more description in ROI.

$$f(x) = \sum_{i=0}^{|\mathcal{V}|} w_i U_i(x), \quad \text{or simply,} \quad \mathbf{f} = \mathbf{U}\mathbf{w}, \tag{1}$$

where $\mathbf{w} = (w_0, w_1, ..., w_{|\mathcal{V}|})^T = \mathbf{U}^{-1}\mathbf{f}$ is a column vector of harmonic weights. When $\mathbf{U}$ is truncated, we compute the first k coefficients with: $\mathbf{w} = (\mathbf{U}^T\mathbf{U})^{-1}\mathbf{U}^T\mathbf{f}$.

Focused Decomposition. We propose a new focused spectral decomposition in a region of interest by exploiting a graph node weighting as a confidence map. This is of interest to fMRI, where signal is often localized in specific neural areas, such as in the visual cortex for retinotopy (Fig. 3). Node weighting is typically $G = D$, which makes the Graph Laplacian a stochastic matrix. Each node has equal chances of occurring, i.e., row sum of $\mathcal{L}$ is 1. When a confidence map $g(x)$ is used in place, the total node probability is changed with $G = \text{diag}(g(x))$ in $G^{-1}(D-W)$. Nodes are given importance with $g(x)$, and stronger nodes become dominant in the Laplacian matrix. The spectral decomposition consequently becomes focused on these stronger graph nodes, yielding what we call *Focused Harmonics* (Fig. 4). In our experiment on functional data, the map is set as the signal difference in a common area between subjects, i.e., high signal difference between subjects indicates low confidence areas.

Spectral Smoothing. Functions on surfaces can be represented with general, or focused harmonics, $\mathbf{f} = \mathbf{U}\mathbf{w}$. One application is smoothing of meshes or surface functions. For instance, surface point coordinates $f(x) = (x, y, z)$ can be reconstructed using the first k low-frequency harmonics: $(x, y, z) \leftarrow \mathbf{U}\left((\mathbf{U}^T\mathbf{U})^{-1}\mathbf{U}^T(x, y, z)\right)$ where the basis is truncated with $\mathbf{U} = (U_0, ..., U_k)$, and has size $|\mathcal{V}| \times k$. Similarly, surface functions, such as retinotopy, can be smoothed on the surface by reconstructing the original maps with k harmonics. Figure 5 shows such reconstructions and illustrates how geometrical details appear with more harmonics.

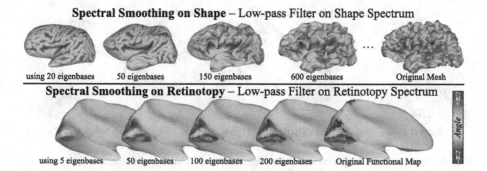

Fig. 5. Spectral Smoothing – *(Top)* Reconstruction of a surface using 20 to 600 eigenbases. Note how the brain convolves with more eigenbases. *(Bottom)* Reconstruction of retinotopy (polar angle map) using 5 to 200 eigenbases. Few focused harmonics are sufficient to reconstruct the polar map.

3 Spectral Transfer

Let us now consider the functions $\mathbf{f} = \mathbf{U}^{(f)}\mathbf{w}^{(f)}$ on a mesh $\mathcal{M}^{(f)}$, and $\mathbf{g} = \mathbf{U}^{(g)}\mathbf{w}^{(g)}$ on a mesh $\mathcal{M}^{(g)}$, and see how their intrinsic geometrical properties are transferred across meshes.

Brain Matching. Conventional spectral matching methods rely on the principle that harmonic bases are *compatible* between meshes. A dense point matching is established via fast nearest-neighbor searches between spectral representations, typically $\mathbf{U}\Lambda^{-\frac{1}{2}}$. However, this approach inherently suffers from the instability of eigenvectors, due to a sign or multiplicity ambiguity in a spectral decomposition. Eigenvectors may even be *mixed* in higher frequencies, which yield incompatible bases between meshes. Spectral methods typically compensate for these issues with a rigid or non-rigid transformation of spectral representations, but fail in addressing the fundamental incompatibility of harmonics between meshes. Recently, a double-layered spectral graph decomposition was proposed in [15], where the graph Laplacian is augmented by incorporating in the same Laplacian matrix, the two original meshes with a correspondence map between them. The decomposition of such joint graph Laplacian produces one unique set of harmonics, common to both surfaces. Correspondence links between such joint Harmonics may be interpreted as shortest random-walk distances between surfaces [15].

Brain Transfer. We propose a new approach for brain matching, where intrinsic geometrical properties are transferred across brains instead of being matched. This transfer addresses the inherent issues on eigenvector incompatibility in spectral methods. It was shown earlier that intrinsic geometrical properties of shapes or functions are captured in harmonic weights, and that shapes and functions can be reconstructed using such weights. However, harmonic weights are

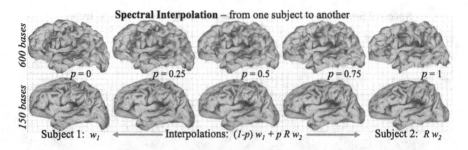

Fig. 6. Spectral Interpolation – Reconstructions of surfaces using interpolation of harmonic weights, from $p = 0$ (left, subject 1), $p = 0.5$ (middle, synthetic average) to $p = 1$ (right, subject 2): Using a common eigenbasis with $\mathbf{w} = (2 - p)\mathbf{w}^{(1)} + pR\mathbf{w}^{(2)}$. Smoothing occurs by removing harmonic coefficients (600 vs. 150 eigenbases).

not directly interchangeable between meshes. Figure 2-b shows an invalid direct transfer with $\mathbf{U}^{(g)}\mathbf{w}^{(f)}$, which does not produce the excepted shape of $\mathcal{M}^{(f)}$. Central to our method is the ability to transfer intrinsic geometrical information between brains, via an optimal spectral transformation of harmonic weights. We assume there exists a spectral transformation $R^{(f \to g)}$ between $\mathbf{U}^{(f)}$ and $\mathbf{U}^{(g)}$ [22–24]. This corresponds to a change of basis $R = (\mathbf{U}^{(g)})^{-1}\mathbf{U}^{(f \circ c)}$, where c is an unknown correspondence map that matches rows of $\mathbf{U}^{(f \circ c)}$ with equivalent rows of $\mathbf{U}^{(g)}$. Such transformation permits the spectral transfer of $\mathbf{w}^{(f)}$ between meshes, such that $\mathbf{U}^{(f)}\mathbf{w}^{(f)}$ becomes equivalent to $\mathbf{U}^{(g)}R\mathbf{w}^{(f)}$, which uses a different basis. In practice, only $k < 20$ coefficients $\mathbf{w} = (w_0, ..., w_k)^T$ are required in brain matching. The $k \times k$ spectral transformation matrix from $\mathcal{M}^f$ to $\mathcal{M}^g$ is computed with the truncated basis $\mathbf{U}^{(f)}$ and $\mathbf{U}^{(g)}$:

$$R^{(f \to g)} = \left((\mathbf{U}^{(g)})^T \mathbf{U}^{(g)} \right)^{-1} \left((\mathbf{U}^{(g)})^T \mathbf{U}^{(f \circ c)} \right), \tag{2}$$

such that $\mathbf{U}^{(f \circ c)}\mathbf{w}^{(f)}$ becomes equivalent to $\mathbf{U}^{(g)} R^{(f \to g)}\mathbf{w}^{(f)}$.

Optimization. The optimal spectral transformation requires solving for the point mapping c from $\mathcal{M}^{(f)}$ to $\mathcal{M}^{(g)}$. In effect, this correspondence minimizes several criteria, such as transferred functions across shapes: $E_u^{(f \to g)} = \|\mathbf{U}^{(f \circ c)}\mathbf{w}^{(f)} - \mathbf{U}^{(g)}R^{(f \to g)}\mathbf{w}^{(f)}\|^2$, or surface data, such as a sulcal depth map $\mathbf{s}$ on the surface, and/or its gradient: $E_{\text{data}}^{(f \to g)} = \|\mathbf{s}^{(f \circ c)} - \mathbf{s}^{(g)}\|^2 + \|\nabla\mathbf{s}^{(f \circ c)} - \nabla\mathbf{s}^{(g)}\|^2$. Symmetry is enforced in adding the inverse mapping, c^{-1} from $\mathcal{M}^{(g)}$ to $\mathcal{M}^{(f)}$, in the energy:

$$E^{(\text{sym})}(f, g, c) = E^{(f \to g)}(f \circ c, g) + E^{(g \to f)}(g, f \circ c^{-1}), \text{where} \tag{3}$$

$$E^{(f \to g)}(f \circ c, g) = \|\mathbf{U}^{(f \circ c)}\mathbf{w}^{(f)} - \mathbf{U}^{(g)}R^{(f \to g)}\mathbf{w}^{(f)}\|^2$$
$$+ \alpha_s \|\mathbf{s}^{(f \circ c)} - \mathbf{s}^{(g)}\|^2 + \alpha_{\nabla s}\|\nabla\mathbf{s}^{(f \circ c)} - \nabla\mathbf{s}^{(g)}\|^2, \tag{4}$$

where α_s ensures that corresponding points between meshes should have similar sulcal depth maps, while $\alpha_{\nabla s}$ ensures that corresponding sides of sulci should be matched. The harmonic weights are set to $\mathbf{w} = \Lambda^{-\frac{1}{2}}$, which favors eigenfunctions in low, rather than high frequency. Global geometrical characteristics are favored over fine details.

The energies in Eq. 3 can be formulated as the L_2 norm of the difference between high-dimensional vectors: $E^{(f \to g)} = \|X^{(f \circ c)} - X^{(f \to g)}\|^2$ and $E^{(g \to f)} = \|X^{(g \circ c^{-1})} - X^{(g \to f)}\|^2$, where: $X^{(f)} = (\mathbf{U}^{(f)} \Lambda^{(f)^{-\frac{1}{2}}}, \alpha_s \mathbf{s}^{(f)}, \alpha_{\nabla_s} \nabla \mathbf{s}^{(f)})$, $X^{(g)} = (\mathbf{U}^{(g)} \Lambda^{(g)^{-\frac{1}{2}}}, \alpha_s \mathbf{s}^{(g)}, \alpha_{\nabla_s} \nabla \mathbf{s}^{(g)})$, $X^{(f \to g)} = (\mathbf{U}^{(g)} R^{(f \to g)} \Lambda^{(f)^{-\frac{1}{2}}}, \alpha_s \mathbf{s}^{(g)}, \alpha_{\nabla_s} \nabla \mathbf{s}^{(g)})$, and $X^{(g \to f)} = (\mathbf{U}^{(f)} R^{(g \to f)} \Lambda^{(g)^{-\frac{1}{2}}}, \alpha_s \mathbf{s}^{(f)}, \alpha_{\nabla_s} \nabla \mathbf{s}^{(f)})$. Each vector is a combination of intrinsic geometrical information and a data term based on sulcal depth. The data term may also consist of functional data, such as polar and eccentricity maps. The mapping c is established with simple nearest-neighbor searches between vectors $X^{(f)}$ and $X^{(f \to g)}$, and c^{-1} is established similarly between $X^{(g)}$ and $X^{(g \to f)}$: $c = \arg\min_c \|X^{(f \circ c)} - X^{(f \to g)}\|^2$ and $c^{-1} = \arg\min_{c^{-1}} \|X^{(g \circ c^{-1})} - X^{(g \to f)}\|^2$.

The correspondences may be further refined by decomposing the joint graph Laplacian formed with c and c^{-1} between $\mathcal{M}^{(f)}$ and $\mathcal{M}^{(g)}$, as used in [15]. This may be interpreted as a random walker wandering between surfaces, with probabilities given by the links formed by c and c^{-1}.

The optimization iteratively alternates between (1) a correspondence map phase, which finds the mapping c and c^{-1} and (2) an update phase, which refines the spectral transformation matrices $R^{(f \to g)}$ and $R^{(g \to f)}$. The iterations are initialized by using a 3×3 identity matrix for R and a truncated $\mathbf{U}$ with 3 eigenfunctions. The number of eigenfunctions is increased at each iteration, up to 20 in our experiments.

– Initialize $R^{(f \to g)}$ and $R^{(g \to f)}$ with identity
– Iterate by increasing $k = 3$ to $k = K$
  (1) Build vectors $X^{(f)}, X^{(f \to g)}$, and $X^{(g)}, X^{(g \to f)}$ with k eigenfunctions
  (2) Find mapping c via nearest-neighbor search between $X^{(f)}$ and $X^{(f \to g)}$
  (3) Find mapping c^{-1} via nearest-neighbor search between $X^{(g)}$ and $X^{(g \to f)}$
  (4) Refine c and c^{-1} with a Joint Graph Laplacian between $\mathcal{M}^{(f)}$ and $\mathcal{M}^{(g)}$
  (5) Update $R^{(f \to g)}$ and $R^{(g \to f)}$ with new c and c^{-1} (Eq. 2)

Spectral Statistics. The harmonic weights $\mathbf{w}$ form a vector space in k dimensions that is spanned by an eigenbasis $\mathbf{U}$. In this context, one may wonder what this space looks like. Let us consider two set of transferred harmonic weights for two surface functions: $R^{(f \to \text{ref})} \mathbf{w}^{(f)}$ and $R^{(g \to \text{ref})} \mathbf{w}^{(g)}$. We define the linear interpolation between them as $\mathbf{w}^{(p)} = (1 - p) R^{(f \to \text{ref})} \mathbf{w}^{(f)} + p R^{(g \to \text{ref})} \mathbf{w}^{(g)}$, where $\mathbf{U}^{(\text{ref})}$ may be either $\mathbf{U}^{(f)}$, $\mathbf{U}^{(g)}$, or else. The average weight would be at midpoint $p = 0.5$. Figure 6 shows the reconstruction of shapes from such interpolated harmonic weights.

The average weights for N surface functions become $\mathbf{w}^{(\mu)} = \frac{1}{N} \sum_{i=1}^{N} R^{(i \to \text{ref})} \mathbf{w}^{(i)}$. The covariance matrix of N transferred harmonic weights is $\Sigma = WW^T$, where $W = (\mathbf{w}^{(1)}, \mathbf{w}^{(2)}, ..., \mathbf{w}^{(N)})^T - \mathbf{w}^{(\mu)^T}$, with the vector

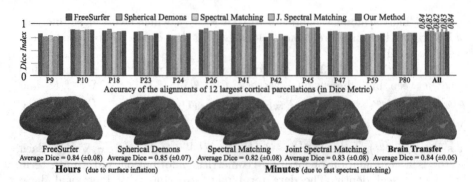

Fig. 7. Accuracy of Shape Alignment – *Top*: Average Dice Index across 240 alignments of cortical parcellations, using FreeSurfer (dark blue, Dice: 0.84), Spherical Demons (light blue, Dice: 0.85), Spectral Matching (light green, Dice: 0.82), Joint Spectral Matching (orange, Dice: 0.83), and our Brain Transfer (dark red, Dice: 0.84) – *Bottom*: One example showing the alignment of 12 major parcellations (light blue for one cortex, light red for aligned second cortex) – Our method yields similar accuracy as compared with the state-of-the-art, with significant speedup(Color figure online).

operator $\mathbf{w}$, linearizing $\mathbf{w}$ into a column vector. At last, the decomposition of $\Sigma = \mathbf{Q}\Lambda_\Sigma\mathbf{Q}^T$ provides the principal modes of variations [28,29] of the harmonic weights (Fig. 7).

4   Results

We evaluate the performance of Brain Transfer in two folds, first, in aligning cortical surfaces, and second, in aligning retinotopy.

4.1   Alignment Using Shape Features

Shape alignment is evaluated with a dataset of 16 cortical surfaces with 109 k to 174 k vertices, each with a manual labeling of cortical parcellations. We align all 240 possible pairs of cortices using FreeSurfer (FS), Spherical Demons (SD), Spectral Matching (SM), Joint Spectral Matching (JSM), and Brain Transfer (BT). The average Dice overlap $(2|A\cap B|/(|A|+|B|))$ for 12 major parcellations, among all pairs, is 0.84 (± 0.08) for FS (timing is 3 hours for one matching), 0.85 (± 0.07) for SD (2 hours), 0.82 (± 0.08) for SM (110 s), 0.83 (± 0.08) for JSM (140 s), and 0.84 (± 0.06) for Brain Transfer (220 s). Running times are measured on a 2.6 GHz Core i7 laptop with 16 GB of RAM. The matching accuracy is arguably similar among all methods with an average Dice score of 0.84. Spectral Methods have, however, a notable speed advantage over conventional methods, from hours to minutes of computation (Fig. 8).

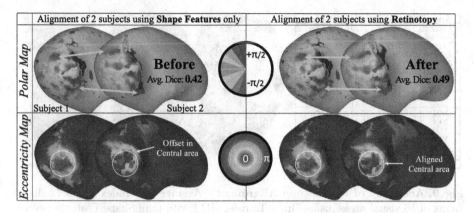

Fig. 8. Alignment of Retinotopy with Brain Transfer – *(Top)* Polar and *(Bottom)* Eccentricity map, before and after use of functional features. Surface maps become non-rigidly warped on surface. Transferred harmonic weights enable map comparisons. Matching accuracy increases by 17%, cpu time is 220sec. Brain shows occipital lobe.

4.2 Alignment Using Functional Features

The advantage of Brain Transfer is better assessed when using focused harmonics on functional data, such as retinotopy on the visual cortex. Our dataset is collected from 9 subjects, each with a polar angle map (θ between $\pm\pi/2$), an eccentricity map (ρ between 0 and π), as well as a manual labeling of 16 visual areas used for evaluation. Data were projected on cortical surfaces of 117k to 164k vertices. We set the graph node weighting with the difference of surface data in the overlapping regions between two shape-aligned cortices: $g(x) = \exp\left(-\beta((\theta^{(1)} - \theta^{(2)})^2 + (\rho^{(1)} - \rho^{(2)})^2)\right)$, where $\beta = 1/2$.

Since Brain Transfer showed an equivalent accuracy as compared with conventional methods in cortical alignment, we use it in order to compare matching with sulcal features only, and with functional data. This reflects the benefit of using functional data via focused harmonics within the same framework. Figure 9 shows the average Dice overlap for all 16 visual areas, using Brain Transfer with shape features only: 0.42, and functional features: 0.49. These alignments reveal the challenges of matching visual cortices, whereas large cortical parcellations, based on anatomy, were used in the previous experiment. The use of functional data, via focused harmonics, shows an increase in matching accuracy, up to 54%, notably in areas that are away from the calcarine fissure [12,30].

4.3 Variability Study of Cortical Shape and Functional Data

Brain Transfer captures intrinsic properties of shapes and functions in harmonic weights. We now provide a Principal Component Analysis (PCA) in order to explore the parameter space spanned by the harmonic weights.

Areas	BT w/Shape	BT w/Function	%Improv.
V1 ventral	0.65	0.70	+8%
V1 dorsal	0.65	0.71	+8%
V2 ventral	0.58	0.67	+18%
V2 dorsal	0.50	0.61	+22%
V3 ventral	0.43	0.57	+31%
V3 dorsal	0.33	0.45	+34%
V3A	0.55	0.62	+12%
V3B	0.38	0.41	+10%
V7	0.45	0.53	+18%
LO1	0.40	0.41	+3%
LO2	0.33	0.33	0%
hV4	0.40	0.54	+37%
VO1	0.23	0.35	+54%
VO2	0.32	0.39	+21%
PHC1	0.22	0.23	+6%
PHC2	0.30	0.27	-8%
Total	0.42	0.49	+17%

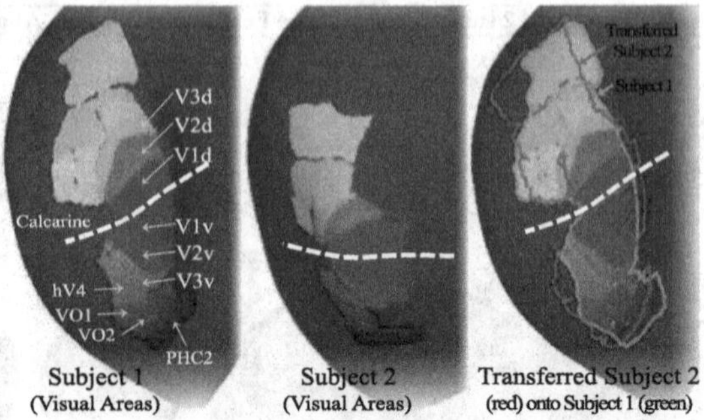

Fig. 9. Accuracy of Retinotopy Alignment – Average Dice Index across 72 alignments of 16 visual areas, using Brain Transfer (BT) with pure Shape Features (sulcal depth), with average Dice: 0.42, and Functional Features (polar and eccentricity maps, with focused harmonics), with Dice: 0.49. An example showing the initial and aligned visual areas using Brain Transfer with functional features (green countour for one subject, red for second subject). Brains show occipital lobe (Color figure online).

Shape Variability. We reuse the harmonic weights computed in the former experiment on cortical alignment. PCA is applied on all 16 transferred harmonic weights, each representing surface point coordinates. The target space is chosen arbitrarily as the harmonic basis of the first subject. Our aim is to explore the variability of weights in a common space, regardless of finding an optimal unbiased space. Figure 10-a shows the reconstruction of cortical surfaces using the average of transferred harmonic weights, and the first 3 principal modes of variations within 2 standard deviations. The first mode appears to capture a global rotation of the cortices, which interestingly, were not initially aligned in space. This indicates that Brain Transfer can correctly handle datasets that are not initially aligned. Further modes capture variabilities in the cortical folds, such as, shape differences in the occipital and temporal lobes.

Functional Variability. We now reuse the harmonic weights computed in the latter experiment on retinotopy alignment. PCA is applied on all 9 transferred harmonic weights, each representing polar and eccentricity maps, expressed in the focused harmonic basis of the first subject. Figure 10-b shows the reconstruction of polar maps using the average of transferred weights, and the first 3 principal modes of variations. The modes capture specific variabilities in the distinct stripped pattern of the polar angle map. The variability study is directly performed on the focused harmonic weights, which captures functional information that is independent from the cortical shape. This contrasts with conventional variability studies where shape and function may be mixed by coupling surface values onto point positions. Statistics are therefore performed directly on intrinsic geometrical properties, rather than on pure surface point values.

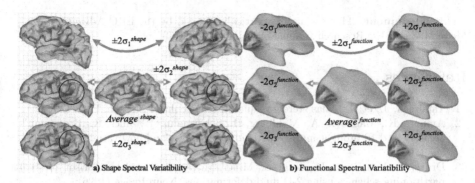

Fig. 10. Variability of Harmonic Weights – PCA on harmonic weights, *(Left)* using shape-based weights (function is point coordinates $f(x) = (x, y, z)$) and, *(Right)* using the functional-based weights (function is retinotopy $f(x) = (\theta, \rho)$), with focused harmonics). Showing the first 3 principal modes of variations $\pm 2\sigma$ from average.

5   Conclusion

Our method, *Brain Transfer*, contributes to the challenging problem of matching shapes and functional data on cortical surfaces. Spectral methods have demonstrated a tremendous speed advantage over conventional cortical matching methods, but remain inherently limited by the instability of the Laplacian eigenvectors. Incompatible surface harmonics typically require to compensate for the sign flip, ordering, and differences of eigenvectors. Our approach ameliorates spectral methods by enabling a natural transfer of intrinsic geometrical properties across surfaces, where harmonic weights are optimally expressed using different surface harmonics. In other words, intrinsic geometrical information travels across surfaces by translating it into the language of a different surface. Functional data is often localized on the cortical surface, such as retinotopy in the visual area. *Focused harmonics* are, therefore, proposed to better capture surface data in regions of interests. Our results show a 17 % improvement in matching visual areas when functional features are used instead of only shape features. *Brain Transfer* also offers a new way to perform statistics across surfaces, by directly analyzing intrinsic geometrical properties of shapes or of surface functions. This analysis on harmonic weights contrasts with conventional approaches where surface values are typically coupled with surface points. Possible extensions to images [31] may be also provide new applications. To conclude, our method, *Brain Transfer*, offers a better formulation for spectral methods by enabling the spectral transfer of intrinsic geometrical properties across surfaces. It also addresses the instability issue of Laplacian eigenvectors. Finally, our improved alignment of functional data may potentially translate into a lower number of required acquisitions in fMRI studies, and still preserve an equivalent statistical power.

Acknowledgment. This research is partically funded by the ERC Advanced Grant MedYMA, and the Research Council of Canada (NSERC).

References

1. Talairach, J., et al.: Atlas stereotaxique du telencephale. Masson, Paris (1967)
2. Amunts, K., Malikovic, A., Mohlberg, H., Schormann, T., Zilles, K.: Brodmann's areas 17 and 18 brought into stereotaxic space-where and how variable? NeuroImage (2000)
3. Drury, H., Van Essen, D., Joshi, S., Miller, M.: Analysis and comparison of areal partitioning schemes using 2-D fluid deformations. NeuroImage (1996)
4. Thompson, P., Toga, A.W.: A surface-based technique for warping three-dimensional images of the brain. TMI (1996)
5. Fischl, B., Sereno, M.I., Tootell, R.B., Dale, A.M.: High-resolution intersubject averaging and a coordinate system for cortical surface. HBM (1999)
6. Fischl, B., Rajendran, N., Busa, E., Augustinack, J., Hinds, O., Yeo, B.T., Mohlberg, H., Amunts, K.: Cortical folding patterns and predicting cytoarchitecture. Cereb Cortex, Zilles (2007)
7. Yeo, T., Sabuncu, M., Vercauteren, T., Ayache, N., Fischl, B., Golland, P.: Spherical demons: fast diffeomorphic landmark-free surface registration. TMI **29**, 650–668 (2010)
8. Beg, F., Miller, M., Trouvé, A., Younes, L.: Computing large deformation metric mappings via geodesic flows of diffeomorphisms. IJCV **61**, 139–157 (2005)
9. Vaillant, M., Glaunès, J.: Surface matching via currents. In: Christensen, G.E., Sonka, M. (eds.) IPMI 2005. LNCS, vol. 3565, pp. 381–392. Springer, Heidelberg (2005)
10. Durrleman, S., Pennec, X., Trouvé, A., Ayache, N.: Statistical models of sets of curves and surfaces based on currents. MedIA **13**, 793–808 (2009)
11. Segonne, F., Pacheco, J., Fischl, B.: Geometrically accurate Topology-Correction of cortical surfaces using nonseparating loops. TMI **26**, 518–529 (2007)
12. Haxby, J.V., et al.: A common, high-dimensional model of the representational space in human ventral temporal cortex. Neuron **72**, 404–416 (2011)
13. Chung, F.: Spectral Graph Theory. AMS (1997)
14. Lombaert, H., Grady, L., Polimeni, J., Cheriet, F.: Feature oriented correspondence using spectral regularization, a method for accurate surface matching. PAMI (2012)
15. Lombaert, H., Sporring, J., Siddiqi, K.: Diffeomorphic spectral matching of cortical surfaces. In: Gee, J.C., Joshi, S., Pohl, K.M., Wells, W.M., Zöllei, L. (eds.) IPMI 2013. LNCS, vol. 7917, pp. 376–389. Springer, Heidelberg (2013)
16. Reuter, M.: Hierarchical shape segmentation and registration via topological features of Laplace-Beltrami eigenfunctions. IJCV (2009)
17. Niethammer, M., Reuter, M., Wolter, F.-E., Bouix, S., Peinecke, N., Koo, M.-S., Shenton, M.E.: Global medical shape analysis using the Laplace-Beltrami spectrum. In: Ayache, N., Ourselin, S., Maeder, A. (eds.) MICCAI 2007, Part I. LNCS, vol. 4791, pp. 850–857. Springer, Heidelberg (2007)
18. Shi, Y., Lai, R., Kern, K., Sicotte, N.L., Dinov, I.D., Toga, A.W.: Harmonic surface mapping with Laplace-Beltrami eigenmaps. In: Metaxas, D., Axel, L., Fichtinger, G., Székely, G. (eds.) MICCAI 2008, Part II. LNCS, vol. 5242, pp. 147–154. Springer, Heidelberg (2008)

19. Mateus, D., Horaud, R., Knossow, D., Cuzzolin, F., Boyer, E.: Articulated shape matching using Laplacian eigenfunctions and unsupervised point registration. In: CVPR (2008)

20. Jain, V., Zhang, H.: Robust 3D Shape Correspondence in the Spectral Domain. In: CSMA (2006)

21. Shi, Y., Lai, R., Wang, D.J.J., Pelletier, D., Mohr, D., Sicotte, N., Toga, A.W.: Metric optimization for surface analysis in the Laplace-Beltrami space. TMI **33**(7), 1447–1463 (2014)

22. Vallet, B., Lévy, B.: Spectral geometry processing with manifold harmonics. CG **27**(2), 251–260 (2008)

23. Ovsjanikov, M., Ben-Chen, M., Solomon, J., Butscher, A., Guibas, L.: Functional maps. ACM Trans. Graph. **31**(4), 30 (2012)

24. Kovnatsky, A., et al.: Coupled quasi-harmonic bases. CG Forum **32**, 439–448 (2013)

25. Chung, R., Dalton, M., Davidson, R., Alexander, A.: Cortical thickness analysis in autism with heat kernel smoothing. NeuroImage, Evans (2005)

26. Anqi, Q., Bitouk, D., Miller, M.I.: Smooth functional and structural maps on the neocortex via orthonormal bases of the Laplace-Beltrami operator. TMI **25**(10), 1296–1306 (2006)

27. Grady, L., Polimeni, J.R.: Discrete Calculus: Analysis on Graphs. Springer, Heidelberg (2010)

28. Styner, M., Oguz, I., Xu, S., Brechbühler, S., et al.: Framework for the statistical shape analysis of brain structures using SPHARM-PDM. Insight (2006)

29. Gao, Y., Riklin, R.-R., Bouix, S.: Shape analysis, a field in need of careful validation. HBM (2014)

30. Wang, L., Mruczek, R.E.B., Arcaro, M.J., Kastner, S.: Probabilistic maps of visual topography in human cortex. Cerebral Cortex (2014)

31. Lombaert, H., Grady, L., Pennec, X., Ayache, N., Cheriet, F.: Spectral Demons – image registration via global spectral correspondence. In: Fitzgibbon, A., Lazebnik, S., Perona, P., Sato, Y., Schmid, C. (eds.) ECCV 2012, Part II. LNCS, vol. 7573, pp. 30–44. Springer, Heidelberg (2012)

Finding a Path for Segmentation Through Sequential Learning

Hongzhi Wang$^{(\boxtimes)}$, Yu Cao, and Tanveer F. Syed-Mahmood

IBM Almaden Research Center, San Jose, USA
hongzhiw@us.ibm.com

Abstract. Sequential learning techniques, such as auto-context, that applies the output of an intermediate classifier as contextual features for its subsequent classifier has shown impressive performance for semantic segmentation. We show that these methods can be interpreted as an approximation technique derived from a Bayesian formulation. To improve the effectiveness of applying this approximation technique, we propose a new sequential learning approach for semantic segmentation that solves a segmentation problem by breaking it into a series of simplified segmentation problems. Sequentially solving each of the simplified problems along the path leads to a more effective way for solving the original segmentation problem. To achieve this goal, we also propose a learning-based method to generate simplified segmentation problems by explicitly controlling the complexities of the modeling classifiers. We report promising results on the 2013 SATA canine leg muscle segmentation dataset.

1 Introduction

Medical image segmentation is the problem of locating anatomical structures from medical images. The gold standard segmentation is typically defined based on manual segmentation protocols. For automatic segmentation, classification-based machine learning techniques have been widely applied for medical image segmentation, e.g. [10]. Given pre-labeled training images and pre-selected feature descriptors, one can directly train classifiers, e.g. AdaBoost or random forest, to discriminate different tissue classes based on extracted training samples.

The recent work on auto-context learning [9] and stacked hierarchical learning [7] applies a sequential learning strategy, where the output of an intermediate classifier is applied as contextual features for its subsequent classifier. The advantage of this strategy is that it propagates and integrates local image features such that long-range structural context can be more effectively captured for semantic segmentation. Our first contribution is to show that these sequential learning methods can be interpreted as an approximation technique derived from a Bayesian formulation. To ensure that the approximation is accurate, our study gives a strong motivation for an intuitive strategy that solving a difficult segmentation problem by breaking it into a series of simplified segmentation problems, i.e. problems that can be solved with less ambiguity than the original segmentation problem, and then solving them sequentially. If we interpret

© Springer International Publishing Switzerland 2015
S. Ourselin et al. (Eds.): IPMI 2015, LNCS 9123, pp. 488–500, 2015.
DOI: 10.1007/978-3-319-19992-4_38

each of the simplified segmentation problem as a *step* towards solving the original segmentation problem, then the series of simplified problems define a *path*. Sequentially learning classifiers to solve each of the simplified problem along the path leads to a more effective way for solving the original segmentation problem.

To apply this approach, our second contribution is a learning-based method for automatically deriving simplified segmentation problems. In a related work, [7] builds simplified segmentation problems through a coarse-to-fine hierarchical decomposition of regions for images using low level segmentation. However, this method does not address the complexities in learning models for solving these problems. Hence, there is no guarantee that the generated hierarchical segmentation problems can be more easily solved than the original problem. This limitation is addressed in our work by explicitly controlling the complexities of classifiers learned for modeling the simplified segmentation problem.

We applied our method on the canine leg muscle segmentation dataset from the SATA segmentation challenge [1]. Our technique produced significant improvement over the auto-context technique and significantly improved the state of the art performance on the challenge category using standard registration.

2 Method

2.1 A Probabilistic View for Image Segmentation

Image segmentation can be formulated as a conditional probability estimation problem $p(S|I)$, where I is an observed image and S is a segmentation for I. Given a target segmentation protocol and training images, for which the gold standard segmentation has been produced following the protocol, automatic segmentation can be achieved by estimating the conditional probability $p(S|I)$ through classification techniques. A common technique directly estimate the posterior probability of assigning label l to a location x in I based on image features, i.e. $p(l|I,x)$. Under a conditional independent assumption, the problem can be addressed by $p(l|I,x) = p(l|I(\mathcal{N}(x)))$ and $p(S|I) = \prod_x p(S(x)|I(\mathcal{N}(x)))$, where $\mathcal{N}(x)$ is a neighborhood surrounding x and $I(\mathcal{N}(x))$ is the image features extracted from the neighborhood. Given the estimated probabilities, the maximum a posterior (MAP) segmentation can be derived as $S(x) = \text{argmax}_l p(l|I(\mathcal{N}(x)))$.

2.2 Complexity of Image Segmentation

Under the probabilistic view, each segmentation problem can be modeled by classifiers learned from training data. Hence, the complexity of a segmentation problem can be measured by the complexity of the corresponding classification problem. We define the complexity of a segmentation problem as follows:

$$H(D) = H(D;C) + H(D|C) \tag{1}$$

where $D = (F, Y)$ are data extracted from training images with $F = \{f_1, ..., f_n\}$ specifying feature representations of n samples and $Y = \{y_1, ..., y_n\}$ specifying the segmentation labels. C is a classifier. $H(D; C)$ is the information about the segmentation problem captured by C. $H(D|C)$ is the residual information not captured by classifier C, which can be defined as:

$$H(D|C) = \frac{1}{n} \sum_{i=1}^{n} - \log p(y_i | f_i, C) \qquad (2)$$

where $p(y_i | f_i, C)$ is the label posterior computed by C using feature f_i.

In the literature, classifier complexity $H(C)$ is often described as the complexity of decision boundaries. Many factors may affect classifier complexity. The most influential factors include features and the learning model, e.g. linear or nonlinear. When a classifier accurately models a classification problem, $H(D) = H(D; C) = H(C)$. Due to overfitting, it is common that $H(D; C) < H(C)$ and $H(D|C) > 0$. When overfitting is minimized, e.g. through techniques such as cross-validation, the complexities of two segmentation problems can be approximately compared by the residual terms, given that the modeling classifiers for the two problems have similar complexities, e.g. both trained by the same learning model using same image features. If $p(l|f, C)$ is narrowly peaked around its maximum for each data, there is little residual information. In contrast, if the distribution is flat or multiple modes are widely scattered, the segmentation problem is more complex as more residual information is not captured by C.

2.3   Bayesian Approximation

Under the Bayesian rule, the posterior label probability distribution of a target segmentation can be computed as:

$$p(l|I, x) = \int_{S'} p(S'|I, C^1) p(l|I, S', x) \qquad (3)$$

S' index through all possible segmentations for I. $p(S'|I, C^1)$ is the probability of a segmentation given the observed image I as modeled by classifier C^1.

Although it is intractable to enumerate all feasible segmentations in (3), accurate approximation exists when certain conditions are satisfied. When $p(S'|I, C^1)$ is narrowly peaked around its maximum, a commonly applied approximation is based on the MAP segmentation, e.g. [11]:

$$p(l|I, x) \sim p(S^1|I, C^1) p(l|I, S^1, x) \propto p(l|I, S^1, x) \qquad (4)$$

where S^1 is the MAP segmentation derived from C^1. The condition also means that the underlying segmentation problem modeled by C^1 can be reliably solved by C^1. If the condition is not satisfied, the MAP solution has larger variations, which results in greater mismatch between features extracted from S^1 during training and testing. This limitation makes learning more easily prone to overfitting, reducing the benefit of adding S^1 as additional features. Since $p(S^1|I, C^1)$ is a constant scale factor, to solve the original segmentation problem, we only need to estimate $p(l|I, S^1, x)$. As shown in [6,9,13], when S^1 is correlated with the target segmentation, it provides contextual information, such as shape or spatial relations between neighboring anatomical regions, that is not captured by local image features.

The above approximation has an intuitive interpretation. A segmentation problem may be solved through transferring it into a simpler segmentation problem that can be solved with less ambiguity. Solving the simplified segmentation problem first may help solving the original segmentation problem.

A Case Study: Corrective learning [13] applies classification techniques to correct systematic errors produced by a *host* segmentation method with respect to some gold standard segmentation. In our context, the segmentation produced by the host method is a MAP solution. In corrective learning, the classifiers trained for making corrections aim to estimate label posteriors given the observation of the image and the segmentation produced by the host method, i.e. $p(l|I, S^1, x)$. Hence, corrective learning is in fact an application of the MAP approximation (4). The fact that corrective learning achieves better performance than learning purely based on image features on some previous studies indicates the effectiveness of the MAP-based approximation. Our study suggests that corrective learning may work even more effectively when the host method aims to solve a simplified segmentation problem derived from the target segmentation problem.

2.4 Iterative Extension: Finding a Path to Segmentation

The approximation in (4) can be recursively expanded. Hence, we have:

$$p(l|I, x) \sim p(S^1|I, C^1)p(l|I, S^1, x) \tag{5}$$
$$\sim p(S^1|I, C^1)p(S^2|I, S^1, C^2)p(l|I, S^1, S^2, x) \tag{6}$$
$$\sim p(S^1|I, C^1)\ldots p^n(S^n|I, S^1, \ldots, S^{n-1}, C^n)p(l|I, S^1, \ldots, S^n, x) \tag{7}$$
$$\propto p(l|I, S^1, \ldots, S^n, x) \tag{8}$$

C^i are trained classifiers and S^i is the MAP solution derived from C^i.

For this approximation to be accurate, a necessary condition is that for each $1 < i \leq n$, S^i can be computed with little ambiguity with C^i given the image I and the MAP segmentations obtained from previous iterations, i.e. $\{S^1, \ldots, S^{i-1}\}$. To allow solving the original segmentation problem benefit from this approximation, an additional requirement is that each S^i must provide additional information about the desired segmentation that is not already captured by I and $\{S^1, \ldots, S^{i-1}\}$. In other words, S^i should be more similar to the desired segmentation as i increases. Under these requirements, $(C^1, \ldots, C^n)$ defines a path for solving the original segmentation problem. Each C^i aims to accurately solve a simplified segmentation problem. As i increases, the complexity of the problem solved by C^i also increases.

2.5 The Path Learning Algorithm

To implement the sequential learning model in (7), we propose an iterative extension to the corrective learning method [13]. The motivation for building the implementation based on corrective learning is that corrective learning is designed to be more effective in utilizing segmentation results produced in previous iterations for building stronger segmentation classifiers.

Algorithm 1. Path sequential learning algorithm

1: INPUT: A set of training images with segmentations $\{(I_i, L_i), i = 1, ..., m\}$.

2: **for** $t = 1$ to T **do**

3:    Take the images and the segmentation results produced for each image in previous iterations, i.e. MAP segmentations $(S^1, ..., S^{t-1})$ + label posterior maps, as feature images, derive a simplified segmentation problem for the original segmentation problem, i.e. $\{(I_i, L_i^t), i = 1, ..., m\}$ (see details in Sect. 2.6).

4:    Train classifier C^t using all training images to solve the simplified problem.

5:    For the next iteration, produce MAP segmentation S_i^t and label posterior maps for solving the simplified problem for each image using cross-validation.

6: **end for**

7: Train classifier C^{T+1} using all training images to solve the original segmentation problem with images and the segmentation results produced above as features.

8: Returns the sequence of trained classifiers $(C^1, C^2, ..., C^T, C^{T+1})$.

For step 4 at each iteration t, we train AdaBoost classifiers [4] to solve the simplified segmentation. First, we define a working region of interest (ROI) for each label by performing dilation to the set of all voxels assigned the label in the MAP segmentation produced in the previous iteration, i.e. S^{t-1}. Using instances uniformly sampled within a label's working ROI, one AdaBoost classifier is trained to identify voxels assigned to this label against voxels assigned to other labels in the target segmentation within the ROI. To apply these classifiers on a testing image, each classifier is applied to evaluate the confidence of assigning the corresponding label to each voxel within the label's working ROI. If a voxel belongs to the ROI of multiple labels, the label whose classifier gives the maximal posterior at the voxel is chosen for the voxel. At the first iteration, if no segmentation has been produced yet, the AdaBoost classifiers are trained without using working ROIs.

Three types of features are applied to describe each voxel, including spatial, appearance, and contextual features. The spatial features are computed as the relative coordinate of each voxel to the ROI's center of mass. The appearance features are derived from the voxel's neighborhood patch from the training image(s). The contextual features are extracted from the voxel's neighborhood patch from all MAP segmentations and spatial label probability maps produced in previous iterations. To enhance spatial correlation, the joint spatial-appearance and joint spatial-contextual features are also included by multiplying each spatial feature with each appearance and contextual feature, respectively. If no segmentation has been produced yet, only the appearance features will be applied.

Stacking Learning: Another issue we need to address is that sequential learning is more prone to the overfitting problem. Due to overfitting, the intermediate segmentation results produced for a testing image may be different from those produced for training images. Since these segmentation results are applied as features in subsequent iterations, this training/testing mismatch will compromise the performance of the classifiers learned in subsequent iterations. To alleviate this problem, we apply the stacking technique [3,7,15] (at step 5 in the above algorithm). For training, the MAP segmentation produced for each training image is produced from cross-validation.

Relation to Auto-context Learning: The key difference from the auto-context technique is that our technique reduces the approximation error by predicting a simplified segmentation problem at each iteration, while auto-context always tries to predict the original segmentation problem. The other difference is that auto-context does not apply the Stacking technique. Both improvements in our algorithm allow our method to retain performance gains through more iterations.

2.6   Generating Simplified Segmentation Problems

A crucial requirement for the above algorithm to be applicable is the ability to define simplified segmentation problems for any given segmentation problem. For this task, we propose a learning-based approach.

[7] proposed to break a segmentation problem into stacked hierarchical segmentation problems. Given an image, a coarse-to-fine hierarchical decomposition of regions for the image is first created using low level segmentation methods. For each decomposition of regions in the hierarchy, a new probabilistic segmentation problem is created by generating label distributions for each region according to the original segmentation. With the hierarchical representation, the stacked hierarchical segmentation problem is solved by sequentially solving the coarse-to-fine segmentation problems. The results produced at each level is passed as contextual features to assist solving the next finer level segmentation problem. This approach has one key limitation. Since the problems at various hierarchical levels are defined based on low level segmentation, without considering the difficulty in learning models for predicting them, there is no guarantee that any coarser level probabilistic segmentation problem can be solved with less ambiguity than solving finer level segmentation problems or the original segmentation problem. Hence, the accuracy of applying (7) still may be compromised.

We propose to generate simplified segmentation problems directly from learning by controlling the complexity of their modeling classifiers. In this work, we apply the AdaBoost classifier. AdaBoost is an ensemble learning technique that iteratively builds a strong classifier from linearly combining complimentary weak classifiers [4]. Typically, as training iteration increases, training error decreases and the learned classifier can model more complex decision boundaries to better fit the training data. To generate simplified segmentation problems, given feature images and target segmentations, we train AdaBoost classifiers (as described in Sect. 2.5) to predict the target segmentation using all training images. When training errors are greater than zero, simplified segmentations can be generated by applying the trained classifiers to segment the training images. This approach works by setting the residual information to zero in (1)(2). By varying the iterations of AdaBoost training, the complexity of the simplified segmentation problem can be controlled as well.

By reducing the complexity of the modeling classifiers, we ensure that the simplified segmentation problem can be more easily predicted than the original segmentation problem, making the MAP segmentation based approximations (4)(7) better conditioned. Furthermore, through AdaBoost training, the learned classifiers may encode non-linear contextual relations between the applied features into the simplified segmentation protocol, making the simplified segmentation problem useful for predicting the target segmentation.

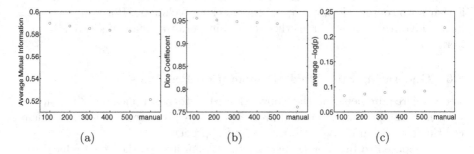

(a)   (b)   (c)

Fig. 1. (a) average mutual information between feature images and various segmentation protocols, including manual segmentation and simplified segmentation obtained with 100, 200, 300, 400, and 500 AdaBoost training iterations, respectively; b) Prediction accuracy (measured in Dice coefficient) for various segmentation protocols; (c) The prediction uncertainty for various segmentation protocols. (see text for detail)

Empirical Justification: To verify its effectiveness, we conducted an experimental study using the canine leg muscle data (see more details about the data description in Sect. 3.1). 22 training subjects were applied. For each subject, two MR images are available. The manual segmentation for seven muscle types are provided for each training subject. For each subject, an automatic segmentation produced by multi-atlas joint label fusion [5, 8, 12] is produced by using the remaining training subjects as atlases. In this study, we applied the corrective learning technique to train AdaBoost classifiers for predicting manual segmentation using all training subjects, with both the MR images and the multi-atlas segmentation applied as feature images. To generate segmentations with various complexities, we produced simplified segmentation for each training subject using the AdaBoost classifiers trained with 100, 200, 300, 400, and 500 iterations, separately. Hence, five simplified segmentation problems were produced.

Figure 1.(a) shows the average mutual information measured between each of the feature images, i.e. two MR images and the multi-atlas segmentation, and each of the segmentation protocols, i.e. the manual segmentation and the five simplified segmentations, respectively. The feature images contain higher mutual information for simplified segmentations than for manual segmentation, indicating less uncertainty in predicting the simplified segmentation protocols using

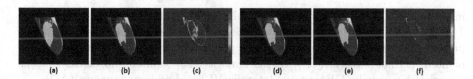

Fig. 2. (a) Manual segmentation for one subject. (d) The simplified segmentation produced by AdaBoost training with 500 iterations. (b)(e) MAP segmentation produced for manual and the simplified segmentation, respectively, in the leave-one-out experiment. (c)(f) MAP probability map produced for manual and the simplified segmentation, respectively. (see text for details and better viewed with colors) (Colour figure online).

the feature images. As expected, since simplified segmentations produced using more AdaBoost training iterations are more similar to manual segmentation, the feature images also contain less mutual information for them.

To verify that predicting simplified segmentation problems indeed can be achieved with less uncertainty than predicting manual segmentation, we conducted a leave-one-out cross-validation experiment. For each training subject, we applied the remaining training subjects to train another set of AdaBoost classifiers using the feature images to predict the manual segmentation and each of the five simplified segmentations, respectively. Figure 1.(b) summarizes the segmentation performance. The simplified segmentation problems can be estimated with higher accuracy, $\sim$0.95 average Dice coefficient, than manual segmentation, $\sim$0.75 Dice coefficient. To quantify the uncertainty in predicting different segmentation problems, we apply the following function $U(C, I) = \frac{\sum_x -log(p(l(x)|I,x,C))}{N}$, where $l(x)$ is the MAP label derived by classifier C and N is the number of processed voxels in I. This function measures the averaged uncertainty over the image. When $p(l(x)|I, x, C)) = 1$ for every x, there is no uncertainty and the uncertainty measure is zero, otherwise the uncertainty measure is greater than zero. Figure 1.(c) shows the average uncertainty produced for each segmentation problem in the leave-one-out experiment. Figure 2 shows one example of the MAP probability map, i.e. $p(l(x)|I, x, C)$, produced for predicting manual segmentation and the simplified segmentation obtained using 500-iteration AdaBoost learning, respectively. Clearly, there is less uncertainty in predicting the simplified segmentation problem than predicting manual segmentation.

3   Experiments

3.1   Data

The dataset used in this study is the canine leg muscle data from the SATA segmentation challenge [1]. So far, this dataset has been mostly applied for evaluating multi-atlas label fusion techniques. The dataset contains 45 canine leg MR scans (22 for training and 23 for testing). For each dog, images were acquired with two MR modalities: a T2-weighted image sequence was acquired using a variable-flip-angle turbo spin echo (TSE) sequence and a T2-weighted fat-suppressed images (T2FS) sequence was then acquired using the same variable-flip-angle TSE sequence with the same scanning parameters except that a fat saturation preparation was applied. Seven proximal pelvic limb muscles were manually segmented: cranial sartorius(CS), rectus femoris(RF), semitendinosus(SE), biceps femoris(BF), gracilis(GR), vastus lateralis(VL) and adductor magnus(AD).

To make the comparison between different label fusion methods invariant to the performance of image registration, the challenge provides standard registration results produced by using the ANTs registration software [2] between each training subject and each of the remaining (training and testing) subjects. We report performance based on these standard registrations.

3.2   Experimental Setup

For the canine leg muscle segmentation challenge using standard registration, so far the best published results were produced by using the joint label fusion (**JLF**) method [12] combined with non-iterative corrective learning [1]. To facilitate our comparison with the current state of the art method, we took the same joint label fusion method as the host method in our study. We applied joint label fusion with the parameters reported in [14], i.e. patch radius $r_p = 2$, searching radius $r_s = 4$ and model parameter $\beta = 0.5$, to produce the initial segmentation for each image. For each training image, its joint label fusion result was produced by using the remaining training images as the atlases. For the tested learning algorithms, we applied a one-voxel dilation to define working ROIs and a cubic neighborhood of size $5 \times 5 \times 5$ to compute appearance and contextual features. For our method, we applied AdaBoost with 500 training iterations for deriving simplified segmentation problems at each iteration.

We compare with **Auto-context** learning. In our experiment, Auto-context is implemented through extending corrective learning as well. The only differences from our Path algorithm is that 1) no simplified segmentation problems are defined in each iteration; 2) the Stacking technique is not applied. To evaluate the effectiveness of each component, we also tested a **Stacked** method, where the Auto-context algorithm is implemented with the Stacking technique, but still without defining simplified segmentation problems at each iteration.

We conducted two experiments. The first experiment is a four-fold cross-validation on the 22 training subjects. In this test, the 22 training subjects were randomly divided into four non-overlapping groups. For cross-validation, each group was applied for testing once and the remaining groups were applied for training. In the second experiment, all training subjects were applied to train each method and the performance was evaluated on the 23 testing subjects. The evaluation results on the testing subjects were computed by the online evaluation system provided by the challenge organizer.

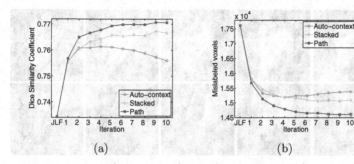

(a)   (b)

Fig. 3. The performance of the joint label fusion and the performance of Auto-context, Stacked, Path at each iteration on the 4-fold cross-validation experiment. The performance is reported in Dice coefficient (a) and average number of mislabeled voxels (b).

Table 1. Segmentation performance produced in the 4-fold cross-validation experiment for each anatomical region by joint label fusion, Auto-context, Stacked, and Path after 10 iterations, respectively. Results are measured using the Dice similarity coefficient.

Anatomical region	JLF	Auto-context	Stacked	Path
CS	0.564±0.168	0.589±0.208	**0.606±0.198**	0.595±0.208
RF	0.664±0.162	0.717±0.149	0.730±0.168	**0.736±0.169**
SE	0.855±0.062	0.870±0.074	0.871±0.065	**0.875±0.068**
BF	0.805±0.095	0.798±0.108	0.814±0.102	**0.822±0.103**
GR	0.832±0.052	0.863±0.036	0.865±0.034	**0.870±0.035**
VL	0.774±0.135	0.800±0.138	0.810±0.128	**0.821±0.121**
AD	0.646±0.142	0.654±0.158	0.667±0.149	**0.675±0.153**

3.3   Results

Figure 1 shows the overall segmentation performance produced in the four-fold cross-validation experiment by Auto-context, Stacked and Path, respectively. The performance of joint label fusion is given as a baseline. Note that the first iteration produced the most improvement for all three methods. The subsequent iterations produced further improvement but with diminishing improvement gains as iteration increases. We observed a performance drop for Auto-context after 4 iterations, which indicates overfitting. In contrast, Stacked and Path showed more consistent improvement as iteration increases. One interesting finding is that the results produced by Auto-context and Stacked at the first iteration are slightly worse than those produced by Path. At the first iteration, each method has the same feature images and the only difference is that Path tries to predict a simplified segmentation problem, while Auto-context and Stacked try to predict the original manual segmentation. Hence, this result shows that employing a simplified segmentation problem actually improves the performance for predicting the original manual segmentation as well. A possible explanation is that the simplified

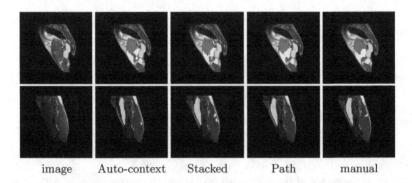

image   Auto-context   Stacked   Path   manual

Fig. 4. Segmentation produced by Auto-context, Stacked and Path after 10 iterations on the 4-fold cross-validation experiment.

Table 2. Segmentation performance on the testing data produced by JLF, JLF+corrective learning, and Auto-context/Stacked/Path after 10 iterations, respectively. Results are reported in mean(median) Dice coefficient over all anatomical labels.

Method	JLF	JLF+CL	Auto-context	Stacked	Path
Dice	0.731(0.768)	0.762(0.797)	0.782(0.815)	0.793(0.818)	0.800(0.829)

segmentation problem may be less noisy than manual segmentation, which allows the learning algorithm to reach more optimal solution. Table 1 gives more details on the segmentation accuracy for each anatomical label produced by each method after 10 iterations. The improvement over Auto-context produced by Stacked and Path both are statistically significant, with $p < 0.01$ and $p < 0.0001$ on the paired Students t-test, respectively. The improvement over Stacked produced by Path is statistically significant with $p < 0.02$ on the paired Students t-test. Figure 4 shows some segmentation results.

Table 2 shows the segmentation performance produced for the 23 testing subjects by Auto-context, Stacked, and Path after 10 iterations, respectively. The results produced by combining joint label fusion and corrective learning is so far the best published results on the canine leg muscle data using standard registration, which is provided as a baseline. Overall, Auto-context produced prominent improvement over the baseline, with 2 % improvement in Dice coefficient. The proposed method produced 1.8 % improvement over Auto-context.

4   Conclusions and Discussion

We showed that sequential learning based semantic segmentation methods can be interpreted as an approximation technique derived from a Bayesian formulation. To improve the effectiveness of applying this approximation technique, we proposed a Path algorithm that solves a segmentation problem by sequentially solving a series of simplified segmentation problems. To achieve this goal, we also proposed a learning-based method to generate simplified segmentation problems by explicitly controlling the complexities of the modeling classifiers.

The complexity of the simplified segmentation problem at each iteration is a free parameter, which is controlled by AdaBoost training iteration in our method. Low complexity reduces the risk of inaccurate approximation caused by using the MAP solution to replace the Bayesian integration. However, it also makes the contextual features provided from solving the simplified problem less useful for solving the original problem. Hence, an optimal complexity is expected to balance the two considerations, which will be studied in future work.

References

1. Asman, A., Akhondi-Asl, A., Wang, H., Tustison, N., Avants, B., Warfield, S.K., Landman, B.: MICCAI 2013 segmentation algorithms, theory and applications (SATA) challenge results summary. In: MICCAI 2013 Challenge Workshop on Segmentation: Algorithms, Theory and Applications. Springer (2013)
2. Avants, B., Epstein, C., Grossman, M., Gee, J.: Symmetric diffeomorphic image registration with cross-correlation: evaluating automated labeling of elderly and neurodegenerative brain. Med. Image Anal. **12**(1), 26–41 (2008)
3. Cohen, W.W., Carvalho, V.R.: Stacked sequential learning. In: Proceedings of the 19th International Joint Conference on Artificial Intelligence, Edinburgh, Scotland, pp. 671–676 (2005)
4. Freund, Y., Schapire, R.E.: A desicion-theoretic generalization of on-line learning and an application to boosting. In: Vitányi, P.M.B. (ed.) EuroCOLT 1995. LNCS, vol. 904, pp. 23–37. Springer, Heidelberg (1995)
5. Heckemann, R., Hajnal, J., Aljabar, P., Rueckert, D., Hammers, A.: Automatic anatomical brain MRI segmentation combining label propagation and decision fusion. NeuroImage **33**, 115–126 (2006)
6. Montillo, A., Shotton, J., Winn, J., Iglesias, J.E., Metaxas, D., Criminisi, A.: Entangled decision forests and their application for semantic segmentation of CT images. In: Székely, G., Hahn, H.K. (eds.) IPMI 2011. LNCS, vol. 6801, pp. 184–196. Springer, Heidelberg (2011)
7. Munoz, D., Bagnell, J.A., Hebert, M.: Stacked hierarchical labeling. In: Daniilidis, K., Maragos, P., Paragios, N. (eds.) ECCV 2010, Part VI. LNCS, vol. 6316, pp. 57–70. Springer, Heidelberg (2010)
8. Rohlfing, T., Brandt, R., Menzel, R., Russakoff, D.B., Maurer Jr., C.R.: Quo vadis, atlas-based segmentation? In: Suri, J.S., Wilson, D.L., Laxminarayan, S. (eds.) Volume III: Registration Models. Topics in Biomedical Engineering International Book Series, pp. 435–486. Springer, US (2005)
9. Tu, Z., Bai, X.: Auto-context and its application to high-level vision tasks and 3D brain image segmentation. IEEE Trans. on PAMI **32**(10), 1744–1757 (2010)
10. Tu, Z., Zheng, S., Yuille, A., Reiss, A., Dutton, R., Lee, A., Galaburda, A., Dinov, I., Thompson, P., Toga, A.: Automated extraction of the cortical sulci based on a supervised learning approach. IEEE TMI **26**(4), 541–552 (2007)
11. Van Leemput, K., Benner, T., Bakkour, A., Wiggins, G., Wald, L., Augustinack, J., Dickerson, B., Golland, P., Fischl, B.: Automated segmentation of hippocampal subfields from ultra-high resolution in vivo mri. Hippocampus **19**, 549–557 (2009)
12. Wang, H., Suh, J.W., Das, S., Pluta, J., Craige, C., Yushkevich, P.: Multi-atlas segmentation with joint label fusion. IEEE Trans. on PAMI **35**(3), 611–623 (2013)

13. Wang, H., Das, S.R., Suh, J.W., Altinay, M., Pluta, J., Craige, C., Avants, B.B., Yushkevich, P.A.: A learning-based wrapper method to correct systematic errors in automatic image segmentation: Consistently improved performance in hippocampus, cortex and brain. Neuroimage **55**(3), 968–985 (2011)

14. Wang, H., Yushkevich, P.A.: Multi-atlas segmentation with joint label fusion and corrective learning - an open source implementation. Front. neuroinformatics **7**, 27 (2013)

15. Wolpert, D.H.: Stacked generalization. Neural netw. **5**(2), 241–259 (1992)

Pancreatic Tumor Growth Prediction with Multiplicative Growth and Image-Derived Motion

Ken C.L. Wong[1], Ronald M. Summers[1], Electron Kebebew[2], and Jianhua Yao[1(✉)]

[1] Radiology and Imaging Sciences, Clinical Center, NIH, Bethesda, MD, USA
ken.wong@nih.gov, jyao@cc.nih.gov
[2] Endocrine Oncology Branch, National Cancer Institute, NIH, Bethesda, MD, USA

Abstract. Pancreatic neuroendocrine tumors are abnormal growths of hormone-producing cells in the pancreas. Different from the brain in the skull, the pancreas in the abdomen can be largely deformed by the body posture and the surrounding organs. In consequence, both tumor growth and pancreatic motion attribute to the tumor shape difference observable from images. As images at different time points are used to personalize the tumor growth model, the prediction accuracy may be reduced if such motion is ignored. Therefore, we incorporate the image-derived pancreatic motion to tumor growth personalization. For realistic mechanical interactions, the multiplicative growth decomposition is used with a hyperelastic constitutive law to model tumor mass effect, which allows growth modeling without compromising the mechanical accuracy. With also the FDG-PET and contrast-enhanced CT images, the functional, structural, and motion data are combined for a more patient-specific model. Experiments on synthetic and clinical data show the importance of image-derived motion on estimating physiologically plausible mechanical properties and the promising performance of our framework. From six patient data sets, the recall, precision, Dice coefficient, relative volume difference, and average surface distance were $89.8 \pm 3.5\,\%$, $85.6 \pm 7.5\,\%$, $87.4 \pm 3.6\,\%$, $9.7 \pm 7.2\,\%$, and $0.6 \pm 0.2\,\mathrm{mm}$, respectively.

1 Introduction

Pancreatic neuroendocrine tumors are abnormal growths of hormone-producing cells in the pancreas [4]. They are slow growing and usually not treated until reaching a certain size threshold. Similar to most tumors, pancreatic tumor growth is associated with cell invasion and mass effect [6]. In cell invasion, tumor cells migrate as a group and penetrate to the surrounding tissues. Mass effect is the result of expansive growth which increases the tumor volume, and the outward pushing may displace the tumor cells and surrounding tissues. Mass effect also contributes to and enhances cell invasion.

The rights of this work are transferred to the extent transferable according to title 17 U.S.C. 105.

© Springer International Publishing Switzerland 2015
S. Ourselin et al. (Eds.): IPMI 2015, LNCS 9123, pp. 501–513, 2015.
DOI: 10.1007/978-3-319-19992-4_39

In image-based macroscopic tumor growth modeling, tumor cell invasion is mostly modeled through reaction-diffusion equations [3,7,9,12,18]. The differences among these models are usually the choices between isotropic and anisotropic diffusion, Gompertz and logistic cell proliferation, or with and without considering treatment effects. Because of the highly deformable nature of the pancreas, we concentrate on mass effect and tumor mechanical properties in this paper. Most works have modeled mass effect by explicitly enforcing tumor size change or by exerting tumor-density-induced forces to a mechanical model [3,7,13,18]. In [3,13], the mass effects of the brain glioma and its surrounding edema were modeled differently based on their physiological characteristics. In [3], the volume change of the bulk tumor core was modeled as an exponential function, and a penalty method was used to enforce the volume change via homogeneous pressure. For the edema, internal stresses proportional to the local tumor cell densities were introduced, thus the tumor and its surrounding structures are displaced by tumor-density-induced forces proportional to the negative gradients of the local tumor densities. In [13], the expansive force of the bulk tumor was approximated by constant outward pressure acting on the tumor boundary, and the growth of the edema was modeled as an isotropic expansive strain. In [7], using the edema model of [3], the tumor-density-induced forces were applied to the entire brain glioma. The forces were converted to velocities through a linear mechanical model, which were used in the advection term of a reaction-advection-diffusion equation to displace the tumor cell densities. In [18], the tumor-density-induced forces were adopted to model the mass effect of pancreatic tumor growth using finite element methods (FEM).

Despite the promising results, these models were mostly developed for brain tumors and may be inappropriate for pancreatic tumor growths. Different from the brain in the skull, the pancreas in the abdomen can be largely deformed by the body posture and its surrounding organs [5]. Therefore, the tumor shape difference observable from images is not only driven by the tumor growth, but also the motion of the pancreas. As images at different time points are used to infer the tumor growth properties during model personalization, the prediction accuracy may be reduced if such motion is not properly considered. For the approaches using tumor-density-induced forces [7,18], the tumor volume change could not be explicitly modeled. These approaches, together with those converting the volume change into pressure [3,13], modeled the tumor growth as stress-strain relation in continuum mechanics. First of all, this contradicts the nearly incompressible nature of most solid tumors, and thus the incompressibility of the mechanical model has to be compromised. Secondly, for the mechanical models with nonlinear constitutive laws, the tumor stiffness increases with its elastic volume change regardless of the underlying physiology, and this reduces the model accuracy.

In view of these limitations, here we adopt the multiplicative growth decomposition for mass effect, which was initially introduced to study residual stresses in soft tissues [11,15]. In this approach, the continuous deformation field of a body after growth can be decomposed into its growth and elastic parts (Fig. 1). The intermediate growth configuration can be stress-free but incompatible,

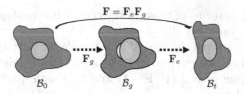

Fig. 1. Multiplicative growth decomposition. The original configuration $\mathcal{B}_0$ comprises the tumor (cyan) and its surrounding tissues (blue) before growth. The growth deformation gradient $\mathbf{F}_g$, which grows the tumor only, leads to an intermediate incompatible configuration $\mathcal{B}_g$. With the elastic deformation gradient $\mathbf{F}_e$ applied, the final configuration $\mathcal{B}_t$ is compatible (Color figure online).

which may have holes, overlaps, or other discontinuities. To maintain the continuity of the structure in reality, elastic deformation which generates residual stresses is applied to the growth deformation. With this decomposition, tumor growth can be modeled separately from the elastic part using explicit growth functions. This preserves the accuracy of the elastic response, and anisotropic mass effect can be easily incorporated. Moreover, with the relation between the growth and elastic parts, the deformation exerted by the surrounding structures on the tumor can be naturally included through displacement boundary conditions.

In this paper, the tumor growth model accounting for both cell invasion and mass effect is personalized using medical images. The tumor cell invasion is modeled as a reaction-diffusion equation. The mass effect is modeled through multiplicative growth decomposition [11], with the growth part modeled as orthotropic stretches with logistic functions, and the elastic part modeled using a hyperelastic constitutive law [8]. The tumor growth prediction is achieved through model parameter estimation using derivative-free optimization. Following [18], 2-[^{18}F]-fluoro-2-deoxy-D-glucose positron emission tomographic (FDG-PET) images are used to compute the proliferation rates, and contrast-enhanced computed tomographic (CT) images are used to provide the local tumor cell densities. We also incorporate the displacements derived from post-contrast CT images to account for the pancreatic motion. Experiments were performed on synthetic and clinical data to compare the differences between using different models of mass effect and between with and without imaged-derived motion.

2 Multiplicative Growth with Hyperelastic Mechanical Model

Let $\mathbf{X}$ be the coordinates in the original configuration ($\mathcal{B}_0$) and $\mathbf{x}$ be the corresponding coordinates in the final (deformed) configuration ($\mathcal{B}_t$) (Fig. 1). To model mass growth, the deformation gradient $\mathbf{F} = \partial\mathbf{x}/\partial\mathbf{X}$, which maps the original configuration to the final configuration as $d\mathbf{x} = \mathbf{F}d\mathbf{X}$, can be decomposed into its elastic part ($\mathbf{F}_e$) and growth part ($\mathbf{F}_g$) as $\mathbf{F} = \mathbf{F}_e\mathbf{F}_g$ [11]. Inhomogeneous growth can result in gaps or overlaps in the intermediate configuration ($\mathcal{B}_g$), and the system equation cannot be solved therein. Therefore, we need to reformulate the quantities in $\mathcal{B}_g$ in terms of those in the compatible configuration $\mathcal{B}_0$ for the total-Lagrangian formulation [2].

In multiplicative growth decomposition, the elastic part is governed by the strain energy function which provides the stress-strain relation. The Green-Lagrange strain tensor $\boldsymbol{\epsilon} = \frac{1}{2}\left(\mathbf{F}^\mathrm{T}\mathbf{F} - \mathbf{I}\right)$ and its elastic part ($\boldsymbol{\epsilon}_e$) and growth part ($\boldsymbol{\epsilon}_g$) are related as:

$$\boldsymbol{\epsilon}_e = \mathbf{F}_g^{-\mathrm{T}}\left(\boldsymbol{\epsilon} - \boldsymbol{\epsilon}_g\right)\mathbf{F}_g^{-1} \tag{1}$$

With tissue growth, the changes of mass and density need to be considered for accurate stress-strain relation. Let $^t m$ be the grown mass in $\mathcal{B}_t$, and $^0 V$ and $^g V$ be the volumes in $\mathcal{B}_0$ and $\mathcal{B}_g$, respectively[1]. The densities of the grown mass with respect to different configurations are given as $^t_0\rho = \mathrm{d}^t m/\mathrm{d}^0 V$ and $^t_g\rho = \mathrm{d}^t m/\mathrm{d}^g V$, with relation $^t_0\rho = {}^t_g\rho J_g$ ($J_g = \det \mathbf{F}_g = \mathrm{d}^g V/\mathrm{d}^0 V$ indicates the volume ratio). Therefore, the second Piola-Kirchhoff (PKII) stress tensor in $\mathcal{B}_g$ is given as:

$$\mathbf{S}_e = \frac{\partial({}^t_g\rho\psi)}{\partial\boldsymbol{\epsilon}_e} = \frac{1}{J_g}\frac{\partial({}^t_0\rho\psi)}{\partial\boldsymbol{\epsilon}_e} \tag{2}$$

where ψ is the strain energy per unit grown mass, and thus $^t_g\rho\psi$ and $^t_0\rho\psi$ are the strain energy per unit intermediate and original volume, respectively. Thus the PKII stress tensor in $\mathcal{B}_0$ is given as:

$$\mathbf{S} = \frac{\partial({}^t_0\rho\psi)}{\partial\boldsymbol{\epsilon}_e} : \frac{\partial\boldsymbol{\epsilon}_e}{\partial\boldsymbol{\epsilon}} = \mathbf{F}_g^{-1}\frac{\partial({}^t_0\rho\psi)}{\partial\boldsymbol{\epsilon}_e}\mathbf{F}_g^{-\mathrm{T}} = J_g\mathbf{F}_g^{-1}\mathbf{S}_e\mathbf{F}_g^{-\mathrm{T}} \tag{3}$$

and the corresponding fourth-order elasticity tensor is given as:

$$\mathbb{C} = \frac{\partial\mathbf{S}}{\partial\boldsymbol{\epsilon}} = \frac{\partial J_g\mathbf{F}_g^{-1}\mathbf{S}_e\mathbf{F}_g^{-\mathrm{T}}}{\partial\boldsymbol{\epsilon}} = J_g\left(\mathbf{F}_g^{-1}\bar{\otimes}\mathbf{F}_g^{-1}\right) : \mathbb{C}_e : \left(\mathbf{F}_g^{-\mathrm{T}}\bar{\otimes}\mathbf{F}_g^{-\mathrm{T}}\right) \tag{4}$$

with the non-standard dyadic product $[\mathbf{A}\bar{\otimes}\mathbf{B}]_{ijkl} = [\mathbf{A}]_{ik}[\mathbf{B}]_{jl}$ and $\mathbb{C}_e = \partial\mathbf{S}_e/\partial\boldsymbol{\epsilon}_e$. Note that when there is no growth (i.e. $\mathbf{F}_g = \mathbf{I}$), $\mathbf{S} = \mathbf{S}_e$ and $\mathbb{C} = \mathbb{C}_e$.

To model the highly deformable pancreas, the modified Saint-Venant-Kirchhoff (hyperelastic) constitutive law is used [8]:

$$^t_g\rho\psi(\boldsymbol{\epsilon}_e) = \frac{1}{2}\lambda(J_e - 1)^2 + \mu\mathrm{Tr}(\bar{\boldsymbol{\epsilon}}_e^2) \tag{5}$$

where $\bar{\boldsymbol{\epsilon}}_e$ is the isovolumetric part of $\boldsymbol{\epsilon}_e$ and $J_e = \det\mathbf{F}_e$. The first and second term of (5) account for the volumetric and isochoric elastic response, respectively, and thus λ is the bulk modulus and μ is the shear modulus.

Therefore, given $\mathbf{F}_g$ from a growth model, and $\mathbf{F}$ the existing deformation, $\boldsymbol{\epsilon}_e$ can be computed by (1). $\mathbf{S}_e$ and $\mathbb{C}_e$ can then be computed using (5) and converted to $\mathbf{S}$ and $\mathbb{C}$ by (3) and (4) for the total-Lagrangian formulation. The system is solved by FEM with Newton-Raphson iterations for the final geometry [2].

---

[1] The left superscript and subscript represent the measuring time and reference configuration.

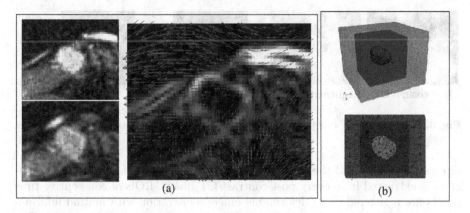

Fig. 2. (a) Image-derived pancreatic motion. Left: the ROIs of the post-contrast CT images at the earlier (top) and later (bottom) time points. Right: the 3D deformation field from the earlier to the later time point obtained by deformable image registration, overlapping with the gradient magnitude image at the earlier time point. Only the displacements of the salient features are used. (b) The 3D linear FEM mesh and its middle slice. The green zone is the segmented tumor, which can freely grow into the blue zone. The red zone is for enforcing image-derived displacements (Color figure online).

2.1 Orthotropic Growth

The growth deformation $\mathbf{F}_g$ can be modeled using explicit functions. Although tissue structure is unavailable in our data, orthotropic mass growth is adopted [11]:

$$\mathbf{F}_g = \vartheta_1 \mathbf{v}_1 \otimes \mathbf{v}_1 + \vartheta_2 \mathbf{v}_2 \otimes \mathbf{v}_2 + \vartheta_3 \mathbf{v}_3 \otimes \mathbf{v}_3 \qquad (6)$$

with ϑ_1, ϑ_2, and ϑ_3 the stretch ratios along the orthonormal vectors $\mathbf{v}_1$, $\mathbf{v}_2$, and $\mathbf{v}_3$, respectively. All $\vartheta_i > 0$. As tumor growth slows down after a certain size as nutrients are limited, we model the stretch ratios as logistic functions:

$$\vartheta_i(t) = \frac{\bar{\vartheta}_i}{1 + \left(-1 + \frac{\bar{\vartheta}_i}{\vartheta_i(t_0)}\right) e^{-\varrho_i(t-t_0)}}, \quad i = 1, 2, 3 \qquad (7)$$

with ϱ_i the proliferation rate, $\vartheta_i(t_0)$ the initial stretch ratio, and $\bar{\vartheta}_i$ the maximum stretch ratio. As $\vartheta_i(t_0)$ is relative and cannot be measured from a single image, we assume $\vartheta_i(t_0 = 0) = 1$ at the first measurement time point. The maximum stretch ratio is computed as the maximum allowable tumor size to the initial tumor size. In [10], the largest pancreatic neuroendocrine tumor size without metastasis is 5 cm.

2.2 Image-Derived Pancreatic Motion

The tumor shape difference observable from images is caused by both the tumor growth and the deformation exerted by the surrounding structures. To incorporate such deformation for more realistic model personalization, the region of

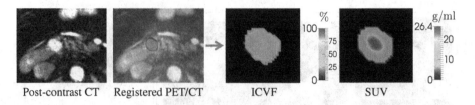

Post-contrast CT   Registered PET/CT   ICVF   SUV

Fig. 3. ICVF and SUV computed from contrast-enhanced CT and FDG-PET images.

interest (ROI) around the tumor which covers the salient features of the pancreas is extracted from every post-contrast CT image. ROIs of consecutive time points are registered using deformable image registration with mutual information to provide the displacements of the salient features [14] (Fig. 2(a)). The displacements are enforced as boundary conditions to deform the grown tumor through the hyperelastic constitutive law, and this allows more accurate comparison with the measurements during model personalization. To avoid interfering the tumor growth, a 3D FEM mesh is constructed from the ROI with three zones: the tumor, its surroundings for growth, and the outer zone (Fig. 2(b)). The image-derived displacements are only applied at the outer zone.

3   Tumor Cell Invasion by Reaction-Diffusion Equation

With the mass effect modeled by multiplicative growth decomposition and image-derived motion, the tumor cell invasion is modeled by a reaction-diffusion equation [18]:

$$\frac{\partial c}{\partial t} = \mathrm{div}(\mathbf{D}\nabla c) + \rho c\,(1-c) \tag{8}$$

where the first and second term account for the tumor invasion and logistic cell proliferation, respectively. $c \in [0,1]$ is the intracellular volume fraction (ICVF) which is equivalent to the number of tumor cells (N) divided by the carrying capacity (K) as the number of cells is proportional to the space they occupy. ICVF can be computed from contrast-enhanced CT images to provide the initial conditions of (8) and the measurements for model personalization (Fig. 3). $\mathbf{D}$ is the anisotropic diffusion tensor, which is a diagonal matrix with components D_x, D_y, and D_z regardless of the tissue structure, characterizing the invasive property. ρ is the proliferation rate, which can be computed from FDG-PET images for better subject-specificity.

3.1   Computing Intracellular Volume Fractions from CT Images

An intravenously-administered iodine-based contrast agent is used to produce contrast-enhanced CT images. The contrast agent causes greater absorption and scattering of x-ray in the target tissue, thereby producing contrast enhancement [1]. As the enhancement is proportional to the extracellular space, ICVF (c) of the tumor is given as [18]:

$$c = 1 - \frac{HU_{\text{post\_tumor}} - HU_{\text{pre\_tumor}}}{E[HU_{\text{post\_blood}} - HU_{\text{pre\_blood}}]}(1 - Hct) \qquad (9)$$

where $HU_{\text{post\_tumor}}$, $HU_{\text{pre\_tumor}}$, $HU_{\text{post\_blood}}$, and $HU_{\text{pre\_blood}}$ are the Hounsfield units of the post- and pre-contrast CT images at the segmented tumor and blood pool (aorta), respectively. Hct is the hematocrit which can be obtained from blood samples, thus the ICVF of the tumor is computed using the ICVF of blood (Hct) as a reference.

3.2   Computing Proliferation Rates from FDG-PET Images

The energy flow rate (B) provided to tissue can be consumed to maintain existing cells or create new cells [17], which can be represented as:

$$B = B_c Kc + E_c K \frac{\partial c}{\partial t} \qquad (10)$$

with B_c the metabolic rate of a cell and E_c the metabolic energy to create a cell. Assuming logistic growth, we substitute $\frac{\partial c}{\partial t} = \rho c (1 - c)$ and (10) becomes:

$$\rho = \frac{\alpha SUV - \beta c}{c(1 - c)}; \quad \text{with } \alpha SUV = \frac{B}{E_c K} \text{ and } \beta = \frac{B_c}{E_c} \qquad (11)$$

where SUV is the standardized uptake value computed from FDG-PET images, which indicates metabolic activity. $\alpha > 0$ is an unknown scalar to be estimated, and $\beta \approx 0.02$ day^{-1} [17]. $B = \alpha E_c K SUV$ indicates that the energy flow rate (B) is proportional to SUV. Therefore, the proliferation rate (ρ) can be approximated from FDG-PET and CT images (Fig. 3). With (8), (9) and (11), physiologically meaningful quantities can be computed from images and combined to produce a more patient-specific model.

4   Gradient-Free Model Personalization

The model personalization is achieved by parameter estimation. The simulation with model parameters $\boldsymbol{\theta}$ is rasterized into an ICVF image by using the CT image at the same time point as a reference, and then the following objective function is computed:

$$f(\boldsymbol{\theta}) = \sqrt{E\left[(\bar{c} - c(\boldsymbol{\theta}))^2\right]} + (1 - recall + 1 - precision); \qquad (12)$$

$$recall = TPV/V_m; \quad precision = TPV/V_s$$

where TPV is the true positive volume, the overlapping volume between the simulated tumor volume (V_s) and the measured (segmented) tumor volume (V_m). $\bar{c}$

and $c(\boldsymbol{\theta})$ are the respective measured and simulated ICVF within TPV. Therefore, the objective function accounts for both the ICVF root-mean-squared error and volume difference.

As the gradient of the objective function is difficult to derive analytically, we adopt the gradient-free direct search method SUBPLEX (SUBspace-searching simPLEX) for parameter estimation [16], which is a generalization of the Nelder-Mead simplex method (NMS). A simplex in n-dimensional space is a convex hull of $n+1$ points, such as a tetrahedron in 3D. In NMS, a simplex moves through the objective function space, changing size and shape, and shrinking near the minimum. SUBPLEX improves NMS by decomposing the searching space into subspaces for better computational efficiency, so that the model personalization can be performed with intact model nonlinearity.

Not all parameters are estimated in our current framework. In (11), with known c and SUV from images, ρ is a plane function of α and β, and any α and β on the same contour contribute to the same proliferation rate. Therefore, we fix $\beta = 0.02$ day^{-1} from [17]. For the mechanical parameters in (5), λ in all regions are set to 5 kPa for tissue incompressibility. As a result, the parameters to be estimated are $\boldsymbol{\theta} = \{D_x, D_y, D_z, \alpha, \varrho_x, \varrho_y, \varrho_z, \mu_{\text{normal}}, \mu_{\text{tumor}}\}$, with μ_{tumor} and μ_{normal} the shear moduli of the tumor and its surrounding tissues, respectively.

5   Experiments

Three frameworks were tested on synthetic and clinical data to study the differences between with and without image-derived motion, and between using multiplicative growth decomposition and tumor-density-induced forces:

- **MG-IM:** the proposed framework with multiplicative growth decomposition (MG) and image-derived motion (IM).
- **MG:** using multiplicative growth decomposition without image-derived motion.
- **F-IM:** using tumor-density-induced forces (F), $\mathbf{f}_b = -\gamma \nabla c$, for the mass effect, with γ a scalar to be estimated [18]. Image-derived motion was used.

5.1   Experimental Setups

Measurements at three time points were used in each experiment, which comprised both FDG-PET and contrast-enhanced CT images. From each post-contrast CT image, the tumor was segmented by a level set algorithm with region competition [19]. A ROI of the post-contrast CT image around the tumor was selected manually, which covered the salient features of the pancreas (Fig. 2(a)). ROIs of consecutive time points were registered to provide image-derived displacements (Fig. 2(a)), which were enforced to the outer region of the FEM mesh (Fig. 2(b), Sect. 2.2). ICVF and SUV were also computed from the contrast-enhanced CT and FDG-PET images for the reaction-diffusion equation (Sects. 3.1 and 3.2).

Table 1. Synthetic data. Estimated parameters and prediction performances. Simulations with $\varrho_x = 1.0, 2.0, 3.0, 4.0 \times 10^{-4}$ day^{-1} were used to study the performances at different growth rates.

	D_x,D_y,D_z(mm²/day,10⁻³)			α(mm³/g/day)	ϱ_y,ϱ_z(day⁻¹,10⁻⁴)		μ_{normal},μ_{tumor}(kPa)	
Ground truth	1.0	0.5	0.5	0.6	2.0	1.0	1.0	5.0
MG-IM	1.0±0.0	0.5±0.0	0.5±0.0	0.6±0.0	1.9±0.1	1.0±0.0	1.0±0.0	5.0±0.1
MG	1.3±0.1	0.5±0.1	0.2±0.2	0.6±0.0	1.0±1.0	0.4±0.1	0.6±0.2	0.6±0.1
F-IM	0.9±0.2	0.5±0.2	0.3±0.2	0.6±0.1	-	-	1.1±0.1	5.2±0.4

Ground truth ϱ_x	1.0 2.0 3.0 4.0		Recall(%)	Precision(%)	Dice(%)	RVD(%)	ASD(mm)	RMSE(%)
MG-IM ϱ_x	0.9 2.0 2.9 3.9	MG-IM	99.4±0.2	99.7±0.1	99.6±0.2	0.3±0.2	0.0±0.0	0.2±0.1
MG ϱ_x	0.6 0.0 2.4 0.0	MG	89.2±2.0	91.5±1.8	90.3±0.6	3.8±2.1	0.6±0.1	6.9±0.6
F-IM γ(kPa)	0.5 0.6 0.7 0.0	F-IM	92.4±1.6	98.2±3.1	95.2±1.1	6.1±3.8	0.3±0.2	3.6±1.5

In each experiment, simulation was performed on the FEM mesh at the first time point, with the ICVF, SUV, and image-derived motion providing the initial conditions, proliferation rates, and displacement boundary conditions, respectively. This simulation was rasterized and compared with the measured ICVF and tumor volume at the second time point to evaluate the objective function for parameter estimation. Prediction was performed by simulating the tumor growth using the personalized parameters, with the mesh, ICVF, SUV, and image-derived motion at the second time point. The prediction performance was evaluated using the measurements at the third time point, and was represented as recall, precision, Dice coefficient, relative volume difference (RVD), average surface distance (ASD), and ICVF root-mean-squared error (RMSE) (Dice $= 2 \times TPV/(V_s + V_m)$ and RVD $= |V_s - V_m|/V_m$).

5.2 Synthetic Data

Using the FEM mesh and image-derived information of a patient at the first time point (Day 0, Fig. 4(a)), the second time point (Day 300) was simulated with the ground-truth model parameters using the proposed model (Table 1). This FEM simulation was rasterized into an ICVF image to provide the measurement input to the experiments. The estimated parameters were then used to predict the tumor growth at the third time point (Day 600) and compared with the simulated ground truth. Ground truths with $\varrho_x = 1.0, 2.0, 3.0, 4.0 \times 10^{-4}$ day^{-1} were simulated to study the prediction performance at different multiplicative growth rates. Identical settings were used in all tests.

Figure 4(b) shows the strain of the simulated ground truth with $\varrho_x = 3.0 \times 10^{-4}$ day^{-1}. Only the strain along the x-axis is shown due to space limitation. The growth strain ($\epsilon_{xx(g)}$) of the normal tissues was zero as we modeled no growth in that region. As the tumor was five times as stiff as the surrounding tissues (Table 1), the tumor region had almost no elastic strain ($\epsilon_{xx(e)}$) with the enforced image-derived displacements. The final strain (ϵ_{xx}) comprised the features of both the growth and elastic parts. These demonstrate the characteristics of the multiplicative growth decomposition.

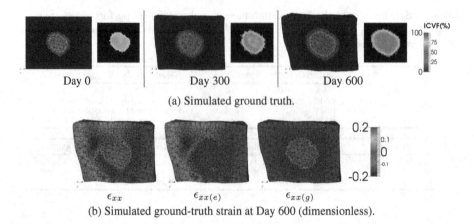

Day 0   Day 300   Day 600

(a) Simulated ground truth.

ϵ_{xx} $\epsilon_{xx(e)}$ $\epsilon_{xx(g)}$

(b) Simulated ground-truth strain at Day 600 (dimensionless).

Fig. 4. Synthetic data ($\varrho_x = 3.0 \times 10^{-4}$ day^{-1}). (a) The simulated ground truth at three time points. Left: FEM simulation. Right: rasterized image. (b) The ground-truth strain along the x-axis (ϵ_{xx}) and its elastic ($\epsilon_{xx(e)}$) and growth ($\epsilon_{xx(g)}$) parts at Day 600.

Table 1 shows the estimated parameters and the prediction performances. As discretization noise and information loss were introduced during image rasterization, the parameter estimation was nontrivial. The proposed MG-IM framework had the best overall performance as it used the same model as the ground truth with the image-derived motion. The MG and F-IM frameworks could not precisely estimate the diffusion parameters (D_i), but the estimated degrees of anisotropy were similar to those of the ground truth. Without the image-derived motion, the MG framework underestimated the shear moduli (μ_{normal}, μ_{tumor}), and thus the multiplicative growth rates (ϱ_i) could not be accurately estimated. On the other hand, although the ground-truth values of the force scalar (γ) of the F-IM framework were unknown, they mostly increased with the increase of ϱ_x because of the better estimation of μ_{normal} and μ_{tumor}. The F-IM framework performed better than the MG framework in general.

5.3   Clinical Data

Images from six patients (five males and one female) with diagnosed pancreatic neuroendocrine tumors were studied. The average age and weight of the patients at the first time point were 46.5±14.0 years and 89.6±17.7 kg, respectively. Each data set had three time points of images spanning three to four years, and the pixel sizes were less than $0.94 \times 0.94 \times 1.00$ mm^3 for CT and $4.25 \times 4.25 \times 3.27$ mm^3 for PET. Fig. 5(a) shows an example of the measurements. Identical settings were used in all tests.

Table 2 shows the estimated parameters and prediction performances. The MG-IM framework had similarly good prediction performance with the MG framework, while that of the F-IM framework was the worst. The diffusion

Table 2. Clinical data. Estimated parameters and prediction performances.

	D_x,D_y,D_z(mm²/day,10⁻³)			α(mm³/g/day)	$\varrho_x,\varrho_y,\varrho_z$(day⁻¹,10⁻⁴)			μ_{normal},μ_{tumor}(kPa)		γ(kPa)
MG-IM	0.0±0.0	0.0±0.0	0.0±0.0	0.4±0.4	4.7±3.2	4.2±3.2	4.6±4.7	0.6±0.3	40.4±10.1	-
MG	0.0±0.0	0.0±0.0	0.0±0.0	0.5±0.3	8.2±8.6	6.9±5.1	6.2±7.3	3.5±1.9	1.6±1.3	-
F-IM	0.0±0.1	0.1±0.2	0.3±0.8	0.5±0.5	-	-	-	0.8±0.9	44.3±13.1	2.4±3.8

	Recall(%)	Precision(%)	Dice(%)	RVD(%)	ASD(mm)	RMSE(%)
MG-IM	89.8±3.5	85.6±7.5	87.4±3.6	9.7±7.2	0.6±0.2	9.6±5.0
MG	90.1±5.2	87.9±6.6	88.7±2.9	9.2±8.6	0.5±0.2	9.2±5.4
F-IM	84.1±9.1	91.6±6.0	87.2±3.7	14.3±7.4	0.5±0.2	11.4±5.1

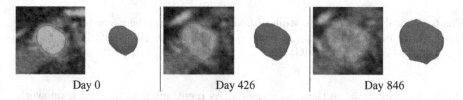

| Day 0 | Day 426 | Day 846 |

(a) Measurements at different time points.

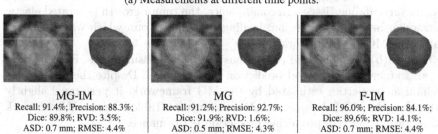

MG-IM	MG	F-IM
Recall: 91.4%; Precision: 88.3%;	Recall: 91.2%; Precision: 92.7%;	Recall: 96.0%; Precision: 84.1%;
Dice: 89.8%; RVD: 3.5%;	Dice: 91.9%; RVD: 1.6%;	Dice: 89.6%; RVD: 14.1%;
ASD: 0.7 mm; RMSE: 4.4%	ASD: 0.5 mm; RMSE: 4.3%	ASD: 0.7 mm; RMSE: 4.4%

(b) Predictions at the third time point (Day 846).

Fig. 5. Clinical data. (a) The segmented tumor volumes at different time points, and the corresponding contours overlapping with the post-contrast CT images. (b) The prediction results at the third time point, with red and green represent measurements and predictions, respectively (Color figure online).

parameters (D_i) of the MG-IM and MG frameworks were close to zero, which means that the tumor size changes were mainly governed by the mass effect. Similar to the synthetic data, the μ_{tumor} estimated by the MG framework were relatively small, which on average even smaller than μ_{normal}. As this is physiologically implausible for solid tumors, this shows the importance of using image-derived motion on estimating plausible mechanical parameters.

Figure 6 compares the predicted strains between the MG-IM and MG frameworks. As the image-derived motion was relatively small in this example, the elastic strains ($\epsilon_{xx(e)}$) caused by the tumor growth were more obvious. The negative elastic strains around the tumor indicate the outward pushing of the tumor and the resistance of its surrounding tissues. These negative elastic strains reduced

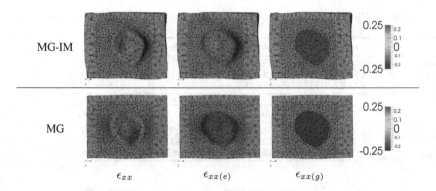

Fig. 6. Clinical data. Predicted strains (dimensionless) along the x-axis (ϵ_{xx}) and their elastic ($\epsilon_{xx(e)}$) and growth ($\epsilon_{xx(g)}$) parts at the third time point. MG-IM: μ_{normal} = 0.4 kPa, μ_{tumor} = 26.5 kPa. MG: μ_{normal} = 3.9 kPa, μ_{tumor} = 1.1 kPa.

the final strains (ϵ_{xx}) in the tumor region. As mentioned, as the MG framework had the estimated μ_{tumor} smaller than μ_{normal}, the tumor was more deformable than its surrounding tissues. In consequence, the tumor growth generated elastic contraction in the tumor region, leading to a final strain which was similar to that of the MG-IM framework.

Figure 5(b) compares the predictions with the measurements. For this data set, all frameworks had good prediction performances. Despite the implausible mechanical properties estimated by the MG framework, it performed slightly better than the MG-IM framework. Consistent with Table 2, the F-IM framework had the worst but still promising prediction performance.

6   Conclusion

In this paper, we have presented a pancreatic tumor growth prediction framework with multiplicative growth decomposition and image-derived pancreatic motion. By combining the multiplicative decomposition with a hyperelastic mechanical model, the expansive growth can be modeled by explicit functions without compromising the accuracy of the elastic response. With also the contrast-enhanced CT and FDG-PET images, the structural, functional, and motion information can be combined for more patient-specific models. Experiments on synthetic data show that image-derived motion is important for estimating physiologically plausible mechanical properties. Experiments on clinical data show that the framework can achieve promising prediction performance.

References

1. Bae, K.T.: Intravenous contrast medium administration and scan timing at CT: considerations and approaches. Radiology **256**(1), 32–61 (2010)
2. Bathe, K.J.: Finite Element Procedures. Prentice Hall, Upper Saddle River (1996)

3. Clatz, O., Sermesant, M., Bondiau, P.Y., Delingette, H., Warfield, S.K., Malandain, G., Ayache, N.: Realistic simulation of the 3D growth of brain tumors in MR images coupling diffusion with biomechanical deformation. IEEE Trans. Med. Imaging **24**(10), 1334–1346 (2005)

4. Ehehalt, F., Saeger, H.D., Schmidt, C.M., Grützmann, R.: Neuroendocrine tumors of the pancreas. Oncologist **14**(5), 456–467 (2009)

5. Feng, M., Balter, J.M., Normolle, D., Adusumilli, S., Cao, Y., Chenevert, T.L., Ben-Josef, E.: Characterization of pancreatic tumor motion using cine MRI: surrogates for tumor position should be used with caution. Int. J. Radiat. Oncol. Biol. Phys. **74**(3), 884–891 (2009)

6. Friedl, P., Locker, J., Sahai, E., Segall, J.E.: Classifying collective cancer cell invasion. Nat. Cell Biol. **14**(8), 777–783 (2012)

7. Hogea, C., Davatzikos, C., Biros, G.: An image-driven parameter estimation problem for a reaction-diffusion glioma growth model with mass effects. J. Math. Biol. **56**(6), 793–825 (2008)

8. Holzapfel, G.A.: Nonlinear Solid Mechanics: A Continuum Approach for Engineering. John Wiley & Sons Inc, Chichester (2000)

9. Konukoglu, E., Clatz, O., Menze, B.H., Stieltjes, B., Weber, M.A., Mandonnet, E., Delingette, H., Ayache, N.: Image guided personalization of reaction-diffusion type tumor growth models using modified anisotropic eikonal equations. IEEE Trans. Med. Imaging **29**(1), 77–95 (2010)

10. Libutti, S.K., Choyke, P.L., Bartlett, D.L., Vargas, H., Walther, M., Lubensky, I., Glenn, G., Linehan, W.M., Alexander, H.R.: Pancreatic neuroendocrine tumors associated with von Hippel Lindau disease: diagnostic and management recommendations. Surgery **124**(6), 1153–1159 (1998)

11. Lubarda, V.A., Hoger, A.: On the mechanics of solids with a growing mass. Int. J. Solids Struct. **39**(18), 4627–4664 (2002)

12. Menze, B.H., Van Leemput, K., Honkela, A., Konukoglu, E., Weber, M.A., Ayache, N., Golland, P.: A generative approach for image-based modeling of tumor growth. In: Székely, G., Hahn, H.K. (eds.) IPMI 2011. LNCS, vol. 6801, pp. 735–747. Springer, Heidelberg (2011)

13. Mohamed, A., Davatzikos, C.: Finite element modeling of brain tumor mass-effect from 3D medical images. In: Duncan, J.S., Gerig, G. (eds.) MICCAI 2005. LNCS, vol. 3749, pp. 400–408. Springer, Heidelberg (2005)

14. Pluim, J.P.W., Maintz, J.B.A., Viergever, M.A.: Mutual-information-based registration of medical images: a survey. IEEE Trans. Med. Imaging **22**(8), 986–1004 (2003)

15. Rodriguez, E.K., Hoger, A., McCulloch, A.D.: Stress-dependent finite growth in soft elastic tissues. J. Biomech. **27**(4), 455–467 (1994)

16. Rowan, T.: Functional Stability Analysis of Numerical Algorithms. Ph.D. thesis, University of Texas at Austin (1990)

17. West, G.B., Brown, J.H., Enquist, B.J.: A general model for ontogenetic growth. Nature **413**(6856), 628–631 (2001)

18. Wong, K.C.L., Summers, R., Kebebew, E., Yao, J.: Tumor growth prediction with hyperelastic biomechanical model, physiological data fusion, and nonlinear optimization. In: Golland, P., Hata, N., Barillot, C., Hornegger, J., Howe, R. (eds.) MICCAI 2014, Part II. LNCS, vol. 8674, pp. 25–32. Springer, Heidelberg (2014)

19. Yushkevich, P.A., Piven, J., Hazlett, H.C., Smith, R.G., Ho, S., Gee, J.C., Gerig, G.: User-guided 3D active contour segmentation of anatomical structures: significantly improved efficiency and reliability. NeuroImage **31**(3), 1116–1128 (2006)

IMaGe: Iterative Multilevel Probabilistic Graphical Model for Detection and Segmentation of Multiple Sclerosis Lesions in Brain MRI

Nagesh Subbanna[✉], Doina Precup, Douglas Arnold, and Tal Arbel

McGill University, Montreal, QC, Canada
nagesh@cim.mcgill.ca

Abstract. In this paper, we present IMaGe, a new, iterative two-stage probabilistic graphical model for detection and segmentation of Multiple Sclerosis (MS) lesions. Our model includes two levels of Markov Random Fields (MRFs). At the bottom level, a regular grid voxel-based MRF identifies potential lesion voxels, as well as other tissue classes, using local and neighbourhood intensities and class priors. Contiguous voxels of a particular tissue type are grouped into regions. A higher, non-lattice MRF is then constructed, in which each node corresponds to a region, and edges are defined based on neighbourhood relationships between regions. The goal of this MRF is to evaluate the probability of candidate lesions, based on group intensity, texture and neighbouring regions. The inferred information is then propagated to the voxel-level MRF. This process of iterative inference between the two levels repeats as long as desired. The iterations suppress false positives and refine lesion boundaries. The framework is trained on 660 MRI volumes of MS patients enrolled in clinical trials from 174 different centres, and tested on a separate multi-centre clinical trial data set with 535 MRI volumes. All data consists of T1, T2, PD and FLAIR contrasts. In comparison to other MRF methods, such as [5,9], and a traditional MRF, IMaGe is much more sensitive (with slightly better PPV). It outperforms its nearest competitor by around 20 % when detecting very small lesions (3–10 voxels). This is a significant result, as such lesions constitute around 40 % of the total number of lesions.

1 Introduction

Multiple Sclerosis (MS) is an inflammatory, demyelinating disease of the Central Nervous System (CNS)[1]. Establishing patient lesion load, through counts and volume measurements, provides important measures of disease progression and drug efficacy [1]. Current clinical practice involves manual labelling of MS lesions by experts, a task that is time-consuming, expensive and subject to inter- and intra-rater variability. Automatic MS lesion detection and segmentation are particularly challenging tasks, as lesions display wide variability in terms of shape, size, appearance, and location throughout the white matter (WM) (and possibly grey matter (GM)) of the brain. Normalization of different field strengths,

S. Ourselin et al. (Eds.): IPMI 2015, LNCS 9123, pp. 514–526, 2015.
DOI: 10.1007/978-3-319-19992-4_40

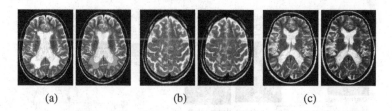

(a)   (b)   (c)

Fig. 1. (left) Brain images of MS patients with (right) lesions segmented by experts. We show (a) a volume with heavy peri-ventricular lesion load, (b) volume with supra-ventricular lesions, and (c) volume with juxta-cortical lesions. The different shapes, sizes, positions and intensities make lesion segmentation challenging.

acquisition sequences and different scanner types yields subtle differences in the appearances and absolute intensities of the lesions. These variabilities are further dependent on disease stage [2]. Figure 1 shows some lesion examples.

Although various automatic approaches have been developed for the segmentation of MS lesions, their adoption into real clinical practice has been limited. This is primarily due to strong simplifying assumptions, which restrict the robustness to variability displayed in large clinical datasets [2]. For example, techniques that define lesions as outliers of healthy class distributions [3,7] risk missing a large set of subtle lesions located throughout the brain, for which these assumptions are violated. Techniques based on topological features and template matching (e.g. [10]) presume that lesion shape can easily be modelled by a set of candidate lesion shapes, which is difficult to achieve in practice. Finally, most techniques are tested on synthetic lesion data, or on the limited MICCAI Challenge dataset [4,7], neither of which reflects the variability present in large clinical datasets.

Various MRF techniques have been proposed for pathology segmentation [3,11] but typically only class relationships are reflected in the priors (e.g. Ising models). However, traditional MRFs tend to smooth class labels excessively, and hence may lead to the removal of smaller MS lesions. To alleviate this problem, a modified MRF [9] has been proposed, which models both voxel intensities and intensity differences in the cliques. However, a local model of a voxel and its neighbourhood is insufficient for this task, and a more global view of context is necessary for accurate classification. Recently, several different, multi-level graphical models have been introduced for segmentation of pathologies [12,13]. However, none have been designed for the unique context of MS lesion segmentation.

In this work, we present IMaGe, a new, iterative, two-stage, probabilistic, graphical model for the detection and segmentation of MS lesions in multi-channel MRI. The goal of this architecture is to take advantage of both local information, as well as global context, in order to remove false assertions and refine boundaries. The lower level consists of nodes associated with each voxel, and models the intensities of healthy tissues and lesions, as in [9]. It produces a set of lesion candidates, passed to the higher level, whose goal is to determine which of these candidates are indeed lesions, by looking at a larger context

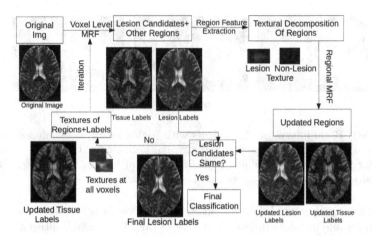

Fig. 2. Flowchart of the proposed approach. The multimodal MRI are processed by a 2 stage iterative MRF. At the bottom level, a voxel based MRF identifies potential lesion voxels, as well as other tissue classes. Contiguous voxels of a particular tissue type are grouped into regions. A higher, non-lattice based MRF is then constructed, in which each node corresponds to a region, and edges are defined based on neighbourhood relationships between regions. Regional features such as textures are extracted from each region. The goal of this MRF is to evaluate the probability of candidate lesions, based on group intensity, texture, and neighbouring regions. If the resulting labels have changed at this stage, the labels and textures are then propogated back down to the voxel-level MRF. This process of iterative inference continues until convergence.

around each region. The higher level consists of a non-lattice based MRF (whose structure is not a regular, uniform grid). Each node corresponds to a contiguous region of voxels currently labelled with the same class, and nodes are connected if the corresponding regions have at least one voxel adjacent to the other region. Each region is modelled using both intensity and textural features, and the relations between different regions are also considered. The class label computed based on this information, as well as the texture information, is then passed to the lower level. Inference alternates between the two levels, until a consensus is reached about the lesion candidates, or a given number of iterations has elapsed. Figure 2 illustrates this process.

IMaGe is trained on 660 MS patient MRI volumes from a clinical trial involving 174 centres. In order to test the robustness of the framework to different trial data, testing was performed on a different clinical trial data set of 535 MRI MS patient volumes from 128 centres. Both datasets include T1, T2, PD and FLAIR contrasts. We compared IMaGe to a recent MRF technique based on FLAIR [5], a traditional MRF, and the result of the voxel-based MRF [9]. IMaGe outperformed the competitors based on sensitivity and Positive Predictive Value, particularly in the context of smaller lesion detection (i.e. in the 3–10 voxel range), comprising around 40 % of the clinical trial dataset. These small lesions often constitute a very small portion of the total volume of the lesions, but it is important to detect them in clinical settings since the activity of the disease is measured by the number of lesions, both large and small.

2   Methodology

Given a multichannel MRI volume, the task is to identify the voxels corresponding to MS lesions. The proposed hierarchical MRF technique identifies potential
lesion candidates at the lower level, and the validity of the candidates is inferred
at the higher level, where the lesion boundaries are also refined. We describe in
detail the framework in Fig. 2.

2.1   Voxel-Level MRF

Traditional voxel level MRFs [8,11] are typically lattice-based and infer the class
of a voxel using observations local to that voxel (such as intensity) and the classes
of the neighbouring voxels. However, this process tends to smooth over small
patches of voxels whose class differs from their neighbours. This is problematic
for MS lesions, which tend to be very small (3–10 voxels). To alleviate this
problem, we employ a modified MRF at the voxel level, as in [9], which uses at
each voxel the contrast of the local observation with those of the neighbours.
Specifically, at each node we consider the observation to include the intensity
difference between the corresponding voxel and its neighbours.

The MRF is structured as a regular lattice, with a node for each voxel and
connectivity as depicted in Fig. 3. Let Q be the number of voxels in the volume, and $\mathbf{I}_i$ denote the vector of multimodal intensities at voxel i and N_i denote
i's neighbourhood (Fig. 3). The goal is to infer the class label C_i, corresponding to voxel i's tissue type (lesion, white matter (WM), grey matter (GM),
cerebro-spinal fluid (CSF) or partial volume[1] (PV)). Let $\mathbf{I}_{N_i}$ denote the vector
of intensities of the voxels in N_i and $\mathbf{C}_{N_i}$ denote the vector of class labels for
these voxels. Let $\mathbf{C} = (C_0, C_1, \ldots, C_{Q-1})$ be the collection of all class labels
for the corresponding voxels in the volume, and $\mathbf{I} = (\mathbf{I}_0, \mathbf{I}_1, \ldots, \mathbf{I}_{Q-1})$ be the
corresponding intensities. The goal is to compute $P(\mathbf{C} \mid \mathbf{I})$, which in an MRF is
given by:

$$P(\mathbf{C} \mid \mathbf{I}) \propto e^{-U(\mathbf{C} \mid \mathbf{I})}, \tag{1}$$

where $U(\mathbf{C} \mid \mathbf{I})$ is the energy of the configuration. Following [9], the posterior
probability of class C_i is given by:

$$P(C_i \mid \mathbf{I}_i, \mathbf{I}_{N_i}) = \sum_{\mathbf{C}_{N_i}} P(C_i, \mathbf{C}_{N_i} \mid \mathbf{I}_i, \mathbf{I}_{N_i}) = \sum_{\mathbf{C}_{N_i}} \frac{P(\mathbf{I}_{N_i}, \mathbf{I}_i \mid C_i, \mathbf{C}_{N_i}) P(C_i, \mathbf{C}_{N_i})}{P(\mathbf{I}_i, \mathbf{I}_{N_i})}$$

$$\propto \sum_{\mathbf{C}_{N_i}} P(\mathbf{I}_{N_i} \mid \mathbf{I}_i, C_i, \mathbf{C}_{N_i}) P(\mathbf{I}_i \mid \mathbf{C}_{N_i}, C_i) P(\mathbf{C}_{N_i} \mid C_i) P(C_i).$$

$$\tag{2}$$

where the sums marginalize over all combinations of class labels that can be
assigned to the neighbourhood voxels. In Eq. (2), $P(C_i)$ is the prior probability

---

[1] Partial volume denotes the class ascribed to voxels which are a mix of GM and CSF.
  This class is created in order to reduce the number of false negatives at the edges of
  the ventricles.

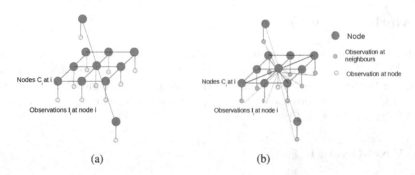

Fig. 3. (a) The regular MRF model and (b) the MRF model used in [9]. Note that the neighbouring intensities are considered in the computation of the label at every node i in this model.

at voxel i, $P(\mathbf{C}_{N_i} \mid C_i)$ represents the probability of class transitions in the neighbourhood, $P(\mathbf{I}_i|C_i)$ is the likelihood of $\mathbf{I}_i$ given class C_i and $P(\mathbf{I}_{N_i}|\mathbf{C}_{N_i}, C_i, \mathbf{I}_i)$ models the likelihood of the intensity of the neighbouring voxels, given their classes and the information at voxel i.

Let $\mathbf{\Delta I}_{N_i}$ be defined as the intensity difference between $\mathbf{I}_i$ and $\mathbf{I}_{N_i}$ in the clique (see Sect. 3.1 for details on computing intensity differences). Since $\mathbf{I}_{N_i}$ can be computed deterministically from $\mathbf{\Delta I}_{N_i}$ and $\mathbf{I}_i$, in Eq. 2, we replace $P(\mathbf{I}_{N_i} \mid \mathbf{I}_i, C_i, \mathbf{C}_{N_i})$ with $P(\mathbf{\Delta I}_{N_i} \mid \mathbf{I}_i, \mathbf{C}_i, \mathbf{C}_{N_i})$. We can also assume that the difference in intensity between a voxel and its neighbours depends on the classes in the neighbourhood, but not on the absolute intensity of the voxel itself, and hence we can replace $P(\mathbf{\Delta I}_{N_i} \mid \mathbf{I}_i, \mathbf{C}_{N_i}, C_i)$ with $P(\mathbf{\Delta I}_{N_i} \mid \mathbf{C}_{N_i}, C_i)$. Furthermore, we assume that the intensity of a voxel is conditionally independent of the neighbourhood classes, given the class label at the voxel. Hence, we can replace $P(\mathbf{I}_i \mid C_i, \mathbf{C}_{N_i})$ with $P(\mathbf{I}_i \mid C_i)$. With these assumptions, Eq. (2) simplifies to:

$$P(C_i \mid \mathbf{I}_i, \mathbf{I}_{N_i}) \approx P(\mathbf{I}_i \mid C_i)P(C_i) \sum_{\mathbf{C}_{N_i}} P(\mathbf{\Delta I}_{N_i} \mid C_i, \mathbf{C}_{N_i})P(\mathbf{C}_{N_i} \mid C_i). \quad (3)$$

Using Eqs. 1 and 3, the Gibbs energy function is given by: $P(\mathbf{C} \mid \mathbf{I}) \propto \prod_{i=0}^{Q-1} e^{-U(C_i|\mathbf{I}_i,\mathbf{I}_{N_i})}$. To infer the class labels, the total energy must be minimised. The energy at each voxel i can be expressed as:

$$U(C_i|\mathbf{I}_i, \mathbf{I}_{N_i}) = -\log P(\mathbf{I}_i|C_i) - \log P(C_i)$$
$$- \sum_{k \in \text{Cliques}(N_i)} \sum_{j \in k} (\log P(\mathbf{\Delta I}_{i,j}|C_i, \mathbf{C}_j) - \alpha m(\mathbf{C}_j, C_i)), \quad (4)$$

where k indexes over all the possible cliques in N_i and j indexes over all the possible elements of clique k, $m(\mathbf{C}_j, C_i)$ is the potential associated with the relationship between C_i and the vector of classes in the jth clique, $\mathbf{C}_j$, and α is a weighting parameter used to handle the differences between inter-slice and intra-slice distances.

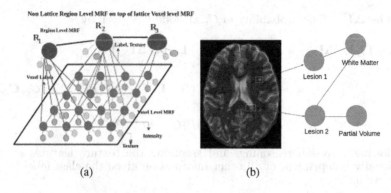

(a)   (b)

Fig. 4. In (a), the schematic diagram of the hierarchical MRF and the features used at each level are shown. Red nodes represent the classes at each voxel. Light blue nodes are the derived textures, and yellow are the intensities. The voxels with the same labels are merged into regions and moved into the higher level MRF. In (b), all the different classes of a volume in one slice are marked. All the links of the two lesions (highlighted with yellow rectangles) are shown. Lesion 1 has only one neighbour, white matter (seen in blue in the MRI). Lesion 2 has two neighbours, partial volume (seen in magenta on the MRI) and white matter (Color figure online).

In order to estimate the lesion candidates, we run inference in the MRF until convergence. The parameters of the voxel-based MRF have been trained so as to obtain high sensitivity in lesion detection, at the expense of a higher false positive rate, as pruning of the false positives will occur at the region level. All voxels for which the lesion class probability is higher than a certain threshold are labelled as lesions. For all the other voxels, the label is the MAP class. The value of the lesion threshold is also chosen to ensure high sensitivity.

2.2 Region-Level MRFs

The goal of the region level MRF is to adjust the class labels by taking larger scale contextual information into account. The region level MRF is non-lattice-based and is constructed adaptively based on the labels assigned by the voxel-level MRF (depicted in Fig. 4). A region is defined as a set of voxels that have been assigned the same class by the voxel-based MRF and that are connected in 3D. Each region is represented by a node in the MRF. The nodes corresponding to two regions r and q have an edge between them if there are at least two voxels $i \in r, j \in q$ which are adjacent. Due to this process, regions correspond to different numbers of voxels and have different shapes. The region based MRF aims to assign classes to the voxels in each region based on the intensities of the voxels in the region and in the neighbouring regions, as well as based on texture information obtained from the voxels in each region. A region's class will be inferred as the class of its corresponding MRF voxel.

Let $\mathbf{T}_r$ denote the vector of texture features at node r. Let the intensity of the region be $\mathbf{I}_r$ and intensity difference between the region r and its neighbouring regions be $\boldsymbol{\Delta I}_{N_r}$. The probability of C_r at node r is given by

$$P(C_r \mid \mathbf{T}_r, \mathbf{I}_r, \boldsymbol{\Delta I}_{N_r}) = \sum_{\mathbf{C}_{N_r}} P(C_r, \mathbf{C}_{N_r} \mid \mathbf{I}_r, \mathbf{T}_r, \boldsymbol{\Delta I}_{N_r})$$

$$\propto \sum_{\mathbf{C}_{N_r}} P(\boldsymbol{\Delta I}_{N_r} \mid \mathbf{T}_r, \mathbf{I}_r, C_r, \mathbf{C}_{N_r}) P(\mathbf{T}_r \mid \mathbf{I}_r, C_r, \mathbf{C}_{N_r})$$

$$P(\mathbf{I}_r \mid C_r, \mathbf{C}_{N_r}) P(\mathbf{C}_{N_r} \mid C_r) P(C_r) \tag{5}$$

Following Bayesian reasoning, and assuming the texture features are also conditionally independent of all other information given the class label for any node r, we have:

$$P(C_r \mid \mathbf{I}_r, \mathbf{T}_r, \mathbf{I}_{N_r}) \approx P(\mathbf{T}_r|C_r)P(\mathbf{I}_r|C_r)P(C_r) \sum_{\mathbf{C}_{N_r}} P(\boldsymbol{\Delta I}_{N_r} \mid C_r, \mathbf{C}_{N_r})P(\mathbf{C}_{N_r}| C_r) \tag{6}$$

The MRF energy equation, corresponding to Eq. (6) is given by $P(\mathbf{C} \mid \mathbf{I}, \mathbf{T}) \propto \prod_{r=0}^{R-1} e^{-U(\mathbf{C}_r|\mathbf{I}_r, \mathbf{I}_{N_r}, \mathbf{T}_r)}$, where R is the total number of regions in the volume. By reasoning similar to Eq. (3), and assuming that we consider cliques of size 2 at maximum, we obtain:

$$U(C_r \mid \mathbf{I}_r, \mathbf{I}_{N_i}, \mathbf{T}_r) = -\log P(\mathbf{I}_r \mid C_r) - \log P(\mathbf{T}_r \mid C_r) - \log(C_r)$$

$$- \sum_{s \in \text{Cliques}(N_r)} (\log P(\boldsymbol{\Delta I}_{r,s} \mid C_r, C_s) - \alpha m(C_s, C_r)), \tag{7}$$

where s indexes over all possible cliques of size 2. The inference process in the MRF minimizes the energy in this model, and re-labels all the regions. The result of this process is typically an elimination of false positives from the voxel-based MRF.

2.3   Iterations

After the region-level inference, the result is compared to the low-level MRF. If there are discrepancies in the lesion voxel labelling, further iterations are needed. In this case, the information computed by the region-level MRF has to be communicated to the voxel-level. Two types of information are transmitted: the class labels that are inferred for each region, and the texture information that was computed. Each voxel $i \in r$ will initially have $C_i = C_r$ meaning that all the labels in the region are moved back down to their corresponding voxels to initiate the process. Similarly, there is a voxel- associated texture $\mathbf{T}_i$ (whose computation is described in Sect. 2.2). At this stage, further refinement of boundaries is performed.

The voxel-level MRF is exactly as described in Sect. 2.1, except it also uses the texture information $\mathbf{T}_i$, Using the same assumptions as in Eq. (3) and assuming that $\mathbf{T}_i$ is conditionally dependent only on C_i, we get

$$P(C_i \mid \mathbf{I}_i, \mathbf{T}_i, \mathbf{I}_{N_i}) = \sum_{\mathbf{C}_{N_i}} P(\boldsymbol{\Delta I}_{N_i} \mid C_i, \mathbf{C}_{N_i})P(\mathbf{T}_i \mid C_i)P(\mathbf{I}_i \mid C_i)P(\mathbf{C}_{N_i} \mid C_i)P(C_i) \tag{8}$$

and the corresponding energy at voxel i given a particular configuration of classes is given by:

$$U(C_i|\mathbf{I}_i, \mathbf{I}_{N_i}) = -\log P(C_i) - \log P(\mathbf{I}_i|C_i) - \log P(\mathbf{T}_i|C_i)$$
$$- \sum_{k \in \text{Cliques}_{N_i}} \sum_{j \in k} (\log P(\Delta\mathbf{I}_{i,j}|C_i, \mathbf{C}_j) - \alpha m(\mathbf{C}_j, C_i)), \quad (9)$$

where, again, k indexes over all possible cliques in N_i and j indexes over all the possible elements of clique k. Once the MRF inference has been run to convergence at the voxel level, inferring new class labels C_i, and the process is iterated.

3 Experiments and Results

We used two proprietary clinical trial data sets of patients with Relapsing Remitting MS for training and testing. The training data set consisted of 660 MS patients from 174 centres. The test data set contained 535 MS patients' MRI volumes from 128 centres. The test data and training data come from entirely different clinical trials. Both data sets included semi-manual lesion segmentations by trained experts following a strict protocol. All volumes consisted of four contrasts: T1, T2, FLAIR (T2w fluid attenuation inversion recovery), and PD (proton density). All volumes underwent bias-field inhomogeneity correction using N3 [14], intra-subject registration of multispectral volumes [15], extraction of non-brain regions from the MRI (brain parenchyma) [16], and intensity range normalization [17]. Intra-subject registration of volumes involves registering contrasts to stereotactic space before any further processing is done.

In our experiments, we compare our results against 3 different methods. The first [5] is an MRF which categorizes lesions based on outliers in $T1$ and labels them in $FLAIR$. The second is a traditional MRF, which encapsulates class relations using priors and similar classes in the neighbourhood. The last is the modified MRF from [9], where classification is based on modelling both intensities and intensity differences, as well as class similarities in the neighbourhood.

3.1 Implementation of IMaGe

Computation of Intensity Difference $\Delta\mathbf{I}_{N_i}$: For a 2 voxel clique, we have the node and one of its neighbours. Assume that the intensity of the node is $\mathbf{I}_1$ and that of the neighbour is $\mathbf{I}_2$. The $\Delta\mathbf{I}_{1,2}$ is computed simply by $[\mathbf{I}_1 - \mathbf{I}_2]$. For a 3 voxel clique, we have the node and two of its neighbours. Assuming that the intensity of the node is $\mathbf{I}_1$ and that of the neighbours are $\mathbf{I}_2$ and $\mathbf{I}_3$, we have $\mathbf{I}_{1,2,3}$ given by

$$\Delta\mathbf{I}_{1,2,3} = \begin{bmatrix} \mathbf{I}_1 - \mathbf{I}_2 \\ \mathbf{I}_1 - \mathbf{I}_3 \end{bmatrix}. \quad (10)$$

The computation of intensity differences for 4 and 5 node cliques follows similarly.

Voxel Level MRF: There are two stages in the technique. In the training stage, all the models are learned from the expert labelled volumes.

Training: The intensities and intensity differences of both the healthy tissues and the lesions are modelled using multivariate Gaussian Mixture Models, with two components per contrast since all tissue classes are either unimodal or bimodal [8]. The neighbourhood contains the 8 in plane neighbours and the two corresponding voxels in the slices above and below. We generate the intensity difference models for all the cliques possible (2, 3, 4 and 5 voxel cliques for the neighbourhood chosen). The method models combinations of labels in cliques, not the order (position) in which they occur. The spatial transition probabilities between the different classes are learned from the frequency of co-occurrence in the labelled training volumes.

Classification: In the classification stage, the prior probabilities required for healthy tissues $P(C_i)$ are taken from an ICBM152 healthy brain atlas registered non-linearly to the volumes. The lesion probabilities are taken from a proprietary lesion atlas, built manually from over 3000 MS patients from different clinical trials (separate from the training and testing data sets), non-linearly registered to the volume being classified. If the lesion posterior probability $P(C_i \mid \mathbf{I}_i, \mathbf{I}_{N_i})$ of a voxel i is above a particular threshold, it is considered a potential lesion candidate. Iterated Conditional Modes are used to minimze the total energy at this stage.

Regional MRF: Here, $\mathbf{I}_r$ is computed as the mean intensity of all voxels associated with region r. $\Delta\mathbf{I}_{N_r}$ is computed based on the 'border' voxels of the two regions, as:

$$\Delta\mathbf{I}_{N_r} = \frac{1}{S_r} \sum_{i \in r} \sum_{j \in s, j \mathrm{adj} i} (\mathbf{I}_j - \mathbf{I}_i) \tag{11}$$

where S_r is the number of edges connecting voxels i in r with voxels j in s, and denotes adjacency of i and j.

Texture can be modelled in many ways, and the approach proposed can accommodate any choice of texture features. Here, we use multi-window Gabor textures. Multi-window Gabor coefficients are very flexible, and can be customized to problems since the analysis and synthesis windows are de-coupled [6]. To compute $\mathbf{T}_r$, at every voxel i in the region r, we choose the first Gabor window at a particular orientation centred at i that completely crosses the boundary of the region r before the Gabor coefficient value falls to a thousandth of the peak. This gives the value of $\mathbf{T}_r$ at the voxel i. The mean texture $\mathbf{T}_r$ is obtained for each Gabor window for the class using the textures at all the individual voxels in the region. Gabor texture computation for every region has been described in detail in [18] for the case of brain tumours.

Training and classification: Gabor textures $\mathbf{T}_r$, the regional intensities $\mathbf{I}_r$ and the intensity differences $\Delta\mathbf{I}_r$ are all modelled as Gaussian mixtures. Regional class transition probabilities are computed from the frequency of co-occurrence of the classes. During classification, we consider only cliques of size 2. We start with labels obtained by the voxel-based MRF and apply ICM for the inference.

Iterations. We compare the lesions estimated from the voxel level MRF and the region level MRF. If the difference between the two is less than a threshold (in number of voxels), then iterations are stopped. Otherwise, the iterations proceed in the same fashion, using the currently estimated parameters. The textures for each voxel obtained at the region level MRF and the labels of each region are passed down to the voxel level MRF and the process iterates as described in Eq. (9). In some cases, it is possible that the iterations will oscillate between the solution of voxel-level MRF and the regional level MRF. To account for such cases, we set a maximum number of iterations. The solution obtained at the end of the number of maximum iterations is taken to be the final answer. The maximum time taken by the technique on a Dell Optiplex 980 I7 machine is 40 minutes per volume.

3.2 Qualitative Results

Juxta-cortical lesions, often resembling grey matter in intensity, are hard to detect with just voxel level information. When lesion candidates are chosen (Fig. 5c), not only are all lesions detected by experts in Fig. 5b chosen as lesion candidates, but some additional false positive lesions are also chosen (Fig. 5c). Final results by IMaGe (Fig. 5d) show false positive regions removed iteratively, and true positive boundaries refined.

3.3 Quantitative Results

The clinical goal of this work is to detect all lesions accurately, rather than attain high precision in lesion boundaries, particularly given that there is little agreement regarding boundaries among expert raters. In clinical trials, detection accuracy is crucial, as lesion counts are used to assess if a treatment is working, and even one new lesion can indicate that the disease is active. Hence,

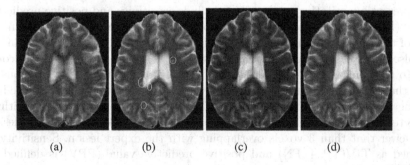

Fig. 5. Qualitative results on T2 slices of patient (a) Original unlabelled volume (b) Expert classification (lesions circled), (c) Lesion Candidates from first level of IMaGe, and (d) Final classification by IMaGe. In all images, red=true positive, blue=false positive lesions (Color figure online).

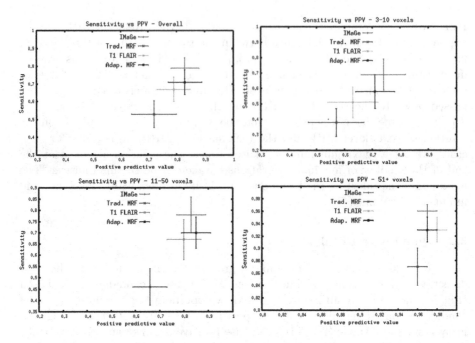

Fig. 6. Sensitivity against PPV for the overall data set, and broken down according to lesion size ranges in voxels. Lesion breakdown: Small lesions (3–10 voxels) 39 % (12737 lesions), moderate lesions (11–50 voxels) 36 % (11767 lesions), and large lesions (51+ voxels) 25 % (8124 lesions). IMaGe outperforms competing approaches in terms of sensitivity, particularly for small lesions of size 3–10 voxels, and shows some sensitivity and PPV improvements for all lesion sizes. In the figures, Trad. MRF refers to a standard Potts model MRF, Adap. MRF refers to the technique used in [9], and T1-FLAIR refers to the method used in [5]

metrics that consider false positives and false negatives with respect to the number of lesions in the volume are the best way to measure the algorithm's efficacy. We present quantitative results which include sensitivity and positive predictive value (PPV) at the lesion level. We use positive predictive value, since the number of true negative regions is very small and consequently, the relative number of false positives is better reflected by using PPV instead of specificity. According to the clinical protocol, a lesion is a set of 3 or more voxels, contiguous in 3D, that are labelled as lesion by the expert. An expert lesion is counted as a true positive (TP) when 3 or more of its voxels overlap with the algorithm-detected lesion. Otherwise, it is a false negative (FN). A false positive (FP) lesion has fewer that than 3 voxels overlapping with the expert lesion. Sensitivity is defined as TP/(TP + FN) and positive predictive value (PPV) is defined as TP/(TP+FP).

In Fig. 6, there is an overall improvement in sensitivity by 11.26 % compared to the next closest competitor, with the largest gain obtained for smaller lesion detection. The sensitivity for small lesions (3–10 voxels) is 18.96 % higher than for the closest competitor, and for moderate lesions (11–50) voxels, it is 11.42 %

higher. For large lesions, (51+ voxels), all methods have sensitivities greater than 0.9.

In our test data set, small lesions (between 3–10 voxels) accounted for 39 % of total lesions. Hence, overlap metrics such as Dice statistics, which do not properly penalize missing smaller lesions [2], are not as appropriate as lesion-based metrics. However, since most results in MS lesion segmentation literature are in terms of Dice similarity values, we also provide the equivalent Dice similarity coefficient values for all 4 techniques. The Dice similarity for Standard MRFs is 0.48, for Adaptive MRFs is 0.67, for T1-FLAIR is 0.63 and for IMaGe is 0.69. IMaGe results in a slightly higher Dice value, but its real advantage is in its ability to provide accurate detection of smaller lesions.

4   Conclusion and Future Work

In this paper, we introduced IMaGe, a new, iterative, multi-level probabilistic graphical model for the detection and segmentation of MS lesions. The method leverages both local and global, contextual information. Training and experimental validation are based on two, large, clinical trial datasets of relapsing remitting MS patients, in which multi-channel MRI data was recorded. The proposed method outperforms other state-of-the-art graphical models, providing much higher sensitivity for the detection of small lesions, with a slight improvement in PPV. In the future, we plan to explore more expressive models for the different classes, as well as alternative optimization techniques, in order to improve the computational speed and further improve the method's accuracy.

References

1. MacDonald, I.W., et al.: Recommended diagnostic criteria for multiple sclerosis: guidelines from the international panel on the diagnosis of multiple sclerosis. Ann. Neurol. **50**(1), 121–127 (2001)
2. Garcia-Lorenzo, D., et al.: Review of automatic segmentation methods of multiple sclerosis white matter lesions on conventional magnetic resonance imaging. Med. Image Anal. **17**(1), 1–18 (2013)
3. von Leemput, K., et al.: Automated segmentationo of multiple sclerosis lesions by model outlier detection. IEEE Trans. Med. Imag. **20**(8), 677–688 (2001)
4. Souplet, J., et al.: An automatic segmentation of T2-FLAIR Multiple Sclerosis lesions. In: Midas Jounal (2008)
5. Schmidt, P., et al.: An automated tool for detection of FLAIR-hyperintense white-matter lesions in multiple sclerosis. NeuroImage **59**, 3774–3783 (2012)
6. Subbanna, N., et al.: Existence conditions for non canonical multiwindow gabor functions. Trans. Signal Process. **55**(11), 5112–5117 (2007)
7. Weiss, N., Rueckert, D., Rao, A.: Multiple sclerosis lesion segmentation using dictionary learning and sparse coding. In: Mori, K., Sakuma, I., Sato, Y., Barillot, C., Navab, N. (eds.) MICCAI 2013, Part I. LNCS, vol. 8149, pp. 735–742. Springer, Heidelberg (2013)
8. Harmouche, R., et al.: Bayesian MS Lesion classification modelling regional and local spatial information. In: Proceedings of ICPR 2006, pp. 984–987 (2006)

9. Subbanna, N., et al.: Adapted MRF Segmentation of MS Lesions uisng Local Contextual Information. In: Proceedings of MIUA 2011, pp. 445–450 (2011)
10. Wu, Y., et al.: Automated segmentation of multiple sclerosis subtypes with multichannel MRI. NeuroImage **32**, 1205–1215 (2006)
11. Khayati, R., et al.: Fully automatic segmentation of multiple sclerosis lesions in brain MR FLAIR images using adaptive mixtures method and Markov Random field model. Comput. Bio. Med. **38**, 379–390 (2008)
12. Karimaghaloo, Z., Rivaz, H., Arnold, D.L., Collins, D.L., Arbel, T.: Adaptive voxel, texture and temporal conditional random field for detection of gad-enhancing multiple sclerosis lesions in brain MRI. In: Mori, K., Sakuma, I., Sato, Y., Barillot, C., Navab, N. (eds.) Proceedings MICCAI 2013, Part I. LNCS, vol. 8149, pp. 543–550. Springer, Heidelberg (2013)
13. Subbanna, N.K., Precup, D., Collins, D.L., Arbel, T.: Hierarchical probabilistic gabor and MRF segmentation of brain tumours in MRI volumes. In: Mori, K., Sakuma, I., Sato, Y., Barillot, C., Navab, N. (eds.) MICCAI 2013, part i. LNCS, vol. 8149, pp. 751–758. Springer, Heidelberg (2013)
14. Sled, J.G., Pike, G.B.: Correction for b(1) and b(0) variations in quantitative T(2) measurements using MRI. Magn. Reson. Med. **43**(4), 589–593 (2000)
15. Collins, D.L., et al.: Automatic 3D model based neuro-anatomical segmentation. Hum. Brain Mapp. **3**, 190–208 (1995)
16. Smith, S.M.: Fast robust automated brain extraction. Hum. Brain Mapp. **17**(3), 143–155 (2002)
17. Nyl, L.G., et al.: New variants of a method of MRI scale standardization. IEEE Trans. Med. Imag. **19**(2), 143–150 (2000)
18. Subbanna, N., et al.: Iterative multilevel MRF leveraging context and voxel information for brain tumour segmentation in MRI. In: Proceedings of Computer Vision and Pattern Recognition 2014, Columbus, June 2014

Moving Frames for Heart Fiber Reconstruction

Emmanuel Piuze[1]([⊠]), Jon Sporring[2], and Kaleem Siddiqi[1]

[1] School of Computer Science and Centre for Intelligent Machines,
McGill University, Montreal, QC, Canada
emman.piuze@gmail.com
[2] eScience Center, Department of Computer Science, University of Copenhagen,
Copenhagen, Denmark

Abstract. The method of moving frames provides powerful geometrical tools for the analysis of smoothly varying frame fields. However, in the face of missing measurements, a reconstruction problem arises, one that is largely unexplored for 3D frame fields. Here we consider the particular example of reconstructing impaired cardiac diffusion magnetic resonance imaging (dMRI) data. We combine moving frame analysis with a diffusion inpainting scheme that incorporates rule-based priors. In contrast to previous reconstruction methods, this new approach uses comprehensive differential descriptors for cardiac fibers, and is able to fully recover their orientation. We demonstrate the superior performance of this approach in terms of error of fit when compared to alternate methods. We anticipate that these tools could find application in clinical settings, where damaged heart tissue needs to be replaced or repaired, and for generating dense fiber volumes in electromechanical modelling of the heart.

1 Introduction

The method of moving frames (MMF), armed with the machinery of exterior calculus, offers tools for the analysis of smoothly varying frame fields. This approach provides useful geometrical descriptors which generalize the concepts of curvature and torsion for space curves, and the shape operator for surfaces [6]. Various problems can be analyzed from a moving frame perspective, including fluid flows in computational mechanics, equivalence and symmetry problems in physics [4], and invariant geometrical features in computer vision. The latter includes the geometry and evolution of curves in the euclidean, affine and projective planes [5], the differential geometry of motion paths [7] and the classical structure from motion problem [3].

In applications that involve acquired or fitted frame data, regions with missing measurements require data reconstruction. Although there exists a literature on the inpainting of 1D and 2D signals [11], the case of 3D frame fields is relatively unexplored. Here we consider the reconstruction of such frame fields fit to cardiac diffusion magnetic resonance imaging (dMRI) data. Prior work has shown that for normal hearts such frames rotate smoothly in the myocardium, lending them to moving frame analysis [9,12]. The presence of pathologies can

© Springer International Publishing Switzerland 2015
S. Ourselin et al. (Eds.): IPMI 2015, LNCS 9123, pp. 527–539, 2015.
DOI: 10.1007/978-3-319-19992-4_41

upset this organization and impair the ability of the heart muscle to operate efficiently. Modern treatments of such conditions include tissue engineering, where a synthetic material or stem cell therapy is used to mimic cardiomyocyte growth to restore cardiac contractile muscle properties in vitro [14], and mechanical ventricular restoration techniques that involve reconstruction, cauterization, and/or ablation of impaired or necrotic regions. Clinical studies have demonstrated that these techniques effectively improve ventricular function [1]. However, at present no formal rigorous geometrical constraints are used to guide or validate the reconstruction process. Among the presently available techniques for recovering missing information in dMRI are the interpolation of the diffusion tensor or the diffusion signal itself [15] and the application of rule-based methods [2].

Motivated by the recovery of fiber differential signatures using atlas-based methods in [8], we consider a new approach where moving frame analysis is combined with an intrinsic diffusion inpainting scheme that also allows for the inclusion of cardiac image priors. In contrast to [8] where only differential signatures were recovered, this new approach also recovers the local fiber direction, which is critical for most applications such as electromechanical modelling and guidance [2]. We demonstrate the use of our method for reconstruction in test settings simulating prototypical dMRI volumes and show that it achieves low error compared to other alternatives. Our key contributions include the development of a novel closed-form method for connection forms in 3D frame fields, and its use in a frame field inpainting scheme.

The paper is organized as follows. In Sect. 2 we review basic principles of cardiac fiber anatomy. In Sect. 3 we derive differential descriptors for three-dimensional frame fields, following which we present methods for computing them in Sect. 4 and a frame field inpainting scheme in Sect. 5. These tools are then adapted to reconstructing frame fields derived from cardiac dMRI data in Sect. 6. We conclude and review our main contributions in Sect. 7.

2   Cardiac Fiber Anatomy

To situate our work we provide a brief review of cardiac anatomy based on [13]. The heart is a hollow, fibromuscular organ with a truncated ellipsoidal shape. Its orientation is determined by a well-defined lower extremity, the *apex*, and an ill-defined upper part, the *base*. The heart can be divided in four distinct chambers: the left (LV) and right (RV) ventricles, a pair of synchronized valved muscular pumps, respectively connect with the left (LA) and the right (RA) atria. Structurally, the LV is considerably larger and thicker than the RV, since it pumps oxygenated blood to the entire body. The bulk of the heart muscle is called *myocardium*. It is principally composed of elongated muscle cells called *cardiomyocytes* which measure approximately 10–20 μm in diameter and 50–100 μm in length. Their primary function is to produce mechanical tension during ejection, but certain specialized cells also serve to conduct electrical activation of the heart muscle. Cardiomyocytes are densely and smoothly packed within a three-dimensional extracellular matrix principally made of connective tissue.

The term *myofiber* is often used as a proxy for localized parallel groups of cardiomyocytes, although they do not exist at a microscopic level. Histological and medical imaging studies have established certain key geometrical properties of cardiac myofibers: (1) they form a smoothly varying medium which wraps around each ventricle, (2) this wrapping generates the truncated ellipsoidal shape of the myocardium, (3) focusing on the LV, the *helix angle*, which is the angle of cardiomyocyte orientation taken with respect to the short-axis plane smoothly rotates from outer to inner wall by a total amount of approximately 120 degrees.

3   Moving Frames in $\mathbf{R}^3$

Let a point $\boldsymbol{x} = \sum_i x_i \boldsymbol{e}_i \in \mathbf{R}^3$ be expressed in terms of $\boldsymbol{e}_1, \boldsymbol{e}_2, \boldsymbol{e}_3$, the natural basis for $\mathbf{R}^3$. We define a right-handed orthonormal frame field $\boldsymbol{f}_1, \boldsymbol{f}_2, \boldsymbol{f}_3 : \mathbf{R}^3 \rightarrow \mathbf{R}^3$. Each frame axis can be expressed by the rigid rotation $\boldsymbol{f}_i = \sum_j a_{ij} \boldsymbol{e}_j$, where $A = \{a_{ij}\} \in \mathbf{R}^{3 \times 3}$ is a differentiable attitude matrix such that $A^{-1} = A^T$. Treating $\boldsymbol{f}_i$ and $\boldsymbol{e}_j$ as symbols, we can write [6]

$$[\boldsymbol{f}_1 \, \boldsymbol{f}_2 \, \boldsymbol{f}_3]^T = A \, [\boldsymbol{e}_1 \, \boldsymbol{e}_2 \, \boldsymbol{e}_3]^T. \tag{1}$$

Since each $\boldsymbol{e}_i$ is constant, the differential geometry of the frame field is completely characterized by A. Taking the exterior derivative on both sides, we have

$$\mathrm{d} [\boldsymbol{f}_1 \, \boldsymbol{f}_2 \, \boldsymbol{f}_3]^T = (\mathrm{d}A) \, A^{-1} [\boldsymbol{f}_1 \, \boldsymbol{f}_2 \, \boldsymbol{f}_3]^T = C \, [\boldsymbol{f}_1 \, \boldsymbol{f}_2 \, \boldsymbol{f}_3]^T, \tag{2}$$

where d denotes the exterior derivative, and $C = (\mathrm{d}A) \, A^{-1} = \{c_{ij}\} \in \mathbf{R}^{3 \times 3}$ is the Maurer-Cartan matrix of connection forms c_{ij}. Writing $\boldsymbol{f}_i$ as symbols, (2) is to be understood as $\mathrm{d}\boldsymbol{f}_i = \sum_j c_{ij} \boldsymbol{f}_j$. The Maurer-Cartan matrix is skew symmetric [6], hence we have

$$C = \begin{bmatrix} 0 & c_{12} & c_{13} \\ -c_{12} & 0 & c_{23} \\ -c_{13} & -c_{23} & 0 \end{bmatrix}, \tag{3}$$

such that there are at most 3 independent, non-zero 1-forms: c_{12}, c_{13}, and c_{23}. 1-forms operate on tangent vectors through a process denoted *contraction*, written as $\mathrm{d}w\langle \boldsymbol{v} \rangle \in \mathbf{R}$ for a general 1-form $\mathrm{d}w = \sum_i w_i \mathrm{d}e_i$ and tangent vector $\boldsymbol{v}$ on $\mathbf{R}^3$, which yields $\mathrm{d}w\langle \boldsymbol{v} \rangle = \sum_i w_i \mathrm{d}e_i \langle \sum_j v_j \boldsymbol{e}_j \rangle = \sum_i w_i v_i$, since $\mathrm{d}e_i \langle \boldsymbol{e}_j \rangle = \delta_{ij}$, where δ_{ij} is the Kronecker delta.

The space of linear models for smooth frame fields is fully parametrized by the 1-forms c_{ij}. This space can be explored by considering the motion of $\boldsymbol{f}_i$ in a direction $\boldsymbol{v} = \sum_k v_k \boldsymbol{f}_k$, using the first order terms of a Taylor series centered at $\boldsymbol{x}_0$:

$$\tilde{\boldsymbol{f}}_i(\boldsymbol{x}_0 + \boldsymbol{v}) = \boldsymbol{f}_i + \mathrm{d}\boldsymbol{f}_i\langle \boldsymbol{v} \rangle + \mathcal{O}(\|\boldsymbol{v}\|^2) \approx \boldsymbol{f}_i + \sum_{j \neq i} \boldsymbol{f}_j \sum_k v_k c_{ijk}, \tag{4}$$

where $\boldsymbol{f}_i$ and $\mathrm{d}\boldsymbol{f}_i$ are evaluated at $\boldsymbol{x}_0$, and $c_{ijk} \equiv c_{ij}\langle \boldsymbol{f}_k \rangle$ are the *connection forms* of the local frame. Since only 3 unique non-zero combinations of c_{ij} are possible, there are in total 9 connections c_{ijk}. These coefficients express the rate of turn of the frame vector $\boldsymbol{f}_i$ towards $\boldsymbol{f}_j$ when $\boldsymbol{x}$ moves in the direction $\boldsymbol{f}_k$. Figure 1 illustrates the behavior of the frame field described by c_{ijk}. For example, with $\boldsymbol{f}_1$ taken to be the local orientation of a fiber and $\boldsymbol{f}_3$ taken to be the component of the heart wall normal orthogonal to $\boldsymbol{f}_1$, c_{131} measures the circumferential curvature of a fiber and c_{123} measures the change in its helix angle [9].

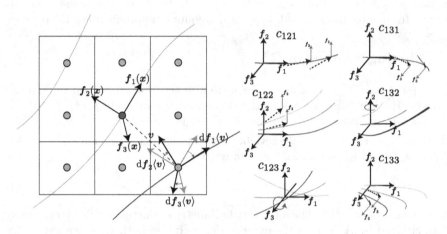

Fig. 1. (Left) Turning of frame axes at $\boldsymbol{x}$ expressed in the local basis $\boldsymbol{f}_1, \boldsymbol{f}_2, \boldsymbol{f}_3$ when $\boldsymbol{x}$ moves in the direction $\boldsymbol{v}$. (Right) frame field variation characterized by the connections c_{ijk} for $i = 1$ (c_{23k} are not shown).

4   Computation of Connection Forms

A first order generator for frame fields using (4) requires knowledge of the underlying connection forms c_{ijk}. We shall explore three ways of computing these: (1) a direct estimate based on finite differences, (2) a regularized optimization scheme, and (3) a novel closed-form computation which yields exact results on linear manifolds. In Sect. 4.4 we discuss conditions under which each method could be used, and later in Sect. 5 we use various combinations of these for inpainting 3D frame fields.

4.1   Connections via Finite Differentiation

In smooth frame fields, the connection 1-forms c_{ij} can be directly obtained using (2), i.e., $\mathrm{d}\boldsymbol{f}_i \cdot \boldsymbol{f}_k = \left(\sum_j^3 c_{ij}\boldsymbol{f}_j\right) \cdot \boldsymbol{f}_k = \sum_j^3 c_{ij}\delta_{jk} = c_{ik}$. The differentials $\mathrm{d}\boldsymbol{f}_i$ can be computed by applying the exterior derivative for a function, i.e., for the k'th component of $\boldsymbol{f}_i$, $\boldsymbol{f}_{ik} : \mathbf{R}^3 \to \mathbf{R}$, $\mathrm{d}\boldsymbol{f}_{ik} = \sum_l^3 \frac{\partial f_{ik}}{\partial x_l}\mathrm{d}e_l$,

$$\mathrm{d}\boldsymbol{f}_i \cdot \boldsymbol{f}_j \langle \boldsymbol{v} \rangle = \boldsymbol{f}_j^T \mathrm{d}\boldsymbol{f}_i \langle \boldsymbol{v} \rangle = \sum_k^3 \sum_l^3 f_{jk} \frac{\partial f_{ik}}{\partial x_l}\mathrm{d}e_l \langle \boldsymbol{v} \rangle = \boldsymbol{f}_j^T \mathbf{J}_i \boldsymbol{v}, \qquad (5)$$

where $\mathbf{J}_i = \left[\frac{\partial f_{ip}}{\partial x_q}\right] \in \mathbf{R}^{3\times 3}$ is the Jacobian matrix of partial derivatives of $\boldsymbol{f}_i$. Setting $\boldsymbol{v} = \boldsymbol{f}_k$, we obtain

$$c_{ijk} = \boldsymbol{f}_j^T \mathbf{J}_i \boldsymbol{f}_k. \tag{6}$$

The Jacobian matrix $\mathbf{J}_i$ can be approximated to first order using, e.g., finite differences on $\boldsymbol{f}_i$ with a spacing of size δx: $\frac{\partial f_{ij}}{\partial x_k}(\boldsymbol{x}) \approx \frac{f_{ij}(\boldsymbol{x}+e_k)-f_{ij}(\boldsymbol{x})}{\delta x}$.

4.2   Connections via Energy Minimization

The connection forms c_{ijk} at a point $\boldsymbol{x}_0$ can also be obtained as the minimizer of an extrapolation energy $\mathcal{E}$ contained within a neighborhood Ω:

$$c_{ijk}^*(\boldsymbol{x}_0) = \underset{c_{ijk}}{\arg\min}\, \mathcal{E}(\boldsymbol{x}_0, \Omega) + \lambda\,|c_{ijk}|, \tag{7}$$

where λ is a regularization weight used to penalize high curvature. Denoting $\tilde{\boldsymbol{f}}_i$ as the normalized approximation to $\boldsymbol{f}_i$ at $\boldsymbol{x}_0 + \boldsymbol{v}$ using (4), we follow [8] and choose $\mathcal{E}$ to minimize the angular error between $\tilde{\boldsymbol{f}}_i$ and $\boldsymbol{f}_i$: $\mathcal{E}(\boldsymbol{x}_0, \Omega) = \frac{1}{|\Omega|}\sum_{v\in\Omega}\sum_i^3 \varepsilon_i(\boldsymbol{x}_0 + \boldsymbol{v})$, with $\varepsilon_i(\boldsymbol{x}_0 + \boldsymbol{v}) = \arccos\left(\boldsymbol{f}_i(\boldsymbol{x}_0 + \boldsymbol{v})\cdot\tilde{\boldsymbol{f}}_i(\boldsymbol{x}_0 + \boldsymbol{v})\right)$.

4.3   Closed-Form Connections in Linear Space

A disadvantage of using the previous energy minimization approach is that coupling between the connections c_{ijk} is not explicitly enforced, i.e., the requirement that $c_{ij}\langle\boldsymbol{v}\rangle = \sum_k c_{ijk}v_k$. Thus it may lead to non-integrable differential descriptors. We now develop a novel way of computing connection forms that is based on trigonometrical considerations in the first-order structure of 3D frame fields and which enforces that coupling. This method also provides exact c_{ijk} measurements in manifolds that have low second-order curvatures ($\mathrm{d}^2\boldsymbol{f}_i \to 0$). Given a local basis $\boldsymbol{f}_i$ and data-driven neighboring bases $\boldsymbol{f}_i(\boldsymbol{v}\in\Omega)$, the 1-forms $c_{ij}\langle\boldsymbol{v}\rangle$ can be solved for using linear least-squares. We begin by expanding (4),

$$\boldsymbol{f}_i(\boldsymbol{v}) = \boldsymbol{f}_i + c_{ij}\langle\boldsymbol{v}\rangle\boldsymbol{f}_j + c_{ik}\langle\boldsymbol{v}\rangle\boldsymbol{f}_k \tag{8}$$

and analyze this expression geometrically using Fig. 2. Let $\boldsymbol{f}_i^j(\boldsymbol{v})$ denote the projection of $\boldsymbol{f}_i(\boldsymbol{v})$ in the $\boldsymbol{f}_i$-$\boldsymbol{f}_j$ plane, i.e., $\boldsymbol{f}_i^j(\boldsymbol{v}) = \boldsymbol{f}_i(\boldsymbol{v})-(\boldsymbol{f}_i(\boldsymbol{v})\cdot\boldsymbol{f}_k)\boldsymbol{f}_k$, $k \in (1,2,3) \neq i \neq j$, and let $\theta_{ij}(\boldsymbol{v})$ denote the *signed angle* between $\boldsymbol{f}_i$ and $\boldsymbol{f}_i^j(\boldsymbol{v})$ with positive values assigned to $\theta_{ij}(\boldsymbol{v})$ rotating $\boldsymbol{f}_i$ towards $\boldsymbol{f}_j$, obtained as

$$\theta_{ij}(\boldsymbol{v}) = \mathrm{sgn}\left(\boldsymbol{f}_i^j(\boldsymbol{v})\cdot\boldsymbol{f}_j\right)\cdot\arccos\left(\left|\boldsymbol{f}_i\cdot\boldsymbol{f}_i^j(\boldsymbol{v})/\|\boldsymbol{f}_i^j(\boldsymbol{v})\|\right|\right). \tag{9}$$

Using trigonometry, we obtain

$$\tan\left(\theta_{ij}(\boldsymbol{v})\right) = \frac{c_{ij}\langle\boldsymbol{v}\rangle}{\|\boldsymbol{f}_i\|} = c_{ij}\langle\boldsymbol{v}\rangle \quad \text{since } \boldsymbol{f}_i \text{ is a unit vector.} \tag{10}$$

Expanding the contraction $c_{ij} \langle v \rangle$:

$$c_{ij} \langle v \rangle = (v \cdot f_1) c_{ij1} + (v \cdot f_2) c_{ij2} + (v \cdot f_3) c_{ij3} \tag{11}$$

$$= v_1 c_{ij1} + v_2 c_{ij2} + v_3 c_{ij3} \quad \text{with } v_k \equiv v \cdot f_k \tag{12}$$

$$\Rightarrow \begin{bmatrix} c_{12} \langle v \rangle & c_{13} \langle v \rangle & c_{23} \langle v \rangle \end{bmatrix} = \begin{bmatrix} v_1 & v_2 & v_3 \end{bmatrix} \begin{bmatrix} c_{121} & c_{131} & c_{231} \\ c_{122} & c_{132} & c_{232} \\ c_{123} & c_{133} & c_{233} \end{bmatrix} \tag{13}$$

and substituting in (10), we get a linear system in the 9 unknowns c_{ijk}:

$$\begin{bmatrix} v_1 \\ v_2 \\ v_3 \end{bmatrix}^T \begin{bmatrix} c_{121} & c_{131} & c_{231} \\ c_{122} & c_{132} & c_{232} \\ c_{123} & c_{133} & c_{233} \end{bmatrix} = \begin{bmatrix} \tan(\theta_{12}(v)) \\ \tan(\theta_{13}(v)) \\ \tan(\theta_{23}(v)) \end{bmatrix}^T . \tag{14}$$

Aggregating n measurements $v_i \in \Omega(x)$, we have

$$\underbrace{\begin{bmatrix} v_{11} & v_{12} & v_{13} \\ & \vdots & \\ v_{i1} & v_{i2} & v_{i3} \\ & \vdots & \\ v_{n1} & v_{n2} & v_{n3} \end{bmatrix}}_{V \in \mathbf{R}^{n \times 3}} \underbrace{\begin{bmatrix} c_{121} & c_{131} & c_{231} \\ c_{122} & c_{132} & c_{232} \\ c_{123} & c_{133} & c_{233} \end{bmatrix}}_{C \in \mathbf{R}^{3 \times 3}} = \underbrace{\begin{bmatrix} \tan(\theta_{12}(v_1)) & \tan(\theta_{13}(v_1)) & \tan(\theta_{23}(v_1)) \\ & \vdots & \\ \tan(\theta_{12}(v_i)) & \tan(\theta_{13}(v_i)) & \tan(\theta_{23}(v_i)) \\ & \vdots & \\ \tan(\theta_{12}(v_n)) & \tan(\theta_{13}(v_n)) & \tan(\theta_{23}(v_n)) \end{bmatrix}}_{\tilde{C} \in \mathbf{R}^{n \times 3}} \tag{15}$$

We need $n \geq 3$ otherwise the system will be undetermined. In general, $v_i \cdot v_j \neq 0$ such that V is not full row rank. A QR factorization or singular value decomposition (SVD) pseudoinverse can be used to solve for $C = \left(V^T V \right)^{-1} V^T \tilde{C}$.

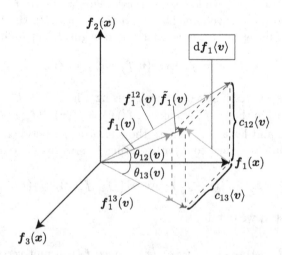

Fig. 2. Differential of the frame axis $f_1(x)$ expressed in local coordinates.

4.4   Method Comparison

We compare the three previous methods by computing mean connection forms along with fitting errors in a neighborhood containing 50 K voxels in Fig. 3. The frame field data is from a healthy rat heart, taken from [12], where f_1 is the fiber direction, f_3 is approximately normal to the heart wall, and $f_2 = f_3 \times f_1$. For the energy-minimizing approach we experimented with Nelder-Mead (NM) and BOBYQA (BQ) [10] optimizers[1] to solve the energy term in (7). Here, all connection forms are estimated in an isotropic neighborhood of size 3^3, seeds are obtained using (6), and $\lambda = 0.0001$. On an SSD quad-core 2.5 GHz machine, fitting 1 k voxels takes about 3 ms using finite differentiation, 100 ms using 200 Nelder-Mead iterations, 30 ms using closed-form estimation, and 1 s using BOBYQA optimization. Seeded NM computations converge faster than unseeded, and reach comparable values at about 150 iterations. BOBYQA yields a slightly lower error but is impractical due its large time complexity. Our closed-form method yields a slightly larger global error than both optimizers beyond 100 iterations but has the advantage of being considerably faster, and, unlike the other methods, offers the theoretical advantage of enforcing integrability of the reconstructed frame field while being exact to first order.

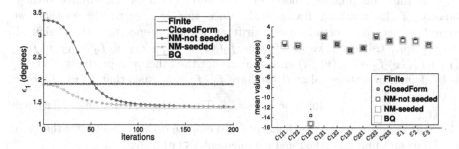

Fig. 3. (Left) Mean f_1 fitting error ϵ_1 (radians), and (right) mean connection forms and errors (radians) for different c_{ijk} estimation techniques in 50 k voxels.

5   Frame Field Reconstruction

We now describe our frame field inpainting procedure. Here, Ω is a region where frame field data is available, and A is a reconstruction domain. Starting with $A^0 = A$, each iteration propagates information on the boundary ∂A^n such that $\partial A^{n+1} = \partial A^n \oplus B_r$ is eroded with a ball element B_r of radius $r = 1$ and c_{ijk} is updated in Ω and ∂A^{n+1} until $A^{n+1} = \emptyset$. Frames f_i are transported from $x \in \partial A^n$ in a direction v across ∂A using a neighbor accumulation of (4),

$$\tilde{f}_i^{n+1}|_{x+v} = \sum_{x \in \partial A^n} (f_i^n|_x + \sum_{j \neq i} f_j^n|_x \sum_k c_{ijk}(x+v) \cdot f_k^n|_x), \qquad (16)$$

---

[1] See [10] for these and other optimization strategies.

which is then normalized. c_{ijk} at $x \in \partial A^n$ are obtained by combining the methods described in Sect. 4, using the following heuristics[2], where $\kappa = \|V^{-1}\|_F \|V\|_F$ is the condition number of V in (15) and F is the Frobenius norm:

$$c_{ijk}(x) = \begin{cases} \text{Closed-form of (15)} : x \text{ has } > N \text{ neighbors, and } \kappa < \kappa_0 \\ \text{Energy of (7) with } \lambda = 0.0001 \text{ and seeding with (6)} : \text{else,} \end{cases} \quad (17)$$

where $N = \frac{1}{2}(2r+1)^3$ and $\kappa_0 = 3$ were determined empirically and offer a good tradeoff between neighborhood connectivity and well-conditioning of V, although these should be tailored to the application at hand. Unrealistically large c_{ijk} values can still arise in spite of the regularization. To see this, make $f_1(x+v)$ parallel to $f_2(x)$ in a neighboring voxel. Using (4), we have $\tilde{f}_1(v) \approx f_1 + c_{12}\langle v\rangle f_2 + c_{13}\langle v\rangle f_3$, such that $f_1(v)\backslash\backslash f_2 \Rightarrow c_{12}\langle v\rangle \to \infty$. When necessary, we thus apply a hard threshold on $\mathcal{E}$ and c_{ijk} in (17). We set $c_{ijk} = 0$ if $\mathcal{E} > \frac{\pi}{4}$, or if c_{ijk} exceeds bounds obtained as follows. Using discrete forward differences, the frame differential $df_i = d(f_{i1}e_1 + f_{i2}e_2 + f_{i3}e_3)$ is bounded since $\left|\frac{\partial f_i}{\partial x_k}\right| \approx \frac{1}{2}|f_{ij}(x+e_k) - f_{ij}(x)| \leq 1$ and $\|f_i\| = 1$. Thus, $|c_{ij}\langle v\rangle| = |f_j^T \, \mathcal{J}_{f_i}(x_1, x_2, x_3) \, v| \leq f_j^T \cdot [\|v\|_1 \|v\|_1 \|v\|_1]^T \leq \|v\|_1$, and $c_{ijk} = \min(c_{ijk}, \|v\|_1)$.

The diffusion process guided by (16) and (17) does not enforce orthogonality of the resulting frame field. Since this is a first-order method we expect to see some orthogonality drift as we get deeper into the region A. To see this, using (8) we get $f_1(v) \cdot f_2(v) = (f_1 + c_{12}\langle v\rangle f_2 + c_{13}\langle v\rangle f_3) \cdot (f_2 + c_{21}\langle v\rangle f_1 + c_{23}\langle v\rangle f_3)$ and similarly for the other axis products. Since f_i is by definition orthogonal at 0, we have $f_i \cdot f_j = \delta_{ij}$ such that $f_i(v) \cdot f_j(v) = \begin{cases} 1 + c_{ij}^2 + c_{ik}^2 : i = j \\ c_{ik}c_{jk} \quad : i \neq j \end{cases}$ for $k \neq i, k \neq j$. The extrapolated frame $f_i(v)$ will therefore never be exactly orthonormal. To enforce orthonormality we therefore fix $f_1(v)$ and find its orthogonal complement $f_2^\perp(v)$ using

$$f_2^\perp(v) = f_2 - (f_1(v) \cdot f_2(v))f_1(v) \quad (18)$$
$$= (-c_{12} - c_{13}c_{23})f_1 + (1 - c_{13}c_{23}c_{12})f_2 + (c_{23} - c_{13}^2 c_{23})f_3, \quad (19)$$

where c_{ij} is taken as $c_{ij}\langle v\rangle$. We proceed similarly for $f_3^\perp(v)$.

6 Application to Cardiac Fiber Reconstruction

Given a partial volume Ω of fiber orientations f_1 in a mask H of the heart, we now explore the problem of reconstructing f_1 everywhere in $A = H - \Omega$.

6.1 Rule-Based Orientation Priors

Our inpainting procedure is guided by rule-based priors for fiber orientations based on H and estimated heart wall normals: one relating to the circumferential arrangement of myofibers and the other to their helix angle turning.

---

[2] When Jacobian matrix computations are available using a combination of backward, central, and forward differences, we seed (7) using (6) which improves convergence.

Estimating the Circumferential Component. Using a smoothing kernel G_σ, the Euclidean distance transforms $G_\sigma * D_+$ and $G_\sigma * D_-$ to the outer and inner walls are first computed. From the average $D = \frac{1}{2}(D_+ - D_-)$ local wall normal directions are computed using $\hat{f}_3 = \nabla D$. The apex ξ_0 and an upward unit direction as $\hat{u}$ are identified, and used to obtain heart centerline measurements ξ_t parametrized over t steps along $\hat{u}$, $\xi_t = \frac{\sum_x w(x)\Xi(x)x}{\sum_x w(x)\Xi(x)}$, where $\Xi(x) = \mathrm{sgn}\left(|(x - \xi_0 - t\hat{u}) \cdot \hat{u}|\right)$, i.e., $\Xi(x)$ is 1 in the current short axis plane and 0 elsewhere, and $w(x)$ is 1 if x is in the myocardium and is 0 otherwise. A smooth heart centerline is then obtained as $L(t) = G_\sigma * \xi_t$. We can now obtain a local long-axis direction f_L using $f_L = \frac{\partial L(t)}{\partial t}$ and finally estimate the circumferential direction f_c from the cross product of f_L and the local wall normal $\hat{f}_3$ as $f_c = f_L \times f_3$.

Estimating the Helical Component. We use a rule-based helix angle variation prior from α^+ to α^- from outer to inner wall, similarly to the work of [2]. A voxel x is first parametrized over the local depth of the heart wall in the range $[0, 1]$, where 0 indicates that the voxel is lying on the outer wall and 1 on the inner wall, using $\gamma(x) = \frac{D_+}{D_+ + D_-}(x) = \left(1 + D_- D_+^{-1}\right)^{-1}(x) \in [0, 1]$. Then, the local

Table 1. Reconstructed volumes and errors using our frame inpainting for (left) a damaged portion of a rat short axis slab, and (right) a sparse (93 % damage) rule-based synthetic field (without rule-based priors). In comparison, vector interpolation yields $(20.6 \pm 10.7, 4.5 \pm 5.3)$, vector diffusion yields $(18.6 \pm 9.9, 3.7 \pm 3.5)$, and rule-based yields $(14.66 \pm 4.8, -)$ degrees respectively for ϵ_1(a,b). Color-coding is based on the helix angle, from -90 (blue) to $+90$ (red) degrees (Color figure online).

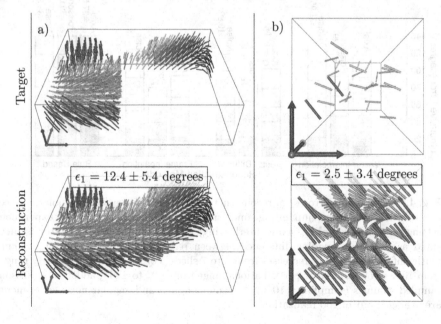

Table 2. (Top) Mean angular reconstruction error ϵ_1 between reconstructed fibers and the ground truth (top) for increasingly Poisson-sparse volumes (s is the percentage of available data) using our frame inpainting methods. 100 realizations were performed, one of which is shown. (Bottom) Reconstruction for increasingly interleaved volumes (s is the number of slices available), in a long-axis cutout. Available data slices are marked with blue arrows (Color figure online).

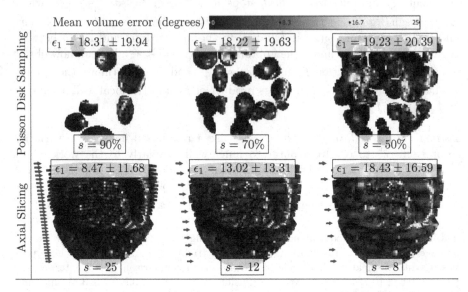

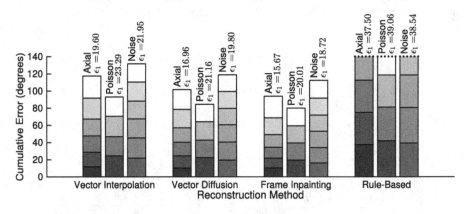

Fig. 4. Mean volume error ϵ_1 of reconstruction (degrees) for vector interpolation, vector diffusion, our frame inpainting, and rule-based methods, for various experiment settings: Poisson sampling, axial interleaving, and angular noise. The error is measured as the mean angular difference between reconstructed fibers and the ground truth. Interleaving values increases from 2 to 7 slices; Poisson sampling sparsity ranges from 10 % to 50 %; angular perturbations range from $\pm 2°$ to $\pm 11°$, added to a Poisson-sampled volumes (sampling = 10 %). Poisson sampling and angular noise experiments are averaged out of 100 realizations.

helix angle at x is linearly interpolated using $\alpha(x) = (\alpha_+ - \gamma\alpha_+ + \gamma\alpha_-)(x)$. Finally, the helix fiber direction $\hat{f}_1$ is obtained using a helical rotation of f_c about the local transmural axis $\hat{f}_3$ from the axis angle $\langle \hat{f}_3, \alpha \rangle$ using Rodrigues' formula, $\hat{f}_1 = \cos\alpha f_c + \sin\alpha(\hat{f}_3 \times f_c) + (1 - \cos\alpha)(\hat{f}_3 \cdot f_c)\hat{f}_3$.

Coupling Rule-based Prior and Diffusion. Each diffusion pass $n+1$ combines current frame field estimates $\tilde{f}_i$, differentials df_i and rule-based priors $\hat{f}_i$ using

$$\tilde{f}_1^{n+1} = \phi_1 f_1(x) + (1 - \phi_1) \sum_{y \in \partial A} \left(\tilde{f}_1^{\,n} + c_{12} \langle v \rangle \tilde{f}_2^{\,n} + c_{13} \langle v \rangle \tilde{f}_3^{\,n} \right)$$

$$\tilde{f}_3^{n+1} = \phi_3 \left(\hat{f}_3 - \left(\hat{f}_3 \cdot \tilde{f}_1^{\,n} \right) \tilde{f}_1^{\,n} \right) + (1 - \phi_3)\tilde{f}_3^{\,n}(x), \quad \tilde{f}_2^{n+1} = \tilde{f}_3^{n+1} \times \tilde{f}_1^{n+1}.$$

Here, $v = x - y$, $\partial\Omega(x)$ denotes the current (diffused) boundary around x from which data is inpainted, and $\phi_1 = 0.1$ and $\phi_3 = 0.7$ are prior weights determined empirically. The higher the confidence in the rule-based model, the larger these coefficients should be. Each $\tilde{f}_i^{\,n+1}$ is normalized after each diffusion pass.

6.2 Experiments

Damaged diffusion volumes were simulated using Poisson disk stochastic sampling, where each sample point p satisfies a minimum distance constraint to others. At p, an ellipsoid with random semi-axis lengths (range = 1 to 10 voxels) is carved out. A prototypical synthetic *in vivo* mask was also obtained by regularly slicing H along its long-axis. We applied these corruptions to a dMRI volume of a healthy rat heart from [12]. We compared our frame inpainting method against a standard vector interpolation scheme based on spatial distance weighting, against a pure vector diffusion scheme using (16) with $c_{ijk} = 0$, and against a ruled-based model similar to [2] and described in Sect. 6.1. We also tested robustness to noise by combining Poisson sampling (10 % sparsity) and random angular perturbations to f_1, prior to reconstruction. Table 1 shows the reconstruction of cardiac fibers in a short axis slab near the mid-section from which a chunk of tissue was removed, and from a synthetic transmural cardiac sample obtained using a rule-based helix angle variation (total turning 120 degrees). Our reconstruction method shows a significantly reduced angular error compared to other methods. Table 2 shows Poisson and slicing error maps using our method. Error increases with the amount of damage, and is higher near boundaries. Figure 4 shows that our frame inpainting outperforms compared methods in minimizing the reconstruction error in all corruption scenarios, and also shows comparable robustness to noise.

7 Conclusion

We proposed a cardiac fiber inpainting method based on the theory of moving frames, which makes use of a novel closed-form computation for connection forms in 3D frame fields, and incorporates rule-based cardiac priors. We demonstrated its use by recovering fiber orientations in highly sparse and damaged volumes, and showed that it achieves low error compared to other alternatives, and is robust to noise. We anticipate that the application of these tools could aid computer-assisted guidance and repair of damaged heart walls, and the super-resolution of fiber volumes. Future work includes validation with real *in vivo* beating hearts, and extending our work with higher order and temporal parameterizations of connection forms along with the development of atlas-based cardiac differential priors.

References

1. Athanasuleas, C.L., Buckberg, G.D., Stanley, A.W., Siler, W., Dor, V., Di Donato, M., Menicanti, L., de Oliveira, S.A., Beyersdorf, F., Kron, I.L., et al.: Surgical ventricular restoration in the treatment of congestive heart failure due to post-infarction ventricular dilation. J. Am. Coll. Cardiol. **44**(7), 1439–1445 (2004)
2. Bayer, J., Blake, R., Plank, G., Trayanova, N.: A novel rule-based algorithm for assigning myocardial fiber orientation to computational heart models. Ann. Biomed. Eng. **40**(10), 2243–2254 (2012)
3. Boutin, M., Bazin, P.L.: Structure from motion: a new look from the point of view of invariant theory. SIAM J. Appl. Math. **64**(4), 1156–1174 (2004)
4. Calabi, E., Olver, P.J., Shakiban, C., Tannenbaum, A., Haker, S.: Differential and numerically invariant signature curves applied to object recognition. Int. J. Comput. Vis. **26**(2), 107–135 (1998)
5. Faugeras, O.: Cartan's moving frame method and its application to the geometry and evolution of curves in the euclidean, affine and projective planes. In: Mundy, J.L., Zisserman, A., Forsyth, D. (eds.) AICV 1994. LNCS, vol. 825, pp. 9–46. Springer, Heidelberg (1994)
6. Flanders, H.: Differential Forms with Applications to the Physical Sciences. Courier Dover Publications, Mineola (2012)
7. Flash, T., Handzel, A.A.: Affine differential geometry analysis of human arm movements. Biol. Cybern. **96**(6), 577–601 (2007)
8. Piuze, E., Lombaert, H., Sporring, J., Siddiqi, K.: Cardiac fiber inpainting using cartan forms. In: Mori, K., Sakuma, I., Sato, Y., Barillot, C., Navab, N. (eds.) MICCAI 2013, Part II. LNCS, vol. 8150, pp. 509–517. Springer, Heidelberg (2013)
9. Piuze, E., Sporring, J., Siddiqi, K.: Moving frames for heart fiber geometry. In: Gee, J.C., Joshi, S., Pohl, K.M., Wells, W.M., Zöllei, L. (eds.) IPMI 2013. LNCS, vol. 7917, pp. 524–535. Springer, Heidelberg (2013)
10. Rios, L.M., Sahinidis, N.V.: Derivative-free optimization: a review of algorithms and comparison of software implementations. J. Global Optim. **56**(3), 1247–1293 (2013)
11. Sapiro, G.: Geometric Partial Differential Equations and Image Analysis. Cambridge University Press, Cambridge (2006)
12. Savadjiev, P., Strijkers, G.J., Bakermans, A.J., Piuze, E., Zucker, S.W., Siddiqi, K.: Heart wall myofibers are arranged in minimal surfaces to optimize organ function. Proc. Nat. Acad. Sci. U.S.A. **109**(24), 9248–9253 (2012)
13. Sengupta, P.P., Korinek, J., Belohlavek, M., Narula, J., Vannan, M.A., Jahangir, A., Khandheria, B.K.: Left ventricular structure and function: basic science for cardiac imaging. J. Am. Coll. Cardiol. **48**(10), 1988–2001 (2006)

14. Song, K., Nam, Y.J., Luo, X., Qi, X., Tan, W., Huang, G.N., Acharya, A., Smith, C.L., Tallquist, M.D., Neilson, E.G., et al.: Heart repair by reprogramming non-myocytes with cardiac transcription factors. Nature 485(7400), 599–604 (2012)

15. Toussaint, N., Sermesant, M., Stoeck, C.T., Kozerke, S., Batchelor, P.G.: In vivo human 3D cardiac fibre architecture: reconstruction using curvilinear interpolation of diffusion tensor images. In: Jiang, T., Navab, N., Pluim, J.P.W., Viergever, M.A. (eds.) MICCAI 2010 Part I. LNCS, vol. 6361, pp. 418–425. Springer, Heidelberg (2010)

Detail-Preserving PET Reconstruction with Sparse Image Representation and Anatomical Priors

Jieqing Jiao[1]([✉]), Pawel Markiewicz[1], Ninon Burgos[1], David Atkinson[2], Brian Hutton[3], Simon Arridge[4], and Sebastien Ourselin[1,5]

[1] Translational Imaging Group, CMIC, University College London, London, UK
jieqing.jiao@gmail.com
[2] Centre for Medical Imaging, University College London, London, UK
[3] Institute of Nuclear Medicine, University College London, London, UK
[4] Centre for Medical Image Computing, University College London, London, UK
[5] Dementia Research Centre, Institute of Neurology,
University College London, London, UK

Abstract. Positron emission tomography (PET) reconstruction is an ill-posed inverse problem which typically involves fitting a high-dimensional forward model of the imaging process to noisy, and sometimes undersampled photon emission data. To improve the image quality, prior information derived from anatomical images of the same subject has been previously used in the penalised maximum likelihood (PML) method to regularise the model complexity and selectively smooth the image on a voxel basis in PET reconstruction. In this work, we propose a novel perspective of incorporating the prior information by exploring the sparse property of natural images. Instead of a regular voxel grid, the sparse image representation jointly determined by the prior image and the PET data is used in reconstruction to leverage between the image details and smoothness, and this prior is integrated into the PET forward model and has a closed-form expectation maximisation (EM) solution. Simulations show that the proposed approach achieves improved bias versus variance trade-off and higher contrast recovery than the current state-of-the-art methods, and preserves the image details better. Application to clinical PET data shows promising results.

Keywords: PET · Image reconstruction · Image prior · Supervoxels · EM

1 Introduction

Position Emission Tomography (PET) is a unique *in vivo* functional imaging technique which provides the most sensitive non-invasive molecular assay of human body. The photons emitted from radioactively labelled molecules (tracer) in a subject are collected by the PET detectors. With the photon data, the spatio-temporal distribution of the tracer can be estimated by image reconstruction.

© Springer International Publishing Switzerland 2015
S. Ourselin et al. (Eds.): IPMI 2015, LNCS 9123, pp. 540–551, 2015.
DOI: 10.1007/978-3-319-19992-4_42

The PET image reconstruction can be considered as a problem of fitting a high-dimensional model (in terms of the number of unknowns, for example the intensity values of millions of voxels in a modern PET scanner) to noisy projection data where the photon emission is a random process greatly affected by the amount of tracer reached to the imaging target. The measured projection data can be highly undersampled due to the detector configuration when there are only a fraction of counts collected by the scanner (which is the motivation for developing the ultra-sensitive total-body PET scanner http://explorer.ucdavis.edu/). The fitting of a high-dimensional forward model to this undersampled and noisy data would result in overfitting of the noise and unreliable image reconstruction.

Given this ill-posed problem of PET image reconstruction with low-count projection data, in the maximum likelihood (ML) PET reconstruction framework, penalised likelihood (PL) reconstruction (or equivalently maximum *a posteriori*, *MAP*) has been extensively studied [1–7]. Such methods involve adding a regularisation (penalty) term to the log likelihood function, and thus the effective forward model complexity can be controlled by changing the weight of this regularisation. Ideally the effective complexity should be reduced to match the size of the measured data to avoid overfitting. However the appropriate model complexity is usually unknown for a particular clinical task, and this is a general problem of using penalised likelihood framework. Two other problems are how to formulate the penalty model and how to solve the corresponding MAP problem. When there is no regularisation, the ML problem can be solved by the expectation maximisation (EM) algorithm iteratively with a closed form update equation [8]. For some of the penalty models, the optimisation transfer technique can be applied to derive a closed form update from the surrogate functions of the original penalised likelihood function [9]. However such penalty models are usually not edge-preserving and would result in undesirable oversmooth on the edges and fine features in the image. When the closed-form solution does not exist, a modified EM solution may be found for some of the penalty models. The one-step-late (OSL) algorithm [1] gives one such solution by using the gradient of the penalty term evaluated at the previous image estimation, however OSL does not guarantee convergence or non-negativity, depending on the penalty and penalty weight. Realistic penalty models which preserve the image details are usually non-smooth and non-convex, making the optimisation mathematically and computationally challenging. Among the penalty models, anatomical images acquired by high-resolution magnetic resonance (MR) or X-ray computed tomography (CT) from the same subject are considered useful, as they provide the prior information on the underlying structures. Recent reviews on using anatomical prior information for PET image reconstruction can be found in [5,6,10], and the Bowsher method [4] which encourages PET image smoothness over the neighbour voxels selected from the anatomical image, was found to achieve better performance while being relatively efficient computationally compared to other methods [5]. Apart from the penalised likelihood PET reconstruction frameworks, very recently an alternative perspective of using the image-derived prior was proposed in [11], by incorporating the prior information into the image representation via kernel functions, and the regularisation was applied to the PET forward model. This leads to a very elegant kernelised EM solution and achieves better performance.

In this work, we propose a novel perspective on constraining the ill-posed PET reconstruction with low-count projection data by exploring the sparsity in natural images [12,13]. Instead of using a regular voxel grid, the PET image is represented by a reduced number of supervoxels of various sizes and shapes so that the complexity of the PET forward model (in terms of the number of unknowns) is reduced to match the low-count data. The sparse image representation is jointly derived from the anatomical prior image and the PET data, preserving the edges and anatomical details without degradation of the structures only present in the PET image. This approach can be considered as a segmentation-based reconstruction method which is potentially able to eliminate the partial volume effect and it is more flexible than the method proposed in [3]. The prior information is integrated in the image representation as in [11], and therefore the regularisation operates in the forward model instead of in the additive penalty term, so the reconstruction is directly solved by the EM algorithm. Experiments using simulated and clinical data show promising results.

2   Methods

2.1   Sparse Image Representation Using Supervoxels

Supervoxels can be defined as an over-segmentation of an image into perceptually meaningful regions that preserves the image details. Using such supervoxels instead of the voxels defined on a regular grid leads to a more compact and sparse image representation which greatly reduces the image redundancy with little loss of the details. A visual demonstration of this concept can be found in [14].

In this work the supervoxel clustering was conducted using the *simple linear iterative clustering* (SLIC) method proposed in [15] for its computational efficiency and good performance to adhere to boundaries. The supervoxels were generated by an adapted k-means clustering of the voxels (with limited search region instead of the whole image) based on multi-dimensional Euclidean distance $D_{i,j}$ between two points i and j in the image domain, defined by

$$D_{i,j} = \sqrt{d_f^2 + \left(\frac{d_s}{S}\right)^2 m^2}, \tag{1}$$

$$d_s = \sqrt{(x_i - x_j)^2 + (y_i - y_j)^2 + (z_i - z_j)^2},$$

$$d_f = \sqrt{(f_i - f_j)^2},$$

where d_s is the spatial Euclidean distance, d_f is the image intensity similarity, and these two different measures are combined into a single one with $S = \sqrt[3]{(N/K)}$ (N the number of voxels and K the number of supervoxels) being the mean spatial distance within a supervoxel as a normalisation factor, and m being a weight between the intensity similarity and spatial proximity. Note that the intensity similarity d_f can be extended to include additional dimensions when there are a group of images or multi-channel information for clustering.

It can be seen that SLIC does not explicitly enforce connectivity, therefore in this work, connected-component labelling [16] was performed after SLIC supervoxel clustering to assign the originally disconnected groups of voxels within the same supervoxel to new supervoxels where all the voxels within the same supervoxel are spatially connected. Also the supervoxels generated by SLIC of extremely small size due to image noise were considered as "orphans" and were merged into the nearest supervoxels.

The over-segmentation generated by the supervoxel clustering leads to a sparse image representation when the number of supervoxels K is greatly smaller than the number of voxels N. Let $\mathbf{A}$ denote the representation matrix in the image domain, $\mathbf{A}$ is binary and sparse, which determines whether a voxel i belongs to a given supervoxel j, that is

$$A_{i,j} = \begin{cases} 1, & i \in j \\ 0, & i \notin j. \end{cases}$$

Then from the supervoxel intensity values s, the original image f on the voxel grid can be established by $f = \mathbf{A}s$ where $f \in \mathbb{R}^{N \times 1}$ and $s \in \mathbb{R}^{K \times 1}$. In PET reconstruction, using the image representation $f = \mathbf{A}s$ with a given $\mathbf{A}$ (not a square matrix) transfers the reconstruction of the original image f to the estimation of s with less number of the unknowns when $K < N$, without losing the image details preserved in $\mathbf{A}$. The joint determination of $\mathbf{A}$ from both the anatomical prior images and the PET data will be discussed in Sect. 2.3. Notably, in contrary to embedding the anatomical information within a Bayesian reconstruction framework based on solely the image intensity such as joint entropy or mutual information, the proposed method avoids the potential bias by using the image geometry instead.

2.2   PET Reconstruction with Sparse Image Representation

The sparse image representation can be directly integrated into the forward model of PET reconstruction

$$\bar{g} = \mathbf{PA}s + r, \tag{2}$$

where $\bar{g}$ is the expected projection data, $\mathbf{P}$ is the system information matrix of the detection probabilities, and r is the expected scatter and random events.

Within the maximum likelihood (ML) reconstruction framework, the estimate of the image f (here $f = \mathbf{A}s$) is found by maximising the Poisson log likelihood [17]

$$L(g|\bar{g}) = \sum_i g_i \log \bar{g}_i - \bar{g}_i \tag{3}$$

with observed projection data g

$$\hat{s} = \arg\max_{s \geq 0} L(g|\mathbf{A}s). \tag{4}$$

The iterative update to find the solution can be directly derived by the expectation-maximisation (EM) algorithm [8]

$$s^{n+1} = \frac{s^n}{\mathbf{A}^T\mathbf{P}^T\mathbf{1}}\mathbf{A}^T\mathbf{P}^T\frac{g}{\mathbf{PA}s^n + r}, \tag{5}$$

where T denotes the matrix transpose and n denotes the iteration number.

With prior images, it is possible to have the sparse image representation matrix $\mathbf{A}$ defined on a denser voxel grid that does not match the PET imaging system characterised by $\mathbf{P}$. Instead of downsampling the prior images to match the PET imaging resolution, in this work a resampling operator is introduced into the forward model to maintain the image at higher spatial resolution to avoid the loss of the edges and other image details. Let $\mathbf{R}$ denote the matrix form of the resampling operator in the image domain, then the forward model becomes $\bar{g} = \mathbf{PRA}s + r$, and the iterative update becomes

$$s^{n+1} = \frac{s^n}{\mathbf{A}^T\mathbf{R}^T\mathbf{P}^T\mathbf{1}}\mathbf{A}^T\mathbf{R}^T\mathbf{P}^T\frac{g}{\mathbf{PRA}s^n + r}. \tag{6}$$

So far it has been demonstrated the use of the sparse image representation in reconstructing PET images. For dynamic PET data, directly reconstruct the parametric images from the raw projection data can achieve improved accuracy and robustness [9,18,19]. The sparse image representation is directly applicable to dynamic PET data as it is a linear operation in the image domain. For dynamic PET data, the sparse representation matrix $\mathbf{A}$ is consistent for all time frames, and in $f = \mathbf{A}s$, f and s are expanded so that $f \in \mathbb{R}^{N \times nt}$ and $s \in \mathbb{R}^{K \times nt}$ where nt is the number of time frames. Using a linearised kinetic model [20], s can be described as $s = \theta\mathbf{B}$, where $\mathbf{B} \in \mathbb{R}^{nk \times nt}$ are the temporal basis functions and $\theta \in \mathbb{R}^{K \times nk}$ are the kinetic parameters for all supervoxels, with nk being the number of kinetic parameters for each supervoxel. The direct estimation of the kinetic parameters θ can be solved by applying the optimisation transfer technique [9] to obtain a closed-form update equation with improved convergence performance.

2.3   Aggregation of Multi-layer Supervoxels and Joint Clustering

A single layer of supervoxels provides a sparse representation of the image which is affected by the algorithm and parameters used to generated the over-segmentation. As suggested in [21], aggregation of multi-layer supervoxels generated by different algorithms with varying parameters can improve the performance of capturing the diverse and multi-scale visual features in a natural image. For PET reconstruction, to eliminate the bias introduced by a specific algorithm or parameter, the aggregation can be performed as an average of multiple PET images reconstructed from the same projection data and prior images using different over-segmentations generated by varying the supervoxel clustering algorithm and/or the parameters. In this work the multi-layer supervoxels were generated by varying the number of supervoxels N and the weight m between the intensity similarity and spatial proximity in the SLIC algorithm.

One contribution of this work is the joint determination of the sparse image representation $\mathbf{A}$ from both the PET data and the prior image. It is widely acknowledged that the use of an anatomical prior can introduce bias and artefacts in PET image reconstruction when there is signal mismatch between the prior image and true PET image. In this work the over-segmentations derived from the prior images and from the PET data are combined to avoid missing the PET signal absent from the prior image. Also since the proposed sparse image representation is an image geometry constraint rather than an image intensity one, the structures shown in the prior images but not in the true PET image will not explicitly bias the PET image reconstruction. The additional over-segmentation information from PET data is derived from the gradient of the log likelihood in Eq. 3 with respect to the image f at $f = f_{prior} = \mathbf{A}_{prior} s_{prior}$, $s_{prior} = \arg\max_{s \geq 0} L(g | \mathbf{A}_{prior} s)$, where f_{prior} is the PET image determined by only the sparse representation matrix $\mathbf{A}_{prior}$ derived from the prior image. The gradient $\frac{\partial L}{\partial f}$ is derived as

$$\frac{\partial L}{\partial f} = \frac{\partial L}{\partial \bar{g}} \frac{\partial \bar{g}}{\partial f}, \quad \frac{\partial L}{\partial f_j} = \sum_i p_{i,j} \left(\frac{g_i}{\bar{g}_i} - 1 \right), \tag{7}$$

and it is the back-projection of the mismatch of the measured projection data g and the expected projection data $\bar{g}$ generated by the forward model with the current image estimation, so apart from the noise it indicates the difference between the true image and the estimated image, and can be used to modify the over-segmentation to account for the PET-only structures. In this work, the supervoxel clustering method SLIC was used to create from this gradient image new voxel clusters that were then separated from the clusters generated from the prior images as new supervoxels to update the sparse representation matrix $\mathbf{A}$.

3   Experiements

3.1   Simulation Study

Firstly the proposed approach was validated using simulated PET data and compared with the several existing algorithms. [18F]FDG scans were simulated using a 3D brain phantom from the *BrainWeb* database (http://brainweb.bic. mni.mcgill.ca/brainweb/). The associated T1-weighted MR image was used as the anatomical prior with no additional noise. Theoretical [18F]FDG uptake value was used for the activity in white matter (8452.8 Bq/cc) and grey matter (22986.2 Bq/cc). 6 lesions with various sizes and uptake values were added to the PET phantom which were absent from the MR image, as shown in Fig. 1.

The activity image was defined on a grid of $218 \times 218 \times 187$ voxels and used to generate PET projection data (5 mm FWHM resolution). A 20 % uniform background was added as the mean scatter and randoms, and Poisson noise was then introduced. Simulations were conducted at both low-count level (10 million) and high-count level (100 million), with 10 noise realisations for each.

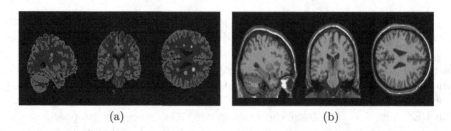

(a)   (b)

Fig. 1. Simulated brain phantom with lesions (voxel size $1 \times 1 \times 1$ mm^3). (a) the *BrainWeb* brain phantom composed of grey matter, white matter and 6 lesions (various sizes and uptake values); (b) the corresponding T1-weighted MR image used as the anatomical prior.

PET reconstruction was performed with pre-reconstruction correction for attenuation, and the estimated scatter and randoms were incorporated in the forward model. The maximum likelihood-expectation maximisation method with no prior [8] (*MLEM*), the bowsher method [4] (*Bowsher*), the kernelised EM method [11] (*KEM*) and the proposed reconstruction algorithm using sparse image representation (*SIR*) were performed for reconstruction. All the methods used the same resampling operator $\mathbf{R}$ in Eq. 6, and the same T1-weighted MR image shown in Fig. 1(b) as the anatomical prior except *MLEM*. For *KEM* and *Bowsher*, 50 nearest neighbours in a $5 \times 5 \times 5$ local neighbourhood were used. The reconstructed PET images are shown in Fig. 2.

For quantitative comparison of the reconstruction methods, the ensemble mean squared bias $Bias^2$ and variance Var were calculated from the reconstructed images. In addition, the contrast recovery coefficient (CRC) was calculated for the lesions. The definitions of $Bias^2$, Var and CRC in [11] were used. The bias and variance images are shown in Fig. 3.

Figure 4 compares the ensemble mean squared bias verse ensemble variance trade-off of the four PET reconstruction algorithms, achieved either by changing the iteration number (*MLEM*, *KEM* and *SIR*) or by varying the penalty weight (*Bowsher*).

Figure 5 compares the contrast recovery coefficient (CRC) ratios versus the background noise trade-off for the 6 lesions. The white matter was used to compute background noise standard deviation. The proposed *SIR* method achieved higher CRCs with lower background noise.

3.2   Clinical Data

The proposed algorithm was also applied to reconstruct clinical [^{18}F]Choline data from a patient scanned with a Siemens Biograph mMR scanner. The T1-weighted MR image (3T 3D GR/IR TR = 1800 ms TE = 2.67 ms FA = 9°) shown in Fig. 6(a) was used as the anatomical prior image after bias field correction using FreeSurfer (http://freesurfer.net/) and denoising with a non-local mean filter [22]. For PET reconstruction, the attenuation map was calculated from a pseudo CT image synthesised from the subject's T1-weighted MR image acquired

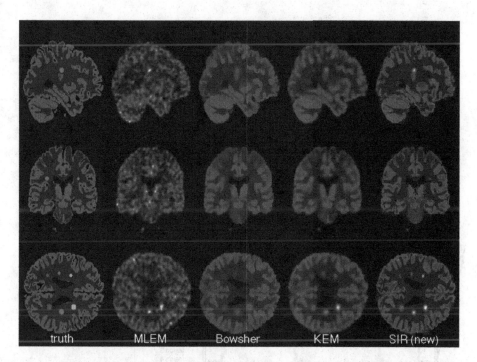

Fig. 2. PET images reconstructed by *MLEM* (no prior), *Bowsher*, *KEM* and the proposed *SIR* at low-count level (1e7) with the same colour scale. *Bowsher* oversmooths the lesions, whereas *KEM* and *SIR* reduce the noise while recovering the lesion contrast and the proposed *SIR* shows improved edge preservation.

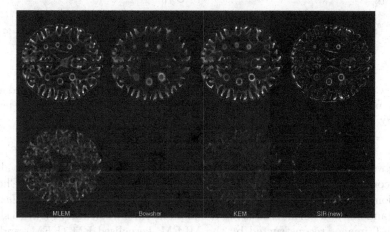

Fig. 3. Bias images (top, with the same colour scale) and variance images (bottom, with the same colour scale) achieved by *MLEM* (no prior), *Bowsher*, *KEM* and the proposed *SIR* at low-count level (1e7). *SIR* achieved reduced bias. Note that the mismatch between the PET phantom and MR image, and the MR partial volume effect also contribute to the bias.

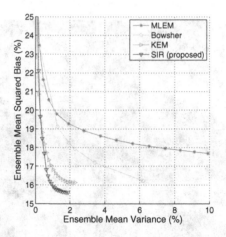

Fig. 4. Ensemble mean squared bias verse ensemble variance trade-off achieved by *MLEM* (no prior), *Bowsher*, *KEM* and the proposed *SIR* at low-count level (1e7).

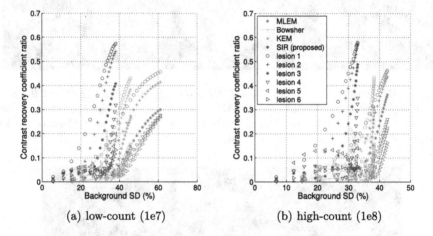

(a) low-count (1e7)   (b) high-count (1e8)

Fig. 5. Contrast recovery coefficient (CRC) ratios of the lesions verse background noise. A CRC ratio is the CRC value normalised to the ground truth CRC, and 1 is the perfect recovery.

in the same imaging session using http://cmictig.cs.ucl.ac.uk/niftyweb/ based on the work in [23]. [^{18}F]Choline PET projection data of 27 s was used to evaluate the reconstruction performance. The data started from 150 s after [^{18}F]Choline injection, and was corrected for dead-time, scatter (based on the synthesised CT), randoms and normalised using the manufacturer's software. Figure 6 shows the PET images reconstructed by the MLEM, kernelised EM (KEM) and the proposed sparsity-based method, along with the T1-weighted MR image used as the anatomical prior image, and the gadolinium-enhanced T1-weighted MR image which supported the identification of a lesion and it was not used as the anatomical prior. It shows that the image reconstructed by MLEM is too noisy for lesion detection, and the KEM and the proposed methods reduced noise and improved the lesion identification from low-count PET projection data. Note that for the proposed method, the image reconstructed using a single layer of supervoxels is presented here to show its potential.

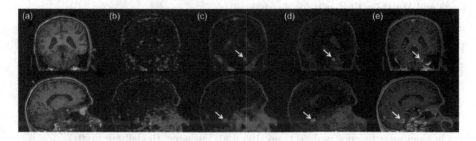

Fig. 6. Reconstruction of low-count clinical [^{18}F]Choline data by (b) *MLEM* (no prior), (c) *KEM* and (d) the proposed *SIR* method shown with the same colour scale. (a) the T1w MR used as the image prior and (e) the gadolinium-enhanced T1w MR showing the lesion (not used as the prior).

4 Conclusion and Discussion

In this work we have provided a novel perspective of solving the ill-posed problem in PET reconstruction, by exploring the sparse nature of images to reduce the complexity of PET forward projection model to fit noisy photon count data. The PET image is reconstructed on the basis of supervoxels of various sizes and shapes instead of the voxels defined on a regular grid, using a sparse image representation derived from an over-segmentation in the image domain which provides a lower-dimensional representation with little loss of image details. The supervoxel clustering is derived from the anatomical prior images and the log likelihood gradient image computed from the PET data. Multiple layers of supervoxels are used to eliminate the bias introduced by the clustering algorithm and parameters. Unlike in the MAP framework, this regularisation is directly integrated into the PET forward projection model and achieves a very efficient EM solution, and it is directly applicable to direct parametric reconstruction of dynamic PET data. The results of experiments on simulated data show improved bias versus variance trade-off and higher contrast recovery over the current state-of-the-art methods. The application to clinical [^{18}F]Choline data shows promising results of identifying a brain lesion from low-count projection data.

The proposed approach is readily applicable for incorporating multiple prior images, such as MR images (for example T1-weighted, T2-weighted, FLAIR). It can be seen that the over-segmentation is a key factor that affects the final reconstructed PET image, in this work a state-of-the-art supervoxel clustering algorithm was used, and the optimisation specific to a given clinical problem and the strategy of aggregating multi-layer supervoxels will be explored to further improve the performance. Applications to whole-body imaging will also be explored in the future.

Acknowledgement. EPSRC (EP/H046410/1, EP/J020990/1, EP/K005278), the MRC (MR/J01107X/1), the NIHR Biomedical Research Unit (Dementia) at UCL and the National Institute for Health Research University College London Hospitals Biomedical Research Centre (NIHR BRC UCLH/UCL High Impact Initiative). Mattias Heinrich, Benjamin Irving, Carole Sudre, Michael Hütel, M. Jorge Cardoso, Pankaj Daga and Matthias Ehrhardt for discussions.

References

1. Green, P.: Bayesian reconstructions from emission tomography data using a modified em algorithm. IEEE Trans. Med. Imaging **9**(1), 84–93 (1990)
2. Leahy, R., Yan, X.: Incorporation of anatomical MR data for improved functional imaging with PET. In: Colchester, A., Hawkes, D. (eds.) IPMI 1991. Lecture Notes in Computer Science, vol. 511, pp. 105–120. Springer, Heidelberg (1991)
3. Baete, K., Nuyts, J., Van Paesschen, W., Suetens, P., Dupont, P.: Anatomical-based FDG-PET reconstruction for the detection of hypo-metabolic regions in epilepsy. IEEE Trans. Med. Imaging **23**(4), 510–519 (2004)
4. Bowsher, J., Yuan, H., Hedlund, L., Turkington, T., Akabani, G., Badea, A., Kurylo, W., Wheeler, C., Cofer, G., Dewhirst, M., Johnson, G.: Utilizing MRI information to estimate F18-FDG distributions in rat flank tumors. In: Conference Record of the 2004 Nuclear Science Symposium, vol. 4, pp. 2488–2492. IEEE (Oct 2004)
5. Vunckx, K., Atre, A., Baete, K., Reilhac, A., Deroose, C., Van Laere, K., Nuyts, J.: Evaluation of three MRI-based anatomical priors for quantitative pet brain imaging. IEEE Trans. Med. Imaging **31**(3), 599–612 (2012)
6. Bai, B., Li, Q., Leahy, R.M.: Magnetic resonance-guided positron emission tomography image reconstruction. Semin. Nucl. Med. **43**(1), 30–44 (2013)
7. Wang, G., Qi, J.: Edge-preserving PET image reconstruction using trust optimization transfer. IEEE Trans. Med. Imaging **34**(4), 930–939 (2015)
8. Shepp, L., Vardi, Y.: Maximum likelihood reconstruction for emission tomography. IEEE Trans. Med. Imaging **1**(2), 113–122 (1982)
9. Wang, G., Qi, J.: Direct estimation of kinetic parametric images for dynamic PET. Theranostics **3**(10), 802–815 (2013)
10. Nguyen, V.G., jin Lee, S.: Incorporating anatomical side information into PET reconstruction using nonlocal regularization. IEEE Trans. Image Process. **22**(10), 3961–3973 (2013)
11. Wang, G., Qi, J.: PET image reconstruction using kernel method. IEEE Trans. Med. Imaging **34**(1), 61–71 (2015)
12. Olshausen, B.A., Field, D.J.: Emergence of simple-cell receptive field properties by learning a sparse code for natural images. Nature **381**(6583), 607–609 (1996)
13. Ren, X., Malik, J.: Learning a classification model for segmentation. In: Proceedings of the Ninth IEEE International Conference on Computer Vision, vol. 1, pp. 10–17, October 2003
14. Heinrich, M.P., Jenkinson, M., Papież, B.W., Glesson, F.V., Brady, S.M., Schnabel, J.A.: Edge- and detail-preserving sparse image representations for deformable registration of chest MRI and CT volumes. In: Gee, J.C., Joshi, S., Pohl, K.M., Wells, W.M., Zöllei, L. (eds.) IPMI 2013. LNCS, vol. 7917, pp. 463–474. Springer, Heidelberg (2013)

15. Achanta, R., Shaji, A., Smith, K., Lucchi, A., Fua, P., Süsstrunk, S.: Slic superpixels compared to state-of-the-art superpixel methods. IEEE Trans. Pattern Anal. Mach. Intell. **34**(11), 2274–2282 (2012)

16. Dillencourt, M.B., Samet, H., Tamminen, M.: A general approach to connected-component labeling for arbitrary image representations. J. ACM **39**(2), 253–280 (1992)

17. Qi, J., Leahy, R.M.: Iterative reconstruction techniques in emission computed tomography. Phys. Med. Biol. **51**(15), R541–R578 (2006)

18. Tong, S., Shi, P.: Tracer kinetics guided dynamic PET reconstruction. In: Karssemeijer, N., Lelieveldt, B. (eds.) IPMI 2007. LNCS, vol. 4584, pp. 421–433. Springer, Heidelberg (2007)

19. Gao, F., Liu, H., Jian, Y., Shi, P.: Dynamic dual-tracer PET reconstruction. In: Prince, J.L., Pham, D.L., Myers, K.J. (eds.) IPMI 2009. LNCS, vol. 5636, pp. 38–49. Springer, Heidelberg (2009)

20. Gunn, R.N., Gunn, S.R., Cunningham, V.J.: Positron emission tomography compartmental models. J. Cereb. Blood Flow Metab. **21**(6), 635–652 (2001)

21. Li, Z., Wu, X.M., Chang, S.F.: Segmentation using superpixels: A bipartite graph partitioning approach. In: 2012 IEEE Conference on Computer Vision and Pattern Recognition (CVPR), pp. 789–796, June 2012

22. Buades, A., Coll, B., Morel, J.M.: A non-local algorithm for image denoising. In: 2005 IEEE Computer Society Conference on Computer Vision and Pattern Recognition, CVPR 2005, vol. 2, pp. 60–65, June 2005

23. Burgos, N., Cardoso, M., Thielemans, K., Modat, M., Pedemonte, S., Dickson, J., Barnes, A., Ahmed, R., Mahoney, J., Schott, J., Duncan, J., Atkinson, D., Arridge, S., Hutton, B., Ourselin, S.: Attenuation correction synthesis for hybrid pet-mr scanners: application to brain studies. IEEE Trans. Med. Imaging **33**(12), 2332–2341 (2014)

Automatic Detection of the Uterus and Fallopian Tube Junctions in Laparoscopic Images

Kristina Prokopetc[(✉)], Toby Collins, and Adrien Bartoli

Image Science for Interventional Techniques (ISIT), UMR 6284 CNRS,
Université d' Auvergne, Clermont-Ferrand, France
prokopec.kristina@mail.ru,
{toby.collins,adrien.bartoli}@gmail.com

Abstract. We present a method for the automatic detection of the uterus and the Fallopian tube/Uterus junctions (FU-junctions) in a monocular laparoscopic image. The main application is to perform automatic registration and fusion between preoperative radiological images of the uterus and laparoscopic images for image-guided surgery. In the broader context of computer assisted intervention, our method is the first that detects an organ and registration landmarks from laparoscopic images without manual input. Our detection problem is challenging because of the large inter-patient anatomical variability and pathologies such as uterine fibroids. We solve the problem using learned contextual geometric constraints that statistically model the positions and orientations of the FU-junctions relative to the uterus' body. We train the uterus detector using a modern part-based approach and the FU-junction detector using junction-specific context-sensitive features. We have trained and tested on a database of 95 uterus images with cross validation, and successfully detected the uterus with Recall = 0.95 and average Number of False Positives per Image (NFPI) = 0.21, and FU-junctions with Recall = 0.80 and NFPI = 0.50. Our experimental results show that the contextual constraints are fundamental to achieve high quality detection.

1 Introduction

An ongoing research objective in medical imaging is to perform inter-modal registration of organs during laparoscopic surgery. The main motivation is to provide Augmented Reality (AR) by visualizing the position of important subsurface structures such as tumors and blood vessels. This has the potential to significantly improve intraoperative resection planning. The registration problem falls into two main categories depending on whether the non-optical modality is captured preoperatively *e.g.* [5,11,12,15,18] or simultaneously and intraoperatively *e.g.* [17]. The registration problem is considerably more challenging in the first category because the transform between modalities is not usually rigid. This is due to changes in the organ's shape between capture times, and caused

© Springer International Publishing Switzerland 2015
S. Ourselin et al. (Eds.): IPMI 2015, LNCS 9123, pp. 552–563, 2015.
DOI: 10.1007/978-3-319-19992-4_43

mainly by the patient lying in different positions, abdominal insufflation and interventional incisions. All the methods for registering laparoscopic and preoperative images of an organ use anatomical landmarks, which are locations on the organ that are visible in both modalities. A limitation of the above methods is that the landmarks are found manually by a human operator. This is not ideal because it requires the operator to be on hand during surgery and is not practical for locating landmarks in laparoscopic videos. The development of systems to automatically locate landmarks is therefore an important research direction. A second important problem that is also overlooked is organ detection. In previous work the organ is assumed to be visible in the laparoscopic images, so the detection problem is avoided. However, a fully-automatic registration system should detect when the organ is visible, and then instantiate registration. Automatic organ detection also has other important applications, including surgical video parsing and video summarization.

In the context of uterine laparoscopic surgery, it was recently shown that FU-junctions are good landmarks, which are normally formed either sides of the uterus body (Fig. 1). However in [5] FU-junctions were detected manually, and the uterus was assumed to be visible in all laparoscopic images. We present a system for fully automatic detection of the uterus and FU-junctions (with all parameters trained), which brings us a step closer to automatic AR to assist uterine surgeries such as myomectomy and endometriosis.

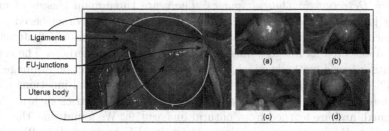

Fig. 1. Laparoscopic images of the uterus. FU-junctions are shown in blue and green for left and right respectively. The detection difficulty comes from ligament junctions, variation in the Fallopian tube orientations and their width. Images (*a-d*) illustrate inter-patient appearance variation.

2   Background and Related Work

Registering Preoperative Images in Laparoscopic Surgery. Existing methods for tackling this problem follow a common pipeline. First the organ is semi-automatically segmented in the preoperative image and a mesh model of its surface is constructed. A deformable model is also constructed to model the non-rigid 3D transform that maps points in the organ to their positions in the laparoscope's coordinate frame. Most methods require stereo laparoscopic images [11,12,18] because these can provide intraoperative 3D surface information. Recently methods have been proposed for monocular laparoscopes [5].

The registration problem is considerably more challenging with monocular laparoscopes. However the application is broader because the overwhelming majority of laparoscopic surgery is performed with monocular laparoscopes. All methods require a suitable deformation model to constrain the organ's shape. These have included biomechanical models [11,12], 3D splines or affine transforms [5]. Organs which have been studied include the liver [12], kidney [11] and uterus [5]. A limitation with all the above methods is that they assume the organ is visible in the laparoscopic images and that there is a manual operator on hand to locate anatomical landmarks.

Detecting Objects in Optical Images. Detecting objects in optical images is a long-standing problem in computer vision that spans several decades of research. In recent years Deformable Part Models (DPMs) have emerged as the best-performing general-purpose object detector [3,9]. DPMs work by modeling the shape variation of an object class with a set of simple parts that are linked with geometric constraints. Each part models the appearance of the object within a local region. The parts can move to handle geometric variation caused by shape and viewpoint changes. DPMs currently are the best performing detectors in the Pascal Challenge dataset [8], and have been used successfully in other areas of medical imaging such as lung nodule classification [20] and fetal nuchal translucency [7]. However their application to organ detection in laparoscopic images has not yet been investigated.

Junction Detection in Optical Images. There are three main classes of methods for junction detection in optical images. The first are corner-based methods which measure 'cornerness' using the image structure tensor [13]. Junctions are then detected as image points with high degree of cornerness. The second are contour-based methods which detect junctions as intersection of image contours [2]. The third are template-based methods which model junctions with a set of templates that correspond to specific junction geometries such as 'Y' or 'T'-shaped, and are learned from natural images [19]. We found that the above classes of methods are not suitable for detecting FU-junctions (Fig. 2). This is for two reasons: *(i)* they are not discriminative enough to separate FU-junctions from other junctions, such as vascular bifurcations, so they give many false positives and *(ii)* they cannot handle well the appearance variation of FU-junctions (Fig. 1).

3 Detection Framework

We propose a learning-based fully-automatic system to detect the uterus and FU-junctions. This is based on four concepts: *(i)* the uterus can be detected prior to FU-junction detection. *(ii)* FU-junctions are too difficult to be detected with generic corner detectors such as [2,13,19], so they should be detected with a learned model. *(iii)* FU-junctions are always located close to tube-like structures, so we can filter out many incorrect FU-junction locations if they exist far from tube-like structures. *(iv)* There exist contextual constraints between the

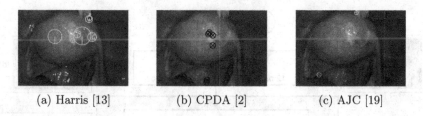

(a) Harris [13]   (b) CPDA [2]   (c) AJC [19]

Fig. 2. Failure of generic junction detectors to detect FU-junctions.

uterus body and FU-junctions. We use two types of contextual constraints. The first models the conditional probability of an FU-junction occurring at a position in the image given the uterus center. Given a uterus detection we can eliminate pixel locations which have low conditional probability giving us Regions of Interest (ROIs) for the locations of FU-junctions. The second contextual constraint encodes the fact that FU-junctions are on the uterus surface, which means there should usually exist a path in the image that connects them to the uterus center which does not cross an object boundary.

Automatically detecting the uterus and FU-junctions is not an easy problem to solve due to large inter-patient anatomic variability (both in shape and texture) (Fig. 1). We restrict the scope of the problem to images of the uterus before resection. This means that the uterus has not changed topologically by surgical incisions. We also assume the uterus is not significantly occluded by surgical tools. In uterine surgery the laparoscope is nearly always held in upright position, so our detectors do not need to be invariant to high degrees of rotations about the laparoscope's optical axis.

We outline the full proposed detection process in Fig. 3. This consists of two main steps: *(i)* uterus detection and *(ii)* FU-junction detection. We use a trained DPM model to detect the whole uterus, its center and its bounding box. We then proceed to detect the FU-junctions using contextual constraints and a number of processing steps which reduce the search space for FU-junction locations. We then compute local and contextual features for all candidate locations and perform classification with a sparse linear SVM.

3.1   The Uterus Detector

Given an input laparoscopic image (Fig. 3 (a)) we use a trained DPM model to detect the uterus body. This is achieved with an open-source implementation of [10] and a set of annotated uterus images (details of the dataset are given in Sect. 4.1). The detector scans the image at multiple scales and positions and returns bounding boxes (Fig. 3 (b)) around positive detections and their corresponding detection scores. We select the bounding box with the highest detection score τ_u, and if τ_u is greater than an acceptance threshold τ_u' the detection is kept (Fig. 3 (c)), otherwise it is rejected (details for computing τ_u' are in Sect. 4.1). We use $u_w \in \mathbb{R}$, $u_h \in \mathbb{R}$ and $\mathbf{u}_p \in \mathbb{R}^2$ to denote the uterus bounding box width, height and center outputted from the DPM uterus detector. We then proceed to detect the FU-junctions.

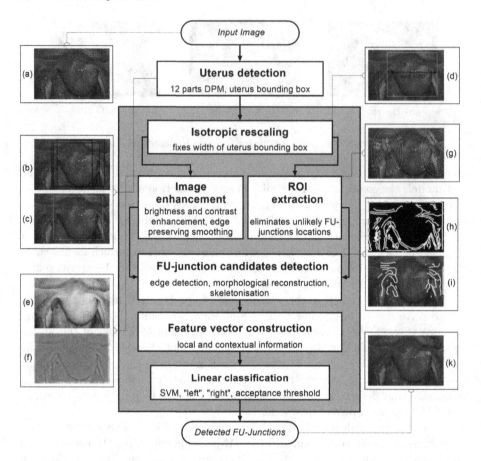

Fig. 3. Diagram of the main pipeline of the proposed detection process.

3.2 The FU-junction Detector

Step 1: Isotropic Rescaling. First the image is isotropically rescaled so the bounding box of the uterus has a default width of $u_w = 200$ pixels (Fig. 3 (d)). This fixes the scale of the uterus and allows us to detect FU-junctions without requiring detection at multiple scales. This has the benefit of increasing computation speed and reducing false positives.

Step 2: Image Enhancement. We enhance the image with contrast stretching on the red channel (Fig. 3 (e)). We perform coarse illumination correction to remove uneven illumination with low pass filtering. We then perform edge preserving smoothing using the guided filter method from Matlab (Fig. 3 (f)). We use only the red channel because it is mostly insensitive to the uterus' natural texture variation (unlike the green and blue channels [4]). This means that strong edges in the red channel are highly indicative of object boundaries.

Step 3: ROI Extraction. We filter out highly improbable locations for the left and right FU-junctions. For each pixel $\mathbf{p} \in \mathbb{R}^2$ in the image we compute the conditional probability $P_L(\mathbf{p}|\mathbf{u}_p) \in \mathbb{R}^+$ of the left junction occurring at $\mathbf{p}$ given $\mathbf{u}_p$. This is a contextual constraint that we model with a Gaussian Mixture Model (GMM):

$$P_L(\mathbf{p}|\mathbf{u}_p) \overset{\text{def}}{=} \sum_{k=1}^{K} w_k^L G(\mathbf{p} - \mathbf{u}_p; \boldsymbol{\mu}_k^L, \boldsymbol{\Sigma}_k^L) \tag{1}$$

where K is the number of GMM components and $\{w_k^L, \boldsymbol{\mu}_k^L, \boldsymbol{\Sigma}_k^L\}$ are the GMM parameters. We keep $\mathbf{p}$ as a left junction candidate if $P_L(\mathbf{p}|\mathbf{u}_p) \geq c$, where c is a small probability threshold. For the right FU-junction we also use a GMM to model the conditional probability $P_R(\mathbf{p}|\mathbf{u}_p)$ of the FU-junction occurring at $\mathbf{p}$. To train the GMM parameters we exploit the fact that the FU-junctions have strong bilateral symmetry about the uterus body (Fig. 1). Because the laparoscope is normally in upright position this implies the FU-junctions are horizontally symmetric. We therefore propose to simplify the model with $\mu_k^R(1) = -\mu_k^L(1)$, $w_k^R = w_k^L$ and $\boldsymbol{\Sigma}_k^R = \boldsymbol{\Sigma}_k^L$. The advantage of doing this is that we effectively double the amount of training data. This is because each training example can now be used to train P_L and P_R by reflecting its position horizontally relative to $\mathbf{u}_p$. Training is performed with the standard K-means/EM algorithm on the training set. We set c using a training dataset (see Sect. 4.1) at the 99 % percentile cut-off point. We select K automatically such that it minimizes the cross-validation error using a hold-out training set (see Sect. 4.1). We then compute two ROIs (Fig. 3 (g)), R_l and R_r for the left and right FU-junctions respectively, with

$$R_l(\mathbf{p}) = \begin{cases} 1 & \text{if } P_L(\mathbf{p}|\mathbf{u}_p) \geq c \\ 0 & \text{otherwise} \end{cases} \qquad R_r(\mathbf{p}) = \begin{cases} 1 & \text{if } P_R(\mathbf{p}|\mathbf{u}_p) \geq c \\ 0 & \text{otherwise} \end{cases} \tag{2}$$

Step 4: Detecting FU-junction Candidates. We then detect candidate FU-junction locations using the ROIs from Step 3 (Fig. 3 (h)). This uses the fact that FU-junctions occur close to the medial axis of the Fallopian tubes. We find tube like structures by performing edge detection on the enhanced image computed in Step 2, using the Canny detector with automatic thresholding. Because we use the enhanced image strong edges are highly indicative of object boundaries. We then compute a skeleton S of the edge - map within the region $R_l \cup R_r$ (Fig. 3 (h)) using the implementation of Contour-Pruned Skeletonization from [14], where $S(\mathbf{p}) = 1$ if $\mathbf{p}$ is on the skeleton and $S(\mathbf{p}) = 0$ otherwise. As we see from Fig. 3 (i) the skeleton can be computed quite robustly despite of imperfect edge map. We take all pixels for which $S(\mathbf{p}) = 1$ as a candidate FU-junction locations.

Step 5: Feature Vector Computation. For each candidate location $\mathbf{p}$ we compute three types of local features (we denote these by x_h, x_θ and x_w). The first x_h are HOG features [6] to encode image gradient patterns around FU-junctions. We extract HOG features within a local window of w pixels using default HOG parameters, giving x_h 81 dimensions. We have conducted experiments with different window sizes and found a default of $w = 15$ pixels well. The second local feature $x_\theta \in [0, \pi]$ encodes the orientation of the Fallopian tube as it enters the uterus (Fig. 1). This is computed from the skeleton edge map, by fitting a line to the 5 nearest-neighbors in the skeleton edge map and keeping its slope. The third feature $x_w \in \mathbb{R}^+$ encodes the width of the Fallopian tube as it enters the uterus. This is approximated by twice the distance between $\mathbf{p}$ and the closest edge in the edge map. The reason why we use both HOG and edge-based features is that they complement one another. HOG features do not require computing edge or skeleton maps, which makes them very robust particularly when the contrast between the uterus and background structures is low (even after enhancement). However, HOG features also include gradient information from background structures within the HOG window. On the other hand, edge-based features require edge detection, which makes them less robust. Nevertheless, the benefit of using edge-based features is that if the edges have been computed well, then the edge features encode only the shape of the FU-junction and not structures in the background. We compute two types of contextual features (we denote these by x_g, x_c). The first x_g is computed from the position and direction of $\mathbf{p}$ relative to the uterus center $\mathbf{u}_p$ in the rescaled image:

$$x_g = \left[d_x, d_y, d_x^2, d_y^2, \alpha \right]^\top, \ [d_x, d_y] \stackrel{\text{def}}{=} \mathbf{p} - \mathbf{u}_p, \ \alpha \stackrel{\text{def}}{=} \text{atan}\,(d_x/d_y) \qquad (3)$$

The second contextual feature x_c encodes the fact that FU-junctions lie on the uterus. Assuming uterus is not occluded by a tool, this means there should exist a path in the image between points $\mathbf{p}$ and $\mathbf{u}_p$ that does not cross the bounding contour of the uterus (Fig. 1). To evaluate this exactly we would need to segment the uterus, which is hard to achieve automatically. Instead we exploit the fact that the uterus body is mostly convex. This means that with high probability the straight line segment between $\mathbf{p}$ and $\mathbf{u}_p$ will not cross the bounding contour of the uterus. In our dataset this assumption holds in all cases, including pathological cases such as uteri with fibroids. We evaluate x_c as the number of times the line segment between $\mathbf{p}$ and $\mathbf{u}_p$ crosses an edge in the edge map. Typically we find that when $\mathbf{p}$ is a correct FU-junction location then $x_c = 0$, however this is not always the case because some spurious edges may exist in the edge map which are caused by high-contrast texture variation.

Step 6: Linear Classification. The features are combined into a feature vector which is passed to two trained classifiers. We use one classifier for the left and one for the right FU-junctions. We use linear SVM classifiers with an L1 sparse prior, which are known to work well for detectors with HOG features and small datasets of order $\mathcal{O}(10^2)$. We then take the candidates with the highest detection scores for the left and right FU-junctions, and output positive detections (Fig. 3 (k)) if their scores are above an acceptance threshold τ_j' (details for computing τ_j' are in Sect. 4.1).

4   Dataset, Training and Performance Evaluation

4.1   Dataset and Training

We have not find any large publicly available collection of laparoscopic uterus images. We therefore constructed the dataset from various sources. This has a total of 95 uterus images from 38 different individuals. 45 images were collected from internet image search engine queries; 26 of which were obtained from 3 publicly available surgical videos. The image resolution of these varied from 311×217 to 1377×1011 pixels. We collected 50 images from 13 videos of different individuals recorded with monocular HD laparoscopes at a partner local hospital. The image resolution of these varied from 553×311 to 817×556. 77 images in the database were of healthy uteri and 18 were of abnormal uteri with fibroids. All images were annotated manually with uterus bounding box and junction locations. We obtained a negative dataset of 100 images from the 13 videos where the uterus was not visible. These were randomly chosen frames in the time period from insufflation to when the surgeon begun incising the uterus. We divided the dataset into training and test sets using k-fold cross validation with $k = 7$. To guarantee that we measure patient-independent performance, we ensured that images of the same patient were not in training and test sets. At most 4 images of each individual were put in the test set, which was done to keep test performance results balanced across the population. The detection thresholds τ'_u and τ'_j were computed for each fold as the best 'cut-off' point on the recall vs. NFPI curve that was closest to $[0,1]$ (Figs. 4 (b) and 6).

4.2   Uterus Detection

To evaluate the performance of the uterus detector we adopted the PASCAL VOC challenge protocol to generate Receiver Operating Curves (ROC). A predicted bounding box was considered a true positive if it overlapped more than 50 % with the ground-truth bounding box, otherwise it was considered a false positive. Two types of performance have been computed. The first is recall vs. precision and the second is precision vs. Number of False Positives Per Image (NFPI). The most important free parameter of the DPM detector is the number of parts, which we varied from 1 to 12. The evaluation curves shown in Fig. 4 illustrate a general performance gain with increased number of parts. For

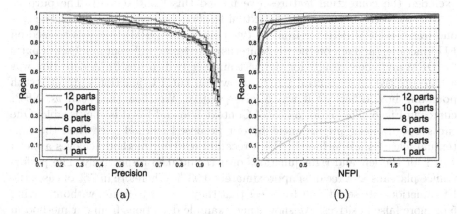

(a)   (b)

Fig. 4. Uterus detection performance. The Precision/Recall curves are shown in (a) and the NFPPI/Recall curves are presented in (b) with different number of parts.

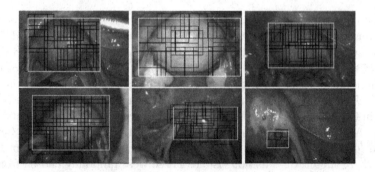

Fig. 5. Examples of uterus' detections. Bounding boxes of the uteri are shown in green and the bounding boxes of the parts are shown in blue (Color figure online).

Table 1. Comparison statistics (in pixels) for the three methods in the second experiment with the best method highlighted.

<table>
<tr><td colspan="6">Left FU-Junction</td><td colspan="6">Right FU-junction</td></tr>
<tr><td></td><td>mean</td><td>median</td><td>min</td><td>max</td><td>std</td><td></td><td>mean</td><td>median</td><td>min</td><td>max</td><td>std</td></tr>
<tr><td>Proposed</td><td>27.16</td><td>10.26</td><td>0.25</td><td>381.47</td><td>56.45</td><td>Proposed</td><td>25.46</td><td>16.12</td><td>0.80</td><td>117.76</td><td>24.95</td></tr>
<tr><td>Context-free</td><td>77.96</td><td>40.69</td><td>0.97</td><td>479.17</td><td>95.61</td><td>Context-free</td><td>44.23</td><td>24.41</td><td>0.52</td><td>415.80</td><td>65.66</td></tr>
<tr><td>DPM</td><td>51.60</td><td>23.63</td><td>2.12</td><td>477.25</td><td>78.87</td><td>DPM</td><td>54.99</td><td>29.84</td><td>0.31</td><td>373.20</td><td>82.73</td></tr>
</table>

a precision of 0.90, the recall of the 12-parts modes was 0.86, and the recall of the 6-part model was 0.78. We show some representative detection results in Fig. 5. Typical correct detections are shown in the five top left images while the bottom-right shows a failure due to it being mostly out of frame.

4.3 FU-junction Detection

We compared the performance of our FU-junction detector against two other approaches. The first was a context-free version of our detector where we excluded the contextual features (we named this Context-free). The purpose was to reveal the benefit that contextual features had on the problem. The second was the DPM detector from [9] (we named this DPM) that was trained on FU-junctions (and not on the whole uterus). We tested different numbers of parts for DPM and show results for the best number (which was 6). A detection was a true positive if its central point was within the FU-junction's ground-truth bounding box, otherwise it was a false positive. We show the recall *vs.* NFPI curves in Fig. 6. The performance of Context-free and DPM is comparable. One can see a dramatic improvement by our proposed method (*i.e.* when the contextual features are included). For a recall of 0.80 our method achieves a mean NFPI for the left and right junctions of 0.47 and 0.53 respectively. The performance plateaus at a recall of approximately 0.93 %. Therefore in 7 % of cases the FU-junctions are so difficult to detect that they cannot be found without having 5 or more false positives. We show some example detections from our method in Fig. 7. The examples show results with normal uteri (second row) and abnormal

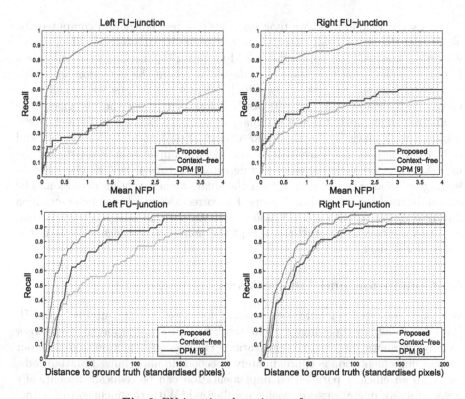

Fig. 6. FU-junction detection performance.

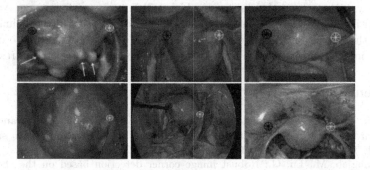

Fig. 7. Examples of detected FU-junctions. Left FU-junction is shown in blue and right in green. Arrows in the top left image show multiple small fibroids (Color figure online).

uteri with fibroids (first row). The images show the ability to handle significant variation in orientation of the Fallopian tubes. In Fig. 7 bottom left we show a test image where only the right FU-junction was visible (the left FU-junction was occluded by the uterus body). A failure is given in the bottom right image, where there was confusion with the round ligament junctions.

In a second experiment we took each positive test image and computed the distance of the best-scoring detection to the ground-truth position. The purpose was to see how well the approaches could localize FU-junctions when they were forced to make a hard decision (*i.e.* the point where the detection score was maximal). Because the test images had different resolutions we rescaled the images to a default width of 640 pixels before computing the distances. The results are shown in Fig. 6 and summary of statistics is given in Table 1. For a distance of 25 pixels our method had a recall of 0.73 and 0.64 for the left and right FU-junctions respectively. If we consider the application of registering the uterus, it therefore makes sense for our detector to return a small number of high-scoring detections rather than return the single highest-scoring detection. The set can be used for registration because the correct detection may be determined during registration with *e.g.* softassign [16]. We see that our proposed method performs the best in all statistics except the minimum distance (although it is still under a pixel).

5   Conclusion and Future Work

We have presented an automatic system for detecting the uterus and FU-junctions in laparoscopic images. This work brings us an important step closer to fully automatic inter-modal registration. The average detection time with our current implementation is approximately 8 seconds in unoptimized Matlab code, but with an efficient parallelized implementation can be reduced dramatically because many operations are easily parallelized. With the inclusion of a tool detector *e.g.* [1] the assumption about absence of tool occlusion can be relaxed. We also want to extend the database which will improve performance. Another direction is to extend the detector to stereo images, and it will be valuable to know if the depth data helps detection performance. The possibility to exploit multiple images and/or motion information is also promising for further research.

References

1. Allan, M., Ourselin, S., Thompson, S., Hawkes, D.J., Kelly, J., Stoyanov, D.: Toward detection and localization of instruments in minimally invasive surgery. IEEE Trans. Biomed. Eng. **60**(4), 1050–1058 (2013)
2. Awrangjeb, M., Lu, G.: Robust image corner detection based on the chord-to-point distance accumulation technique. IEEE Trans. Multimedia **10**(6), 1059–1072 (2008)
3. Bouchard, G., Triggs, B.: Hierarchical part-based visual object categorization. In: CVPR (2005)
4. Collins, T., Pizarro, D., Bartoli, A., Canis, M., Bourdel, N.: Realtime wide-baseline registration of the uterus in laparoscopic videos using multiple texture maps. In: Liao, H., Linte, C.A., Masamune, K., Peters, T.M., Zheng, G. (eds.) MIAR 2013 and AE-CAI 2013. LNCS, vol. 8090, pp. 162–171. Springer, Heidelberg (2013)
5. Collins, T., Pizarro, D., Bartoli, A., Canis, M., Bourdel, N.: Computer-assisted laparoscopic myomectomy by augmenting the uterus with pre-operative MRI data. In: ISMAR (2014)

6. Dalal, N., Triggs, B.: Histograms of oriented gradients for human detection. In: CVPR (2005)
7. Deng, Y., Wang, Y., Chen, P.: Automated detection of fetal nuchal translucency based on hierarchical structural model. In: ICBMS (2010)
8. Everingham, M., Van Gool, L., Williams, C.K.I., Winn, J., Zisserman, A.: The PASCAL Visual Object Classes Challenge 2010 (VOC2010) Results
9. Felzenszwalb, P., Girshick, R., McAllester, D., Ramanan, D.: Object detection with discriminatively trained part-based models. Pattern Anal. Mach. Intell. 32(9), 1627–1645 (2010)
10. Girshick, R.B.: From rigid templates to grammars: object detection with structured models. Ph.D. thesis, University of Chicago (2012)
11. Hamarneh, G., Amir-Khalili, A., Nosrati, M., Figueroa, I., Kawahara, J., Al-Alao, O., Peyrat, J.-M., Abi-Nahed, J., Al-Ansari, A., Abugharbieh, R.: Towards multi-modal image-guided tumour identification in robot-assisted partial nephrectomy. In: MECBME (2014)
12. Haouchine, N., Dequidt, J., Peterlik, I., Kerrien, E., Berger, M.-O., Cotin, S.: Image-guided simulation of heterogeneous tissue deformation for augmented reality during hepatic surgery. In: ISMAR (2013)
13. Harris, C., Stephens, M.: A combined corner and edge detector. In: Fourth Alvey Vision Conference (1988)
14. Howe, N.R.: Kontour-Pruned Skeletonization (2006). http://cs.smith.edu/~nhowe/research/code/Skeleton.zip. Accessed 23 September 2014
15. Plantefève, R., Haouchine, N., Radoux, J.-P., Cotin, S.: Automatic alignment of pre and intraoperative data using anatomical landmarks for augmented laparoscopic liver surgery. In: Bello, F., Cotin, S. (eds.) ISBMS 2014. LNCS, vol. 8789, pp. 58–66. Springer, Heidelberg (2014)
16. Rangarajan, A., Chui, H., Bookstein, F.L.: The softassign procrustes matching algorithm. In: Information Processing in Medical Imaging (1997)
17. Simpfendorfer, T., Baumhauer, M., Muller, M., Gutt, C.N., Meinzer, H.-P., Rassweiler, J.J., Guven, S., Teber, D.: Augmented reality visualization during laparoscopic radical prostatectomy. J. Endourol. 25, 1841–1845 (2011)
18. Su, L.-M., Vagvolgyi, B.P., Agarwal, R., Reiley, C.E., Taylor, R.H., Hager, G.D.: Augmented reality during robot-assisted laparoscopic partial nephrectomy: toward real-time 3D-CT to stereoscopic video registration. Urology 73(4), 896–900 (2009)
19. Xia, G.-S., Delon, J., Gousseau, Y.: Accurate junction detection and characterization in natural images. Int. J. Comput. Vision 106(1), 31–56 (2014)
20. Zhang, F., Song, Y., Cai, W., Lee, M.-Z., Zhou, Y., Huang, H., Shan, S., Fulham, M., Feng, D.: Lung nodule classification with multilevel patch-based context analysis. IEEE Trans. Biomed. Eng. 61(4), 1155–1166 (2014)

A Mixed-Effects Model with Time Reparametrization for Longitudinal Univariate Manifold-Valued Data

J.-B. Schiratti[1,3]([⊠]), S. Allassonnière[3], A. Routier[1], the Alzheimers Disease Neuroimaging Initiative, O. Colliot[1,2], and S. Durrleman[1]

[1] Inria Paris-Rocquencourt, Inserm U1127, CNRS UMR 7225,
Sorbonne Universités UPMC Univ Paris 06 UMRS 1127,
Institut du Cerveau et de la Moelle épinière, ICM, 75013 Paris, France
jean-baptiste.schiratti@cmap.polytechnique.fr
[2] AP-HP, Pitié-Salpêtrière Hospital, Departments of Neurology and Neuroradiology,
75013 Paris, France
[3] Ecole Polytechnique, Palaiseau, France

Abstract. Mixed-effects models provide a rich theoretical framework for the analysis of longitudinal data. However, when used to analyze or predict the progression of a neurodegenerative disease such as Alzheimer's disease, these models usually do not take into account the fact that subjects may be at different stages of disease progression and the interpretation of the model may depend on some implicit reference time. In this paper, we propose a generative statistical model for longitudinal data, described in a univariate Riemannian manifold setting, which estimates an average disease progression model, subject-specific *time shifts* and *acceleration factors*. The *time shifts* account for variability in age at disease-onset time. The *acceleration factors* account for variability in speed of disease progression. For a given individual, the estimated time shift and acceleration factor define an affine reparametrization of the average disease progression model. This statistical model has been used to analyze neuropsychological assessments scores and cortical thickness measurements from the Alzheimer's Disease Neuroimaging Initiative database. The numerical results showed that we can distinguish between slow versus fast progressing and early versus late-onset individuals.

1 Introduction

The Alzheimer's disease (AD), and most neurodegenerative diseases alike, is a slowly progressive neurodegenerative disorder and a growing public health issue as the number of people diagnosed with AD is steadily increasing over the years, partly due to an increasing ageing population. The progressive loss of cognitive functions, such as memory, language and reasoning, are the observable consequences of pathological processes which started to affect the brain several years

© Springer International Publishing Switzerland 2015
S. Ourselin et al. (Eds.): IPMI 2015, LNCS 9123, pp. 564–575, 2015.
DOI: 10.1007/978-3-319-19992-4_44

before. In [1], Clifford R. Jack et al. proposed a widely accepted hypothetical model which describes the temporal evolution of the AD biomarkers in which the decline in cognitive functions and memory loss occur in the late stages of the disease. The impairment of the cognitive functions is preceded by decreasing cerebrospinal fluid (CSF) amyloid-$\beta 42$ ($A\beta_{1-42}$) peptide, increasing CSF tau protein and neurodegeneration, characterized by cerebral atrophy and neuron loss. In order to increase the chances of success of a given treatment, the need for an early diagnosis and the need to understand the progression of the disease are crucial.

Longitudinal data, which consists in repeated observations of a given individual or group of individuals over time, allows to study the progression of a disease and the statistical analysis of longitudinal data may provide useful informations to help diagnose AD in its early phase. Mixed effects models provide a rich framework to analyze longitudinal measurements. The fixed (and respectively random) effects allow to describe the model at the group (respectively subject) level and the distribution of the random effects accounts for inter-subject variability. A particular case of the linear mixed-effects models introduced by Laird and Ware in [5] can be used to model a linear relationship between univariate longitudinal measurement and the times of observation : the random slope and intercept model. If $y_{i,j}$ denotes the j-th observation of the i-th subject associated to time $t_{i,j}$, the random slope and intercept model would write : $y_{i,j} = (\overline{a} + a_i)(t_{i,j} - t_0) + (\overline{b} + b_i) + \varepsilon_{i,j}$, where $\varepsilon_{i,j}$ denotes a Gaussian noise with zero mean. The fixed effects $\overline{a}$ and $\overline{b}$ respectively correspond to the slope and intercept of an average trajectory $\overline{D}(t) = \overline{a}(t - t_0) + \overline{b}$ whereas t_0 plays the role of a reference time. The subject-specific slope a_i and b_i correspond to the slope and intercept of the trajectory of the i-th individual.

If the longitudinal observations arise, for example, from developmental studies, breeding studies or pharmacological studies, there is a natural choice for the baseline time t_0, which may represent the time of birth, beginning of the study or time at which a certain drug has been administered. In those situations, the baseline time is known and is therefore not estimated along with the parameters of the model. However, in studies on neurodegenerative diseases, such as Alzheimer's disease, there may be no natural choice for the reference time. As pointed out by Yang et al. in [4] and Delor et al. in [3], the disease-onset time is probably different for every individual and, at a given age, two individuals may be at very different stages of disease progression. When the baseline (or disease-onset) time is unknown, one may consider it as a fixed effect of the given model. In [2], the authors proposed an interesting mixed-effect model for scalar measurements but the model did not account for the difference in stages progression among individuals. Yang et al. [4] and Delor et al. [3] addressed this issue by including time shifts in their models but Yang et al. did not estimate the time shifts in a statistical framework. In Delor et al., the observations of a given individual were shifted in time before the estimation of a disease-onset time. In both situations, the reference time was not estimated. In [8], Singh et al. proposed an interesting model for longitudinal manifold-valued observations using parallel transport. However, if the model is written for univariate longitudinal data, the model does include a random effect to account for the variability in speed of disease progression.

When the time reference time t_0 is considered unknown, the linear model given above is not identifiable and there is a relation between the distribution of the intercept random effect b_i and the fixed effect t_0, which makes the interpretation of the distribution of the intercept random effect b_i difficult.

To address the issues we pointed out, we propose to replace the intercept random effect b_i, which characterizes the distribution of the measurement values at time t_0, by a time shift τ_i which measures the delay (or advance) in disease progression. We therefore consider the model : $y_{i,j} = v_0 \alpha_i (t_{i,j} - t_0 - \tau_i) + \varepsilon_{i,j}$ where α_i is a random effect log-normally distributed with mean equal to 1 and τ_i is the time shift random effect normally distributed with mean 0. The fixed effect v_0 correspond to the slope of the mean trajectory and is the fixed effect associated to α_i whereas t_0 is now the fixed effect associated to the random effect τ_i. If D denotes the straight line $D(t) = v_0(t - t_0)$, the model writes : $y_{i,j} = D(\alpha_i(t_{i,j} - t_0 - \tau_i) + t_0) + \varepsilon_{i,j}$. As a consequence, the random effects α_i and τ_i allow to define a subject-specific affine reparametrization of the straight line D, which can be thought of as an average trajectory. The *acceleration factor* α_i and the time shift τ_i of the affine subject-specific reparametrization provide informations on the dynamical evolution of a given subject with respect to the average model: the *acceleration factor* will determine whether an individual is progressing faster than the individual trajectory. The *time shift* determines whether the individual is lagging behind or ahead of the average model. Therefore, the random effects of the model will allow to determine, among a group of individuals, who are fast or slow progressing individuals and whether a given individual might develop the disease earlier (early-onset) or later (late-onset) than the estimated reference time t_0.

Moreover, since the subject-specific trajectories are affine reparametrizations of an average trajectory, this model can easily be generalized to longitudinal measurements on a Riemannian manifold. The average trajectory may be replaced with a geodesic of the manifold and the subject-specific trajectories will remain geodesics on the manifold. As a matter of fact, longitudinal measurements arising from neuroimaging, neuropsychological tests or clinical examinations may belong to nonlinear spaces. The scores to a neuropsychological test often belong to a bounded interval. Riemannian manifolds offer a very flexible framework which includes the previous examples. The generalization of this statistical model to Riemannian manifold-valued observations could be used either to analyze shapes, cortical thickness measurements or neuropsychological assessment scores. After a proper renormalization, the ADAS-Cog 13 scores belong to the open unit inverval $(0, 1)$ which, equipped with a specific metric, can be seen as a univariate Riemannian manifold. For this metric, the geodesics are logistic curves. The models presented in [2] and [3] do not generalize to manifold-valued data. In [9], Lorenzi et al. used Riemannian manifold techniques to estimate a model of the brain's normal ageing from healthy individuals T1 MR scans. The model was used to compute a time shift, called *morphological age shift*, which corresponds to the actual anatomical age of the subject with respect to an estimated average age for healthy subjects. However, the subject-specific time shifts were not estimated as parameters of a statistical model. In [7], Datar et al. generalized a particular linear mixed-effects model to longitudinal shape analysis but the proposed model did not include time shifts to account for the variability in stages of disease progression among the population. Even though the model is used to analyze shapes (given by a set of points), the model is not described in a Riemannian manifold setting.

The work presented herein will generalize the model written above to a Riemannian manifold included in $\mathbb{R}$. In Sect. 2, we will introduce our model and we will present two particular cases of this model : the *straight lines model* and the *logistic curves model*. We also explain how the parameters of the model are estimated. In Sect. 3, the straight lines model and logistic curves model were used to analyze longitudinal ADAS-Cog and cortical thickness measurements from the ADNI database. We show that the estimated random effects of the model allowed to distinguish between slow versus fast progressing individuals and early versus late-onset individuals.

2 A Mixed-Effects Model with Time Reparametrization for Manifold-Valued Observations

2.1 Model Description

Let us assume that we observe p different individuals. For each individual, we have n_i observations, obtained at times $t_{i,1} < \ldots < t_{i,n_i}$ and the observations of the i-th individual are denoted by $y_{i,1}, \ldots, y_{i,n_i}$. We assume that each observation $y_{i,j}$ is a point on a one-dimensional Riemannian manifold (M, g) included in $\mathbb{R}$. In addition to this, we assume that the geodesics of M are defined on the entire real line.

Let p_0 be a point in M, t_0 in $\mathbb{R}$ and $v_0 \in T_{p_0}M$, a tangent vector to M at the point p_0. The triplet (p_0, t_0, v_0) allows to define an *average trajectory* γ_{p_0,t_0,v_0}, the geodesic of M which passes through the point $p_0 \in M$ at time t_0 and with the velocity $v_0 \in T_{p_0}M \simeq \mathbb{R}$. This average trajectory summarises the progression of all the individuals and could be interpreted as the evolution of an "average subject". While the average subject passes through the point p_0 at time t_0 with the velocity v_0, we assume that the trajectory of the i-th subject is the geodesic γ_i which passes through the point p_0 at time $t_0 + \tau_i$ with velocity $\alpha_i v_0$. The parameters (p_0, t_0, v_0) will be the fixed effects of the model whereas α_i and τ_i will be the random effects of the model. The point p_0 in M can be understood as an *observation point*. A simplistic interpretation of the role played by α_i and τ_i is the following : an observer standing at the point p_0 in M and aware that the average subject passes through the point at the time t_0, with velocity v_0, will be able to tell whether the i-th subject passes through this point earlier or later than the average subject and whether he passes faster or slower. More precisely,

τ_i is a time shift which will provide an information on whether the progression of the i-th trajectory is ahead of the average trajectory or not and α_i provides the information on whether the i-th subject is evolving faster or slower than the average subject. As a consequence, the random effects α_i and τ_i take into account the fact that two different subjects may be at very different stages of disease progression and allow for inter-subjects comparaisons. The description above makes the assumption that every subject-specific trajectory of disease progression will eventually reach a common value p_0. This assumption does not make sense in a higher-dimensional Riemannian manifold. In order to generalize the proposed model to a higher-dimensional setting, one would need to add another random effect, associated to the fixed effect p_0.

For a point $p_0 \in M$ and $t_0 \in \mathbb{R}$, $v_0 \in T_{p_0}M$, we define $\gamma_{p_0,t_0,v_0} := \mathrm{Exp}_{t_0,p_0}(\alpha_i v_0)(\cdot)$ as the geodesic which passes through the point p_0 at time t_0 with velocity $v_0 : \gamma_{p_0,v_0,t_0}$ is the unique curve, drawn on M and defined on $\mathbb{R}$, which satisfies $\nabla_{\dot{\gamma}_{p_0,t_0,v_0}} \dot{\gamma}_{p_0,t_0,v_0} = 0$ and $\gamma_{p_0,t_0,v_0}(t_0) = p_0$, $\dot{\gamma}_{p_0,t_0,v_0}(t_0) = v_0$. For the dataset $(t_{i,j}, y_{i,j})$ $(1 \leq i \leq p$ and $1 \leq j \leq n_i)$, we assume the following model :

$$y_{i,j} = \mathrm{Exp}_{t_0+\tau_i,p_0}(\alpha_i v_0)(t_{i,j}) + \varepsilon_{i,j} \tag{1}$$

where $\alpha_i = \exp(\eta_i)$ and :

$$\begin{cases} \eta_i \sim \otimes_{i=1}^p \mathcal{N}(0,\sigma_\eta^2) \\ \tau_i \sim \otimes_{i=1}^p \mathcal{N}(0,\sigma_\tau^2) \\ \varepsilon_{i,j} \sim \otimes_{i,j} \mathcal{N}(0,\sigma^2). \end{cases}$$

The random variables $(\eta_i)_{1 \leq i \leq p}$ and $(\tau_i)_{1 \leq i \leq p}$ are assumed independent. The vector $\theta = (p_0, t_0, v_0, \sigma_\eta, \sigma_\tau, \sigma)^\top$ is the vector of the parameters of the model. We will discuss later how this vector is estimated from the data.

An important feature of the model (1) is that in can be written as follows :

$$y_{i,j} = \gamma_{p_0,t_0,v_0}(\alpha_i v_0(t_{i,j} - t_0 - \tau_i)) + \varepsilon_{i,j} \tag{2}$$
$$= \gamma_i(t_{i,j}) + \varepsilon_{i,j}. \tag{3}$$

The subject-specific trajectory of the i-th subject, the geodesic γ_i, therefore appears as an affine reparametrization of the average trajectory γ_{p_0,t_0,v_0}. As a consequence, in order to compare the progression of a given individual with respect to the average trajectory (respectively compare two given subjects together), one only need to compare the affine reparametrization $t \mapsto \alpha_i v_0(t-t_0-\tau_i)$ with the identity map $t \mapsto t$ (respectively, compare the slopes and intercepts of the two subject-specific affine reparametrization). We can observe that these reparametrization play the same role as the *time warps* which were introduced by Durrleman et al. in [11] and [10], in the context of longitudinal shape analysis. The time warps considered in those papers were diffeomorphisms of the real line which accounted for the different rates of shape changes and were constructed using the LDDMM framework : the diffeomorphism was obtained by integration of a time-varying vector field which belongs to a Gaussian reproducing kernel Hilbert space. The affine reparametrizations (with non-zero intercept) are also diffeomorphisms but only model a constant rate of progression. However, with only two random effects, we are able to describe the progression of a given subject in a realistic and easily interpretable manner.

Considering p_0 as a fixed effect of the model and estimating p_0 along with the other fixed effects ensures that the estimated p_0 will be the best observation point possible. It should be noted that the model does not depend on a reference time because if the observations $(t_{i,j}, y_{i,j})$ are transformed into $(t_{i,j} + t'_0, y_{i,j})$ then, only the estimated value of t_0 will change whereas the variance parameters will remain the same. Therefore, the interpretation of the random effects (and between-subjects or subjects-average comparaisons) do not depend on the timeline.

2.2   The Straight Lines Model

In this section, we will illustrate the flexibility of the model we introduced in the previous section. The choice of the Riemannian metric on M determines the shape of the geodesics of M. By taking the canonical metric on $\mathbb{R}$, the geodesics will be straight lines.

When $M = \mathbb{R}$ is equipped with the canonical metric, M is a geodesically complete Riemannian manifold and the geodesics of M are of the form $t \mapsto p + tv$. In this case, (1) writes :

$$y_{i,j} = p_0 + \alpha_i v_0(t_{i,j} - t_0 - \tau_i) + \varepsilon_{i,j}. \tag{4}$$

Even though the model is called "linear", (4) does not belong to the class of linear mixed-effects models introduced in [5].

2.3   The Logistic Curves Model

The situation when $M = (0,1)$ may arise when the observations are naturally bounded. For example, neuropsychological assessments such as ADAS-Cog or MMSE produce positive scores which are bounded above by a maximum score. The 13 questions ADAS-Cog assessment test is marked out of 85 points. Therefore, a typical ADAS-Cog score is a number in $[0, 85]$. By a proper renormalization, the score values can be considered as points in the interval $(0, 1)$. Fitting a linear model to such observations might not be such a good idea since the fitted trajectories will not always remain in the domain $(0, 1)$. On the other hand, $(0, 1)$ corresponds to the range of logistic curves with asymptote equal to 1. In order to equip the open interval $(0, 1)$ with a Riemannian manifold structure, we must give a Riemannian metric. At a point $p_0 \in (0, 1)$, the tangent space $T_{p_0}M$ is isomorphic to $\mathbb{R}$. For all p_0 in M, we define g_{p_0} to be the following inner product : $\forall (u, v) \in T_{p_0}M$, $g_{p_0}(u, v) = uM(p_0)v$ where $M(p_0) = \frac{1}{p_0^2(1-p_0)^2}$. The mapping $p_0 \mapsto g_{p_0}$ is smooth on M and defines a Riemannian metric on M. In this particular setting, the geodesic equation $\nabla_{\dot{\gamma}}\dot{\gamma} = 0$ writes : $\ddot{\gamma}(t) + \Gamma^1_{1,1}(\gamma(t))(\dot{\gamma}(t))^2 = 0$ where $\Gamma^1_{1,1}$ is the Christoffel symbol determined by

the only coefficient $g_{1,1}(t) = M(t)$ of the metric. The geodesic equation writes :
$\ddot{\gamma}(t) - \left(\frac{1}{\gamma(t)} + \frac{1}{\gamma(t)-1}\right)(\dot{\gamma}(t))^2 = 0$, or equivalently : $\gamma(\gamma - 1)\ddot{\gamma} - (2\gamma - 1)(\dot{\gamma})^2 = 0$.
Solving for this differential equation allows to determine that the geodesics of M
are logistic curves of the form $t \mapsto \frac{1}{1+a\exp(-rt)}$ with $a > 0$ and $r \in \mathbb{R}$. The geodesics are defined on $\mathbb{R}$ and therefore ensure that M is a geodesically complete
Riemannian manifold. In this case, (1) writes :

$$y_{i,j} = \frac{1}{1 + \left(\frac{1}{p_0} - 1\right)\exp\left(-\frac{\alpha_i v_0}{p_0(1-p_0)}(t_{i,j} - t_0 - \tau_i)\right)} + \varepsilon_{i,j}. \tag{5}$$

2.4   Estimation of the Parameters of the Model

The satistical model described in (1) is a nonlinear mixed-effects model with
gaussian random effects. Such models have been extensively studied in the lit-
terature and several methods exist for maximum likelihood estimation. The esti-
mation of the parameters $(p_0, t_0, v_0, \sigma_\eta, \sigma_\tau, \sigma)$ was coded into the SAS software
(SAS Institute) using the Gauss-Hermite quadrature approximation with one
quadrature point. This quadrature approximation method is equivalent to the
Laplace approximation of the observed likelihood. During the estimation procedure, the objective function resulting from the Laplace approximation was
minimized using the Newton-Raphson algorithm or the Nelder-Mead simplex
algorithm. It should be mentioned that these estimation procedures were quite
sensitive to the choice of starting values. However we observed that this method
was more efficent and more robust than the Alternating Algorithm, proposed by
Lindstrom and Bates in [13] or Pinheiro and Bates in [12], and implemented in
other softwares.

3   Results

3.1   Data

We used data from the Alzheimer's Disease Neuroimaging Initiative (ADNI)
database [15]. The ADAS-Cog scores we used were collected for 1391 individuals enrolled in the ADNI1, ADNIGO and ADNI2 phases and cortical thickness
measurements for 725 individuals from the ADNI1 database. The longitudinal
follow-up of these individuals ranges from 18 months to 4 years. Diagnoses were
recorded for every individual and at each visit. These subject-specific sequences
of diagnoses allowed to classify the individuals into 4 groups of interest : stable controls (329 individuals), stable mild cognitive impairment, also denoted as
stable MCI (471 individuals), stable Alzheimer patients (248 individuals) and
converters MCI (282 subjects). Cortical thickness measurements were available
for 194 stable controls, 182 stable MCI, 170 converters MCI and 162 Alzheimer
patients. The individuals who reverted to control or MCI were not included in
these groups.

3.2   Experimental Results

The ADAS-Cog scores were normalized by 85, which corresponds to the maximum possible score, and analyzed using the logistic curves model. For each individual, a couple of random variables (α_i, τ_i) where $\alpha_i = \exp(\eta_i)$ were estimated along with the parameters of the model. We recall that α_i (and respectively τ_i) account for the change in speed of disease progression (and respectively delay in disease progression) of a given individual with respect to the average disease progression trajectory. The couples (η_i, τ_i) have been plotted in Fig. 1.

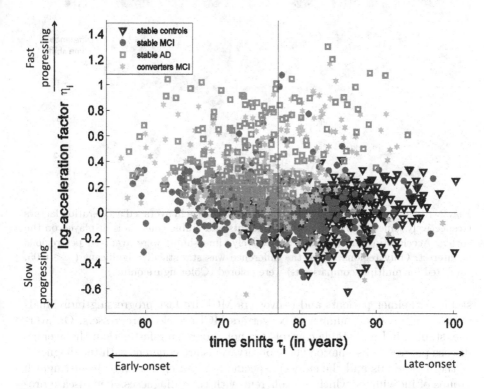

Fig. 1. Log-acceleration factors η_i plotted against the time shifts τ_i for the 1391 individuals with ADAS-Cog measurements. An horizontal line was plotted at the level $\eta_i = 0$ (no change in speed with respect to the average trajectory) and at $\tau_i = t_0 = 77.17$ (the estimated reference time t_0).

The results presented in Fig. 1 allow to compare the informations provided by (η_i, τ_i) across the groups of interest we previously mentioned. We can observe that stable controls have larger time shifts than other groups. The stable controls can be considered as late-onset individuals who are not, on average, evolving faster than the average disease progression trajectory. On the other hand, stable Alzheimer patients and MCI individuals tend to have smaller time shifts than stable controls. A portion of the stable MCI and most of the stable Alzheimer patients can be considered as early-onset individuals. It appears clearly that

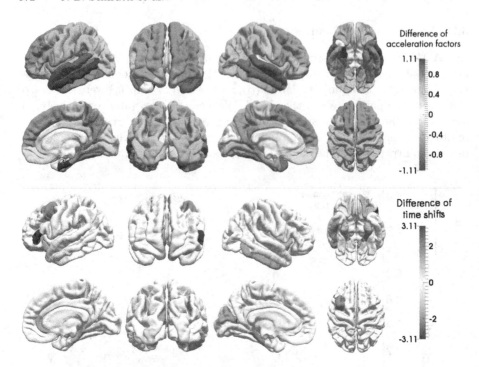

Fig. 2. At the top (respectively bottom) : the difference in averaged acceleration factors (respectively time shifts) between AD patients and stable controls is displayed on the cortex. Acceleration factors (and respectively time shifts) were averaged per regions of interest. Only regions where the difference was statistically significant ($p < 0.05$, corrected for multiple comparisons) were colored (Color figure online).

stable Alzheimer patients and converters MCI are fast progressing individuals even though a small number of converters MCI are slow-progressers. On average, stable MCI and stable controls are not progressing faster than the average disease progression scenario. These observations are coherent with the diagnoses of the individuals and the subject- specific random effects allow to distinguish groups of individuals which are coherent with their diagnoses. The disease progression for Alzheimer patients and converters MCI is faster and started earlier than for stable controls. The Alzheimer patients are quite clearly separated from the stable controls. In the model, the random effects η_i and τ_i are assumed independent, therefore uncorrelated. For this experiment, we computed the estimated covariance matrix of the random effects. For stable controls, we find that $\mathrm{Corr}(\eta_i, \tau_i) = 0.20$, for stable MCI : $\mathrm{Corr}(\eta_i, \tau_i) = -0.17$, for stable AD : $\mathrm{Corr}(\eta_i, \tau_i) = 0.12$ and for converters MCI : $\mathrm{Corr}(\eta_i, \tau_i) = 0.18$. These results seem coherent with the shape of the point clouds in the log-acceleration-time-shift plane, especially for stable controls and stable MCI.

The cortical thickness measurements (computed with Freesurfer) were averaged within 34 regions of interest defined with the Desikan-Killiany [19]

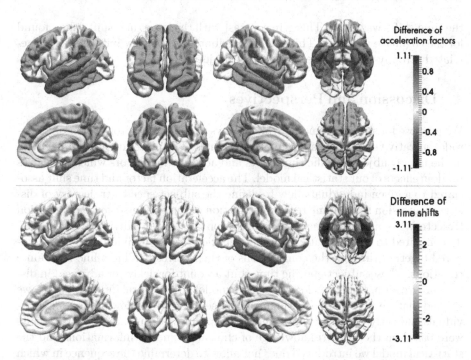

Fig. 3. At the top (respectively bottom) : the difference in averaged acceleration factors (respectively time shifts) between converters MCI and stable MCI is displayed on the cortex. Acceleration factors (and respectively time shifts) were averaged per regions of interest. Only regions where the difference was statistically significant ($p < 0.05$, corrected for multiple comparisons) were colored (Color figure online).

cortical atlas. The averaged cortical thickness measurements were analyzed using the straight lines model. For each subject, time shifts and acceleration factors were estimated and the corresponding values were displayed on the cortical surface. The differences in the estimated time shifts and acceleration factors were compared between Alzheimer patients and controls (Fig. 2), and between converters MCI and stable MCI (Fig. 3). Significance level was set at 0.05, corrected for multiple comparisons using Bonferroni correction. Alzheimer patients present accelerated gray matter loss compared to stable controls in a large number of regions, with highest speed in temporal (including entorhinal cortex, parahippocampal gyrus, superior and middle temporal gyri), parietal associative (including precuneus) and frontal regions. A similar topographical pattern was found for converters MCI compared to stable MCI but with smaller accelerations than in AD patients. On the contrary, primary motor and sensitive as well as visual cortices were spared. These results are highly consistent with the spatial-temporal progression patterns of neurodegeneration evidenced in histopathological studies [16,17]. Furthermore, accelerated atrophy has also been recently shown to coincide with disease-onset [18]. On the other hand, the estimated time shifts were not significantly different for the vast majority of regions. In the few significant regions, the magnitude of the time-shifts was small. This is in contrast with the large time-shift values found for the cognitive variables. This can be attributed to the slow but consistent age-related atrophy that is present in control subjects.

4   Discussion and Perspectives

We proposed a statistical model which allows to model the progression of a neurodegenerative disease for a group of individuals. The power of our approach lies in the use of subject-specific time shifts and acceleration factors which appear as random effects of our statistical model. The acceleration factor and time shift associated to a given individual allow to define the subject-specific trajectory of disease progression as an affine reparametrization of the average disease-progression trajectory. As a consequence, the progression of a given individual can be easily compared to the estimated average scenario and two individuals can be compared together through the comparisons of their corresponding affine reparametrizations. These subject-specific time shift account for delay (or advance) in disease progression. Using the logistic curves model and the straight lines model, we showed that we were able to distinguish between fast versus slow progressing individuals and early versus late onset individuals. However, our experimental results were based on the a priori knowledge of clinical diagnostic informations and the statistical model we introduced does not allow to determine the sequence in which biomarkers reach pathological levels. Fonteijn et al. proposed such an event-based model in [14]. Finally, our model was described in a Riemannian manifold setting which ensures that the model can be applied to data of varying complexity. This also paves the way for a generalization of this model to a multivariate framework.

Acknowledgments. This work was partially supported by the FMJH (Governement Program: ANR-10-CAMP-0151-02). The research leading to these results has received funding from the program Investissements davenir ANR-10-IAIHU-06.

References

1. Jack Jr., C.R., Knopman, D.S., Jagust, W.J., Shaw, L.M., Aisen, P.S., Weiner, M.W.: Hypothetical model of dynamic biomarkers of the Alzheimer's pathological cascade. Lancet Neurol. **9**(1), 119–128 (2010)
2. Samtani, M.N., Raghavan, N., Shi, Y., Novak, G., Farnum, M., Lobanov, V.: Disease progression model in subjects with mild cognitive impairment from the Alzheimer's disease neuroimaging initiative: CSF biomarkers predict population subtypes. Brit. J. Clin. Pharmacol. **75**(1), 146–161 (2013)
3. Delor, I., Charoin, J.E., Gieschke, R., Retout, S., Jacqmin, P.: Modeling Alzheimers disease progression using disease onset time and disease trajectory concepts applied to cdr-sob scores from ADNI. CPT Pharmacometrics Syst. Pharmacol. **2**(10), e78 (2013)
4. Yang, E., Farnum, M., Lobanov, V., Schultz, T., Raghavan, N., Samtani, M.N.: Quantifying the pathophysiological timeline of Alzheimer's disease. J. Alzheimer's Dis. **26**(4), 745–753 (2011)

5. Laird, N.M., Ware, J.H.: Random-effects models for longitudinal data. Biometrics **38**, 963–974 (1982)
6. DoCarmo, M.P.: Riemannian Geometry. Springer, Hiedelberg (1992)
7. Datar, M., Muralidharan, P., Kumar, A., Gouttard, S., Piven, J., Gerig, G., Whitaker, R., Fletcher, P.T.: Mixed-effects shape models for estimating longitudinal changes in anatomy. In: Durrleman, S., Fletcher, T., Gerig, G., Niethammer, M. (eds.) STIA 2012. LNCS, vol. 7570, pp. 76–87. Springer, Heidelberg (2012)
8. Singh, N., Hinkle, J., Joshi, S., Fletcher, P.T.: A hierarchical geodesic model for diffeomorphic longitudinal shape analysis. In: Gee, J.C., Joshi, S., Pohl, K.M., Wells, W.M., Zöllei, L. (eds.) IPMI 2013. LNCS, vol. 7917, pp. 560–571. Springer, Heidelberg (2013)
9. Lorenzi, M., Pennec, X., Frisoni, G.B., Ayache, N.: Alzheimer's disease neuroimaging initiative: disentangling normal aging from alzheimer's disease in structural magnetic resonance images. Neurobiol Aging **31**(8), 1443–1451 (2015)
10. Durrleman, S., Pennec, X., Trouvé, A., Braga, J., Gerig, G., Ayache, N.: Toward a comprehensive framework for the spatiotemporal statistical analysis of longitudinal shape data. IJCV **103**(1), 22–59 (2013)
11. Durrleman, S., Pennec, X., Trouvé, A., Gerig, G., Ayache, N.: Spatiotemporal atlas estimation for developmental delay detection in longitudinal datasets. In: Yang, G.Z., Hawkes, D., Rueckert, D., Noble, A., Taylor, C. (eds.) MICCAI 2009. LNCS, pp. 297–304. Springer, Heidelberg (2009)
12. Pinheiro, J.C.: Mixed-effects models in S and S-PLUS. Springer, Heidelberg (2000)
13. Lindstrom, M.J., Bates, D.M.: Nonlinear mixed effects models for repeated measures data. Biometrics **46**, 673–687 (1990)
14. Fonteijn, H.M., Modat, M., Clarkson, M.J., Barnes, J., Lehmann, M., Hobbs, N.Z., Alexander, D.C.: An event-based model for disease progression and its application in familial Alzheimer's disease and Huntington's disease. NeuroImage **60**(3), 1880–1889 (2012)
15. The Alzheimer's Disease Neuroimaging Initiative. https://ida.loni.usc.edu/
16. Braak, H., Braak, E.: Staging of Alzheimer's disease-related neurofibrillary changes. Neurobiol Aging **16**(3), 271–278 (1995)
17. Delacourte, A., David, J.P., Sergeant, N., Buee, L., Wattez, A., Vermersch, P., Di Menza, C.: The biochemical pathway of neurofibrillary degeneration in aging and Alzheimer's disease. Neurology **52**(6), 1158–1165 (1999)
18. Benzinger, T.L., Blazey, T., Jack, C.R., Koeppe, R.A., Su, Y., Xiong, C., Morris, J.C.: Regional variability of imaging biomarkers in autosomal dominant Alzheimer's disease. Proc. Natl. Acad. Sci. USA **110**(47), 18982–18987 (2013)
19. Desikan, R.S., Ségonne, F., Fischl, B., Quinn, B.T., Dickerson, B.C., Blacker, D., Killiany, R.J.: An automated labeling system for subdividing the human cerebral cortex on MRI scans into gyral based regions of interest. Neuroimage **31**(3), 968–980 (2006)

Prediction of Longitudinal Development of Infant Cortical Surface Shape Using a 4D Current-Based Learning Framework

Islem Rekik, Gang Li, Weili Lin, and Dinggang Shen[✉]

Department of Radiology and BRIC, University of North Carolina at Chapel Hill,
Chapel Hill, NC, USA
dinggang_shen@med.unc.edu

Abstract. Understanding the early dynamics of the highly folded human cerebral cortex is still an actively evolving research field teeming with unanswered questions. Longitudinal neuroimaging analysis and modeling have become the new trend to advance research in this field. However, this is challenged by a limited number of acquisition timepoints and the absence of inter-subject matching between timepoints. In this paper, we propose a novel framework that unprecedentedly solves the problem of predicting the dynamic evolution of infant cortical surface shape solely from a single baseline shape based on a spatiotemporal (4D) current-based learning approach. Specifically, our method learns from longitudinal data both the geometric (vertices positions) and dynamic (temporal evolution trajectories) features of the infant cortical surface, comprising a training stage and a prediction stage. *In the training stage*, we first use the current-based shape regression model to set up the inter-subject cortical surface correspondences at baseline of all training subjects. We then estimate for each training subject the diffeomorphic temporal evolution trajectories of the cortical surface shape and build an empirical mean spatiotemporal surface atlas. *In the prediction stage*, given an infant, we first warp all training subjects onto its baseline cortical surface. Second, we select the most appropriate learnt features from training subjects to *simultaneously* predict the cortical surface shapes at all later timepoints from its baseline cortical surface, based on closeness metrics between this baseline surface and the learnt baseline population average surface atlas. We used the proposed framework to predict the inner cortical surface shape at 3, 6 and 9 months from the cortical shape at birth in 9 healthy infants. Our method predicted with good accuracy the spatiotemporal dynamic change of the highly folded cortex.

1 Introduction

The highly folded human cerebral cortex nests vital cognitive and decision-making functions that control our behavior. Analyzing cortical morphometrics from neuroimages opens a wide widow to pinpoint population and individual based cortical growth patterns [1]. In particular, characterizing the morphological dynamics of the cerebral cortex as it matures will enable us to examine their

© Springer International Publishing Switzerland 2015
S. Ourselin et al. (Eds.): IPMI 2015, LNCS 9123, pp. 576–587, 2015.
DOI: 10.1007/978-3-319-19992-4_45

relationship with functional dynamics and thereby advance our understanding of how the cerebral cortex grows and what modulates its development [2]. Besides, quantifying cortical morphological dynamics at an early stage of cortical growth will help unravel early developing brain disorders [3]. More importantly, the possibility of predicting cortical morphological changes will eventually help improve prognosis for infants with neurodevelopmental brain disorders.

However, despite their importance, modeling approaches for examining the early postnatal human brain morphometrics and dynamics using longitudinal neuroimaging data are scarce. In [4], a computational mechanical cortical growth model was developed to simulate the dynamics of cortical folding from longitudinal data in the first year of life, during which the cortical surface area increase by 76 % [3]. Although promising, this method requires the use of cortical surfaces at all later timepoints of the same infant to guide the growth model and also will gradually lose its accuracy and informative potential as the number of data acquisition timepoints decreases. Ideally, a cortical growth model should be able to accurately and dynamically predict the highly convoluted shape of the cortical surface from one or a very limited number of input surfaces. By *cortical dynamic prediction*, we imply the estimation of the spatiotemporal cortex shape deformation in the future (i.e. the evolution trajectories of the shape) using a set of existing observations and measurements. Recently developed methods [5–8] proposed various geodesic shape regression models to estimate smooth diffeomorphic evolution trajectories; however, they were implemented for image time-series change tracking. A non-linear mixed effect dynamic prediction model was proposed in [9] to estimate temporal change trajectories of radial diffusivity images derived from diffusion tensor imaging (DTI) of early brain development. However, its application was only limited to estimate region-level changes in the image space, and also it required a predefined complex parametric form of the development trajectory.

This paper proposes a learning-based framework that predicts the dynamic postnatal cortical shape from a single baseline cortical surface at birth using a recently developed spatiotemporal (4D) diffeomorphic surface growth model based on the theory of 'measuring' a surface as a current [10,11]. The theory of currents elegantly and generically represents a shape as a current without the need to establish the point-to-point surface landmark correspondence on the longitudinal and cross-sectional shapes. Furthermore, piece-wise geodesic current deformation trajectories can be estimated from disparately spaced-out measurements in time for 0-currents (set of points), 1-currents (curves), 2-currents (surfaces) and 3-currents (volumes) using a robust converging numerical scheme developed in [10]; thereby facilitating the integration of multidimensional shapes from multimodal images in a unified statistical framework for data analysis. Specifically, our approach is composed of a training stage and a prediction stage. *In the training stage*, the proposed framework learns both geometric (vertices positions) and dynamic (smooth and invertible evolution trajectories) features of cortical surface growth for each infant using the available acquisition timepoints. We then estimate the mean empirical spatiotemporal atlas at the

most commonly shared timepoints among the training subjects to simultaneously initialize the cortical surface shapes at all later timepoints for prediction.
In the prediction stage, for each new subject, we refine this initialization by
jointly moving some vertices based on different closeness metrics between the
baseline cortical shape and the baseline cortical atlas. Once the baseline vertices positions are updated, they form together a *virtual* baseline shape, which
is proximal to the ground truth baseline cortical shape. Finally, retrieving the
corresponding learnt smooth deformation trajectory for every vertex belonging
to the constructed virtual shape predicts the cortical shape up to the last time-
point in the training dataset. Of note, the proposed method requires neither
predefined prarametric forms of the cortical developmental trajectories nor the
guidance from the later time points of the same subject.

2   Current-Based Learning of Shape Growth Model

2.1   Spatiotemporal Current-Based Atlas Building (Training Stage)

We first present the key mathematical ingredients for 'measuring' a surface as a
current. In this context, the current metric is used for building a diffeomorphic
regression model that matches a set of shapes $S = \{S_0, \ldots, S_N\}$ with high
accuracy as demonstrated in [11]. More details can be found in [10,11].

Cortical Surface Representation Using Currents. The concept of representing a surface as a current derives from Faraday's law of induction in physics,
which states that the variation of any magnetic vector field W through a surface
S induces a current in the space W^* within a wire loop delimiting S [10]. The
intensity of the current is proportional to the variation of the flux of this magnetic field, which mathematically translates as an integration of the vector field
elements $\omega \in W$ along the shape unit normal vectors n: $S = \int \omega(x)^t n(x) d\lambda(x)$,
where $d\lambda$ denotes Lebesgue measure on the surface. Hence, a surface can be
geometrically defined as the collection of local fluxes for all possible vector fields
traversing it. In this regard, W is defined as a Reproducing Kernel of Hilbert
Space (RKHS) spanned by convolutions between a square integrable vector field
and a Gaussian smooth kernel $K(x, y) = exp(-|x - y|^2/\sigma_W^2)$. The rate of decay
of the kernel σ_W denotes the scale under which the geometric details of the
surface –when converted into a current– are overlooked.

A vector $\omega \in W$ can be measured at a location x for any fixed points y
and vectors α as a convolution between the kernel K^W and vectors α: $\omega(x) =
K^W(x, y)\alpha(y)$, where the couple (x, α) is called a momentum. On the other
hand, the space of currents W^* is defined as a vector space containing the set
of all continuous linear maps from W to $\mathbb{R}$ (i.e. the dual space of W). Any
current in W^* is then defined as: $\omega \mapsto \delta_x^n(\omega) = n^t\omega(x)$, where δ_x^n defines a Dirac
delta current. Although it is scale-dependent, W enables to *densely* 'convert' the
surface S into a current by locally measuring these localized Dirac delta currents
and summing them up: $S = \sum_k \delta_{x_k}^{\alpha_k}$; thus S becomes fully parameterized by its
meshes (triangles) k and normals n_k located at each center of these meshes and
approximated using the Dirac delta currents located at the center of each of its

meshes k (Fig. 1). Hence, any surface can be decomposed into an infinite sum of Dirac delta currents which act as basis vectors in the space of currents W^*. More importantly, the current space W^* is endowed with a metric that enables us to measure the distance between two shapes (i.e. two currents): $< S, S' >_W^* = \sum_i \sum_j \alpha_i^t K^W(x_i, x_j)\beta_j$ where $S = \sum_i \delta_{x_i}^{\alpha_i}$ and $S' = \sum_j \delta_{x_j}^{\beta_j}$, thereby elegantly paving the way to formulate and solve geodesic surface matching problems.

Spatiotemporal Diffeomorphic Current-based Surface Regression Model. Considering a set of longitudinal cortical surfaces $\mathcal{S} = \{S_0, \ldots, S_N\}$ acquired at different timepoints t_i, $i \in [0, N]$, we estimate a spatiotemporal surface growth model that successively deforms the baseline shape S_0 onto the consecutive shapes: $S(t) = \xi_t(S_0)$. This deformation process is guided by the diffeomorphic mapping ξ_t, which identifies for each mesh the optimal evolution trajectory as a solution of the following flow equation:

$$\begin{cases} \frac{d\xi_t(x)}{dt} = v_t(\xi_t(x)), & t \in [0, T] \\ \xi_0 = Id. \end{cases}$$

Here $v_t \in V$ denotes the time-dependent deformation velocity. To guarantee the smoothness and the invertibility of the estimated deformation trajectory ξ_t, the velocity field V is defined as a RKHS with a Gaussian kernel K^V. The deformation kernel decays at a rate σ_V denoting the scale under which deformations are locally similar to the identity map (no deformation). The time-dependent velocity writes as $v_t(x) = \sum_{k=1}^{M} K^V(x_k(t), x)\alpha_k(t)$, with M the number of meshes in the baseline shape S_0 [10]. For a static shape S_0, the vector field W associated with it is closely spanned by the momenta (x, n). To cause S_0 to become dynamic and warp it onto different shapes, an external momentum (x_k, α_k) of the deformation field locally acts on its Dirac delta currents $\delta_{x_k}^{n_k}$ to geodesically deform it into the consecutive observed shapes. The estimation of the momenta $(x_k(t), \alpha_k(t))$ fully defines the surface deformation process from $t = 0$ to $t = T$. This is achieved through conjugate gradient descent algorithm minimizing the following energy:

$$E = \int_0^1 ||v_t||_V^2 dt + \frac{1}{\gamma} \sum_{j \in \{1, \ldots, N\}} ||\xi_{t_j}^v \cdot S_0 - S_j||_{W^*}^2$$

Where γ denotes a trade-off parameter between the total kinetic energy of the deformation (first term) and the similarity measure between the deformed baseline shape and the consecutive ground truth observations (second term).

Current-Based Geometric and Dynamic Features Learning. In the training stage, we estimate a cortical surface growth scenario for each infant in our training dataset using the available MR acquisition timepoints. We first register all the baseline surfaces of the training subjects into a common space. Then, for each warped baseline shape in this space, we estimate its temporal evolution trajectory. Both of these steps are achieved using the current-based deformation model, thereby providing a normalized current space, where all subjects' longitudinal shapes become 'linked' in space and time. This facilitates inter-subject comparison of deformation features estimated at any timpoint falling in the in-between obervations interval $]t_i, t_{i+1}[$. At this point, we introduce the notion

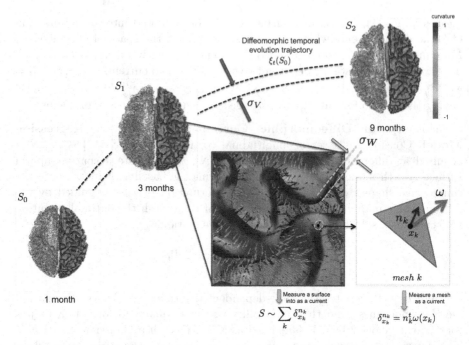

Fig. 1. *Geodesic longitudinal shape regression using currents.* Each cortical surface S_i is represented by the sum of the Dirac delta currents $\delta_{x_k}^{n_k}$ with x_k being the center of the mesh k (triangle) and n_k as its normal (illustrated in the left hemispheres).

of a *cloud* $\mathcal{C}$, which is composed of points $c(x,t) = (x, \xi(x,t))$ with x a vertex belonging to any baseline shape S_0 in the training data and $\xi(x,t)$ as its corresponding temporal deformation trajectory. In other words, a point $c(x,t)$ in the cloud locates the new position $\xi(x,t)$ of any baseline vertex x at a specific timepoint t. Here, the 3D position of any baseline vertex x defines the *geometric feature* and its evolution trajectory $c(x,t)_{t\in[0,T]}$ defines the *dynamic feature* of the learnt model. We will exploit both of these features to predict the evolution trajectory for a new baseline shape.

Cortical Spatiotemporal Atlas Estimation. For each of the most commonly shared acquisition timepoints $t_{i\{i\in0,\dots,N\}}$, we build an empirical mean atlas $\mathcal{A}_i$ by computing the mean 3D position of the spatiotemporally aligned training subjects. We also include the estimated shapes using the current-based surface growth model for the atlas building *if* these shapes were acquired at $\pm1-$month gap from the ground-truth shape (Fig. 2). Indeed, at $\pm1-$month gap, the current-model recovers neighboring information with high accuracy (mean $\pm$ std $= 1.05\pm$ $0.16mm$). One could intuitively explain this by recalling the principle of the least action in a classical mechanical Lagrangian framework, which grounds the diffeomorphic geodesic surface deformation framework. This strategy allows us to include more data into building the temporal atlas $\{\mathcal{A}_t\}$ with $t \in \{t_0,\dots,t_N\}$ and to better capture inter-subject variability.

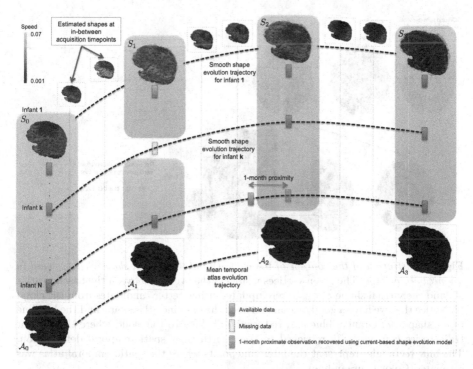

Fig. 2. *An overview of the proposed framework for learning dynamic cortical surface growth (training stage).* We estimate a smooth temporal trajectory for each of the baseline cortical shapes in the training dataset. Here we overlay the ground truth shapes (transparent gray) with the estimated ones. A spatiotemporal atlas is built at the most commonly shared acquisition timepoints in the training subjects. We also include the *estimated* cortical surface if it is $\pm 1-$month distant from the ground truth in the atlas building process.

2.2   Prediction Using the Learnt Geometric And dynamic Features

To predict the evolution of the cortical surface for a new infant, the only information we need is the shape of the baseline cortical surface S_0 (at the first acquisition timepoint). Here we propose two different methods that exploit S_0 to select geometric and dynamic features from the cloud. The extracted features will define the temporal evolution of the cortical surface up to the last common acquisition timepoint in the training dataset. Both methods are based on the intuitive idea that vertices in the baseline ground truth shape dynamically behave in a way that is similar to their *nearest* neighboring vertices in the cloud. Subsequently, we introduce the concept of a *virtual* shape that explores the learnt shape features to find the closest shape in the cloud to the baseline shape S_0. The prediction framework for the spatiotemporal evolution of the ground truth surface S_0 is composed of two main steps:

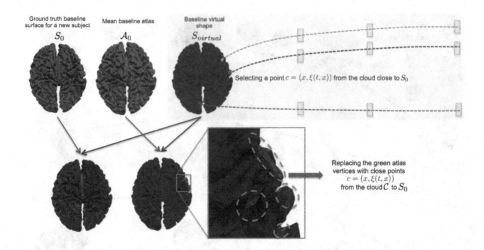

Fig. 3. *Illustration of the concept of the cloud C and the virtual shape $S_{virtual}$ used in the prediction stage.* The green vertices visible in the overlap between the baseline atlas A_0 and the virtual shape $S_{virtual}$ were updated using better candidates from the cloud C. Notice that we have a good overlap between the baseline atlas shape and the baseline input shape S_0. Orange, blue and red vertices belong to the cloud where their learnt trajectories can be easily retrieved to track forth their spatiotemporal deformation. The blue rectangles represent the later timepoints where the spatiotemporal atlas was estimated(Color figure online).

- **Step 1: Virtual shape construction for simultaneous shape prediction at all late timepoints.** First, we define a *virtual shape $S_{virtual}$* as the ensemble of baseline vertices from the cloud C that are close to the ground truth baseline shape S_0 (Fig. 3). We initialize the virtual shape as the baseline atlas shape A_0 and also the shapes to predict $\{\tilde{S}_i\}$ as the mean atlases A_i at the timepoint t_i. If the error distance between any vertex in the mean atlas shape A_0 and its corresponding baseline vertex in S_0 is smaller than ϵ, then we keep this vertex unmoved. Otherwise, we seek the closest vertex from the cloud that is within an ϵ-neighborhood of the current vertex. If the ϵ-closest vertex exists, then the position of the current vertex in $S_{virtual}$ is updated accordingly. Otherwise, for vertices in $S_{virtual}$ having no closest vertex in the $\epsilon-$range in the baseline shape, we propose two closeness metrics to construct the virtual shape $S_{virtual}$:

1. **The Mahalanobis distance from the cloud (Metric 1):** We use the Mahalanobis metric to update vertices in $S_{virtual}$ that are $> \epsilon-$further from the baseline shape S_0. More specifically, we select vertices from the cloud C that are closer to S_0 and fall within the $\epsilon-$neighborhood.
   $S_{virtual} = \{v_i\}_{\{i=1,...,M\}} = argmin_{v_k \in C_j; j \in \{0,...N\}} (v_i - v_k)^t \Sigma_j^{-1} (v_i - v_k)$
   C_j is the points of the cloud C that belong to the jth subject in the training dataset. Σ_j is the covariance matrix of the vertices in the cloud C_j.
   Finally, for each vertex in the virtual shape, we retrieve its dynamic feature $c(x,t)_{t \in [0,T]}$ from the cloud. This ultimately defines the smooth temporal

trajectory for every vertex in the constructed virtual shape and predicts its shape at any later timepoint.

2. **The $k-$closest neighbors from the cloud (Metric 2):** We update the position of a *virtual* vertex x that is $> \epsilon-$far from S_0 by computing the mean position of the k-closest vertices in the cloud to x using Euclidean distance. We compute the mean evolution trajectory $\bar{\xi}$ over the k retrieved trajectories. This mean spatially smoothed trajectory predicts the growth of the input baseline surface S_0.

These key steps are briefly stated in Algorithm 1.

Algorithm 1. Prediction of cortical surface shape evolution from a baseline shape

---

1: **INPUTS:**
   The learnt mean atlases $\mathcal{A}_{t_i}$
   The learnt cloud C
   The baseline ground truth shape S_0
2: Initialize $S_{virtual} \leftarrow \mathcal{A}_0$.
3: Initialize $\tilde{S}_i \leftarrow \mathcal{A}_i$ for $i \in \{1, \ldots, N\}$
4: Initialize ϵ as the mean distance between S_0 and $\mathcal{A}_0$ plus its standard deviation
5: **for** every vertex x in the *virtual shape* $S_{virtual}$ that is located outside the $\epsilon-$neighborhood from S_0 **do**
   Update its position using the closeness metric (1 or 2)
   Retrieve (or update if using Metric 2) its dynamic feature (evolution trajectory) $c(x,t)_{t \in [0,T]}$
   $\tilde{S}_i(x) = c(x, t_i)$
6: **end for**
7: Estimate the geodesic current-based *baseline shape* evolution using $\{S_0, \{\tilde{S}_i\}\}$ by minimizing:
   $\tilde{E} = \int_0^1 ||v_t||_V^2 dt + \frac{1}{\gamma} \sum_i ||\tilde{S}_i - \phi_{t_i}^v \cdot S_0||_{W^*}$
8: **OUTPUT:**
   Set of predicted surfaces $\{\tilde{S}_i\}$ at timepoints t_i with $i \in \{0, \ldots, N\}$
   Set of smooth temporal evolution trajectories for vertices in S_0 for $t \in [0, t_N]$

• *Step 2: Estimation of a geodesic evolution of the cortical shape for a new subject.* Once the set of shapes $\{\tilde{S}_i\}$ are predicted at later timepoints, we minimize the energy $\tilde{E}$ (Algorithm 1) to estimate the spatiotemporal deformation trajectory of the baseline shape S_0.

3   Results

3.1   Data and Parameters Setting

We evaluated the proposed framework on longitudinal inner cortical surfaces of 9 infants randomly selected from 17 healthy infants, each with 4 serial MRI scans acquired at around birth, 3 months, 6 months and 9 months of age. After rigid alignment of longitudinal and cross-sectional infant MR images and brain tissue segmentation, we reconstructed the cortical surfaces with correct topology and geometry using the method proposed in [12]. We used the current-based geodesic shape regression model with parameters $\gamma = 10^{-5}$, $\sigma_W = 5$, and set σ_V as half size the bounding box confining the surface at the last acqustion timepoint [10,11].

3.2   Cortical Shape Prediction Evaluation

We built three spatiotemporal atlases using alternatively selected 14 different training subjects from the dataset, while leaving 3 subjects for testing to predict the inner cortical surface shape at 3, 6 and 9 months from the cortical surface shape at birth.

Spatiotemporal Mean Population Atlas Building. We set the inter- and intra-subject cortical correspondences using the current-based shape regression model, so we can easily navigate from any subject at any timepoint to a different subject at a different timepoint. We then built spatiotemporal mean atlases at 0, 3, 6 and 9 months. Each spatiotemporal atlas $\{A_0, A_1, A_2, A_3\}$ was estimated using 14 infants, while leaving 3 infants out for testing.

Cortical Shape Prediction From the Baseline Cortical Surface S_0. We implemented Algorithm 1 using the two proposed closeness metrics to construct the virtual shape for each of the 9 testing infants. The parameter ϵ was fixed as the mean distance between S_0 and A_0 plus its standard deviation. We chose $k = 4$ closest neighbors for the second metric. We display in Table 1 a comparison between the prediction surface distance error for the two different metrics. Clearly, the prediction method based on Metric 2 shows a more promising performance in decreasing the prediction errors at later timepoints, compared with Metric 1 (Table 1). One could intuitively explain this observation as a result of including more vertices (here $k = 4$ closest neighbors) from the cloud to contribute into building more robust baseline virtual shape $S_{virtual}$. This in turn allows to stretch the neighborhood of vertices formed when shooting $S_{virtual}$ to the next missing timepoint by tracking their temporal evolution trajectories. In other words, this leads to better capture inter-subject spatial variability at later timepoints. Therefore, Metric 2 was used to build the spatiotemporal evolution of the baseline shape S_0.

We show in Fig. 4 the vertex-wise distance error map between the predicted $\{\tilde{S}_i\}$ and the ground truth shapes $\{S_i\}$ at 3, 6 and 9 months (top row) and their spatial overlap (bottom row) for one representative testing infant. The prediction error gradually increases as the shape to predict becomes very distant in time from S_0.

Figure 5 (a) and (b) shows the mean value and standard deviation prediction errors over the 9 testing infants in each cortical region defined in [13] at 3, 6 and 9 months. The average distance errors over two hemispheres and across all 36 ROIs are $0.811mm$, $0.953mm$ and $1.011mm$ at 3, 6, and 9 months, respectively. As we

Table 1. *Shape prediction errors (mm) from a single baseline cortical surface for 9 infants.* Mean ± standard deviation and median distance between the predicted shape and the ground truth shape were computed using metrics 1 (Mahalanobis distance) and 2 (k-closest vertices, $k = 4$).

Timepoint	Mean error 1	Median error 1	Mean error 2	Median error 2
3 months	1.279 ± 1.692	0.912	**1.235 ± 1.604**	**0.865**
6 months	1.324 ± 1.551	0.967	**1.296 ± 1.615**	**0.925**
9 months	3.347 ± 8.313	1.414	**1.695 ± 3.205**	**1.147**

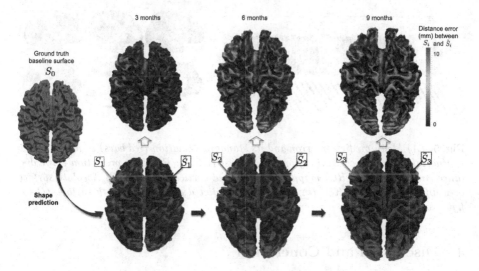

Fig. 4. *Spatiotemporal shape prediction in one representative infant.* (Top row) The 3D surface distance error map between the ground truth shape (in red) and the predicted shape (in blue) from the baseline shape S_0 (Color figure online).

can see, the distance errors are quite small, although they gradually increase from 3 to 9 months. Besides, the mean prediction error across the 9 subjects peaks at $0.86mm$ (in the right and left temporal poles), $1.11mm$ (in the right and left superior temporal gyri) and $1.05mm$ (in the right and left superior temporal gyri) successively for 3, 6 and 9 months. We also observe regionally non-uniform error maps, which is most likely caused by the spatially variable inter-subject variations in terms of cortical folding and its development. We also report the percentage of surface area difference in each ROI between the ground truth and the predicted cortical surfaces in Fig. 5 (c). The average surface area difference across all ROIs are 7.8 %, 12.9 % and 15.4 % at 3, 6, and 9 months, respectively, further demonstrating the good performance of the proposed method.

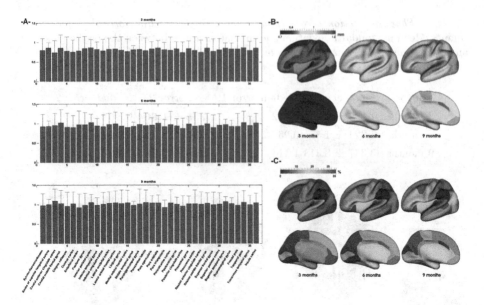

Fig. 5. *(A) Mean prediction error and its standard deviation (red bars) in mm across 9 testing infants in 36 cortical regions of interest (ROI). (B) Mean prediction error distance (in mm) of each ROI mapped onto inflated cortical surface. (C) Absolute surface area difference in each ROI (in %) between predicted and ground truth surfaces(Color figure online).*

4   Discussion and Conclusion

We presented the first prediction model for dynamic cortical surface evolution in infants during the first year based solely on a single baseline cortical shape. We used the diffeomeorphic 4D current-based shape regression model to learn both geometric and dynamic features of cortical surface shape growth for shape prediction at later timepoints. Although the infant cortical shape is very challenging to model due to its highly convoluted foldings and dynamic growth, the proposed framework showed promising prediction results. We would like to note that the proposed learning framework is generic and can also be applied to a new infant that has a limited set of measurements. In our future work, we would further boost up its performance by including more than one input shape and also additional morphological features (e.g. surface thickness or gyrification index) for predicting the shape evolution in space, time and morphology. Furthermore, exploring the recently developed unbiased approaches for 3D shape atlas building may also increase the prediction accuracy [14].

Acknowledgments. We kindly thank Deformetrica research team [11] for making their source code available at www.deformetrica.org.

References

1. Huttenlocher, P.: Morphometric study of human cerebral cortex development. Neuropsychologia **28**, 517–527 (1990)
2. Fischl, B., Rajendran, N., Busa, E., Augustinack, J., Hinds, O., Yeo, B., Mohlberg, H., Amunts, K., Zilles, K.: Cortical folding patterns and predicting cytoarchitecture. Cereb. Cortex **18**, 1973–1980 (2008)
3. Lyall, A., Shi, F., Geng, X., Woolson, S., Li, G., Wang, L., Hamer, R., Shen, D., Gilmore, J.: Dynamic development of regional cortical thickness and surface area in early childhood. Cereb. Cortex **2014**, 46–56 (2014)
4. Nie, J., Li, G., Wang, L., Gilmore, J., Lin, W., Shen, D.: A computational growth model for measuring dynamic cortical development in the first year of life. Cereb. Cortex **22**, 2272–2284 (2012)
5. Fletcher, P.: Geodesic regression and the theory of least squares on riemannian manifolds. Int. j. Comput. vis. **105**, 171–185 (2013)
6. Niethammer, M., Huang, Y., Vialard, F.-X.: Geodesic regression for image time-series. In: Fichtinger, G., Martel, A., Peters, T. (eds.) MICCAI 2011, Part II. LNCS, vol. 6892, pp. 655–662. Springer, Heidelberg (2011)
7. Singh, N., Hinkle, J., Joshi, S., Fletcher, P.: A vector momenta formulation of diffeomorphisms for improved geodesic regression and atlas construction. In: 2013 IEEE 10th International Symposium on Biomedical Imaging (ISBI), pp. 1219–1222 (2013)
8. Singh, N., Hinkle, J., Joshi, S., Fletcher, P.: A hierarchical geodesic model for diffeomorphic longitudinal shape analysis. Inf. Process. Med. Imaging **23**, 560–571 (2013)
9. Sadeghi, N., Fletcher, P., Prastawa, M., Gilmore, J., Gerig, G.: Subject-specific prediction using nonlinear population modeling: application to early brain maturation from DTI. Med. Image Comput. Comput. Assist. Interv. **17**, 33–40 (2014)
10. Durrleman, S.: Statistical models of currents for measuring the variability of anatomical curves, surfaces and their evolution. Ph.D. thesis. Université de Nice-Sophia Antipolis (2010)
11. Durrleman, S., Prastawa, M., Charon, N., Korenberg, J., Joshi, S., Gerig, G., Trouvé, A.: Morphometry of anatomical shape complexes with dense deformations and sparse parameters. Neuroimage **101**, 35–49 (2014)
12. Li, G., Wang, L., Shi, F., Lin, W., Shen, D.: Simultaneous and consistent labeling of longitudinal dynamic developing cortical surfaces in infants. Med. Image. Anal. **18**, 1274–1289 (2014)
13. Desikan, R., Segonne, F., Fischl, B., Quinn, B., Dickerson, B., Blacker, D., Buckner, R., Dale, A., Maguire, R., Hyman, B., Albert, M., Killiany, R.: An automated labeling system for subdividing the human cerebral cortex on mri scans into gyral based regions of interest. Neuroimage **31**, 968–980 (2006)
14. Gori, P., Colliot, O., Worbe, Y., Marrakchi-Kacem, L., Lecomte, S., Poupon, C., Hartmann, A., Ayache, N., Durrleman, S.: Bayesian atlas estimation for the variability analysis of shape complexes. Med. Image Comput.Comput. Assist. Interv. **16**, 267–274 (2013)

Multi-scale Convolutional Neural Networks for Lung Nodule Classification

Wei Shen[1], Mu Zhou[3], Feng Yang[2(✉)], Caiyun Yang[1], and Jie Tian[1(✉)]

[1] Key Laboratory of Molecular Imaging of Chinese Academy of Sciences,
Institute of Automation, Chinese Academy of Sciences, Beijing, China
[2] School of Computer and Information Technology, Beijing Jiaotong University,
Beijing, China
fengyang@bjtu.edu.cn
[3] Department of Computer Science and Engineering,
University of South Florida, Tampa, USA
tian@ieee.org

Abstract. We investigate the problem of diagnostic lung nodule classification using thoracic Computed Tomography (CT) screening. Unlike traditional studies primarily relying on nodule segmentation for regional analysis, we tackle a more challenging problem on directly modelling raw nodule patches without any prior definition of nodule morphology. We propose a hierarchical learning framework—Multi-scale Convolutional Neural Networks (MCNN)—to capture nodule heterogeneity by extracting discriminative features from alternatingly stacked layers. In particular, to sufficiently quantify nodule characteristics, our framework utilizes multi-scale nodule patches to learn a set of class-specific features simultaneously by concatenating response neuron activations obtained at the last layer from each input scale. We evaluate the proposed method on CT images from Lung Image Database Consortium and Image Database Resource Initiative (LIDC-IDRI), where both lung nodule screening and nodule annotations are provided. Experimental results demonstrate the effectiveness of our method on classifying malignant and benign nodules without nodule segmentation.

Keywords: Lung nodule classification · Computed Tomography (CT) Imaging · Convolutional Neural Networks · Computer-Aided Diagnoses (CAD)

1 Introduction

Lung cancer is notoriously aggressive with a low long-term survival rate [1]. Quantitative analysis in lung nodules using thoracic Computed Tomography (CT) has been a central focus for early cancer diagnosis, where CT phenotype provides a powerful tool to comprehensively capture nodule characteristics [2].

W. Shen and M. Zhou—These authors contributed equally.

© Springer International Publishing Switzerland 2015
S. Ourselin et al. (Eds.): IPMI 2015, LNCS 9123, pp. 588–599, 2015.
DOI: 10.1007/978-3-319-19992-4_46

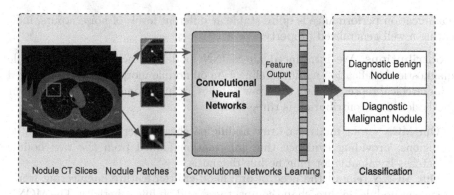

Fig. 1. An overview of the MCNN. Our approach first extracts multiple nodule patches to capture the wide range of nodule variability from input CT images. The obtained patches are then fed into the networks simultaneously to compute discriminative features. Finally, our approach applies a classifier to label the input nodule malignancy.

The importance of diagnostically classifying malignant and benign nodules using CT images is to facilitate radiologists for nodule staging assessment and individual therapeutic planning. Despite different approaches proposed for nodule analysis such as parametric texture feature extraction [4,8,13], they are problematic in finding well-suited parameters for robust analysis. It comes without doubt that, technical challenges still remain in defining and extracting quantitative features from clinical images for improving image-guided disease diagnosis. Furthermore, prior studies mostly focused on nodule morphology [5,19], which may not be able to provide an accurate description of the nodule. For example, the definition of nodule boundaries is obscure and subjective—inter-reader variability from radiologists makes precise nodule delineation a challenging task. In view of these challenges, the following specific questions arise: (a) What should be done to learn discriminative features from heterogeneous nodule data for representing different diagnostic groups? (b) How could one design a robust framework that is capable of extracting quantitative features from *original* nodule patches—instead of *segmented nodules*—that is advantageous in completely eliminating onerous preprocessing steps such as a nodule segmentation?

In this paper, we study the problem of lung nodule diagnostic classification based on thoracic CT scans. In contrast to the current methods primarily relying on nodule segmentation and textural feature descriptors for the classification task, we propose a hierarchical learning framework to capture the nodule heterogeneity by utilizing Convolutional Neural Networks (CNN) to extract features (as illustrated in Fig. 1). The learned features can be readily combined with state-of-the-art classifiers (e.g., Support Vector Machine (SVM) and Random Forest (RF)) for related Computer-Aided Diagnoses (CADs). Our method achieves 86.84 % accuracy on nodule classification using only nodule patches. We also observe that the proposed method is robust against noisy corruption—the classification performance is quite stable at different levels of noise inputs, indicating a well generalized property.

Contributions. We introduced an MCNN model to tackle the lung nodule diagnostic classification without delineation on nodule morphology and explored a hierarchical representation from raw patches for lung nodule classification. Our methodological contribution is three-fold:

- Our MCNN take multi-scale raw nodule patches, rather than the segmented regions, providing evidence that information gained from the raw nodule patches is valuable for lung nodule diagnosis.
- Our MCNN remove the need of any hand-crafted feature engineering work, such as nodule texture, shape compactness, and nodule sphericity. The MCNN can automatically learn the discriminative features.
- Although it is challenging to directly deal with noisy data in nodule CT, we show that the proposed MCNN model is effective in capturing nodule characteristics in nodule diagnostic classification even with a high-level noisy corruption.

Related Work. Image-based lung nodule analysis is normally performed with nodule segmentation [5], feature extraction [2], and labelling nodule categories [8,17,19]. Way et al. [19] first segmented the nodules and then extracted texture features to train a linear discriminant classifier. El-Baz et al. [5] used shape analysis for diagnosing malignant lung nodules. Han et al. [8] used 3-D texture feature analysis for the diagnosis of pulmonary nodules by considering extended neighbouring structures. However, all of these mentioned methods relied on nodule segmentation as a prerequisite for nodule feature extraction. Notably, automated nodule segmentation can affect classification since segmentation usually depends on initialization, such as region growing and level set methods. Working on these segmented regions may yield inaccurate features that lead to erroneous outputs.

Descriptors of Histogram of Oriented Gradients (HOG) [4] and Local Binary Patterns (LBP) [13] are widely used for feature representation in medical image analysis. However, it is known that they are domain agnostic [15]. In other words, the required hyper-parameters make these approaches sensitive to specific tasks. For example, a repetitious parameter tuning is needed for the neighbourhood points in LBP and the size of the cell window in HOG.

Our work is conceptually similar to the massive training artificial neural network [17], which suggested a feasibility on learning knowledge from artificial neural networks. However, the work was an integrated classifier that required extra support from a 2-D Gaussian distribution for the decision-making, where an image-to-image mapping based on local pixels was learned. Our approach, without knowing any extra distributions, aims at feature extraction globally from the original nodule image space through stacked convolutional operations and max-pooling selections. In contrast to [17], our work is more computationally effective in reducing the feature dimensionality and resulting in highly discriminative features from hierarchical layers.

2   Learning Multi-scale Convolutional Neural Networks

Given a lung nodule CT image, our goal is to discover a set of globally discriminative features using the proposed MCNN model, which captures the essence of class-specific nodule information. The challenge is that the image space is extremely heterogeneous since both healthy tissues and nodules are included. In this work, we make full use of the CNN to learn discriminative features, and build three CNN in parallel to extract multi-scale features from nodules with different sizes. Details are given in this section.

2.1   Convolutional Neural Networks Architecture

Our Convolutional Neural Networks contain two convolutional layers, both of which are followed by a max-pooling layer, and a fully connected layer which represents the final output feature. The detailed structure of the network is shown in Fig. 2. From the input nodule patch to the final feature layer, the sizes of feature maps keep decreasing, which helps remove the potential redundant information in the original nodule patch and obtains discriminative features in nodule classification.

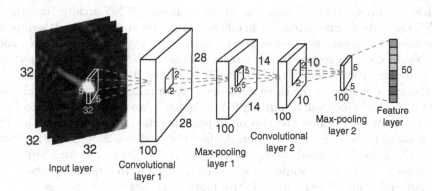

Fig. 2. The structure of the Convolutional Neural Networks learned in our work. The numbers along each side of the cuboid indicate the dimensions of the feature maps. The inside cuboid represents the 3D convolution kernel and the inside square stands for the 2D pooling region. The number of the hidden neurons in the final feature layer is marked aside.

The network starts from a convolutional layer, which convolves the input feature map with a number of convolutional kernels and yields a corresponding number of output feature maps. Formally, the convolution operation between an input feature map f and a convolutional kernel h is defined by:

$$y = \max\left(0, \sum_c f_c * h_c + b\right), \tag{1}$$

where f_c and h_c denote the cth slice from the feature map and that from the convolutional kernel respectively, and b is the bias scalar. $*$ is the convolution operation. Both h and b are continuously learned in the training process. In order to perform a non-linear transformation from the input to the output space, we adopt the rectified linear unit (ReLu) non-linearity in Eq. 1 for each convolution [11]. It is expressed as $y = \max(0, x)$, where x is the convolution output.

Following the convolutional layer, a max-pooling layer is introduced to select feature subsets. It is formulated as

$$y_{(i,j)} = \max_{0 \le m,n \le s} \{x_{(i \cdot s+m, j \cdot s+n)}\}, \tag{2}$$

where s is the pooling size and x denotes the output of the convolutional layer. An advantage of using the max-pooling layer is its translation invariability which is especially helpful when different nodule images are not well-aligned.

2.2   Multi-scale Nodule Representation

Our idea of the multi-scale sampling strategy is motivated from the clinical fact that nodule sizes vary remarkably, ranging from less than 3 mm to more than 30 mm in the Lung Image Database Consortium and Image Database Resource Initiative (LIDC-IDRI) [3] datasets. In the proposed MCNN architecture, three CNN that take nodule patches from different scales (as shown in Fig. 3) as inputs are assembled in parallel. We briefly refer to the three CNN as CNN_0, CNN_1, and CNN_2. In order to reduce the parameters of the MCNN, we follow the setting in [6] to share parameters among all the CNN. The resulting output of our MCNN is the concatenation of the three CNN outputs, forming the final discriminative feature vector, which will be directly fed to the final classifier without any feature reduction. We also follow the idea of deeply supervised networks (DSN) in [12] to construct our objective function. Unlike the traditional objective function in CNN, DSN introduced "companion objectives" [12] into the final objective function to alleviate the vanishing gradients problem so the training process can be fast and stable. The entire objective function is thus represented as

$$F(W) = P(W) + Q(W), \tag{3}$$

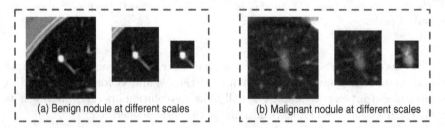

(a) Benign nodule at different scales   (b) Malignant nodule at different scales

Fig. 3. Nodule slice examples from a benign nodule patch (a) and a malignant nodule patch (b). The scales are $96 \times 96 \times 96$, $64 \times 64 \times 64$, and $32 \times 32 \times 32$ in pixel respectively.

In our work, $P(W) = LOSS(W, w^{(out)})$ is the overall hinge loss function for the concatenated feature layer, and $Q(W) = \sum_{m=1}^{M} \alpha_m loss(W, w^{(m)})$ is the sum of the companion hinge loss functions from all CNN. α_m is the coefficient for the mth CNN. W denotes the combination of the weights from all of the CNN, while $w^{(m)}$ and $w^{(out)}$ are the weights of the feature layer of the mth CNN and the weights of the final concatenated feature layer respectively. In this way, $F(W)$ keeps each network optimized and also makes the assembly sensible. Figure 4 shows the concatenated features projected into a 2-D subspace. It shows that the proposed MCNN model is able to remove the redundant information in the original images and extract discriminative features.

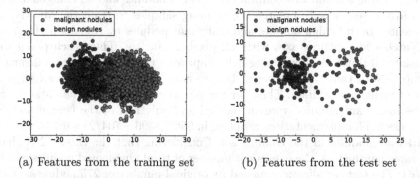

(a) Features from the training set   (b) Features from the test set

Fig. 4. Feature visualization. The learned features by the MCNN from both training set (a) and test set (b) are illustrated by projecting them into a 2-D subspace with principal component analysis (PCA) [10].

3 Experiments

3.1 Datasets and Setup

We evaluated our method on the LIDC-IDRI datasets [3]. It consists of 1010 patients with lung cancer screening thoracic CT scans as well as mark-up annotated lesions. The nodules are rated from 1 to 5 by four experienced thoracic radiologists, indicating an increasing degree of malignancy (1 denotes low malignancy and 5 is high malignancy). In this study, we included nodules along with their annotated centers from the nodule report[1]. We chose the averaged malignancy rating for each nodule as in [8]. For those with an average score lower than 3, we labelled them as benign nodules; for those with an average score higher than 3, we labelled them as malignant nodules. We removed nodules with ambiguous IDs and those with an average score of 3. Overall, there were 880 benign nodules and 495 malignant nodules. Since the resolution of the images varied, we resampled those images to set the resolution to a fixed 0.5 mm/pixel

---

[1] http://www.via.cornell.edu/lidc/.

along all three axes. Thus, the effect of resolution on the classification performance was removed. Then each nodule patch is cropped from the resampled CT image based on the marked nodule centers. The three scale inputs are $32 \times 32 \times 32$, $64 \times 64 \times 64$, and $96 \times 96 \times 96$ in pixels. Patches are all resampled to $32 \times 32 \times 32$ so that they can be uniformly fed into each CNN.

3.2   Implementation Details

We used a 5-fold cross validation for evaluating classification performance based on features learned from the MCNN. During each round of validation, there were originally 1100 nodules (704 benign nodules and 396 malignant nodules) in the training set and 275 nodules (176 benign nodules and 99 malignant nodules) in the test set. To enlarge the training samples to train the MCNN, we augmented both benign nodules and malignant nodules by translating the nodule patches along three axes with ± 2 pixels as in [16]. Thus, each patch was translated 6 times. Such a setting helps capture a range of translation invariant features. Note that the number of benign nodules is almost twice as large as that of malignant nodules. Thus, for the purpose of balancing the datasets, all of the malignant nodules were augmented and only half of the benign nodules were selected for augmentation, resulting in 5588 $((396 + 704/2) \times 6 + 396 + 704)$ multi-scale nodules in the training set. Considering that the three CNN share the same parameters, the equivalent number of total augmented nodules can be 16,764. The test set always remained its original number of 275 nodule samples at each validation round.

To systematically evaluate the performance of the MCNN, we covered different network configurations, i.e. different numbers of convolutional kernels of each convolutional layer and that of the hidden neurons in the feature layer. The numbers of the convolutional kernels were $n_1 = \{50, 100\}, n_2 = \{50, 100\}$ for the first and second layer and the number of neurons in the hidden layer was $n_3 = \{20, 50\}$. Therefore, there were 8 configurations in total for the MCNN. Note that we set $\alpha_m = 0.001$ for all m as found best in [12]. The convolutional kernel size is $5 \times 5 \times k$ which is quite typical in traditional CNN. k represents the third dimension of the input feature map. The pooling size was fixed to a 2×2 window. We added L2 norm weight decay during the training process to relieve overfitting. Two classifiers were used in experiments including SVM with a Radial Basis Function (RBF) kernel and RF. The hyper-parameters in both SVM and RF were obtained via a grid search on the training set.

We compared our results with two competing methods including HOG and LBP descriptors. For the HOG descriptor, we included different cell window sizes, $s_w = \{8, 16, 32\}$ with the number of orientations $n_o = 8$. For the LBP descriptor, the uniform LBP descriptor was computed with different neighbourhood points $n_{pt} = \{8, 16, 24\}$. Computation was done on all three scales of nodule patches for both descriptors.

Speaking of time complexity, although training deep networks often takes time, we choose a strategy of off-line training and on-line testing. In other words, once the network is finely trained off-line, it will be fast when a new sample comes in. In our study, using the NVIDIA Tesla K40 GPU, the test time for a single nodule patch was within 0.1 s. The CNN implementation used in this work was the deep learning toolkit CAFFE [9]. The classifiers of SVM and RF were from the scikit-learn package [14]. The HOG descriptor and the uniform LBP descriptor were from the scikit-image package [18].

3.3   Binary Nodule Classification Results

In this section, we evaluated the binary nodule classification. We used the average accuracy to observe the classification performance, i.e. the average ratio of corrected classified nodules from both classes from a 5-fold cross validation. Note that in the test set during each round of cross validation, 176 benign nodules and 99 malignant nodules made a baseline accuracy of 64 % by voting the majority class. From Fig. 5, it was immediately observed that the proposed MCNN showed competitive results above **84 %** with different configurations. The highest classification accuracy was obtained with the RF classifier with 86.84 % under the configuration of $n_1 = 100$, $n_2 = 100$ and $n_3 = 50$ (see Fig. 2). The overall performance of both classifiers suggested that our method can achieve promising results. The advantages can be ascribed to a factor that the hierarchical learning strategy selected high-level features, eliminating a number of redundant features. As already proven in [7], convolutional networks can produce useful dimensional reduction that is very helpful for image-related classification.

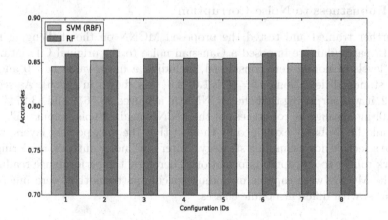

Fig. 5. The classification performance of SVM with the RBF kernel and RF based on features from the MCNN using 8 different configurations. Each configuration is assigned to a unique ID for display convenience.

Accuracy of the HOG and LBP descriptors are shown in Table 1 (numbers in bold denote the best results in columns). It was apparent that the HOG descriptor was quite sensitive to the size of the cell window (s_w). The results of the HOG descriptor dropped and were even worse than the baseline when s_w expanded, indicating that the information gained is minimal when the size was becoming larger. For the LBP descriptor, we observed that the number of neighbourhood points (n_{pt}) was positively related to the performance since sophisticated neighbourhood structures led to better results. However, when comparing best results among different approaches, our MCNN outperformed HOG and LBP descriptors with 10.91 % and 13.17 %, respectively. Overall, our observation confirmed that parametric textural descriptors were sensitive to parameters.

Table 1. Performance using the HOG and LBP descriptors with different s_w and n_{pt}.

Classifier	Scales	HOG			LBP		
		$s_w = 8$	$s_w = 16$	$s_w = 32$	$n_{pt} = 8$	$n_{pt} = 16$	$n_{pt} = 24$
SVM	32	74.18 %	63.27 %	49.82 %	64.58 %	66.40 %	67.35 %
	64	66.69 %	66.40 %	56.15 %	49.24 %	59.93 %	59.20 %
	96	64.07 %	65.16 %	56.58 %	36.00 %	52.22 %	54.84 %
RF	32	**75.93 %**	67.71 %	60.07 %	**71.27 %**	**72.07 %**	**73.67 %**
	64	73.16 %	**67.78 %**	**62.84 %**	62.54 %	62.25 %	66.55 %
	96	67.56 %	64.58 %	61.75 %	60.07 %	60.15 %	62.84 %

3.4 Robustness to Noise Corruption

We further trained and tested the proposed MCNN on the challenging noisy data. In particular, we imposed a Gaussian noise to the original CT data. Different levels of noises were considered, including a mean value $\mu = 0$ and different standard deviations $\sigma = \{0.5, 1.0, 2.0\}$ (as shown in Fig. 6). As seen in Table 2, it was surprising that the MCNN still achieved 83.56 % and 83.27 % with $\sigma = 2.0$, indicating the robustness of the MCNN against noisy inputs. The success could be probably explained by the fact that the max-pooling layers, which use the selective downsampling strategy, "filter out" noisy outliers, rendering the network robust to corrupted information. Therefore, the performance reaffirmed that the MCNN were capable of finding specific patterns that were inherently associated with different nodule classes.

3.5 Discussion

We have shown promising results of the proposed MCNN framework on classifying diagnostic nodule classes. Convolutional network is a powerful tool for image analysis because its capacities can be easily adjusted to a specific task and it makes strong and mostly correct assumptions about the nature of images [11]. In our study, although it suggested a clear need to further investigate the appropriate scales of nodules that lead to improved performance, we experimentally found that even with a single scale, the results remained competitive (for CNN_0,

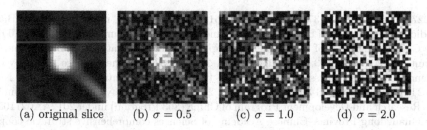

(a) original slice   (b) $\sigma = 0.5$ (c) $\sigma = 1.0$ (d) $\sigma = 2.0$

Fig. 6. Slice demonstration with different levels of noise. Gaussian noises with a mean value $\mu = 0$ and different standard deviations were imposed.

Table 2. Performance of the MCNN under different levels of noise

Classifier	$\sigma = 0.5$	$\sigma = 1.0$	$\sigma = 2.0$
SVM	85.82 %	84.22 %	83.56 %
RF	85.60 %	85.24 %	83.27 %

CNN_1, and CNN_2, it achieved 86.12 %, 83.88 %, and 79.00 % respectively). However, using the multi-scale strategy eliminated the careful designing of the patch sizes, which could be a tedious work. Rather than using isotropic kernels, we kept the third dimension of the kernels to be the same with the dimension of the input feature map which is quite common in the intermediate layers of conventional CNN. It also enabled us to directly use CAFFE out of the box.

4   Conclusion

In this paper, we proposed a Multi-scale Convolutional Neural Networks (MCNN) architecture to tackle the challenging problem on learning from lung nodule patches for nodule diagnostic classification. We demonstrated that the learned compact features are able to capture nodule heterogeneity. It is particularly promising that the MCNN model is robust against noisy inputs, which is valuable in the medical image analysis field. Extensive experiments showed that our method achieved 86.84 % for nodule classification and outperformed competing benchmark textural descriptors. In future work, we plan to expand data inclusion for a large-scale evaluation, and we will perform an investigation to seek appropriate scales for improving image-guided nodule analysis.

Acknowledgments. The authors acknowledge the National Cancer Institute and the Foundation for the National Institutes of Health, and their critical role in the creation of the free publicly available LIDC/IDRI Database used in this study. We also gratefully acknowledge the support of NVIDIA Corporation with the donation of the Tesla K40 GPU used for this research. This paper is supported by the Chinese Academy of Sciences Key Deployment Program under Grant No. KGZD-EW-T03, the National Basic Research Program of China (973 Program) under Grant 2011CB707700, the National Natural Science Foundation of China under Grant No.

81227901, 61231004, 81370035, 81230030, 61301002, 61302025, major projects of Biomedicine Department of Shanghai Science and Technology Commission (13411950100), the Chinese Academy of Sciences Fellowship for Young International Scientists under Grant No. 2010Y2GA03, 2013Y1 GA0004, 2013Y1GB0005, the Chinese Academy of Sciences Visiting Professorship for Senior International Scientists under Grant No. 2012T1G0036, 2010T2G 36, 2012T1G0039, 2013T1G0013, the National High Technology Research and Development Program of China (863 Program) under 2012AA021105, the Guangdong Province-Chinese Academy of Sciences comprehensive strategic cooperation program under 2010A090100032 and 2012B090400039, the NSFC-NIH Biomedical collaborative research program under 81261120414, the National Science and Technology Supporting Plan under 2012BAI15B08, the Beijing Natural Science Foundation under Grant No. 4132080, the Fundamental Research Funds for the Central Universities under Grant No. 2013JBZ014.

References

1. Aberle, D.R., Adams, A.M., Berg, C.D., Black, W.C., Clapp, J.D., Fagerstrom, R.M., Gareen, I.F., Gatsonis, C., Marcus, P.M., Sicks, J.: Reduced lung-cancer mortality with low-dose computed tomographic screening. N. Engl. J. Med. **365**(5), 395–409 (2011)
2. Aerts, H.J., Velazquez, E.R., Leijenaar, R.T., Parmar, C., Grossmann, P., Cavalho, S., Bussink, J., Monshouwer, R., Haibe-Kains, B., Haibe-Kains, D., Rietveld, D., Hoebers, F., Rietbergen, M.M., Leemans, C.R., Dekker, A., Quackenbush, J., Gillies, R.J., Lambin, P.: Decoding tumour phenotype by noninvasive imaging using a quantitative radiomics approach. Nat. Commun. **5**, Article No. 4006 (2014). doi:10.1038/ncomms5006
3. Armato III, S.G., McLennan, G., Bidaut, L., McNitt-Gray, M.F., Meyer, C.R., Reeves, A.P., Zhao, B., Aberle, D.R., Henschke, C.I., Hoffman, E.A., et al.: The lung image database consortium (LIDC) and image database resource initiative (IDRI): a completed reference database of lung nodules on CT scans. Med. phys. **38**(2), 915–931 (2011)
4. Dalal, N., Triggs, B.: Histograms of oriented gradients for human detection. In: IEEE Computer Society Conference on Computer Vision and Pattern Recognition (CVPR 2005), vol. 1, pp. 886–893 (2005)
5. El-Baz, A., Nitzken, M., Khalifa, F., Elnakib, A., Gimel'farb, G., Falk, R., El-Ghar, M.A.: 3D shape analysis for early diagnosis of malignant lung nodules. In: Székely, G., Hahn, H.K. (eds.) IPMI 2011. LNCS, vol. 6801, pp. 772–783. Springer, Heidelberg (2011)
6. Farabet, C., Couprie, C., Najman, L., LeCun, Y.: Learning hierarchical features for scene labeling. IEEE Trans. Pattern Anal. Mach. Intell. **35**(8), 1915–1929 (2013)
7. Hadsell, R., Chopra, S., LeCun, Y.: Dimensionality reduction by learning an invariant mapping. IEEE Comput. Soc. Conf. Comput. Vis. Pattern Recognit. **2**, 1735–1742 (2006)
8. Han, F., Zhang, G., Wang, H., Song, B., Lu, H., Zhao, D., Zhao, H., Liang, Z.: A texture feature analysis for diagnosis of pulmonary nodules using LIDC-IDRI database. In: IEEE International Conference on Medical Imaging Physics and Engineering, pp. 14–18 (2013)
9. Jia, Y., Shelhamer, E., Donahue, J., Karayev, S., Long, J., Girshick, R., Guadarrama, S., Darrell, T.: Caffe: Convolutional architecture for fast feature embedding (2014). arXiv preprint arXiv:1408.5093

10. Jolliffe, I.: Principal Component Analysis. Wiley Online Library, Chichester (2005)
11. Krizhevsky, A., Sutskever, I., Hinton, G.E.: Imagenet classification with deep convolutional neural networks. In: Advances in Neural Information Processing Systems, pp. 1097–1105 (2012)
12. Lee, C.Y., Xie, S., Gallagher, P., Zhang, Z., Tu, Z.: Deeply-supervised nets (2014). arXiv preprint arXiv:1409.5185
13. Ojala, T., Pietikainen, M., Maenpaa, T.: Multiresolution gray-scale and rotation invariant texture classification with local binary patterns. IEEE Trans. Pattern Anal. Mach. Intell. **24**(7), 971–987 (2002)
14. Pedregosa, F., Varoquaux, G., Gramfort, A., Michel, V., Thirion, B., Grisel, O., Blondel, M., Prettenhofer, P., Weiss, R., Dubourg, V., Vanderplas, J., Passos, A., Cournapeau, D.: Scikit-learn: machine learning in python. J. Mach. Learn. Res. **12**, 2825–2830 (2011)
15. Prasanna, P., Tiwari, P., Madabhushi, A.: Co-occurrence of Local Anisotropic Gradient Orientations (CoLlAGe): distinguishing tumor confounders and molecular subtypes on MRI. In: Golland, P., Hata, N., Barillot, C., Hornegger, J., Howe, R. (eds.) MICCAI 2014, Part III. LNCS, vol. 8675, pp. 73–80. Springer, Heidelberg (2014)
16. Roth, H.R., Lu, L., Seff, A., Cherry, K.M., Hoffman, J., Wang, S., Liu, J., Turkbey, E., Summers, R.M.: A new 2.5D representation for lymph node detection using random sets of deep convolutional neural network observations. In: Golland, P., Hata, N., Barillot, C., Hornegger, J., Howe, R. (eds.) MICCAI 2014, Part I. LNCS, vol. 8673, pp. 520–527. Springer, Heidelberg (2014)
17. Suzuki, K., Li, F., Sone, S., Doi, K.: Computer-aided diagnostic scheme for distinction between benign and malignant nodules in thoracic low-dose ct by use of massive training artificial neural network. IEEE Trans. Med. Imaging **24**(9), 1138–1150 (2005)
18. van der Walt, S., Schönberger, J.L., Nunez-Iglesias, J., Boulogne, F., Warner, J.D., Yager, N., Gouillart, E., Yu, T.: Scikit-image: Image processing in python. Technical report, PeerJ PrePrints (2014)
19. Way, T.W., Hadjiiski, L.M., Sahiner, B., Chan, H.P., Cascade, P.N., Kazerooni, E.A., Bogot, N., Zhou, C.: Computer-aided diagnosis of pulmonary nodules on CT scans: segmentation and classification using 3D active contours. Med. Phys. **33**(7), 2323–2337 (2006)

Tractography-Driven Groupwise Multi-scale Parcellation of the Cortex

Sarah Parisot[1]([✉]), Salim Arslan[1], Jonathan Passerat-Palmbach[1],
William M. Wells III[2], and Daniel Rueckert[1]

[1] Biomedical Image Analysis Group, Department of Computing,
Imperial College London, London, UK
s.parisot@imperial.ac.uk
[2] Surgical Planning Laboratory, Brigham and Women's Hospital,
Harvard Medical School, Boston, USA

Abstract. The analysis of the connectome of the human brain provides key insight into the brain's organisation and function, and its evolution in disease or ageing. Parcellation of the cortical surface into distinct regions in terms of structural connectivity is an essential step that can enable such analysis. The estimation of a stable connectome across a population of healthy subjects requires the estimation of a groupwise parcellation that can capture the variability of the connectome across the population. This problem has solely been addressed in the literature via averaging of connectivity profiles or finding correspondences between individual parcellations a posteriori. In this paper, we propose a groupwise parcellation method of the cortex based on diffusion MR images (dMRI). We borrow ideas from the area of cosegmentation in computer vision and directly estimate a consistent parcellation across different subjects and scales through a spectral clustering approach. The parcellation is driven by the tractography connectivity profiles, and information between subjects and across scales. Promising qualitative and quantitative results on a sizeable data-set demonstrate the strong potential of the method.

1 Introduction

Understanding the brain's organisation and function remains an elusive goal and a very active research subject. There seems to be an agreement amongst scientists that the brain's cortical surface can be separated or parcellated into functionally and structurally distinct regions. Many approaches have sought to identify those regions over the years, principally relying on anatomical properties. Nonetheless, while some anatomical parcellations are widely known and relied upon [8,18], they do not properly reflect the brain's structural connectivity which is key to understanding its function and the impact of neurological diseases. Structural brain connectivity or *connectome* studies typically rely on anatomical or random parcellations to build connectivity graphs from diffusion MRI (dMRI) and tractography. However, such parcellations introduce a bias in the way the network is constructed and can lead to erroneous connections and conclusions

S. Ourselin et al. (Eds.): IPMI 2015, LNCS 9123, pp. 600–612, 2015.
DOI: 10.1007/978-3-319-19992-4_47

[17]. This issue can be addressed via the construction of tractography driven parcellations that will identify distinct regions in terms of connectivity, and enable more meaningful connectome analysis.

A significant amount of effort has been focused on the complementary task of resting-state functional MRI (fMRI) driven parcellation [4,7]. Recently, dMRI-driven parcellation has gained interest as well. Several methods have focused on parcellation of brain substructures [2,10], modelling the task as a clustering problem driven by the correlation between connectivity profiles. Aiming at whole brain parcellation makes the task harder, since the high dimensionality of the data prevents the direct use of common clustering techniques.

Clarkson et al. [5] proposed to refine an anatomical parcellation by introducing information from dMRI and iteratively updating labels. The method is also extended to groupwise parcellation through averaging of the connectivity profiles. Its main drawback is the strong bias introduced by the initial anatomical parcellation. Roca et al. [15] proposed an iterative approach that aims to reduce the dimensionality of the data. In each iteration, the cortical surface is divided into a set of Voronoi cells on which k-medoids clustering is performed. Parcels that respect certain size and boundary constraints are excluded from the domain for the subsequent iterations. Only a subset of the cortical surface (regions that are strongly connected) is parcellated. The method was later extended to a group parcellation [16] through averaging of the different subjects' connectivity profiles. A hierarchical clustering based parcellation method was presented in [13]. Despite the appeal of obtaining consistent parcellations across resolutions (i.e. number of parcels), hierarchical clustering is at risk of propagating errors from low resolution clusterings and does not circumvent the need of selecting a number of parcels for further analysis.

While individual parcellations are the most faithful to a given subject's connectivity, they can be sensitive to noise and unreliable. Furthermore, they make group studies difficult as there are no direct correspondences across subjects. Such studies are however essential if one seeks to identify a common connectome across healthy subjects (a connectome "backbone"), which could later enable to evaluate the impact of a disease on the brain's organisation. Both issues can be overcome through a groupwise parcellation approach. Existing groupwise methods either seek a matching across subjects after independent parcellations [13] relying on possible noisy results, or perform a groupwise parcellation after constructing an average connectivity profile [5,16] which prevents from obtaining single subject parcellations. In this paper, we propose a whole brain groupwise parcellation method that directly estimates matching parcels across subjects without the need for averaging. We borrow ideas from the concept of cosegmentation [12] and design a multi-scale and multi-subjects spectral clustering method driven by correlation between connectivity profiles. Here, consistency across scales (so-called supervertex parcellations of the cortical surface) and subjects is enforced via a set of links embedded in a constraint matrix. We tackle the challenge of evaluating brain parcellations by computing group consistency and information loss based measures, which provide sensible quantitative com-

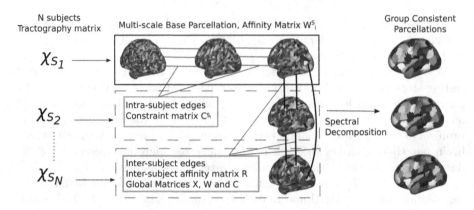

Fig. 1. Illustration of the proposed method. Each subject S_i is associated with a connectivity matrix χ_{S_i} that drives the construction of a multi-scale base parcellation. Intra-subject edges (between base parcellation resolutions) and inter-subject edges (between all pairs of subjects at the coarsest parcellation resolution) are built to allow a common spectral decomposition of the affinity matrix (connectivity profiles correlation).

parisons across methods and distinct groups. Qualitative evaluation shows how correspondences between subject-dependent parcels are obtained within a group, as well as achieving strong consistency across different groups.

2   Groupwise Multi-scale Parcellation

In this section, we describe the method for obtaining a group parcellation of the cortical surface of a set of N different subjects into K parcels. We represent these surfaces as a triangular mesh made of N_v vertices, and assume all surfaces to be registered to the same reference [9]. As a result, all surface vertices have direct correspondence across all subjects. Furthermore, we consider that a $N_v \times N_v$ tractography matrix χ_{S_i} has been computed from diffusion data for each subject S_i. Each row of this matrix $\chi_{S_i}(\mathbf{v})$ describes how a vertex $\mathbf{v}$ is connected to the rest of the cortical surface.

The proposed method is illustrated in Fig 1. For each subject, a set of high resolution parcellations is constructed for L different resolution layers (base parcellation). These parcellation layers then serve as the basis of a multi-scale groupwise spectral clustering problem, where the affinity between vertices is described by the tractography matrix, and edges across resolutions and subjects force the parcellations to be consistent.

2.1   Base Parcellation

The first step towards building our groupwise parcellation is to capture structural connectivity information at multiple scales through the construction of *supervertices* at different resolutions. Similarly to superpixels [1], supervertices can be seen as an initial over-segmentation of the cortical surface based on connectivity information such that vertices within a supervertex have very similar connectivity profiles. We rely on the geodesic distance between vertices to obtain spatially contiguous supervertices, while the correlation between their connectivity profiles enforces homogeneous connectivity.

We are inspired by the method proposed in [14] that relies on Fast Marching to compute geodesic distances for surface segmentation. In this setting, the computation of the geodesic distance $d(\mathbf{v_0}, \mathbf{v}) = U(\mathbf{v})$ from vertex $\mathbf{v_0}$ can be reformulated as a front propagation problem, where U follows the Eikonal equation $\|\nabla U\| F = 1$ which can be solved using the Fast Marching algorithm. F is the speed function characterising the front propagation. We can compute a correlation dependent geodesic distance by defining a correlation weighted speed function: $F(\mathbf{v}) = \exp\left(\mu\rho(\chi_{S_i}(\mathbf{v_0}), \chi_{S_i}(\mathbf{v}))\right)$. Here, $\rho(.,.)$ is the Pearson's correlation coefficient between the vertices' connectivity profiles $\chi_{S_i}(\mathbf{v})$ and μ is a weighting parameter. In this setting, the front will propagate faster towards vertices that have a high correlation (i.e. similar connectivity profiles) with the source vertex $\mathbf{v_0}$.

Each supervertex resolution is computed through an iterative approach. Given a specified number of N_l supervertices, we initialise by uniformly sampling N_l seeds across the brain's cortical surface. At each iteration, we first compute the correlation weighted geodesic distance from each seed to the rest of the surface, and build supervertices by assigning a vertex to its closest seed. We then reevaluate the seeds by selecting, for each supervertex, the vertex that has the highest correlation with the rest of the cluster. This process is iterated until convergence for the L different levels.

Each base parcellation level is associated to a $N_l \times N_l$ merged connectivity matrix, constructed by adding the fibre counts across vertices. The level's affinity matrix W_l is defined as the Pearson's correlation coefficient between those merged connectivity profiles. In order to obtain spatially contiguous parcels, correlation weighted edges are only constructed between supervertices that are adjacent.

Our next step is to build connections between the different base parcellation levels, so as to recover a common partition of the cortical surface across resolutions.

2.2 Intra-subject Connections Between Resolutions

We seek coherence across resolutions by enforcing supervertices that are in similar locations on the cortical surface to be assigned to the same parcels through the construction of inter-resolutions edges.

For a given resolution level l, each supervertex is connected to a supervertex at the finer level $l-1$ if they share vertices on the original cortical surface. The strength of the edge is defined by the amount of overlapping vertices, so that the same parcellation result is imposed on supervertices that are the most similar. The intra-subject, inter-resolutions links can be written as:

$$C_{l-1,l}(j,k) = \frac{|s_l^j \cap s_{l-1}^k|}{|s_l^j|} \tag{1}$$

where s_l^j is the set of vertices at the original resolution that belong to the j-th supervertex at resolution level l and $|s_l^j|$ is the number of vertices in s_l^j.

In this setting, we can estimate a parcellation for a single subject S_i that is consistent across resolutions using the multi-scale normalised cut approach [19]. For each level l, we aim at finding a K-way parcellation matrix $X_l \in \{0,1\}^{N_v \times K}$ defined as:

$$X_l(i,j) = \begin{cases} 1 & \text{if } s_l^i \in \text{parcel } j \\ 0 & \text{otherwise} \end{cases} \tag{2}$$

The multi-scale parcellation and affinity matrices can then be constructed as follows:

$$X^{S_i} = \begin{pmatrix} X_1 \\ \vdots \\ X_L \end{pmatrix}, W^{S_i} = \begin{pmatrix} W_1 & & 0 \\ & \ddots & \\ 0 & & W_L \end{pmatrix} \tag{3}$$

Finally, we build a constraint matrix that encodes the inter-resolution links and ensures consistency of the recovered parcellation across resolutions:

$$C^{S_i} = \begin{pmatrix} C_{1,2} & -I_{N_2} & & 0 \\ & \ddots & \ddots & \\ 0 & & C_{L-1,L} & -I_{N_L} \end{pmatrix} \tag{4}$$

Here, I_{N_l} is the $N_l \times N_l$ identity matrix and N_l is the number of supervertices at scale l. This matrix forces the obtained parcellation to be consistent across scales through the following constraint equation:

$$CX = 0 \tag{5}$$

Optimisation of the multi-scale normalised cut criterion, subject to the inter-resolution constraint [19], yields a single subject parcellation that captures local connectivity information at different scales. Comparing the obtained parcellations within a group is however a very challenging task as there are no direct matches between parcels, and anatomical variability (as well as registration errors) can cause different subjects to have very different parcel boundaries. This issue can be addressed by performing a concurrent parcellation of all the subjects within the group to directly obtain correspondences between parcels.

2.3   Inter-subject Connections

Spectral clustering offers the possibility to integrate different subjects in the same framework in a very natural manner. A group consistent parcellation can be obtained through a joint estimation of the parcellation matrix X across subjects. The groupwise parcellation, affinity and constraint matrices are defined as:

$$X = \begin{pmatrix} X^{S_1} \\ \vdots \\ X^{S_N} \end{pmatrix}, W = \begin{pmatrix} W^{S_1} & & R \\ & \ddots & \\ R^T & & W^{S_N} \end{pmatrix}, C = \begin{pmatrix} C^{S_1} & & 0 \\ & \ddots & \\ 0 & & C^{S_N} \end{pmatrix} \qquad (6)$$

Matching parcellations are enforced by adding inter-subject connections encoded in the matrix R. Following [12], we only connect the coarsest resolution layers. This step is essential in our case as it relaxes the need for a precise registration in addition to allowing individual differences at the highest resolution.

Let us consider that all subjects have been registered to a common surface mesh. Similarly to the multi-scale parcellation approach, we seek a common parcellation across subjects by forcing supervertices in similar locations to belong to the same parcel. To this end, a supervertex from subject i is connected to a supervertex from subject j if they share the highest amount of overlapping surface vertices and have the strongest correlated connectivity profiles. We define the inter-subject edges between matching supervertices as follows:

$$R(s^i(S_1), s^j(S_2)) = \alpha\rho(s^i(S_1), s^j(S_2)) \qquad (7)$$

where $\rho(s^i(S_1), s^j(S_2))$ is the correlation between the connectivity profiles of the two different subjects' supervertices and α is a weighting parameter. Correlation weighted edges enable accounting for differences in anatomy and possible errors in registration by decreasing the strength of the edges in non matching regions.

2.4 Optimisation

The joint parcellation is eventually recovered by optimising the multi-scale normalised cut objective criterion [6]:

$$\text{maximise} \quad E(X) = \frac{1}{K} \sum_{l=1}^{K} \frac{X_l^T W X_l}{X_l^T D X_l}$$
$$\text{subject to} \quad X \in \{0,1\}^{N \times K}, \qquad (8)$$
$$X 1_k = 1_N,$$
$$CX = 0$$

A near global-optimal solution to this NP-complete problem can be estimated in a two-step approach. First by finding the global optimum of the relaxed continuous problem Z^*, and second by solving a discretisation problem to project this continuous optimum to the discrete space.

We define the normalised affinity matrix $P = D^{-\frac{1}{2}} W D^{-\frac{1}{2}}$, and the projector matrix Q that integrates the constraint matrix:

$$Q = I - D^{-\frac{1}{2}} C^T (C D^{-1} C^T)^{-1} C D^{-\frac{1}{2}} \qquad (9)$$

We solve the continuous problem following the Rayleigh Ritz theorem [20], through computation and normalisation of the K largest eigenvectors of the matrix QPQ. This solution is then discretised through an iterative process [19] by seeking the closest solution to Z^* that satisfies the constraints of the discrete problem.

3   Experimental Evaluation

Evaluation of cortical parcellations remains a very challenging task due to the lack of a ground truth parcellation. In this section, we evaluate the quality of our parcellations based on two main ideas: group consistency and fidelity to each individual's connectivity matrix. We are seeking to observe similarities in connectivity within and across groups, while preserving individual variability.

3.1   Data Acquisition and Preprocessing

We evaluated our method on 100 different subjects (age range 22–35 years old) from the latest release of the Human Connectome Project (HCP)[1]. The HCP dMRI have been acquired using a multi-shell approach, with three shells at b-values 1000, 2000, and $3000\,s/mm^2$ and 90 gradient directions per shell. The structural and diffusion data of all subjects have been preprocessed following the HCP's minimum processing pipeline [9]. The cortical surfaces of all subjects are registered and represented as a triangular mesh of 32 k vertices per hemisphere. Vertices corresponding to the medial wall are excluded from parcellations. The tractography matrix is obtained on the native mesh representing the gray/white matter interface using FSL's bedpostX and probtrackX methods [3,11] which estimate the fibres orientation at each voxel with a ball and stick model, and perform probabilistic tractography respectively. Following [11], we fitted three fibre compartments per voxel. 5000 streamlines were sampled from each of the mesh vertices. Each entry $\chi(\mathbf{v}, \mathbf{q})$ counts the number of streamlines sampled from the surface vertex $\mathbf{v}$ that reach vertex $\mathbf{q}$. The groupwise parcellation was performed on the left hemisphere of two disjoint groups of 50 randomly selected subjects with a base parcellation of 3 levels of 2000, 1000 and 500 super-vertices and parameter μ heuristically set to 3.

3.2   Parameter Selection

The weighting parameter α has a large influence on the obtained parcellation and its consistency across subjects. We evaluate the quality of our parcellations and the impact of this parameter via an intra-subject information loss measure and a group consistency measure. Both measures are estimated on the connectivity graph rather than the parcellation itself. This is particularly relevant for group consistency, where the parcellations are expected to have different boundaries, but the merged connectivity graphs should be similar.

Our main objective is to obtain parcellations that summarise the structural connectivity maps faithfully. In other words, we seek to lose as little information

---

[1] Human Connectome Project Database, https://db.humanconnectome.org/.

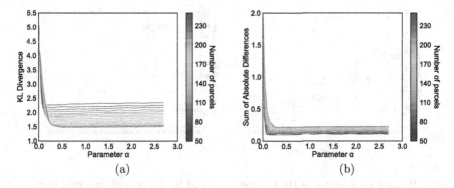

Fig. 2. Evolution of the average KL divergence (a) and the SAD (b) across subjects depending on the value of the parameter α and the number of parcels.

as possible when merging the connectivity profiles of several vertices into one entity. The first measure we are computing aims to evaluate this information loss through the Kullback Leibler (KL) divergence. Each subject's $K \times K$ merged connectivity matrix is converted into a $N_v \times N_v$ matrix $\chi_{S_i}^{clus}$ that should be as similar as possible to the $N_v \times N_v$ matrix χ_{S_i} prior to clustering. The matrix $\chi_{S_i}^{clus}$ is constructed by assigning the same connectivity profile to all the vertices that belong to the same cluster. The KL divergence is then computed between the matrices χ_{S_i} and $\chi_{S_i}^{clus}$, that are normalised to be probability mass functions. The idea is to evaluate how much information is lost when $\chi_{S_i}^{clus}$ is used to approximate χ_{S_i}. Second, we evaluate group consistency using the sum of absolute differences (SAD). After parcellation, an average $K \times K$ connectivity matrix is constructed from all the subjects' merged connectivity matrices. The deviation of each subject from the average is then evaluated by computing the SAD between the average matrix and the subject's matrix. We compute those measures for a range of 50 to 250 parcels and the weighting parameter α ranging from 0.1 to 3. The obtained results are shown in Fig. 2. Intuitively, the KL divergence should decrease when the number of parcels increases, as the averaging of connectivity profiles is reduced. Conversely, the SAD is expected to increase with the number of parcels, as more individual information is maintained. Both measures show a rapid decrease, then stabilise when α is increased. This can be explained by the fact that when α is low enough, the parcellations are not constrained to be in accordance. Hence, the K clusters will be spread across subjects, leading to different parcellations and different numbers of parcels. However, both SAD and KL tend to increase slowly after reaching a minimum as constraints that are too strong can force identical parcellations, while isolated supervertices start to appear. Our main goal is to obtain parcellations that are as faithful as possible to the subjects connectivity profiles, we therefore select the value of α that minimises the KL divergence. The two groups we tested our method on show the same behaviour, and require α to be increased with the number of parcels (from 0.1 to 0.5 in our setting). Figure 4 shows examples of parcellations obtained with the optimal value of α for 160 parcels. We can observe a

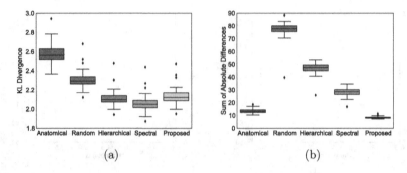

Fig. 3. Boxplot comparison of the proposed method to anatomical, random, hierarchical and spectral parcellations for the KL divergence (a) and SAD (b).

strong consistency, but also the different shapes and boundaries of the parcels across subjects.

3.3 Method Evaluation

We have compared the proposed groupwise parcellation method to (a) multiscale individual spectral clustering (described in Sect. 2.2), (b) hierarchical clustering of the finest supervertex resolution level, (c) anatomical parcellations from the Destrieux atlas [8], and (d) Poisson disk sampling random parcellations. We computed the KL divergence and SAD for the five different methods for 75 parcels (anatomical parcellation granularity). In the absence of existing matching across the subjects clusterings, the clusters that had the highest overlap were matched. This matching is not optimal, but highlights one of the main drawbacks of individual parcellations. Results are shown in Fig. 3. While it is expected that a groupwise parcellation would not perform as well as individual parcellations in terms of information loss, the increase in KL remains very limited and faithful to the data in comparison with random or anatomical parcellation. The SAD score is significantly ouperforming all methods.

3.4 Group Comparisons

Finally, we compared the consistency across our two groups' parcellations. Given the sizeable data-set, both groups should reflect common connectivity properties

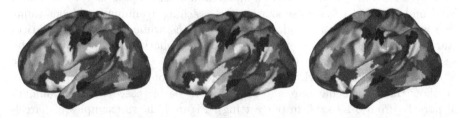

Fig. 4. Example parcellations (160 parcels) of subjects within the same group.

and be essentially free of inter-subject variability. The average parcellations obtained through majority voting are compared by computing the Dice score between all highest matching parcels. We obtain a mean Dice score of 72 ± 5 % across all numbers of parcels. It is as expected lower than the average intra group pairwise dice score of $79 \pm 7\%$ but significantly outperforms the average pairwise dice scores between independent parcellations ($57 \pm 3\%$). The strong similarity between the two groups' parcellations is shown in Fig. 5. We also computed the SAD score between average connectivity profiles after matching the parcels. Its mean value of 0.20 ± 0.05 is on par with intra group SAD scores (individual vs. average connectivity matrices, mean value 0.16 ± 0.07) and outperforms the SAD scores between individual parcellations (mean 0.48 ± 0.1).

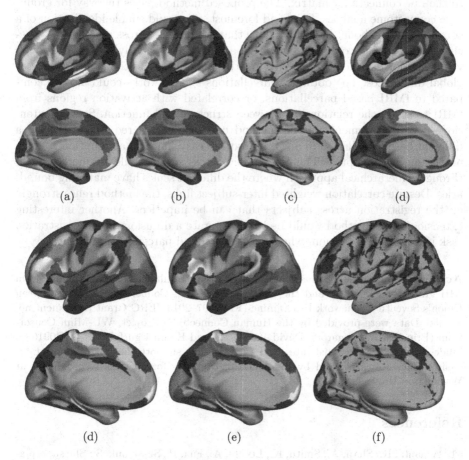

(a)   (b)   (c)   (d)

(d)   (e)   (f)

Fig. 5. Average parcellations for 70 (a,b,c) and 130 parcels (e,f,g). (a,e) and (b,f) show parcellations from two different groups of normal subjects, while (c,g) shows the disagreement between both groups. Each group contains 50 subjects. The average 75 clusters anatomical parcellation (d) is shown as comparison to our proposed 70 clusters parcellation.

Inter-group comparisons for other methods are not performed here as the high within group variability does not allow the construction of a meaningful average parcellation.

4   Discussion

We presented a groupwise multi-scale parcellation method of the brain's cortical surface that is driven by structural connectivity. Our proposed spectral clustering approach allows the recovery of consistent parcellations across subjects and scales without averaging raw connectivity profiles. It shows great consistency across and within groups as well as limited information loss with respect to the raw connectivity matrix. The proposed method paves the way for groupwise connectome analysis. First and foremost, this could enable idenfication of a connectome backbone, *i.e.* connections that are present across populations. Specific groups studies could consequently be considered (healthy vs. disease, young vs. ageing for instance) in order to identify possible connectivity disruptions or global differences. The obtained parcellations and networks could also be compared to fMRI based parcellations, or correlated with activation regions from fMRI to study the relationship between structure and function. Several extensions and improvements of the method could be considered. Incorporating a different base parcellation in our framework is easy, since no assumption is made on the method adopted. The consistency across scales would be more natural through a hierarchical approach where the different scales have matching boundaries. Despite correlation weighted inter-subject links, the method relies strongly on the registration across subjects that can be imperfect. Another interesting extension of the method would be to incorporate a diffusion driven registration task in an iterative fashion, where registration and parcellation alternate.

Acknowledgements. The research leading to these results has received funding from NIH grant P41EB015902 and the European Research Council under the European Union's Seventh Framework Programme (FP/2007–2013)/ERC Grant Agreement no. 319456. Data were provided by the Human Connectome Project, WU-Minn Consortium (Principal Investigators: David Van Essen and Kamil Ugurbil; 1U54MH091657) funded by the 16 NIH Institutes and Centers that support the NIH Blueprint for Neuroscience Research; and by the McDonnell Center for Systems Neuroscience at Washington University.

References

1. Achanta, R., Shaji, A., Smith, K., Lucchi, A., Fua, P., Susstrunk, S.: Slic superpixels compared to state-of-the-art superpixel methods. IEEE Trans. Pattern Anal. **34**, 2274–2282 (2012)
2. Anwander, A., Tittgemeyer, M., von Cramon, D.Y., Friederici, A.D., Knösche, T.R.: Connectivity-based parcellation of Broca's area. Cereb. Cortex **17**(4), 816–825 (2007)

3. Behrens, T., Berg, H.J., Jbabdi, S., Rushworth, M., Woolrich, M.: Probabilistic diffusion tractography with multiple fibre orientations: what can we gain? NeuroImage **34**(1), 144–155 (2007)
4. Blumensath, T., Jbabdi, S., Glasser, M.F., Van Essen, D.C., Ugurbil, K., Behrens, T.E., Smith, S.M.: Spatially constrained hierarchical parcellation of the brain with resting-state fmri. NeuroImage **76**, 313–324 (2013)
5. Clarkson, M.J., Malone, I.B., Modat, M., Leung, K.K., Ryan, N., Alexander, D.C., Fox, N.C., Ourselin, S.: A framework for using diffusion weighted imaging to improve cortical parcellation. In: Jiang, T., Navab, N., Pluim, J.P.W., Viergever, M.A. (eds.) MICCAI 2010, Part I. LNCS, vol. 6361, pp. 534–541. Springer, Heidelberg (2010)
6. Cour, T., Bnzit, F., Shi, J.: Spectral segmentation with multiscale graph decomposition. In: CVPR (2), pp. 1124–1131. IEEE Computer Society (2005)
7. Craddock, R.C., James, G.A., Holtzheimer, P.E., Hu, X.P., Mayberg, H.S.: A whole brain fmri atlas generated via spatially constrained spectral clustering. Hum. Brain Mapp. **33**, 1914–1928 (2012)
8. Destrieux, C., Fischl, B., Dale, A., Halgren, E.: Automatic parcellation of human cortical gyri and sulci using standard anatomical nomenclature. NeuroImage **53**(1), 1–15 (2010)
9. Glasser, M.F., Sotiropoulos, S.N., Wilson, J.A., Coalson, T.S., Fischl, B., Andersson, J.L., Xu, J., Jbabdi, S., Webster, M., Polimeni, J.R., Essen, D.C.V., Jenkinson, M.: The minimal preprocessing pipelines for the human connectome project. NeuroImage **80**, 105–124 (2013)
10. Jbabdi, S., Woolrich, M.W., Behrens, T.E.: Multiple-subjects connectivity-based parcellation using hierarchical dirichlet process mixture models. NeuroImage **44**, 373–384 (2009)
11. Jbabdi, S., Sotiropoulos, S.N., Savio, A.M., Graa, M., Behrens, T.E.J.: Model-based analysis of multishell diffusion MR data for tractography: how to get over fitting problems. Magn. Reson. Med. **68**(6), 1846–1855 (2012)
12. Kim, E., Li, H., Huang, X.: A hierarchical image clustering cosegmentation framework. In: CVPR, pp. 686–693. IEEE (2012)
13. Moreno-Dominguez, D., Anwander, A., Knösche, T.R.: A hierarchical method for whole-brain connectivity-based parcellation. Hum. Brain Mapp. **35**, 5000–5025 (2014)
14. Peyré, G., Cohen, L.D.: Surface segmentation using geodesic centroidal tesselation. In: 3DPVT, pp. 995–1002. IEEE Computer Society (2004)
15. Roca, P., Rivière, D., Guevara, P., Poupon, C., Mangin, J.-F.: Tractography-based parcellation of the cortex using a spatially-informed dimension reduction of the connectivity matrix. In: Yang, G.-Z., Hawkes, D., Rueckert, D., Noble, A., Taylor, C. (eds.) MICCAI 2009, Part I. LNCS, vol. 5761, pp. 935–942. Springer, Heidelberg (2009)
16. Roca, P., Tucholka, A., Rivière, D., Guevara, P., Poupon, C., Mangin, J.-F.: Inter-subject connectivity-based parcellation of a patch of cerebral cortex. In: Jiang, T., Navab, N., Pluim, J.P.W., Viergever, M.A. (eds.) MICCAI 2010, Part II. LNCS, vol. 6362, pp. 347–354. Springer, Heidelberg (2010)
17. Sporns, O.: The human connectome: a complex network. Ann. NY Acad. Sci. **1224**, 109–125 (2011)

18. Tzourio-Mazoyer, N., Landeau, B., Papathanassiou, D., Crivello, F., Etard, O., Delcroix, N., Mazoyer, B., Joliot, M.: Automated anatomical labeling of activations in spm using a macroscopic anatomical parcellation of the mni mri single-subject brain. NeuroImage **15**(1), 273–289 (2002)
19. Yu, S.X., Shi, J.: Multiclass spectral clustering. In: ICCV (2). IEEE (2003)
20. Yu, S.X., Shi, J.: Segmentation given partial grouping constraints. IEEE Trans. Pattern Anal. **26**(2), 173–183 (2004)

Illumination Compensation and Normalization Using Low-Rank Decomposition of Multispectral Images in Dermatology

Alexandru Duliu[1(✉)], Richard Brosig[1], Saahil Ognawala[1],
Tobias Lasser[1], Mahzad Ziai[2], and Nassir Navab[1]

[1] Computer Aided Medical Procedures (CAMP),
Technische Universität München, Munich, Germany
duliu@in.tum.de
[2] Department of Dermatology and Allergology,
Klinikum Rechts der Isar, Munich, Germany

Abstract. When attempting to recover the surface color from an image, modelling the illumination contribution per-pixel is essential. In this work we present a novel approach for illumination compensation using multispectral image data. This is done by means of a low-rank decomposition of representative spectral bands with prior knowledge of the reflectance spectra of the imaged surface. Experimental results on synthetic data, as well as on images of real lesions acquired at the university clinic, show that the proposed method significantly improves the contrast between the lesion and the background.

1 Introduction

When acquiring images with a color camera, spatial distribution of the incoming illumination and geometry of an object have a great impact on image formation. In applications, such as lesion classification in dermatology, the actual color (diffuse spectral reflectance or albedo) of the tissue is the main point of interest, and not how its surface has interacted with the illumination. As intensity values of the image pixels only store how the surface has interacted with the incoming illumination, we are looking for a way to separate the albedo A from the illumination L in an image I:

$$I = A \odot L \tag{1}$$

where I, A are multi-channel images, L is a single-channel image (same size as I and A), and $\odot$ is the component-wise product of the pixel values.

Multispectral imaging is a powerful tool for tissue classification, due to its improved spectral resolution compared to conventional RGB imaging, with the latter only approximating the subjective color perception of the human eye. This improved spectral resolution allows for better tissue discrimination, however this is hampered by the presence of large illumination changed across the image. As lesion classification methods [3] rely on many features that can be observed on a lesion, such as color and fine structures, they are quite sensitive to illumination

© Springer International Publishing Switzerland 2015
S. Ourselin et al. (Eds.): IPMI 2015, LNCS 9123, pp. 613–625, 2015.
DOI: 10.1007/978-3-319-19992-4_48

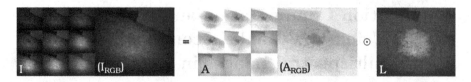

Fig. 1. Example of separating a multispectral image I into albedo A and illumination L (false-colors) using our method. I_{RGB} and A_{RGB} are projections of their respective multispectral images, I and A, onto RGB space. Here and in all following figures, a heat color-map is used to visualize the illumination L (Color figure online).

changes. Our motivation is to exploit the additional information of multispectral imaging, in order to compensate for such illumination changes, while preserving both morphological and colorimetric (spectral) features of the lesions.

In applications that recover the albedo or just compensate for illumination for detail enhancement [1,10], it is common practice to acquire multiple images while keeping the viewpoint fixed and varying the illumination. The assumption is made that the albedo remains the same while the illumination changes. In our work we also acquire multiple images under a fixed viewpoint, however we do not vary the illumination but the spectral range for each image channel. We assume that it is the spatial distribution of the illumination that remains constant and that the albedo varies.

We introduce a two step approach based on low-rank decomposition of the multispectral image I in order to approximate a per-pixel illumination map L which enables the recovery of the diffuse albedo A. We evaluate the method on multispectral images of synthetic lesions on volunteers and of real lesions of patients.

2   Related Work

When considering Eq. (1), the image I cannot be separated into A and L without additional information.

Photometric stereo methods [10] acquire multiple images, while keeping the viewpoint fixed. In each image, the scene is illuminated from a different calibrated direction. Here, both the the surface geometry and albedo are estimated together. More recently [1], the requirement for calibrated illumination has been relaxed, only assuming the light sources to be sufficiently distant. Although multispectral imaging can be adapted to such multi-light acquisitions [9] (which considerably increases acquisition times), our focus is on illumination compensation from a single multispectral image.

Similar data as in [1] (fixed viewport multi-light images) is used by image enhancement methods [6,14] which, rather than removing the illumination altogether, focus on minimizing its influence, while preserving fine features, that would otherwise be lost without illumination cues. Fattal *et al.* [6] propose an image decomposition method for multi-light image sequences that removes large illumination artefacts (like shadows) while enhancing small surface details due

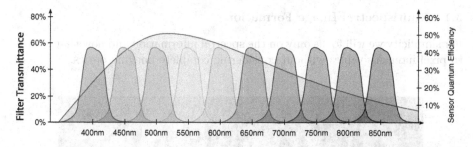

Fig. 2. Example transmission spectra of band-pass filters (colored functions), and example spectral sensitivity of image sensor (larger gray function) (Color figure online).

to shading. Such methods have a simpler model than photometric stereo of how light interacts with the scene as they only focus on image enhancement.

These methods [1,6,10,14] all exploit variations in illumination in order to recover the albedo. This is not unlike our method, we however make the reverse assumption, that the albedo varies and that the illumination stays the same.

Influences of illumination can also be modeled in single images when enough assumptions can be made about the scene. Shi *et al.* [11] propose an adaptive linear function that estimates the background of historical documents, compensating for uneven shading due to paper geometry and non-uniform illumination. For robust face recognition, Chen *et al.* [2] propose an illumination normalization approach based on a Discrete Cosine Transform in the logarithmic domain. Although not exactly modeling illumination, the methods focuses on preserving application relevant features while removing most image illumination.

Vogel *et al.* [13] present a radiometrically calibrated multispectral imaging system to assess tissue vasculature. The authors model both the distribution of the illumination across the image and the geometry of the subject. The former is mostly corrected for by the radiometric calibration of the camera and the calibrated illumination, leaving only the influence of the geometry. Assumptions are made about the geometry of the object and a simple curvature model is fitted to the data in order to compensate for the remaining shading. This method has the most similar input data and hardware to our own, however, most of the influences of illumination are corrected through a calibrated and controlled acquisition environment. Unlike Vogel *et al.* [13] we make no assumptions about either the distribution of light intensity or the geometry of the scene.

3   Methods

Our method exploits the increased spectral resolution of multispectral images in order to distinguish between the most important spectra that influence image formation: illumination, background and foreground. As this method was initially developed for dermatology, the background is the skin and the foreground is the lesion we are investigating. The method can also be used on multiple foreground and/or background spectra as long as certain criteria are met (see Sect. 3.2).

3.1   Multispectral Image Formation

For simplicity we will focus only on the spectral information and how that relates to pixel intensity values without considering complete imaging optics.

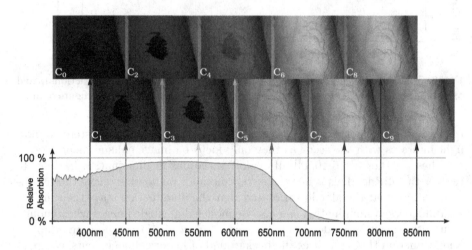

Fig. 3. Example multispectral image of a forearm marked with a red dye that has a similar absorption spectrum as an erythemous lesion (Fig. 1). Above 700 nm the dye is no longer distinguishable from the skin, just as its relative absorption spectrum would indicate (relative to skin) (Color figure online).

The basic layout of a multispectral camera is analogous to that of most RGB camera: lens, filters and gray-scale sensor. Where a RGB camera has a *color filter array* (CFA) consisting of tiny red, green and blue filters mounted directly on the sensor, a multispectral camera can have different designs in order to support a considerably larger number of filters. Although we will only focus on filter-wheel cameras[1], our method can be applied on images acquired with any type multispectral camera.

Sensors used in multispectral cameras have a wide spectral sensitivity (Fig. 2), however they cannot distinguish the wavelength of the photons they detect. The transmission spectra (Fig. 2) of the camera filters act as windowing functions, letting only a certain part of the spectrum through. This is how both RGB and multispectral cameras are able to distinguish between different parts of spectrum of the incoming light: they use the filters to select what wavelengths reach the sensor. Therefore the intensity value $C_{i,p}$ for a pixel p of channel i is:

$$C_{i,p} = \int Sl_p(\lambda) \cdot St_i(\lambda) \cdot Ss(\lambda) \, d\lambda \tag{2}$$

---

[1] *Filter-wheel multispectral cameras* sequentially acquires multiple images of different spectral bands, each time exposing the sensor through a different filter.

with Sl_p the spectrum of the light entering the camera, St_i the transmission spectrum of the ith channel, Ss the sensitivity spectrum of the sensor and wavelength λ. Considering that we store the spectra as discrete vectors, Eq. (2) can also be written as:

$$C_{i,p} = (Sl_p \odot St_i) \cdot Ss \qquad (3)$$

3.2 Modeling Illumination

Illumination compensation can be viewed as reversing image formation in order to separate the multispectral diffuse reflectance A from the illumination L. Handling a multispectral image $\mathbf{I} \in \mathbb{R}^{m \times n \times k}$ consisting of k channels ($I = (C_i)_{i=1}^{k}$), can be simplified by linearizing all channels. Therefore a channel $C_i \in \mathbb{R}^{nm}$ can be described by:

$$C_i = A_i \odot (L \cdot f_i) \qquad (4)$$

with the global illumination term $f \in \mathbb{R}^k$ and the local illumination term $L \in \mathbb{R}^{nm}$ and a channel and pixel dependant albedo $A_i \in \mathbb{R}^{nm}$. The reshaped I can be modeled as the component-wise multiplication of A with the *outer product* between L and f:

$$I = A \odot (L \cdot f^T) \qquad (5)$$

Modeling this problem like this makes several assumptions

The emission spectrum is the same for all light sources. The concept of the channel-wise multiplicative factor f in Eq. (5) holds only for a globally constant emission spectrum. This generally applies to indoor environments, with similar light bulbs and no sunlight. If this were not the case, the illumination would vary spatially across the image depending on the observed channel. It would even be possible to measure this factor beforehand, however since our method is estimating this factor (see Sect. 3.3) this is not necessary.

The bidirectional reflectance distribution function (BRDF) of both background and foreground does not vary with the wavelength. This assumption is key in our

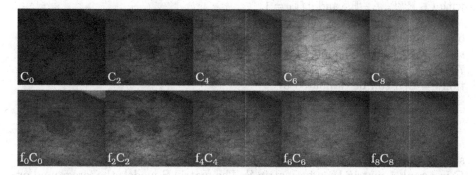

Fig. 4. Selected channels of the multispectral image (detail view of lesion from Fig. 1): C_i before (top row) and $f_i C_i$ after (bottom row) global illumination correction/normalization.

formulation of the local illumination term L, enabling us to consider it the same for all channels and as such the low-rank component.

The foreground spectrum is not completely distinguishable from the background spectrum; this is to say that in certain channels the reflectance of the foreground (lesion) is identical to that of the background (skin), see Fig. 3. We select the channels where this is the case as they only contain the background and illumination. This requires either prior knowledge about the reflectance spectra of both foreground and background or manual selection of the channels. When estimating the local illumination term L, the low-rank decomposition is only performed on these channels.

3.3   Low-Rank Decomposition

We consider I as a set of k channels $C_i \in \mathbb{R}^{mn}$, $i \in \{1, \ldots, k\}$ that show the same scene under different acquisition conditions (here, different spectral bands) and compute the correction factors.

We differentiate between two illumination effects. *Global* and *local*. First, the *global* illumination $f \in \mathbb{R}^k$ is a channel wise multiplicative factor correcting global properties like filter permeability or the lamp spectrum. Therefore the set of k channels (C_i) of the same image I are linearly dependent, excluding noise and non-multiplicative foreground denoted as S. Consequently, the matrix $C \in \mathbb{R}^{mn \times k}$, containing the linearized images as columns, has to have rank one. However, assuming noisy images or foreground structures, which do not have the same spectral response, we are searching for a rank-1 matrix L with

$$C = S + L, \tag{6}$$

where S accommodates the non-multiplicative residuals. Based on Eq. (6), the global, multiplicative illumination correction factors f can be recovered by the unique decomposition of

$$L = lf^T, \tag{7}$$

with $l \in \mathbb{R}^{mn}$, $f \in \mathbb{R}^k$ and $\|f\|_1 = 1$.

In the second step, we calculate the *local* illumination correction. It is based on the same principle, but additionally exploits properties of multispectral acquisition. We take the channels C_i, corresponding to acquisitions in the range over 700 nm, and stack them column-wise in $\tilde{C}$. Hence, the vectorized *local* illumination $\tilde{l} = L(:)$ can be estimated by

$$\tilde{C} = \tilde{S} + \tilde{L} = \tilde{S} + \tilde{l}f^T \tag{8}$$

For both matrix decompositions in Eqs. (6) and (8), we use an algorithm similar to the one of Cui *et al.* [4]. Revising formula (6), we want to decompose C in a rank-1 matrix L and a matrix S. The matrix S models the foreground or noise, and thus should be sparse. This leads to following objective

$$\min \|S\|_0 \quad \text{s.t.} \quad C = S + L \quad \text{and} \quad \text{rank}(L) = 1 \tag{9}$$

Similar to [4], we relax $\|\cdot\|_0$ to $\|\cdot\|_{2,0}$ norm, which is a row-wise 2-norm followed by column wise 0-norm. Both are optimized with an greedy algorithm, which alternately optimizes for the rank-1 condition and the sparsity condition. Obtaining a rank-1 approximation is achieved by Singular Value Decomposition (SVD). For the sparsity approximation, we enforce $\|\mathbf{S}\|_{2,0} < \alpha$, by setting $\mathbf{S}_{ij} = 0$ except for the α largest rows in the $\|\cdot\|_2$ norm, therefore α is an upper bound on the number of non-zero rows. The threshold α is roughly set to the number of foreground pixels.

Finally, the albedo A_i is reconstructed using Eq. (4) by replacing L with a reshaped l from Eq. (8) and plugging in the estimate f_i from Eq. (7),

$$A_i = f_i \cdot C_i \oslash L = f_i \cdot C_i \oslash \tilde{\mathbf{l}} \quad \forall i \in \{1, \dots, k\} \tag{10}$$

where $\oslash$ denotes the component-wise division.

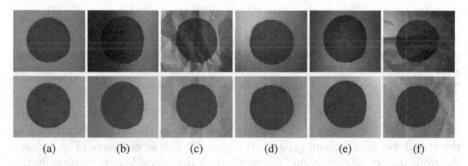

(a)   (b)   (c)   (d)   (e)   (f)

Fig. 5. Red dye on paper under varying illumination conditions: (a,b,c) uniform light from the right, (d,e,f) spot light. The paper was: flat (a,d), bent (b,e) and crumpled (c,f). Top row depicts the original images and the bottom row the corrected images (Color figure online).

4 Experiments

We have acquired multispectral images in order to evaluate our method under multiple scenarios. We start with simple scenarios, where both the scene and the illumination are controlled and move on to images of real lesions of actual patients under varying lighting conditions.

Synthetic Lesions on Paper: Our most simple test scenario involves images of red dye on white paper (Fig. 5). Here we vary both the illumination and the geometry of the paper. The first three images (Fig. 5a–c) are acquired under uniform illumination (same light intensity across the image) from the right, while varying the geometry of the paper: flat (a), bent (b) and crumpled (c). The other three images are acquired under a non-uniform illumination (light is more bright

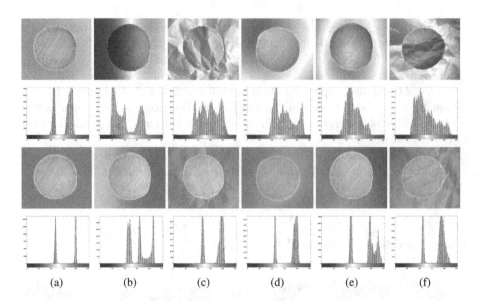

Fig. 6. The grayscale version of the images from Fig. 5 are accentuated with false colors (divergent color-map: blue/white/red) to visualize the drop in image variance after correction (bottom two rows). The histograms also reflect this, clearly showing the two regions (red dye and background) (Color figure online).

in some regions of the image than others), while under the same deformations as the first three: flat (d), bent (e) and crumpled (f). The second row of Fig. 5 shows the same images after applying our method. A considerable improvement in the contrast between foreground and background can be observed, with shading caused by illumination almost completely removed.

Figure 6 shows false color images representing grayscale versions of the same images from Fig. 5: top two rows before and bottom rows after applying our method. Additionally the histogram of each image is also shown in Fig. 6, visualizing how the two areas (red foreground and white background) are much better defined.

Synthetic Lesions on Skin: Images were taken of the forearms of multiple volunteers, with ages ranging from 22 to 34 years (Fig. 7). Red dye was painted on the skin and the images were acquired under uniform illumination, which was provided by multiple halogen lamps behind diffuser curtains (to improve uniformity).

Since the dye was applied uniformly, we can also use this set to validate the performance of our illumination compensation. As can be observed in Fig. 8, the spectra of pixels (both dye and skin) vary considerably less after *local illumination compensation*. It can also be observed that the shape of the spectra, which dictates their color, has not changed. This shows that our method preserves the spectral signature of the tissue.

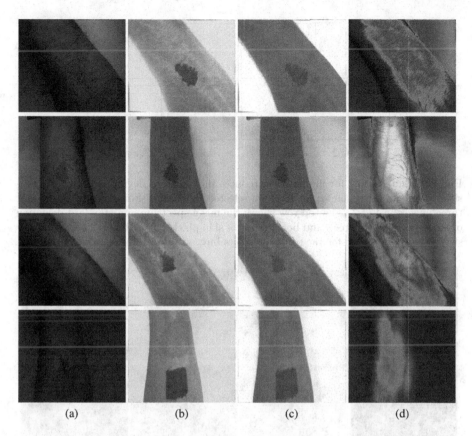

Fig. 7. Each row depicts a synthetic lesion of a different volunteer, with: (a) original image, (b) both local and global illumination compensated, (c) only local illumination compensated without global compensation and (d) illumination map L (false colors).

Psoriasis Lesions: Images were acquired at the university clinic during regular consultation hours of patients with confirmed diagnosis of *psoriasis vulgaris*, with ages between 19 and 74 years. All patients were undergoing treatment with positively responding lesions that were reducing in size. Illumination was provided by a regular halogen examination lamp that had to be repositioned depending on the location of the lesion on the patients body (Fig. 9 column-wise: lower leg, elbow, upper arm and left wrist).

5   Discussion

In Sect. 3.2 we have stated three assumptions essential to our method, with the latter two dictating how we estimate the illumination map L. We will now discuss two special cases, where we observed that these assumptions do not hold completely.

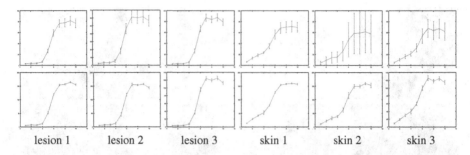

| lesion 1 | lesion 2 | lesion 3 | skin 1 | skin 2 | skin 3 |

Fig. 8. Compensating for illumination reduces the standard deviation of pixels intensities from similar tissue types. Here we selected lesion and skin pixels from the first three images in Fig. 7. The top row shows the mean spectrum and standard deviation of lesion pixles (left three), and bottom row of skin pixels (right three). The second row shows the same metric for the same pixel sets but, after local illumination correction.

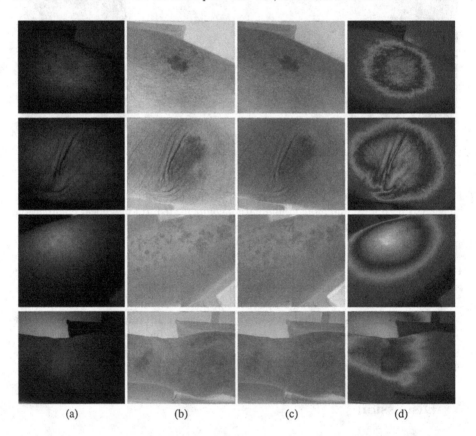

| (a) | (b) | (c) | (d) |

Fig. 9. Each row depicts a different psoriasis lesion(s) (lower leg, elbow, upper arm and left wrist), with: (a) original image, (b) both local and global illumination compensated, (c) only local illumination compensated without global compensation and (d) illumination map L (false colors).

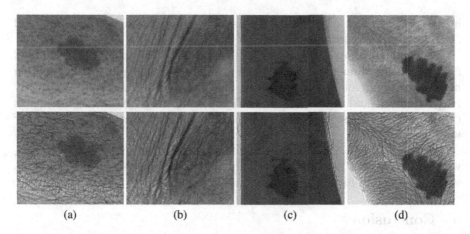

(a)   (b)   (c)   (d)

Fig. 10. Normalized albedo of several lesions (psoriasis and red dye) with the top row using unprocessed illumination maps, and the bottom processing the illumination map with a bilateral filter before albedo recovery. Due to their similar size, specular highlights on fine geometric details are introduced and can be observed in the bottom row. Bilateral filtering of L has no impact on the global normalization. These are magnified regions of images shown in Figs. 7 and 9 (Color figure online).

Although we assume the BRDF of both skin and lesions to be constant across the visible spectrum, which it mostly is, we could observe in Fig. 7 that subjects of rows 1 and 3 had clearly visible blood vessels under the skin. Above 750 nm, skin becomes increasingly translucent, potentially revealing underlying blood vessels which are then included in the illumination map L. This introduced bias brightens the areas where the blood vessels are visible, however the spectrum of the tissue is still preserved. We assume two factors to be responsible for this: the relative young age of the subjects in this test, and that all measurements were taken of the inside forearm, where blood vessels are especially prominent. We could not observe this for patients with psoriasis lesions.

We could also observe that the reflectance spectrum of hair does not conform to our assumption (see Sect. 3.2) regarding the distinguishability of the foreground and background spectra. Hair has a spectrum clearly distinguishable from both lesions and skin, and is often included in L. This distinction can be observed in both Figs. 3 and 4, where the hair is clearly black across all images, thus different from both lesion and skin.

Removing the hair from the illumination map would imply to restoring it to the corrected image, and thus the albedo A. Although we could employ a specialized method to remove the hair from L (such as described in [8]), we believe a more generalized approach would be better suited, as it could also encompass fine geometric details.

The task then becomes the removal of local features from L, while preserving the larger scale illumination. We believe this to be similar to the principle of local adaptation, used for tonemapping high dynamic range images [5,7]. As discussed in Sect. 2, Fattal *et al.* [6] use a multiscale decomposition based on bilateral filtering to preserve local features.

We employ a simplified implementation [12] with only one level of bilateral filtering, with parameters tuned to preserve larger features in the illumination map, such as skin folds, while removing fine ones, such as hair. Hairs are clearly removed from L and restored to A (see Fig. 10), and although some halo artefacts can be observed, these are considerably less pronounced than if a Gaussian filter were used.

Although L approximates the distribution of illumination across the image, we can observe that treating hair as illumination has the benefit of reducing its visibility in A and further improving image quality.

6 Conclusion

We presented a novel illumination normalization method for use on multispectral images in dermatology to better distinguish between lesions and their background. The spatial distribution of illumination in an image can be recovered by exploiting differences between the spectra of the materials (tissues) being imaged and that of the incoming light. We achieve this by means of a low-rank decomposition that estimates the local variations in illumination as well as global variations across the spectrum. Experimental results on both synthetic and clinical data show significant improvements in image quality.

Acknowledgements. This work was partially funded by the TUM Graduate School of Information Science in Health.

References

1. Basri, R., Jacobs, D., Kemelmacher, I.: Photometric stereo with general, unknown lighting. Int. J. Comput. Vis. **72**(3), 239–257 (2007)
2. Chen, W., Er, M.J., Wu, S.: Illumination compensation and normalization for robust face recognition using discrete cosine transform in logarithm domain. IEEE Trans. Syst. Man Cybern. Part B Cybern. **36**(2), 458–466 (2006)
3. Cheng, Y.I., Swamisai, R., Umbaugh, S.E., Moss, R.H., Stoecker, W.V., Teegala, S., Srinivasan, S.K.: Skin lesion classification using relative color features. Skin Res. Technol. **14**(1), 53–64 (2008)
4. Cui, X., Huang, J., Zhang, S., Metaxas, D.N.: Background subtraction using low rank and group sparsity constraints. In: Fitzgibbon, A., Lazebnik, S., Perona, P., Sato, Y., Schmid, C. (eds.) ECCV 2012, Part I. LNCS, vol. 7572, pp. 612–625. Springer, Heidelberg (2012)
5. Durand, F., Dorsey, J.: Fast bilateral filtering for the display of high-dynamic-range images. ACM Trans Graph. (TOG). **21**, 257–266 (2002)
6. Fattal, R., Agrawala, M., Rusinkiewicz, S.: Multiscale shape and detail enhancement from multi-light image collections. ACM Trans. Graph. **26**(3), 51 (2007)
7. Li, Y., Sharan, L., Adelson, E.H.: Compressing and companding high dynamic range images with subband architectures. ACM Trans. Graph. (TOG). **24**, 836–844 (2005)

8. Nguyen, N.H., Lee, T.K., Atkins, M.S.: Segmentation of light and dark hair in dermoscopic images: a hybrid approach using a universal kernel. In: SPIE Medical Imaging. p. 76234N, International Society for Optics and Photonics (2010)

9. Park, J.I., Lee, M.H., Grossberg, M.D., Nayar, S.K.: Multispectral imaging using multiplexed illumination. In: IEEE 11th International Conference on Computer Vision, ICCV 2007, pp. 1–8 (2007)

10. Samaras, D., Metaxas, D., Fua, P., Leclerc, Y.G.: Variable albedo surface reconstruction from stereo and shape from shading. In: Proceedings of IEEE Conference on Computer Vision and Pattern Recognition. vol. 1, pp. 480–487. IEEE (2000)

11. Shi, Z., Govindaraju, V.: Historical document image enhancement using background light intensity normalization. In: Proceedings of the 17th International Conference on Pattern Recognition, ICPR 2004, vol. 1, pp. 473–476. IEEE (2004)

12. Tomasi, C., Manduchi, R.: Bilateral filtering for gray and color images. In: Sixth International Conference on Computer Vision, 1998, pp. 839–846. IEEE (1998)

13. Vogel, A., Chernomordik, V.V., Demos, S.G., Pursley, R., Little, R.F., Tao, Y., Gandjbakhche, A.H., Yarchoan, R., Riley, J.D., Hassan, M., et al.: Using noninvasive multispectral imaging to quantitatively assess tissue vasculature. J. Biomed. Opt. **12**(5), 051604–051604 (2007)

14. Zheng, J., Li, Z., Rahardja, S., Yao, S., Yao, W.: Collaborative image processing algorithm for detail refinement and enhancement via multi-light images. In: IEEE International Conference on Acoustics Speech and Signal Processing (ICASSP), pp. 1382–1385. IEEE (2010)

Efficient Gaussian Process-Based Modelling and Prediction of Image Time Series

Marco Lorenzi[1]([⊠]), Gabriel Ziegler[2], Daniel C. Alexander[1], and Sebastien Ourselin[1] for ADNI

[1] Centre for Medical Image Computing, CMIC, UCL, London, UK
m.lorenzi@ucl.ac.uk
[2] Wellcome Trust Centre for Neuroimaging, UCL, London, UK

Abstract. In this work we propose a novel Gaussian process-based spatio-temporal model of time series of images. By assuming separability of spatial and temporal processes we provide a very efficient and robust formulation for the marginal likelihood computation and the posterior prediction. The model adaptively accounts for local spatial correlations of the data, and the covariance structure is effectively parameterised by the Kronecker product of covariance matrices of very small size, each encoding only a single direction in space. We provide a simple and flexible framework for within- and between-subject modelling and prediction. In particular, we introduce the Hoffman-Ribak method for efficient inference on posterior processes and its uncertainty. The proposed framework is applied in the context of longitudinal modelling in Alzheimer's disease. We firstly demonstrate the advantage of our non-parametric method for modelling of within-subject structural changes. The results show that non-parametric methods demonstrably outperform conventional parametric methods. Then the framework is extended to optimize complex parametrized covariate kernels. Using Bayesian model comparison via marginal likelihood the framework enables to compare different hypotheses about individual change processes of images.

1 Introduction

Modelling longitudinal changes in organs is fundamental for the understanding of biological and pathological processes. For instance the development of a spatio-temporal model of disease progression in Alzheimer's disease (AD) from time series of magnetic resonance images (MRIs) would be highly valuable for the fundamental understanding of the disease process, for diagnostic purposes and

---

G. Ziegler—Joint first author.

Data used in preparation of this article were obtained from the Alzheimer's Disease Neuroimaging Initiative (ADNI) database (http://adni.loni.usc.edu/). As such, the investigators within the ADNI contributed to the design and implementation of ADNI and/or provided data but did not participate in analysis or writing of this report.

S. Ourselin et al. (Eds.): IPMI 2015, LNCS 9123, pp. 626–637, 2015.
DOI: 10.1007/978-3-319-19992-4_49

individual predictions, and for testing the efficacy of disease modifying drugs in clinical trials.

The consistent modelling and prediction of spatio-temporal changes in longitudinal MRI is still an important challenge from both methodological and computational perspectives. In fact, flexible modelling instruments are required in order to robustly capture meaningful pathological accelerations specific to sensitive brain regions. Moreover, since a biological model of local brain changes is often unknown, it is important to develop optimal models in terms of statistical complexity.

Many of the previous works on spatio-temporal modelling of image time series are based on non-linear image registration, describing signal differences between images as local spatial transformations [2,3,9,10]. However, statistical inference in registration models is often limited, due to the computational complexity, and since image-registration is generally not flexible enough to perform model comparisons and clinical prediction, to account for covariates and for the within- and between subjects heterogeneity.

A statistical focus on the modeling of image time series is commonly provided by parametric linear modelling frameworks (GLM) [5]. However, GLM approaches are often limited by the choice of arbitrary model complexity and spatial resolution at which the data is analyzed. Even though flexible non-parametric models have been proposed for the analysis of spatio-temporal signals in brain images [4,7], their computational complexity still prevents the straightforward application in time series of high-resolution MRIs. Non-parametric Gaussian process (GP) models have emerged as a flexible and elegant Bayesian approach for prediction and modelling in manifold applications [11], and have been recently successfully introduced to the field of neuroimaging, e.g. in the context of single-case inference in aging [13]. However, the application of GPs to the voxel-wise modelling of image time series is to date very challenging, since the specification of the joint covariance structure of the image features is in general computationally prohibitive.

In this work we introduce a generative model of spatio-temporal changes based on GPs, to provide a flexible and computationally efficient approach to the analysis of aligned image time series by accounting for spatial and temporal correlation. In particular, by assuming a local spatial correlation model and the separability between spatial and temporal changes, we introduce a very efficient formulation based on a covariance structure parameterized by the Kronecker product of small size covariance matrices [12]. The proposed model extends GLM approaches by providing a flexible and efficient statistical tool for the analysis of image features from spatially aligned time series, for instance by allowing statistical inference on the model parameters.

The paper is organized as follows. In Sect. 2 we propose our generative model of longitudinal changes in image time series, while in Sect. 3 we provide computationally tractable optimization and prediction schemes. We also introduce a novel computational scheme based on the Hoffman-Ribak method for the statistical inference in high dimensional GP-based spatio-temporal models. Finally, in Sects. 4 and 5, we apply the model in the context of longitudinal data from from the Alzheimer's Disease Neuroimaging Initiative (ADNI) for (1) within-subject modelling and prediction of local and regional brain longitudinal changes, and (2) group-wise joint modelling of local ventricle growth rates based on socio-demographics, genetic factors, and clinical scores.

2   A Generative Model for Within-Subject Image Time Series

Let $u = (x, y, z)$ be the 3-dimensional spatial coordinate system and t the temporal dimension. We consider the image time series I as a discretely sampled spatio-temporal signal of dimensions $N \times N \times N \times N_T$, where N is the dimension of the sampling grid on a single spatial axis, and N_T is the number of time points[1]. In the following sections we represent the image time-series I as a single dimensional array of dimensions $N^3 N_T$. We model the image time series $I(u, t)$ as a realization of a latent spatio-temporal process $f(u, t)$ with additive noise:

$$I(u, t) = f(u, t) + \epsilon(u, t). \tag{1}$$

The true signal will be modelled as a GP with zero mean and covariance Σ, while ϵ is assumed to be i.i.d. Gaussian distributed measurement noise $\epsilon(u, t) \sim \mathcal{N}(0, \sigma^2)$. Here we first assume that spatial and temporal processes are *separable*, and thus that the covariance matrix Σ can be factorised in the Kronecker product of independent spatial and temporal covariance matrices: $\Sigma = \Sigma_S \otimes \Sigma_T$.

This is a valid modeling assumption when the temporal properties of the signal are similar across space; for instance, when analyzing within-subject time series of brain MRIs in AD the expected pathological change rates are generally mild and slowly varying across the brain. Second, a central assumption made in this paper is that the spatial dependencies of the signal are *local*, i.e. that the image intensities are smoothly varying and correlated within a spatial neighborhood of radius l_s. We note that our assumptions about separability and stationarity are compatible with the spatio-temporal correlation models commonly assumed by registration-based approaches.

A reasonable choice for such a local spatial covariance structure is a negative squared exponential model $\Sigma_S(u_1, u_2) = \lambda_s \exp(-\frac{\|u_1 - u_2\|^2}{2l_s})$, where λ_s is the global spatial amplitude parameter, and l_s is the length-scale of the Gaussian spatial neighborhood. We observe that such a covariance structure is *stationary* with respect to the space parameters. Furthermore we can exploit the separability properties of the negative exponential function to note that given two separate spatial locations $u_1 = (x_1, y_1, z_1)$ and $u_2 = (x_2, y_2, z_2)$ we have

$$\Sigma_S(u_1, u_2) = \lambda_s \exp(-\frac{(x_1 - x_2)^2}{2l_s}) \exp(-\frac{(y_1 - y_2)^2}{2l_s}) \exp(-\frac{(z_1 - z_2)^2}{2l_s}).$$

---

[1] For simplicity we focus on an even sampling across spatial directions, even though the generalization of the proposed model to the uneven case is straightforward.

For this reason the covariance matrix Σ_S can be further decomposed as the Kronecker product of covariance matrices of 1-dimensional processes: $\Sigma = K_x \otimes K_y \otimes K_z \otimes \Sigma_T$. We observe that the model is here conveniently represented by the product of independent covariances of significantly smaller size, and is completely identified by the spatial, temporal and noise parameters. In particular the proposed model is flexible with respect to the temporal covariance matrix Σ_T, which can be expressed in terms of complex mixed-effects structure, and can account for covariates and different progression models. For instance, in this work the matrix Σ_T is first specified in order to model the temporal progression observed in time series of images (Sect. 4), and then is used to model the influence of anatomical, genetic, clinical, and sociodemographic covariates on individual atrophy rates modelled by non-linear registration (Sect. 5).

3   Inference in Gaussian Processes with Kronecker Structure

The GP-based generative model with Kronecker covariance structure outlined in this work provides a powerful and efficient framework for prediction using image time series. Here we provide the main results concerning the marginal likelihood computation, the hyper-parameter optimization and the posterior prediction.

Let $(U_{K_x}, S_{K_x} = \mathrm{diag}(\lambda_1^x, \ldots, \lambda_N^x))$ and $(U_T, S_T = \mathrm{diag}(\lambda_1^t, \ldots, \lambda_{N_T}^t))$ be the eigenvectors and eigenvalues associated to the one-dimensional spatial and temporal covariance matrices K_x and Σ_T. This eigendecomposition problem can be easily and efficiently solved beforehand offline. We further introduce the shortform notation $\bigotimes A = A_x \otimes A_y \otimes A_z$.

Log-Marginal Likelihood. The marginal likelihood of the model (1) is the following:

$$\log \mathcal{L} = -\frac{1}{2} \sum_{i,j,k,l} \log(\lambda_i^x \lambda_j^y \lambda_k^z \lambda_l^t + \sigma^2) - \frac{1}{2} V_I^T (\bigotimes S_K \otimes S_T + \sigma^2 Id)^{-1} V_I + const,$$

$$(2)$$

with $const = -\frac{N^3 N_T}{2} \log(2\pi)$, $V_I = \mathrm{vec}\left[(U_{K_z}^T \otimes U_T^T)\tilde{I}(U_{K_x} \otimes U_{K_y})\right]$, and where $\tilde{I}$ is the matricization of I into a 2 dimensional matrix of dimension $N^2 \times NN_T$, and $\lambda_i^x, \lambda_j^y, \lambda_k^z$ and λ_l^t are the eigenvalues of respectively K_x, K_y, K_z and Σ_t. The computation of the vector V_I requires the storage and multiplication of matrices of relatively small sizes, respectively $N^2 \times N^2$, $N^2 \times NN_T$ and $NN_T \times NN_T$. The product $(\bigotimes S_K \otimes S_T + \sigma^2 Id)^{-1} V_I$ can be finally computed as the solution of the linear system $(\bigotimes S_K \otimes S_T + \sigma^2 Id)\mathbf{X} = V_I$, which is straightforward since $(\bigotimes S_K \otimes S_T + \sigma^2 Id)$ is diagonal.

Hyperparameter Optimization. The derivative of the log-likelihood (2) with respect to the model parameters $\boldsymbol{\theta}$ is:

$$\frac{\mathrm{d}}{\mathrm{d}\boldsymbol{\theta}} \log \mathcal{L} = -\frac{1}{2} Tr \left((\bigotimes K \otimes \Sigma_T + \sigma^2 Id)^{-1} \frac{\mathrm{d}}{\mathrm{d}\boldsymbol{\theta}} (\bigotimes K \otimes \Sigma_T + \sigma^2 Id) \right)$$
$$- \frac{1}{2} \frac{\mathrm{d}}{\mathrm{d}\boldsymbol{\theta}} I^T (\bigotimes K \otimes \Sigma_T + \sigma^2 Id)^{-1} I. \tag{3}$$

It can be shown that formula (3) can be efficiently computed with respect to each model parameters. For instance, the gradient with respect to the noise parameter can be expressed in the form:

$$\frac{\mathrm{d}}{\mathrm{d}\sigma^2} \log \mathcal{L} = -\frac{1}{2} \sum_{i,j,k,l} (\lambda_i^x \lambda_j^y \lambda_k^z \lambda_l^t + \sigma^2)^{-1} + \frac{1}{2} V_I^T (\bigotimes S_K \otimes S_T + \sigma^2 Id)^{-2} V_I. \tag{4}$$

Prediction. A major strength of a GP framework for image time series is that it easily enables probabilistic predictions based on given observations. The proposed generative model allows us to consider the predictive distributions of the latent spatio-temporal process at any testing locations u^* and timepoints t^*. Given image time series $I(u,t)$, we now aim at predicting the image I^* at $N^* \times N_T^*$ testing coordinates $\{u^*, t^*\}$. Let us define $\Sigma_{I,I^*} = \Sigma(u,t,u^*,t^*)$ the cross-covariance matrix of training and testing data, and $\Sigma_{I^*,I^*} = \Sigma(u^*,t^*,u^*,t^*)$ the covariance evaluated on the new coordinates. The joint GP model of training and testing data is:

$$\begin{pmatrix} I(u,t) \\ I^*(u^*,t^*) \end{pmatrix} \sim \mathcal{N} \left[\begin{pmatrix} 0 \\ 0 \end{pmatrix}, \begin{pmatrix} \Sigma + \sigma^2 Id & \Sigma_{I,I^*} \\ \Sigma_{I^*,I} & \Sigma_{I^*,I^*} + \sigma^2 Id \end{pmatrix} \right], \tag{5}$$

and it can be easily shown that the posterior distribution of I^* conditioned on the observed time series I and parameters $\boldsymbol{\theta}$ is [11]:

$$I^* | I, \{u^*, t^*\}, \boldsymbol{\theta} \sim \mathcal{N} \left(\mu^*, \Sigma^* \right), \text{ where } \mu^* = \Sigma_{I,I^*} \Sigma^{-1} I$$
$$\text{and } \Sigma^* = \Sigma_{I^*,I^*} - \Sigma_{I,I^*} \Sigma^{-1} \Sigma_{I^*,I} + \sigma^2 Id. \tag{6}$$

From the practical perspective, we notice that by definition the new covariance matrices still have a Kronecker product form: $\Sigma_{I,I^*} = K_{x,x^*} \otimes K_{y,y^*} \otimes K_{z,z^*} \otimes \Sigma_{t,t^*}$, and $\Sigma_{I^*,I^*} = K_{x^*,x^*} \otimes K_{y^*,y^*} \otimes K_{z^*,z^*} \otimes \Sigma_{t^*,t^*}$. The predicted mean μ^* at coordinates $\{u^*, t^*\}$ is then

$$\mu^* = \left(K_{x,x^*} U_{K_x} \otimes K_{y,y^*} U_{K_y} \otimes K_{z,z^*} U_{K_z} \otimes \Sigma_{t,t^*} U_T \right) (\bigotimes S_K \otimes S_T + \sigma^2 Id)^{-1} V_I,$$

which can be computed efficiently by noting that the matrix to be inverted is diagonal and by using the product rule of the Kronecker operator. While the posterior form (6) can also be used to evaluate the posterior marginal covariance, certain considerations are necessary for a tractable approach. Indeed, the covariance matrix Σ^* is computed from Σ, Σ_{I^*,I^*} and $\Sigma_{I^*,I}$, which are evaluated on different sets of spatial and temporal coordinates. In particular, the Kronecker structure is lost and in the absence of further assumptions the matrix Σ^* must therefore be explicitly computed, generally leading to impractical solutions.

Hoffman-Ribak Method for Posterior Sampling. We propose to compute the *sample distribution* of (6) using the Hoffman-Ribak method (HR) introduced in the late 1990s in the astrophysics literature [8]. Given the Gaussian distribution (5) partitioned into training (observed) and testing (unobserved) components, the HR method provides a computationally efficient and exact algorithm for sampling from (6) consisting of the following two steps:

- Sample a random observation (Y, Y^*) from the joint distribution (5),
- Compute a sample Z of the marginal posterior (6) according to $Z = Y^* + \Sigma_{I^*,I}(\Sigma + \sigma^2 Id)^{-1}Y$.

Despite its simple formulation, the HR method cannot be straightforwardly applied in our case as sampling from the very high dimensional joint distribution is generally prohibitive. Therefore, instead of focusing on predicting time series at arbitrary spatial and temporal coordinates, we provide here an efficient scheme for spatio-temporal prediction at arbitrary time points $T^* = \{t^*\}$ evaluated in the same spatial coordinates of the training image time-series I. Under this assumption the matrices Σ, Σ_{I^*,I^*} and $\Sigma_{I^*,I}$ differ in the temporal part only,

$$\Sigma = \Sigma_S \otimes \Sigma_T + \sigma^2 Id; \quad \Sigma_{I^*,I^*} = \Sigma_S \otimes \Sigma_{T^*,T^*}; \quad \Sigma_{I^*,I} = \Sigma_S \otimes \Sigma_{T^*,T} + \sigma^2 Id,$$

and it is simple to show that the joint covariance is $\Sigma^{joint} = P(\Sigma_S \otimes \Sigma_{T^j} + \sigma^2 Id)P^T$, where P is a structured permutation matrix, and $\Sigma_{T^j} = \begin{pmatrix} \Sigma_T & \Sigma_{t,t^*} \\ \Sigma_{t^*,t} & \Sigma_{t^*,t^*} \end{pmatrix}$. A sample Z from the joint distribution can thus be easily computed as $Z = P(U\Lambda)X$, where X is a standard multivariate normal distributed vector, and $U\Lambda^2 U^T$ is the eigen-decomposition of the covariance $(\Sigma_S \otimes \Sigma_{T^j} + \sigma^2 Id)$. Eigen-decomposition and matrix multiplication can be efficiently computed by virtue of the properties of the Kronecker product.

In the following sections, after validating the proposed framework in a controlled setting, we provide a modelling application in the context of longitudinal modelling in AD.

4   Model Validation

Estimation of the Spatio-temporal Properties in Synthetic Data. Here, we test the ability of the proposed GP model to correctly estimate the underlying spatial and temporal properties prescribed in synthetic data. We chose a time-series of brain MRIs composed of 6 aligned longitudinal gray matter (GM) segment images of an example ADNI patient, and we applied Gaussian smoothing to obtain synthetic samples of a spatio-temporal process with predefined spatial correlation and signal to noise ratio. Moreover we generated synthetic longitudinal progressions of increasing temporal complexity following respectively voxel-wise linear, quadratic and cubic functions of time estimated through a general linear model (GLM). Furthermore, longitudinal changes in the synthetic time series were modelled with the proposed GP model. We applied a squared exponential model for the temporal covariance parameterized by the temporal length-scale l_t. A maximum-a-posteriori (MAP) estimate of the parameters was obtained by using Gauss-Newton optimization scheme of the log-hyperparameters, using multivariate uninformative Gaussian hyperprior with log-hyperparameters $\mu_h = [-2, -2, 0, 3]$ and $\Sigma_h = \text{diag}([5, 5, 1, 5])$ for respectively $(\sigma^2, l_s, \lambda_s, l_t)$.

Table 1 shows the relationship between the spatio-temporal properties of the synthetic data and the MAP estimates of the GP parameters. Noticeably, the estimated spatial length-scale closely resembles the global smoothness parameter of the synthetic data, adaptively accounting for image smoothness properties. Additionally, we observed that the estimated temporal length-scale decreased when modeling longitudinal progressions of higher order models. Thus, the model also correctly denotes the increased complexity of the temporal changes.

Table 1. Estimation of the global spatial and temporal properties. The estimated spatial length-scale l_s closely correspond to the global smoothness of the synthetic data, while the noise term and the signal amplitude decrease with increasingly smoother data. The estimated temporal length-scale is inversely proportional to the underlying complexity of the temporal progression.

Spatial smoothness (mm)	l_s	σ^2	λ_s
0	0.09	9e-6	0.7
0.5	0.81	5e-6	0.64
1	1.2	3e-6	0.53
2	2.3	1e-6	0.5
3	3.3	3e-10	0.48
4	4.3	7e-11	0.47

Temporal progression	l_t (log-values)
linear	4.3
quadratic	1.79
cubic	1.72

Within-Subject Modelling and Prediction of Longitudinal Changes.
We chose high-resolution longitudinal images of 10 AD patients, 10 patients with mild cognitive impairment (MCIc) subsequently converting to AD, and 10 healthy controls from the ADNI dataset. AD patients and healthy controls (HC) had 4 images per participant, corresponding to baseline, 6 months, 1 and 2 years scans, while for MCIc patients additional images corresponding to 3 or 4 years were available. The images were processed according to established procedures consisting of joint bias correction, tissue segmentation, alignment to the within-subject average anatomy, and non-linear normalization to a group-wise anatomical reference [1]. The final image size was of 100^3 cubic voxels with isotropic resolution of 1.5 mm.

The longitudinal changes in the resulting time series of processed gray matter density maps were modelled according to the proposed GP model. The model was estimated for each subject by using 3 training images corresponding to baseline, 6 months and 1 year scans. In order to capture meaningful non-linear trends during disease progression to AD, we also applied the GP model in the MCIc group by using 4 and 5 training images, corresponding to the time range from baseline to respectively 2 and 3 years follow-up.

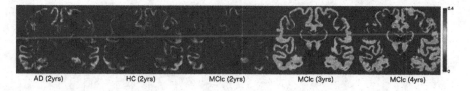

Fig. 1. Group-wise average absolute differences between extrapolated images and real ones. The GP model was trained on scans from 3 time points corresponding to baseline, 6 months and 1 year. Errors were generally found to be proportional to the extrapolation time.

We applied the optimization scheme illustrated in Sect. 4 while imposing an informative prior on the temporal length-scale parameter with log-mean and -variance of 3 and 0.1 respectively. This choice was done in virtue of the experimental results illustrated in Table 1 in order to promote a moderately non-linear behaviour of the GP model, and at the same time avoid overfitting on the limited number of within-subject observations. The resulting computational time for the parameter estimation was of about 5 min per subject on a standard PC (with 2.6 GHz, QuadCore, 16 GB RAM). The predictive accuracy of the model was then tested by voxel-wise comparison of the extrapolated image series with respect to the corresponding ground truth follow-up images, and compared with respect to a standard linear and quadratic voxel-by-voxel model using within-subject GLM. The group-wise average voxel-wise absolute differences between extrapolated images and real ones are shown in Fig. 1. Errors were generally found to be proportional to the extrapolation time. Table 2 shows that the results of the GP model are comparable to those obtained by linear modelling when training on 3 time points only. However, the prediction of the GP model significantly improves the linear one when using more training points. This result indicates that the GP model is able to capture meaningful accelerations of the time process when sufficient data is provided, while it stays essentially linear otherwise. Figure 2 shows the mean hippocampal progression and associated confidence interval from the posterior latent process for a MCIc patient.

Table 2. Mean absolute error (averaged over the whole brain and subjects) between predicted extrapolated image and real one (values are scaled by a factor 1e3). The proposed GP model significantly outperformed predictions obtained from GLM when trained on 4 and 5 time points, from baseline to 2–3 years follow-up (* for statistically significant difference, $p < 0.05$, paired t-test).

	AD	HC	MCI	
N train points	3	3	4	5
GP	1.9	1.9	2.9*	2.5*
GLM linear	1.9	2	3.1	2.7
GLM quadratic	6.7	2.6	8.7	5.4

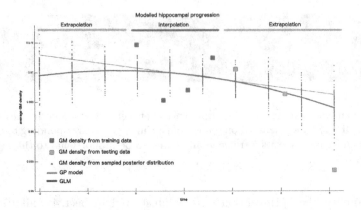

Fig. 2. Predicted hippocampal progression for a sample MCIc patient. The model was estimated from 4 image time points (baseline to 2 years) in a bounding region including the hippocampus. The longitudinal sample distribution (gray dots) and mean prediction (red line) are estimated according to the marginal GP posterior of Sect. 3 by using the Hoffman-Ribak method (Colour figure online).

We observe that the GP-based model of hippocampal loss is non-linear and fairly predicts the acceleration of volume loss observed in the follow-up testing images.

5   Application: Between-Subjects Prediction of Individual Rates of Ventricle Growth Using Multi-kernel Learning

In this second application, we exploit the flexibility of our model to make covariate-based predictions of individual rates of atrophy in elderly subjects. In contrast to typical multivariate models which predict or classify scalar values, our GP framework allows prediction of images. In particular, we here focus on predicting the rate of volumetric growth in the lateral ventricle regions.

Firstly, we used computational morphometry to obtain the rates of atrophy in a large sample from the ADNI longitudinal dataset. To obtain these features for training and testing, we used 1143 and 569 MRI scans of 206 and 105 elderly subjects respectively (ages 59–91, age mean ± std: 76.0 ± 6.0 years). In order to enable predictions across a broad range of clinical states, the sample was pooled across clinical groups. It contained 111 healthy elderly and 108 subjects with stable and 92 subjects with progressive MCI. After longitudinal registration, tissue segmentation and inter-subject alignment [1], we calculated each subject's ventricle growth rate from registered CSF images using a linear model.

Secondly, using the preprocessed images as features we considered a special case of generative model (1) to implement a prediction model based on individual subject's covariates, e.g. age, cognitive scores, etc. This is realized by a different choice of covariance function Σ_T compared to the above within-subject application. In order to enable a prediction based on multiple available covariate sets e.g. genes, clinical scores, etc. we used an additive multi-kernel learning covariance

$$\Sigma_T = \sum_{r=1}^{4} K_r, \quad \text{with} \quad K_r(c_1, c_2) = \alpha_r \exp(-\frac{1}{2}(c_1 - c_2)^T M_r(c_1 - c_2)) \quad (7)$$

using a sum of (up to four) squared exponential covariances K_r with amplitudes α_r, and c_1, c_2 denoting pairs of covariate vectors from each of (up to four) covariate sets. The symmetric matrices M_r were chosen to be either $M_{ISO} = \ell^{-2}Id$ or $M_{ARD} = \text{diag}(\ell)^{-2}$. Like in typical GP regression applications, using (7) explicitly models covariance of (latent) observations f as a function of similarity of inputs c (here the covariate vectors of subjects). That implements the idea that subjects with similar covariates are expected to have similar rates of atrophy. In particular, the choice of $M_r = M_{ISO}$ parametrizes an isotropic covariance assuming equal length-scale for different covariates of the same covariate set. An alternative choice of $M_r = M_{ARD}$ implements automatic relevance determination (ARD) with separate length-scales estimated for each variable. We compared

Table 3. Log marginal likelihood (ml) of Gaussian process covariance using M_{ISO} and M_{ARD} for prediction of ventricle growth rate maps based on sets of subject's covariates. Hyperparameters were optimized in 206 subjects training sample. Column 3 shows mean absolute error (mae) averaged across voxels in prediction of unseen 105 test subjects from independent test sample.

Model	ml - ISO	ml - ARD	mae - ARD
1	1.6697	1.6769	0.0059
2	2.4309	2.0249	0.0058
3	2.4356	2.0513	0.0080
4	2.2768	2.4434	0.0057

successively complex prediction models using (1) only global brain volumes (tgmv, twmc, tcsv) or (2) additionally using demography (age, sex, education, marital status, year of retirement), or (3) also including genetic risk in terms of the number of ApoE4 allele and (4) finally also using the clinical neuropsychological test scores MMSE, ADAS, and CDR. The models (1)–(4) step-by-step increased the amount of subject-specific information to predict maps of rates of ventricle growth. Comparison across models was performed using log marginal likelihood balancing model fit and model complexity with varying numbers of hyperparameters. We found an increasing marginal likelihood for more complex models using ARD covariance (see Table 3) and decreased model evidence for model 4 under ISO covariance. Highest marginal likelihood was observed for ARD model 4 including all predictors. This trend is also reflected in terms of mean absolute error maps demonstrating increased prediction accuracy and generalization ability during testing in an independent test sample of 105 subjects

(Fig. 3A). Results also showed a correlation of up to 0.52 of predicted and true growth rates (Fig. 3B).

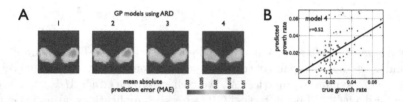

Fig. 3. (A) Mean absolute error (MAE) of prediction maps in an independent testing sample of 105 subjects show increasingly better predictions using more predictor sets and Gaussian process models with ARD. (B) Predicted over true growth rates using model 4 in an example voxel showing correlation of $r = 0.52$.

6   Conclusions

We presented a novel framework for modelling and prediction of spatio-temporal processes in image time series. It is flexible and computationally efficient thanks to the proposed Kronecker structure of the covariance, and to the use of the Hoffman-Ribak method for efficient sampling from the posterior. Our model provided promising results when tested in very different experimental scenarios concerning longitudinal modelling in AD, and opens the path to the effective use of GPs for the generative modeling of neuroimaging data. The strength of the framework relies on assuming separability of spatial and temporal processes. We show that this assumption leads to meaningful results when applied to the longitudinal modeling in AD, where the expected pathological changes are generally mild and slowly varying across brain regions. This assumption might be relaxed in future work in order to also model spatially varying processes that might underlie biological progressions with different properties. It may be indeed possible to further extend the framework to allow non-stationary correlations and noise models without compromising the computational efficiency, by accounting for local smoothly varying stationary processes as previously proposed in geostatistics [6]. Finally, further extensions of the proposed work will be devoted to the group-wise non-parametric mixed-effect modeling of disease progression in clinical cohorts such as ADNI, by exploiting the flexibility of the proposed spatio-temporal covariance structure in accounting for subject and group-specific progressions and confounders.

Acknowledgements. Marco Lorenzi is grateful to Prof. John Ashburner, for his help in finalizing this work, and to Dr. Richard Turner, for his precious suggestions on the train toward London. Sebastien Ourselin receives funding from the EPSRC (EP/H046410/1, EP/J020990/1, EP/K005278), the MRC (MR/J01107X/1), the EU-FP7 project VPH-DARE@IT (FP7-ICT-2011-9-601055), the NIHR Biomedical Research Unit (Dementia) at UCL and the National Institute for Health

Research University College London Hospitals Biomedical Research Centre (NIHR BRC UCLH/UCL High Impact Initiative- BW.mn.BRC10269). Gabriel Ziegler is supported in part by the German Academic Exchange Service (DAAD). The Wellcome Trust Centre for Neuroimaging is supported by core funding from the Wellcome Trust [grant number 091593/Z/10/Z].

References

1. Ashburner, J., Friston, K.: Unified segmentation. NeuroImage **26**, 839–851 (2005)
2. Ashburner, J., Ridgway, G.: Symmetric diffeomorphic modeling of longitudinal structural MRI. Frontiers Neurosci. **6**(197) (02 2013)
3. Davis, B.C., Fletcher, P.T., Bullitt, E., Joshi, S.C.: Population shape regression from random design data. IJCV **90**(2), 255–266 (2010)
4. Flandin, G., Penny, W.D.: Bayesian fMRI data analysis with sparse spatial basis function priors. NeuroImage **34**(3), 1108–1125 (2007)
5. Friston, K.J., Holmes, A., Worsley, K.J.: Statistical parametric maps in functional imaging: a general linear approach. Hum. Brain Mapp. **2**, 189–210 (1995)
6. Gelfand, A., Fuentes, M., Guttorp, P., Diggle, P.: Handbook of Spatial Statistics. Chapman & Hall/CRC Handbooks of Modern Statistical Methods. Taylor & Francis, London (2010)
7. Harrison, L.M., Green, G.G.: A Bayesian spatiotemporal model for very large data sets. NeuroImage **50**(3), 1126–1141 (2010)
8. Hoffman, Y., Ribak, E.: Constrained realizations of Gaussian fields -a simple algorithm. Astrophys. J. Lett. **380**, L5–L8 (1991)
9. Lorenzi, M., Ayache, N., Frisoni, G.B., Pennec, X.: The Alzheimer's disease neuroimaging initiative: mapping the effects of $A\beta_1 - 42$ levels on the longitudinal changes in healthy aging: hierarchical modeling based on stationary velocity fields. In: Fichtinger, G., Martel, A., Peters, T. (eds.) MICCAI 2011, Part II. LNCS, vol. 6892, pp. 663–670. Springer, Heidelberg (2011)
10. Niethammer, M., Huang, Y., Vialard, F.-X.: Geodesic regression for image timeseries. In: Fichtinger, G., Martel, A., Peters, T. (eds.) MICCAI 2011, Part II. LNCS, vol. 6892, pp. 655–662. Springer, Heidelberg (2011)
11. Rasmussen, C.E., Williams, C.K.I.: Gaussian Processes for Machine Learning. The MIT Press, Cambridge (2005)
12. Stegle, O., Lippert, C., Mooij, J.M., et al.: Efficient inference in matrix-variate gaussian models with iid observation noise. In: Shawe-Taylor, J., Zemel, S., Bartlett, P.L., Pereira, F.C.N., Weinberger, K.Q. (eds.) Advances in Neural Information Processing Systems 24, pp. 630–638. Second Life, Granada (2011)
13. Ziegler, G., Ridgway, G.R., Dahnke, R., Gaser, C.: Individualized Gaussian process-based prediction and detection of local and global gray matter abnormalities in elderly subjects. NeuroImage **97**, 333–348 (2014)

A Simulation Framework for Quantitative Validation of Artefact Correction in Diffusion MRI

Mark S. Graham[✉], Ivana Drobnjak, and Hui Zhang

Centre for Medical Image Computing and Department of Computer Science,
University College London, London, UK
mark.graham.13@ucl.ac.uk

Abstract. In this paper we demonstrate a simulation framework that enables the direct and quantitative comparison of post-processing methods for diffusion weighted magnetic resonance (DW-MR) images. DW-MR datasets are employed in a range of techniques that enable estimates of local microstructure and global connectivity in the brain. These techniques require full alignment of images across the dataset, but this is rarely the case. Artefacts such as eddy-current (EC) distortion and motion lead to misalignment between images, which compromise the quality of the microstructural measures obtained from them. Numerous methods and software packages exist to correct these artefacts, some of which have become de-facto standards, but none have been subject to rigorous validation. The ultimate aim of these techniques is improved image alignment, yet in the literature this is assessed using either qualitative visual measures or quantitative surrogate metrics. Here we introduce a simulation framework that allows for the direct, quantitative assessment of techniques, enabling objective comparisons of existing and future methods. DW-MR datasets are generated using a process that is based on the physics of MRI acquisition, which allows for the salient features of the images and their artefacts to be reproduced. We demonstrate the application of this framework by testing one of the most commonly used methods for EC correction, registration of DWIs to b = 0, and reveal the systematic bias this introduces into corrected datasets.

1 Introduction

Diffusion-weighted magnetic resonance (DW-MR) imaging is a powerful, non-invasive technique that allows us to probe the microstructure of biological tissue. The technique is well suited to the brain, and is used by clinicians and researchers studying its structure in health and disease.

A DW measurement is made by applying a diffusion-sensitising gradient in a particular direction across a sample, before acquiring an MR image. The image contains information on the diffusion of water in this direction. This diffusion is influenced by the underlying microstructure, and by acquiring a range of images with varying gradient strength and direction we can probe this structure.

© Springer International Publishing Switzerland 2015
S. Ourselin et al. (Eds.): IPMI 2015, LNCS 9123, pp. 638–649, 2015.
DOI: 10.1007/978-3-319-19992-4_50

Many techniques, both model-based [1] and model-free [2] use the rich information provided by such datasets to characterise brain microstructure.

Unfortunately images acquired with DW-MRI are susceptible to a number of artefacts [3]. For example, B_0 field inhomogeneities and the uneven magnetisation of the brain due to its magnetic susceptibility can lead to spatial displacements of several pixels. This prevents comparison between these images and others that do not contain these artefacts, such as T1- and T2-weighted images. Some artefacts lead to spatial offsets between the DW-MR images in a dataset, which compromises their anatomical correspondence and undermines the estimates of microstructure obtained from them. For example, motion can lead to rigid offsets between images, and eddy currents lead to a shear, scaling and translation of the image in the phase encoding (PE) direction that varies according to the amount of diffusion sensitisation used (typically summarised by the b-value) and the direction it is applied in.

Techniques for dealing with these artefacts can broadly be divided into those implemented at acquisition time, involving either some modification to the acquisition process or the collection of supplementary data, and post-processing methods implemented after acquisition time. Post-processing techniques are the most widely used, as they have several advantages: they can be applied retrospectively to already acquired data, a user can revert to the original data if the technique does not work as hoped, and they don't require additional scan-time, which is often expensive.

The literature contains a vast body of post-processing techniques and software packages for correcting artefacts in DW-MRI [4–6]. Ideally their corrections would be validated by comparison to the ground truth, i.e. a map of the spatial deformations caused by the artefacts, but these cannot be obtained for real data. As a result the literature relies on either qualitative visual assessments of image alignment [7], or quantitative assessments of surrogate measures of alignment that have questionable validity, such as tract length [8], or reduced residuals from fits to microstructural models [9]. The lack of an objective ground truth means existing techniques cannot be systematically assessed, preventing end-users from making an informed choice. The development of new methods is also hindered, as any improvements over existing ones are difficult to demonstrate.

Simulation could provide us with a ground truth that would enable us to assess methods objectively, allowing researchers to make informed decisions when selecting post-processing methods. Simulation systems exist for MRI [10,11] but there is nothing satisfactory for DW-MRI. Several systems are designed to simulate DWIs of white matter bundles [12] but these are unable to generate the full brain images required for the assessment of post-processing methods. Methods that do attempt to simulate full-brain DWIs exhibit at least one of two serious limitations. The first is the failure to model the full process of image acquisition [13], i.e. the recording of a signal in frequency space which is Fourier transformed to generate a spatial image, which precludes the inclusion of realistic artefacts. The second is the use of a heavily simplified model to create the DW contrast, which means the simulations do not capture some of the features of DWIs that makes their processing uniquely challenging, such as the variation of contrast with the direction of diffusion weighting [14].

In this work we introduce a simulation framework that allows for realistic DW-MR images to be generated, enabling the effectiveness of correction techniques to be assessed objectively and directly. The framework simulates the physics of MRI acquisition by solving Bloch's and Maxwell's equations, which ensures the images and their artefacts capture the key features of their real-world counterparts. The complexity of diffusion contrast is captured using a model-based approach. The framework is flexible, and allows for a range of artefacts to be modelled including EC, motion, B_0 inhomogeneities and magnetic susceptibility. We demonstrate an application of this framework to EC artefacts, by providing a quantitative assessment of the most commonly used correction technique, registration of all DWIs to $b = 0$.

2 Methods

In this section we describe our simulation framework for producing realistic DW-MR images, and discuss its application to validating eddy-current correction schemes. An overview of the framework is discussed in Sect. 2.1, our implementation of it in Sect. 2.2 and its application in Sect. 2.3.

2.1 Simulation Framework

The framework (Fig. 1) combines a physics-based approach to the MR image acquisition process with a model-based representation of diffusion in order to simulate realistic DW-MR datasets. To provide a meaningful validation a simulation must capture the key characteristics of DW-MR images and their artefacts. Many of the artefacts are introduced during the acquisition of the MR signal in k-space, so it is necessary to reproduce this process for a faithful simulation.

The framework takes four main inputs. The first is a geometric object that specifies the proton density and location of white matter (WM), grey matter (GM) and cerebrospinal fluid (CSF) along with their T1 and T2 values. The second is a representation of diffusion-weighting. These two inputs are combined to produce a geometric object with its proton density reduced by an attenuation factor determined by the diffusion model. The third input is a pulse sequence, detailing the RF pulses and gradients. The fourth are details of any artefacts to be included, e.g. motion. The effects of eddy currents are included in the pulse sequence. The MR simulator takes the attenuated object, pulse sequence and artefacts and solves Bloch's and Maxwell's equations at each point in the object, summing the resultant signal in order to generate the k-space measurements. This is Fourier transformed to produce the output DWI.

2.2 Implementation

A full-brain segmentation was used as the geometric object input. It was created with T1- and T2-weighted images from a single subject from the WU-Minn HCP

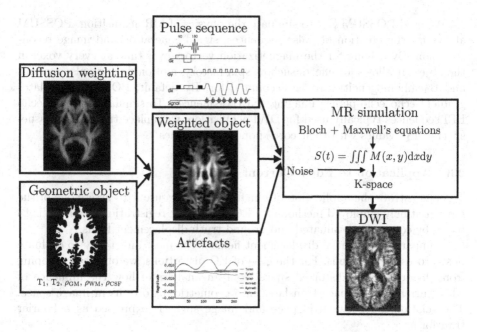

Fig. 1. The pipeline for simulating DWIs.

dataset [15], using FSL's FAST [16]. Diffusion weighting was achieved using the diffusion tensor (DT) [17]. Although the DT can not faithfully represent complex WM anatomy, such as crossing fibres, empirically we find it adequate for capturing the main features that make the processing of DWIs particularly challenging: the contrast between WM, GM and CSF, as well as the variation of signal with both the direction and strength of diffusion weighting (see Fig. 3). To account for the departure from Gaussian diffusion at higher b-values, separate tensors were fit to the b $= 1000$ s mm^{-2} and b $= 2000$ s mm^{-2} DWIs in the HCP dataset using FSL's DTIFIT. The tensor from the b $= 1000$ s mm^{-2} shell was used to predict attenuation for simulated DWIs with $b \leq 1000$ s mm^{-2}, and the tensor from the b $= 2000$ s mm^{-2} shell was used for simulations with b-values above this.

Eddy currents were added to the pulse sequence using the method in [14], by superposing a sum of decaying exponentials on each gradient field:

$$G_{x,y,z}^{E} = \sum_{i} \pm \varepsilon \, G_{x,y,z}^{\text{diff}} \exp\left[-(t - t_i)/\tau\right] \tag{1}$$

where t_i corresponds to the time each diffusion gradient is turned on or off, τ is the decay time, ε is a constant determining the relationship between the strength of eddy and diffusion gradients and a $+$ or $-$ is selected depending on whether the gradient is being turned on or off. We performed simulations with $G^{\text{diff}} = 40$ m T m^{-1}, and selected $\varepsilon = 0.006$ and $\tau = 100$ ms to represent typical values found in a clinical scanner [9].

We used POSSUM [11] to simulate the physics of MR acquisition. POSSUM allows for the creation of pulse sequences, signal generation and image reconstruction. By solving for the magnetization vectors over time at every voxel in the object it allows for effects such as spin history, motion during pulse readout and B_0 inhomogeneities to be accounted for. By default, POSSUM simulates gradient-echo echo-planar imaging (EPI) sequences. To simulate the spin-echo EPI sequences typically used for DWI acquisition, we replace the default tissue-specific $T_2{}^*$ values with their corresponding T_2 values.

2.3   Application to Eddy-Current Artefacts

To demonstrate the application of our framework we use it to assess one of the most routinely employed methods for EC correction, registration of all DWIs to $b = 0$, by comparing evaluated and ground truth displacement fields.

Comparison of spatial displacement fields is the most direct way to evaluate post-processing methods. For the case of EC distortions, we obtain a mapping from distorted to undistorted space from an analysis of how the influence of eddy currents on k-space translates into geometric distortions in image space. The relationship between k-space and image space is expressed as a Fourier transform:

$$\rho(x, y) = \iint S(k_x, k_y) \exp\left(ik_x x\right) \exp\left(ik_y y\right) \, \mathrm{d}k_x \, \mathrm{d}k_y \tag{2}$$

where $k_i = \int \bar{\gamma} G_i(t) \, \mathrm{d}t$, $\bar{\gamma}$ is the gyromagnetic ratio, G_x and G_y are the imaging gradients applied, $S(k_x, k_y)$ is the MR signal in k-space, and $\rho(x, y)$ is the image in real space. In the presence of eddy currents, our imaging gradients are modified by additional gradients $\left(G_x^E, G_y^E, G_z^E\right)$ and a spatially invariant term ϵ_0, causing our phase term to become modified. Assuming the phase-encoding (PE) direction is aligned with the y-axis, our signal equation becomes [9]:

$$\rho(x, y) = \iint S(k_x, k_y) \exp\left(ik_x x\right) \exp\left(ik_y y'\right) \, \mathrm{d}k_x \, \mathrm{d}k_y \tag{3}$$

where

$$y' = \left[\left(1 + \frac{\Delta k_y^E}{k_y}\right) y + \frac{\Delta k_x^E}{k_y} x + \frac{\Delta k_z^E}{k_y} z + \frac{\Delta k_0}{k_y}\right] \tag{4}$$

Neglecting the decay of the EC field, which we have found has a negligible effect on our obtained displacement fields, the ratios $\frac{\Delta k_i}{k_y}$ are constants. As a result the effects of EC induced gradients is to introduce two shears and a scaling which correspond to displacements along the PE direction in image space, as shown in Fig. 2. For any given slice z is constant, so we observe these deformations as a shear, scaling and translation of the image. The simulation framework allows us to find the EC induced offsets $\frac{\Delta k_i}{k_y}$ and thus obtain the transformations they lead to in image space; this gives us a ground truth displacement field that we can compare to the output of each EC correction tool.

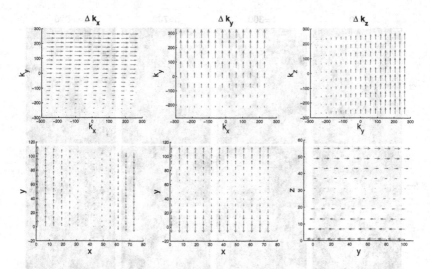

Fig. 2. The top row shows the k-space offsets that occur when EC induced gradients are added to the x-, y- and z-gradient channels, and their corresponding image space shifts are shown in the bottom row. K-space displacements are obtained from the simulation framework, and the image space displacement fields calculated according to the analytical relationship described in Sect. 2.3.

3   Experiments and Results

In this section we explain our experiment design and show results for our validation of the simulation framework (Sect. 3.1) and its application to assessing registration to b = 0 for EC correction (Sect. 3.2).

3.1   Validation of the Framework

We first assess how well the simulated images capture the most important characteristics of real images. POSSUM has been shown to provide realistic MR simulation without diffusion weighting [11,18], so here we focus on assessing the simulation of diffusion weighting. In the case of DW-MR the key characteristic is the variation in contrast as the strength and direction of diffusion weighting changes. To test this we compared a real and a simulated, artefact-free dataset with identical parameters: a 3 T scanner with three shells, $b = 300/700/2000\,\mathrm{s}$ mm^{-2}, 8/32/64 directions with 1/4/8 $b = 0$ images, TR/TE = 3000/109 ms. Figure 3a compares the changes in contrast with varying b-value. Figure 3b compares changes in contrast with varying direction of b-vector.

3.2   Application to Eddy-Current Artefacts

To assess the effectiveness of registration to b = 0 as a method for eddy correction we applied three techniques to a simulated dataset. The first is FSL's

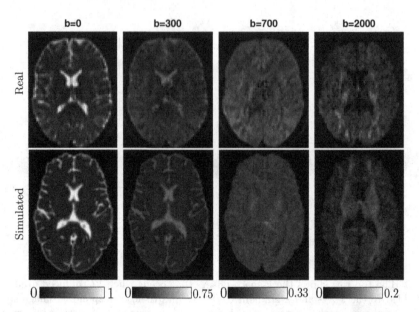

(a) Variation in contrast with respect to b-value. Both real and simulated datasets normalised against their respective $b=0$ images. The direction of diffusion weighing is the same for both datasets.

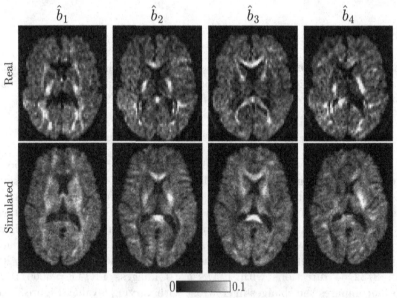

(b) Variation in contrast with respect to direction of diffusion weighting. Each column represents an image acquired at $b=2000\,\mathrm{s}\,\mathrm{mm}^{-2}$ with a different b-vector, $\hat{b}_1$-$\hat{b}_4$. Real and simulated datasets are normalised against their respective $b=0$ images and shown on one intensity scale.

Fig. 3. Comparison of real and simulated data.

eddy_correct, which performs registration of each DWI to b = 0. To provide some comparison we also used a method designed to circumvent registration to b = 0, proposed by Zhuang et al. [8]. Zhuang's technique assumes eddy-distortions are a function of the applied diffusion gradients and obtains this relationship by only registering DWIs with similar contrast. It predicts a shear, scaling and translation parameter for every slice of each volume. Zhuang's technique is tailored to ECs, and uses a constrained, 3 degree of freedom (DOF) registration algorithm, whilst eddy_correct uses a full 12 DOF. To control for this, our third method registers each DWI to b = 0 using the same constrained, 3 DOF registration algorithm used by Zhuang.

The simulated dataset consisted of two shells, $b = 700/2000\,\mathrm{s}\ \mathrm{mm}^{-2}$, 32/64 directions with 4/8 $b = 0$ images, TR/TE = 3000/90 ms, 78×110×60 with isotropic voxel size 1.85 mm. Rician noise was added to give SNR = 20. EC gradients were added to the pulse sequences according to the model in Sect. 2.2. No other artefacts were added.

The three correction methods were also applied to a real dataset, to see if the findings from simulation manifest themselves in real data. The dataset was acquired on a 3T Siemens scanner with similar parameters to the simulated dataset: $b = 700/2000\,\mathrm{s}\ \mathrm{mm}^{-2}$, 32/64 directions with 4/8 $b = 0$ images, TR/TE = 7500/103 ms, 96×96×55 with isotropic voxel size 2.5 mm. To test the effectiveness of correction an outline was drawn around the b = 0 image for the dataset, which is not affected by EC distortions, and then superposed on the corrected DWIs. This allows for a visual assessment of correction.

Figure 4 reports the mean error in the displacement fields predicted by the three eddy correction methods. Figure 5 shows the spatial distribution of these errors for a typical slice from one gradient of the $b = 2000\,\mathrm{s}\ \mathrm{mm}^{-2}$ shell. Figure 6 shows the results for correction on a real dataset.

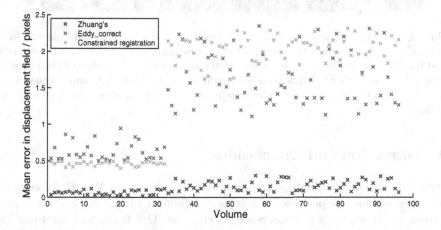

Fig. 4. Mean error in displacement field across the brain. The ground truth displacement was calculated from k-space shifts as described in Sect. 2.3. The first 32 volumes have $b = 700\,\mathrm{s}\ \mathrm{mm}^{-2}$, the remaining 64 $b = 2000\,\mathrm{s}\ \mathrm{mm}^{-2}$.

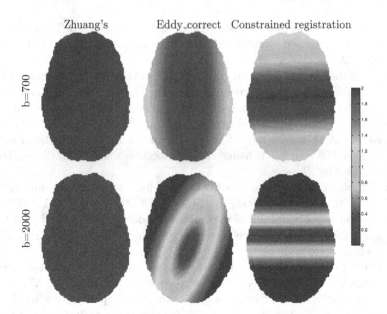

Fig. 5. Spatial distribution of errors in displacement fields in pixels, shown for one slice of a single gradient direction.

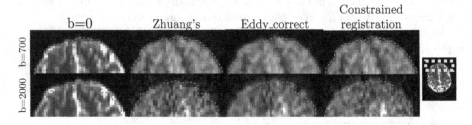

Fig. 6. Correction applied to real data. Anterior portion of the brain shown. Red outlines were drawn on the b = 0 images. Note these outline are different for the b = 700 and b = 2000 images as the CSF in the b = 0 has been cut out in the b = 2000 image. This is because the CSF rim is attenuated fully in the b = 2000 data and this needs to be reflected in the outline for it to be a useful guide for testing alignment (Color figure online).

4   Discussion and Conclusions

We have presented a simulation framework that allows for DW-MR datasets to be generated for the purposes of testing, providing an objective and quantitative means of assessing post-processing techniques. Our framework improves on previous attempts at simulation in two key areas. Firstly, our simulated images are able to provide a much more realistic representation of the contrast differences found across DW-MR datasets. This is demonstrated in Fig. 3a, which shows that the signal attenuation with increasing b-value is well matched to the attenuation found in real data, and Fig. 3b, which shows that variations in contrast with varying b-vector are captured, particularly noticeable in the white matter. Previous simulations have used a single representative mean diffusivity or diffusion tensor for each tissue type to provide diffusion-weighting [13,14], which leads to vastly oversimplified contrast which will bias assessments of correction schemes. The second improvement comes from our modelling of the MR acquisition process. Some attempts at simulations have modelled artefacts by applying geometric transforms in the spatial domain [13]. These distortions are not fully realistic, and furthermore without simulating the full image generation process certain artefacts cannot be introduced, such as those caused by motion during the read-out phase. Our approach extends both the range and realism of artefacts that can be simulated.

The simulation framework allowed us to quantitatively assess registration to $b=0$ as a method for correcting eddy currents. Figure 4 shows that registration to $b=0$ performs poorly for both $b=700$ and $b=2000$ shells. In the $b=700$ shell the displacement fields obtained from eddy_correct are off by 0.5-1 pixels, and this rises to 1-2.5 pixels for the $b=2000$ images. By contrast Zhuang's scheme, which explicitly avoids registration to $b=0$, is able to provide correction with mean errors of less than 0.5 pixel for both shells. This performance cannot be attributed to Zhuang's method explicitly modelling the two shears and one scaling that ECs gives rise to because results from the constrained, 3 DOF registration to $b=0$ were poor, particularly for the $b=2000$ shell where it performed worse than eddy_correct. It is notable that the constrained registration performed slightly better than eddy_correct for the $b=700$ shell and slightly worse for the $b=2000$ shell. This is likely because the registration used by eddy_correct is better optimised which allows it to cope better with the decreased SNR in the $b=2000$ shell. Figure 5 shows how these errors are spatially distributed in the brain. As expected, these errors are largest at the edges of the brain, where the scalings have the largest effect.

The results from simulation corroborate with our findings on real data. Figure 6 shows that data corrected by the two methods for registration to $b=0$ overscaled the images, causing them to overlap with the $b=0$ outlines. This effect is particularly noticeable for the $b=2000$ shell, where overlaps of more than two pixels are clear, in agreement with our findings on simulated data.

These results are important in the context of techniques that use DW-MR data. Data is most commonly acquired at $b=1000$, and our results indicate we can expect errors of more than 0.5 pixels in such images if they are corrected using registration to $b=0$. These are enough to cause anatomical misalignment in regions of partial volume, such as the boundaries between grey matter and CSF which will compromise any information on microstructure obtained from such data. Our results demonstrate this effect will be even more severe for data acquired at $b=2000$, which is becoming more common with the increasing popularity of high angular resolution (HARDI) techniques.

Future work will focus on further development of the framework. A more realistic model of diffusion could be used, such as NODDI [1], to prevent the need to fit multiple diffusion tensors. Currently a single T1 and T2 value is used for each tissue type, which could be replaced by spatial maps which will allow for variations within tissue types. The inclusion of spatially varying EC gradients will allow for higher order effects to be modelled, allowing us to model artefacts at much higher b-values.

Using the simulation framework, we can quantitatively assess the effectiveness of artefact correction schemes. In demonstrating the framework's application to ECs, we have shown that one of the most commonly used correction techniques introduces a systematic error that is significant enough to undermine any analysis performed on data corrected using this scheme. The framework is flexible and allows for simulation of the full range of artefacts found in DW-MR, including motion, susceptibility and B_0 inhomogeneities. We hope that this framework will become a key aspect of the validation of any post-processing schemes, which will allow users to make decisions on their choice of processing techniques that are informed by objective, quantitative evidence.

Acknowledgements. MG is supported by the EPSRC (EP/L504889/1). MG and HZ are supported by the Royal Society International Exchange Scheme with China. HZ is additionally supported by the EPSRC (EP/L022680/1) and the MRC (MR/L011530/1). ID is supported by the Leverhulme Trust.

References

1. Zhang, H., Schneider, T., Wheeler-Kingshott, C.A., Alexander, D.C.: NODDI: practical in vivo neurite orientation dispersion and density imaging of the human brain. NeuroImage **61**(4), 1000–1016 (2012)
2. Tournier, J., Calamante, F., Gadian, D.G., Connelly, A., et al.: Direct estimation of the fiber orientation density function from diffusion-weighted MRI data using spherical deconvolution. NeuroImage **23**(3), 1176–1185 (2004)
3. Le Bihan, D., Poupon, C., Amadon, A., Lethimonnier, F.: Artifacts and pitfalls in diffusion MRI. J. Magn. Reson. Imaging **24**(3), 478–488 (2006)
4. Oguz, I., Farzinfar, M., Matsui, F., Budin, F., Liu, Z., Gerig, G., Johnson, H.J., Styner, M.: DTIPrep: quality control of diffusion-weighted images. Front. neuroinformatics. **8**, 1–11 (2014)
5. Jenkinson, M., Smith, S.: A global optimisation method for robust affine registration of brain images. Med. Image Anal. **5**(2), 143–156 (2001)
6. Andersson, J.L.R., Skare, S., Ashburner, J.: How to correct susceptibility distortions in spin-echo echo-planar images: application to diffusion tensor imaging. Neuroimage **20**(2), 870–888 (2003)
7. Mangin, J.-F., Poupon, C., Clark, C., Le Bihan, D., Bloch, I.: Distortion correction and robust tensor estimation for MR diffusion imaging. Med. Image Anal. **6**(3), 191–198 (2002)
8. Zhuang, J., LU, Z.-L., Vidal, C.B., Damasio, H.: Correction of eddy current distortions in high angular resolution diffusion imaging. J. Magn. Reson. Imaging **37**(6), 1460–1467 (2013)

9. Jezzard, P., Barnett, A.S., Pierpaoli, C.: Characterization of and correction for eddy current artifacts in echo planar diffusion imaging. Magn. Reson. Med. **39**(5), 801–812 (1998)
10. Kwan, R.K.-S., Evans, A.C., Pike, G.B.: MRI simulation-based evaluation of image-processing and classification methods. IEEE Trans. Med. Imaging **18**(11), 1085–1097 (1999)
11. Drobnjak, I., Gavaghan, D., Süli, E., Pitt-Francis, J., Jenkinson, M.: Development of a functional magnetic resonance imaging simulator for modeling realistic rigid-body motion artifacts. Magn. Reson. Med. **56**(2), 364–380 (2006)
12. Neher, P.F., Laun, F.B., Stieltjes, B., Maier-Hein, K.H.: Fiberfox: Facilitating the creation of realistic white matter software phantoms. Magn. Reson. Med. **72**(5), 1460–1470 (2013)
13. Bastin, M.E.: Correction of eddy current induced artefacts in MR diffusion iterative cross-correlation. Magn. Reson. Imaging **17**(7), 1011–1024 (1998)
14. Nunes, R.G., Drobnjak, I., Clare, S., Jezzard, P., Jenkinson, M.: Performance of single spin-echo and doubly refocused diffusion-weighted sequences in the presence of eddy current fields with multiple components. Magn. Reson. Imaging **29**(5), 659–667 (2011)
15. Van Essen, D.C., Ugurbil, K., et al.: The human connectome project: a data acquisition perspective. Neuroimage **62**(4), 2222–2231 (2012)
16. Zhang, Y., Brady, M., Smith, S.: Segmentation of brain MR images through a hidden markov random field model and the expectation-maximization algorithm. IEEE Trans. Med. Imaging **20**(1), 45–57 (2001)
17. Basser, P.J., Mattiello, J., LeBihan, D.: Estimation of the effective self-diffusion tensor from the NMR spin echo. J. Magn. Reson. Imaging **103**, 247–254 (1994)
18. Drobnjak, I., Pell, G.S., Jenkinson, M.: Simulating the effects of time-varying magnetic fields with a realistic simulated scanner. Magn. Reson. Imaging **28**(7), 1014–1021 (2010)

Towards a Quantified Network Portrait
of a Population

Birkan Tunç[1]([✉]), Varsha Shankar[1], Drew Parker[1],
Robert T. Schultz[2,3], and Ragini Verma[1]

[1] Center for Biomedical Image Computing and Analytics,
University of Pennsylvania, Philadelphia, USA
`Birkan.Tunc@uphs.upenn.edu`
[2] Center for Autism Research, Children's Hospital of Philadelphia,
Philadelphia, USA
[3] Departments of Pediatrics and Psychiatry, University of Pennsylvania,
Philadelphia, USA

Abstract. Computational network analysis has enabled researchers to investigate patterns of interactions between anatomical regions of the brain. Identification of subnetworks of the human connectome can reveal how the network manages an interplay of the seemingly competing principles of functional segregation and integration. Despite the study of subnetworks of the human structural connectome by various groups, the level of expression of these subnetworks in each subject remains for the most part largely unexplored. Thus, there is a need for methods that can extract common subnetworks that together render a network portrait of a sample and facilitate analysis of the same, such as group comparisons based on the expression of the subnetworks in each subject. In this paper, we propose a framework for quantifying the subject-specific expression of subnetworks. Our framework consists of two parts, namely subnetwork detection and reconstructive projection onto subnetworks. The first part identifies subnetworks of the connectome using multi-view spectral clustering. The second part quantifies subject specific manifestations of these subnetworks by nonnegative matrix decomposition. Positivity constraint is imposed to treat each subnetwork as a structure depicting the connectivity between specific anatomical regions. We have assessed the applicability of the framework by delineating a network portrait of a clinical sample consisting of children affected by autism spectrum disorder (ASD), and a matched group of typically developing controls (TDCs). Subsequent statistical analysis on the intra- and inter-subnetwork connections, revealed decreased connectivity in ASD group between regions of social cognition, executive functions, and emotion processing.

Keywords: Subnetwork · Meso-scale · Group difference · ASD

1 Introduction

Identifying patterns of structural and functional connectivity in the human brain aids in the understanding of the neural substrates of the mind, its cognitive computations and its outward expressions in behavior [1]. Hence, research on the human connectome,

© Springer International Publishing Switzerland 2015
S. Ourselin et al. (Eds.): IPMI 2015, LNCS 9123, pp. 650–661, 2015.
DOI: 10.1007/978-3-319-19992-4_51

with a goal of identifying interpretable motifs of interactions between anatomical regions has drawn extensive attention in the neuroscience community. Methodologies developed for computational network analysis [2] have enabled researchers to investigate the overall communication design of the human brain by defining networks over a set of anatomical regions and their connections. This was established by advances in in vivo imaging techniques such as functional MRI and diffusion MRI, in conjunction with improvement in tools depicting connectivity between anatomical regions such as tractography [3].

While the overall attention directed to network analysis has increased at every level of study [4–6], studies performed at meso-scale currently form the main line of investigation. Meso-scale structures refer to grouping of anatomical regions based on their distinctive connectivity patterns. In brain networks, the identification of meso-scale structures can reveal how the network manages an interplay of seemingly competing principles of functional segregation and integration [7], thereby how specific communication pathways between set of regions contribute to behavior. One of the best known examples of a meso-scale structure is a module [8]. In the context of this paper, we adopt the term *subnetwork* instead of module since it has a broader scope that encompasses any cluster of anatomical regions with a distinctive connectivity pattern. Henceforth, the term *meso-scale architecture* will refer to decomposition of connectome into subnetworks, rendering a *network portrait* of a subject or a sample.

Although the extraction of subnetworks of the human connectome has been studied by various groups [6, 7, 9, 10], subsequent studies on identified subnetworks suffer from a common methodical deficiency. That is, the subnetworks are determined with the goal of architectural characterization i.e. characterizing the overall aggregation/segregation of regions. Other than a few exceptions [4, 11], the expression of these subnetworks in each subject followed by their quantification and subsequent comparison, remains for the most part largely unexplored. Thus, there is a need for methods that can extract the meso-scale architecture of a sample and facilitate analysis of the same, such as group comparisons based on the magnitude of expression of subnetworks in subjects.

In this paper, we propose a framework for quantifying the subject-specific expression of subnetworks, by decomposing connectomes into a basis set that is explicitly defined by these subnetworks. This is an important advancement since the proposed framework not only extracts subnetworks, but also quantifies their presence in a subject, enabling subsequent statistical comparison of individuals and different groups of individuals (e.g., cases *vs.* controls). Similar approaches have been explored in [4, 11], with critical differences in the way subnetworks were extracted and defined. In [11], the authors extracted subnetworks that corresponded to the most dominant sets of connections that were not spatially/anatomically correlated. This approach is useful for identifying important connections, but does not lend itself well to identify how anatomical regions contribute to function by their segregation and integration. This was improved in [4] where a subnetwork (or hub as the authors refer to it) consists of a set of anatomical regions and their intra-connections. However, subnetworks are not necessarily defined by sparse sets of regions and a thresholding is required to determine the final membership of regions to subnetworks.

Our framework separates the stage of subnetwork identification from the stage of quantification of their expression in each subject. Hence, subnetworks that are extracted by different approaches such as community detection [8] or clustering [10] can be incorporated into our framework, making it a generic methodology for network analysis. The result is a quantified network portrait of a sample that renders a comprehensive low dimensional representation that is common to each subject, facilitating population studies. Additionally, subnetworks and their corresponding weights are estimated under non-negativity constraints, leading to easily interpretable results since each subnetwork is a connectivity matrix on its own.

We assessed the applicability of this framework by first identifying subnetworks in a clinical sample consisting of children affected by autism spectrum disorder (ASD), and a matched group of typically developing controls (TDCs). The coefficients that quantify the expression of these subnetworks in each subject were estimated. Subsequent statistical analysis on these coefficients revealed group differences between TDC and ASD groups, in terms of differing connectivity patterns.

2 Method and Materials

The proposed methodology consists of two parts, namely subnetwork detection and reconstructive projection onto subnetworks. The first part identifies subnetworks of the connectome by assigning anatomical regions into different clusters based on their connectivity. We use multi-view spectral clustering [12] to extract a meso-scale architecture that is common to all subjects of a group. This facilitates a decomposition of the connectome into common subnetworks. The second part quantifies subject specific manifestations of these subnetworks. This is achieved by nonnegative matrix decomposition [13] to calculate the strength of expression of each subnetwork. Positivity constraint is imposed to get nonnegative components and coefficients so that each subnetwork is a connectivity matrix on its own. This enables us to treat each subnetwork as a structure depicting the connectivity between specific anatomical regions. The output is a subject specific vector of coefficients corresponding to weights of identified subnetworks in this subject (depicting both intra- and inter-connectivity). These coefficients, inherently, can be used for subsequent statistical analyses such as group differences.

2.1 Multi Subject Subnetwork Detection

Subnetwork detection in the human connectome aims at finding grouping of anatomical regions depicting the meso-scale architecture of the brain [4]. Each group consists of several regions that are densely connected to each other and sparsely connected to regions outside their group. Several methods have been proposed to extract subnetworks in the human connectome either by utilizing algorithms specifically developed for complex network analysis such as modularity maximization [8] or by using domain general clustering algorithms such as spectral clustering [10]. Recently, a few approaches have been also proposed to extract structures that are common to a group of subjects [10, 14, 15]. In this work, we adapt multi-view spectral clustering approach [12] that identifies both common clusters and subject-level variations, to extract subnetworks from a sample.

The classical spectral clustering for a single subject starts with the construction of the normalized (or un-normalized) Laplacian (L) of the connectivity (adjacency) matrix A of the subject. A is a symmetric matrix where the element A_{ij} is the connectivity between the regions i and j. Then, a simple clustering technique such as k-means is used on the eigenvectors (U) corresponding to the smallest k eigenvalues of L to determine groupings of nodes. This can be formulated as the following minimization problem:

$$\min_U tr(U^T L U), \text{ subject to } U^T U = I. \tag{1}$$

Solution of (1) is to choose the aforementioned eigenvectors of L. The centroid based co-regularization approach as proposed by Kumar et al. [12] formulates the problem of finding a common architecture among multiple subjects, by minimizing the disagreement between subject specific subnetworks and the common subnetworks. Similar to the formulation of spectral clustering, we have the following minimization problem:

$$\min_{U_1,\dots,U_N,U_c} \sum_{s=1}^{N} tr(U_s^T L_s U_s) - \sum_{s=1}^{N} \lambda_s tr(U_s U_s^T U_c U_c^T), \tag{2}$$

where the centroid eigenvector matrix U_c encodes the common set of subnetworks. Eigenvector matrices U_s correspond to individual subnetworks of subjects ($s = 1\dots N$). λ_s's are the weights of each regularization term. Once this problem is solved for U_c, k-means clustering is applied on U_c to get the common k subnetworks. The solution is obtained by a two-step iterative scheme after initializing U_c: (a) solve for U_s by fixing U_c and (b) solve for U_c by fixing U_s. This is repeated until convergence is achieved for U_c. Given U_c, U_s are determined by solving

$$\min_{U_1,\dots,U_N} \sum_{s=1}^{N} tr(U_s^T (L_s - \lambda_s U_c U_c^T) U_s). \tag{3}$$

This is equivalent to calculating eigenvectors corresponding to the smallest k eigenvalues of the modified Laplacian $\tilde{L}_s = L_s - \lambda_s U_c U_c^T$. Then by fixing U_s, U_c is determined by solving

$$\max_{U_c} \sum_{s=1}^{N} \lambda_s tr(U_s U_s^T U_c U_c^T), \tag{4}$$

that is again equivalent to finding the eigenvectors corresponding to the largest k eigenvalues of $\sum_{s=1}^{N} \lambda_s U_s U_s^T$.

2.2   Reconstructive Projection onto Subnetworks

Subnetwork detection determines membership of each anatomical region to a specific subnetwork. Based on these memberships, a connectivity matrix of a subject can be decomposed into blocks (after reordering rows and columns), each corresponding to connections in a subnetwork or between two subnetworks. This is illustrated in Fig. 1. The block structure of a connectivity matrix, as illustrated in Fig. 1, naturally defines a generative model for the multiple subject case: for each block we define a common basis (M_{ij}) that includes connections in a subnetwork or between two subnetworks, and subject specific coefficients (α_{ij}^s).

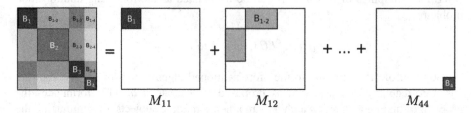

$$M_{11} \qquad\qquad M_{12} \qquad\qquad M_{44}$$

Fig. 1. Decomposition of a connectivity matrix into blocks corresponding to connections in a single subnetwork (B_1, B_2, B_3, B_4) or between two subnetworks $(B_{1-2}, B_{1-3}, \dots)$. Each matrix M_{ij} includes zeros everywhere except at the region corresponding to the encoded block. Note that in case of a single subject, this decomposition defines an exact reconstruction of the original connectivity matrix.

Then the connectivity matrix A^s of a subject s is assumed to be generated as

$$A^s = \alpha_{11}^s M_{11} + \alpha_{12}^s M_{12} + \dots + \alpha_{22}^s M_{22} + \dots + \alpha_{kk}^s M_{kk}, \qquad (5)$$

where M_{ij} (corresponding to a block in Fig. 1) defines a common basis of connections in the subnetwork i (if $i = j$) or between subnetworks i and j (if $i \neq j$), including zeros everywhere except at the region corresponding to the connections encoded by M_{ij}. The coefficients α_{ij}^s are subject specific weights. The estimation of each M_{ij} can be done independently since they do not share any connection. Thus, each basis component and corresponding coefficients are determined by solving

$$\min_{m,p} f(m,p) = \left\| X - mp^T \right\|_F^2, \quad \text{subject to} \quad m > 0, p > 0 \qquad (6)$$

where the sth column of matrix X has the elements of matrix A^s in the block corresponding to M_{ij}. m is a vector including only non-zero elements of M_{ij}. p is a vector including the coefficient α_{ij}^s as its sth element. This is solved independently for each M_{ij} by a projected gradient descent algorithm for nonnegative matrix factorization [13]. The solution is found iteratively by updating the current estimate of parameters $\theta^t \equiv (m^t, p^t)$ as

$$\theta^{t+1} = P[\theta^t - \beta^t \nabla_\theta f(\theta^t)], \qquad (7)$$

$$P[x] \underline{\underline{\mathrm{def}}} \begin{cases} x & if \ l < x < u, \\ u & if \ x \geq u, \\ l & if \ x \leq l, \end{cases} \tag{8}$$

$$\nabla_\theta f \underline{\underline{\mathrm{def}}} \left((mp^T - X)p, m^T(mp^T - X) \right). \tag{9}$$

The step size parameter β^t is selected so that the following inequality is satisfied.

$$f(\theta^{t+1}) - f(\theta^t) \leq \sigma \nabla_\theta f(\theta^t)^T (\theta^{t+1} - \theta^t), \tag{10}$$

where σ is any value between $0 - 1$. The projection function $P[x]$ projects the value of x into the range defined by the lower and upper bounds l, u.

2.3 Population Studies

The coefficients of generative model (5), α_{ij}^s, are subject-specific and encode the overall strength of connections in a subnetwork or between subnetworks. These coefficients that provide a comprehensive low dimensional representation of each subject facilitate population studies. Similar to edge-wise comparison of groups [5], we can compare two groups, such as controls vs. Patients, on a subnetwork-wise basis i.e. we can identify which group has higher/lower expression of a subnetwork or connections of an inter-subnetwork communication. This approach also increases statistical power by lowering the dimensionality of the comparison. Instead of comparing each edge individually, we divide the connectome into subnetworks and compare only coefficients that depict the overall communication pattern of these subnetworks, reducing the problem of multiple comparisons.

2.4 Dataset

Our clinical sample consists of 172 male participants, including 97 children (age: 12.6 ± 2.9 years) affected by autism spectrum disorder (ASD), and a matched group of typically developing controls (TDCs) (age: 12.2 ± 3.3 years). Participants with a community diagnosis of an ASD were recruited in part through autismMatch (https://autismmatch.org), and diagnoses were confirmed using diagnostic instruments and expert consensus clinical judgment by two independent psychologists following Collaborative Programs of Excellence in Autism (CPEA) diagnostic guidelines.

Diffusion tensor imaging was acquired in two epochs on the same scanner with different scanner parameters. In the first set, DTI was acquired using a mono-polar+ sequence, with repetition time (TR)/echo time (TE) = 11000/75 ms, resolution = $2 \times 2 \times 2$ mm, collecting 30 directions with b-value = 1000 s/mm2 and 1 b = 0 image on a Siemens Verio 3T scanner. In the second epoch, DTI TR/TE was 11000/76 ms using a monopolar sequence. DTI measures of FA and MD were verified not to vary between scans within the two epochs. T1-weighted (TR/TE = 1900/2.54) MRI images with resolution 0.4 × 0.4 × 0.9 mm were also acquired. The T1 image of each subject was segmented into 95 anatomical regions of interest (ROIs) of the Desikan atlas [16] using Freesurfer [17]. FSL's bedpostx was fit to each voxel in the DTI image, and FSL's probtrackx was used to perform tractography seeded from each of the 95 ROIs and going to the others [18]. A 95 × 95 connectivity matrix A was created for each subject, where $A_{ij} = (S_{ij}/S_i) \cdot R_i$. In this formula, S_{ij} represents the number of fibers connecting seed region i to target j, and S_i represents the total number of fibers emanating from region i. R_i, the surface area of region i, accounts for the different sizes of the 95 ROIs.

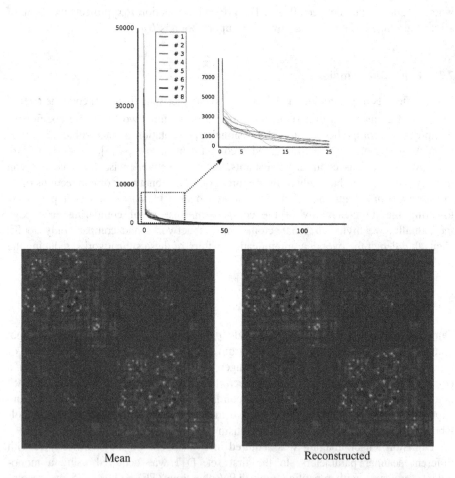

Mean   Reconstructed

Fig. 2. Top: Singular values of X in Eq. (6), for eight subnetworks. For each subnetwork, we have one clearly dominant singular value. Bottom left: Mean connectivity matrix of our clinical sample. Bottom right: Reconstructed mean connectivity matrix using (5). Similarity between the two is easily noticeable, illustrating the reliability of reconstruction.

3   Results

Here, we first review our projection approach introduced in Sect. 2.2. Then, experimental results for group comparison will be presented. In the generative model (5), we assume a single common basis M_{ij} for each block of the connectivity matrix (see Fig. 1). Estimating M_{ij} in (6) corresponds to finding a single basis for connections that are included in M_{ij}. The feasibility of this assumption can be easily validated by observing singular values[1] of the matrix X in (6). This is illustrated in Fig. 2 (top) where our dataset was used to identify eight common subnetworks. The matrix X for each subnetwork has only one dominant singular value and the remaining singular values diminish quickly. One expects to have even clearer dominance as the number of subnetworks increases, since with increasing number of subnetworks, variation of connection strength in each subnetwork tends to decrease. In Fig. 2 (bottom left and right), the connectivity matrix that was reconstructed by the estimated components M_{ij} and mean coefficients α_{ij}^s is compared to the average connectivity matrix of our dataset. Overall agreement between two matrices, thereby the quality of reconstruction is clear.

In order to use our framework for group comparisons, we first extracted the meso-scale architecture of the sample. We created several network portraits consisting of different numbers of subnetworks. The actual choice of the number depends on the level of detail required for the hypothesis being investigated. Figure 3 illustrates two network portraits consisting of 8 and 12 subnetworks that are common to all subjects, to provide a representation of how subnetworks are formed at different resolutions. Statistical analysis was performed on the coefficients α_{ij}^s that describe the expression of these subnetworks in each of the subjects. Figure 4 shows sets of connections that differ significantly between TDC and ASD groups ($p < 0.01$), when the 12-subnetwork portrait was used to describe the population. For the remainder of the paper where we discuss extracted subnetworks, we refer to the subnetworks of the 12-subnetwork portrait, unless otherwise stated.

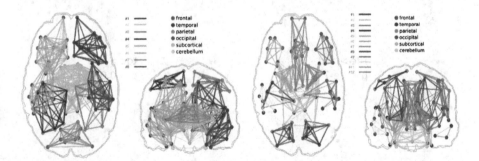

Fig. 3. Common meso-scale architectures of our clinical sample, depicting network portraits of 8 (left) and 12 (right) subnetworks. Only intra-subnetwork connections are displayed (Color figure online).

---

[1] Note that X is not a square matrix; hence, we cannot speak of its eigenvalues.

Overall symmetry of the meso-scale architectures in Fig. 3 conforms to previously published findings on the structural core of human connectome [9]. Meso-scale architectures (both for 8 and 12 subnetworks) define spatially correlated subnetworks, each characterized mostly by local (short-range) connections. This is consistent with the fact that cortical communication in the human brain is dominantly characterized by short-range connections [19]. Inter-hemispheric connections (Subnetworks #2 and #12) exist between bilateral temporal lobes and sub-cortical regions (Subnetwork #2), or within frontal lobe (Subnetwork #12). We should note that the meso-scale architectures illustrated in Fig. 3 only shows intra-subnetwork connections. More inter-hemispheric connections appear when statistically analyzing the inter-subnetwork communication.

Four sets of connections related to inter-subnetwork communication were found to be significantly lower in ASD group (Fig. 4). Lower structural connectivity supports the underconnectivity hypothesis for ASD [20]. Specifically, connections related to the regions involved in social cognition such as amygdala, insula, caudate (Subnetworks #6 and #7) [21] and regions involved in executive functions as well as social cognition such as left orbitofrontal cortex and left middle frontal cortex (Subnetwork #5) [20], [22] were found to be lower in the ASD group. In addition, connections related to the regions involved in emotion processing such as right superior temporal and supra-marginal cortex (Subnetwork #3) [23] were significantly lower in the ASD group. Accordingly, identified group differences revealed decreased connectivity

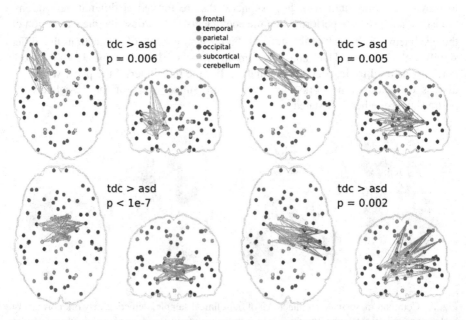

Fig. 4. Connections with significant (p < 0.01) group differences between TDC and ASD samples, for the 12 subnetwork case. Colors of edges correspond to the subnetworks that they are part of (see Fig. 3). They are all two-colored since they are connections between two subnetworks. Connections that are significantly different are between subnetworks #3 (brown), #5 (blue), #6 (green), and #7 (pink) (Color figure online).

between regions of social cognition, executive functions, and emotion processing, which is very consistent with common conceptualization of ASD [24].

4 Conclusion

We have developed a framework for creating a quantified network portrait of a population. Our framework quantifies the subject-specific expression of subnetworks, by decomposing connectomes into a basis set that is explicitly defined by these subnetworks. The approach introduced here separates the subnetwork extraction that is usually performed with community detection or clustering methods from the stage of quantification of identified subnetworks in each subject. Hence, subnetworks that are extracted by different approaches can be incorporated. Our framework provides a novel way of identifying subnetworks, and subsequent analysis both at the population and subject level. Subject level coefficients can be correlated with clinical measures to identify the imaging correlates of clinical manifestations.

The resulting meso-scale architecture of the sample renders a comprehensive low dimensional representation that is common to each subject, facilitating population studies. This approach also increases statistical power since we divide the connectome into subnetworks and compare only coefficients that depict the overall communication pattern of these subnetworks, instead of comparing each edge individually, alleviating the problem of multiple comparisons.

The applicability of the framework was assessed on a clinical sample consisting of children affected by ASD and a matched group of TDCs. The extracted meso-scale architecture of the sample was consistent with previously published findings on the structural core of human connectome. Subsequent statistical analysis on the intra- and inter-subnetwork connections revealed decreased connectivity between regions of social cognition, executive functions, and emotion processing. Overall, the results support the underconnectivity hypothesis for ASD.

Group differences at the level of meso-scale structures reveal important changes in integration/segregation of anatomical regions, which would not be possible with traditional edge-wise analyses. Our results provide insights on how overall communication between cortical clusters pertaining to different faculties such as social cognition, executive functions, and emotion changes between TDC and ASD groups.

References

1. Friston, K.: Beyond phrenology: what can neuroimaging tell us about distributed circuitry? Annu. Rev. Neurosci. **25**, 221–250 (2002)
2. Sporns, O., Chialvo, D.R., Kaiser, M., Hilgetag, C.C.: Organization, development and function of complex brain networks. Trends Cogn. Sci. **8**(9), 418–425 (2004)
3. Basser, P.J., Pajevic, S., Pierpaoli, C., Duda, J., Aldroubi, A.: In vivo fiber tractography using DT-MRI data. Magn. Reson. Med. **44**(4), 625–632 (2000)

4. Ghanbari, Y., Bloy, L., Shankar, V., Edgar, J.C., Roberts, Timothy P.L., Schultz, R., Verma, R.: Functionally driven brain networks using multi-layer graph clustering. In: Golland, P., Hata, N., Barillot, C., Hornegger, J., Howe, R. (eds.) MICCAI 2014, Part III. LNCS, vol. 8675, pp. 113–120. Springer, Heidelberg (2014)

5. Ingalhalikar, M., Smith, A., Parker, D., Satterthwaite, T.D., Elliott, M.A., Ruparel, K., Hakonarson, H., Gur, R.E., Gur, R.C., Verma, R.: Sex differences in the structural connectome of the human brain. Proc. Natl. Acad. Sci. U. S. A. 111(2), 823–828 (2014)

6. Bassett, D.S., Wymbs, N.F., Porter, M.A., Mucha, P.J., Carlson, J.M., Grafton, S.T.: Dynamic reconfiguration of human brain networks during learning. Proc. Natl. Acad. Sci. U. S. A. 108(18), 7641–7646 (2011)

7. Schwarz, A.J., Gozzi, A., Bifone, A.: Community structure and modularity in networks of correlated brain activity. Magn. Reson. Imaging 26(7), 914–920 (2008)

8. Girvan, M., Newman, M.E.J.: Community structure in social and biological networks. Proc. Natl. Acad. Sci. U. S. A. 99(12), 7821–7826 (2002)

9. Hagmann, P., Cammoun, L., Gigandet, X., Meuli, R., Honey, C.J., Wedeen, V.J., Sporns, O.: Mapping the structural core of human cerebral cortex. PLoS Biol. 6(7), e159 (2008)

10. Ozdemir, A., Mahyari, A.G., Bernat, M.E., Aviyente. S.: Multiple subject analysis of functional brain network communities through co-regularized spectral clustering. In: IEEE Engineering in Medicine and Biology Society, pp. 5992–5995 (2014)

11. Ghanbari, Y., Smith, A.R., Schultz, R.T., Verma, R.: Connectivity subnetwork learning for pathology and developmental variations. Med. Image Comput. Comput. Interv. 16(Pt 1), 90–97 (2013)

12. Kumar, A., Rai, P., Daume, H.: Co-regularized multi-view spectral clustering. In: Advances in Neural Information Processing Systems, pp. 1413–1421 (2011)

13. Lin, C.-J.: Projected gradient methods for nonnegative matrix factorization. Neural Comput. 19(10), 2756–2779 (2007)

14. Bolaños, M.E., Bernat, E.M., Aviyente, S.: Multivariate synchrony modules identified through multiple subject community detection in functional brain networks. IEEE Eng. Med. Biol. Soc. 2011, 2534–2537 (2011)

15. Chen, H., Li, K., Zhu, D., Jiang, X., Yuan, Y., Lv, P., Zhang, T., Guo, L., Shen, D., Liu, T.: Inferring group-wise consistent multimodal brain networks via multi-view spectral clustering. IEEE Trans. Med. Imaging 32(9), 1576–1586 (2013)

16. Desikan, R.S., Segonne, F., Fischl, B., Quinn, B., Dickerson, B., Blacker, D., Buckner, R., Dale, A., Maguire, R., Hyman, B., Albert, M., Killiany, R.: An automated labeling system for subdividing the human cerebral cortex on MRI scans into gyral based regions of interest. Neuroimage 31(2), 968–980 (2006)

17. Fischl, B., Sereno, M.I., Dale, A.M.: Cortical surface-based analysis. II: Inflation, flattening, and a surface-based coordinate system. Neuroimage 9(2), 195–207 (1999)

18. Behrens, T.E.J., Berg, H.J., Jbabdi, S., Rushworth, M.F.S., Woolrich, M.W.: Probabilistic diffusion tractography with multiple fibre orientations: What can we gain? Neuroimage 34(1), 144–155 (2007)

19. Markov, N.T., Ercsey-Ravasz, M., Van Essen, D.C., Knoblauch, K., Toroczkai, Z., Kennedy, H.: Cortical high-density counterstream architectures. Science 342(6158), 1238406 (2013)

20. Pelphrey, K.A., Shultz, S., Hudac, C.M., Vander Wyk, B.C.: Constraining heterogeneity: the social brain and its development in autism spectrum disorder. J. Child Psychol. Psychiatry 52(6), 631–644 (2011)

21. Adolphs, R.: The social brain: neural basis of social knowledge. Annu. Rev. Psychol. 60, 693–716 (2009)

22. Blakemore, S.-J., Choudhury, S.: Development of the adolescent brain: implications for executive function and social cognition. J. Child Psychol. Psychiatry **47**(3–4), 296–312 (2006)
23. Alaerts, K., Woolley, D.G., Steyaert, J., Di Martino, A., Swinnen, S.P., Wenderoth, N.: Underconnectivity of the superior temporal sulcus predicts emotion recognition deficits in autism. Soc. Cogn. Affect. Neurosci. **9**(10), 1589–1600 (2014)
24. Levy, S.E., Mandell, D.S., Schultz, R.T.: Autism. Lancet **374**(9701), 1627–1638 (2009)

Segmenting the Brain Surface from CT Images with Artifacts Using Dictionary Learning for Non-rigid MR-CT Registration

John A. Onofrey[1]([✉]), Lawrence H. Staib[1,2,3], and Xenophon Papademetris[1,3]

[1] Departments of Diagnostic Radiology, Yale University,
New Haven, CT 06520, USA
[2] Electrical Engineering, Yale University,
New Haven, CT 06520, USA
[3] Biomedical Engineering, Yale University,
New Haven, CT 06520, USA
{john.onofrey,lawrence.staib,xenophon.papademetris}@yale.edu

Abstract. This paper presents a dictionary learning-based method to segment the brain surface in post-surgical CT images of epilepsy patients following surgical implantation of electrodes. Using the electrodes identified in the post-implantation CT, surgeons require accurate registration with pre-implantation functional and structural MR imaging to guide surgical resection of epileptic tissue. In this work, we use a surface-based registration method to align the MR and CT brain surfaces. The key challenge here is not the registration, but rather the extraction of the cortical surface from the CT image, which includes missing parts of the skull and artifacts introduced by the electrodes. To segment the brain from these images, we propose learning a model of appearance that captures both the normal tissue and the artifacts found along this brain surface boundary. Using clinical data, we demonstrate that our method both accurately extracts the brain surface and better localizes electrodes than intensity-based rigid and non-rigid registration methods.

Keywords: Segmentation · Dictionary learning · Skull stripping · Computed-tomography · Non-rigid registration · Multi-modal · Image-guided surgery

1 Introduction

Epilepsy is a neurological disorder in which brain function is temporarily disrupted by seizures. For certain patients who do not respond favorably to medication, surgical resection of ictal tissue, *e.g.* tissue involved in the generation of the seizures, can be an effective method to reduce or eliminate seizures. As part of a diagnostic procedure, neurosurgeons sometimes perform a craniotomy and surgically implant electrodes on the brain surface (intra-cranial) and in the brain (depth) throughout regions of the brain suspected to be causing the seizures. Clinicians monitor brain activity from these electrodes to localize ictal

© Springer International Publishing Switzerland 2015
S. Ourselin et al. (Eds.): IPMI 2015, LNCS 9123, pp. 662–674, 2015.
DOI: 10.1007/978-3-319-19992-4_52

events [15]. However, before performing a resection, surgeons must determine if the electrode locations correspond to functionally eloquent brain tissue, e.g. motor, sensory, and language regions, which may be identified by pre-operative imaging, including anatomical magnetic resonance imaging (MRI) and functional imaging modalities such as functional MRI (fMRI), PET, and SPECT. Therefore, accurate localization of the electrodes with respect to this pre-operative imaging is crucial for surgical planning.

The current best method to co-register the implanted electrodes and the pre-implantation imaging involves acquisition of both an anatomical MRI and an X-ray computed tomography (CT) image after implantation. The electrodes are easily identified in the post-implantation CT images and can be interactively labeled by a trained technologist. While the post-op CT image can easily be fused with the post-op MRI using intensity-based registration methods to visualize electrodes within the post-op MRI [2] (negligible non-rigid deformations occur between the two image acquisitions), we ultimately want to visualize electrodes with respect to intra-subject, multi-modal, pre-implantation imaging in order to integrate this information into the surgical plan. However, the post-op CT image cannot easily be registered with the pre-op MRI because the surgical procedure can result in non-rigid deformations of the brain surface often larger than 1 cm [8]. Intensity-based registration of pre-op MRI and post-op CT is difficult because of (i) CT's poor soft tissue contrast lacking salient anatomical structure, (ii) missing anatomical correspondences, such as removal of the skull during surgery, and (iii) imaging artifacts and intensity inhomogeneities caused by the presence of the implanted electrodes. Therefore, the CT image is first rigidly registered to the post-op MRI, and then the post-op MRI is non-rigidly registered to the pre-op MRI image to compensate for the post-surgical deformations. While the post-op MRI also contains artifacts caused by the implanted electrodes, the excellent soft tissue contrast provided by MRI makes enough anatomical structure clearly visible that accurate non-rigid registration to the relatively high quality pre-op MRI is possible. The identified electrodes are then transformed to the pre-implantation imaging space and may be co-visualized with the multi-modal pre-implantation image studies.

Unfortunately, acquiring a post-implantation MRI presents both an inconvenience for the patient, who has electrode wires sticking out of their head, and an additional potential source of infection for the patient as they are moved about the hospital and scanner, as well as an additional expense. Thus, the post-implantation MRI is not available at all institutions. A method for accurate non-rigid registration of post-op CT to the pre-op CT is necessary and remains an open area of research. Intensity-based registration of pre-op MRI and post-op CT is difficult because the post-op CT is of poor quality due to artifacts and relatively poor soft tissue contrast. With these confounding factors, non-rigid registration was actually shown to perform worse than rigid registration in terms of electrode localization error [10]. Onofrey et al. [10] attempt to bypass this post-op MRI by building a statistical modeled of non-rigid procedure-induced deformation to directly register the post-op CT image to the pre-op MRI.

While this method successfully reduced electrode localization errors, it relies upon registration of all images to a common reference space to model the statistical deformations, which makes it complex for clinical use. In this work, we propose using a surface-based registration scheme to directly non-rigidly register the post-op CT and pre-op MRI.

The key challenge in registering the post-implantation CT and the pre-implantation MRI is not the registration itself, as numerous surface-based registration methods exist [4,11]. Instead, the extraction of the cortical surface from the CT image presents a challenge due to (i) the absence of parts of the boundary at some points, e.g. sections where the skull was removed for craniotomy; and (ii) the presence of imaging artifacts, e.g. due to implanted electrodes. Well-tested methods exist for extracting the brain surface from MRIs [14], but no tool exists yet to accurately extract the brain surface from post-implant CT images, where the appearance of the border is varied and likely non-Gaussian. To extract the brain surface from post-implantation CT images, we propose learning a sparse representation of the brain cortical surface appearance in a data-driven manner. Huang et al. [9] use a dictionary-learning framework to model textural appearance both inside and outside cardiac boundaries for intra-subject tracking of those contours in time sequence ultrasound images. In Sect. 2.2 we adopt this methodology to train two dictionaries that model the appearance of regions inside and outside the brain surface. This work differs from Huang et al. [9] in that we propose using locally oriented image patches along the surface, as opposed to image patches canonically aligned with the image axes, to provide a more invariant model of appearance relative to the surface of interest. Brown et al. [3] made use of locally oriented image patches for image matching, but our method differs in that we use the geometry of our estimated surface segmentation to orient the patches instead of using image intensity information to determine the orientation. We also train our dictionary appearance model for inter-subject segmentation by building the appearance dictionaries using a set of clinical training data, and estimate the surface differently. Section 2.3 details how we use these appearance dictionaries to classify points along the brain surface as belonging to either inside or outside the brain surface and use this information to extract the cortical surface. We then describe how we use the segmented cortical surface to non-rigidly register post-implantation CT images with pre-implantation MR images in Sect. 2.4. Figure 1 illustrates and summarizes our proposed training, segmentation, and registration framework. Finally, Sect. 3.1 presents our results demonstrating accurate segmentation of the cortical surface from post-implantation CT images. Section 3.2 then shows improved registration performance using this segmented surface to directly register post-op CT and pre-op MRI compared to intensity-based registration.

2 Methods

From a clinical database of $N = 18$ epilepsy patients at our institution, we have a set of images $\mathcal{I} = \left\{ I^1_{\mathrm{MR},i}, I^2_{\mathrm{MR},i}, I^2_{\mathrm{CT},i} | i = 1, \ldots, N \right\}$, where $I^t_{m,i}$ denotes pre-op images acquired at time $t = 1$ and post-op images acquired at time $t = 2$

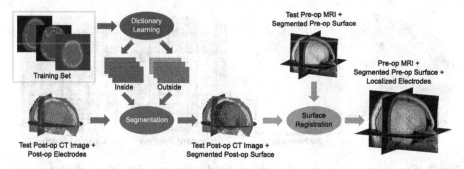

Fig. 1. Dictionary-based appearance learning and segmentation of post-surgical cortical brain surface in CT images for direct non-rigid registration of with pre-surgical MRI. We use a training set of post-implantation CT image to learn two models of image appearance, one inside the cortical surface and one outside. We then use these models to segment the cortical surface from test CT images. Using the extracted post-op surface, we perform surface-based registration with the pre-op MRI in order to co-visualize post-implantation electrodes with pre-op imaging data.

using imaging modality m for patient i. Following the current practice, for each patient we (i) create pre-op and post-op brain surfaces S_i^1 and S_i^2 from the MR images by extracting isosurfaces of the brain masks generated by using the Brain Extraction Tool (BET) [14], (ii) rigidly register $I_{\mathrm{CT},i}^2$ to $I_{\mathrm{MR},i}^2$ to produce the transformation $T_{\mathrm{CT}\to\mathrm{MR},i}$ by maximizing the normalized mutual information (NMI) similarity metric [16], and (iii) non-rigidly register $I_{\mathrm{MR},i}^2$ to $I_{\mathrm{MR},i}^1$ using a free-form deformation (FFD) [13] with 30 mm B-spline control point spacing and maximizing their NMI to produce the transformation $T_{\mathrm{MR}\rightsquigarrow\mathrm{MR},i}$. We make use of this data to train our model of brain surface appearance in post-surgical CT images.

2.1 Oriented Local Image Appearance

Let $I : \Omega_I \subset \mathbb{R}^3 \mapsto \mathbb{R}$ be the 3D image that maps points from the spatial domain Ω_I to image intensity values. We define the set of intensities in an orientable local image patch Φ centered about $\mathbf{u} \in \Omega_I$:

$$\Phi(\mathbf{u}, \sigma) = \{I(\mathbf{u} + \sigma\mathbf{R}\mathbf{t})| \quad \forall \mathbf{t} \in \Theta\}. \tag{1}$$

Here, $\mathbf{R} \in \mathbb{R}^{3\times3}$ is a rotation matrix consisting of a set of orthonormal basis vectors and Φ is a set of d image intensity values sampled at patch template points $\Theta = \{\mathbf{t}_i | \mathbf{t}_i \in \mathbb{R}^3, i = 1, \ldots, d\}$, whose physical size is controlled by a scale term $\sigma \in \mathbb{R}$. Typically, *standard* image patches are aligned with the image axes such that $\mathbf{R}$ uses the standard basis $\mathbf{R} = \mathbf{I}$, the identity matrix, and Φ consists of an isotropic grid of sample points centered about the patch origin. For example, a $5 \times 5 \times 5$ isotropic image patch Φ consists of $d = 125$ sample points Θ arranged in a grid about the patch origin.

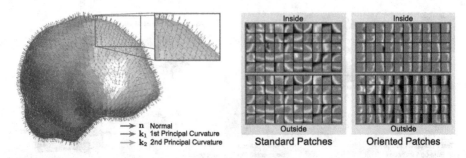

Fig. 2. Examples of local oriented image patches compared to their corresponding standard local image patches oriented along the image axes. For the surface S, the local surface normal $\mathbf{n}$ and directions of principal curvature $\mathbf{k}_1, \mathbf{k}_2$ define a local orthonormal basis by which we orient the image patches. We show patch examples from both inside and outside the cortical surface.

In this work, we use *oriented* image patches, where the orientation of the patch $\mathbf{R}$ is determined by the data. Since we are interested in building a model of image appearance both inside and outside the brain surface, we orient image patches according to local surface geometry. For each point on the surface of interest $\mathbf{u} \in S$, we compute the local surface normal $\mathbf{n} \in \mathbb{R}^3$ and the directions of principal curvature $\mathbf{k}_1, \mathbf{k}_2 \in \mathbb{R}^3$ [6]. These normalized vectors form an orthonormal basis $\mathbf{R} = [\mathbf{n}|\mathbf{k}_1|\mathbf{k}_2]$ with which we orient the patch $\Phi(\mathbf{u})$ in (1). Figure 2 provides an illustrative comparison between standard and oriented patches at corresponding points along a surface $\mathbf{u} \in S$. By orienting the patches in this manner, the texture patterns in our patches exhibit greater invariance to changes in location along the surface S.

2.2   Training the Cortical Surface Appearance Model

To learn our model of brain boundary appearance, we first map the segmented post-op brain surface to the post-op CT image space, $S_i^{2'} = T_{\mathrm{CT} \to \mathrm{MR},i}^{-1} \circ S_i^2$, where $\circ$ is the transformation operator. We then create a sparse representation model $\mathbf{D}_{\mathrm{in}}$ (dictionary) of the intensities inside of the brain and a model $\mathbf{D}_{\mathrm{out}}$ of the region just outside the brain [9]. These dictionaries will capture the varieties of textural appearance found near the brain surface boundary. We create these models by extracting a training set of overlapping local image patches inside, $\Phi_{\mathrm{in}}(\mathbf{u} - \alpha\mathbf{n})$, and outside, $\Phi_{\mathrm{out}}(\mathbf{u} + \alpha\mathbf{n})$, points on the surface $\mathbf{u} \in S_i^{2'}$, where $\mathbf{n}$ is the outward facing local surface normal and $0 < \alpha \leq 3.0\mathrm{mm}$ defines a narrow band region. As in Sect. 2.1, we use the local surface geometry at $\mathbf{u}$ to orient the image patches.

For each appearance class $c = \{\mathrm{in}, \mathrm{out}\}$, we create appearance vectors $\mathbf{p}_c \in \mathbb{R}^d$ for each image patch by concatenating the patch values from the set Φ_c, where d is the sample dimensionality determined by the chosen patch sampling template Θ in Sect. 2.1, and normalize $\mathbf{p}_c$ to have unit length. Then, we model the distribution of $\mathbf{p}_c$'s from all N training images using an overcomplete dictionary

$\mathbf{D}_c \in \mathbb{R}^{d \times n}$ such that $\mathbf{p}_c \approx \mathbf{D}_c \boldsymbol{\gamma}$ [1]. Here, n is the number of dictionary atoms and $\boldsymbol{\gamma}$ is the sparse dictionary weighting coefficients. To reconstruct a given appearance sample $\mathbf{p}$ (normalized to have unit length) from the dictionary with a given target sparsity constraint Γ_0, we solve the sparse coding problem

$$\min_{\boldsymbol{\gamma}} \|\mathbf{p} - \mathbf{D}\boldsymbol{\gamma}\|_2^2 \text{ s.t. } \|\boldsymbol{\gamma}\|_0 \leq \Gamma_0, \tag{2}$$

using an orthogonal matching pursuit (OMP) algorithm [12]. Next, we define the residual error

$$R_c(\mathbf{p}) = \|\mathbf{p} - \mathbf{D}_c \boldsymbol{\gamma}\|_2 \tag{3}$$

for both the inside and outside region classes. Using normalized appearance vectors, $0 \leq R_c(\mathbf{p}) \leq 1$, where values of 0 correspond to perfect signal reconstruction (strong membership to class c) and values of 1 indicate $\mathbf{p}$ could not be reconstructed by $\mathbf{D}_c$ (poor membership to class c). Intuitively, $R_{in}(\mathbf{p}) < R_{out}(\mathbf{p})$ for points inside the cortical surface boundary. In contrast to Huang et al. [9]'s multi-scale modeling where multi-scale data is concatenated into appearance vectors, we perform this sampling and training procedure individually for each level $k = 1, \ldots, K$ in a multi-resolution Gaussian image pyramid, which means that we train K dictionary pairs $\{\mathbf{D}_{in}^k, \mathbf{D}_{out}^k\}$.

2.3   Segmenting the Cortical Surface in Post-implantation CT Images

Given a new pair of pre-implantation MRI and post-implantation CT test images not in the training set $I_{MR}^1, I_{CT}^2 \notin \mathcal{I}$, we perform an initial brain surface segmentation estimate $\hat{S}$ using an intensity-based rigid registration of I_{MR}^1 and I_{CT}^2 and transforming the segmented MR surface S^1 to post-op imaging space, i.e. $\hat{S} = T_{MR \to CT} \circ S^1$. For a point on the estimated surface $\mathbf{u} \in \hat{S}$, we extract the oriented local image patch $\Phi(\mathbf{u})$ to create the appearance vector $\mathbf{p}$, and then compute the difference of the appearance model residuals from (3) such that

$$D(\mathbf{p}) = R_{out}(\mathbf{p}) - R_{in}(\mathbf{p}). \tag{4}$$

Intuitively, if $\mathbf{u}$ lies within the true boundary of the cortical surface in the CT image then $D(\mathbf{p}) > 0$, and if $\mathbf{u}$ is outside the true boundary then $D(\mathbf{p}) < 0$. Thus, the cortical surface boundary is located at the point $\mathbf{u}$ where $D(\mathbf{p}) = 0$. We therefore seek the surface that minimizes the objective function

$$\hat{S} = \min_S \int_S \|D\|_2 dS. \tag{5}$$

To solve this optimization problem, we proceed to segment the brain from I_{CT}^2 by iteratively updating the surface in a greedy manner. At each iteration t, our surface update follows

$$\mathbf{u}_{t+1} = \mathbf{u}_t + \sigma D(\mathbf{p}_t)\mathbf{n}_t + \mathbf{r}_t, \quad \forall \mathbf{u}_t \in \hat{S}_t \tag{6}$$

where $\sigma \in \mathbb{R}_{>0}$ is a scale term determined by the image resolution, and $\mathbf{r}_t$ is a regularization update vector that maintains surface smoothness with respect to the local surface curvature as done by BET [14]. As the surface estimate approaches the true boundary of the cortical surface, $\|\sigma D(\mathbf{p_t})\mathbf{n_t}\|$ tends to zero, and the algorithm converges. Because $-1 \leq D(\mathbf{p}) \leq 1$ from (3), this update in the direction of the surface normal $\mathbf{n}_t$ can have a maximum magnitude σ. We update the surface estimate starting at the lowest level of resolution in our multi-resolution Gaussian image pyramid representation of I^2_{CT} and proceed for a fixed number of iterations before switching to the next higher resolution level. Proceeding in this multi-resolution manner, the algorithm first updates the surface with large changes to the surface and then successively refines the results at high levels of resolution until converging.

2.4   Non-rigid MR-CT Registration

Once we have a final estimate of the cortical brain surface $\hat{S}$ in the post-implantation CT image I^2_{CT} , we then seek to non-rigidly register this image to the pre-implantation MR image I^1_{MR} with previously segmented surface S^1. To do so, we use a non-rigid robust point matching (RPM) algorithm [4,11] that uses a free-form deformation (FFD) model for surface-based registration of $\hat{S}$ to S^1. We choose RPM for this task because the RPM metric allows for fuzzy correspondences between points on the two surfaces and can accommodate outlier points, which makes the algorithm robust to small segmentation errors that could exist in the reference and transform surfaces. The RPM registration algorithm results in a transformation $T_{\mathrm{CT}\rightsquigarrow\mathrm{MR}}$ with which we can then directly warp the post-implantation CT image data back to the pre-op MR image space $I_{\mathrm{CT}\rightsquigarrow\mathrm{MR}} = T_{\mathrm{CT}\rightsquigarrow\mathrm{MR}} \circ I^2_{\mathrm{CT}}$.

3   Results

To validate our proposed approach, we selected 18 patients with pre-op and post-op MR images, and post-op CT images from a clinical database of epilepsy patients who had electrodes surgically implanted. A trained technician segmented the pre-op and post-op MR brain masks using BET [14], and performed manual corrections, if necessary, according to our clinical protocol. For computational efficiency, we resampled all images to have $1\mathrm{mm}^3$ isotropic resolution. All images had different volume dimensions. In this work, we parameterized each of our surfaces S as a triangulated mesh. We performed 6-fold cross-validation, where we partitioned the 18 datasets into 6 subsets of $N = 15$ subjects for training and 3 subjects for testing. We quantitatively evaluated segmentation accuracy between two surface points A and B using the following metrics: (i) Dice overlap

$$\mathrm{DICE}(A, B) = \frac{2V_A \cap V_B}{V_A + V_B},$$

where V_S is the volume enclosed by surface S; (*ii*) Hausdorff Distance

$$\text{HD}(A, B) = \max\left\{\max_{\mathbf{a}\in A} d(\mathbf{a}, B), \max_{\mathbf{b}\in B} d(\mathbf{b}, A)\right\};$$

and (*iii*) Mean Absolute Distance

$$\text{MAD}(A, B) = \frac{1}{2}\left\{\frac{1}{N_A}\sum_{\mathbf{a}\in A} d(\mathbf{a}, B) + \frac{1}{N_B}\sum_{\mathbf{b}\in B} d(\mathbf{b}, A)\right\},$$

where $d(\mathbf{a}, B) = \min_{\mathbf{b}\in B}\|\mathbf{b} - \mathbf{a}\|_2$. Additionally, we specifically quantified segmentation errors at the identified electrode locations $\mathbf{x}_e \in E \subset \Omega_I$. We define the Mean Electrode to Surface Distance

$$\text{MESD}(E, S) = \frac{1}{N_E}\sum_{\mathbf{x}_e\in E} d(\mathbf{x}_e, S)$$

to be a measure of the distribution of electrode distances from the given surface S. We expect implanted intra-cranial cortical electrodes to lie on the surface of the brain, thus the MESD metric quantifies how close the electrodes are to the surface S. High MESD values indicate that the distribution of electrodes is far from the surface, which means they could appear as floating above the surface or sunk within. To calculate MESD, we extracted only the largest 8×8 electrode grids (64 total electrodes per patient) from each patient's set of electrodes as these grids lie on the surface closest to the craniotomy location where we expect the largest amount of brain deformation [7].

3.1 CT Cortical Surface Segmentation

For each fold in our cross-validation study, we tested how our proposed cortical boundary learning (Sect. 2.2) and segmentation (Sect. 2.3) performed using oriented local image patches (Sect. 2.1) by comparing our results to those found using local image patches using standard orientation, *e.g.* $\mathbf{R} = \mathbf{I}$ in (1). For each of these two methods, we used a multi-resolution Gaussian image pyramid with $K = 3$ levels. For each level, we created appearance dictionaries of size $n = 256$ with sparsity constraint $\Gamma_0 = 2$. Local image patches $\Phi(\mathbf{u}, \sigma)$ used point sample templates Θ with $5\times 5\times 5$ isotropic grids centered around each surface vertex $\mathbf{u} \in S$, thus the appearance samples had dimensionality $d = 125$. We adjusted the spacing between the Θ sample points for each resolution level k, *e.g.* $k = 1, 2, 3$ had scales $\sigma = 1, 2, 4$mm, respectively. By doing so, image patches at high image scales have larger physical sizes. The training surface meshes $S_i^{2'}$ had on average 2685 ± 188 vertices, and we extracted 3 times this many patch samples from the N training CT images to train the inside and outside dictionaries in Sect. 2.2.

To segment the 3 test images in each cross-validation fold using the method described in Sect. 2.3, we set the number of update iterations to $t = 150$ for each resolution level k. The testing surface meshes $\hat{S}$ used in Sect. 2.3 had on average

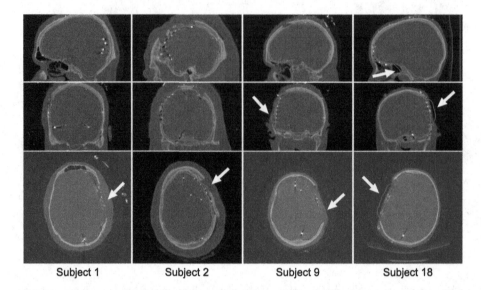

Subject 1   Subject 2   Subject 9   Subject 18

Fig. 3. Cortical surface segmentation results using (*i*) our proposed appearance method using local image patches oriented by the surface estimate's geometry (orange contour), and (*ii*) the standard appearance method using local image patches oriented along the image axes (blue contour). Sagittal (top row), coronal (middle row), and axial (bottom row) slice of 4 example subjects. Arrows highlight areas where our approach better identified the cortical surface(Color figure online).

2740 ± 197 vertices. Figure 3 shows example qualitative segmentation results from 4 subjects using both the standard patch orientation and our proposed oriented patches. Segmentation using oriented patches appeared to extract the cortical surface better than using standard image patches as the standard patch method had trouble correctly localizing the cortical surface in areas where the skull was removed.

To quantify how well our proposed method extracted the cortical surface, we evaluated our segmented surface estimate $\hat{S}_i$ with respect to the rigidly registered post-op MR surface $S_i^{2'}$ as a gold-standard. For each subject i, we computed our 3 surface evaluation measures comparing our surface estimate $\hat{S}_i$ with the reference surface $S_i^{2'}$. We compared three different estimated test surfaces $\hat{S}_i$: (*i*) the initial, rigidly registered pre-op surface, *i.e.* no segmentation updates; (*ii*) the surface estimate using standard image patch orientation; and (*iii*) the surface estimate using oriented image patches. Table 1 summarizes the distribution of these results. Using oriented image patches provided significantly better segmentation results (two-tailed paired t-test $p < 0.05$) in terms of higher $\mathrm{DICE}(\hat{S}_i, S_i^{2'})$, and lower $\mathrm{HD}(\hat{S}_i, S_i^{2'})$, $\mathrm{MAD}(\hat{S}_i, S_i^{2'})$, and $\mathrm{MESD}(E_i, \hat{S}_i)$ values on average. Figure 4 shows an example comparing these 3 surface estimates along with electrodes identified in the CT images to illustrate how our proposed method estimates a more physically plausible surface on which the electrodes lie.

Table 1. Segmentation evaluation quality measures for cortical surface segmentation using our proposed method compared to the initial surface and dictionary-based segmentation using standard images patches. Values are expressed as Mean±SD. †,‡ and ⋆ indicate statistically significant results (two-tailed paired t-test $p < 0.05$) between the two methods indicated by the symbol.

Method	Dice (%)	HD (mm)	MAD (mm)	MESD (mm)
▨ Initial	$93.38 \pm 2.34^{\dagger,\ddagger}$	$17.29 \pm 8.20^{\ddagger}$	3.22 ± 0.91	$3.16 \pm 1.15^{\ddagger}$
▪ Standard	$94.24 \pm 1.38^{\dagger,\star}$	$16.84 \pm 5.06^{\star}$	$3.32 \pm 0.53^{\star}$	$2.83 \pm 1.57^{\star}$
▪ Oriented	$\mathbf{95.08 \pm 0.82^{\ddagger,\star}}$	$\mathbf{13.21 \pm 5.16^{\ddagger,\star}}$	$\mathbf{2.99 \pm 0.36^{\star}}$	$\mathbf{0.95 \pm 0.25^{\ddagger,\star}}$

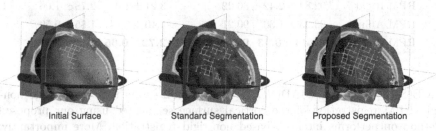

Initial Surface   Standard Segmentation   Proposed Segmentation

Fig. 4. Visualizing electrodes on the segmented cortical brain surface mesh. In this example (subject 2), (left) the electrodes initially appear embedded within the surface, and (middle) using the standard segmentation approach only partially corrects the surface. Our proposed method (right) correctly segments the cortical surface and the electrodes appear to sit correctly on the surface.

We implemented the training and segmentation algorithms in MATLAB. The running time for the segmentation using oriented patches was 11.46 ± 0.82 minutes on average, and 2.94 ± 0.31 minutes on average using standard patch orientation. The main reason for the increase in computation time using oriented patches is computation of the principal curvatures.

3.2   Non-rigid MR-CT Registration

Using the CT brain surface segmentation results $\hat{S}_i$ found by our proposed algorithm, we registered the post-implantation CT image I_{CT}^2 directly to the pre-implantation MRI I_{MR}^1 with a robust point matching (RPM) surface registration algorithm (Sect. 2.4). We compared our results to intensity-based registration where we registered the post-op CT image to the pre-op MRI using (i) rigid, (ii) affine, and (iii) non-rigid free-form deformation (FFD) [13] transformations T_i. Both the non-rigid RPM and non-rigid intensity FFDs had isotropic B-spline control point spacing set to 30 mm. The intensity registration methods used a multi-resolution image pyramid and conjugate gradient optimization to maximize the normalized mutual information (NMI) similarity metric [16].

We evaluated registration performance with respect to the pre-op MR brain surface S_i^1 and the transformed post-op CT surface estimate $T_i \circ \hat{S}_i$ by calculating

Table 2. Registration evaluation quality measures for direct non-rigid registration of post-op CT images to pre-op MRI. We computed rigid, affine, and non-rigid registration results using (i) RPM registration of the CT brain surface (found using our proposed segmentation method) to the segmented MR brain surface, and (ii) intensity-based registration of the two images. Values are expressed as Mean±SD.

Method	Dice (%)	Min. Dice (%)	MAD (mm)	MESD (mm)
Intensity Rigid	93.40 ± 2.36	87.27	3.02 ± 0.99	3.12 ± 1.16
Intensity Affine	92.69 ± 2.89	84.48	3.21 ± 1.15	3.56 ± 1.17
Intensity FFD	93.25 ± 3.45	82.72	3.07 ± 1.37	2.31 ± 0.91
RPM Rigid	92.84 ± 2.42	86.22	3.21 ± 1.05	2.78 ± 1.06
RPM Affine	93.23 ± 1.36	90.21	3.10 ± 0.84	1.85 ± 0.59
RPM Non-rigid	$\mathbf{94.44 \pm 0.93}$	**92.08**	$\mathbf{2.72 \pm 0.65}$	$\mathbf{1.55 \pm 0.37}$

DICE($S_i^1, T_i \circ \hat{S}_i$) and MAD($S_i^1, T_i \circ \hat{S}_i$). Table 2 shows that on average non-rigid RPM registration of the cortical surface segmented using our proposed method outperforms intensity-based non-rigid registration. More importantly, our proposed method had a much smaller standard deviation of Dice values and greater minimum Dice value, 92.08 for our method compared to 82.72 for intensity FFD. Interestingly, intensity FFD had worse minimum performance than intensity-based rigid and affine registration. Non-rigid RPM registration also had lower mean MAD performance than intensity FFD (two-tailed paired t-test $p = 0.13$). Additionally, we quantified how close the electrodes E_i identified in the CT image were to the MR brain surface after registration, *i.e.* MESD($T_i \circ E_i, S_i^1$). Table 2 shows that electrodes were significantly closer to the segmented pre-op MR surface using non-rigid RPM than the intensity-based registration methods (two-tailed paired t-test $p < 0.05$). These results were to be expected given that the RPM registration explicitly seeks to align the two surfaces, while intensity-based registration does not enforce such a constraint.

4   Conclusion

The method proposed in this paper can be used to solve an actual clinical problem using imperfect clinical data. Our proposed method accurately extracts the brain surface from post-electrode implantation CT images that contain many artifacts, distortions, and missing anatomical features. By orienting local images, we create a dictionary-based model of the brain boundary's appearance that is more invariant to image orientation changes in comparison to appearance models that use local image patches aligned with the image axes. The resulting appearance model, when used with our proposed surface estimation method, significantly improves segmentation performance (Table 1). Then, using this brain surface estimate, we demonstrate improved non-rigid registration of post-implantation CT images to pre-implantation MRI in comparison to intensity-based registration methods. Further testing is necessary with respect to the algorithm parameters, in particular, the size of the dictionaries, the sparsity constraint term, and the local image patch size, in order to determine optima settings. Furthermore, our segmentation method does not incorporate any prior information regarding the shape of the brain surface. In the future, we aim to combine our locally oriented appearance model with a statistical model of brain shape [5] to better constrain the surface estimation process. The approach presented in this paper could be applied to segment other anatomical structures of interest whose appearance has a highly non-Gaussian distribution, e.g. due to post-surgical appearance changes caused by scar tissue or implants.

References

1. Aharon, M., Elad, M., Bruckstein, A.: K -SVD: an algorithm for designing over-complete dictionaries for sparse representation. IEEE Trans. Sig. Process. **54**(11), 4311–4322 (2006)
2. Azarion, A.A., Wu, J., Davis, K.A., Pearce, A., Krish, V.T., Wagenaar, J., Chen, W., Zheng, Y., Wang, H., Lucas, T.H., Litt, B., Gee, J.C.: An open-source automated platform for three-dimensional visualization of subdural electrodes using CT-MRI coregistration. Epilepsia (2014)
3. Brown, M., Szeliski, R., Winder, S.: Multi-image matching using multi-scale oriented patches. In: CVPR, vol. 1, pp. 510–517 (2005)
4. Chui, H., Rangarajan, A.: A new point matching algorithm for non-rigid registration. Comput. Vis. Image Underst. **89**(2–3), 114–141 (2003)
5. Cootes, T., Taylor, C., Cooper, D., Graham, J.: Active shape models-their training and application. Comput. Vis. Image Underst. **61**(1), 38–59 (1995)
6. do Carmo, M.P.: Differential Geometry of Curves and Surfaces, vol. 2. Prentice-Hall, Englewood Cliffs (1976)
7. Hartkens, T., Hill, D., Castellano-Smith, A., Hawkes, D., Maurer, C.R., Martin, A.J., Hall, W., Liu, H., Truwit, C.: Measurement and analysis of brain deformation during neurosurgery. IEEE TMI **22**(1), 82–92 (2003)
8. Hill, D.L., Maurer, C.R.J., Maciunas, R.J., Barwise, J.A., Fitzpatrick, M.J., Wang, M.Y.: Measurement of intraoperative brain surface deformation under a craniotomy. Neurosurgery **3**, 514–526 (1998)
9. Huang, X., Dione, D.P., Compas, C.B., Papademetris, X., Lin, B.A., Bregasi, A., Sinusas, A.J., Staib, L.H., Duncan, J.S.: Contour tracking in echocardiographic sequences via sparse representation and dictionary learning. Med. Image Anal. **18**(2), 253–271 (2014)
10. Onofrey, J.A., Staib, L.H., Papademetris, X.: Learning nonrigid deformations for constrained multi-modal image registration. In: Mori, K., Sakuma, I., Sato, Y., Barillot, C., Navab, N. (eds.) MICCAI 2013, Part III. LNCS, vol. 8151, pp. 171–178. Springer, Heidelberg (2013)
11. Papademetris, X., Jackowski, A.P., Schultz, R.T., Staib, L.H., Duncan, J.S.: Computing 3D Non-rigid brain registration using extended robust point matching for composite multisubject fMRI analysis. In: Ellis, R.E., Peters, T.M. (eds.) MICCAI 2003. LNCS, vol. 2879, pp. 788–795. Springer, Heidelberg (2003)
12. Rubinstein, R., Zibulevsky, M., Elad, M.: Efficient implementation of the K-SVD algorithm using batch orthogonal matching pursuit. Technical Report, Technion (2008)

13. Rueckert, D., Sonoda, L., Hayes, C., Hill, D., Leach, M., Hawkes, D.: Nonrigid registration using free-form deformations: application to breast MR images. IEEE TMI **18**(8), 712–721 (1999)
14. Smith, S.M.: Fast robust automated brain extraction. Hum. Brain Mapp. **17**(3), 143–155 (2002)
15. Spencer, S.S., Sperling, M., Shewmon, A.: Intracranial electrodes. In: Engel Jr., J., Pedley, T.A. (eds.) Epilepsy, a Comprehensive Textbook, pp. 1719–1748. Lippincott-Raven, Philadelphia (1998)
16. Studholme, C., Hill, D., Hawkes, D.: An overlap invariant entropy measure of 3D medical image alignment. Pattern Recogn. **32**(1), 71–86 (1999)

AxTract: Microstructure-Driven Tractography Based on the Ensemble Average Propagator

Gabriel Girard[1,2]([✉]), Rutger Fick[1], Maxime Descoteaux[2],
Rachid Deriche[1], and Demian Wassermann[1]

[1] Athena Project-Team, INRIA Sophia Antipolis - Méditerranée,
Sophia Antipolis, France
[2] Sherbrooke Connectivity Imaging Lab (SCIL) Computer Science Department,
Université de Sherbrooke, Sherbrooke, Canada
gabriel.p.girard@usherbrooke.ca

Abstract. We propose a novel method to simultaneously trace brain white matter (WM) fascicles and estimate WM microstructure characteristics. Recent advancements in diffusion-weighted imaging (DWI) allow multi-shell acquisitions with b-values of up to $10,000\,\mathrm{s/mm^2}$ in human subjects, enabling the measurement of the ensemble average propagator (EAP) at distances as short as $10\,\mu m$. Coupled with continuous models of the full 3D DWI signal and the EAP such as Mean Apparent Propagator (MAP) MRI, these acquisition schemes provide unparalleled means to probe the WM tissue *in vivo*. Presently, there are two complementary limitations in tractography and microstructure measurement techniques. Tractography techniques are based on models of the DWI signal geometry without taking specific hypotheses of the WM structure. This hinders the tracing of fascicles through certain WM areas with complex organization such as branching, crossing, merging, and bottlenecks that are indistinguishable using the orientation-only part of the DWI signal. Microstructure measuring techniques, such as AxCaliber, require the direction of the axons within the probed tissue before the acquisition as well as the tissue to be highly organized. Our contributions are twofold. First, we extend the theoretical DWI models proposed by Callaghan et al. to characterize the distribution of axonal calibers within the probed tissue taking advantage of the MAP-MRI model. Second, we develop a simultaneous tractography and axonal caliber distribution algorithm based on the hypothesis that axonal caliber distribution varies smoothly along a WM fascicle. To validate our model we test it on *in silico* phantoms and on the HCP dataset.

1 Introduction

Diffusion-weighted (DW) magnetic resonance imaging (MRI) has empowered the analysis of the brain's white matter (WM) anatomy and its relationship with function and pathologies in recent years. DWI has provided great tools to advance the study of neuroscience and neuropathology. However, the relationship between the measures obtained from the DWI signal and their underlying

© Springer International Publishing Switzerland 2015
S. Ourselin et al. (Eds.): IPMI 2015, LNCS 9123, pp. 675–686, 2015.
DOI: 10.1007/978-3-319-19992-4_53

biological process is still unclear. In this work, we build upon current advances in DWI acquisition and signal modelling to develop a new technology to trace WM fascicles while simultaneously characterizing the distribution of axonal calibers (i.e. diameters) within the fascicle. In doing this, we expect to provide better tools to characterize the WM. Examples of these possible applications could be pathology-oriented, for instance through the detection of axonal swelling and quantification of the connectivity between two cortical areas; or neuroscience oriented, as axonal caliber has been shown to be closely related to the efficiency of electrical signal propagation within the axons [12].

Despite recent advances in axonal caliber quantification from DWI, to the best of our knowledge, none of them has been used to improve tractography at the moment of the tract tracing process. Two approaches to combine microstructure information and tractography have been proposed [9,14]. To solve complex WM areas (e.g. branching, crossing, merging, and bottlenecks), these approaches reject tracts from a full brain tractography based on microstructure information. This is sensitive to the choice of the tractography algorithm used, since this requires all plausible configurations of tracts inside the complex region. Our novel tractography algorithm, AxTract, addresses the complex configuration problem differently. AxTract incorporates the axonal caliber estimation in the tractography algorithm and uses it during the tracing process. This produces tracts with embedded microstructure information and enables the possibility of solving the tracing through WM areas using axonal calibers information.

In developing AxTract to be useful for reasonably long DWI acquisitions, we base our model solely on the ensemble average propagator (EAP) [11] at a fixed gradient separation time. This relaxes the requirements of axonal caliber estimation techniques such as AxCaliber [3] and ActiveAx [1] which focus on the signal attenuation and need a sampling over different gradient separation times. Our approach has the main advantage of simultaneously modelling, through the Fourier slice theorem, all measurements on the perpendicular plane to the cylinder population. To prove the soundness of our model, we developed the first contribution of this work: a generalized return-to-axis probability (RTAP) measure [11] showing that even at gradient separation times used in current clinical protocols, axonal caliber can be quantified. This enabled our second contribution: the AxTract algorithm which estimates axonal caliber during the tractography process using it as a prior for the traced tract.

2   Theory

The DWI signal within a voxel measures diffusion of water particles within different compartments, such as axons and astrocytes. It is possible to characterize the diffusion process as the displacement probability density of water particles within these compartments, the ensemble average propagator (EAP) [11]:

$$\bar{P}(\boldsymbol{r} - \boldsymbol{r}'; \Delta) = \sum_{c \in C} \rho_c(\boldsymbol{r}') \int_{\mathbb{R}^3} P_0(\boldsymbol{r}'; c) P_c(\boldsymbol{r}; \boldsymbol{r}', \Delta) d\boldsymbol{r}' \qquad (1)$$

where r', r are the particle's start and end positions; Δ the diffusion time; C is the set of compartments; $\rho_c(r')$ is the probability of r' being inside compartment c; P_0 the probability of the initial position in c; and P_c the compartment-specific propagator. The EAP is related to the attenuation of the DWI signal by the Fourier transform:

$$E(q; \Delta) = \mathcal{F}_{r-r'} \{\bar{P}(r - r'; \Delta)\} (q) \tag{2}$$

Within the study of the human brain WM, the axons present a specific interest. Within a voxel, axons can be modelled as cylindrical segments, for which specific formulations of P and E exist [6]. In compartments where diffusion takes place within a set of cylinders oriented along direction $r_\parallel$ with negligible tortuosity and permeability, the displacement $r - r'$ is decomposable in the parallel and perpendicular directions to the cylinder [4]. We write this as $r - r' = (r_\parallel - r'_\parallel) + (r_\perp - r'_\perp)$ leading to separable formulations of P and E [4]:

$$\bar{P}(r - r'; \Delta) = \bar{P}(r_\parallel - r'_\parallel; \Delta) \, \bar{P}(r_\perp - r'_\perp; \Delta)$$

$$= \int_{\mathbb{R}} P_0(r'_\parallel) P_{c_\parallel}(r_\parallel - r'_\parallel; \Delta) dr'_\parallel \int_{\mathbb{R}^2} P_0(r'_\perp) P_{c_\perp}(r_\perp - r'_\perp; \Delta) dr'_\perp$$

$$E(q; \Delta) = E(q_\parallel; \Delta) \, E(q_\perp; \Delta). \tag{3}$$

This decomposition enables the use of theoretical models for P_c [6]. If the propagator P_c is measured at a cylinder of cross-sectional area A and it's filled with water with diffusion coefficient D, we derive the following expressions [6]:

$$P_{cyl_\parallel}(r_\parallel; r'_\parallel, \Delta) = \frac{e^{-\frac{\|r_\parallel - r'_\parallel\|^2}{4D\Delta}}}{\sqrt{2\pi D \Delta}} \tag{4a}$$

$$P_{cyl_\perp}(r_\perp; r'_\perp, \Delta, A) = \sum_{nk} 2^{1_{n=0}} \left(e^{-\frac{\pi \gamma_{nk}^2 D\Delta}{A}} \frac{\gamma_{nk}^2}{J_n(\gamma_{nk}^2)(\gamma_{nk}^2 - n^2)A} \right.$$

$$\left. J_n \left(\frac{\sqrt{\pi}\gamma_{nk}\|r_\perp\|}{\sqrt{A}} \right) J_n \left(\frac{\sqrt{\pi}\gamma_{nk}\|r'_\perp\|}{\sqrt{A}} \right) \cos(n\theta) \cos(n\theta') \right) \tag{4b}$$

where $1_{n=0}$ is the indicator function for $n = 0$, θ and θ' are the respective angles of $r_\perp$ and $r'_\perp$ when expressed in polar coordinates, J_n is the n-th cylindrical Bessel function and γ_{kn} the k-th the root of its derivative: $J'_n(\gamma_{km}) = 0$.

Having a specific model for cylindrical compartments, i.e. axons, we can derive the theory to estimate the axonal cross-sectional area. Different techniques to capitalize the theoretical model in Eq. (4) for cylinder compartments and measure axonal radii have been proposed. The main exponents of these are AxCaliber [3]; ActiveAx [1] and the Return-to-Axis-Probability (RTAP) [11]. However, the applicability of these techniques is limited, even in current state-of-the-art whole human brain acquisitions such as the HCP project: AxCaliber relies on a relatively dense sampling along the q and Δ dimensions; ActiveAx estimates a single-parameter which experimentally correlates with the mean caliber without an explicit formal relationship to it; and RTAP which needs very large diffusion times (Δ) for the perpendicular EAP to become [11]

$$\bar{P}_{cyl_\perp}(\boldsymbol{r}_\perp; A, \Delta) \xrightarrow{\Delta \to \infty} \frac{4\cos^{-1}\left(\frac{\|\boldsymbol{r}_\perp\|\sqrt{\pi}}{2\sqrt{A}}\right) - \frac{\|\boldsymbol{r}_\perp\|\sqrt{\pi}}{2\sqrt{A}}\sqrt{4 - \frac{\|\boldsymbol{r}_\perp\|^2 \pi}{A}}}{2\pi A}$$

and converge to the reciprocal of the cross-sectional area of the axonal population

$$\mathrm{RTAP}(\Delta) = \int_{\mathbb{R}^2} E_\perp(\boldsymbol{q}_\perp; \Delta)d\boldsymbol{q}_\perp = \bar{P}_\perp(\boldsymbol{0}, \Delta) \xrightarrow{\Delta \to \infty} A^{-1}.$$

The first contribution of our work is to prove that, even at small Δ values, the propagator along the cylinder has a specific relationship with the distribution of cross-sectional areas in a cylinder population. **We base our model on the EAP as opposed to the AxCaliber and RTAP approaches which focus on the signal attenuation.** This has the main advantage of simultaneously modelling, through the Fourier slice theorem, all measurements on the perpendicular plane to the cylinder population. We start our model in the style of AxCaliber and "infinite Δ" RTAP, we attach a density to the cross-sectional area of a cylinder population. Our density is based on three hypotheses given by Özarslan et al. [11]. First, each particular cylinder's contribution to the overall signal is proportional to the ratio of water particles in it, which is in direct relationship with the cylinder's cross-sectional area. Second, the cylinder population is Gamma-distributed [3]. This leads to specific EAP formulation, Eq. (1), for N cylinders:

$$\bar{P}(\boldsymbol{r} - \boldsymbol{r}'; \Delta, \alpha, \beta, N) = \sum_{i=1}^{N} \frac{A_i}{\sum_j^N A_j} \bar{P}_{cyl}(\boldsymbol{r} - \boldsymbol{r}'; \Delta, A), \quad A_i \sim \Gamma(\alpha, \beta), \quad (5)$$

where each A_i is an independent and identically distributed random variable with Gamma distribution, of shape α and rate β, of the cross-sectional area. Finally, our third hypothesis assumes that the population is large enough to be approximated by an infinite number of cylinders. Combining Equations (1) and (5)

$$\bar{P}(\boldsymbol{r} - \boldsymbol{r}'; \Delta, \alpha, \beta) = \lim_{N \to \infty} \bar{P}(\boldsymbol{r} - \boldsymbol{r}'; \Delta, \alpha, \beta, N) =$$

$$\int_0^\infty \frac{A f(A; \alpha, \beta)}{\alpha \beta^{-1}} \bar{P}_{cyl}(\boldsymbol{r} - \boldsymbol{r}'; \Delta, A)\, dA \tag{6}$$

where the integral over A takes in account all possible cross-sectional areas; $f(A; \alpha, \beta)$ is the probability density function of a Gamma distribution with shape α and rate β; and $\alpha\beta^{-1}$ is the average cross-sectional area under the distribution $\Gamma(\alpha, \beta)$. By using the separability of the EAP (see Eq. (3)) and assuming a uniform probability of finding a water particle within the cylinder population, we marginalize Eq. (6) for the return-to-axis probability, i.e. $\boldsymbol{r}'_\perp = \boldsymbol{r}_\perp$,

$$\bar{P}_\perp(\boldsymbol{0}; \Delta, \alpha, \beta) = \int_0^\infty \frac{A f(A; \alpha, \beta)}{\alpha \beta^{-1}} \int_{\mathbb{R}^2} P_0(\boldsymbol{r}; A) P_{cyl_\perp}(\boldsymbol{r}; \boldsymbol{r}, \Delta, A)\, d\boldsymbol{r} dA \tag{7}$$

where $P_0(\boldsymbol{r}; A)$ is the uniform distribution of $\boldsymbol{r}$ within the disc of surface A.

Then, replacing Eq. (4) into Eq. (7), we reach our first result

$$\bar{P}_\perp(0; \Delta, \alpha, \beta) = \frac{(D\Delta\pi)^{\frac{\alpha-1}{2}}}{\beta^{\frac{-1-\alpha}{2}}\Gamma(\alpha)} \sum_{nk} 2^{1_{n=0}} \gamma_{nk}^\alpha \mathrm{K}_{\alpha-1}\left(2\gamma_{nk}\sqrt{D\Delta\pi\beta}\right) \mathrm{R}_n(\gamma_{nk}) \quad (8)$$

$$\mathrm{R}_n(\gamma) \triangleq \frac{\gamma\left(\mathrm{J}_n^2(\gamma) + \mathrm{J}_{n+1}^2(\gamma)\right) - 2n\mathrm{J}_n(\gamma)\mathrm{J}_{n+1}(\gamma)}{\mathrm{J}}^2 (\gamma)(\gamma^2 - n^2)$$

where K is the modified Bessel function. Finally, the calculating $P_\perp(0; \Delta, \alpha, \beta)$ from the 3D signal combining Eqs. (3), (4) and (8) is the same as RTAP

$$\int_0^\infty \bar{P}(\boldsymbol{r}_\parallel r + \boldsymbol{r}_\perp 0)dr = \int_0^\infty \bar{P}_\parallel(r; \Delta)dr\, \bar{P}_\perp(0; \Delta, \alpha, \beta) = \frac{1}{2}\bar{P}_\perp(0; \Delta, \alpha, \beta) \quad (9)$$

This characterization of $P_\perp$ in the case of an axonal population has two main advantages: first, it doesn't depend on a very large Δ for its relationship with the axonal radii to be true; second, as a corollary of the relationship between the EAP $P_\perp$ and the attenuation $E_\perp$, Eq. (8) aggregates information from all measurements perpendicular to the cylinder population and, by using a full 3D model with analytic Fourier transform such as Mean Apparent Propagator (MAP) MRI [11], takes advantage of the full extent of q-space measurements in the acquisition protocol.

3 Methods

3.1 AxTract: Microstructure-Driven Tractography

Model Fitting. The main purpose of our novel tractography algorithm, AxTract, is to simultaneously trace WM fascicle and estimate their axonal caliber. The main hypothesis driving AxTract is that the average caliber of the axons composing a tract varies slowly along its pathway.

To formulate our algorithm we start from the classical equation driving streamline tractography [5]:

$$\frac{dt(s)}{ds} = d(s), \quad t(0) = t_0 \quad (10)$$

where the curve $r(s)$ is the streamline tracing the WM fascicle that traverses t_0, and $d(s)$ is the tangent vector to $t(s)$, and taken to be the eigenvector corresponding to the maximal eigenvalue of the diffusion tensor (DT) at $t(s)$. More generally, using the DTI EAP model, $d(s)$ is equivalent to the direction of maximal diffusion probability

$$d(s) = \arg\max_{\hat{r} \in \mathbb{R}^3, \|\hat{r}\|=1} \mathrm{ODF}(\hat{r}; s) \quad (11)$$

where ODF is the orientation distribution function [17]

$$\mathrm{ODF}(\hat{r}) = \int_0^\infty \bar{P}(\hat{r}r)\rho(r)dr, \quad \hat{r} \in \mathbb{R}^3, \|\hat{r}\| = 1 \quad (12)$$

with $\rho(r)$ a function of the area element of the sphere, such as $\rho(r) = r^2$ [16].

Algorithms based on Eq. (10) rely on the hypothesis that fiber tracts are locally tangent to direction of maximal diffusion probability. Specifically, the DT model cannot express complex geometries such as tract crossings and kissings. Hence, several algorithms have been proposed to extend this algorithm and be able to trace through these geometries [15–17]. These algorithms rely on the same hypothesis of that the direction of maximum probability is enough to trace these tracts and add, in one way or another, a new hypothesis of preservation of the previous tracking direction.

With AxTract, we aim to preserve not only direction but average axonal caliber, adding a biologically-driven hypothesis and enabling to traverse complex structures with more confidence on the results. At each point along the tract, we fit a model of the EAP based on the theoretical models presented in Sect. 2. We develop a multi-compartment fitting model to separate the EAP data corresponding to a particular population from other compartments. Hence, we assign to each ODF peak an EAP formulation for a cylindrical population and we add to the whole ensemble an isotropic tensor representing the combination of extracellular water and spherical compartments such as astrocytes. The formulation of our tract-point model

$$\bar{P}_{fit}(\boldsymbol{r}; D, f_1, \ldots, f_N, A_1, \ldots, A_N, d_1, \ldots, d_N) =$$
$$\sum_i^N f_i \bar{P}_{cyl}(\boldsymbol{r}; A_i, d_i) + (1 - \sum_i^N f_i)\bar{P}_{ec}(\boldsymbol{r}; D), \quad \sum_i^N f_i \le 1, f_i \in [0, 1] \quad (13)$$

where N is the number of non-collinear tracts crossing that point, namely of ODF peaks; A_i the average calibers; d_i the tract orientation; $\bar{P}_{cyl}$ the propagator of a cylindrical ensemble, where for implementation speed, we assume a large diffusion time. $\bar{P}_{ec}(\boldsymbol{r}, D)$ is the extra-cylindrical compartment propagator:

$$\bar{P}_{ec}(\boldsymbol{r}, D) = \frac{\exp\left(-\frac{1}{4D\tau}\boldsymbol{r}^T\boldsymbol{r}\right)}{\sqrt{2\pi D\tau}^3}, \quad D \in \mathbb{R}_{>0} \quad (14)$$

and f are the mixing factors.

Then, for a given an EAP $\bar{P}(\boldsymbol{r})$, we fit our model in Eq. (13) by minimizing the squared loss function with combined global-local optimisers

$$\underset{D,f_1,\ldots,f_N,A_1,\ldots,A_N}{\operatorname{argmin}} = \int_{\mathbb{R}^3} [\bar{P}(\boldsymbol{r}) - \bar{P}_{fit}(\boldsymbol{r}; D, f_1, \ldots, f_N, A_1, \ldots, A_N, d_1, \ldots, d_N)]^2 d\boldsymbol{r}$$
(15)

To fit Eq. (15) and to extract the ODF peaks, we use a continuous representation of $\bar{P}$ which is analytically estimated from the DWI signal attenuation, MAP-MRI [11]. This provides us with the means to obtain the ODF peaks and optimize our objective function over a dense sampling on $\boldsymbol{r}$.

Tractography. Streamlines propagate in a WM volume and stop when a position outside the volume is reached [15]. The tracking process propagates a seed from the initial position (placed within the volume) following diffusion properties. To obtain these properties, the signal at the tracking position is obtained with trilinear interpolation of the DWIs. Then, MAP-MRI is used to represent the signal locally [11], from which the ODF peaks are extracted. Using the peak directions and the signal representation from MAP-MRI, AxTract estimates each peak's caliber (see Eq. (15)). The streamline propagation follows the peak with the estimated axonal caliber closest to the median caliber of the current streamline. The estimated streamline caliber is given by median caliber over previous tracking directions for a fixed maximum distance of 5 mm. Peaks forming an angle greater than $\theta = 75°$ with the previous tracking direction are discarded from the selection to enforce smoothness in streamline reconstruction [15]. The tracking stops if no peaks are available. The initial tracking direction is set to the direction associated with the maximum value of the ODF locally. Once the tracking stops, it is re-initiated in the opposite initial direction to form the complete streamline. Additionally, we fixed the tracking discrete step size to 0.5 mm.

4   Dataset

4.1   Human Dataset

We used the Human Connectome Project (HCP) MGH adult diffusion dataset (subject mgh1010) [13]. The diffusion acquisition scheme consists of 552 volumes with b-values ranging from 1000 to 10,000 s/mm^2 ($\delta = 12.9ms$, $\Delta = 21.8ms$). The data were acquired using at 1.5 mm isotropic voxel size using a Spin-echo EPI sequence (TR/TE 8800/57 ms).

4.2   Synthetic Dataset

We used Phantomas [7] to generate *in silico* data using the acquisition scheme of the HCP dataset. The DWI signal is simulated in each voxel based on the Numerical Fiber Generator [8]. The simulated signal is obtained using a hindered and restricted diffusion model [2], and adding Rician noise. Synthetic data with signal-to-noise ratio (SNR) of 20 and 100 are used in this study.

5   Results

Figure 1 shows the error in caliber estimation using Eq. (15), varying the axon population caliber. Figure 1 (a, b) shows the caliber estimation in a single axon population per voxel. Figure 1 (c, d) shows caliber etimation of two axon populations crossing at 90° in a voxel (SNR=100, 20), with a constant axon caliber of 12 μm for the second axon population. Figure 2 shows estimated calibers in the corpus callosum (CC) on *in vivo* data. The algorithm is able to recover various calibers that are consistent locally, with lower caliber in the genu and in the splenium than in the body of the CC (see Fig. 2(b)).

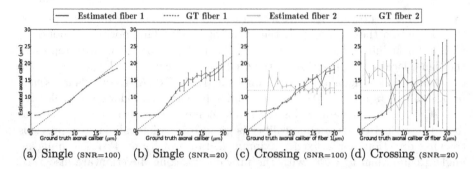

(a) Single (SNR=100) (b) Single (SNR=20) (c) Crossing (SNR=100) (d) Crossing (SNR=20)

Fig. 1. Error on synthetic fiber calibers estimation using Eq. (15). (a, b) Single fiber caliber estimation. The ground truth caliber is shown by the dashed blue line. (b, d) 90° crossing fibers caliber estimation. The second fiber has a constant caliber of 12 μm shown by the dashed green line.

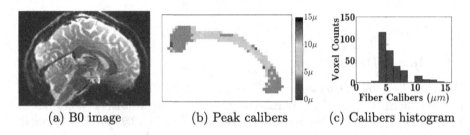

(a) B0 image   (b) Peak calibers   (c) Calibers histogram

Fig. 2. Axonal caliber estimation in the CC using HCP data. Caliber was estimated in the maximum direction of the ODF. Calibers are lower in the genu and in the splenium than in the body of the CC.

We further test Eq. (15) in kissing configuration. Figure 3 (a-c) shows the synthetic kissing dataset. The right fiber (4μm) is predominant on the ODFs image (see Fig. 3 (a)). This can also be observed in the EAP at low radius (Fig. 3 (b)). At higher radii (Fig. 3 (c)), both fibers are visible in crossing regions. However, when both fiber crosses at less than 20°, only one peak appears and it is biased in the direction of the fiber with the smallest axonal caliber. ODFs peaks are shown in Fig. 3 (d). Figure 3 (e, f) shows in each voxel the peak with the highest and lowest caliber value. This can be observed quantitatively in Fig. 4 on the histogram of peaks caliber and on the caliber map, for both SNR=100 and SNR=20.

Figure 5 shows a comparison of deterministic ODF tractography and AxTract on a synthetic kissing configuration. All streamlines connecting valid fascicle extremities are shown in blue (left fiber fascicle) or green (right fiber fascicle) and other streamlines (invalid or incomplete) are shown in red. The deterministic tractography is not able reconstruct the fascicle on the left side. Streamlines are deviated in the right fascicle which has higher diffusion properties. Single peak voxel tends to be biased in the direction the fiber with the lowest caliber,

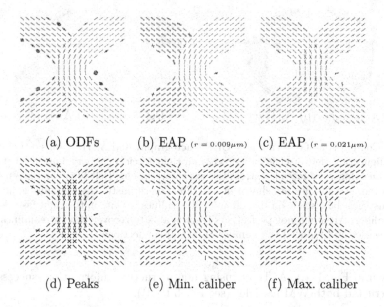

(a) ODFs   (b) EAP $(r = 0.009\mu m)$ (c) EAP $(r = 0.021\mu m)$

(d) Peaks   (e) Min. caliber   (f) Max. caliber

Fig. 3. Synthetic kissing configuration dataset at SNR=20. The fiber on the left has a caliber of $12\,\mu$m and the fiber on the right has a caliber of $4\,\mu$m. (a) ODFS, (b, c) EAP value at fixed radii r, (d) peaks extracted from ODFs, (e, f) peaks with the minimum, respectively the maximum, caliber in each voxel.

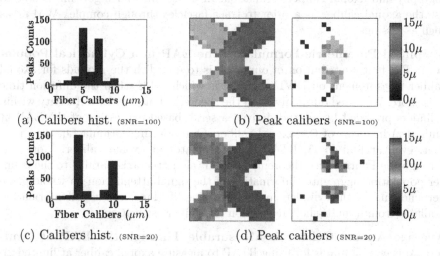

(a) Calibers hist. (SNR=100)   (b) Peak calibers (SNR=100)

(c) Calibers hist. (SNR=20)   (d) Peak calibers (SNR=20)

Fig. 4. Peaks caliber estimation using Eq. (15). The fiber on the left has a caliber of $12\,\mu$m and the fiber on the right has a caliber of $4\,\mu$m. (a, c) Histograms of estimated calibers for all peaks, (b, d) spacial maps of peaks with lowest caliber estimated on the left and the highest caliber on the right.

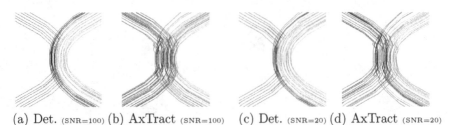

(a) Det. (SNR=100) (b) AxTract (SNR=100)   (c) Det. (SNR=20) (d) AxTract (SNR=20)

Fig. 5. Comparison of deterministic ODF tractography and AxTract on synthetic kissing configuration (left fascicle caliber=12 μm, right fascicle caliber=4 μm). All streamlines connecting valid fascicle extremities are shown in blue (left fiber) and green (right fiber), other streamlines are shown in red. The deterministic tractography is not able to reconstruct the fascicle on the left side. Streamlines deviate in the right fascicle with lower caliber. Although not perfect, AxTract is able to recover valid streamlines from both fascicles and reduced the number of invalid connections.

as shown in Fig. 3 (d). AxTract, using microstructure information, successfully reconstructed both WM fascicles (see Fig. 5 (b,d)).

6   Discussion and Conclusion

In this paper, we introduced a novel algorithm to simultaneously perform tractography and axonal caliber estimation. In doing this, our algorithm is able to use the axonal caliber as a prior to trace fascicles through complex WM areas such as kissings.

Simplified Parametric Formula for the EAP in a Cylindrical Population: The first contribution of our work is to establish the grounds for axonal caliber measurement on DWI acquisitions which holds when the diffusion time Δ is short. We based our analysis on the theoretical models for diffusivity within cylinders provided by [6] and derived a series-based expression of the EAP at limited Δ in terms of the axonal caliber. Our resulting formula Eq. (8) shows that, even at limited Δ, RTAP is an estimator of axonal caliber. Moreover, through the Fourier slice theorem, the EAP along the axis parallel to the cylinder population aggregates information of the signal attenuation on whole plane perpendicular to the cylinders, providing a simplified mean to use all information available from a multi-shell acquisition for caliber estimation.

Average Axonal Caliber is Measurable Through the EAP at Limited Δ: Having grounds for using RTAP to measure axonal caliber at limited Δ, we proceeded to test its sensitivity in different scenarios. Figure 1 (a) showed, in synthetic experiments, that RTAP clearly distinguishes various axonal calibers in single axon population cases. This is further supported by Fig. 2 where various calibers are recovered in the human corpus callosum. As show by McNab et al. [10], the recovered calibers are generally higher in the body of the CC than in the genu and the splenium of the CC. However, no axonal calibers difference was observed between the genu and the splenium of the CC in this single subject. Further investigation is required to quantify the difference between AxCaliber axonal caliber estimation and AxTract. Nevertheless, Fig. 2 shows that axon populations with various caliber can be identified *in vivo*, which can be used within the choice of the propagation direction of the tractography.

AxTract Effectively Solves Kissings Using Axonal Caliber as a Prior: In fiber crossing regions, AxTract distinguishes axonal caliber population, specially at low noise level (see Figs. 1 and 4). Even though the estimation is not as accurate as in single population cases, it showed improvements in the streamline reconstruction, both at SNR=20 and SNR=100 (Fig. 5). The median caliber estimated locally seems to be robust to misestimation of the caliber at some of the tracking steps. We can observe in Fig. 5 that the tractography needs in some cases to follow peaks with higher local deviations to keep following the fascicle with the closest caliber. Always following peaks with the lowest local deviation, as with deterministic peak tractography, leads to error in the kissing configuration reconstruction. A smaller tracking step size would help following the fascicle tangent direction and reduce the maximum deviation angle θ parameter, thus producing a smoother WM pathway reconstruction. AxTract allows the streamline propagation to follow pathways otherwise not explored by the deterministic tractography. Those results are preliminary, but expose a potential use of the microstructural information in tractography to properly reconstruct complex WM architectures such as kissing and branching configurations. Future work on full brain WM reconstruction is planned. The main limitation of the current implementation is the computational requirements.

To conclude, in this work we presented AxTract, a novel algorithm that uses simultaneous axonal caliber estimation and tractography to resolve WM fascicle tracking through areas of complex WM con figurations. In order to develop this algorithm, we provided mathematical grounds for the feasibility of caliber estimation and evidence for both *in silico* and human data. Finally, we tested our tractography algorithm which was able to tract through a fiber kissing using a priori information of the traced fascicle which was previously not possible.

Acknowledgments. Human brain data were provided by the Human Connectome Project (HCP; Principal Investigators: Bruce Rosen, M.D., Ph.D., Arthur W. Toga, Ph.D., Van J. Weeden, MD). HCP funding was provided by the National Institute of Dental and Craniofacial Research, the National Institute of Mental Health, and the National Institute of Neurological Disorders and Stroke.

References

1. Alexander, D.C., Hubbard, P.L., Hall, M.G., Moore, E.A., Ptito, M., Parker, G.J., Dyrby, T.B.: Orientationally invariant indices of axon diameter and density from diffusion MRI. NImg **42**, 1374–1389 (2010)
2. Assaf, Y., Basser, P.J.: Composite hindered and restricted model of diffusion (CHARMED) MR imaging of the human brain. NImg **27**(1), 48–58 (2005)

3. Assaf, Y., Blumenfeld-Katzir, T., Yovel, Y., Basser, P.J.: AxCaliber: a method for measuring axon diameter distribution from diffusion MRI. MRM **59**, 1347–1354 (2008)
4. Assaf, Y., Freidlin, R.Z., Rohde, G.K., Basser, P.J.: New modeling and experimental framework to characterize hindered and restricted water diffusion in brain white matter. MRM **52**, 965–978 (2004)
5. Basser, P.J., Pajevic, S., Pierpaoli, C., Duda, J., Aldroubi, A.: In vivo fiber tractography using DT-MRI data. MRM **44**, 625–632 (2000)
6. Callaghan, P.: Pulsed-Gradient Spin-Echo NMR for planar, cylindrical, and spherical pores under conditions of wall relaxation. J. Magn. Reson. Series A **13**, 53–59 (1995)
7. Caruyer, E., Daducci, A., Descoteaux, M., Houde, J.C., Thiran, J.P., Verma, R.: Phantomas: a flexible software library to simulate diffusion MR phantoms. In: International Symposium on Magnetic Resonance in Medicine (2014)
8. Close, T.G., Tournier, J.D., Calamante, F., Johnston, L.A., Mareels, I., Connelly, A.: A software tool to generate simulated white matter structures for the assessment of fibre-tracking algorithms. NImg **47**(4), 1288–1300 (2009)
9. Daducci, A., Dal Palu, A., Alia, L., Thiran, J.P.: COMMIT: convex optimization modeling for micro-structure informed tractography. IEEE Trans. Med. Imaging **34**, 246–257 (2014)
10. McNab, J.A., Edlow, B.L., Witzel, T., Huang, S.Y., Bhat, H., Heberlein, K., Feiweier, T., Liu, K., Keil, B., Cohen-Adad, J., Tisdall, M.D., Folkerth, R.D., Kinney, H.C., Wald, L.L.: The human connectome project and beyond: initial applications of 300 mT/m gradients. NImg **80**, 234–245 (2013)
11. Özarslan, E., Koay, C.G., Shepherd, T.M., Komlosh, M.E., İrfanoğlu, M.O., Pierpaoli, C., Basser, P.J.: Mean apparent propagator (MAP) MRI: a novel diffusion imaging method for mapping tissue microstructure. NImg **78**, 16–32 (2013)
12. Ritchie, J.M.: On the relation between fibre diameter and conduction velocity in myelinated nerve fibres. In: Proceedings of the Royal Society of London. Series B, Containing papers of a Biological character. Royal Society (Great Britain) 217(1206), 29–35 (1982)
13. Setsompop, K., Kimmlingen, R., Eberlein, E., Witzel, T., Cohen-Adad, J., McNab, J., Keil, B., Tisdall, M., Hoecht, P., Dietz, P., Cauley, S., Tountcheva, V., Matschl, V., Lenz, V., Heberlein, K., Potthast, A., Thein, H., Horn, J.V., Toga, A., Schmitt, F., Al, E.: Pushing the limits of in vivo diffusion MRI for the human connectome project. NImg **80**, 220–233 (2013)
14. Sherbondy, A.J., Rowe, M.C., Alexander, D.C.: MicroTrack: an algorithm for concurrent projectome and microstructure estimation. In: International Conference on Medical Image Computing and Computer-Assisted Intervention, pp. 183–190 (2010)
15. Tournier, J.D., Calamante, F., Connelly, A.: MRtrix: diffusion tractography in crossing fiber regions. Int. J. Imaging Syst. Technol. **22**(1), 53–66 (2012)
16. Tristán-Vega, A., Westin, C.F., Aja-Fernández, S.: Estimation of fiber orientation probability density functions in high angular resolution diffusion imaging. NImg **47**, 638–650 (2009)
17. Tuch, D.: Q-ball imaging. MRM **52**, 1358–1372 (2004)

Sampling from Determinantal Point Processes for Scalable Manifold Learning

Christian Wachinger[1,2]($\boxtimes$) and Polina Golland[1]

[1] Computer Science and Artificial Intelligence Lab, MIT, Cambridge, USA
wachinger@csail.mit.edu
[2] Massachusetts General Hospital, Harvard Medical School, Boston, USA

Abstract. High computational costs of manifold learning prohibit its application for large datasets. A common strategy to overcome this problem is to perform dimensionality reduction on selected landmarks and to successively embed the entire dataset with the Nyström method. The two main challenges that arise are: (i) the landmarks selected in non-Euclidean geometries must result in a low reconstruction error, (ii) the graph constructed from sparsely sampled landmarks must approximate the manifold well. We propose to sample the landmarks from determinantal distributions on non-Euclidean spaces. Since current determinantal sampling algorithms have the same complexity as those for manifold learning, we present an efficient approximation with linear complexity. Further, we recover the local geometry after the sparsification by assigning each landmark a local covariance matrix, estimated from the original point set. The resulting neighborhood selection based on the Bhattacharyya distance improves the embedding of sparsely sampled manifolds. Our experiments show a significant performance improvement compared to state-of-the-art landmark selection techniques on synthetic and medical data.

1 Introduction

Spectral methods are central for a multitude of applications in medical image analysis, computer vision, and machine learning, such as dimensionality reduction, classification, and segmentation. A limiting factor for the spectral analysis on large datasets is the computational cost of the eigen decomposition. To overcome this limitation, the Nyström method [21] is commonly applied to approximate the spectral decomposition of the Gramian matrix. A subset of rows/columns is selected and based on the eigen decomposition of the resulting small sub-matrix, the spectrum of the original matrix can be approximated. While the Nyström extension is the standard method for the matrix reconstruction, the crucial challenge is the subset selection. In early work [21], uniform sampling without replacement was proposed. This was followed by numerous alternatives including K-means clustering [22], greedy approaches [12] , and volume sampling [3,9]. A recent comparison is presented in [16].

Of particular interest for subset selection is volume sampling [9], equivalent to determinantal sampling [3], because reconstruction error bounds exist. It is,

© Springer International Publishing Switzerland 2015
S. Ourselin et al. (Eds.): IPMI 2015, LNCS 9123, pp. 687–698, 2015.
DOI: 10.1007/978-3-319-19992-4_54

however, not used in practice because of the high computational complexity of sampling from the underlying distributions [16]. Independently, determinantal point processes (DPPs) have been proposed recently for tracking and pose estimation [15]. They were originally designed to model the repulsive interaction between particles. DPPs are well suited for modeling diversity in a point set. A sampling algorithm for DPPs was presented in [14, 15], which has complexity $\mathcal{O}(n^3)$ for n points. Since this algorithm has the same complexity as the spectral analysis, it cannot be directly used as a subset selection scheme.

In this paper, we focus on nonlinear dimensionality reduction for large datasets via manifold learning. Popular manifold learning techniques include kernel PCA, Isomap [19], and Laplacian eigenmaps [5]. All of these methods are based on a kernel matrix of size $\mathcal{O}(n^2)$ that contains the information about the pairwise relationships between the input points. The spectral decomposition of the kernel matrix leads to the low-dimensional embedding of the points. For large n, one seeks to avoid the explicit construction and storage of the matrix. In contrast to general rank-k matrix approximation, this is possible by taking the nature of the non-linear dimensionality reduction into account and relating the entries of the kernel matrix directly to the original point set.

We propose to perform DPP sampling on the original point set to extract a diverse set of landmarks. Since the input points lie in a non-Euclidean space, ignoring the underlying geometry leads to poor results. To account for the non-Euclidean geometry of the input space, we replace the Euclidean distance with the geodesic distance along the manifold, which is approximated by the shortest path distance on the graph. Due to the high complexity of DPP sampling, we derive an efficient approximation that runs in $\mathcal{O}(ndk)$ with input dimensionality d and subset cardinality k. The algorithm restricts the updates to be local, which enables sampling on complex geometries. This, together with its low computational complexity, makes the algorithm well suited for the subset selection in large scale manifold learning.

A consequence of the landmark selection is that the manifold is less densely sampled than before, making its approximation with neighborhood graphs more difficult. It was noted in [2], as a critical response to [19], that the approximation of manifolds with graphs is topologically unstable. In order to improve the graph construction, we retain the local geometry around each landmark by locally estimating the covariance matrix on the original point set. This allows us to compare multivariate Gaussian distributions with the Bhattacharyya distance for neighborhood selection, yielding improved embeddings.

2   Background

We assume n points in high dimensional space $x_1, \ldots, x_n \in \mathbb{R}^d$ and let $X \in \mathbb{R}^{d \times n}$ be the matrix whose i-th column represents point x_i. Non-linear dimensionality reduction techniques are based on a positive semidefinite kernel K, with a typical choice of Gaussian or heat kernel $K_{i,j} = \exp(-\|x_i - x_j\|^2 / 2\sigma^2)$. The resulting kernel matrix is of size $\mathcal{O}(n^2)$. The eigen decomposition of the kernel matrix is necessary for spectral analysis. Unfortunately, its complexity is $\mathcal{O}(n^3)$. Most techniques require only the top k eigenvectors. The problem can therefore also be viewed as finding the best rank-k approximation of the matrix K, with the optimal solution $K_k = \sum_{i=1}^{k} \lambda_i u_i u_i^\top$, where λ_i is the i-th largest eigenvalue and u_i is the corresponding eigenvector.

2.1 Nyström Method

Suppose $J \subseteq \{1,\ldots,n\}$ is a subset of the original point set of size k and $\bar{J}$ is its complement. We can reorder the kernel matrix K such that

$$K = \begin{bmatrix} K_{J \times J} & K_{J \times \bar{J}} \\ K_{\bar{J} \times J}^\top & K_{\bar{J} \times \bar{J}} \end{bmatrix}, \qquad \tilde{K} = \begin{bmatrix} K_{J \times J} & K_{J \times \bar{J}} \\ K_{\bar{J} \times J}^\top & K_{\bar{J} \times J}^\top K_{J \times J}^{-1} K_{J \times \bar{J}} \end{bmatrix} \qquad (1)$$

where $\tilde{K}$ is the matrix estimated via the Nyström method [21]. The Nyström extension leads to the approximation $K_{\bar{J} \times \bar{J}} \approx K_{\bar{J} \times J}^\top K_{J \times J}^{-1} K_{J \times \bar{J}}$. The matrix inverse is replaced by the Moore-Penrose generalized inverse in the case of rank deficiency. The Nyström method leads to the minimal kernel completion [3] conditioned on the selected landmarks and has been reported to perform well in numerous applications [8,13,18]. The challenge lies in finding landmarks that minimize the reconstruction error

$$\|K - \tilde{K}\|_{\mathrm{tr}} = \mathrm{tr}(K_{\bar{J} \times \bar{J}}) - \mathrm{tr}(K_{\bar{J} \times J}^\top K_{J \times J}^{-1} K_{J \times \bar{J}}). \qquad (2)$$

The trace norm $\|.\|_{\mathrm{tr}}$ is applied because results only depend on the spectrum due to its unitary invariance.

2.2 Annealed Determinantal Sampling

A large variety of methods have been proposed for selecting the subset J. For general matrix approximation, this step is referred to as row/column selection of the matrix K, which is equivalent to selecting a subset of points X. This property is important because it avoids explicit computation of the $\mathcal{O}(n^2)$ entries in the kernel matrix K. We focus on volume sampling for subset selection because of its theoretical advantages [9]. We employ the factorization $K_{J \times J} = Y_J^\top Y_J$, which exists because K_J is positive semidefinite. Columns in Y_J can be thought of as feature vectors describing the selected points. Based on this factorization, the volume $\mathrm{Vol}(\{Y_i\}_{i \in J})$ of the simplex spanned by the origin and the feature vectors Y_J is calculated, which is equivalent to the volume of the parallelepiped spanned by Y_J. The subset J is then sampled proportionally to the squared volume. This is directly related to the calculation of the determinant with $\det(K_{J \times J}) = \det(Y_J^\top Y_J) = \det(Y_J)^2 = \mathrm{Vol}^2(\{Y_i\}_{i \in J})$. These ideas were further generalized in [3] based on annealed determinantal distributions

$$p^s(J) \propto \det(K_{J \times J})^s = \det(Y_J^\top Y_J)^s = \det(Y_J)^{2s}. \qquad (3)$$

This distribution is well defined because the principal submatrices of a positive semidefinite matrix are themselves positive semidefinite. Varying the exponent

$s \geq 0$ results in a family of distributions, modeling the annealing behavior as used in stochastic computations. For $s = 0$ this is equivalent to uniform sampling [21]. In the following derivations, we focus on $s = 1$. It was shown in [9] that for $J \sim p(J), |J| = k$

$$\mathbb{E}\left[\|K - \tilde{K}\|_{\mathrm{tr}}\right] \leq (k + 1)\|K - K_k\|_F^2, \tag{4}$$

where $\tilde{K}$ is the Nyström reconstruction of the kernel based on the subset J, K_k the best rank-k approximation achieved by selecting the largest eigenvectors, and $\|.\|_F$ the Frobenius norm. It was further shown that the factor $k + 1$ is the best possible for a k-subset. Related bounds were presented in [4].

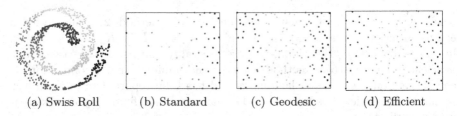

(a) Swiss Roll   (b) Standard   (c) Geodesic   (d) Efficient

Fig. 1. DPP sampling from 1,000 points lying on a manifold. We show results for standard DPP sampling, geodesic DPP sampling, and efficient DPP sampling. Note that the sampling is performed in 3D, but we can plot the underlying 2D manifold by reversing the construction of the Swiss roll. Geodesic and efficient sampling yields a diverse subset from the manifold.

3   Method

We first analyze the sampling from determinantal distributions on non-Euclidean geometries. We then introduce an efficient algorithm for approximate DPP sampling on manifolds. Finally, we present our approach for robust graph construction on sparsely sampled manifolds.

3.1   DPP Sampling on Manifolds

As described in Sect. 2.2, sampling from determinantal distributions is used for row/column selection. Independently, determinantal point processes (DPPs) were introduced for modeling probabilistic mutual exclusion. They present an attractive scheme for ensuring diversity in the selected subset. Here we work with the construction of DPPs based on L-ensembles [7]. Given a positive semi-definite matrix $L \in \mathbb{R}^{n \times n}$, the likelihood for selecting the subset $J \subseteq \{1, \ldots, n\}$ is

$$P_L(J) = \frac{\det(L_{J \times J})}{\det(L + I)}, \tag{5}$$

where I is the identity matrix and $L_{J \times J}$ is the sub-matrix of L containing the rows and columns indexed by J. By associating the L-ensemble matrix L with the kernel matrix K, we can apply DPPs to sample subsets from the point set X.

To date, applications using determinantal point processes have assumed Euclidean geometry [15]. For non-linear dimensionality reduction, we assume that the data points lie in a non-Euclidean space, such as the Swiss roll in Fig. 1(a). To evaluate the performance of DPPs on manifolds, we sample from the Swiss roll. Since we know the construction rule in this case, we can invert it and display the sampled 3D points in the underlying 2D space. The result in Fig. 1(b) shows that the inner part of the roll is almost entirely neglected, as a consequence of not taking the manifold structure into account. A common solution is to use geodesic distances [19], which can be approximated by the graph shortest path algorithm. We replace the Euclidean distance $\|.\|$ in the construction of the kernel matrix K with the geodesic distance $K_{i,j} = \exp(-\|x_i - x_j\|_{\text{geo}}^2 / 2\sigma^2)$ to obtain the result in Fig. 1(c). We observe a clear improvement in the diversity of the sampling, now also including points in the interior part of the Swiss roll.

3.2 Efficient Approximation of DPP Sampling on Manifolds

While it is possible to adapt determinantal sampling to non-Euclidean geometries and to characterize the error for the subset selection, we are missing an efficient sampling algorithm for handling large point sets. In [9], an approximative sampling based on the Markov chain Monte Carlo method is proposed to circumvent the combinatorial problem with $\binom{n}{k}$ possible subsets. Further approximations include sampling proportionally to the diagonal elements K_{ii} or their squared version K_{ii}^2, leading to additive error bounds [4,11]. In [10], an algorithm is proposed that yields a $k!$ approximation to volume sampling, worsening the approximation from $(k+1)$ to $(k+1)!$.

Algorithm 1. DPP sampling equivalent to [15]

Require: Eigen decomposition of K: $\{(v_i, \lambda_i)\}_{i=1}^{n}$
1: Initialize $V = \varnothing$
2: **for** i = 1 to n **do**
3:     Add eigenvector v_i with probability $\frac{\lambda_i}{\lambda_i + 1}$ to V
4: **end for**
5: $B = V^{\mathsf{T}}$
6: **for** 1 to $|V|$ **do**
7:     Select $i \in 1 \dots n$ with probability $P(i) \propto \|B_i\|^2$
8:     $J \leftarrow J \cup i$
9:     $B_j \leftarrow \text{Proj}_{\perp B_i} B_j$ for all $j \in \{1, \dots, n\}$
10: **end for**
11: **return** J

An exact sampling algorithm for DPPs was presented in [14,15], which requires the eigen decomposition of $K = \sum_{i=1}^{n} \lambda_i v_i v_i^{\mathsf{T}}$. Algorithm 1 states an equivalent formulation of this sampling approach. First, eigenvectors are selected proportionally to the magnitude of their eigenvalues and stored as columns in V. Assuming m vectors are selected, $V \in \mathbb{R}^{n \times m}$. By setting $B = V^\top$, we use $B_i \in \mathbb{R}^m$ to denote the rows of V. In each iteration, we select one of the n points where point i is selected proportionally to the squared norm $\|B_i\|^2$. The selected point is added to the subset J. After the selection of i, all vectors B_j are projected to the orthogonal space of B_i. Since $\mathrm{Proj}_{\perp B_i} B_i = 0$, the same point is almost surely not selected twice. The update formulation differs from [15], where an orthonormal basis of the eigenvectors in V perpendicular to the i-th basis vector $e_i \in \mathbb{R}^n$ is constructed. Both formulations are equivalent but provide a different point of view on the algorithm. This modification is essential to motivate the proposed efficient sampling procedure. The following proposition characterizes the behavior of the update rule in the algorithm.

Proposition 1. *Let* $B_i, B_j \in \mathbb{R}^m \setminus \{0\}$ *be two non-zero vectors in* $\mathbb{R}^m$, *and* $\theta = \angle(B_i, B_j)$ *be the angle between them. Then*

$$\|\mathrm{Proj}_{\perp B_i} B_j\|^2 = \|B_j\|^2 \sin^2 \theta, \tag{6}$$

where $\mathrm{Proj}_{\perp B_i} B_j$ *is the the projection of* B_j *on the subspace perpendicular to* B_i. *For* $B_i \neq 0$ *and* $B_j = 0$ *the projection is* $\|\mathrm{Proj}_{\perp B_i} B_j\|^2 = 0$.

Sampling from a determinantal distribution is not only advantageous because of the presented error bounds but it also makes intuitive sense that a selection of a diverse set of points yields a more accurate matrix reconstruction. The computational complexity of Algorithm 1 is, however, similar or even higher than that of manifold learning because the spectral decomposition of a dense graph is required, whereas Laplacian eigenmaps operate on sparse matrices. An approach for efficient sampling proposed in [15] works with the dual representation of $K = Y^\top Y$ to obtain $Q = YY^\top$, with Q hopefully smaller than the matrix K. Considering that we work with a Gaussian kernel matrix, this factorization corresponds to the inner product in feature space $\phi(x_i)^\top \phi(x_j)$ of the original points x_i, x_j. The Gaussian kernel corresponds to an infinite dimensional feature space. Since we work with symmetric, positive definite matrices, we can calculate a Cholesky decomposition. In this case, the dual representation has the same size as the original matrix and therefore yields no improvement.

To overcome the high computational costs of exact DPP sampling, we present an efficient approximation in Algorithm 2. The computational complexity is $\mathcal{O}(ndk)$. Vector $D \in \mathbb{R}^n$ models the probabilities for the selection of points as does $\|B_i\|^2$ in the original DPP sampling algorithm. The algorithm proceeds by sampling k points. At each iteration we select one point x_i with probability $p(i) \propto D_i$. Next we compute distances $\{\Delta_j\}_{j=1...n}$ of the selected point x_i to all points in X. Based on these distances we identify a local neighborhood $\mathcal{N}_i$ of m nearest neighbors around the selected point x_i. The update of the probabilities D is restricted to the neighborhood $\mathcal{N}_i$, which proves advantageous for sampling on manifolds. In contrast, Algorithm 1 updates probabilities for all points. If we seek a similar behavior to Algorithm 1, the local neighborhood should include

---

Algorithm 2. Efficient approximation of DPP sampling

Require: Point set X, subset cardinality k, nearest neighbor count m, update function f
1: Initialize $D = \mathbf{1}_n$ and $J = \varnothing$
2: **for** 1 to k **do**
3:     Select $i \in 1 \ldots n$ with probability $p(i) \propto D_i$
4:     $J \leftarrow J \cup \{i\}$
5:     Compute $\Delta_j = \|x_i - x_j\|$, $\forall j \in 1 \ldots n$
6:     Set m nearest neighbors of x_i as neighborhood $\mathcal{N}_i$ based on $\{\Delta_j\}_{j=1 \ldots n}$
7:     $D_j \leftarrow D_j \cdot f(\Delta_j)$, $\forall j \in \mathcal{N}_i$
8:     Optional: Compute covariance C_i in local neighborhood $\mathcal{N}_i$ around x_i
9: **end for**
10: **return** J and optionally $\{C_i\}_{i \in J}$

---

all points. The update function f takes distances Δ as input, where we consider $f(\Delta) = \sin^2(\Delta/\tau)$ and $f(\Delta) = (1 - \exp(-\Delta^2/2\sigma^2))$, as motivated below. In subsequent iterations of the algorithm, points close to x_i are selected with lower probability.

We initialize the vector $D = \mathbf{1}_n$, since it was noted in [15] that the squared norm of the vectors $\|B_i\|^2$ gives rise initially to a fairly uniform distribution because no points have yet been selected. For the update step, Proposition 1 implies that the update of the probabilities of selecting specific points acts as $\sin^2(\theta)$. The angle $\theta = \angle(B_i, B_j)$ correlates strongly with the distance $\|B_i - B_j\|$, since $\|B_j\|$ and $\|B_i\|$ are initially the same. In Algorithm 1, the largest eigenvalues are selected with high probability. We can therefore draw the analogy to multidimensional scaling (MDS) [20] with a Gaussian kernel, where MDS selects the top eigenvectors. Consequently, vectors B_i correspond to low-dimensional embeddings produced by multidimensional scaling of original points x_i. MDS preserves pairwise distances between the original space and the embedding space, enabling the approximation $\|B_i - B_j\| \approx \|x_i - x_j\|$. We approximate the update based on the distance of points in the original space, $\sin^2(\theta) \approx \sin^2(\|x_i - x_j\|/\tau)$. The scaling factor τ ensures that values are in the range $[-\pi/2; \pi/2]$. This update is similar to the Welsch function $(1 - \exp(-\|x_i - x_j\|^2/2\sigma^2))$, which is directly related to the weights in the kernel matrix and is commonly used in machine learning. For subsequent iterations of the algorithm, the assumption of a similar norm of all vectors B_i is violated, because the projection on the orthogonal space changes their lengths. However, this change is locally restricted around the currently selected point. Since this region is less likely to be sampled in the subsequent iterations, the assumption still holds for parts of the space that contain most probability.

Remark. The proposed algorithm bears similarities to K-means++ [1], which replaces the initialization through uniform sampling of K-means by a new seeding algorithm. K-means++ seeding is a heuristic that samples points based on their distance to the closest selected landmark. Initially, when only one landmark is selected, our algorithm has a nearly identical update rule for a maximal neighborhood $\mathcal{N}_i$. In later iterations, the algorithms differ because K-means++ bases the selection only on the distance to the nearest landmark, while all landmarks influence the probability space in our algorithm. Consequently, our approach potentially yields subsets with higher diversity.

3.3 Robust Landmark-Based Graph Construction

After selecting the landmarks, the next step in the spectral analysis consists of building a graph that approximates the manifold. Common techniques for the graph construction include selection of nearest neighbors or ε-balls around each node. Both approaches require the setting of a parameter, either the number of neighbors or the size of the ball, which is crucial for the performance. Setting the parameter too low leads to a large number of disconnected components, while for many applications one is interested in having all points connected to obtain a consistent embedding of all points. Choosing too high values of the parameters leads to shortcuts, yielding a poor approximation of the manifold. The appropriate selection of the parameters is more challenging on sparsely sampled manifolds, obtained after the subset selection.

To address this issue, we propose a new technique for graph construction that takes the initial distribution of the points into account. For each landmark x_i, we estimate the covariance matrix C_i around this point from its nearest neighbors $\mathcal{N}_i$, as indicated as optional step in Algorithm 2. This step implies a multivariate Gaussian distribution $\mathcal{G}(x_i, C_i)$ centered at the landmark x_i. A commonly used distance to compare distributions is the Bhattacharyya distance, which in case of Gaussian distributions corresponds to

$$B(\mathcal{G}_i, \mathcal{G}_j) = \frac{1}{8}(x_i - x_j)^\top C^{-1}(x_i - x_j) + \frac{1}{2}\ln\left(\frac{|C|}{\sqrt{|C_i||C_j|}}\right), \qquad (7)$$

with $C = \frac{C_i + C_j}{2}$. This distance is less likely to produce shortcuts across the manifold because points that fit the local geometry appear much closer than points that appear as outliers from the local geometry. Consequently, we replace the Euclidean distance for neighborhood selection in manifold learning with the Bhattacharyya distance. Space requirements of this step are $\mathcal{O}(d^2 k)$. An alternative for limited space and large d is to only use the diagonal entries of the covariance matrix, requiring $\mathcal{O}(dk)$ space.

4 Experiments

In our first experiment, we show that the proposed efficient DPP sampling algorithm is well suited for subset selection in non-Euclidean spaces. The algorithm restricts the update of the sampling probability D to a local neighborhood $\mathcal{N}_i$ around the current point x_i. This is in line with the motivation of many manifold learning algorithms that assume that the space behaves locally like a Euclidean

Table 1. Average reconstruction errors over 50 runs for several sampling schemes with subset sizes varying from 25 to 100. Best results are highlighted in bold face.

Sampling	25	50	60	70	80	90	100
Uniform	70.384	8.006	4.838	2.785	1.676	0.731	0.442
K-means Uniform	28.124	3.848	2.319	1.393	0.756	0.403	0.235
K-means++ Seeding	50.114	5.832	3.033	1.655	1.013	0.683	0.347
K-means++	**24.954**	3.575	1.915	1.018	0.711	0.383	0.222
Efficient DPP	33.036	**3.371**	**1.466**	**0.844**	**0.488**	**0.312**	**0.202**

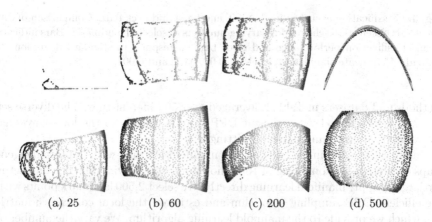

(a) 25   (b) 60   (c) 200   (d) 500

Fig. 2. Selection of 2,500 landmarks from a set of 10 million points. Embedding of landmarks into 2D with Laplacian eigenmaps. Results for Euclidean (first row) and Bhattacharyya neighborhood selection (second row) are shown.

space. In our experiment, we set the local neighborhood $\mathcal{N}_i$ to be the 20 nearest neighbors around the selected point x_i. The sampling result is shown in Fig. 1(d). We obtain a point set with high diversity, covering the entire manifold. This illustrates that the proposed algorithm provides diversity on complex geometries and is therefore appropriate for subset selection in the context of non-linear dimensionality reduction.

In our second experiment, we quantify the reconstruction error for matrix completion as formulated in Eq. (2). We compare the efficient DPP sampling result with uniform sampling [21] and K-means clustering with uniform seeding [22], which represents current state-of-the-art [16]. Moreover, we compare to selecting the subset with the K-means++ seeding and the K-means++ algorithm, which we have not been used for landmark selection before. We construct a Gaussian kernel matrix from 1,000 points on a Swiss roll (Fig. 1). We select subsets of varying size between 25 and 100 and set the parameters $\sigma = 1$ and $m = 30$ for the Swiss roll. Note that a further improvement can be achieved by adapting these parameters to the size of the subset. For smaller subsets, larger σ and m lead to improvements. We report the reconstruction error for the different

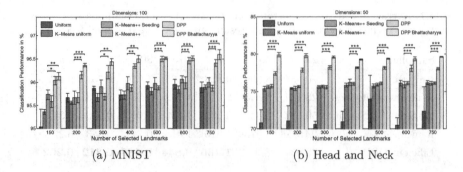

(a) MNIST   (b) Head and Neck

Fig. 3. Classification accuracy for MNIST and head and neck data. Comparison of different subset selection schemes for varying numbers of selected landmarks. Bars indicate mean classification performance and error bars correspond to standard deviation. *, **, and *** indicate significance levels at 0.05, 0.01, and 0.001.

methods and datasets in Table 1, averaged over 50 different runs. The diverse set of landmarks selected with efficient DPP sampling leads to the lowest average reconstruction errors in almost all settings.

In our third experiment, we perform manifold learning with Laplacian eigenmaps on a point set consisting of 10 million points on a Swiss roll. The dataset is too large to apply manifold learning directly. We select 2,500 landmark points with the efficient DPP sampling algorithm and estimate the local covariance matrices, which we provide to the manifold learning algorithm. We vary the number of nearest neighbors in the graph from 25 to 500. We compare the graph construction with Euclidean and Bhattacharyya neighborhood selection with embedding results shown in Fig. 2. The results show that the Bhattacharyya based neighborhood selection is more robust with respect to the number of neighbors.

4.1 Image Data

After having evaluated each of the steps of the proposed approach separately, we now present results for scalable manifold learning on image data. We work with two datasets, one consisting of handwritten digits and a second one consisting of patches extracted from 3D medical images. Each dataset is too large to apply manifold learning directly. Consequently, we select landmarks with the discussed method, perform manifold learning on the landmarks with the Bhattacharyya distance, and use the Nyström method to embed the entire point set. We only consider the diagonal entries of the covariance matrices due to space limitations. The exact formula for the out-of-sample extension with the Nyström method for Laplacian eigenmaps is derived in [6]. To evaluate the quality of the embedding, we use the labels associated to the image data to perform nearest neighbor classification in the low dimensional space. We expect advantages for the DPP landmark selection scheme because a diverse set of landmarks spreads the entire point set in the embedding space and helps the classification.

We avoid sophisticated pre-processing of the data, since we are only interested in the relative performances across the different landmark selection methods.

We evaluate the method on the MNIST dataset [17], consisting of 60,000 binary images of handwritten digits for training and 10,000 for testing with a resolution of 28×28 pixels, and on CT scans with a resolution of $512 \times 512 \times 145$ voxels. The CT scans were acquired for radiation therapy of patients with head and neck tumors. The figure on the right shows one cross sectional slice with segmentations of three structures of risk: left parotid (red), right parotid (blue), and brainstem (green). The segmentation of these structures during treatment planning is of 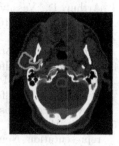 high clinical importance to ensure that they obtain a low radiation dose. We extract image patches from the left and right parotid glands, the brainstem and the surrounding background. We aim to classify patches into these four groups, where the outcome can readily serve in segmentation algorithms. We work with patches of size $7 \times 7 \times 3$ to reflect the physical resolution of the data which is $0.98 \times 0.98 \times 2.5$ mm^3. This results in roughly 150,000 patches extracted from three scans. 80,000 patches are used for training and the remaining ones for testing. We set $m = 5000$ and $\sigma = 5$ in this experiment. We embed the images into 100 dimensional space with Laplacian eigenmaps. Figure 3 reports classification results over 20 repetitions for several landmark selection schemes across different numbers of landmarks k, as well as the Bhattacharyya based graph construction. The results suggest that the K-means++ seeding outperforms the uniform initialization and K-means++ cannot further improve the initialization. Moreover, we observe a significant improvement in classification performance for approximate DPP sampling compared to K-Means++ seeding. Finally, the Bhattacharyya based graph construction further improves the results. In addition to the significant improvement, our runtime measurements showed that our unoptimized Matlab code for efficient DPP sampling runs approximately 15 % faster than an optimized MEX version of K-means.

5   Conclusion

We have presented contributions for two crucial issues of scalable manifold learning in large datasets: (i) efficient sampling of diverse subsets from manifolds and (ii) robust graph construction on sparsely sampled manifolds. We analyzed the sampling from determinantal distributions in non-Euclidean spaces and proposed an efficient approximation of DPP sampling. Furthermore, we proposed the local covariance estimation around landmarks to capture the local geometry of the space. This enabled a more robust graph construction with the Bhattacharyya distance and yielded low dimensional embeddings of higher quality.

Acknowledgements. This work was supported by the Humboldt foundation, the National Alliance for Medical Image Computing (U54-EB005149), the NeuroImaging Analysis Center (P41-EB015902), and the Wistron Corporation.

References

1. Arthur, D., Vassilvitskii, S.: k-means++: The advantages of careful seeding. In: SODA, pp. 1027–1035 (2007)
2. Balasubramanian, M., Schwartz, E.L.: The Isomap algorithm and topological stability. Science **295**(5552), 7 (2002)
3. Belabbas, M., Wolfe, P.: On landmark selection and sampling in high-dimensional data analysis. In: PNAS (2009)
4. Belabbas, M., Wolfe, P.: Spectral methods in machine learning and new strategies for very large datasets. PNAS **106**(2), 369–374 (2009)
5. Belkin, M., Niyogi, P.: Laplacian eigenmaps for dimensionality reduction and data representation. Neural Comput. **15**(6), 1373–1396 (2003)
6. Bengio, Y., Paiement, J., Vincent, P., Delalleau, O., Le Roux, N., Ouimet, M.: Out-of-sample extensions for lle, isomap, mds, eigenmaps, and spectral clustering. In: NIPS (2004)
7. Borodin, A.: Determinantal point processes. In: Akemann, G., Baik, J., Francesco, P.D. (eds.) The Oxford Handbook of Random Matrix Theory, pp. 231–249. Oxford University Press, Oxford (2011)
8. Chen, W., Song, Y., Bai, H., Lin, C., Chang, E.: Parallel spectral clustering in distributed systems. TPAMI **33**(3), 568–586 (2011)
9. Deshpande, A., Rademacher, L., Vempala, S., Wang, G.: Matrix approximation and projective clustering via volume sampling. In: SODA (2006)
10. Deshpande, A., Vempala, S.S.: Adaptive sampling and fast low-rank matrix approximation. In: Díaz, J., Jansen, K., Rolim, J.D.P., Zwick, U. (eds.) APPROX 2006 and RANDOM 2006. LNCS, vol. 4110, pp. 292–303. Springer, Heidelberg (2006)
11. Drineas, P., Mahoney, M.W.: On the nyström method for approximating a gram matrix for improved kernel-based learning. JMLR **6**, 2153–2175 (2005)
12. Farahat, A., Ghodsi, A., Kamel, M.: A novel greedy algorithm for nyström approximation. In: IASTATS (2011)
13. Fowlkes, C., Belongie, S., Chung, F., Malik, J.: Spectral grouping using the nyström method. TPAMI **26**(2), 214–225 (2004)
14. Hough, J., Krishnapur, M., Peres, Y., Virág, B.: Determinantal processes and independence. Probab. Surv. **3**, 206–229 (2006)
15. Kulesza, A., Taskar, B.: Structured determinantal point processes. In: NIPS (2010)
16. Kumar, S., Mohri, M., Talwalkar, A.: Sampling techniques for the nystrom method. J. Mach. Learn. Res. **13**, 981–1006 (2012)
17. LeCun, Y., Bottou, L., Bengio, Y., Haffner, P.: Gradient-based learning applied to document recognition. Proc. IEEE **86**(11), 2278–2324 (1998)
18. Talwalkar, A., Kumar, S., Rowley, H.: Large-scale manifold learning. In: CVPR (2008)
19. Tenenbaum, J., Silva, V., Langford, J.: A global geometric framework for nonlinear dimensionality reduction. Science **290**(5500), 2319–2323 (2000)
20. Williams, C.: On a connection between kernel PCA and metric multidimensional scaling. In: NIPS, pp. 675–681 (2001)
21. Williams, C., Seeger, M.: Using the nyström method to speed up kernel machines. In: NIPS, pp. 682–688 (2001)
22. Zhang, K., Tsang, I., Kwok, J.: Improved nyström low-rank approximation and error analysis. In: ICML, pp. 1232–1239. ACM (2008)

Model-Based Estimation of Microscopic Anisotropy in Macroscopically Isotropic Substrates Using Diffusion MRI

Andrada Ianuş[✉], Ivana Drobnjak, and Daniel C. Alexander

Centre for Medical Image Computing,
University College London, London, UK
a.ianus.11@ucl.ac.uk

Abstract. Non-invasive estimation of cell size and shape is a key challenge in diffusion MRI. Changes in cell size and shape discriminate functional areas in the brain and can highlight different degrees of malignancy in cancer tumours. Consequently various methods have emerged recently that aim to measure the microscopic anisotropy of porous media such as biological tissue and aim to reflect pore eccentricity, the simplest shape feature. However, current methods assume a substrate of identical pores, and are strongly influenced by non-trivial size distribution. This paper presents a model-based approach that provides estimates of pore size and shape from diffusion MRI data. The technique uses a geometric model of randomly oriented finite cylinders with gamma distributed radii. We use Monte Carlo simulation to generate synthetic data in substrates consisting of randomly oriented cuboids with various size distributions and eccentricities. We compare the sensitivity of single and double pulsed field gradient (sPFG and dPFG) sequences to the size distribution and eccentricity and further compare different protocols of dPFG sequences with parallel and/or perpendicular pairs of gradients. The key result demonstrates that this model-based approach can provide features of pore shape (specifically eccentricity) that are independent of the size distribution unlike previous attempts to characterise microscopic anisotropy. We show further that explicitly accounting for size distribution is necessary for accurate estimates of average size and eccentricity, and a model that assumes a single size fails to recover the ground truth values. We find the most accurate parameter estimates for dPFG sequences with mixed parallel and perpendicular gradients, nevertheless all other sequences, including sPFG, show sensitivity as well.

1 Introduction

Diffusion weighted magnetic resonance imaging (DW-MRI) is a non-invasive probe of molecular displacement, providing structural information at the microscopic level. Cellular membranes in the tissue restrict the diffusion of water molecules so that the measured signal is sensitive to cellular architecture. Accurate estimation of pore size and eccentricity from diffusion data is a key challenge in DW-MRI, with potential applications to cancer imaging to discern differences

© Springer International Publishing Switzerland 2015
S. Ourselin et al. (Eds.): IPMI 2015, LNCS 9123, pp. 699–710, 2015.
DOI: 10.1007/978-3-319-19992-4_55

in tumour microstructure [1], white matter imaging to map axon diameter in the presence of orientation dispersion [2] and undulation [3], grey matter imaging to discriminate cytoarchitectures [4], and muscle imaging to assess the degree of injury [5].

The single pulsed field gradient (sPFG) sequence is the standard pulse sequences for acquiring diffusion MRI data. A collection of sPFG measurements is sensitive to pore-size distribution in isotropic pores or coherently oriented anisotropic pores [1,6–8]. However it fails to discriminate between more complex systems, such as isotropic pores with a size distribution and randomly oriented anisotropic pores. More sophisticated pulse sequences, in particular those that have varying gradient orientation within one measurement such as double PFG [9] can remove this ambiguity [10]. This observation has led to various measures of microscopic anisotropy from contrasting dPFG measurements with different combinations of gradient orientation, such as the microscopic anisotropy MA index [11] or fractional eccentricity FE [12]. Similarly, [13] used a combination of gradient waveforms which provide isotropic diffusion weighting, to a arrive at a similar metric. Nevertheless, such indices lack a quantitative interpretation, as they depend on sequence parameters and are not invariant to pore size distributions.

Here we explore a model-based approach to estimate microscopic anisotropy, which offers the key benefit of providing estimates of intrinsic tissue parameters independent of the acquisition protocol. Previously, a model of identical pores featuring microscopic anisotropy (finite cylinders) [14] has been employed to show differences between isotropic substrates in the special cases of spherical pores or randomly oriented cylindrical pores [15]. We demonstrate in simulation the feasibility of using such an approach to provide more quantitative information on compartment shape that is invariant to size distribution for a wide range of substrates. First, we show that standard indices of microscopic anisotropy confound different configurations of pores. We construct a signal model for both sPFG and dPFG assuming restricting geometry of randomly oriented finite cylinders with gamma distributed radii to analyse synthetic diffusion data provided by Monte Carlo (MC) simulations. We use it to recover size and shape parameters from MC simulated data from substrates consisting of randomly oriented cuboids with various size distribution and eccentricities. The experiments further allow us to compare the ability of sPFG and dPFG sequences to recover the ground truth parameters.

2   Background

This section provides some context for the new method we propose and reviews techniques for estimating microscopic anisotropy.

2.1   Microstructure Imaging

The most common diffusion MRI technique is diffusion tensor imaging (DTI) which provides familiar indices, such as fractional anisotropy (FA) and mean diffusivity (MD) that inform tissue micro-architecture. However, these indices lack specificity, as many different microstructural features (cell size, density, shape, orientation distribution, and permeability) affect FA and MD, so contrast in these indices is hard to assign to specific mechanisms. Microstructure imaging uses mathematical models to relate tissue features directly to the signal and thus supports estimates of specific tissue parameters from combinations of diffusion MRI measurements. For example the CHARMED model in AxCaliber [6] estimates axon diameter distribution and density from diffusion measurements perpendicular to white matter tracts. ActiveAx [7] adapts the modelling technique and acquisition protocol to recover these indices in a rotationally invariant framework. Later work [16] extends the model to include fibre dispersion and a comprehensive list of possible white matter models is compared in [8]. VERDICT [1] extends the modelling approach to characterise cancerous tissue and has successfully recovered tumour specific microstructural indices such as cell size and density, vascular volume fraction and cellularity. These techniques all use protocols of simple sPFG measurements.

2.2 dPFG Sequences and Indices of Microscopic Anisotropy

The double pulsed-field gradient (dPFG) sequence [9] concatenates two sPFG sequences separated by a mixing time. dPFG sequences probe the correlation of water displacement at different time scales and in different directions, which can provide sensitivity to features less visible to sPFG, such as pore shape or exchange rate. In practice, protocols of dPFG measurements cover different subsets of the full measurement space depending on what tissue features they intend to investigate. For example, in the limit of short pulses, long diffusion time and short mixing time, pairs of diffusion gradients with the same amplitude and varying orientations have been used to estimate pore size [17]. In the long mixing time regime, the dependence of diffusion signal on the angle between the two gradients reflects pore eccentricity [10,14]. Based on the difference between dPFG measurements with parallel and perpendicular gradients, recent work proposes a model free approach to disentangle microscopic anisotropy from macroscopic anisotropy [11,12].

We briefly present the technique from [12] which keeps the first 4 terms in the cumulant expansion of the dPFG signal. We use this method in the first experiment described in Sect. 3 to illustrate that FE depends on pore size distribution, given a set of sequence parameters, but the same observation holds for similar indices presented in [11,13]. For a macroscopically isotropic substrate:

$$\log(S_\parallel) - \log(S_\perp) = q^4 \epsilon, \tag{1}$$

where $S_\parallel$ is the signal for the dPFG sequence with parallel gradients, $S_\perp$ is the signal for the dPFG sequence with perpendicular gradients, $q = \gamma G \delta$ is the wavenumber, γ the gyromagnetic ratio, G the gradient strength, δ the pulse duration and ϵ depends on pore size and eccentricity. For spherical pores $\epsilon = 0$. To normalize ϵ with respect to size, [12] introduced the fractional eccentricity index FE which varies between 0 (isotropic pores) and 1 (elongated pores):

$$FE = \sqrt{\frac{\epsilon}{\epsilon + 3\Delta^2 ADC^2/5}} \qquad (2)$$

where Δ is the diffusion time (see Fig. 1) and ADC is the apparent diffusion coefficient which reflects the length scale of the substrate.

3   Methods

This section presents the simulations and models we use in this paper to illustrate the feasibility of estimating pore shape and size distribution from diffusion MRI data using a model-based approach.

3.1   Data Synthesis

To synthesize diffusion data we use the MC simulator in Camino [18] with a mesh-based substrate. The mesh consists of 200 randomly oriented cuboids with two equal sides ($l_x = l_y$) and a gamma distribution of sizes, as illustrated in Fig. 1b. We choose a different geometric model to synthesize the data in order to emphasize the robustness of our approach when the geometry is not a perfect match. We prefer cuboids over ellipsoids due to the reduced computational complexity of the mesh. The parameters of the model are the mean width of the cuboid l_x, the ratio between the height and width $E = l_z/l_x$ (eccentricity), which is the same for all sizes, the gamma distribution shape parameter a and the diffusivity constant D. We construct separate substrates for each combination the following parameter values: $l_x = \{2, 4, ..., 12\}\,\mu\text{m}$, $E = \{1, 1.5, 2, 2.5, 3\}$, $a = \{2.5, 10, \infty\}$ ($a \to \infty$ yields identical pores) and $D = 2E - 9$ s/m^2. The MC simulation has 1000 time steps and 20000 walkers, all located inside the pores. Noise, with a Rician distribution and a signal-to-noise ratio (SNR) of 50 was added to the data to create 10 different data sets for each substrate.

3.2   Measurement Protocols

For the model based approach, we compare four different measurement protocols constructed from basic sPFG and dPFG sequences shown in Fig. 1a. As we are interested in a wide range of pore sizes, we construct a rich protocol for each sequence type. For a fair comparison we choose sequence parameters that yield the same maximum diffusion weighting (b-value) and number of measurements in each protocol. The protocols are:

1. **sPFG** protocol has the following parameters: pulse duration $\delta = \{5, 10, ..., 25\}$ ms, time interval between the beginning of the first and second gradients $\Delta = \delta + \{5, 10, 20, 30, 40\}$ ms and gradient strength $G = \{25, 50, 75, 100, 300, 500\}\sqrt{2}$ mT/m. The $\sqrt{2}$ factor ensures the same b-values for all protocols.
2. **dPFG$_\parallel$** protocol has dPFG sequences with parallel gradients of equal amplitudes. The other parameters are: $\delta = \{5, 10, ..., 25\}$ ms, $\Delta = \delta + \{5, 10, 20, 30, 40\}$ ms, mixing time $t_m = \Delta$ and $G = \{25, 50, 75, 100, 300, 500\}$ mT/m.

3. **dPFG$_\perp$** protocol - has dPFG sequences with perpendicular gradients of equal amplitudes. The rest of the parameters are the same as for **dPFG$_\parallel$**.
4. **dPFG$_{\parallel\&\perp}$** protocol has dPFG sequences with both parallel and perpendicular gradients. To have the same number of measurements we keep every other parameter combination from **dPFG$_\parallel$**.

For investigating the dependence of FE on pore eccentricity we choose a subset of the measurements used for model fitting which is the closest to the theoretical requirement of short pulse duration and long diffusion and mixing times: $\delta = 5\,\text{ms}$, $\Delta = t_m = 45\,\text{ms}$ and $G = 500\,\text{mT/m}$.

3.3   Signal Model and Fitting

We construct two signal models for estimating parameters of size and eccentricity by fitting to data from protocols defined in Sect. 3.2. Each assumes macroscopically isotropic signal, but with microscopic anisotropy. The model are:

1. **Finite astro-cylinders** (FAC) consists of randomly oriented identical finite cylinders and is illustrated in Fig. 1c. This model has three parameters: cylin-

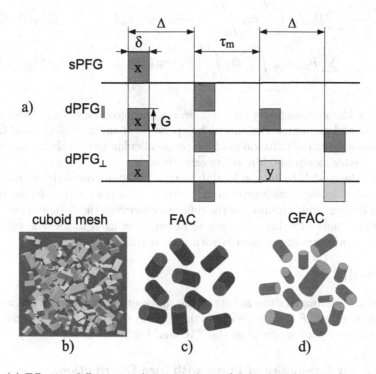

Fig. 1. (a) Effective diffusion gradient waveforms (accounting for the effect of 180° rf pulses) for sPFG, dPFG with parallel gradients and with perpendicular gradients. (b) Mesh based diffusion substrate for MC simulations ($l_x = 6\,\mu\text{m}$, $E = 2$, $a = 10$). (c) Schematic representation of the FAC model. (d) Schematic representation of the GFAC

der radius R, ratio between cylinder length and diameter E (eccentricity) and diffusivity constant D.

2. **Gamma finite astro-cylinders** (GFAC) consists of randomly oriented finite cylinders with a gamma distribution of radii, so explicitly accounts for a size distribution, as illustrated in Fig. 1d. This model has four parameters: D, mean radius $\bar{R}$, the gamma distribution shape parameter a and eccentricity E which is the same across all sizes.

For fast signal computation, we extend the GPD approximation [19] for dPFG sequences and a restriction model of randomly oriented finite cylinders with various sizes. This provides analytical expressions of the signal $S(\mathbf{u}, R)$ for a finite cylinder with orientation $\mathbf{u}$, radius R and length $2RE$, which we then numerically integrate over orientation and size distribution weighted by volume, to obtain the overall signal $S = \int_{\mathbf{u}} \int_0^\infty \mathcal{P}(R)S(\mathbf{u}, R)d\mathbf{u}R^3 dR$. $\mathcal{P}(R)$ is the probability distribution of radii and the factor R^3 arises because the diffusion MRI signal from each pore depends on the amount of spins it contains and in our model the length of the cylinder is proportional to the radius. Assuming independence of parallel and perpendicular displacements [20], the signal for one cylinder is then $S(\mathbf{u}, R) = S_{\perp,\mathbf{u}}S_{\|,\mathbf{u}}$ with

$$\ln S_{\perp,\mathbf{u}} = \frac{\gamma^2}{2} \sum_n B_{cyl,n} \int_0^{TE} dt_1 \int_0^{TE} dt_2 \exp\left(-\lambda_{cyl,n}D|t_2 - t_1|\right) \mathbf{G}_\perp(t_1) \cdot \mathbf{G}_\perp(t_2)$$

$$\ln S_{\|,\mathbf{u}} = \frac{\gamma^2}{2} 2 \sum_n B_{plane,n} \int_0^{TE} dt_1 \int_0^{TE} dt_2 \exp\left(-\lambda_{plane,n}D|t_2 - t_1|\right) \mathbf{G}_\|(t_1) \cdot \mathbf{G}_\|(t_2)$$

$$(3)$$

where γ is the gyromagnetic ratio B_n and λ_n are geometry related factors for cylindrical and planar restriction which depend on R and E [21], $\mathbf{G}_\perp$ and $\mathbf{G}_\|$ are the components of the diffusion gradient perpendicular and parallel, respectively, to the cylinder axis $\mathbf{u}$ and TE is the echo time.

We fit the models to data in Matlab using a two-step procedure: a grid search of predefined values, which gives rough estimates of parameters, followed by a gradient descent which minimizes the difference between the data and the model given Rician noise. During all stages of fitting D is fixed to its true value and all other parameters are estimated with no constraints.

4   Results

This section summarizes the results of the different experiments. First we show the dependence of FE on pore eccentricity, then we present the estimation of microstructural parameters from the FAC and GFAC models.

4.1 FE for Ensembles of Pores with Size Distribution

Figure 2 plots the FE from Eq. 2 against cuboid eccentricity in the range $E \in [1, 3]$ for substrates of various mean sizes $l_x = \{4, 8, 12\}\,\mu m$ and size distribution $a = \{2.5, 10, \infty\}$. It confirms that indices such as FE do not provide a truly quantitative measure of pore shape, because they are not invariant to pore size distribution, although the FE does increase monotonically with cuboid eccentricity. Figure 2 also shows that FE is highly noise sensitive, which arises from its dependence on the 4th order term of the cumulant expansion. This can be most clearly seen for pores with $l_x = 4\,\mu$m and small eccentricity, as the signal attenuation is very low in this case and the difference between the dPFG sequences with parallel and perpendicular gradients is small and prone to noise.

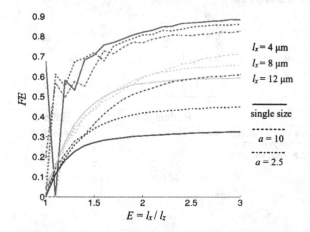

Fig. 2. Dependence of FE on pore eccentricity. Different colours represent different sizes and different line styles represent different shapes of the gamma distribution (Color figure online).

4.2   Parameter Estimation from the FAC Model

Figure 3a shows the parameter estimates (R and E) from the FAC model as a function of the ground truth values used in the MC simulation for sPFG and dPFG$_{\parallel \& \perp}$ protocols. The results show that, if the diffusion substrate consists of identical pores, then a simple model of microscopic anisotropy, such as FAC, can be used to measure average size and eccentricity. For most substrates the maximum difference between the estimated radius and the corresponding ground truth value is less than 15 % and between the estimated eccentricity and the ground truth value is less than 20 %, for all sequences considered. The parameter estimates are more noisy for the substrates with $l_x = 2\,\mu$m, because the size reaches the lower bound of sensitivity with $G_{max} = 500\,$mT/m [22]. A key observation is that, for these simple substrates, the estimates based on sPFG sequences have similar accuracy to those from dPFG sequences. This happens because, for the subset of identical pores, a size distribution in any given direction is generated solely by pore elongation. Figure 3b illustrates the parameter estimates from the FAC model (R and E) for a substrate with a gamma distribution of sizes, with shape parameter $a = 2.5$. The results are presented for sPFG

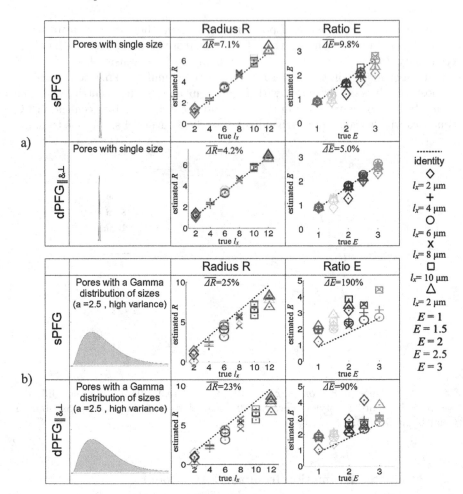

Fig. 3. Estimated parameters (R and E) of the FAC model as function of ground truth values in MC simulations, for (a) a substrate with identical pores and (b) a gamma distribution of sizes. The values were computed as the mean estimates over 10 noise trials with the standard deviation smaller than the size of the symbols. The average relative errors ($\overline{\Delta R}$ and $\overline{\Delta E}$) are also provided. The identity line provides a match between the parameters for cuboids and finite cylinders in a way that ensures the same volume. Thus, for a cuboid with width l_x and $E = l_z/l_x$, the corresponding radius of a finite cylinder is $l_x/\sqrt{\pi}$ and eccentricity is $E\sqrt{\pi}/2$. In addition to this correction, in (b) the identity line also accounts for a volume weighted average.

and dPFG$_{\|\&\perp}$ sequences. The figure shows that, in the presence of a distribution of sizes, the FAC model does not give consistent size and eccentricity estimates from either protocol. The volume weighted average radius is underestimated and the pore eccentricity is overestimated for all diffusion protocols.

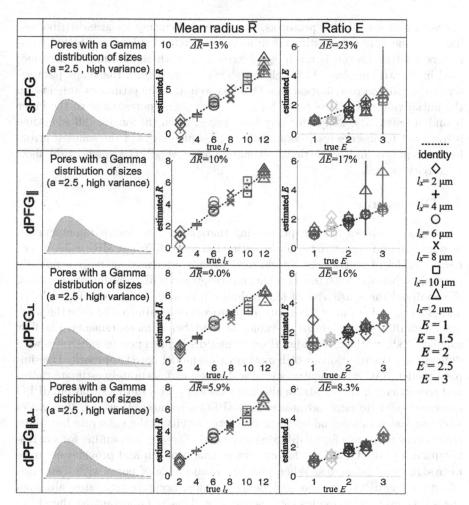

Fig. 4. Estimated parameters ($\bar{R}$ and E) of the GFAC model as a function of ground truth values in MC simulations, for a substrate with a gamma distribution of sizes ($a = 2.5$). The values were computed as the mean estimates over 10 trials of noise with the standard deviation smaller than the size of the symbols, unless otherwise depicted. The average relative errors, excluding outliers, ($\overline{\Delta R}$ and $\overline{\Delta E}$) are also provided. The identity line provides a match between the parameters for cuboids and finite cylinders in a way that ensures the same volume. Thus, for a cuboid with width l_x and $E = l_z/l_x$, the corresponding radius of a finite cylinder is $l_x/\sqrt{\pi}$ and eccentricity is $E\sqrt{\pi}/2$. The volume weighting of the signal is accounted for in the GFAC model.

4.3   Parameter Estimation from the GFAC Model

Figure 4 illustrates $\bar{R}$ and E estimates of the GFAC model for gamma distributed pores with a shape parameter $a = 2.5$ which yields the largest variance considered in this study. The results, including the average relative errors, are presented for all four protocols. Explicitly accounting for size distribution, improves the parameter estimates in more complicated substrates. Fitted parameters from all protocols are in good agreement with the ground truth values used in the MC meshes. Although not shown in the figure, the shape parameter of the gamma distribution was fitted as well and the estimates are close to the initial values. Outliers occur for either very small pores, close to the lower bound of sensitivity [22], or for very large pores, when the longest diffusion time is too short to observe restriction. $dPFG_{\parallel\&\perp}$ sequences yield the smallest errors for both radius and eccentricity estimates, however sPFG sequences do show sensitivity as well.

5 Discussion

This work is a proof of concept showing that microstructural parameters such as pore size and eccentricity can be estimated from diffusion MRI using a geometric model of restriction. Specifically, we are interested in macroscopically isotropic substrates with microscopic anisotropy and a distribution of pore sizes. We analysed the sensitivity of four different protocols: sPFG, $dPFG_{\parallel}$, $dPFG_{\perp}$ and $dPFG_{\parallel\&\perp}$. For fair comparison, all protocols were adjusted to have the same maximum diffusion weighting (b-value) and number of measurements. The first simulation shows that FE index alone cannot distinguish porous substrates with different size distributions, which motivates the model-based approach. The simplest model, FAC which features identical pores, can accurately estimate radius and eccentricity if the substrate also has identical pores. In this situation, dPFG sequences offer no clear advantage over sPFG sequences. However, this model underestimates radius and overestimates eccentricity if the substrate has a distribution of pore sizes for all diffusion sequences. Directly accounting for size distribution, i.e. the GFAC model, overcomes this problem and provides accurate microstructural estimates. When probing an ensemble of pores with a size distribution, the $dPFG_{\parallel\&\perp}$ protocol yields the most accurate estimates, although the sPFG protocol provides clear sensitivity. This is important as the sPFG sequence is much simpler to implement in practice and generally returns higher signal by keeping the echo time shorter. The differences in performance among the protocols are small and further work is required to quantify the sensitivity of the protocols. During fitting, D was fixed to its ground truth value, however, additionally fitting for D does not significantly affect the parameters estimates, but increases the computation time 10 fold.

The models we propose describe a complex tissue architecture, however they include only intracellular diffusion. A first step towards using such models in practical applications is to account for signal from the extracellular space. A simple extracellular model has free diffusion while more complicated ones account for a time-dependent diffusivity which reflects the length scale of restriction [5]. Compartment models, as in [1,6–8], can separate extracellular signal from intracellular but the presence of extracellular signal reduces the sensitivity to the parameters we estimate here. Another limitation is that we focused on macroscopically isotropic substrates. In grey matter for example, anisotropic pores have neither uniform nor coherent orientation, but Watson or Bingham distributions can provide a good model [16]. We can extend the models here similarly, which will further require high angular resolution diffusion imaging in a similar way to [7]. For the proof of concept, we constructed comprehensive diffusion protocols in order to have sensitivity over a wide range of diffusion substrates. For instance, the measurements with high gradient strength improve sensitivity to small pore sizes and measurements with low gradient strengths preserve the signal from larger pores. For practical applications, which require a certain scanning time, the protocols need to be adapted accordingly. For example, to avoid significant signal loss due to $T2$ decay at long diffusion times, which was not accounted for in simulations, spin echo sequences can be replaced with stimulated echo. Additionally, to preserve the sensitivity over a wide range of pore sizes for practical situations, rectangular gradients can be replaced with oscillating ones, or if there is prior knowledge of the system, the diffusion protocol can be substantially shortened using numerical optimisation [23].

Acknowledgements. The EPSRC support this work through the following grants: EP/G007748, EP/H046410/01, EP/K020439/1, EP/M020533/1.

References

1. Panagiotaki, E., Walker-Samuel, S., Siow, B., Johnson, S.P., Rajkumar, V., Pedley, R.B., Lythgoe, M.F., Alexander, D.C.: Noninvasive quantification of solid tumor microstructure using verdict MRI. Cancer Res. **74**, 1902–1912 (2014)
2. Savadiev, P., Campbell, J.S.W., Descoteaux, M., Deriche, R., Pike, G.B., Siddiqi, K.: Labeling of ambiguous subvoxel fibre bundle configurations in high angular resolution diffusion MRI. NeuroImage **41**, 58–68 (2008)
3. Nilsson, M., Latt, J., Stahlberg, F., van Westen, D., Hagslätt, H.: The importance of axonal undulation in diffusion MR measurements: a monte carlo simulation study. NMR Biomed. **25**, 795–805 (2012)
4. Kleinnijenhuis, M., Zerbi, V., Küsters, B., Slump, C.H., Barth, M., van Cappellen van Walsum, A.: Layer-specific diffusion weighted imaging in human primary visual cortex in vitro. Cortex **49**, 2569–2582 (2013)
5. Novikov, M., Jensen, J.H., Helpern, J.A., Fieremans, E.: Revealing mesoscopic structural universality with diffusion. Proc. Nat. Acad. Sci. **11**, 5088–5093 (2014)
6. Assaf, Y., Blumenfeld-Katzir, T., Yovel, Y., Basser, P.J.: AxCaliber: a method for measuring axon diameter distribution from diffusion MRI. Magn. Reson. Med. **59**, 1347–1354 (2008)
7. Alexander, D.C., Hubbard, P.L., Hall, M.G., Moore, E.A., Ptito, M., Parker, G.J.M., Dyrby, T.B.: Orientationally invariant indices of axon diameter and density from diffusion MRI. NeuroImage **52**, 1374–1389 (2010)
8. Ferizi, U., Schneider, T., Panagiotaki, E., Nedjati-Gilani, G., Zhang, H., Wheeler-Kingshott, C., Alexander, D.C.: A ranking of diffusion MRI compartment models with in vivo human brain data. Magn. Reson. Med. **72**, 1785–92 (2014)
9. Cory, D.G., Garroway, A.N., Miller, J.B.: Applications of spin transport as a probe of local geometry. Polym. Prepr. **31**, 149–150 (1990)
10. Mitra, P.P.: Multiple wave-vector extensions of the NMR pulsed-field-gradient spin-echo diffusion measurement. Phys. Rev. B **51**(21), 15074–15078 (1995)

11. Lawrenz, M., Koch, M.A., Finsterbusch, J.: A tensor model and measures of microscopic anisotropy for double-wave-vector diffusion-weighting experiments with long mixing times. J. Magn. Reson. **202**, 43–56 (2010)

12. Jespersen, S.N., Lundell, H., Sonderby, C.K., Dyrby, T.B.: Orientationally invariant metrics of apparent compartment eccentricity from double pulsed field gradient diffusion experiments. NMR Biomed. **26**, 1647–1662 (2013)

13. Lasic, S., Szczepankiewicz, F., Eriksson, S., Nilsson, M., Topgaard, D.: Microanisotropy imaging: quantification of microscopic diffusion anisotropy and orientational order parameter by diffusion MRI with magic-angle spinning of the q-vector. Front. Phys. **2** (2014)

14. Ozarslan, E.: Compartment shape anisotropy (CSA) revealed by double pulsed field gradient MR. J. Magn. Reson. **199**, 56–67 (2009)

15. Shemesh, N., Ozarslan, E., Basser, P.J., Cohen, Y.: Accurate noninvasive measurement of cell size and compartment shape anisotropy in yeast cells using double-pulsed field gradient MR. NMR Biomed. **25**, 236–246 (2012)

16. Zhang, H., Hubbard, P.L., Parker, G.J.M., Alexander, D.C.: Axon diameter mapping in the presence of orientation dispersion with diffusion MRI. NeuroImage **56**, 1301–1315 (2011)

17. Komlosh, M.E., Ozarslan, E., Lizak, M.J., Horkay, F., Schram, V., Shemesh, N., Cohen, Y., Basser, P.J.: Pore diameter mapping using double pulsed-field gradient MRI and its validation using a novel glass capillary array phantom. J. Magn. Reson. **208**, 128–135 (2011)

18. Hall, M., Alexander, D.C.: Convergence and parameter choice for Monte-Carlo simulations of diffusion MRI. IEEE Trans. Med. Imaging **28**, 1354–1364 (2009)

19. Neuman, C.H.: Spin echo of spins diffusing in a bounded medium. J. Chem. Phys. **60**, 4508–4511 (1974)

20. Assaf, Y., Freidlin, R.Z., Rohde, G.K., Basser, P.J.: New modeling and experimental framework to characterize hindered and restricted water diffusion in brain white matter. Magn. Reson. Med. **52**, 965–978 (2004)

21. Stepisnik, J.: Time-dependent self-diffusion by NMR spin echo. Phys. B **183**, 343–350 (1993)

22. Dyrby, T.B., Søgaard, L.V., Hall, M.G., Ptito, M., Alexander, D.C.: Contrast and stability of the axon diameter index from microstructure imaging with diffusion MRI. Magn. Reson. Med. **70**, 711–721 (2013)

23. Alexander, D.C.: A general framework for experiment design in diffusion MRI and its application in measuring direct tissue-microstructure features. Magn. Reson. Med. **60**, 439–448 (2008)

Multiple Orderings of Events
in Disease Progression

Alexandra L. Young[1](✉), Neil P. Oxtoby[1], Jonathan Huang[2],
Razvan V. Marinescu[1], Pankaj Daga[1], David M. Cash[1,3], Nick C. Fox[3],
Sebastien Ourselin[1,3], Jonathan M. Schott[3], Daniel C. Alexander[1], and for the
Alzheimers Disease Neuroimaging Initiative

[1] Centre for Medical Image Computing, University College London, London, UK
alexandra.young.11@ucl.ac.uk
[2] Google Inc., Mountain View, CA, USA
[3] Dementia Research Centre, University College London, London, UK

Abstract. The event-based model constructs a discrete picture of disease progression from cross-sectional data sets, with each event corresponding to a new biomarker becoming abnormal. However, it relies on the assumption that all subjects follow a single event sequence. This is a major simplification for sporadic disease data sets, which are highly heterogeneous, include distinct subgroups, and contain significant proportions of outliers. In this work we relax this assumption by considering two extensions to the event-based model: a generalised Mallows model, which allows subjects to deviate from the main event sequence, and a Dirichlet process mixture of generalised Mallows models, which models clusters of subjects that follow different event sequences, each of which has a corresponding variance. We develop a Gibbs sampling technique to infer the parameters of the two models from multi-modal biomarker data sets. We apply our technique to data from the Alzheimer's Disease Neuroimaging Initiative to determine the sequence in which brain regions become abnormal in sporadic Alzheimer's disease, as well as the heterogeneity of that sequence in the cohort. We find that the generalised Mallows model estimates a larger variation in the event sequence across subjects than the original event-based model. Fitting a Dirichlet process model detects three subgroups of the population with different event sequences. The Gibbs sampler additionally provides an estimate of the uncertainty in each of the model parameters, for example an individual's latent disease stage and cluster assignment. The distributions and mixtures of sequences that this new family of models introduces offer better characterisation of disease progression of heterogeneous populations, new insight into disease mechanisms, and have the potential for enhanced disease stratification and differential diagnosis.

1 Introduction

The sequence in which biomarkers become abnormal provides a simple, intuitive description of disease progression, giving insights into the underlying disease biology and a potential mechanism for disease staging. The sequence of biomarker

© Springer International Publishing Switzerland 2015
S. Ourselin et al. (Eds.): IPMI 2015, LNCS 9123, pp. 711–722, 2015.
DOI: 10.1007/978-3-319-19992-4_56

abnormality in sporadic neurodegenerative diseases, e.g. Alzheimer's disease, has been a topic of intense debate amongst neurologists [1]. Reconstructing this sequence for sporadic neurodegenerative diseases is difficult because the position of subjects with respect to the full disease time course is unknown. Typically clinical diagnoses are used as a time proxy, but this limits the temporal resolution of the sequence, e.g. in Alzheimer's disease there are usually only three clinical diagnosis categories: cognitively normal, mild cognitive impairment and Alzheimer's disease [2]. Additional complications arise due to the long disease time course [3] and inherent heterogeneity of sporadic disease datasets. Many different factors contribute to this heterogeneity [4,5], for example genetic disease subtypes, mixed pathology, environmental factors, and misdiagnosed subjects.

The event-based model [6] considers disease progression as a series of events, where each event corresponds to a new biomarker becoming abnormal. By considering cross-sectional patient data as snapshots of a single common event sequence, the event-based model is able to probabilistically reconstruct the ordering of events across subjects, without relying on a-priori disease staging. Taking samples of the posterior probability of this sequence provides insight into the uncertainty in this single event ordering. The application of this model has been demonstrated in familial Alzheimer's disease and Huntington's disease [6] to determine the sequence in which regional brain volumes become abnormal, and in sporadic Alzheimer's disease to determine the sequence in which cerebrospinal fluid (CSF) markers, cognitive test scores, and a limited set of regional atrophy and brain volume biomakers become abnormal [7]. Young et al. [7] found that this sequence is different in APOE4 positive individuals, with increased genetic risk of Alzheimer's disease, compared to the whole population, suggesting that the whole population contains a proportion of subjects who do not follow the single ordering of events encoded by the event-based model.

The assumption made by the event-based model in [6] and [7] of a single ordering of events in all subjects is a major simplification for heterogeneous sporadic disease datasets. In this work we relax this assumption by considering a family of models that allow for multiple and distributed orderings of events. The first is a generalised Mallows model [8], which parameterises the variance in the single ordering, allowing subjects to deviate from the central event sequence. The second is a Dirichlet process mixture model [9], which allows for subgroups of subjects that follow different event sequences. Previous work [10] on generalised Mallows event-based models relied on a well-defined control population and a complete set of biomarkers for each subject. Here we re-formulate this model to remove the reliance on a well-defined control population, allowing the model to be fitted to heterogeneous sporadic disease datasets, and to handle missing data, providing a multi-modal picture of disease progression. We formulate a Gibbs sampling technique that further provides samples of the uncertainty in the model parameters. We additionally introduce a new model: Dirichlet process mixtures of generalised Mallows event-based models, and develop a Gibbs sampler to estimate its parameters [11]. We apply these models to determine the sequence in which FDG-PET, CSF markers, cognitive test scores, and a large set of regional brain volumes become abnormal in sporadic Alzheimer's disease.

2   Models

2.1   The Event-Based Model

The event-based model of disease progression consists of a set of events $\{e_1, \ldots, e_N\}$ and an ordering $\sigma = (\sigma(1), \ldots, \sigma(N))$, where $\sigma(k) = i$ means that event e_i occurs in position k. In practise we only observe a snapshot of the event sequence for each subject, taken at an unknown stage k. If a subject is at stage k in the sequence σ the events $e_{\sigma(1)} \ldots e_{\sigma(k)}$ have occurred and events $e_{\sigma(k+1)} \ldots e_{\sigma(N)}$ have yet to occur. This adduces a partition of the event set, or partial ranking, $\gamma_k = e_{\sigma(1)}, \ldots, e_{\sigma(k)} | e_{\sigma(k+1)}, \ldots, e_{\sigma(N)}$, where the vertical bar indicates that the first set of events precedes the second. The occurence of event e_i in subject j is informed by biomarker measurement x_{ij}. The generative model of the biomarker data is

$$k_j \sim P(k),$$

$$x_{\sigma(i),j} \sim p(x_{\sigma(i),j} | e_{\sigma(i)}) \text{ if } i \le k_j,$$

$$x_{\sigma(i),j} \sim p(x_{\sigma(i),j} | \neg e_{\sigma(i)}) \text{ otherwise.}$$

$p(x|e)$ and $p(x|\neg e)$ are probability density functions on observing biomarker measurement x given that event e has or has not occurred respectively. $P(k)$ is a prior on the disease stage k.

2.2   The Generalised Mallows Event-Based Model

We formulate the generalised Mallows event-based model by using a generalised Mallows model to parameterise the variance in a central event sequence π through the spread parameter $\theta = (\theta_1, \ldots, \theta_{N-1})$. Each subject then has their own latent ordering σ_j, which is assumed to be a sample from a generalised Mallows model. The generative model of the biomarker data in the event-based model is therefore preceded by

$$\pi, \theta \sim P(\pi, \theta | \nu, r),$$

$$\sigma_j \sim GM(\pi, \theta).$$

$GM(\pi, \theta) = \frac{1}{\psi(\theta)} \exp[-d_\theta(\pi, \sigma)]$ is a generalised Mallows distribution with $\psi(\theta) = \prod_{j=1}^{n-1} \psi_{n-j}(\theta_j) = \prod_{j=1}^{n-1} \frac{1-e^{-(n-j+1)\theta_j}}{1-e^{-\theta_j}}$. $d_\theta(\pi, \sigma)$ is the generalised Kendalls tau distance [8], which penalises the number of pairwise disagreements between sequences. $P(\pi, \theta | \nu, r)$ is a conjugate prior over the generalised Mallows distribution parameters of the form $P(\pi, \theta | \nu, r) \propto \exp\left(-\nu \sum_j [\theta_j r_j + \ln \psi_{n-j}(\theta_j)]\right)$ [12].

2.3   Dirichlet Process Mixtures of Generalised Mallows Event-Based Models

Dirichlet process mixtures of generalised Mallows models assume that each subject has their own central ordering π_j and spread parameters $\boldsymbol{\theta}_j$, which are sampled from a discrete distribution G that is drawn from a Dirichlet process [9]. A Dirichlet process mixture is a generative clustering model where the number of clusters is a random variable, meaning that the number of clusters is detected automatically depending on the concentration parameter α. The generative model of the biomarker data in the event-based model is now preceded by the process

$$G \sim DP(\alpha, P(\pi, \boldsymbol{\theta}|\nu, \boldsymbol{r})),$$

$$\pi_j, \boldsymbol{\theta}_j \sim G,$$

$$\sigma_j \sim GM(\pi_j, \boldsymbol{\theta}_j),$$

where $DP(\alpha, P(\pi, \boldsymbol{\theta}|\nu, \boldsymbol{r}))$ is a Dirichlet process [9]. Each data point π_j can be characterised by an association with a cluster label $c_j \in 1, \dots, C$ and each cluster c with a set of generalised Mallows parameters σ_c and $\boldsymbol{\theta}_c$.

3   Inference

3.1   The Event-Based Model

Inference in the event-based model can be performed by taking Markov Chain Monte Carlo (MCMC) samples of $P(\sigma|X) = \frac{P(X|\sigma)P(\sigma)}{P(X)}$ where

$$P(X|\sigma) = \prod_{j=1}^{J} \left[\sum_{k=0}^{K} P(k) \left(\prod_{i=1}^{k} p(x_{\sigma(i),j}|e_{\sigma(i)}) \prod_{i=k+1}^{N} p(x_{\sigma(i),j}|\neg e_{\sigma(i)}) \right) \right]. \quad (1)$$

3.2   The Generalised Mallows Event-Based Model

We use Gibbs sampling to infer the parameters of the generalised Mallows event-based model. This consists of two stages. First, generating a set of sample event sequences $\sigma_{1:J}$. We sample from an augmented model [10], by alternating between sampling a subject's ordering σ_j and disease stage k_j, which are used to deterministically reconstruct their partial ranking γ_j. The Gibbs sampling updates are therefore

$$\sigma^{(j)} \sim P(\sigma|\gamma = \gamma_j, \pi, \boldsymbol{\theta}),$$

$$k^{(j)} \sim P(k|\sigma = \sigma_j, X_j).$$

Second, sampling the model parameters given the set of sample orderings $\sigma_{1:J}$ using the updates

$$\pi \sim P(\pi|\boldsymbol{\theta}, \nu, \boldsymbol{r}, \sigma_{1:J}),$$

$$\theta_k \sim P(\theta_k|\pi, \nu, \boldsymbol{r}, \sigma_{1:J}).$$

3.3   Dirichlet Process Mixtures of Generalised Mallows Event-Based Models

We formulate another Gibbs sampler to infer the parameters of Dirichlet process mixtures of generalised Mallows event-based models. We generate a set of candidate sample orderings $\sigma_{1:J,1:C}$, disease stages $k_{1:J,1:C}$, and partial rankings $\gamma_{1:J,1:C}$, which are conditioned on the parameters for each cluster via the updates

$$\sigma^{(j,c)} \sim P(\sigma|\gamma = \gamma_{jc}, \pi_c, \boldsymbol{\theta}_c),$$

$$k^{(j,c)} \sim P(k|\boldsymbol{\sigma} = \sigma_{jc}, X_j).$$

From these samples we sample the cluster assignment c_j of each subject conditioned on the cluster assignments of the other subjects c_{-j}, where c_{-j} is the set of cluster assignments for all subjects except subject j, the subject's sample ordering for each cluster $\sigma_{j,1:C}$, disease stage $k_{j,1:C}$ and their biomarker data X_j. We then update the generalised Mallows model parameters for each cluster, π_c and $\boldsymbol{\theta}_c$, from the set of subject orderings assigned to each cluster, $\boldsymbol{\sigma}_c$. So we have the updates

$$c^{(j)} \sim P(c|c_{-j}, \sigma_{j,1:C}, \boldsymbol{\theta}, \alpha, \nu, \boldsymbol{r}, X_j, k_{j,1:C}),$$

$$\pi^{(c)} \sim P(\pi|\boldsymbol{\theta} = \boldsymbol{\theta}_c, \nu, \boldsymbol{r}, \boldsymbol{\sigma}_c),$$

$$\theta_k^{(c)} \sim P(\theta_k|\boldsymbol{\pi} = \pi_c, \nu, \boldsymbol{r}, \boldsymbol{\sigma}_c).$$

4   Implementation

4.1   ADNI Dataset

We considered 382 subjects (135 cognitively normal subjects, 149 mild cognitive impairment, 98 Alzheimer's disease) who had a 1.5 T structural MRI (T1) scan at baseline. We calculated the total volume (left plus right hemisphere) of 82 regions in the Neuromorphometrics parcellation (http://neuromorphometrics. org:8080/) for each subject, correcting for head size variance by regressing against total intracranial volume. Segmentation was performed using the Geodesic Information Flow framework [13]. We retained the 35 regions having significant differences between cognitively normal and Alzheimer's disease subjects using the Wilcoxon rank sum test with $p < 0.01$. We downloaded biomarker values from the ADNI database (adni.loni.usc.edu) for CSF markers ($A\beta_{1-42}$, tau, p-tau), cognitive test scores (MMSE, RAVLT, ADAS-Cog), and global FDG-PET metabolism.

4.2   Model Fitting

We compare the result of fitting the event-based model, generalised Mallows event-based model and Dirichlet process mixtures of generalised Mallows event-based models to the ADNI data set for the set of 42 biomarker abnormality events described. Following previous work [6] we model the probability that a biomarker is normal, $p(x|\neg e)$, as a Gaussian distribution, and the probability that a biomarker is abnormal, $p(x|e)$, as a uniform distribution covering the full range of observed values to reflect the range of severity that corresponds to an abnormal biomarker. We use a mixture model to fit these distributions to the data to account for a proportion of outliers in the control population. In subjects that had missing data points we imputed the biomarker values such that $p(x|e) = p(x|\neg e)$, i.e. it is equally probable that the event e has or has not occurred. The prior probability that a subject is at a particular disease stage $P(k)$ is assumed to be uniform. To fit the generalised Mallows model we need to sample σ from $P(\sigma|\gamma, \pi, \boldsymbol{\theta})$. We approximate this by sampling from a generalised Mallows model for each of the event sets in the partial ranking γ separately; the set of events γ_e that have occurred and the set of events $\gamma_{\neg e}$ that have yet to occur. We sample $\sigma_e \sim GM(\pi_{\gamma_e}, \boldsymbol{\theta}_{\gamma_e})$, and $\sigma_{\neg e} \sim GM(\pi_{\gamma_{\neg e}}, \boldsymbol{\theta}_{\gamma_{\neg e}})$. This means that the precedence of events specified by the partial ranking is preserved, and that the central ordering of the generalised Mallows model for each event set, π_{γ_e} and $\pi_{\gamma_{\neg e}}$, has the minimal Kendalls tau distance [8] from the central ordering π of the full generalised Mallows model. We sample k from $P(k|\sigma, X_j)$ using Eq. 1, i.e. $P(k|\sigma, X_j) \propto \prod_{i=1}^{k} p(x_{\sigma(i),j}|e_{\sigma(i)}) \prod_{i=k+1}^{N} p(x_{\sigma(i),j}|\neg e_{\sigma(i)})$. The remaining sampling updates follow the algorithm in [11]. We sample π exactly using a stage-wise algorithm, and $\boldsymbol{\theta}$ using a beta function approximation. We used the Beta-Gibbs algorithm [11] to update the Dirichlet process mixture model cluster assignments c_j, weighting the probability each subject belongs to each cluster by $P(X_j|\sigma_{j,c}, k_{j,c})$, and the generalised Mallows model parameters π_c, $\boldsymbol{\theta}_c$ for each cluster. We fix the priors to be $\nu = 1$, $\boldsymbol{r} = 1$, $\alpha = 1$. We initialise π randomly, γ_e as the set of events with $p(x|e) > p(x|\neg e)$, $\gamma_{\neg e}$ as the set of events with $p(x|e) \leq p(x|\neg e)$, and the Dirichlet process mixture to have 25 clusters.

5   Results and Discussion

5.1   The Event-Based Model

Figure 1 shows a positional variance diagram of the MCMC samples of the single ordering of events returned by the event-based model. We visualise a few key stages of this sequence in the top row of Fig. 3 to show the spatial correspondence of the sequence of regional volume loss estimated by the model. We find that CSF markers are the first to become abnormal, followed by cognitive test scores, then memory-related brain regions, then FDG-PET, and then other Alzheimer's disease-related brain regions. This sequence complements the findings of other studies, but provides a much more detailed picture of the regional progression of volume changes than has been seen previously in sporadic Alzheimer's disease, and a direct comparison of the sequence of regional changes relative to a multi-modal set of biomarkers. Fonteijn et al. [6] looked at the regional progression of volume loss but in familial Alzheimer's disease and using atrophy rates. The results in Young et al. [7] show a multi-modal sequence of biomarker abnormality in sporadic disease but for a small set of regional volumes, and hippocampal

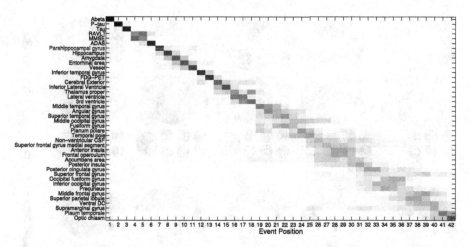

Fig. 1. Central ordering estimated by the event-based model: Positional variance diagram of the MCMC samples of the maximum likelihood event sequence σ. The events on the y-axis are ordered by the maximum likelihood sequence estimated by the model. Each entry of the positional variance diagram represents the proportion of samples in which a particular event appears in a particular position in the central ordering, ranging from 0 in white to 1 in black. A black diagonal corresponds to high certainty in the ordering of events, whereas grey blocks in the diagram mean that the events permute.

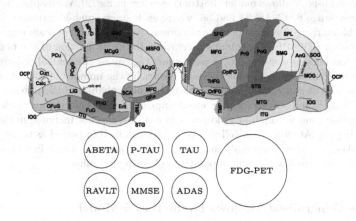

Fig. 2. Key for Figs. 3 and 5, generated using the BrainColorMap software [14].

and whole brain atrophy rates from short-term longitudinal MRI. Here we show the first multi-modal sequence of biomarker abnormality in sporadic Alzheimer's disease, including a large set of regional volumes. We are able to construct this picture from entirely cross-sectional data, and incorporate biomarkers with missing values.

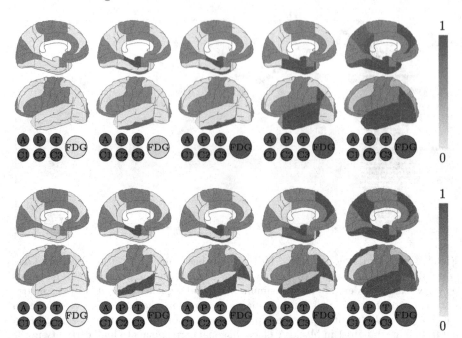

Fig. 3. Comparison of the central ordering estimated by the event-based model (top) with the generalised Mallows model (bottom) (see key in Fig. 2). We display the results for six stages: stage 6, 12, 18, 24 and 36, where each stage number corresponds to the number of biomarkers that have become abnormal. Each biomarker (brain region, CSF, cognitive test or FDG-PET) is coloured according to the proportion of the population in which it has become abnormal by a particular stage along the central ordering. This proportion is estimated for the event-based model by the number of MCMC samples (Fig. 1), and for the generalised Mallows model by the probability (calculated using the central ordering π and spread θ) of an event appearing at or before a particular stage. This proportion ranges from 0 in yellow to 1 in red. Regions not included in the model are shown in grey. At each stage yellow biomarkers can be interpreted as being normal, red biomarkers as being abnormal, and orange biomarkers as varying in whether they have become abnormal across the population (Color figure online).

5.2   The Generalised Mallows Event-Based Model

The generalised Mallows event-based model estimates both the central ordering of the events and the variance in this single event ordering across the population (Fig. 3). Figure 3 compares the central ordering π and variance θ estimated by the generalised Mallows event-based model, i.e. the range of event sequences across the population, with the central ordering estimated by the event-based model. The central event sequence has a similar ordering to the event-based model, but the variance in this central ordering of events increases, as shown by the increase in the number of orange regions in Fig. 3. By using our Gibbs sampling technique we further obtain estimates of the uncertainty in each of the model parameters, as well as the latent variables included in the model, for

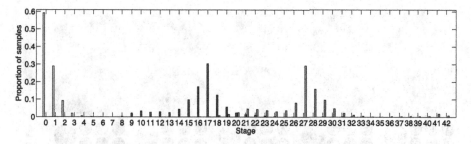

Fig. 4. Estimate of the uncertainty in a subject's disease stage obtained by using Gibbs sampling to fit the generalised Mallows event-based model. We show an estimate of the probability of each stage for an example cognitively normal subject (green), mild cognitive impairment subject (blue), and Alzheimer's disease subject (red). Each stage corresponds to the number of biomarkers in the sequence that have become abnormal.

example a subject's disease stage (Fig. 4). Fitting the generalised Mallows event-based model means that the uncertainty in this stage accounts for the variance in the ordering of the events across the population.

5.3   Dirichlet Process Mixtures of Generalised Mallows Event-Based Models

We fitted a Dirichlet process mixture of generalised Mallows event-based models to allow for clusters of subjects that follow different sequences of events, of which each cluster has its own central ordering π_c and variance θ_c. The Dirichlet process mixture model identifies three main clusters in the data, with an average proportion of 0.48 ($\pm$ 0.02), 0.24 ($\pm$ 0.10), and 0.29 ($\pm$ 0.10) subjects being assigned to each cluster respectively over the Gibbs samples. Figure 5 compares the estimated central ordering and variance for each of the clusters. The first two clusters look more Alzheimer's disease-like than the third cluster, producing a similar event sequence to the event-based model and generalised Mallows model (Fig. 3), with CSF biomarkers and memory-related brain regions becoming abnormal early in the sequence. The third cluster likely captures outliers that do not fit the Alzheimer's disease sequence of events. The ordering of events for the third cluster consists of only mild cognitive deficits and no CSF abnormalities, perhaps representing a normal aging event sequence, or simply reflecting that regional volume loss is a noisy measure on a cross-sectional level. The variance θ_c is greater for the clusters of the Dirichlet process mixture model than the generalised Mallows model (as shown by an increase in the number of orange regions in Fig. 5 compared to Fig. 3), likely because each cluster only contains a proportion of the population, meaning that there are fewer subjects to fit the model to, and due to the uncertainty in the cluster assignment of each subject. Our Gibbs sampling technique returns samples of all of the model parameters. For example, we are able to estimate the uncertainty in the disease stage of each subject for both models, and the cluster assignment of each subject from the Dirichlet process mixture, producing a similar diagram to Fig. 4.

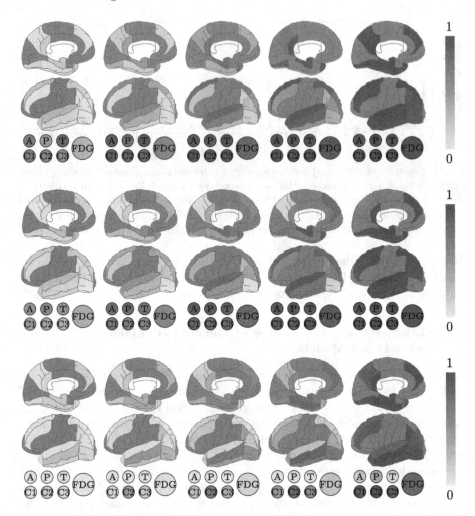

Fig. 5. As Fig. 3 but for the clusters identified by the Dirichlet process mixture of generalised Mallows event-based models (top to bottom: clusters 1 to 3).

6   Conclusions

We proposed a generalised family of event-based models that relax the assumption of a common event sequence over the population in different ways. We formulated these models so that they work for a large multi-modal set of sporadic disease biomarkers, and developed a Gibbs sampler that provides an estimate of the uncertainty on each model parameter. We fitted this family of models to the ADNI dataset to determine the ordering of a much more extensive, multi-modal set of biomarkers than has been seen previously. We find that the generalised Mallows model estimates a similar event sequence to the original event-based model, but with a larger variation across subjects. Fitting a Dirichlet process mixture model detects subgroups of the population with different event sequences.

Many possible extensions are interesting to consider in the future. In their current form these new models do not provide much additional clinical utility, and further validation is required to demonstrate support for the particular event sequences described and increased model complexity. However, these new models have the potential to provide much richer information than the original event-based model. Future work will extend the Dirichlet process model to incorporate data from different disease datasets, allowing the automatic extraction of biomarker orderings in different diseases and mixed pathology. The sampling techniques described naturally extend to incorporate multiple time points within an individual [10]. Extending these models to include longitudinal data will provide richer datasets for characterising the heterogeneity in individual event sequences. The family of models described here have a large number of parameters, developing hierarchical models [15] will reduce the required number of parameters by capturing sections of the sequence that are common or distinct amongst subjects to allow more robust fitting to cross-sectional data.

The family of disease progression models we describe are potentially applicable to any disease or developmental process. The multiple orderings of events described by these models have potential use for outlier detection, differential diagnosis and to characterise disease subtypes for improved patient stratification.

Acknowledgements. The EPSRC support this work with grants EP/J020990/01, EP/M020533/1 and EP/M006093/1. This work was supported by the NIHR Queen Square Dementia Biomedical Research Unit and the Leonard Wolfson Experimental Neurology Centre. The Dementia Research Centre is an ARUK coordination centre. DMC receives funding from an anonymous charitable foundation and support from the Brain Research Trust. SO is partially funded by the EU-FP7 project VPH- DARE@IT (FP7-ICT-2011-9-601055) and the NIHR University College London Hospitals Biomedical Research Centre (NIHR BRC UCLH/UCL High Impact Initiative). JMS acknowledges the support of ARUK, the MRC, and the UCL/H Biomedical Research Centre. Data collection and sharing for this project was funded by the Alzheimer's Disease Neuroimaging Initiative (NIHR Grant U01 AG024904) and DOD ADNI (DOD award number W81XWH-12-2-0012).

References

1. Jack, C.R., Knopman, D.S., Jagust, W.J., Shaw, L.M., Aisen, P.S., Weiner, M.W., Petersen, R.C., Trojanowski, J.Q.: Hypothetical model of dynamic biomarkers of the Alzheimer's pathological cascade. Lancet Neurol. 9(1), 119–128 (2010)
2. McKhann, G., Drachman, D., Folstein, M., Katzman, R., Price, D., Stadlan, E.M.: Clinical diagnosis of Alzheimer's disease: report of the NINCDS-ADRDA Work Group under the auspices of Department of Health and Human Services Task Force on Alzheimer's Disease. Neurology **34**, 939–944 (1984)
3. Villemagne, V.L., Burnham, S., Bourgeat, P., Brown, B., Ellis, K.A., Salvado, O., Szoeke, C., Macaulay, S.L., Martins, R., Maruff, P., Ames, D., Rowe, C.C., Masters, C.L.: Amyloid β deposition, neurodegeneration, and cognitive decline in sporadic Alzheimer's disease: a prospective cohort study. Lancet Neurol. **12**(4), 357–367 (2013)

4. Jack, C.R., Knopman, D.S., Jagust, W.J., Petersen, R.C., Weiner, M.W., Aisen, P.S., Shaw, L.M., Vemuri, P., Wiste, H.J., Weigand, S.D., Lesnick, T.G., Pankratz, V.S., Donohue, M.C., Trojanowski, J.Q.: Tracking pathophysiological processes in Alzheimer's disease: an updated hypothetical model of dynamic biomarkers. Lancet neurology **12**(2), 207–216 (2013)
5. Jack, C.R., Holtzman, D.M.: Biomarker modeling of Alzheimer's disease. Neuron **80**(6), 1347–1358 (2013)
6. Fonteijn, H.M., Modat, M., Clarkson, M.J., Barnes, J., Lehmann, M., Hobbs, N.Z., Scahill, R.I., Tabrizi, S.J., Ourselin, S., Fox, N.C., Alexander, D.C.: An event-based model for disease progression and its application in familial Alzheimer's disease and Huntington's disease. NeuroImage **60**(3), 1880–1889 (2012)
7. Young, A.L., Oxtoby, N.P., Daga, P., Cash, D.M., Fox, N.C., Ourselin, S., Schott, J.M., Alexander, D.C.: A data-driven model of biomarker changes in sporadic Alzheimer's disease. Brain **137**, 2564–2577 (2014)
8. Fligner, M.A., Verducci, J.S.: Distance based ranking models. JSTOR. Ser. B (Methodol.) **48**, 359–369 (1986)
9. Antoniak, C.E.: Mixtures of Dirichlet processes with applications to Bayesian Nonparametric problems. Ann. Stat. **2**, 1152–1174 (1974)
10. Huang, J., Alexander, D.C.: Probabilistic event cascades for Alzheimer's disease. Adv. Neural Inf. Process. Syst. **25**, 3104–3112 (2012)
11. Meila, M., Chen, H.: Dirichlet process mixtures of generalized mallows models. In: Uncertainty in Artificial Intelligence (UAI), pp. 285–294 (2010)
12. Meila, M., Bao, L.: Estimation and clustering with infinite rankings. In: Uncertainty in Artificial Intelligence (UAI), pp. 393–402 (2008)
13. Cardoso, M.J., Wolz, R., Modat, M., Fox, N.C., Rueckert, D., Ourselin, S.: Geodesic information flows. In: Ayache, N., Delingette, H., Golland, P., Mori, K. (eds.) MICCAI 2012, Part II. LNCS, vol. 7511, pp. 262–270. Springer, Heidelberg (2012)
14. Klein, A., Worth, A., Tourville, J., Landman, B., Dal, T., Satrajit, C., David, S.G.: An interactive tool for constructing optimal brain colormaps. **16**, p.84358 (2010)
15. Meek, C., Meila, M.: Recursive inversion models for permutations. Adv. Neural Inf. Process. Syst. **27**, 631–639 (2014)

Construction of An Unbiased Spatio-Temporal Atlas of the Tongue During Speech

Jonghye Woo[1]([⊠]), Fangxu Xing[2], Junghoon Lee[2,3], Maureen Stone[4],
and Jerry L. Prince[2]

[1] Department of Radiology, Massachusetts General Hospital,
Harvard Medical School, Boston, MA, USA
jwoo@mgh.harvard.edu
[2] Department of Electrical and Computer Engineering, Johns Hopkins University,
Baltimore, MD, USA
[3] Department of Radiation Oncology and Molecular Radiation Sciences,
Johns Hopkins University, Baltimore, MD, USA
[4] Department of Neural and Pain Science, University of Maryland,
Baltimore, MD, USA

Abstract. Quantitative characterization and comparison of tongue
motion during speech and swallowing present fundamental challenges
because of striking variations in tongue structure and motion across
subjects. A reliable and objective description of the dynamics tongue
motion requires the consistent integration of inter-subject variability to
detect the subtle changes in populations. To this end, in this work, we
present an approach to constructing an unbiased spatio-temporal atlas
of the tongue during speech for the first time, based on cine-MRI from
twenty two normal subjects. First, we create a common spatial space
using images from the reference time frame, a neutral position, in which
the unbiased spatio-temporal atlas can be created. Second, we transport images from all time frames of all subjects into this common space
via the single transformation. Third, we construct atlases for each time
frame via groupwise diffeomorphic registration, which serves as the initial spatio-temporal atlas. Fourth, we update the spatio-temporal atlas
by realigning each time sequence based on the Lipschitz norm on diffeomorphisms between each subject and the initial atlas. We evaluate and
compare different configurations such as similarity measures to build
the atlas. Our proposed method permits to accurately and objectively
explain the main pattern of tongue surface motion.

Keywords: Spatio-temporal atlas · MRI · Speech · Motion

1 Introduction

Because of the complex interleaved organization of its muscles, the human tongue
is able to create highly variable motions without the benefit of a skeleton, and
this makes it unique among body systems. Despite the capability for variation,

© Springer International Publishing Switzerland 2015
S. Ourselin et al. (Eds.): IPMI 2015, LNCS 9123, pp. 723–732, 2015.
DOI: 10.1007/978-3-319-19992-4_57

there must be common tongue motions in different individuals when they say the same word, since the sound produced is easily recognizable in most cases. To date, however, there has been no method to study the average motion of the tongue as well as its variability in a population of speaking subjects. If such a standard—i.e., a spatio-temporal atlas—were to exist, then it becomes possible to study both the normal variability of tongue motion, perhaps due to variations in shape of the oral cavity, as well as abnormal motion of patients who have undergone treatment for cancer or other diseases such as aphasia caused by brain injury.

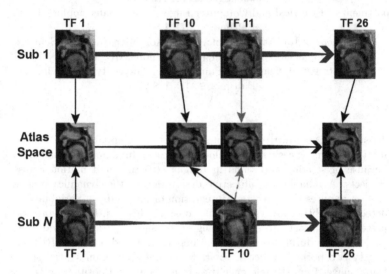

Fig. 1. Illustration of the proposed method. The atlas space is first defined using images of the first time frame (TF). All the time sequences are transformed into the atlas space and the initial spatio-temporal atlas is constructed at each time frame independently. To circumvent the temporal mismatch as shown in TF 10 of subject N, we regroup each time frame based on the Lipschitz norm on diffeomorphisms between each subject and the initial atlas. For example, TF 10 of subject N is included at TF 11 in the final atlas construction. Note that the different widths of the line represent the variations in tongue shape over time.

Recent advances in tongue imaging methods such as magnetic resonance imaging (MRI) have accelerated new advances in image and motion analysis, including segmentation [1,2], motion tracking [3], motion clustering [4], and registration [5,6]. However, despite the popularity of an atlas in other organs (e.g., the brain [7,8] or the heart [9]), research on the tongue or vocal tract atlas is still in its infancy; recently the first vocal tract atlas and statistical model have been published in [10], where structural MRI from normal subjects were used to build the atlas. However, to the best of our knowledge, there has been no spatio-temporal atlas of the tongue during speech or swallowing to date.

In order to create such a spatio-temporal atlas, finding accurate mappings of subjects of a population into a common space is essential. In particular, it is of critical importance to encode both intra-subject motion characteristics and inter-subject difference in the constructed spatio-temporal atlas. Several attempts have been made to address this for the brain and the cardiac applications by performing groupwise registration with kernel regression [8,11] or with an individual subject's growth model [12] or by aligning jointly subject image sequences to a template sequence [13]. In the similar context, Lorenzi et al. [14] presented the Schild's Ladder framework to transport longitudinal deformations in time series of images in a common space using diffeomorphic registration.

In this work, motivated by the works above, we propose to construct an unbiased spatio-temporal atlas of the tongue for the first time to characterize the dynamic tongue motion changes given a specific speech task, based on cine-MRI from eighteen normal speakers. In contrast to the other works above, changes in tongue motion and anatomy are much more variable and complex. Therefore, we develop a framework based on diffeomorphic registration that can capture large and complex deformations in its spatial and temporal tongue shape changes while maintaining topological properties of the tongue. In addition, in our application, the number of time frames for each subject is the same but each time sequence may not be accurately aligned temporally as shown in Fig. 1 (see time frame 10). To address this, the proposed framework consists of multiple steps, which formulates both spatial and temporal alignment problems independently. We attempted to find the minimum distance on diffeomorphisms and proposed an algorithm to solve this problem using the atlas of the reference time frame and the Lipschitz norm on diffeomorphisms, respectively. We evaluated and compared the different configurations such as the similarity measure to build the atlas. We will detail each step and the evaluation in the following sections.

2   Materials and Methods

2.1   Data Acquisition

MRI Instrumentation and Data Collection. In our study, MRI scanning was performed on a Siemens 3.0 T Trim Treo system (Siemens Medical Solutions, Malvern, PA) with a 16-channel head and neck coil. When the subject speaks a pre-trained speech task in repeated utterances, cine MR images were acquired as a sequence of image frames at multiple parallel slice locations that cover a region of interest encompassing the tongue and the surrounding structures. To optimize the spatial resolution in all three planes, the three orthogonal stacks including axial, coronal, and sagittal orientations were acquired. Each dataset had a 1 s duration, 26 time frames per second, 6 mm slice thickness and 1.8 mm in-plane resolution. Other sequence parameters were repetition time (TR) 36 ms, echo time (TE) 1.47 ms, flip angle 6°, and turbo factor 11.

Speech Task. The MRI speech task was "a geese". This phrase begins with a neutral vocal tract configuration (schwa). The tongue body motion is simple because it moves only anteriorly, and the word uses little to no jaw motion, thus increasing the potential for tongue deformation. There are four distinctive frames /ə/, /g/, /i/, and /s/ in this word.

2.2   Preliminaries

Preprocessing. Our study uses T2-weighted multi-slice 2D dynamic cine-MRI at a frame rate of 26 frames per second. To maintain high signal-to-noise ratio (SNR) while minimizing the blurred effect due to involuntary motion such as swallowing, three orthogonal volumes with axial, sagittal, and coronal orientations are acquired one after the other. Each orientation, however, cannot be used directly for further atlas construction. In order to create a single volume with an isotropic resolution, a super-resolution volume reconstruction technique using all three stacks is employed [2,15]. In brief, multiple preprocessing tasks including motion correction, intensity normalization, etc. are carried out, which precedes a region-based Maximum A Posteriori-Markov Random Field (MAP-MRF) method incorporating edge-preserving regularization to reconstruct a single volume termed a super-volume with improved SNR and resolution (1.8 mm × 1.8 mm × 1.8 mm).

Diffeomorphic Image Registration. Diffeomorphic image registration is the key technique to construct the atlas. In particular, we are interested in the well-known Large Deformation Diffeomorphic Metric Mapping (LDDMM) algorithm [16]. The ANTs open source software library [17] is used in our implementation. Let the images $I : \Omega \in \mathbb{R}^3 \to \mathbb{R}$ and $J : \Omega \in \mathbb{R}^3 \to \mathbb{R}$, defined on the open and bounded domain Ω, be the template and target images. We cast image registration as the problem of finding a diffeomorphic transformation, $\phi(\mathbf{x}, t) : \Omega \times t \to \Omega$, parameterized over time, which is a differentiable mapping with a differentiable inverse. The ϕ can be computed by integrating a time-dependent velocity field $v : \Omega \times t \to \mathbb{R}^3$, as given by

$$\frac{d\phi(\mathbf{x}, t)}{dt} = v(\phi(\mathbf{x}, t), t), \phi(\mathbf{x}, 0) = \mathbf{Id}, \tag{1}$$

where the diffeomorphic mapping can be obtained through integration of Eq. (1):

$$\phi(\mathbf{x}, 1) = \phi(\mathbf{x}, 0) + \int_0^1 v(\phi(\mathbf{x}), t)dt. \tag{2}$$

The diffeomorphic, inexact image matching energy functional in a variational framework can be given by

$$\phi^* = \arg\min_\phi \left(\int_0^1 \|v(t)\|_V^2 dt + \lambda \int_\Omega \left\| I \circ \phi^{-1}(\mathbf{x}, 1) - J \right\|_2^2 d\Omega \right), \tag{3}$$

where the energy functional consists of the regularization term (the first term on the right), the data fidelity term or similarity measure (the second term on the right), V is a Reproducing Kernel Hilbert Space (RKHS) of vector fields on the domain Ω, and $\lambda \in \mathbb{R}^+$ is a balancing term. In recent years, new improvements have been made in the original LDDMM formulation [16]. The first is the generalization of the similarity measures to include mutual information (MI) or cross correlation (CC) in order to accommodate intensity differences [7]. The second is the use of a symmetric alternative, utilizing the fact that the diffeomorphism, ϕ, can be decomposed into a pair of diffeormorphisms ϕ_1 and ϕ_2 [7]. The formulation incorporating the two new features is

$$
\begin{aligned}
E(I, J, \phi_1, \phi_2) = \int_0^{0.5} \|v_1(\mathbf{x},t)\|_V^2 + \|v_2(\mathbf{x},t)\|_V^2 dt \\
+ \lambda \int_\Omega \Pi \left(I \circ \phi_1^{-1}(\mathbf{x}, 0.5), J \circ \phi_2^{-1}(\mathbf{x}, 0.5) \right) d\Omega
\end{aligned}
\tag{4}
$$

where Π denotes a similarity measure depending on the considered application. In this work, we use the CC as our similarity metric. The optimal ϕ_1^* and ϕ_2^* can be obtained via minimizing the energy functional from $t=0$ and $t=1$, respectively, thus leading to a symmetric and inverse consistent mapping.

In order to minimize the energy functional above, due to the demanding computational burden, the following gradient descent approach is widely adopted [18]

$$
\nabla\Pi = \frac{\partial}{\partial\phi_i}\Pi\left(I(\phi_1^{-1}(\mathbf{x}, 0.5)), J(\phi_1^{-1}(\mathbf{x}, 0.5))\right), i \in \{1, 2\},
\tag{5}
$$

where the updates of $\phi_1(\mathbf{x}, 0.5)$ and $\phi_2(\mathbf{x}, 0.5)$ at each iteration are given by

$$
\phi_i(x, 0.5) = \phi_i(\mathbf{x}, 0.5) + \alpha(K * \nabla\Pi(\phi_i(\mathbf{x}, 0.5))), i \in \{1, 2\},
\tag{6}
$$

where α represents a step parameter and K is the Gaussian Kernel [18]. The gradient is then mapped back to the original ϕ_1 and ϕ_2. Note that the forward and inverse mappings are guaranteed to be consistent (i.e., $\left\|\phi_i^{-1}(\phi_i) - \mathbf{Id}\right\|^2 < \varepsilon$) in this formulation [18].

2.3 Proposed Approach

One straightforward way to construct an atlas is to perform independently groupwise registration at each time frame. While this provides a spatially aligned atlas over time, it will not take the temporal mismatch into account, thereby leading to the inaccurate spatio-temporal atlas.

To construct an unbiased spatio-temporal atlas, the proposed framework consists of four steps. Let I_i^r $(i=1,\cdots, M)$, where $M=26$, be a time series of images with the reference time frame I_1^r of subject r $(r=1,\cdots, N)$, where $N=18$ in this work. First, we create a common spatial space using images from the first time frame (i.e., neutral position) using groupwise registration given by

$$
\left\{\hat{\phi}_{i,1}^r, \hat{\phi}_{i,2}^r\right\} = \arg\min_{\phi_{i,1}^r, \phi_{i,2}^r} \sum_{p=1}^P E(\bar{I}_i, I_i^p, \phi_{i,1}^p, \phi_{i,2}^p),
\tag{7}
$$

where $E(\bar{I}_i, I_i^p, \phi_{i,1}^p, \phi_{i,2}^p)$ is the energy functional to find the atlas, $\bar{I}_i$ ($i{=}1$), of the first time frame based on Eq. (4). This step produces the unbiased common spatial space without any influence of the temporal mismatch as this time frame presents a neutral vocal tract configuration (schwa). Second, we transport images from all remaining time frames of all subjects into this common space via the single transformation for each subject learnt from the first step. It is worth noting that only a single transformation is needed for each subject to map its image sequence to the atlas space similar to the approaches in [12,14]. This will reduce the potential bias caused by the anatomical differences in each subject while preserving the temporal correspondence. Third, we construct atlases for each time frame, using images deformed to the reference time frame space, via groupwise diffeomorphic registration, which serves as the initial spatio-temporal atlas. Fourth, in order to deal with the potential temporal mismatch across different speakers, we update the initial spatio-temporal atlas by regrouping each time sequence based on the Lipschitz norm on diffeomorphisms between each subject and the resulting atlas [19]. Owing to the Lipschitz continuity to the action of diffeomorphisms, we use the Lipschitz norm as a metric to measure how similar the template image and the target image are after diffeomorphic registration. Let $\varphi_{N_n}^k \in \mathrm{Diff}(\mathbb{R}^2)$ be a diffeomorphism between the time frame k of the initial atlas and the time frame n of subject N. The Lipschitz norm, $\mathrm{Lip}(\varphi, \Omega)$, is then defined by

$$\mathrm{Lip}(\varphi, \Omega) := \inf \left\{ l \in \mathbb{R} : \left\| \varphi^{-1}(x_1) - \varphi^{-1}(x_2) \right\| \le l \|x_1 - x_2\|, x_1, x_2 \in \Omega, x_1 \ne x_2 \right\}. \quad (8)$$

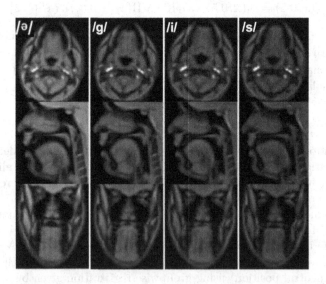

Fig. 2. The spatio-temporal atlas using our method. Four time frames representing /ə/, /g/, /i/, and /s/ are shown from left to right (at time frames 2, 10, 15, and 23, respectively). We used the CC similarity metric to generate this atlas.

We register five adjacent time frames (2D mid-sagittal slice) of each subject with a time frame of interest (2D mid-sagittal slice) of the initial spatio-temporal atlas. Note that we use 2D mid-sagittal slices for computational convenience and the use of full 3D volumes would produce similar results. We then evaluate the Lipschitz norm and find the best candidate time frame from each subject using the formula given by

$$n^* = \underset{n \in \{k-2,k-1,k,k+1,k+2\}}{\arg\min} \mathrm{Lip}(\varphi_{N_n}^k, \Omega). \tag{9}$$

We impose a constraint that the reassignments should be non-decreasing so that the frame reversal should not be allowed. Once regrouping is done, we construct the final atlases for each time frame using the same method in step 3.

3 Experimental Results

The constructed spatio-temporal atlas using our proposed method is shown in Fig. 2, where four representative time points including /ə/, /g/, /i/, and /s/ are illustrated. Since there is no ground truth in the atlas building, we evaluated and compared a set of different similarity measures to build the spatio-temporal atlas. In this experiment, we evaluated the most widely used similarity measures including MI, sum of squared differences (SSD), and CC and the other settings including transformation models and regularization methods remained same. Figure 3 depicts the three atlases at time frame 5 that were generated using different similarity measures. Red arrow indicates the marked differences in the tongue surface, where our proposed method best aligned all the images, thereby creating the sharpest tongue surface among all methods as visually assessed. For quantitative evaluation, we computed two sharpness measures as in [11], namely the intensity variance measure (M1) and the energy of image gradient measure

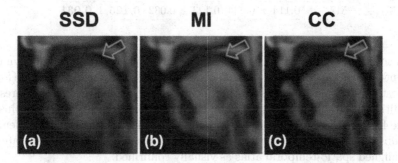

Fig. 3. Comparison of different similarity measures to create the atlas. We used sum of squared differences (SSD), mutual information (MI), and cross correlation (CC) as the similarity measure. Time frame 5 is shown here. Arrows indicate the tongue surface where the most prominent differences were observed and the result using CC provided the most clear tongue surface as visually assessed.

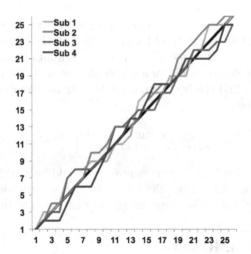

Fig. 4. Illustration of the temporal mismatch of each time sequence compared to the initial spatio-temporal atlas. We used five neighboring time frames of each subject around which to evaluate the Lipschitz norm at time frame of interest of the initial atlas.

(M2) on atlases of ten different time points. Table 1 lists the numerical results of the two measures and CC provided the best results. These results were also consistent with the visual assessment, suggesting that the CC similarity measure is well-suited for this application.

Table 1. Sharpness Measures: M1 and M2 ($n{=}10$)

Metrics	SSD	MI	CC
M1	3.229 ± 0.134	3.378 ± 0.213	**3.415 ± 0.151**
M2	0.114 ± 0.034	0.123 ± 0.032	**0.125 ± 0.031**

In addition, we illustrated the time-alignment step in Fig. 4. Since the dynamic sequences during speech across speakers are not perfectly synchronized, we found the best time frame in each subject that matches the time frame of interest of the initial spatio-temporal atlas using the Lipschitz norm on diffeomorphisms. Figure 4 shows the time-alignment step in four subjects, where different tempos were observed in different subjects. After this step, we were able to generate the time-aligned spatio-temporal atlas as visually confirmed.

4   Discussion and Conclusion

In this work, we presented a novel framework for constructing an unbiased spatio-temporal atlas of the tongue during speech from cine-MRI. The contributions of this work are two-fold. In a spatio-temporal groupwise registration framework, we formulated a spatial and temporal alignment problem independently in contrast to the algorithms used in other applications [9,11], that of finding the minimum distance on diffeomorphisms and we tackled this problem using the atlas of the reference time frame and the Lipschitz norm on diffeomorphisms, respectively. In terms of the similarity measure, CC provided the best performance among other metrics. In a tongue motion/speech analysis context, we created the spatio-temporal atlas for the first time, which opens new vistas to study speech production. The crucial application of this atlas is to allow comparison between subjects in the same coordinate space. This would allow us to address issues of normal speech production, such as whether inter-subject speech motor differences are due to fine tuning, or to entirely different strategies. In studying patients, abnormal behaviors could be better detailed in relation to normal motor variation. Our spatio-temporal atlas was visually assessed and further validations are needed to evaluate the quality of the constructed atlas. For example, we will realign voice recordings and related features of the individual subjects according to the results of our method. The proposed method provides a framework to observe the main pattern of tongue surface motion, which can be potentially used to elucidate speech-related disorders. In our future work, we will apply statistical models (e.g., PCA) to create a statistical atlas for abnormality detection. In addition, we will incorporate multimodal imaging data such as muscles from structural MRI and motion tracking from tagged-MRI into this spatio-temporal atlas. Furthermore, we will apply our method to more complex speech tasks and link our atlas with biomechanics of the muscles of the tongue.

Acknowledgements. We thank reviewers for their comments. This work is supported by NIH/NIDCD R00DC012575.

References

1. Harandia, N.M., Abugharbieh, R., Fels, S.: 3D segmentation of the tongue in MRI: a minimally interactive model-based approach. Computer Methods in Biomechanics and Biomedical Engineering: Imaging & Visualization, pp. 1–11 (2014)
2. Lee, J., Woo, J., Xing, F., Murano, E., Stone, M., Prince, J.: Semi-automatic segmentation for 3D motion analysis of the tongue with dynamic MRI. Comput. Med. Imaging Graph. **38**(8), 714–724 (2014)
3. Parthasarathy, V., Prince, J.L., Stone, M., Murano, E.Z., NessAiver, M.: Measuring tongue motion from tagged cine-MRI using harmonic phase (HARP) processing. J. Acoust. Soc. Am. **121**(1), 491–504 (2007)
4. Woo, J., Xing, F., Lee, J., Stone, M., Prince, J.: Determining functional units of tongue motion via graph-regularized sparse non-negative matrix factorization. In: International Conference on Medical Image Computing and Computer-Assisted Intervention, pp. 146–153, Boston, MA (2014)
5. Woo, J., Stone, M., Prince, J.: Multimodal registration via mutual information incorporating geometric and spatial context. IEEE Trans. Image Process. **24**(2), 757–769 (2015)

6. Kim, J., Lammert, A., Ghosh, P., Narayanan, S.: Co-registration of speech production datasets from electromagnetic articulography and real-time magnetic resonance imaging. J. Acoust. Soc. Am. **135**(2), EL115–EL121 (2014)

7. Avants, B.B., Yushkevich, P., Pluta, J., Minkoff, D., Korczykowski, M., Detre, J., Gee, J.: The optimal template effect in hippocampus studies of diseased populations. Neuroimage **49**(3), 2457–2466 (2010)

8. Serag, A., Aljabar, P., Ball, G., Counsell, S., Boardman, J., Rutherford, M., Edwards, A., Hajnal, J., Rueckert, D.: Construction of a consistent high-definition spatio-temporal atlas of the developing brain using adaptive kernel regression. NeuroImage **59**, 2255–2265 (2012)

9. De Craene, M., Piella, G., Camara, O., Duchateau, N., Silva, E., Doltra, A., D'hooge, J., Brugada, J., Sitges, M., Frangi, A.: Temporal diffeomorphic free-form deformation: application to motion and strain estimation from 3D echocardiography. Med. Image Anal **16**(2), 427–450 (2011)

10. Woo, J., Lee, J., Murano, E., Xing, F., Meena, A., Stone, M., Prince, J.: A high-resolution atlas and statistical model of the vocal tract from structural MRI. Computer Methods in Biomechanics and Biomedical Engineering: Imaging & Visualization, pp. 1–14 (2014)

11. Gholipour, A., Limperopoulos, C., Clancy, S., Clouchoux, C., Akhondi-Asl, A., Estroff, J.A., Warfield, S.K.: Construction of a deformable spatiotemporal MRI atlas of the fetal brain: evaluation of similarity metrics and deformation models. In: International Conference on Medical Image Computing and Computer-Assisted Intervention, pp. 292–299, Boston, MA (2014)

12. Liao, S., Jia, H., Wu, G., Shen, D.: A novel framework for longitudinal atlas construction with groupwise registration of subject image sequences. NeuroImage **59**(2), 1275–1289 (2012)

13. Durrleman, S., Pennec, X., Gerig, G., Trouve, A., Ayache, N.: Spatiotemporal atlas estimation for developmental delay detection in longitudinal datasets. In: International Conference on Medical Image Computing and Computer-Assisted Intervention **59**(2), pp. 297–304 (2009)

14. Lorenzi, M., Ayache, N., Pennec, X.: Schild's ladder for the parallel transport of deformations in time series of images. Inf Process Med Imaging **22**, 463–474 (2011)

15. Woo, J., Murano, E., Stone, M., Prince, J.: Reconstruction of high-resolution tongue volumes from MRI. IEEE Trans Biomed. Eng. **59**(12), 3511–3524 (2012)

16. Beg, M.F., Miller, M.I., Trouv, A., Younes, L.: Computing large deformation metric mappings via geodesic flows of diffeomorphisms. Int. J. Comput. Vision **61**(2), 139157 (2005)

17. Avants, B.B., Tustison, N.J., Song, G., Cook, P.A., Klein, A., Gee, J.C.: A reproducible evaluation of ANTs similarity metric performance in brain image registration. NeuroImage **54**(3), 2033–2044 (2011)

18. Tustison, N., Avants, B.B.: Explicit B-spline regularization in diffeomorphic image registration. Frontiers in Neuroinformatics **7**(39), 1–13 (2013)

19. Bruna, J., Mallat, S.: Invariant scattering convolution networks. IEEE Trans. Pattern Anal. Mach. Intell. **35**(8), 1872–1886 (2013)

Tree-Encoded Conditional Random Fields for Image Synthesis

Amod Jog[1(✉)], Aaron Carass[1], Dzung L. Pham[2], and Jerry L. Prince[1]

[1] Image Analysis and Communications Laboratory,
The Johns Hopkins University, Baltimore, USA
amodjog@jhu.edu
[2] Henry M. Jackson Foundation for the Advancement of Military Medicine,
Bethesda, USA

Abstract. Magnetic resonance imaging (MRI) is the dominant modality for neuroimaging in clinical and research domains. The tremendous versatility of MRI as a modality can lead to large variability in terms of image contrast, resolution, noise, and artifacts. Variability can also manifest itself as missing or corrupt imaging data. Image synthesis has been recently proposed to homogenize and/or enhance the quality of existing imaging data in order to make them more suitable as consistent inputs for processing. We frame the image synthesis problem as an inference problem on a 3-D continuous-valued conditional random field (CRF). We model the conditional distribution as a Gaussian by defining quadratic association and interaction potentials encoded in leaves of a regression tree. The parameters of these quadratic potentials are learned by maximizing the pseudo-likelihood of the training data. Final synthesis is done by inference on this model. We applied this method to synthesize T_2-weighted images from T_1-weighted images, showing improved synthesis quality as compared to current image synthesis approaches. We also synthesized Fluid Attenuated Inversion Recovery (FLAIR) images, showing similar segmentations to those obtained from real FLAIRs. Additionally, we generated super-resolution FLAIRs showing improved segmentation.

Keywords: Magnetic resonance · Image synthesis · Conditional random field

1 Introduction

Image synthesis in MRI is a process in which the intensities of acquired MRI data are transformed in order to enhance the data quality or render them more suitable as input for further image processing. Image synthesis has been gaining traction in the medical image processing community in recent years [6,15], as a useful pre-processing tool for segmentation and registration. It is especially useful in MR brain imaging, where a staggering variety of pulse sequences like Magnetization Prepared Gradient Echo (MPRAGE), Dual Spin Echo (DSE),

© Springer International Publishing Switzerland 2015
S. Ourselin et al. (Eds.): IPMI 2015, LNCS 9123, pp. 733–745, 2015.
DOI: 10.1007/978-3-319-19992-4_58

FLAIR etc. are used to interrogate the various aspects of neuroanatomy. Versatility of MRI is a boon for diagnosticians but can sometimes prove to be a handicap when performing analysis using image processing. Automated image processing algorithms are not always robust to variations in their input [13]. In large datasets, sometimes images are missing or corrupted during acquisition and cannot be used for further processing. Image synthesis can be used as a tool to supplement these datasets by creating artificial facsimiles of the missing images by using the available ones. An additional source of variability is the differing image quality between different pulse sequences for the same subject. An MPRAGE sequence can be quickly acquired at a resolution higher than 1 mm^3, which is not possible for FLAIR. Image synthesis can be used to enhance the resolution of existing low resolution FLAIRs using the corresponding high resolution MPRAGE images, thus leading to improved tissue segmentation.

Previous work on image synthesis has proceeded along two lines, (1) registration-based, and (2) example-based. Registration-based [3,12] approaches register the training/atlas images to the given subject image and perform intensity fusion (in the case of multiple training/atlas pairs) to produce the final synthesis. These approaches are heavily dependent on the quality of registration, which is generally not accurate enough in the cortex and abnormal tissue regions. Example-based approaches involve learning an intensity transformation from known training data pairs/atlas images. A variety of example-based approaches [5,8,15] have been proposed. These methods treat the problem as a regression problem and estimate the synthetic image voxel-by-voxel from the given, available images. The voxel intensities in the synthetic image are assumed to be independent of each other, which is not entirely valid as intensities in a typical MR image are spatially correlated and vary smoothly from voxel-to-voxel.

In this work, we frame image synthesis as an inference problem in a probabilistic discriminative framework. Specifically, we model the posterior distribution $p(\mathbf{y}|\mathbf{x})$, where $\mathbf{x}$ is the collection of known images and $\mathbf{y}$ is the synthetic image we want to estimate, as a Gaussian CRF [10]. Markov random field (MRF) approaches lend themselves as a robust, popular way to model images. However in a typical MRF, the observed data $\mathbf{x}$ are assumed to be independent given the underlying latent variable $\mathbf{y}$, which is a limiting assumption for typical images. A CRF, by directly modeling the posterior distribution allows us to side-step this problem. CRFs have been used in discrete labeling and segmentation problems [9]. A continuous-valued CRF, modeled as a Gaussian CRF, was first described in [17]. Efficient parameter learning and inference procedures of a Gaussian CRF were explored in the Regression Tree Fields concept in [7]. We also model the posterior distribution as a Gaussian CRF, the parameters of which are stored in the leaves of a single regression tree. We learn these parameters by maximizing a pseudo-likelihood objective function given training data. Given a subject image, we build the Gaussian distribution parameters from the learned tree and parameters. The prediction of the synthetic subject image is a maximum a posteriori (MAP) estimate of this distribution and is estimated efficiently using conjugate gradient descent.

We refer to our method as Synthesis with Conditional Random Field Tree or SyCRAFT. We applied SyCRAFT to synthesize T_2-weighted (T_2-w) images from T_1-w (T_1-w) images and showed a superior quality of synthesis compared to state-of-the-art methods. We also applied our method to synthesize FLAIRs from corresponding T_1-w, T_2-w, and P_D-weighted (P_D-w) images and showed that tissue segmentation on synthetic images is comparable to that achieved using real images. Finally, we used our method in an example-based super-resolution framework to estimate a super-resolution FLAIR image and showed improved tissue segmentation. In Sect. 2, we describe our method in detail, followed by experiments and results in Sect. 3 and discussion in Sect. 4.

2 Method

2.1 Model

We start with the definition of a CRF, initially proposed in [10]. A CRF is defined over a graph $G = (V, E)$, V and E are the sets of vertices and edges respectively, of G. In an image synthesis context, the set of all voxels i in the image domain form the vertices of V. A pair of voxels $(i, j), i, j \in V$, that are neighbors according to a predefined neighborhood, form an edge in E. Let $\mathbf{x} = \{\mathbf{x}_1, \ldots, \mathbf{x}_m\}$ be the observed data. Specifically, $\mathbf{x}$ represents the collection of available images from m pulse sequences from which we want to synthesize a new image. Let $\mathbf{y}$ be the continuous-valued random variable over V, representing the synthetic image we want to predict. In a CRF framework, $\mathrm{p}(\mathbf{y}|\mathbf{x})$ is modeled and learned from training data of known pairs of $(\mathbf{x}, \mathbf{y})$. Let $\mathbf{y} = \{y_i, i \in V\}$. Then $(\mathbf{y}, \mathbf{x})$ is a CRF if, conditioned on $\mathbf{x}$, y_i exhibit the Markov property, i.e. $\mathrm{p}(y_i|\mathbf{x}, \mathbf{y}_{V\backslash i}) = \mathrm{p}(y_i|\mathbf{x}, \mathbf{y}_{\mathcal{N}_i})$, where $\mathcal{N}_i = \{j \mid (i, j) \in E\}$, is the neighborhood of i.

Assuming $\mathrm{p}(\mathbf{y}|\mathbf{x}) > 0, \forall \mathbf{y}$, from the Hammersley-Clifford theorem, we can express the conditional probability as a Gibbs distribution. The factorization of $\mathrm{p}(\mathbf{y}|\mathbf{x})$ in terms of association potentials and interaction potentials is given as,

$$\mathrm{p}(\mathbf{y}|\mathbf{x}) = \frac{1}{Z}\exp[-\{\sum_{i \in V} E_{\mathcal{A}}(y_i, \mathbf{x}; \theta) + \lambda \sum_{i \in V}\sum_{j \in \mathcal{N}_i} E_{\mathcal{I}}(y_i, y_j, \mathbf{x}; \theta)\}]. \quad (1)$$

$E_{\mathcal{A}}(y_i, \mathbf{x}; \theta)$ is called an association potential, defined using the parameter set θ, $E_{\mathcal{I}}(y_i, y_j, \mathbf{x}; \theta)$ is called an interaction potential, λ is a weighting factor, and Z is the partition function. If E_A and E_I are defined as quadratic functions of $\mathbf{y}$, we can express this distribution as a multivariate Gaussian as below,

$$\mathrm{p}(\mathbf{y}|\mathbf{x}) = \frac{1}{(2\pi)^{\frac{|V|}{2}}|\boldsymbol{\Sigma}|^{\frac{1}{2}}}\exp(-\frac{1}{2}(\mathbf{y} - \boldsymbol{\mu}(\mathbf{x}))^T \boldsymbol{\Sigma}(\mathbf{x})^{-1}(\mathbf{y} - \boldsymbol{\mu}(\mathbf{x})))$$

$$= \frac{1}{Z}\exp(-\frac{1}{2}(\mathbf{y}^T \mathbf{A}(\mathbf{x})\mathbf{y}) - \mathbf{b}(\mathbf{x})^T\mathbf{y}). \quad (2)$$

The parameters $\mathbf{A}(\mathbf{x})$ and $\mathbf{b}(\mathbf{x})$ are dependent on the association and interaction potential definitions. In most classification tasks involving CRF's the association potential is defined as the local class probability as provided by a generic classifier or a regressor [9]. Image synthesis being a regression task, we chose to model and extract both association and interaction potentials from a single regressor, in our case a regression tree. We define a quadratic association potential as

$$E_{\mathcal{A}}(y_i, \mathbf{x}; \theta) = \frac{1}{2}(a_{L(i)}y_i^2) - b_{L(i)}y_i, \tag{3}$$

where $\{a_{L(i)}, b_{L(i)}\} \in \theta$ are the parameters defined at the leaf $L(i)$. $L(i)$ is the leaf where the feature vector $\mathbf{f}_i(\mathbf{x})$ extracted for voxel i from the observed data $\mathbf{x}$, lands after having been passed through successive nodes of a learned regression tree, Ψ. The features and regression tree construction are described in Sect. 2.2.

The interaction potential usually acts as a smoothing term, but can also be designed in a more general manner. We define interaction potentials for each type of neighbor. A 'neighbor type' $r \in \{1, \ldots, |\mathcal{N}_i|\}$ is given by a voxel i and one of its n ($= |\mathcal{N}_i|$) neighbors. For example, a neighborhood system with four neighbors (up, down, left, right) has four types of neighbors, and hence four types of edges. The complete set of edges E can be divided into non-intersecting subsets $\{E_1, \ldots, E_r, \ldots, E_n\}$ of edges of different types. Let the voxel j be such that $(i, j) \in E$ is a neighbor of type r, that is $(i, j) \in E_r$. Let the corresponding feature vectors $\mathbf{f}_i(\mathbf{x})$ and $\mathbf{f}_j(\mathbf{x})$ land in leaves $L(i)$ and $L(j)$ of the trained tree Ψ, respectively. The interaction potential is modeled as

$$E_{\mathcal{I}}(y_i, y_j, \mathbf{x}; \theta) = \frac{1}{2}(\alpha_{L(i)_r}y_i^2 + \beta_{L(i)_r}y_iy_j + \gamma_{L(i)_r}y_j^2) - \omega_{L(i)_{1r}}y_i - \omega_{L(i)_{2r}}y_j. \tag{4}$$

Let the set of leaves of the regression tree Ψ be $\mathcal{L}_\Psi$. Each leaf $l \in \mathcal{L}_\Psi$ stores the set of parameters $\theta_l = \{a_l, b_l, \alpha_{l1}, \beta_{l1}, \gamma_{l1}, \omega_{l11}, \omega_{l21}, \ldots, \alpha_{ln}, \beta_{ln}, \gamma_{ln}, \omega_{l1n}, \omega_{l2n}\}$. The complete set of parameters is thus, $\theta = \{\theta_l | l \in \mathcal{L}_\Psi\}$. Our approach bears similarity to the regression tree fields concept introduced in [7], where the authors create a separate regression tree for each neighbor type. Thus with a single association potential and a typical 3D neighborhood of 26 neighbors, they would need 27 separate trees to learn the model parameters. Training a large number of trees with large training sets makes the regression tree fields approach computationally expensive. It was especially not feasible in our application with large 3D images, more neighbors, and high dimensional feature vectors. We can however train multiple trees using bagging to create an ensemble of models to create an average, improved prediction. The training of a single regression tree is described in the next section.

2.2 Learning a Regression Tree

As mentioned before, let $\mathbf{x} = \{\mathbf{x}_1, \mathbf{x}_2, \ldots, \mathbf{x}_m\}$ be a collection of co-registered images, generated by modalities $\Phi_1, \ldots, \Phi_m$, respectively. The image synthesis task entails predicting the image $\mathbf{y}$ of a target modality Φ_t. The training data thus consists of known co-registered pair of $\{\mathbf{x}, \mathbf{y}\}$. At each voxel location i, we extract features $\mathbf{f}_i(\mathbf{x})$, derived from $\mathbf{x}$. For our experiments we use two types of features, (1) small, local patches, (2) context descriptors. A small 3D patch, denoted by $\mathbf{p}_i(\mathbf{x}) = [\mathbf{p}_i(\mathbf{x}_1), \ldots, \mathbf{p}_i(\mathbf{x}_m)]$, where the size of the patch is typically $3 \times 3 \times 3$ and provides us with local intensity information.

We construct the context descriptors as follows. The brain images are rigidly aligned to the MNI coordinate system [4] with the center of the brain approximately at the center of the image. Thus for each voxel we can find out the unit vector $\mathbf{u}$ from the voxel i to the origin. We can define 8 directions by rotating the component of $\mathbf{u}$ in the axial plane by angles $\{0, \frac{\pi}{4}, \ldots, \frac{7\pi}{4}\}$. In each of these directions, we select average intensities of cubic regions of cube-widths $\{w_1, w_2, w_3, w_4\}$ at four different radii $\{r_1, r_2, r_3, r_4\}$ respectively. This becomes a 32-dimensional descriptor of the spatial context surrounding voxel i. In our experiments we used $w_1 = 3, w_2 = 5, w_3 = 7, w_4 = 9$ and $r_1 = 4, r_2 = 8, r_3 = 16, r_4 = 32$. These values were chosen empirically. We denote this context descriptor by $\mathbf{c}_i(\mathbf{x})$. The final feature vector is thus $\mathbf{f}_i(\mathbf{x}) = [\mathbf{p}_i(\mathbf{x}), \mathbf{c}_i(\mathbf{x})]$. $\mathbf{f}_i(\mathbf{x})$ is paired with the voxel intensity y_i at i in the target modality image $\mathbf{y}$ to create training data pairs $(\mathbf{f}_i(\mathbf{x}), y_i)$. We train the regression tree Ψ on this training data using the algorithm described in [2]. Once the tree is constructed, we initialize θ_l at each of the leaves $l \in \mathcal{L}_\Psi$. θ_l is estimated by a pseudo-likelihood maximization approach.

2.3   Parameter Learning

An ideal approach to learn parameters would be to perform maximum likelihood using the distribution in Eq. 2. However as mentioned in [7], estimation of the mean parameters Σ and μ, requires calculation of $\mathbf{A}^{-1}$ (see Eq. 2). The size of $\mathbf{A}$ is $|V \times V|$ where $|V|$ is the number of voxels in $\mathbf{y}$ and for large 3D images, $|V|$ is of the order of $\sim 10^6$, which makes the computation practically infeasible. We follow [7] and implement a pseudo-likelihood maximization-based parameter learning.

Pseudo-likelihood is defined as the product of local conditional likelihoods,

$$\hat{\theta}_{\mathrm{MPLE}} = \mathrm{argmax}_\theta \prod_{i \in V} \mathrm{p}(y_i \mid \mathbf{y}_{\mathcal{N}_i}, \mathbf{x}; \theta). \tag{5}$$

The local conditional likelihood can be expanded as

$$\mathrm{p}(y_i \mid \mathbf{y}_{\mathcal{N}_i}, \mathbf{x}; \theta) = \frac{\mathrm{p}(y_i, \mathbf{y}_{\mathcal{N}_i}, \mathbf{x}; \theta)}{\int_{\mathbb{R}} \mathrm{p}(y_i, \mathbf{y}_{\mathcal{N}_i}, \mathbf{x}; \theta) dy_i},$$

$$-\log \mathrm{p}(y_i \mid \mathbf{y}_{\mathcal{N}_i}, \mathbf{x}; \theta) = -\log \mathrm{p}(y_i, \mathbf{y}_{\mathcal{N}_i}, \mathbf{x}; \theta) + \log Z_i, \tag{6}$$

where $Z_i = \int_{\mathbb{R}} \mathrm{p}(y_i, \mathbf{y}_{\mathcal{N}_i}, \mathbf{x}; \theta) dy_i$. Using the CRF definition in Eq. 1, we can write $-\log \mathrm{p}(y_i, \mathbf{y}_{\mathcal{N}_i}, \mathbf{x}; \theta)$ as

$$-\log \mathrm{p}(y_i, \mathbf{y}_{\mathcal{N}_i}, \mathbf{x}; \theta) = E_{\mathcal{A}}(y_i, \mathbf{x}; \theta) + \lambda \sum_{j \in \mathcal{N}_i} E_{\mathcal{I}}(y_i, y_j, \mathbf{x}; \theta)$$

$$= \frac{1}{2} a_{Ci} y_i^2 - b_{Ci} y_i, \tag{7}$$

where we can find a_{Ci}(Eq. 8) and b_{Ci},(Eq. 9) by matching quadratic and linear terms. Equations 8 and 9 show the contribution of interaction potentials induced by the neighbors of voxel i. The $\tilde{r}$ denotes the type of edge which is symmetric to type r. For example, if edges of type r are between voxel i and its right neighbor, then $\tilde{r}$ denotes the type that is between a voxel and its left neighbor.

$$a_{Ci} = a_{L(i)} + \lambda(\sum_{j|(i,j)\in E_r} \alpha_{L(i)_r} + \sum_{h|(h,i)\in E_{\tilde{r}}} \gamma_{L(h)_{\tilde{r}}}) \tag{8}$$

$$b_{Ci} = b_{L(i)} + \lambda(\sum_{j|(i,j)\in E_r} \omega_{L(i)_{1r}} + \sum_{h|(h,i)\in E_{\tilde{r}}} \omega_{L(h)_{2\tilde{r}}}$$
$$- \frac{1}{2}\sum_{j|(i,j)\in E_r} \beta_{L(i)_r} y_j - \frac{1}{2}\sum_{h|(h,i)\in E_{\tilde{r}}} \beta_{L(h)_{\tilde{r}}} y_h). \tag{9}$$

The integral of exponential terms Z_i in Eq. 6, is also known as the log partition term. To optimize objective functions with log partition terms, we express Z_i in its variational representation using the mean parameters $\boldsymbol{\mu}_i = [\mu_i, \sigma_i]$ [18]. The parameter set $\boldsymbol{\theta}_{Ci} = \{b_{Ci}, a_{Ci}\}$ that defines the exponential distribution is known as the canonical parameter set. The conjugate dual function of Z_i is defined as follows,

$$Z_i^*(\mu_i, \sigma_i) = \sup_{\boldsymbol{\theta}_{Ci}} \langle \boldsymbol{\theta}_{Ci}, \boldsymbol{\mu}_i \rangle - Z_i(\boldsymbol{\theta}_{Ci}), \tag{10}$$

where $\langle \rangle$ denotes inner product. Substituting $\boldsymbol{\theta}_{Ci}$ and the expression for $-\log p(y_i, \mathbf{y}_{\mathcal{N}_i}, \mathbf{x}; \theta)$ from Eq. 7, we get the negative pseudo-likelihood contributed by voxel i to be,

$$\text{NPL}_i(\theta) = b_{Ci}(\mu_i - y_i) + \frac{1}{2}a_{Ci}(y_i^2 - \sigma_i) + \log(\sigma_i - \mu_i^2) + \log(2\pi e), \tag{11}$$

where the mean parameters are given by $\mu_i = \frac{b_{Ci}}{a_{Ci}}$ and $\sigma_i = \frac{1}{a_{Ci}} + \mu_i^2$.

Equation 11 is similar to the one in [7], as the overall model is a Gaussian CRF. The objective function is linearly related to θ and is thus convex [7,18]. We minimize $\sum_{i\in V} \text{NPL}_i(\theta)$ using gradient descent. The weighting factor $\lambda = 0.1$, was chosen empirically in our experiments. The regression tree fields concept performed a constrained, projected gradient descent on the parameters to ensure positive definiteness of the final precision matrix ($\mathbf{A}(\mathbf{x})$ in Eq. 1) [7]. We observed that unconstrained optimization in our model and applications generated a positive definite $\mathbf{A}(\mathbf{x})$. Training in our experiments takes about 20–30 min with $\sim 10^6$ samples of dimensionality of the order of $\sim 10^2$ and neighborhood size of 26, on a 12 core 3.42 GHz machine.

2.4   Inference

Given a test image set $\hat{\mathbf{x}} = \{\hat{\mathbf{x}}_1, \ldots, \hat{\mathbf{x}}_m\}$, which are co-registered, we first extract features $\mathbf{f}_i(\hat{\mathbf{x}})$ from all voxel locations i. Next, we apply the learned regression

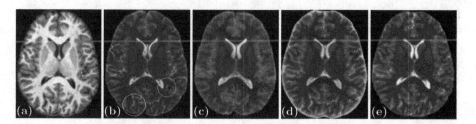

Fig. 1. Shown are (**a**) the input MPRAGE image, (**b**) the true T_2-w image, and the synthesis results from the MPRAGE for each of (**c**) FUSION, (**d**) MIMECS, and (**e**) SyCRAFT (our method). The lesion (green circle) and the cortex (yellow circle) in the true image are synthesized by MIMECS and SyCRAFT, but not by FUSION (Colour figure online).

tree Ψ to each of $\mathbf{f}_i(\hat{\mathbf{x}})$ to determine the leaf node $L(i)$ in Ψ. Using the learned parameters at these leaves, we construct the matrix $\mathbf{A}(\hat{\mathbf{x}})$ and the vector $\mathbf{b}(\hat{\mathbf{x}})$, (see Eq. 2). The diagonal and off-diagonal elements of $\mathbf{A}(\hat{\mathbf{x}})$ are populated by matching the linear and quadratic terms from Eq. 2. The MAP estimate for $p(\mathbf{y}|\hat{\mathbf{x}})$ as well as the conditional expectation $E[\mathbf{y}|\hat{\mathbf{x}}]$ is the mean of the multivariate Gaussian described in Eq. 2. The expression for the mean and hence the estimate $\hat{\mathbf{y}}$ is given by,

$$\hat{\mathbf{y}} = \mathbf{A}(\hat{\mathbf{x}})^{-1}\mathbf{b}(\hat{\mathbf{x}}). \tag{12}$$

$\mathbf{A}(\hat{\mathbf{x}})$ is a large ($\sim 10^6 \times 10^6$), sparse ($\sim 27 \times 10^6$ non-zero entries), symmetric positive definite matrix. Thus, we use an iterative preconditioned conjugate gradient descent method to solve the linear system in Eq. 12. The estimate $\hat{\mathbf{y}}$ is our synthetic image. Estimates from multiple (5 in our experiments) trained models using bagging can also be averaged to produce a final result.

3   Results

3.1   Synthesis of T_2-w Images from T_1-w Images

In this experiment, we used MPRAGE images from the publicly available multimodal reproducibility (MMRR) data [11] and synthesized the T_2-w images of the DSE sequence. The multimodal reproducibility data consists of 21 subjects, each with two imaging sessions, acquired within an hour of each other. Thus there are 42 MPRAGE images. We excluded data of five subjects (ten images), which were used for training and synthesized the remaining 32. We compared SyCRAFT to MIMECS [15] and multi-atlas registration and intensity fusion (FUSION) [3]. We used five subjects as the atlases for FUSION with the parameters $\beta = 0.5$ and $\kappa = 4$ (fuse the four best patch matches).

We used PSNR (peak signal to noise ratio), universal quality index (UQI) [19], and structural similarity (SSIM) [20] as metrics. UQI and SSIM take into account image degradation as observed by a human visual system. Both have values that lie between 0 and 1, with 1 implying that the images

Table 1. Mean and standard deviation (Std. Dev.) of the PSNR, UQI, and SSIM values for synthesis of T_2-w images from 32 MPRAGE scans.

	PSNR Mean (Std)	UQI Mean (Std.)	SSIM Mean (Std)
FUSION	52.73 (2.78)[a]	0.78 (0.02)	0.82 (0.02)
MIMECS	36.13 (2.23)	0.78 (0.02)	0.77 (0.02)
SyCRAFT	49.73 (1.99)	0.86 (0.01)[a]	0.84 (0.01)[a]

[a] Statistically significantly better than either of the other two methods (α level of 0.01) using a right-tailed test.

Subject T_1-w	T_2-w	P_D-w	Synth. FLAIR	True FLAIR

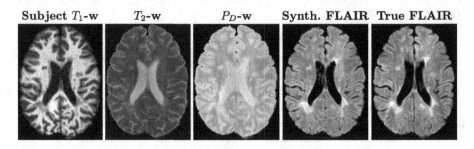

Fig. 2. Subject input images along with the SyCRAFT FLAIR and true FLAIR images.

are equal to each other. SyCRAFT performs significantly better than both the methods for all metrics except PSNR. Figure 1 shows the results for all three methods along with the true T_2-w image. FUSION results (Fig. 1(b)) have the highest PSNR, but produce anatomically incorrect images, especially in the presence of abnormal tissue anatomy (lesions for example) and the cortex. Overall, SyCRAFT produces an image that is visually closest to the true T_2-w image (Table 1).

3.2 Synthesis for FLAIR Images

In this experiment, given atlas P_D-w, T_2-w, T_1-w, and FLAIR images, we trained SyCRAFT and applied it to subject P_D-w , T_2-w, and T_1-w images, to predict the subject synthetic FLAIR image. We used our in-house multiple sclerosis (MS) patient image dataset with 49 subject images, with four training subjects and testing on the remaining 45. We computed average PSNR (20.81, std = 1.19), UQI (0.81, std = 0.03) and SSIM (0.78, std = 0.03), over these 45 subjects. These values indicate that the synthetic FLAIRs are structurally and visually similar to their corresponding real FLAIRs. Figure 2 shows the input images and the synthetic FLAIR image along side the real FLAIR image.

Next, we investigated the segmentations acquired from these synthetic FLAIRs. We would like the segmentation algorithm, LesionTOADS [16], to behave identically for real and synthetic images. LesionTOADS uses a T_1-w and

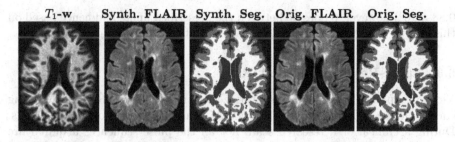

Fig. 3. LesionTOADS segmentations for real and synthetic FLAIRs.

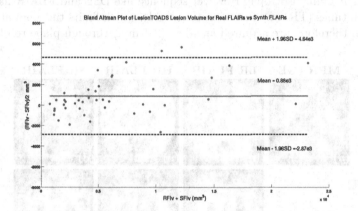

Fig. 4. A Bland-Altman plot of lesion volumes for synthetic FLAIRs vs real FLAIRs.

a corresponding FLAIR to generate a multi-class, topologically correct segmentation in the presence of lesions. We compared the overlap of segmentations obtained using synthetic FLAIRs to those obtained using real FLAIRs in terms of Dice coefficients (averaged over 45 subjects) for white matter (0.97, std = 0.01) (WM), gray matter (0.99, std = 0.01) (GM), cerebrospinal fluid (0.97, std = 0.01) (CSF) and white matter lesions (0.52, std = 0.17) (WML). Figure 3 shows the segmentations by LesionTOADS on real and synthetic FLAIRs. The overlap is very good for WM, GM, and CSF, however it is low for the WML class. The lesions being small and diffuse, even a small difference in the overlap can cause a low value for the Dice coefficient. So, we looked at the overall lesion volumes as provided by the algorithm for real and synthetic FLAIRs. To understand how different the lesion volumes are for the synthetic images as compared to the real images, we created a Bland-Altman [1] plot shown in Fig. 4. Let RFlv be the lesion volumes given by LesionTOADS using real FLAIRs as input. Let SFlv be the lesion volumes using synthetic FLAIRs as input. Bland-Altman plot is a scatter plot of $(RFlv - SFlv)/2$ (y axis) vs. $RFlv + SFlv$ (x axis). The measurements are considered to be interchangeable if 0 lies within $\pm 1.96\sigma$ where σ is the standard deviation of $(RFlv - SFlv)/2$. There is a small bias between RFlv and SFlv (mean =

0.88×10^3) however, 0 does lie between the prescribed limits and hence based on this plot we can say that these two measurements are interchangeable.

3.3   Super-Resolution of FLAIR

Next, we applied SyCRAFT to synthesize super-resolution (SR) FLAIRs using corresponding high resolution (HR) MPRAGE and low resolution (LR) FLAIRs. During a clinical or a research scan, not all the pulse sequences acquired are acquired at the same fixed resolution. Sequences like the T_1-w MPRAGE can be acquired very fast and hence are easy to image at a high resolution–usually higher than $1\,mm^3$ isotropic. However sequence like DSE and FLAIR have long repetition times (TR) and inversion times (TI), which limits the amount of scan time, and therefore, are acquired at a low (2–5 mm) through plane resolution.

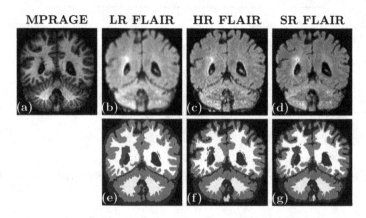

Fig. 5. Coronal slices of LR, HR, and SR FLAIRs along with their corresponding LesionTOADS segmentation are shown. It is evident that using a LR FLAIR affects the segmentation of the lesions and even the cortex.

Our approach can be described as an example-based super-resolution [14] technique. Example-based methods leverage the high resolution information extracted from a HR image—an MPRAGE, for example—in conjunction with a LR input image—corresponding FLAIR image—to generate a SR version of the LR image. We used HR ($1 \times 1 \times 1\,mm^3$) MPRAGE and FLAIR data, and downsampled the HR FLAIR to create a LR ($1 \times 1 \times 4\,mm^3$) FLAIR. The atlas data included an HR MPRAGE + LR FLAIR and we trained SyCRAFT to predict the HR FLAIR. Given a test HR MPRAGE and LR FLAIR, we applied SyCRAFT to synthesize a SR FLAIR. We ran the LesionTOADS [16] segmentation algorithm on three scenarios for each subject: (a) HR MPRAGE + LR FLAIR (b) HR MPRAGE + SR FLAIR (c) HR MPRAGE + HR FLAIR. The last case acting as the ground truth for how the segmentation algorithm should behave on best case data. We aim to show that the tissue segmentation using SR FLAIR is closer to that achieved using HR FLAIR, than using LR

FLAIR. Figure 5(d) shows the super-resolution results, the LR FLAIR image is shown in Fig. 5(b), and the HR FLAIR image in Fig. 5(c). The corresponding LesionTOADS segmentations are shown in Figs. 5(e, f, g), respectively. The lesion boundaries as well as the cortex is overestimated when a LR FLAIR is used. Shown in Fig. 6 are the lesion volumes on 13 subjects for each of the three scenarios.

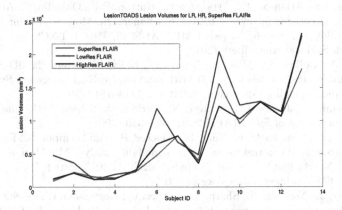

Fig. 6. Shown are the lesion volumes acquired by LesionTOADS on HR FLAIR+HR MPRAGE (black), LR FLAIR+HR MPRAGE (blue), and SR FLAIR+HR MPRAGE (red). Note that the black plot is closer to the red plot than the blue plot for all but one of the subjects (Colour figure online).

4 Conclusion

We have described an image synthesis framework, SyCRAFT, as a learning and inference problem on a Gaussian CRF. The parameters of the Gaussian CRF are built from parameters stored at the leaves of a single regression tree. Parameter learning is done by maximizing a pseudo-likelihood objective function. Our approach is extremely flexible in terms of features it can use to create the initial regression tree. It is also general enough to add larger neighborhoods and long-range relationships among voxels. Adding more neighbors leads to additional parameters, but these can be stored in the same initial tree and we do not need to create any more trees. Our approach is also computationally efficient, training from millions of samples in 20–30 min, and inference taking less than five minutes. We compared SyCRAFT to competitive image synthesis algorithms and showed that the image quality is superior. We also demonstrated practical benefits of using our algorithm to synthesize FLAIRs and validated the synthesis by showing tissue segmentation equivalent to that obtained using real FLAIRs. This shows that our image synthesis algorithm can be used in realistic scenarios, where imaging data is missing and needs to be replaced by a feasible alternative. Finally we also applied our algorithm to enhance the resolution of low resolution FLAIRs and showed improved tissue segmentation as a result.

References

1. Bland, J.M., Altman, D.G.: Statistical Methods For Assessing Agreement Between Two Methods Of Clinical Measurement. The Lancet **327**(8476), 307–310 (1986)
2. Breiman, L., Friedman, J.H., Olshen, R.A., Stone, C.J.: Classification and Regression Trees. Wadsworth Publishing Company, U.S.A (1984)
3. Burgos, N., Cardoso, M.J., Modat, M., Pedemonte, S., Dickson, J., Barnes, A., Duncan, J.S., Atkinson, D., Arridge, S.R., Hutton, B.F., Ourselin, S.: Attenuation correction synthesis for hybrid PET-MR scanners. In: Mori, K., Sakuma, I., Sato, Y., Barillot, C., Navab, N. (eds.) MICCAI 2013, Part I. LNCS, vol. 8149, pp. 147–154. Springer, Heidelberg (2013)
4. Evans, A., Collins, D., Mills, S., Brown, E., Kelly, R., Peters, T.: 3D Statistical Neuroanatomical Models from 305 MRI volumes. In: Nuclear Science Symposium and Medical Imaging Conference, vol. 3, pp. 1813–1817 (1993)
5. Hertzmann, A., Jacobs, C.E., Oliver, N., Curless, B., Salesin, D.H.: Image Analogies. Proceedings of SIGGRAPH **2001**, 327–340 (2001)
6. Iglesias, J.E., Konukoglu, E., Zikic, D., Glocker, B., Van Leemput, K., Fischl, B.: Is synthesizing MRI contrast useful for inter-modality analysis? In: Mori, K., Sakuma, I., Sato, Y., Barillot, C., Navab, N. (eds.) MICCAI 2013, Part I. LNCS, vol. 8149, pp. 631–638. Springer, Heidelberg (2013)
7. Jancsary, J., Nowozin, S., Sharp, T., Rother, C.: Regression Tree Fields; An Efficient, Non-parametric Approach to Image Labeling Problems. In: CVPR, 2376–2383 (2012)
8. Jog, A., Roy, S., Carass, A., Prince, J.L.: Magnetic Resonance Image Synthesis through Patch Regression. In: 10th International Symposium on Biomedical Imaging (ISBI 2013), pp. 350–353 (2013)
9. Kumar, S., Hebert, M.: Discriminative random fields. Int. J. Comput. Vision **68**(2), 179–201 (2006)
10. Lafferty, J.D., McCallum, A., Pereira, F.C.N.: Conditional random fields: probabilistic models for segmenting and labeling sequence data. In: ICML 2001, pp. 282–289 (2001)
11. Landman, B.A., Huang, A.J., Gifford, A., Vikram, D.S., Lim, I.A.L., Farrell, J.A.D., Bogovic, J.A., Hua, J., Chen, M., Jarso, S., Smith, S.A., Joel, S., Mori, S., Pekar, J.J., Barker, P.B., Prince, J.L., van Zijl, P.: Multi-parametric neuroimaging reproducibility: a 3-T resource study. NeuroImage **54**(4), 2854–2866 (2011)
12. Miller, M.I., Christensen, G.E., Amit, Y., Grenander, U.: Mathematical textbook of deformable neuroanatomies. Proc. Natl. Acad. Sci. **90**(24), 11944–11948 (1993)
13. Nyúl, L.G., Udupa, J.K., Zhang, X.: New variants of a method of MRI scale standardization. IEEE Trans. Med. Imag. **19**(2), 143–150 (2000)
14. Rousseau, F.: Brain hallucination. In: Forsyth, D., Torr, P., Zisserman, A. (eds.) ECCV 2008, Part I. LNCS, vol. 5302, pp. 497–508. Springer, Heidelberg (2008)
15. Roy, S., Carass, A., Prince, J.L.: Magnetic resonance image example based contrast synthesis. IEEE Trans. Med. Imag. **32**(12), 2348–2363 (2013)
16. Shiee, N., Bazin, P.L., Ozturk, A., Reich, D.S., Calabresi, P.A., Pham, D.L.: A topology-preserving approach to the segmentation of brain images with multiple sclerosis lesions. NeuroImage **49**(2), 1524–1535 (2010)
17. Tappen, M., Liu, C., Adelson, E., Freeman, W.: Learning gaussian conditional random fields for low-level vision. In: CVPR, pp. 1–8 (2007)
18. Wainwright, M.J., Jordan, M.I.: Graphical models, exponential families, and variational inference. Found. Trends Mach. Learn. **1**(1–2), 1–305 (2008)

19. Wang, Z., Bovik, A.C.: A universal image quality index. IEEE Signal Proc. Letters **9**(3), 81–84 (2002)
20. Wang, Z., Bovik, A.C., Sheikh, H.R., Member, S., Simoncelli, E.P.: Image quality assessment: from error visibility to structural similarity. IEEE Trans. Image Proc. **13**, 600–612 (2004)

Simultaneous Longitudinal Registration with Group-Wise Similarity Prior

Greg M. Fleishman[1,2]([✉]), Boris A. Gutman[2], P. Thomas Fletcher[3], and Paul M. Thompson[2]

[1] Department of Bioengineering, UC Los Angeles, Los Angeles, USA
gfleishman@ucla.edu
[2] Imaging Genetics Center, LONI, Univeristy of Southern California, Los Angeles, USA
[3] Scientific Computing and Imaging Institute, University of Utah, Salt Lake City, USA

Abstract. Here we present an algorithm for the simultaneous registration of N longitudinal image pairs such that information acquired by each pair is used to constrain the registration of each other pair. More specifically, in the geodesic shooting setting for Large Deformation Diffeomorphic Metric Mappings (LDDMM) an average of the initial momenta characterizing the N transformations is maintained throughout and updates to individual momenta are constrained to be similar to this average. In this way, the N registrations are coupled and explore the space of diffeomorphisms as a group, the variance of which is constrained to be small. Our approach is motivated by the observation that transformations learned from images in the same diagnostic category share characteristics. The group-wise consistency prior serves to strengthen the contribution of the common signal among the N image pairs to the transformation for a specific pair, relative to features particular to that pair. We tested the algorithm on 57 longitudinal image pairs of Alzheimer's Disease patients from the Alzheimer's Disease Neuroimaging Initiative and evaluated the ability of the algorithm to produce momenta that better represent the long term biological processes occurring in the underlying anatomy. We found that for many image pairs, momenta learned with the group-wise prior better predict a third time point image unobserved in the registration.

1 Introduction

Nonlinear image registration in brain imaging has progressed to an advanced stage with powerful mathematical tools for sensitive and precise measurements with important theoretical properties. The LDDMM framework establishes a setting wherein constructions like the Fréchet mean and geodesic regression in a space of diffeomorphisms are well defined [7,16]. For some lines of work, the availability of such statistical constructs has promoted a more probabilistic view of transformations. Real image data is noisy, and transformations estimated from it are susceptible to over fitting to this noise. For example, given three images

© Springer International Publishing Switzerland 2015
S. Ourselin et al. (Eds.): IPMI 2015, LNCS 9123, pp. 746–757, 2015.
DOI: 10.1007/978-3-319-19992-4_59

of the same anatomy acquired over time, it is not likely that a geodesic can be drawn in the transformation space that passes through the identity and the optimal transformations for both of the follow up images. (For example, see Fig. 4 in [5].) Hence, an initial momentum characterizing the geodesic between the identity and the optimal transformation for the first or second follow up image does not describe the optimal geodesic that would be obtained from geodesic regression of all three images.

In this paper we attempt to estimate initial momenta from only two images with improved ability to predict future unobserved images, by simultaneously registering many image pairs that share information throughout optimization. Our approach can be viewed in two equivalent ways: we maintain a group level representation of a transformation and constrain individual transformations to be similar to this representation, which is equivalent to compressing the variance of the set of transformations about their mean. Both of these techniques have precedent in the literature. For example in [13], to estimate functional networks from resting state fMRI data, the authors construct a hierarchical Markov Random Field (hMRF) where the highest level of the hierarchy is a group-wise representation of the network estimate. Edges connecting this level to the individual levels represent a group-wise consistency constraint. Shrinkage of the transformations about their mean is also reminiscent of a James-Stein estimator [4], where we have chosen the average momentum as the prior estimate of the true geodesic regression slope. From this perspective, our method can be viewed as an empirical Bayes prior.

This work uses cross-sectional information in a longitudinal study, which also has precedent in the literature. Other works have used statistical information to constrain registration, but more often in the form of a prior learned from a training set as suggested in [8] and implemented in [2]. These authors constrained the strain tensor of an elastic transformation to be similar to an average strain learned from training data. More recently, the authors of [5] use the transformations of normal controls to refine transformations of AD patients for effects due to the disease. Perhaps most similar to our proposal is [9], in which a group level trajectory is jointly estimated with individual trajectories. The group level trajectory is considered a latent generator for the individual trajectories, but unlike the proposed work, deviation from the group level is not explicitly penalized. In all cases, the incorporation of group level information resulted in transformations with features not found without the group level information, and in many cases, these features were shown to be desirable.

2   Methods

Background, the LDDMM Framework: We begin with a brief review of the LDDMM framework for nonlinear image registration [1]. Given $I_0, I_1 \in L^2(\Omega, \mathbb{R})$, the LDDMM energy functional is defined as:

$$E(v, I_0, I_1) = \int_0^1 \|v\|_V dt + \|I_0 \circ \phi_1^{-1} - I_1\|_{L_2} \qquad (1)$$

where $v \in L^2([0,1], V)$ is a time dependent velocity field drawn from the reproducing kernel Hilbert space (RKHS) V. The RKHS is specified by the choice of kernel K, and the inner product in V is then given by $\langle K^{-1}u, u\rangle_{L_2}$ for any $u \in V$. The transformation $\phi(t, x)$ is given by the flow of the velocity $v(t, x)$ through the ODE: $(d/dt)\phi(t, x) = v(t, \phi(t, x))$, with initial condition $\phi(0, x) = x$. $v(t, x)$ and $\phi(t, x)$ will be written as $v_t(x)$ and $\phi_t(x)$. The minimizer of (1) is considered the optimal ϕ for the registration of I_0 and I_1.

The second term on the right hand side of (1) is a quantitative assessment of the similarity between the images $I_0 \circ \phi_1^{-1}$ and I_1, whereas the first term is the geodesic energy of the flow of $v_t(x)$. For suitable choices of K, $\phi_t(x)$ is always a diffeomorphism [10]; hence, (1) defines ϕ_1 to be the transformation that best matches I_0 and I_1 such that ϕ_t is a geodesic in a space of diffeomorphisms specified by the choice of K. As ϕ_t is a geodesic when $E(v, I_0, I_1)$ is optimal, $E(v, I_0, I_1)$ defines a metric distance $d(Id, \phi_1)^2$ in the space of diffeomorphisms. This can also be considered a metric $d(I_0, I_1)^2$ on the orbit given by the group action of the space of diffeomorphisms on the template image I_0.

Background, Geodesic Shooting Algorithm: Several approaches to optimizing (1) have been proposed. In this paper we use the geodesic shooting approach [6,12], which we now review. The kernel K can also be considered a mapping between V^*, the space of linear functionals on V, and V itself. Note that V^* is also a Hilbert space. An Element of V^* is called a momentum. Hence for any momentum $m \in V^*$ there is some $v \in V$ such that $Km = v$ and $K^{-1}v = m$.

An optimal solution to (1) specifies a geodesic, which is uniquely determined by its initial velocity $v_0(x)$, or equivalently, its initial momentum $m_0(x)$. m_t for all t, and hence v_t and ϕ_t, can then be determined by solving the co-adjoint equation [6]: $(\partial/\partial t)m_t = -ad_v^* m_t = -(Dv)^T m_t - Dm_t v - div(v)m_t$, where D denotes the Jacobian operator and $div(.)$ the divergence operator. If the initial momentum is assumed to be proportional to the template image gradient, that is $m_0(x) = p_0(x)\nabla I_0(x)$ for some scalar field p_0, the adjoint equation can be separated into a disjoint system of differential equations for $I_{0,t}$ and p_t respectively [12], where $I_{0,t} = I_0 \circ \phi_t^{-1}$. Considering these equations and the gradient of (1) with respect to v_t, we arrive at a system of partial differential equations that completely specifies ϕ_t given initial conditions I_0 and p_0 ($\star$ denotes convolution):

$$\begin{cases} (\partial/\partial t)p + \nabla \cdot (pv) = 0 \\ (\partial/\partial t)I + \nabla I \cdot v = 0 \\ (\partial/\partial t)v + K \star \nabla I p = 0 \end{cases} \tag{2}$$

With this in mind, (1) is replaced with a functional of the initial momentum exclusively:

$$\mathcal{E}(p_0, I_0, I_1) = \langle p_0 \nabla I_0, K \star p_0 \nabla I_0\rangle_{L_2} + \|I_{0,1} - I_1\|_{L_2}^2 \tag{3}$$

and optimization proceeds within V^* only. In order to optimize (3) by gradient descent, we need the gradient of (3) with respect to p_0, subject to the geodesic shooting constraints (2). This naturally gives way to an optimal control problem. Time dependent Lagrange multipliers $\hat{p}_t$, $\hat{I}_{0,t}$, and $\hat{v}_t$ enable us to write an augmented functional for (3) incorporating the constraints (2):

$$\tilde{\mathcal{E}}(p_0, I_0, I_1) = \mathcal{E} + \int_0^1 \langle \hat{p}_t, (\partial/\partial t)p + \nabla \cdot (pv) \rangle dt \; +$$

$$\int_0^1 \langle \hat{I}_{0,t}, (\partial/\partial t)I + \nabla I \cdot v \rangle dt \; + \tag{4}$$

$$\int_0^1 \langle \hat{v}_t, (\partial/\partial t)v + K \star \nabla I p \rangle dt$$

The first variation of (4) gives the gradient of (3) subject to (2):

$$\nabla_{p_0} \mathcal{E} = \nabla I_0 \cdot K \star p_0 \nabla I_0 - \hat{p}_0 \tag{5}$$

where $\hat{p}_0$ is specified by a system of partial differential equations solved backward in time termed the adjoint system:

$$\begin{cases} (\partial/\partial t)\hat{p} + \nabla \hat{p} \cdot v - \nabla I \cdot K \star \hat{v} = 0 \\ (\partial/\partial t)\hat{I} + \nabla \cdot (Iv) + \nabla \cdot pK \star \hat{v} = 0 \\ (\partial/\partial t)\hat{v} + \hat{I}\nabla I - p\nabla \hat{p} = 0 \end{cases} \tag{6}$$

with initial conditions $\hat{I}_1 = I_1 - I_{0,1}$ and $\hat{p}_1 = 0$. The gradient descent proceeds by solving the system (2) forward in time to acquire p_t, $I_{0,1}$, and v_t for a sufficiently dense sampling of $t \in [0, 1]$, then solving (6) backward in time to acquire $\hat{p}_0$. p_0 is then updated with (5), and the process is repeated until convergence.

Group-wise Similarity Prior: We consider the case where we are given N longitudinal image pairs $I_0^i, I_1^i \in L^2(\Omega, \mathbb{R})$, $i \in [1, 2, ..., N]$, all taken approximately the same time interval apart. We take Ω to be the unit cube with periodic boundary conditions, and the time interval to be $[0, 1]$. Additionally, we are given N transformations ψ^i mapping the initial images I_0^i to a Minimal Deformation Template (MDT) coordinate system, that is, $I_0^k \circ \psi^k \sim I_0^j \circ \psi^j$ for all k and j. To consider all N registrations simultaneously with no modification to the geodesic shooting approach, we could write $\tilde{\mathcal{E}}_{tot} = \sum_{i=1}^N \tilde{\mathcal{E}}_i$ where $\tilde{\mathcal{E}}_i$ is eq. (3) for the ith image pair. The first variation of $\tilde{\mathcal{E}}_{tot}$ with respect to an initial momentum p_0^i will only include terms for the ith pair, that is, the N transformations are decoupled. However, we would like the N transformations to explore the space of diffeomorphisms as a group. We couple them by considering equations of the form:

$$\tilde{\mathcal{E}}_{tot} = \alpha \mathcal{G}(p_1, p_2, ..., p_N) + \sum_{i=1}^N \tilde{\mathcal{E}}_i \tag{7}$$

$\mathcal{G}(.)$ is intended to enforce some criteria that we may think all p_0^i must satisfy. In this paper, we consider longitudinal studies where all N image pairs come from patients in the same diagnostic group, where a predictable distribution of volume change is known to occur. Because V^* is a Hilbert space, we can calculate statistical moments in this space in an ordinary manner, being careful to spatially normalize the p_0^i to a MDT coordinate system using coadjoint transport [15]. First, let $p_0^{mdt,i} = |D\psi^i|p_0^i \circ \psi^i$, be the ith initial momentum in the MDT coordinate system. Let $p_0^{mdt,avg} = (1/N)\sum_{i=1}^N p_0^{mdt,i}$ be the sample average initial momentum in MDT coordinates. Let $p_0^{mdt,cen,i} = p_0^{mdt,i} - p_0^{mdt,avg}$ be the mean centered initial momentum for image pair i in MDT coordinates, and let $A = [p_0^{mdt,cen,1}, p_0^{mdt,cen,2}, ..., p_0^{mdt,cen,N}]^T$ be the mean centered design matrix for all initial momenta in MDT coordinates. We take $\mathcal{G}(.)$ to be:

$$\mathcal{G}(p_1, p_2, ..., p_N) = Trace(AA^T) = \sum_{i=1}^N \|p_0^{mdt,i} - p_0^{mdt,avg}\|_{L_2}^2 \qquad (8)$$

the trace of the sample inner-product matrix for p_0.

First we consider the rightmost form of (8). We see that this term maintains a group-wise average of the initial momentum, and requires that all momenta be close to this average. This is similar to hierarchical latent variable models that maintain a group-wise representation of the data and constrain updates to predictions to be similar to this representation.

Now consider the middle form of (8). The covariance matrix $A^T A$ has the same eigenvalues as the inner-product matrix AA^T. Covariance matrices are symmetric positive-definite, and therefore have all real non-negative eigenvalues. Finally, the trace of a matrix is invariant to rotation. So, considering the canonical form of $A^T A$, we see that $Trace(AA^T) = \sum_{i=1}^N \lambda_i$ where λ_i is the ith eigenvalue of the sample covariance matrix. Each λ_i is a measurement of the magnitude of the corresponding principal axis of the covariance. Hence, by minimizing $\sum_{i=1}^N \lambda_i$, we are compressing the covariance about the mean.

To minimize (8) we need to consider the contribution of $\mathcal{G}(.)$ to the gradient (5). In our implementation, $p_0^{mdt,avg}$ is considered to be constant during any given iteration (see section on gradient descent strategy). Hence, the gradient of $\mathcal{G}(p_1, p_2, ..., p_N)$ with respect to p_0^k for some k in MDT coordinates is simply found to be:

$$\nabla_{p_0^k}\mathcal{G}(p_1, p_2, ..., p_N) = 2\alpha(p_0^{mdt,k} - p_0^{mdt,avg}) \qquad (9)$$

to put this back into individual coordinates, we compose with the appropriate inverse transformation:

$$\nabla_{p_0^k}\mathcal{G}(p_1, p_2, ..., p_N) = 2\alpha|D(\psi^k)^{-1}|(p_0^{mdt,k} - p_0^{mdt,avg}) \circ (\psi^k)^{-1} \qquad (10)$$

and so the complete gradient of (7) with respect to an initial momentum p_0^k in the coordinate system for the kth template image is the sum of Eqs. (5) and (10). The result is that for every update of p_0^k it is pulled in such a way as to map I_0^k to I_1^k by (5), but it is also held close to the group representation of p_0 by (10).

Gradient Descent Algorithms for Optimization of (7): We now consider optimizing (7) with respect to each p_0^i one at a time. Multiple strategies are available for the order in which we update the p_0^i. The most rigorous update would be to use the maximum amount of information possible at each update. That is, for the $(l + 1)$st update of the kth momentum, p_0^{avg} in (10) equals $(1/n) \sum_{i=1}^{k-1} p_0^{i,l+1} \circ \psi^i + (1/n) \sum_{i=k}^{N} p_0^{i,l} \circ \psi^i$. This approach requires the N registrations to be done in series for every iteration and is exceedingly costly in both time and memory.

An alternative is use $(1/n) \sum_{i=1}^{N} p_0^{i,l} \circ \psi^i$ for p_0^{avg} for all N at the $(l + 1)$st iteration. This way, for a given iteration, the N $p_0^{i,l}$ can be updated in parallel. Subsequently, each pair shares its updated value $p_0^{i,l+1}$ to compute $p_0^{avg,l+1} = (1/n) \sum_{i=1}^{N} p_0^{i,l+1} \circ \psi^i$ to be used in the $(l+2)$nd iteration. We used this strategy to compute the results presented in the next section.

3 Results

Experimental Setup: We downloaded screening, 1 year follow up, and 2 year follow up 1.5 Tesla T1-weighted images for 57 participants in the Alzheimer's Disease Neuroimaging Initiative (ADNI). All 57 participants had been diagnosed with Alzheimer's Disease (AD) prior to the acquisition of their screening image. The population consisted of 32 males mean age 75.91 ± 7.85 years and 25 females mean age 75.08 ± 8.15 years. This was the maximum number of individuals we could download from the ADNI 1 cohort that were in the AD group and had screening, year 1, and year 2 follow up images available. All images were corrected for geometric distortion and bias in the static field with GradWarp and N3 before downloading as part of the ADNI preprocessing protocol. Subsequent to downloading, the images were linearly registered to the ICBM template and skull stripped using ROBEX [3]. Transformations ψ^i mapping the template images I_0^i into a MDT coordinate system were computed using a preexisting implementation of [14].

We used a multi-resolution approach for 50, 30, 20, and 5 iterations at 64^3, 80^3, 96^3, and 128^3 resolutions respectively to register the screening images to the year 1 follow up images. We used the second strategy described in the above section to optimize (7) with respect to the initial momenta for the 57 pairs. To test the influence of the group-wise term $\mathcal{G}(.)$, we ran the algorithm over a range of values for α including 0.0 (control), 0.01, 0.025, 0.05, 0.075, 0.1, and 0.5. After completion, we computed and compared the average and variance of the initial momenta for each value of α. We then solved the system (2) over the interval $[0, 2]$, which in this case represents 2 years, and compared the computed image $I_{0,2}$ to the year 2 follow up images for all values of α.

Mean and Variance Images: Coronal slices for the final mean and variance of the initial momenta are shown in Fig. 1 for all values of α. As α increases, both the mean and variance become smaller in magnitude, however the variance falls off at a much faster pace. The primary features of the mean image, including the change in the ventricles and temporal lobes, remain the strongest with increasing α, while individual features fade away with increasing group-wise influence.

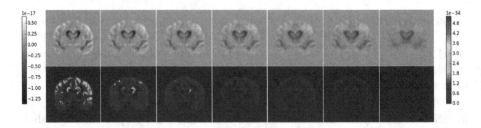

Fig. 1. Mean and variance images for different values of α. Top: Mean images, Bottom: Variance images, Columns correspond to α values from left to right: 0.0, 0.01, 0.025, 0.05, 0.075, 0.1, and 0.5.

The Sum of Squared Difference During Registration: The initial sum of squared difference (SSD) between the screening and year 1 image was retained and used to normalize the SSD at every iteration. This normalized SSD was summed over all 57 image pairs. The results for all values of α are shown in Fig. 2. Clearly, as α increases the total normalized SSD increases for every iteration, which is expected considering the forms of Eqs. (7) and (10). As alpha increases, exact matching to the target is compromised for more coherence with the group-wise representation. The spikes occur where the resolution changes in the multi-scale registration approach.

Prediction of Year 2 Images from Initial Momenta: The momenta learned for all values of α were integrated from $[0, 2]$, representing a 2 year period, and the screening images were transformed with the resulting diffeomorphisms. These images were quantitatively compared to actual year 2 follow up acquisitions. The SSD between the year 2 prediction and actual year 2 image, normalized by its value for $\alpha = 0.0$, is presented in Fig. 3. A value less than one indicates the prediction at a particular α level is closer by SSD than the prediction for $\alpha = 0.0$. Clearly, for many images the prediction improves with increasing α. These images are those for which the true, unobserved, initial momenta lies closer to the group-wise mean. For some images, the prediction becomes worse with increasing α. These images are those for which the true, unobserved, initial momenta does not lie closer to the group-wise mean. An immediate extension of this work to address this issue is to modify (8) to allow for multiple subgroup-wise representations and/or to accommodate outliers.

We performed a one-sided student's t-test to determine if the SSD for predictions with α not equal to zero were significantly different from those with α equal to zero. All values of α except $\alpha = 0.5$ have significantly different SSD values (at a standard significance level of $p = 0.05$) for their predictions. The relevant values are presented in Table 1.

Prediction of Year 2 Images from Average Momenta: The average momentum for all α in MDT coordinates was transformed into individual coordinates for the ith image pair using coadjoint transport through $(\psi^i)^{-1}$. The resulting

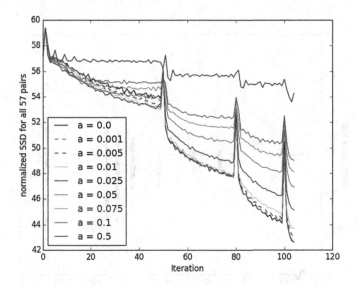

Fig. 2. Normalized SSD throughout optimization for all values of α. The Spikes occur when the resolution changes.

average momenta in individual coordinates were integrated over $[0, 2]$, representing a 2 year period. The screening images were transformed with the resulting diffeomorphisms and the resulting images were compared to the actual year 2 acquisitions. The results are presented in Fig. 4.

We performed a one-sided student's t-test to determine if the SSD for predictions from the average momenta with α not equal to zero were significantly different from those with α equal to zero. All values of α have significantly different SSD values (at a standard significance level of $p = 0.05$) for their predictions. The relevant values are presented in Table 2.

Table 1. t-test results comparing all α not equal to zero with $\alpha = 0$ for SSD between year 2 prediction and acquired year 2 image. μ is the average difference between SSD values for $\alpha = 0$ and $\alpha \neq 0$, σ is the standard deviation, T is the t-statistic, and p is the p-value. Recall, there were 57 image pairs. Significant results are bold.

α	0.001	0.005	0.01	0.025	0.05	0.075	0.1	0.5
μ	13.70	70.21	120.51	222.10	287.75	306.79	324.23	157.03
σ	52.25	143.67	278.01	586.49	953.82	1177.70	1335.04	2066.4
T	1.98	3.70	3.27	2.86	2.28	1.97	1.83	0.57
p	**.026**	**.00025**	**.00092**	**.003**	**.013**	**0.027**	**0.036**	0.29

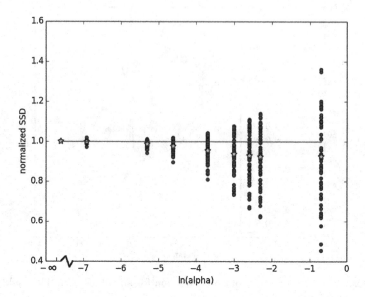

Fig. 3. SSD between year 2 images predicted by integration of initial momenta and actual year 2 image acquisitions for all 57 image pairs and all ln(α) values. The red stars represent the mean.

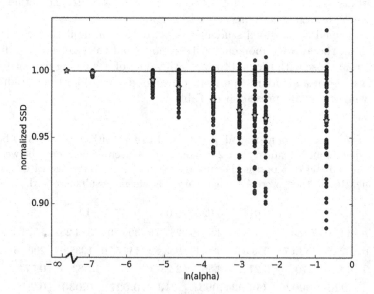

Fig. 4. SSD between year 2 images predicted by integration of average momenta and actual year 2 image acquisitions for all 57 image pairs and all ln(α) values. The red stars represent the mean.

4 Discussion

The first feature of the above presented methods and results to discuss is the obvious compromise between exact image pair matching and group-wise consistency represented by the parameter α. Figure 2 demonstrates the sensitivity of the exact image matching to this parameter. It's interesting to note that the solution trajectory over iterations is very similar in shape for all values of α, though we get less exact matching as α increases as expected. Figure 3 and Table 1 demonstrate the potential advantage to group-wise consistency in learning momenta that more accurately reflect the unobserved long term change. Figure 3 and Table 1 both suggest that there are some values of α that strike a potentially desirable compromise between exact image matching and improved prediction of long term change.

Of course, for some images, the momenta learned with coupling are worse predictors of long term change. As mentioned previously, one avenue to address this is to allow multiple sub-group representations and assign each image pair to the sub-group representation that best approximates it. One interesting question that arises is what is the optimal number of sub-groups for a given population? Additionally, what differences will the sub-group representations encode in them after convergence? Alternatively, the mean is sensitive to outliers, and we could consider replacing the group representation with a different statistic more robust to such variation.

The proposed work has made no effort to normalize temporal misalignment in disease progression across patients. The experimental results suggest that AD disease progression is sufficiently similar at different stages of the disease for group level information to be applicable to individual trajectory estimation. However, this may not be the case for other populations such as the Mild Cognitively Impaired (MCI) or other Neurodegenerative disorders with less well characterized structural changes. Hence, explicit modeling of temporal misalignment in age and disease progression as done in [9] may improve results.

It is important to mention that momenta learned with this technique should not be naively used for statistical tests. We have explicitly minimized the trace covariance of these momenta, so any voxel-wise statistics computed from them

Table 2. t-test results comparing all α not equal to zero with $\alpha = 0$ for SSD between year 2 prediction from average momenta and acquired year 2 image. μ is the average difference between SSD values for $\alpha = 0$ and $\alpha! = 0$, σ is the standard deviation, T is the t-statistic, p is the p-value. Recall, there were 57 image pairs. Significant results are bold.

α	0.001	0.005	0.01	0.025	0.05	0.075	0.1	0.5
μ	10.91	46.26	81.55	148.97	203.29	230.76	246.85	259.22
σ	9.04	37.91	67.28	127.07	179.47	207.67	224.56	249.41
T	9.11	9.21	9.15	8.85	8.55	8.39	8.30	7.85
p	**2.22e-12**	**1.53e-12**	**1.92e-12**	**5.89e-12**	**1.82e-11**	**3.34e-11**	**4.69e-11**	**2.59e-10**

are biased [11]. This issue can be compensated for by determining the null distribution for a particular statistic and establishing significance relative to this learned distribution. However, non-statistical inference applications such as momenta or change map atlas construction and shooting of individual templates via the learned momenta are not affected by this problem.

5   Conclusions

We have presented a mathematical framework for coupling the registration of N image pairs in the geodesic shooting approach for the optimization of the LDDMM energy functional. Individual registrations are coupled by maintaining a group-wise representation of their initial momenta and constraining updates to stay close to this representation. This is an explicit minimization of the variance of the initial momenta in the Lie algebra for the space of diffeomorphisms specified by the choice of metric K. This establishes a trade-off between exact image matching for individual image pairs and group-wise consistency. We've shown that increasing group-wise consistency can improve the prediction of long term change encoded within individual momenta. Finally, we have described some of the strengths and weaknesses of our initial choice for the coupling term $\mathcal{G}(.)$ and suggested methods to address those weaknesses.

References

1. Beg, M.F., Miller, M.I., Trouvé, A., Younes, L.: Computing large deformation metric mappings via geodesic flows of diffeomorphisms. Int. J. Comput. Vis. **61**(2), 139–157 (2005). doi:10.1023/B:VISI.0000043755.93987.aa
2. Brun, C.C., Lepore, N., Pennec, X., Chou, Y.Y., Lee, A.D., de Zubicaray, G.I., McMahon, K., Wright, M.J., Gee, J.C., Thompson, P.M.: A nonconservative lagrangian framework for statistical fluid registration - safira. IEEE Trans. Med. Imaging **30**(2), 184–202 (2011)
3. Iglesias, J., Liu, C., Thompson, P., Tu, Z.: Robust brain extraction across datasets and comparison with publicly available methods. IEEE Trans. Med. Imaging **30**(9), 1617–1634 (2011)
4. James, W., Stein, C.: Estimation with quadratic loss. In: Proceedings of the Fourth Berkeley Symposium on Mathematical Statistics and Probability, vol. 1. Contributions to the Theory of Statistics, pp. 361–379. University of California Press, Berkeley (1961). http://projecteuclid.org/euclid.bsmsp/1200512173
5. Lorenzi, M., Pennec, X., Frisoni, G.B., Ayache, N.: Disentangling normal aging from Alzheimer's disease in structural MR images. Neurobiol. Aging **36**, S42–S52 (2014)
6. Miller, M.I., Trouvé, A., Younes, L.: Geodesic shooting for computational anatomy. J. Math. Imaging Vis. **24**(2), 209–228 (2006)
7. Niethammer, M., Huang, Y., Vialard, F.-X.: Geodesic regression for image time-series. In: Fichtinger, G., Martel, A., Peters, T. (eds.) MICCAI 2011, Part II. LNCS, vol. 6892, pp. 655–662. Springer, Heidelberg (2011)

8. Pennec, X., Stefanescu, R., Arsigny, V., Fillard, P., Ayache, N.: Riemannian elasticity: a statistical regularization framework for non-linear registration. In: Duncan, J.S., Gerig, G. (eds.) MICCAI 2005. LNCS, vol. 3750, pp. 943–950. Springer, Heidelberg (2005)

9. Singh, N., Hinkle, J., Joshi, S., Fletcher, P.T.: A hierarchical geodesic model for diffeomorphic longitudinal shape analysis. In: Gee, J.C., Joshi, S., Pohl, K.M., Wells, W.M., Zöllei, L. (eds.) IPMI 2013. LNCS, vol. 7917, pp. 560–571. Springer, Heidelberg (2013)

10. Trouve, A.: Diffeomorphisms groups and pattern matching in image analysis. Int. J. Comput. Vis. **28**, 213–221 (1998)

11. Tustison, N.J., Avants, B.B., Cook, P.A., Kim, J., Whyte, J., Gee, J.C., Stone, J.R.: Logical circularity in voxel-based analysis: normalization strategy may induce statistical bias. Hum. Brain Mapp. **35**, 745–759 (2012)

12. Vialard, F.X., Risser, L., Rueckert, D., Cotter, C.J.: Diffeomorphic 3D image registration via geodesic shooting using an efficient adjoint calculation. Int. J. Comput. Vis. **97**(2), 229–241 (2012). doi:10.1007/s11263-011-0481-8

13. Wei, L., Awate, S., Anderson, J., Fletcher, T.: A functional network estimation method of resting-state fMRI using a hierarchical markov random field. NeuroImage **100**, 520–534 (2014)

14. Yanovsky, I., Thompson, P.M., Osher, S., Leow, A.D.: Topology preserving log-unbiased nonlinear image registration: theory and implementation. In: CVPR, IEEE Computer Society (2007)

15. Younes, L., Qiu, A., Winslow, R.L., Miller, M.I.: Transport of relational structures in groups of diffeomorphisms. J. Math. Imaging Vis. **32**(1), 41–56 (2008)

16. Zhang, M., Singh, N., Fletcher, P.T.: Bayesian estimation of regularization and atlas building in diffeomorphic image registration. In: Gee, J.C., Joshi, S., Pohl, K.M., Wells, W.M., Zöllei, L. (eds.) IPMI 2013. LNCS, vol. 7917, pp. 37–48. Springer, Heidelberg (2013)

Spatially Weighted Principal Component Regression for High-Dimensional Prediction

Dan Shen[1(✉)] and Hongtu Zhu[2]

[1] Interdisciplinary Data Sciences Consortium, Department of Mathematics
and Statistics, University of South Florida, Tampa, FL, USA
danshen@usf.edu
[2] Department of Biostatistics and Biomedical Research Imaging Center,
University of North Carolina at Chapel Hill, Chapel Hill, NC, USA
htzhu@email.unc.edu

Abstract. We consider the problem of using high dimensional data residing on graphs to predict a low-dimensional outcome variable, such as disease status. Examples of data include time series and genetic data measured on linear graphs and imaging data measured on triangulated graphs (or lattices), among many others. Many of these data have two key features including spatial smoothness and intrinsically low dimensional structure. We propose a simple solution based on a general statistical framework, called spatially weighted principal component regression (SWPCR). In SWPCR, we introduce two sets of weights including importance score weights for the selection of individual features at each node and spatial weights for the incorporation of the neighboring pattern on the graph. We integrate the importance score weights with the spatial weights in order to recover the low dimensional structure of high dimensional data. We demonstrate the utility of our methods through extensive simulations and a real data analysis based on Alzheimer's disease neuroimaging initiative data.

Keywords: Graph · Principal component analysis · Regression · Spatial · Supervise · Weight

1   Introduction

Our problem of interest is to predict a set of response variables $\mathbf{Y}$ by using high-dimensional data $\mathbf{x} = \{\mathbf{x}_g : g \in \mathcal{G}\}$ measured on a graph $\zeta = (\mathcal{G}, \mathcal{E})$, where $\mathcal{E}$ is the edge set of ζ and $\mathcal{G} = \{g_1, \ldots, g_m\}$ is a set of vertexes, in which m is the total number of vertexes in $\mathcal{G}$. The response $\mathbf{Y}$ may include cognitive outcome, disease status, and the early onset of disease, among others. Standard graphs including both directed and undirected graphs have been widely used to build complex patterns [10]. Examples of graphs are linear graphs, tree graphs, triangulated graphs, and 2-dimensional (2D) (or 3-dimensional (3D)) lattices, among many others (Fig. 1). Examples of $\mathbf{x}$ on the graph $\zeta = (\mathcal{G}, \mathcal{E})$ include time series and genetic data measured on linear graphs and imaging data measured on

© Springer International Publishing Switzerland 2015
S. Ourselin et al. (Eds.): IPMI 2015, LNCS 9123, pp. 758–769, 2015.
DOI: 10.1007/978-3-319-19992-4_60

triangulated graphs (or lattices). Particularly, various structural and functional neuroimaging data are frequently measured in a 3D lattice for the understanding of brain structure and function and their association with neuropsychiatric and neurodegenerative disorders [9].

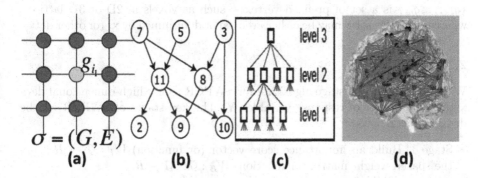

Fig. 1. Illustration of graph data structure $\zeta = (\mathcal{G}, \mathcal{E})$: (a) two-dimensional lattice; (b) acyclic directed graph; (c) tree; (d) undirected graph.

The aim of this paper is to develop a new framework of spatially weighted principal component regression (SWPCR) to use $\mathbf{x}$ on graph $\zeta = \{\mathcal{G}, \mathcal{E}\}$ to predict $\mathbf{Y}$. Four major challenges arising from such development include *ultra-high dimensionality, low sample size, spatially correlation,* and *spatial smoothness.* SWPCR is developed to address these four challenges when high-dimensional data on graphs ζ share two important features including spatial smoothness and intrinsically low dimensional structure. Compared with the existing literature, we make several major contributions as follows:

- (i) SWPCR is designed to efficiently capture the two important features by using some recent advances in smoothing methods, dimensional reduction methods, and sparse methods.
- (ii) SWPCR provides a powerful dimension reduction framework for integrating feature selection, smoothing, and feature extraction.
- (iii) SWPCR significantly outperforms the competing methods by simulation studies and the real data analysis.

2   Spatially Weighted Principal Component Regression

In this section, we first describe the graph data that are considered in this paper. We formally describe the general framework of SWPCR.

2.1   Graph Data

Consider data from n independent subjects. For each subject, we observe a $q \times 1$ vector of discrete or continuous responses, denoted by $\mathbf{y}_i = (\mathbf{y}_{i,1}, \ldots, \mathbf{y}_{i,q})^T$, and a $m \times 1$ vector of high dimensional data $\mathbf{x}_i = \{x_{i,g} : g \in \mathcal{G}\}$ for $i = 1, \ldots, n$. In many cases, q is relatively small compared with n, whereas m is much larger than n. For instance, in many neuroimaging studies, it is common to use ultra-high dimensional imaging data to classify a binary class variable. In this case, $q = 1$, whereas m can be several million number of features. In many applications, $\mathcal{G} = \{g_1, \ldots, g_m\}$ is a set of prefixed vertexes, such as voxels in 2D or 3D lattices, whereas the edge set $\mathcal{E}$ may be either prefixed or determined by $\mathbf{x}_i$ (or other data).

2.2 SWPCR

We introduce a three-stage algorithm for SWPCR to use high-dimensional data $\mathbf{x}$ to predict a set of response variables $\mathbf{Y}$. The key stages of SWPCR can be described as follows.

- Stage 1. Build an importance score vector (or function) $W_I : \mathcal{G} \to R^+$ and the spatial weight matrix (or function) $W_E : \mathcal{G} \times \mathcal{G} \to R$.
- Stage 2. Build a sequence of scale vectors $\{\mathbf{s}_0 = (\mathbf{s}_{E,0}, \mathbf{s}_{I,0}), \cdots, \mathbf{s}_L = (\mathbf{s}_{E,L}, \mathbf{s}_{I,L})\}$ ranging from the smallest scale vector $\mathbf{s}_0$ to the largest scale vector $\mathbf{s}_L$. At each scale vector $\mathbf{s}_\ell$, use generalized principal component analysis (GPCA) to compute the first few principal components of an $n \times m$ matrix $X = (\mathbf{x_1} \cdots \mathbf{x_n})^{\mathbf{T}}$, denoted by $A(\mathbf{s}_\ell)$, based on $W_E(\cdot, \cdot)$ and $W_I(\cdot)$ for $\ell = 0, \ldots, L$.
- Stage 3. Select the optimal $0 \leq \ell^* \leq L$ and build a prediction model (e.g., high-dimensional linear model) based on the extracted principal components $A(\mathbf{s}_{\ell^*})$ and the responses $\mathbf{Y}$.

We slightly elaborate on these stages. In Stage 1, the important scores $w_{I,g}$ play an important feature screening role in SWPCR. Examples of $w_{I,g} = W_I(g)$ in the literature can be generated based on some statistics (e.g., Pearson correlation or distance correlation) between $\mathbf{x}_g$ and $\mathbf{Y}$ at each vertex g. For instance, let $p(g)$ be the Pearson correlation at each vertex g and then define

$$w_{I,g} = -m \log(p(g)) / \left[-\sum_{g \in \mathcal{G}} \log(p(g)) \right]. \tag{1}$$

In Stage 1, without loss of generality, we focus on the symmetric matrix $W_E = (w_{E,gg'}) \in R^{p \times p}$ throughout the paper. The element $w_{E,gg'}$ is usually calculated by using various similarity criteria, such as Gaussian similarity from Euclidean distance, local neighborhood relationship, correlation, and prior information obtained from other data [21]. In Sect. 2.3, we will discuss how to determine W_E and W_I while explicitly accounting for the complex spatial structure among different vertexes.

In Stage 2, at each scale vector $\mathbf{s}_\ell = (\mathbf{s}_{E,\ell}, \mathbf{s}_{I,\ell})$, we construct two matrices, denoted by $Q_{E,\ell}$ and $Q_{I,\ell}$ based on W_E and W_I as follows:

$$Q_{E,\ell} = F_1(W_E, \mathbf{s}_{E,\ell}) \quad \text{and} \quad Q_{I,\ell} = \text{diag}(F_2(W_I, s_{I,\ell})), \tag{2}$$

where $F_1 : R^{p \times p} \times R^+ \to R^{p \times p}$ and $F_2 : R^p \times R^+ \to R^p$ are two known functions. For instance, let $\mathbf{1}(\cdot)$ be an indicator function, we may set

$$F_2(W_I, s_{I,\ell}) = (\mathbf{1}(w_{I,g_1} \geq s_{I,\ell}), \cdots, \mathbf{1}(w_{I,g_m} \geq s_{I,\ell}))^T, \tag{3}$$

to extract 'significant' vertexes. There are various ways of constructing $Q_{E,\ell}$. For instance, one may set $Q_{E,\ell}$ as

$$Q_{E,\ell} = (|w_{E,gg'}|\mathbf{1}(|w_{E,gg'}| \geq s_{E,\ell;1}, D(g,g') \leq s_{E,\ell;2})),$$

where $\mathbf{s}_{E,\ell} = (s_{E,\ell;1}, s_{E,\ell;2})^T$ and $D(g,g')$ is a graph-based distance between vertexes g and g'. The value of $s_{E,\ell;2}$ controls the number of vertexes in $\{g' \in \mathcal{G} : D(g,g') \leq s_{E,\ell;2}\}$, which is a patch set at vertex g [18], whereas $s_{E,\ell;1}$ is used to shrink small $|w_{E,gg'}|$s into zero.

After determining $Q_{E,\ell}$ and $Q_{I,\ell}$, we set $\Sigma_c = Q_{E,\ell}Q_{I,\ell}Q_{I,\ell}^T Q_{E,\ell}^T$ and $\Sigma_r = I_n$ for independent subjects. Let $\widetilde{\mathbf{X}}$ be the centered matrix of $\mathbf{X}$. Then we can extract K principal components through minimize the following objective function given by

$$||\widetilde{\mathbf{X}} - UDV^T||^2 \text{ subject to } U^T\Sigma_r U = V^T\Sigma_c V = I_K \text{ and } \text{diag}(D) \geq 0. \tag{4}$$

If we consider correlated observations from multiple subjects, we may use Σ_r to explicitly model their correlation structure. The solution (U_ℓ, D_ℓ, V_ℓ) of the objective function (4) at $\mathbf{s}_\ell$ is the SVD of $\widetilde{\mathbf{X}}_{R,\ell} = \widetilde{\mathbf{X}}Q_{E,\ell}Q_{I,\ell}$. The we can use a GPCA algorithm to simultaneously calculate all components of (U_ℓ, D_ℓ, V_ℓ) for a fixed K as follows. In practice, a simple criterion for determining K is to include all components up to some arbitrary proportion of the total variance, say 85%.

For ultra-high dimensional data, we consider a regularized GPCA to generate (U_ℓ, D_ℓ, V_ℓ) by minimizing the following objective function

$$||\widetilde{\mathbf{X}}_{R,\ell} - \sum_{k=1}^K d_{k,\ell}\mathbf{u}_{k,\ell}\mathbf{v}_{k,\ell}^T||^2 + \lambda_{\mathbf{u}}\sum_{k=1}^K P_1(d_{k,\ell}\mathbf{u}_{k,\ell}) + \lambda_{\mathbf{v}}\sum_{k=1}^K P_2(d_{k,\ell}\mathbf{v}_{k,\ell}) \tag{5}$$

subject to $\mathbf{u}_{k,\ell}^T\mathbf{u}_{k,\ell} \leq 1$ and $\mathbf{v}_{k,\ell}^T\mathbf{v}_{k,\ell} \leq 1$ for all k, where $\mathbf{u}_{k,\ell}$ and $\mathbf{v}_{k,\ell}$ are respectively the k-th column of U_ℓ and V_ℓ. We use adaptive Lasso penalties for $P_1(\cdot)$ and $P_2(\cdot)$ and then iteratively solve (5) [1]. For each k_0, we define $\mathbf{E}_{\ell,k_0} = \widetilde{\mathbf{X}}_{R,\ell} - \sum_{k \neq k_0} d_{k,\ell}\mathbf{u}_{k,\ell}\mathbf{v}_{k,\ell}^T$ and minimize

$$||\mathbf{E}_{\ell,k_0} - d_{k_0,\ell}\mathbf{u}_{k_0,\ell}\mathbf{v}_{k_0,\ell}^T||^2 + \lambda_{\mathbf{u}}P_1(d_{k_0,\ell}\mathbf{u}_{k_0,\ell}) + \lambda_{\mathbf{v}}P_2(d_{k_0,\ell}\mathbf{v}_{k_0,\ell}) \tag{6}$$

subject to $\mathbf{u}_{k_0,\ell}^T\mathbf{u}_{k_0,\ell} \leq 1$ and $\mathbf{v}_{k_0,\ell}^T\mathbf{v}_{k_0,\ell} \leq 1$. By using the sparse method in [12], we can calculate the solution of (6), denoted by $(\hat{d}_{k_0,\ell}, \hat{\mathbf{u}}_{k_0,\ell}, \hat{\mathbf{v}}_{k_0,\ell})$. In this way, we can sequentially compute $(\hat{d}_{k,\ell}, \hat{\mathbf{u}}_{k,\ell}, \hat{\mathbf{v}}_{k,\ell})$ for $k = 1, \ldots, K$.

In Stage 3, select ℓ^* as the minimum point of the objective function (5) or (6) . let $Q_{F,\ell^*} = Q_{E,\ell^*}Q_{I,\ell^*}V_{\ell^*}D_{\ell^*}^{-1}$ and then K principal components $A(\mathbf{s}_{\ell^*}) = \mathbf{X}Q_{F,\ell^*}$. Moreover, K is usually much smaller than $\min(n,m)$. Then, we build a regression model with $\mathbf{y}_i$ as responses and A_i (the i-th row of $A(\mathbf{s}_{\ell^*})$) as covariates, denoted by $R(\mathbf{y}_i, A_i; \boldsymbol{\theta})$, where $\boldsymbol{\theta}$ is a vector of unknown (finite-dimensional or nonparametric) parameters. Specifically, based on $\{(\mathbf{y}_i, A_i)\}_{i \geq 1}$, we use an estimation method to estimate $\boldsymbol{\theta}$ as follows:

$$\widehat{\boldsymbol{\theta}} = \mathrm{argmin}_{\boldsymbol{\theta}}\{\rho\left(R, \boldsymbol{\theta}, \{(\mathbf{y}_i, A_i)\}_{i \geq 1}\right) + \lambda P_3(\boldsymbol{\theta})\},$$

where $\rho(\cdot, \cdot, \cdot)$ is a loss function, which depends on both the regression model and the data, and $P_3(\cdot)$ is a penalty function, such as Lasso. This leads to a prediction model $R(\mathbf{y}_i, A_i; \boldsymbol{\theta})$. For instance, for binary response $\mathbf{y}_i = 1$ or 0, we may consider a sparse logistic model given by $\mathrm{logit}(P(\mathbf{y}_i = 1|A_i)) = A_i^T \boldsymbol{\theta}$ for $R(\mathbf{y}_i, A_i; \boldsymbol{\theta})$.

Given a test feature vector $\mathbf{x}^*$, we can do predictions from our prediction model as follows:

- Center each component of $\mathbf{x}^*$ by calculating $\tilde{\mathbf{x}}^* = \mathbf{x}^* - \hat{\mu}_\mathbf{x}$, in which $\hat{\mu}_\mathbf{x}$ is the mean and learnt from the training data;
- Optimize an objective function based on $R(\mathbf{y}, \tilde{\mathbf{x}}^{*T} Q_{F,\ell^*}; \widehat{\boldsymbol{\theta}})$ to calculate an estimate of $\mathbf{y}$, denoted by $\hat{\mathbf{y}}^*$.

Our prediction model is applicable to various regression settings for continuous and discrete responses and multivariate and univariate responses, such as survival data and classification problems.

2.3   Importance Score Weights and Spatial Weights

There are two sets of weights in SWPCR including (i) importance score weights enabling a selective treatment for individual features, and (ii) spatial weights accommodating the underlying spatial dependence among features across neighboring vertexes on graph. Below, we propose the strategy of determining both importance score weights and spatial weights.

Importance Score Weights. As discussed in Sect. 2.3, at each vertex g, $w_{I,g}$, such as the Pearson correlation in (1), is calculated based on a statistical model between $\mathbf{x}_g$ and $\mathbf{Y}$ in order to perform feature selection according to each feature's discriminative importance. Statistically, most existing methods use a marginal (or vertex-wise) model by assuming

$$p(\mathbf{x}_i, \mathbf{y}_i) = \prod_{g \in \mathcal{G}} p(\mathbf{x}_{i,g}, \mathbf{y}_i; \boldsymbol{\beta}(g)),$$

where $\boldsymbol{\beta} = (\boldsymbol{\beta}(g) : g \in \mathcal{G})$ and $\boldsymbol{\beta}(g)$ is introduced to quantify the association between $\mathbf{y}_i$ and $\mathbf{x}_{i,g}$ at each vertex $g \in \mathcal{G}$. At the g-th vertex, $w_{I,g}$ is a statistic based on the marginal model $\prod_{i=1}^n p(\mathbf{x}_{i,g}, \mathbf{y}_i; \boldsymbol{\beta}(g))$. However, those $w_{I,g}$s largely ignore complex spatial structure, such as homogenous patches defined below, across all vertexes on graph.

For a graph $\zeta = (\mathcal{G}, \mathcal{E})$, it is common to assume that $\beta(g)$ across all vertexes are naturally clustered into P homogeneous patches, denoted by $\{\mathcal{G}_l : l = 1, \ldots, P\}$, such that $P << m$, $\mathcal{G} = \cup_{l=1}^P \mathcal{G}_l$, and $\beta(g)$ varies smoothly in each $\mathcal{G}_l$. Note that a patch $\mathcal{G}_l$ consists of a set of vertexes that are completely connected through edges in $\mathcal{E}$. That is, if $g, g' \in \mathcal{G}_l$, then there is a sequence of vertexes $g_0 = g, \cdots, g_M = g'$ in $\mathcal{G}_p$ such that $(g_{j-1}, g_j) \in \mathcal{E}$ for all $j = 1, \ldots, M$. It has been shown that for graph data, algorithms based on patch information have led to state-of-the art techniques for classification and denoising. See for example, [18] for overviews of imaging patches.

We propose the strategy to jointly model $\mathbf{x}_i$ and $\mathbf{y}_i$ and simultaneously calculate $w_{I,g}$ across all vertexes, while learning the homogenous patches $\mathcal{G}_l$. The strategy is to model the conditional distribution of $\mathbf{x}_i$ given $\mathbf{y}_i$, denoted by $p(\mathbf{x}_i | \mathbf{y}_i, \beta)$. Then we can learn the patches $\mathcal{G}_l$ in $\mathcal{G}$ from the estimated β.

Here we consider a set of vertexes $\mathcal{G}$ with unknown edge information $\mathcal{E}$. It is important to learn the homogeneous patches $\mathcal{G}_p$ and then form the edge set $\mathcal{E}$. Let $\mathcal{E}_g(h)$ be an edge set at scale h at each vertex g. We consider a sequence of nested edge sets across multiscales h_s such that $h_0 = 0 \leq h_1 \leq \cdots \leq h_S$ and $\mathcal{E}_g(h_0) = \{g\} \subset \cdots \subset \mathcal{E}_g(h_S)$. To learn the homogeneous patches, a general framework of Multiscale Adaptive Regression Model (MARM) developed in [13] is to maximize a sequence of weighted functions as follows:

$$\hat{\beta}(g; h_s) = \operatorname{argmax}_{\beta(g)} \sum_{i=1}^n \sum_{g' \in \mathcal{E}_g(h_s)} \omega(g, g'; h_s) \log p(\mathbf{x}_{i,g'} | \mathbf{y}_i, \beta(g)) \quad \text{for} \quad s = 1, \ldots, S,$$

(7)

where $\omega(g, g'; h)$ characterizes the similarity between the data in vertexes g' and g with $\omega(g, g; h) = 1$. If $\omega(g, g'; h) \approx 0$, then the observations in vertex g' do not provide information on $\beta(g)$. Therefore, $\omega(g, g'; h)$ can prevent incorporation of vertexes whose data do not contain information on $\beta(g)$ and preserve the edges of homogeneous regions. Let $D_1(g, g')$ and $D_2(\hat{\beta}(g; h_{s-1}), \hat{\beta}(g'; h_{s-1}))$ be, respectively, the spatial distance between vertexes g and g' and a similarity measure between $\hat{\beta}(g; h_{s-1})$ and $\hat{\beta}(g'; h_{s-1})$. The $\omega(g, g'; h_s)$ can be defined as

$$\omega(g, g'; h_s) = \mathbb{K}_1(D_1(g, g')/h_s) \cdot \mathbb{K}_2(D_2(\hat{\beta}(g; h_{s-1}), \hat{\beta}(g'; h_{s-1}))/\gamma_n), \quad (8)$$

where $\mathbb{K}_1(\cdot)$ and $\mathbb{K}_2(\cdot)$ are two nonnegative kernel functions and γ_n is a bandwidth parameter that may depend on n. See the detailed algorithm of MARM in [13]. After the iteration h_s, we can obtain $\hat{\beta}(g; h_S)$ and its covariance matrix, denoted by $\operatorname{Cov}(\hat{\beta}(g; h_s))$, across all $g \in \mathcal{G}$ and $\omega(g, g'; h_s)$ for all $g' \in \mathcal{E}_g(h_s)$ and $g \in \mathcal{G}$. Finally, we calculate statistics $w_{I,g}$ based on $\hat{\beta}(g; h_s)$ and $\operatorname{Cov}(\hat{\beta}(g; h_s))$, such as the Wald test, and then we use a clustering algorithm, such as the K-mean algorithm, to group $\{\hat{\beta}(g; h_s) : g \in \mathcal{G}\}$ into several homogeneous clusters, in which $\hat{\beta}(g; h_s)$ varies very smoothly in each cluster. Moreover, each homogenous cluster can be a union of several homogeneous patches.

Spatial Weights. As discussed in Sect. 2.3, $w_{E,gg'}$ often characterizes the degree of certain 'similarity' between vertexes g and g'. The locally spatial weighting matrix consists of non-negative weights assigned to the spatial neighboring vertexes of each vertex. It is assumed that

$$w_{E,gg'} = \frac{\omega(g, g'; h_s)\mathbf{1}(g' \in \mathcal{E}_g(h_s))}{\sum_{g' \in \mathcal{E}_g(h_s)} \omega(g, g'; h_s)\mathbf{1}(g' \in \mathcal{E}_g(h_s))}, \tag{9}$$

in which $\omega(g, g'; h_s)$ is defined in (8). Therefore, $w_{E,gg'} = 0$ for all $g' \notin \mathcal{E}_g(h_s)$ and $\sum_{g' \in \mathcal{G}} w_{E,gg'} = 1$. The weights $\mathbb{K}_1(D_1(g, g')/h_s)$ give less weight to vertex $g' \in \mathcal{E}_g(h_s)$, whose location is far from the vertex g. The weights $\mathbb{K}_2(u)$ downweight the vertex g' with large $D_2(\hat{\boldsymbol{\beta}}(g; h_s), \hat{\boldsymbol{\beta}}(g'; h_s))$, which indicates a large difference between $\hat{\boldsymbol{\beta}}(g'; h_s)$ and $\hat{\boldsymbol{\beta}}(g; h_s)$. Moreover, by following [4,13,15,16], we set $\mathbb{K}_1(x) = (1-x)_+$ and $\mathbb{K}_2(x) = \exp(-x)$. Although m is often much larger than n, the computational burden associated with the local spatial weights is very minor when h_s is relatively small.

3   Simulation Study

In this section, we conducted one set of simulation study corresponding to binary responses, in order to examine the finite-sample performance of SWPCR in the high-dimensional classification analysis. We demonstrate that SWPCR outperforms many state-of-the-art methods for at least in the simulated dataset.

We simulated $20 \times 20 \times 10$ $(x \times y \times z)$ 3D-images from a linear model given by

$$\mathbf{x}_{i,g} = B_0(g) + B_1(g)\mathbf{y}_i + \epsilon_i(g) \quad \text{for} \quad i = 1, \cdots, n, \tag{10}$$

where $\mathbf{y}_i$ is the class label coded as either 0 or 1 and $\epsilon_i(g)$ are random variables with zero mean. The true mean images of class $\mathbf{y}_i = 0$ and class $\mathbf{y}_i = 1$ are

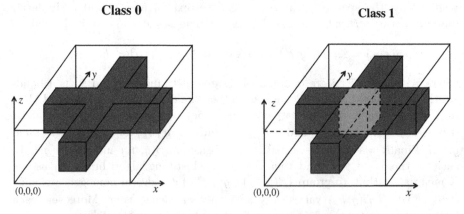

Fig. 2. True mean images for the simulation study: Class 0 in the left panel and Class 1 in the right panel. The white, green, and red colors, respectively, correspond to 0, 1, and 2.

shown in Fig. 2. Voxels in the red cuboid region have the maximum difference 1 between classes 0 and 1. The dimension of red cuboid is $3 \times 3 \times 4$ and contains 36 voxels. In this case, $m = 4,000$ and we set $n = 100$ with 60 images from Class 0 and the rest from Class 1. We consider three types of noise $\epsilon_i(g)$ in (10). First, $\epsilon_i^{(1)}(g)$ were independently generated from a $N(0, 2^2)$ generator across all voxels g. Second, $\epsilon_i^{(2)}(g) = \sum_{\|g'-g\|\leq 1} \epsilon_i^1(g')/m_g$ were generated from $\epsilon_i^{(1)}(g)$ in order to introduce the short range spatial correlation, where m_g is the number of voxels in the set $\{\| g' - g \|\leq 1\}$. Third, to introduce long range spatial correlation, $\epsilon_i^{(3)}(g)$ were generated according to $\epsilon_i^{(3)}(g) = 2\sin(\pi g_1/10)\xi_{i,1} + 2\cos(\pi g_2/10)\xi_{i,2} + 2\sin(\pi g_3/5)\xi_{i,3} + \epsilon_i^{(1)}(g)$, where $\xi_{i,k}$ for $k = 1, 2, 3$ were independenly generated from a $N(0,1)$ generator. Moreover, the noise variances in all voxels of the red cuboid region equal 4, 4/6, and $4\{\sin(\pi g_1/10)^2 + \cos(\pi g_2/10)^2 + \sin(\pi g_3/5)^2\} + 4$ for Type I, II, and III noises, respectively. Therefore, among the three types of noise, Type III noise has the smallest signal-to-noise ratio and Type II noise has the largest one.

Table 1. Classification results for the first set of simulations: comparison between SWPCR and other Classification Methods. sLDA denotes sparse linear discriminant analysis; SPLS denotes sparse partial least squares; SLR denotes sparse logistic regression; SVM denotes support vector machine; ROAD denotes regularized optimal affine discriminant; and PCA denotes principal component analysis.

Noise	sLDA	SPLS	SLR	SVM	ROAD	PCA	SWPCR
Type I	0.28	0.43	0.45	0.38	0.36	0.36	0.10
Type II	0.27	0.08	0.18	0.26	0.08	0.45	0.03
Type III	0.52	0.30	0.61	0.60	0.50	0.35	0.09

We ran the three stages of SWPCR as follows. In Stage 1, let $\{h_\ell = 1.2^\ell, \ell = 0, 1, \ldots, S = 5\}$, and for each $g \in \mathcal{G}$, $w_{I,g} = -m \log(p(g))/\left[-\sum_{g \in \mathcal{G}} \log(p(g))\right]$, where $p(g)$ is the p-value of Wald test $B_1(g) = 0$ in (7) $(\beta(g) = (B_0(g), B_1(g))^T)$ for each voxel g. The spatial weight W_E is given by (9). Here we haven't used the simple Pearson correlation (1) for computing weights because it neglects the spatial correlation of the data set. In Stage 2, for each h_ℓ, we define $Q_{E,\ell} = W_E$ and generate $Q_{I,\ell}$ through (2) and (3), where $s_{I,\ell}$ thresholds out the $w_{I,g}$ with $p(g) < 0.01$. Then we extract different K principal components of GPCA to reconstruct the low dimensional representations of simulated images and then do classification analysis. The results are very stable for different number of principal components and here we let $K = 5$. In Stage 3, we tried different classification methods, including linear regression, k-Nearest Neighbor (k-NN) [11] and support vector machine (SVM) [14], on these low dimensional spaces. Based on the misclassification error for the leave-one-out cross validation, the linear regression is slight better than others. The linear regression uses class label

y_i as dependent variable and principal components as explanatory variables. If the prediction value is less than 0, the image is classified as 0. Otherwise, the image is classified as 1.

We compared SWPCR with other state-of-the-art classification methods. The leave-one-out cross validation is used here to calculate the misclassification rates of the different methods. Other classification methods considered here include sparse linear discriminant analysis (sLDA) [6], sparse partial least squares (SPLS) analysis [5], sparse logistic regression (SLR) [20], SVM, and regularized optimal affine discriminant (ROAD) [8]. These methods are well known for their excellent performance in various simulated and real data sets. Inspecting Table 1 reveal that except SWPCR, all classification methods perform pretty poor, when the signal-to-noise ratio is low in those simulated datasets with Type I and II noises. Except SPLS, PCA, and SWPCR, all other methods are seem to be sensitive to the presence of the long-range correlation structure in Type III noise.

4   Real Data Analysis

4.1   ADNI PET Data

The real data set is the baseline fluorodeoxyglucose positron emission tomography (FDG-PET) data downloaded from the Alzheimer's Disease Neuroimaging Initiative (ADNI) web site (www.loni.ucla.edu/ADNI). The ADNI1 PET data set consists of 196 subjects (102 Normal Controls (NC) and 94 AD subjects). There are three subjects, missing the gender and age information. Among the rest of the subjects, there are 117 males whose mean age is 76.20 years with standard deviation 6.06 years and 76 females whose mean age is 75.29 years with standard deviation 6.29 years.

The dimension of the processed PET images is $79 \times 95 \times 69$. Left panel in Fig. 3 shows some selected slices of the processed PET images from 2 randomly selected AD subjects and 2 randomly selected NC subjects.

4.2   Binary Classification

Our first goal is to apply SWPCR in classifying subjects from ADNI1 to AD or CN group based on their FDG-PET images. Such goal is associated with the second primary objective of ADNI aiming at developing new diagnostic methods for AD intervention, prevention, and treatment. Similar as in Sect. 3 , SWPCR contains the three detailed stages that will not be repeated again. The right panel in Fig. 3 is the three view slices of the weight matrix $Q_{I,\ell}$ at the coordinate $(40, 57, 26)$ in the stage 2 of SWPCR. The red region in three slices corresponds to the large important score weight and contains the most classification information.

We compared SWPCR with six other classification methods including sLDA, SPLS, SLR, SVM, ROAD, and PCA. We used their leave-one-out cross validation rates. Table 2 shows the classification results of all the seven methods. sLDA

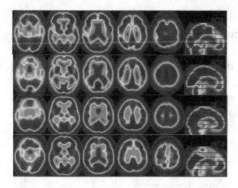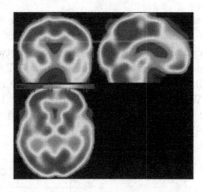

Fig. 3. ADNI1 pet data and the important score weight matrix $Q_{I,\ell}$ in SWPCR. In the left panel, one row sequence of 2-D images belongs to one subject. The first two rows respectively belongs to AD subjects and the rest belongs to NC subjects. In the right panel, the three plots (left -right-bottom) are three view slices of the weight matrix $Q_{I,\ell}$ at the coordinate $(40, 57, 26)$. The red region corresponds to large weight score and contains the most classification information.

performs much worse than all other six methods. ROAD performs slightly better than PCA. SPLS and SVM are comparable with each other, but they outperform SLR and ROAD. SWPCR outperforms all six classification methods. It suggests that the classification performance can be significantly improved by incorporating spatial smoothness and simple dimension reductions methods, such as PCA.

4.3   Age Prediction

Our second goal is to apply SWPCR in predicting subjects' age based on their FDG-PET images. The response variable $\mathbf{y}$ is the age of the subjects and the explanatory variables are the latent scores, extracted from image data. It is very interesting to use memory test scores as the response variable $\mathbf{y}$. However, the data set here contains no such information. The three subjects without the age information are deleted and then we have 193 images left. $\mathbf{y}_i$ in model (10) becomes age of the subjects. Here we will not repeat the detailed stages of SWPCR again, which is similar as in Sect. 3. The slight difference is stage 3. Here we run regression rather than classification methods between age and the SWPCR latent scores.

First, we compared SWPCR with three other dimensional reduction methods including PCA, weighted PCA (WPCA) [17], and supervised PCA (SPCA) [2]. We used the leave-one-out cross validation to compute the prediction errors of

Table 2. Misclassification Rates of Different Methods for ADNI 1 Pet Data

sLDA	SPLS	SLR	SVM	ROAD	PCA	SWPCR
0.255	0.163	0.179	0.168	0.189	0.194	0.117

all the four methods. Let $\hat{\mathbf{y}}_i$ be the fitted response value based on the regression model, and the prediction error is defined as $|\hat{\mathbf{y}}_i - \mathbf{y}_i|/|\mathbf{y}_i|$. Subsequently, we calculated the error difference between SWPCR and all three other methods across different numbers ($K = 5, 7, 10$) of principal components. Panels (a)–(c) in Fig. 4 show the boxplots of the error difference between SWPCR and PCA, WPCA, and SPCA, respectively. The error differences are almost always less than 0 (under the dashed line) and these results show the better performance of SWPCR in dimension reduction.

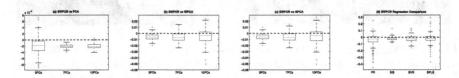

Fig. 4. Performance of SWPCR Regression for ADNI 1 Pet Data. Panels (a)–(c) shows the boxplots of error difference between SWPCR and PCA (WPCA and SPCA). Panel (d) compares SWPCR regression with several other regression methods, including PR, SIS, SVR and SPLS.

Second, we compared SWPCR with several other high-dimensional regression methods including penalized regression (PR) [19], sure independence screening (SIS) regression [7], support vector regression (SVR) [3], and SPLS [5]. Panel (d) in Fig. 4 shows the boxplots of the prediction error difference between SWPCR and all the other regression methods. The analysis results further confirm the better performance of SWPCR in regression.

5 Discussion

SWPCR enables a selective treatment of individual features, accommodates the complex dependence among features of graph data, and has the ability of utilizing the underlying spatial pattern possessed by image data. SWPCR integrates feature selection, smoothing, and feature extraction in a single framework. In the simulation studies and real data analysis, SWPCR shows substantial improvement over many state-of-the-art methods for high-dimensional problems.

Acknowledgements. This work was partially supported by the Startup Fund of University of South Florida, NIH grants MH086633, RR025747, and MH092335 and NSF grants SES-1357666 and DMS-1407655.

References

1. Aharon, M., Elad, M., Bruckstein, A.: K-SVD: an algorithm for designing overcomplete dictionaries for sparse representation. IEEE Trans. Signal Process. **54**, 4311–4322 (2006)

2. Bair, E., Hastie, T., Paul, D., Tibshirani, R.: Prediction by supervised principal components. J. Am. Stat. Assoc. **101**(473), 119–137 (2006)
3. Basak, D., Pal, S., Patranabis, D.C.: Support vector regression. Neural Inf. Process. Lett. Rev. **11**(10), 203–224 (2007)
4. Buades, A., Coll, B., Morel, J.M.: A non-local algorithm for image denoising. In: IEEE Computer Society Conference on Computer Vision and Pattern Recognition, CVPR 2005, vol. 2, pp. 60–65. IEEE (2005)
5. Chun, H., Keles, S.: Sparse partial least squares regression for simultaneous dimension reduction and variable selection. J. Roy. Stat. Soc. Ser. B **72**, 3–25 (2010)
6. Clemmensen, L., Hastie, T., Witten, D., Ersbøll, B.: Sparse discriminant analysis. Technometrics **53**(4), 406–413 (2011)
7. Fan, J., Lv, J.: Sure independence screening for ultrahigh dimensional feature space. J. Roy. Stat. Soc.: Ser. B (Stat. Methodol.) **70**(5), 849–911 (2008)
8. Fan, J., Feng, Y., Tong, X.: A road to classification in high dimensional space: the regularized optimal affine discriminant. J. Roy. Stat. Soc.: Ser. B (Stat. Methodol.) **74**(4), 745–771 (2012)
9. Friston, K.J.: Modalities, modes, and models in functional neuroimaging. Sci. **326**, 399–403 (2009)
10. Grenander, U., Miller, M.I.: Pattern Theory From Representation to Inference. Oxford University Press, New York (2007)
11. Hastie, T., Tibshirani, R., Friedman, J.: The Elements of Statistical Learning: Data Mining, Inference, and Prediction (2nd). Springer, Hoboken (2009)
12. Lee, M., Shen, H., Huang, J.Z., Marron, J.S.: Biclustering via sparse singular value decomposition. Biom. **66**, 1087–1095 (2010)
13. Li, Y., Zhu, H., Shen, D., Lin, W., Gilmore, J.H., Ibrahim, J.G.: Multiscale adaptive regression models for neuroimaging data. J. Roy. Stat. Soc.: Ser. B (Stat. Methodol.) **73**, 559–578 (2011)
14. Lin, Y.: Support vector machines and the bayes rule in classification. Data Min. Knowl. Disc. **6**, 259–275 (2002)
15. Manjón, J.V., Carbonell-Caballero, J., Lull, J.J., García-Martí, G., Martí-Bonmatí, L., Robles, M.: MRI denoising using non-local means. Med. Image Anal. **12**(4), 514–523 (2008)
16. Polzehl, J., Spokoiny, V.G.: Propagation-separation approach for local likelihood estimation. Probab. Theory Relat. Fields **135**, 335–362 (2006)
17. Skočaj, D., Leonardis, A., Bischof, H.: Weighted and robust learning of subspace representations. Pattern Recognit **40**(5), 1556–1569 (2007)
18. Taylor, K.M., Meyer, F.G.: A random walk on image patches. SIAM J. Imaging Sci. **5**, 688–725 (2012)
19. Tibshirani, R.: Regression shrinkage and selection via the lasso. J. Roy. Stat. Soc. Ser B (Methodol.) **58**, 267–288 (1996)
20. Yamashita, O.: Quick manual for sparse logistic regression toolbox ver1.2.1: software at http://www.cns.atr.jp/~oyamashi/SLR_WEB/ (2011)
21. Yan, S., Xu, D., Zhang, B., Zhang, H.J., Yang, Q., Lin, S.: Graph embedding and extensions: a general framework for dimensionality reduction. IEEE Trans. Pattern Anal. Mach. Intell. **29**, 40–51 (2007)

Coupled Stable Overlapping Replicator Dynamics for Multimodal Brain Subnetwork Identification

Burak Yoldemir[1(✉)], Bernard Ng[2,3], and Rafeef Abugharbieh[1]

[1] Biomedical Signal and Image Computing Lab,
The University of British Columbia, Vancouver, BC, Canada
buraky@ece.ubc.ca
[2] Parietal Team, INRIA Saclay, Saclay, France
[3] Functional Imaging in Neuropsychiatric Disorders Lab,
Stanford University, Stanford, CA, USA

Abstract. Combining imaging modalities to synthesize their inherent strengths provides a promising means for improving brain subnetwork identification. We propose a multimodal integration technique based on a sex-differentiated formulation of replicator dynamics for identifying subnetworks of brain regions that exhibit high inter-connectivity both functionally and structurally. Our method has a number of desired properties, namely, it can operate on weighted graphs derived from functional magnetic resonance imaging (fMRI) and diffusion MRI (dMRI) data, allows for subnetwork overlaps, has an intrinsic criterion for setting the number of subnetworks, and provides statistical control on false node inclusion in the identified subnetworks via the incorporation of stability selection. We thus refer to our technique as coupled stable overlapping replicator dynamics (CSORD). On synthetic data, we demonstrate that CSORD achieves significantly higher subnetwork identification accuracy than state-of-the-art techniques. On real data from the Human Connectome Project (HCP), we show that CSORD attains improved test-retest reliability on multiple network measures and superior task classification accuracy.

Keywords: Brain · Connectivity · dMRI · fMRI · Multimodal integration · Overlapping community detection · Replicator dynamics · Stability selection

1 Introduction

Functional magnetic resonance imaging (fMRI) and diffusion MRI (dMRI) are currently the dominant modalities for studying functional connectivity in the brain and the underlying structural substrate, respectively. A prominent approach for understanding the brain's functional architecture is to group brain regions into subnetworks (also referred to as communities). Seed-based correlation [1] and independent component analysis (ICA) [2] have been the primary techniques for identifying subnetworks from fMRI data. Catalyzed by the advances in network science, the graph-theoretic approach for functional subnetwork identification has been gaining popularity, where brain regions are modeled as nodes and their connections as edges [3]. This approach is also

© Springer International Publishing Switzerland 2015
S. Ourselin et al. (Eds.): IPMI 2015, LNCS 9123, pp. 770–781, 2015.
DOI: 10.1007/978-3-319-19992-4_61

becoming widely adopted for subnetwork identification on structural graphs derived from dMRI data [4].

Early studies that jointly examined fMRI and dMRI data have mainly focused on comparing estimates of functional and structural connectivity (FC and SC) [5]. The main findings were that brain areas with high SC typically display high FC but the converse does not always hold [5]. However, recent studies have shown that the correlation between FC and SC estimates is rather low with typical data acquisition schemes [6]. Specifically, FC estimates tend to contain many false positive connections arising from confounds such as head movements, cardiac and respiratory pulsations, and scanner drifts. On the other hand, SC estimates often suffer from false negatives due to premature termination of reconstructed tracts at fiber crossings. These discrepancies may appear as setbacks at first sight, but these inter-modality differences in fact render multimodal integration useful since incorporating SC would reduce the effects of noise-induced FC and vice versa. Benefits from reaping these complementary characteristics of fMRI and dMRI for connectivity estimation are shown in [7–9], but multimodal subnetwork identification remains largely unexplored. For this problem, a multi-view spectral clustering algorithm has been recently adopted in [10], where FC and SC are considered as two views of the brain network. The Laplacian of the similarity matrix of one view is projected onto the eigenspace of the other view in an alternating manner, with spectral clustering subsequently applied on the converged eigenspace to identify subnetworks. A related approach has been used in [11], where the common eigenspace between the similarity matrices of FC and SC is found via joint diagonalization, on which spectral clustering is performed.

A major limitation in most subnetwork identification techniques is the lack of consideration as to whether the subnetworks identified are statistically significant. We argue that this is critical to avoid extracting artifactual subnetworks, such as those commonly assigned as confounds in ICA. Also, allowing for subnetwork overlaps is important, since certain brain regions are known to interact with multiple subnetworks [12]. There exist a few techniques for identifying overlapping brain subnetworks [4, 12], but to the best of our knowledge, none of these permits multimodal integration.

In this paper, we propose a technique based on replicator dynamics (RD) that facilitates integration of fMRI and dMRI data in identifying brain subnetworks. We start by reviewing the properties of RD [13], which only permits unimodal subnetwork identification (Sect. 2.1). We then describe a sex-differentiated formulation of RD [14] (Sect. 2.2) that permits FC and SC to be jointly modeled. In particular, this formulation extracts coupled subnetwork pairs based on fitness measures of both females and males, which in the present context, correspond to FC and SC estimates. We refer to this formulation as coupled RD (CRD). Importantly, we prove that for dense graphs, CRD always selects the same set of nodes for each pair of identified subnetworks (Sect. 2.2). Hence, the effective output of CRD is actually a single set of subnetworks with FC and SC integrated. CRD alone is prone to noise and tends to falsely divide the subnetworks. We thus adopt a graph incrementation scheme [15] to facilitate merging of subnetwork components that might be falsely split and present a procedure for incorporating stability selection [16] to statistically control for inclusion of false nodes arising from noise and overmerging (Sect. 2.3). We refer to this extension of CRD as coupled stable RD (CSRD). Further, we describe how a graph augmentation strategy [12] can be integrated into CSRD to enable overlapping subnetwork identification (Sect. 2.4). In aggregate, the resulting technique: (i) facilitates multimodal integration, (ii) can operate on weighted graphs, (iii) allows for subnetwork overlaps, (iv) has an intrinsic criterion for determining the number of subnetworks, (v) does not force all nodes to be part of a subnetwork, and (vi) statistically controls for false node inclusion. We refer to this technique as coupled stable overlapping RD (CSORD).

2 Methods

2.1 Replicator Dynamics

Let $\mathbf{w}(k)$ be a $d \times 1$ vector with each element being the proportion of an allele persisting in the gene pool during generation k. Further, let $\mathbf{C}$ be a $d \times d$ matrix with each element, $\mathbf{C}_{ij}$, reflecting the fitness of a genotype, i.e. a pair of alleles i and j. Under natural selection, $\mathbf{w}(k + 1)$ is given by the replicator equation [13]:

$$\mathbf{w}(k+1) = \frac{\mathbf{w}(k) \circ \mathbf{Cw}(k)}{\mathbf{w}(k)^T \mathbf{Cw}(k)}, \tag{1}$$

where $\circ$ denotes element-wise multiplication. (1) has been shown to provide local maxima of the following non-convex optimization problem [17]:

$$\max_{\mathbf{w}} \mathbf{w}^T \mathbf{Cw} \quad s.t. \|\mathbf{w}\|_1 = 1, \ \mathbf{w} \geq 0, \tag{2}$$

for real-valued, symmetric, and non-negative $\mathbf{C}$. By construction, $\mathbf{w}$ is constrained to lie on the standard simplex, i.e. $\|\mathbf{w}\|_1 = 1$, $\mathbf{w} \geq 0$, which encourages sparse $\mathbf{w}$ since restricting the l_1 norm induces sparsity. $\mathbf{w}_j(k) \neq 0$ thus indicates that allele j persisted in generation k. The average fitness of the surviving alleles has been proven to be all equal upon convergence of (1) [12]. Thus, in graph-theoretic terms, RD groups nodes based on mutual similarity. The local maximum to which RD converges highly depends on $\mathbf{w}(0)$. In the absence of a priori knowledge, setting $\mathbf{w}(0)$ to $1/d$ provides an unbiased choice that tends to extract the subnetwork with the highest mutual similarity between its nodes [17]. Other subnetworks can be found by reapplying (1) after removing the nodes in the identified subnetworks [18].

2.2 Coupled Replicator Dynamics

Separating $\mathbf{C}$ into $d \times d$ genotype fitness matrices $\mathbf{F}$ for females and $\mathbf{M}$ for males to model sex differences, the survival probabilities of the alleles in the female gene pool, $\mathbf{p}(k)$, and in male gene pool, $\mathbf{q}(k)$, based on natural selection can be estimated using the following multiplicative updates [14]:

$$\mathbf{p}(k+1) = 0.5 \frac{\mathbf{p}(k) \circ \mathbf{Fq}(k) + \mathbf{q}(k) \circ \mathbf{Fp}(k)}{\mathbf{p}(k)^T \mathbf{Fq}(k)}, \tag{3}$$

$$\mathbf{q}(k+1) = 0.5 \frac{\mathbf{q}(k) \circ \mathbf{Mp}(k) + \mathbf{p}(k) \circ \mathbf{Mq}(k)}{\mathbf{p}(k)^T \mathbf{Mq}(k)}. \tag{4}$$

Analogous to RD, $\mathbf{F}$ and $\mathbf{M}$ are assumed to be real, symmetric, and non-negative. The non-negativity constraint enforces $\mathbf{p}(k)$ and $\mathbf{q}(k)$ to be ≥ 0. Also, $\Sigma_j \, \mathbf{p}_j(k) = 1$ since $0.5 \cdot \Sigma_j \, (\mathbf{p}_j(k)(\mathbf{Fq}(k))_j + \mathbf{q}_j(k)(\mathbf{Fp}(k))_j) = 0.5(\mathbf{p}(k)^T \mathbf{Fq}(k) + \mathbf{q}(k)^T \mathbf{Fp}(k)) = 0.5(\mathbf{p}(k)^T \mathbf{Fq}(k) + \mathbf{p}(k)^T \mathbf{Fq}(k)) = \mathbf{p}(k)^T \mathbf{Fq}(k)$, where we have exerted the property that a scalar and its transpose are equal, i.e. $\mathbf{q}(k)^T \mathbf{Fp}(k) = \mathbf{p}(k)^T \mathbf{Fq}(k)$. Similarly, $\Sigma_j \, \mathbf{q}_j(k) = 1$. Thus, by matching the denominator of (3) and (4) with that of (1), one can see that (3) and (4) together form a local maximizer of the following optimization problem:

$$\max_{\mathbf{p},\mathbf{q}} \mathbf{p}^T \mathbf{Fq} + \mathbf{p}^T \mathbf{Mq} \; s.t. \|\mathbf{p}\|_1 = 1, \mathbf{p} \geq 0, \|\mathbf{q}\|_1 = 1, \mathbf{q} \geq 0, \tag{5}$$

where the l_1 constraint on $\mathbf{p}$ and $\mathbf{q}$ enforces sparsity. Since $\mathbf{p}$ is multiplied to both $\mathbf{F}$ and $\mathbf{M}$ in (5), the optimal $\mathbf{p}$ would jointly account for the genotype fitness of both sexes, and the same goes for $\mathbf{q}$. This coupling property of CRD can be more clearly seen by examining (3) and (4). Specifically, information in $\mathbf{M}$ is propagated to $\mathbf{p}$ through $\mathbf{q}$, and vice versa. We note that CRD also uses mutual similarity as the criterion for grouping nodes, which can be proved in a similar manner as in the case of RD. Further, we highlight that the sparsity patterns of $\mathbf{p}$ and $\mathbf{q}$ tend to perfectly match upon convergence for dense graphs. Specifically, assume $\mathbf{p}_i(k) = 0$ upon convergence. Based on (3), this implies $\mathbf{p}_i(k) \circ \mathbf{Fq}_i(k) + \mathbf{q}_i(k) \circ \mathbf{Fp}_i(k) = 0$. $\mathbf{p}_i(k) \circ \mathbf{Fq}_i(k)$ must equal 0 since $\mathbf{p}_i(k) = 0$, thus $\mathbf{q}_i(k) \circ \mathbf{Fp}_i(k)$ must also equal 0. This condition is satisfied only if $\mathbf{q}_i(k) = 0$ or $\mathbf{Fp}_i(k) = 0$. $\mathbf{Fp}_i(k) = 0$ requires $\mathbf{F}_{ij}$ to be exactly zero for each surviving allele j. In both our synthetic and real data, $\mathbf{F}$ is never sparse enough to warrant this condition. Hence, $\mathbf{q}_i(k) \circ \mathbf{Fp}_i(k) = 0$ can only arise by having $\mathbf{q}_i(k) = 0$, which enforces $\mathbf{p}$ and $\mathbf{q}$ to have the same sparsity patterns. The nodes in the identified subnetwork are thus given by the nonzero elements of either $\mathbf{p}$ or $\mathbf{q}$. Again, other subnetworks can be found by reapplying (3) and (4) after removing the nodes of the identified subnetworks from the graphs. However, this strategy modifies the original graph structure, thereby affecting the remaining local maxima. We describe a more principled way of identifying the other subnetworks that permits subnetwork overlaps and preserves the location of the remaining local maxima in Sect. 2.4.

2.3 Coupled Stable Replicator Dynamics

Graph Incrementation. Sparsity of the subnetworks identified by CRD is intrinsically determined based on the mutual similarity among nodes. This property is desirable under the ideal case of noiseless graphs. In practice, such a strict criterion for grouping nodes could easily result in a subnetwork being falsely split into components [19], since even small perturbations to $\mathbf{F}$ and $\mathbf{M}$ would render certain nodes non-mutually connected. To reduce this effect, one strategy is to add a constant, η, to the off-diagonal elements of **F** and **M** [15]. This strategy artificially increases the mutual similarity among all nodes and swamps the differences between elements of **F** (and **M**) that are considerably smaller than η. We can hence adjust the sparsity level of the identified subnetworks by changing η. Choosing the optimal η is non-trivial. Also, noise in **F** and **M** could result in false nodes being included in the subnetworks. To jointly deal with these problems, we present next a procedure for integrating stability selection into CRD.

Stability Selection. The idea behind stability selection is that if we bootstrap the data many times and perform subnetwork identification on each bootstrap sample, nodes that truly belong to the same subnetwork are likely to be jointly selected over a large fraction of bootstrap samples, whereas false nodes are unlikely to be persistently selected [16]. To incorporate stability selection in refining each subnetwork identified by CRD, we first generate a set of matrices $\{F_\eta\}$ by adding η to the off-diagonal elements of **F**. A range of η from 0 to $d \cdot \max_{ij} |F_{ij}|$ at a step size of κ is used, where κ is chosen small enough to ensure that no more than one node is added to a subnetwork at each increment of η. The same procedure is applied to **M** to generate $\{M_\eta\}$. We then apply CRD to each (F_η, M_η) pair with $p(0)$ and $q(0)$ set to the CRD solution of the previous η increment (with $1/d$ added to all elements and renormalized to sum to 1), which enforces CRD to converge to a local maximum in the vicinity of the previous η increment for retaining subnetwork correspondence. We note that adding $1/d$ is critical since zeros in $p(k)$ and $q(k)$ remain as zeros as (3) and (4) are iterated, which prohibits new nodes from being added. We discard subnetworks that contain more than 10 % of the nodes assuming a subnetwork would not span more than 10 % of the brain. Next, we generate 100 bootstrap samples of **F** and **M** (as explained in Sect. 2.5), and compute $\left\{F_\eta^b\right\}$ and $\left\{M_\eta^b\right\}$ from each bootstrap sample F^b and M^b. We then apply CRD on each $\left(F_\eta^b, M_\eta^b\right)$ pair. For each η, we estimate the selection probability of each node as the proportion of bootstrap samples in which the given node attains a nonzero weight [16]. This estimation can be done based on either **p** or **q** since their sparsity patterns perfectly match. Finally, we threshold the selection probabilities to identify nodes that belong to the same subnetwork. A threshold τ that bounds the expected number of false nodes in a subnetwork, E, is given by [16]:

$$\tau \le \left(\frac{q^2}{Ed} + 1\right)\bigg/ 2, \qquad (6)$$

where q is the average number of nodes per subnetwork, which can be estimated as the sum of selection probabilities of all nodes averaged over η. We set E to 1 so that the average number of false nodes included in a subnetwork is statistically controlled to be less than or equal to 1. We declare the set of nodes with selection probabilities higher than the resulting τ for any η to be a subnetwork [16]. We note that each subnetwork identified by CRD is refined independently using the above procedure.

2.4 Coupled Stable Overlapping Replicator Dynamics

Since CRD is deterministic, reapplying it with the same initialization will converge to the same local maximum. Here, we adopt a graph augmentation strategy that enables destabilization of previously-found local maxima without altering the location of the others [12]. Reapplying CRD on this augmented graph would thus converge to one of the remaining local maxima. The required graph augmentation is as follows [20]:

$$
\mathbf{F}_{ij}^{aug} = \begin{cases} \mathbf{F}_{ij} & \text{if } i,j \le d \\ \alpha & \text{if } j > d \text{ and } i \notin S_{j-d} \\ \beta & \text{if } i,j > d \text{ and } i = j \\ \gamma_{ij} & \text{if } i > d \text{ and } j \in S_{i-d} \\ 0 & \text{otherwise} \end{cases}, \tag{7}
$$

$$
\gamma_{ij} = \sigma_{ij} \frac{1}{|S_{i-d}|} \sum_{m \in S_{i-d}} \mathbf{F}_{mj}, \ \sigma_{ij} > 1,
$$

where $\alpha > \beta$, $\beta = \max_{i \ne j} \mathbf{F}_{ij}$, S_l is the set of nodes of the lth identified subnetwork, and $|\cdot|$ denotes cardinality. $\mathbf{M}$ is similarly augmented to generate $\mathbf{M}^{aug}$. In effect, this is equivalent to adding artificial nodes to the graphs by appending $\mathbf{F}$ and $\mathbf{M}$ with new rows and new columns, and extending weighted edges to the original nodes such that the previously-found local maxima provably become unstable. Given S_1 found using CRD and refined by stability selection, finding S_2 proceeds by adding a new row and a new column to $\mathbf{F}$ and $\mathbf{M}$ based on (7), applying CRD on the new ($\mathbf{F}^{aug}$, $\mathbf{M}^{aug}$) pair, and refining the resulting subnetwork using stability selection. Remaining S_l can be similarly extracted. We highlight that an intrinsic criterion for terminating further subnetwork extraction is to stop if after convergence, $\mathbf{p}(k)^T \mathbf{F} \mathbf{q}(k) + \mathbf{p}(k)^T \mathbf{M} \mathbf{q}(k) \le \mathbf{p}(0)^T \mathbf{F} \mathbf{q}(0) + \mathbf{p}(0)^T \mathbf{M} \mathbf{q}(0)$, since this suggests that no further solutions of (5) are present. In practice, we found on synthetic data that using $a \cdot (\mathbf{p}(0)^T \mathbf{F} \mathbf{q}(0) + \mathbf{p}(0)^T \mathbf{M} \mathbf{q}(0))$, $a > 1$, as the stopping criterion is more robust to noisy $\mathbf{F}$ and $\mathbf{M}$. A rigorous way of choosing a is discussed in Sect. 2.5.

2.5 Parameter Selection and Implementation

In the context of brain subnetwork identification, $\mathbf{F}$ and $\mathbf{M}$ correspond to estimates of FC and SC, respectively, and alleles correspond to brain regions of interest (ROIs). Our goal is to find subnetworks of ROIs that are highly inter-connected both functionally and structurally. For $\mathbf{F}$, we use the conventional Pearson's correlation between average ROI time series. To ensure $\mathbf{F}$ is non-negative as required for the properties of CRD to hold, we set negative $\mathbf{F}_{ij}$ to zero given the currently unclear interpretation of negative FC. For $\mathbf{M}$, we use the fiber count between ROIs [5]. The main diagonals of $\mathbf{F}$ and $\mathbf{M}$ are set to zero to avoid self-connections [17]. Given the substantially larger magnitudes in $\mathbf{M}$ compared to $\mathbf{F}$, the subnetwork detection process would be dominated by $\mathbf{M}$. To mitigate this effect, we linearly rescale $\mathbf{M}$ such that the values in $\mathbf{F}$ and $\mathbf{M}$ are in the same range.

An open problem in subnetwork identification is the choice on the number of subnetworks. Although $\mathbf{p}(k)^T \mathbf{F} \mathbf{q}(k) + \mathbf{p}(k)^T \mathbf{M} \mathbf{q}(k) \le \mathbf{p}(0)^T \mathbf{F} \mathbf{q}(0) + \mathbf{p}(0)^T \mathbf{M} \mathbf{q}(0)$ is theoretically justified, noisy $\mathbf{F}$ and $\mathbf{M}$ could lead to spurious subnetworks with $\mathbf{p}(k)^\mathrm{T}\mathbf{Fq}$ $(k) + \mathbf{p}(k)^\mathrm{T}\mathbf{Mq}(k)$ being slightly above the threshold. Hence, there is a need for a stricter threshold, $a\cdot(\mathbf{p}(0)^\mathrm{T}\mathbf{Fq}(0) + \mathbf{p}(0)^\mathrm{T}\mathbf{Mq}(0))$, $a \geq 1$. To set a, we generate 500 synthetic datasets and extract subnetworks over a range of a from 1 to 10. The value of a that minimizes the difference between the number of estimated subnetworks and the ground truth is declared as the optimal a. We note that the synthetic datasets used for selecting a are separate from those used for evaluating the performance of CSORD.

To generate bootstrap samples of $\mathbf{F}$ for applying stability selection, we adopt a parametric bootstrap approach [21] since the spatiotemporal correlation structure of fMRI data would not be retained with regular bootstrap, where time points are independently sampled with replacement. Let $\mathbf{X}$ be a $t \times d$ fMRI time series matrix, where t is the number of time samples. We randomly draw 100 $\mathbf{X}^b$ of size $t \times d$ from a multivariate normal distribution with zero mean and covariance, $\mathbf{F}_\mathrm{pd}$, where $\mathbf{F}_\mathrm{pd}$ is a positive definite approximation of $\mathbf{F}$, computed by setting non-positive eigenvalues of $\mathbf{F}$ to 10^{-16}. $\mathbf{F}^b$ is then computed as the Pearson's correlation of $\mathbf{X}^b$. As for $\mathbf{M}$, one approach for generating bootstrap samples is to randomly select diffusion gradient directions with replacement to generate bootstrapped dMRI volumes and reapply tractography [22], but this is very computationally intensive. Instead, we use the same parametric bootstrap procedure to generate bootstrap samples of $\mathbf{M}$.

3 Materials

Synthetic Data. We generated 500 synthetic datasets that cover a wide variety of network configurations. Each dataset comprised $d = 200$ regions and 4 scans of 1200 time points as in the real data. We set the number of subnetworks, N, in each dataset to a random value between 10 and 20. The number of ROIs in each subnetwork was set to $\lceil d/N \rceil + c$ with c being a random number between 1 and 5, which ensures that the total number of ROIs across subnetworks is greater than d, hence guaranteeing the presence of subnetwork overlaps. ROIs were randomly assigned to subnetworks, and the same ROI was allowed to repeat across subnetworks. Using the resulting network configuration, we generated a $d \times d$ adjacency matrix, Σ, which was taken as the ground truth. Next, we built a noise-free SC matrix, Σ_s, by randomly setting p_1 % of the values in Σ to 0 to model how SC estimates are prone to false negatives, and built a noise-free FC matrix, Σ_f, by randomly setting p_2 % of the values in Σ to 1 to model how FC estimates are prone to false positives. p_1 and p_2 were randomly chosen from [0, 20]. Two sets of time series were then generated by drawing random samples from $N(0, \Sigma_\mathrm{s})$ and $N(0, \Sigma_\mathrm{f})$. Finally, SC and FC matrices were simulated by adding Gaussian noise to the time series with signal-to-noise ratio (SNR) randomly set between -6 and -3 dB, and computing the Pearson's correlation of these noisy time series.

Real Data. Minimally preprocessed resting state fMRI (RS-fMRI), task fMRI data, and dMRI from 40 unrelated healthy adults were obtained from the Human Connectome Project (HCP) database. The acquisition involved two RS-fMRI sessions, a single task fMRI session for each of the seven different tasks (working memory, gambling, motor, language, social cognition, relational processing, and emotional processing), and a single dMRI session. Acquisition details of these datasets can be found in [23].

In addition to the preprocessing already performed [24], we regressed out motion artifacts, white matter and cerebrospinal fluid confounds, and principal components of high variance voxels found using CompCor [25] from the RS-fMRI data. Band-pass filtering (0.01 Hz 0.1 Hz) was subsequently applied. For task fMRI data, we performed similar temporal processing, except a high-pass filter at 1/128 Hz was used. To define ROIs, we functionally divided the brain into $d = 200$ parcels by temporally concatenating RS-fMRI voxel time series across scans of all subjects and applying Ward clustering [26]. This value of d provides higher functional homogeneity than typical anatomical atlases, while maintaining reasonable ROIs to time samples ratio for reliable connectivity estimation. ROI time series were then generated by averaging voxel time series within each ROI. For group-level analysis, ROI time series were concatenated across subjects prior to estimating FC. For subject-level analysis, FC was directly estimated from each subject's ROI time series.

dMRI data were downsampled to 2 mm isotropic resolution prior to analysis to ease the computational load. We applied global tractography on constant solid angle orientation distribution function (ODF) using MITK [27] to reconstruct fiber tracts. To compute the fiber count between ROIs, which were taken as SC estimates, we warped our functionally-derived group parcellation map onto the $b = 0$ volume of each subject. For group-level analysis, individual SC estimates were averaged across subjects.

4 Results and Discussion

Synthetic Data. We compared CSORD against CSRD, CRD, stable RD (SRD), RD, NC [28], and multi-view spectral clustering (MVSC) [10]. SRD is analogous to CSRD, except (1) is used instead of (3) and (4) in finding subnetworks. Among the contrasted techniques, CSORD, CSRD, CRD and MVSC permit multimodal subnetwork identification, whereas SRD, RD, and NC are limited to a single modality. For these unimodal techniques, we focused on their performance in extracting subnetworks from FC estimates. On 500 synthetic datasets, we assessed each contrasted technique by computing the Dice coefficient (DC) between the estimated and ground truth subnetworks as: $DC = 2|S_{est} \cap S_{gnd}|/(S_{est} + S_{gnd})$, where S_{est} is the set of ROIs in an estimated subnetwork, and S_{gnd} is the set of ROIs in the corresponding ground truth subnetwork matched to S_{est} using Hungarian clustering [29]. DC of unmatched subnetworks was set to zero. CSORD achieved significantly higher DC than each contrasted technique at $p = 10^{-40}$ based on Wilcoxon signed rank test (Fig. 1).

Real data. Since ground truth subnetworks are unknown for real data, we based our validation on test-retest reliability and task classification accuracy. We estimated test-retest reliability as the intra-class correlation (ICC) over four graph metrics. Specifically, we first computed the clustering coefficient, transitivity, global efficiency, and local efficiency [30] for each subnetwork extracted from RS-fMRI data (and dMRI data for multimodal methods) of each scan session of a given subject. We then averaged the values of a given metric across each subject's subnetworks for each of the two scan sessions. Collecting these average values of each metric across subjects, we computed the ICC between the two scan sessions. We finally estimated test-retest reliability as the average of resulting four ICC values.

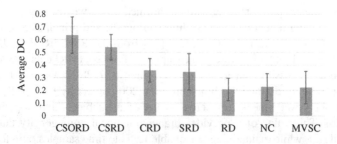

Fig. 1. Subnetwork identification accuracy on synthetic data.

High test-retest reliability is a desired property, but could arise from common noise between scan sessions. We thus additionally assessed the task classification accuracy of the contrasted techniques as follows. We first extracted group subnetworks from RS-fMRI and dMRI data. We then computed $\mathbf{F}$ of each task from each subject's task fMRI dataset, and scaled its elements as: $\mathbf{F}_{ij}^s = \mathbf{F}_{ij} \cdot |m_i \cap m_j| / |m_i \cup m_j|$, where m_i and m_j are the group subnetwork memberships of nodes i and j based on RS-fMRI and dMRI data. This scaling weighs down $\mathbf{F}_{ij}$ if nodes i and j were assigned to different group subnetworks, which in effect, propagates the group subnetwork structure onto $\mathbf{F}$. The weighted degree of each brain region computed from $\mathbf{F}^s$ was taken as a feature, resulting in a $d \times 1$ feature vector for each task. Support vector machine was used for classification. For estimating classification accuracy, we subsampled the data over 100 random splits with 35 subjects used for training and 5 for testing.

We adopted the above scaling scheme of $\mathbf{F}$, which was originally used for extending the definition of modularity to overlapping subnetworks [31], since the notion of within and between subnetwork connections become fuzzy when subnetworks are allowed to overlap. Also, this evaluation scheme ensures the data used for subnetwork identification (RS-fMRI and dMRI data) are independent from the data used for classification performance assessment (task fMRI data). The assumption is that tasks induce only small functional changes to intrinsic brain connectivity. This hypothesis is supported by the strong resemblance between RS and task subnetworks [32], as well as how energy consumption in the brain is mainly for supporting ongoing activity with task-evoked response constituting less than 5 % of the total [33].

Results on test-retest reliability and task classification accuracy are shown in Fig. 2 (a). Comparing RD's and CRD's performance suggests that simply incorporating SC without considering the limitations of RD produces only marginal benefits. In fact, a much larger gain was obtained by controlling for false node inclusions with SRD. Nevertheless, by jointly incorporating SC and controlling for false node inclusion as well as enabling subnetwork overlaps, CSORD achieved the highest task classification accuracy and is on par with the best contrasted techniques in terms of test-retest reliability. We note that average FC has been argued to contain no dynamical information. It is true that average connectivity matrix does not capture dynamical connectivity, but the overlapping structure of subnetworks is well reflected by the relative magnitude of its elements, and can be readily extracted as shown by our results.

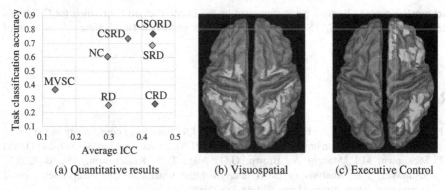

(a) Quantitative results   (b) Visuospatial   (c) Executive Control

Fig. 2. Real data results. (a) CSORD achieved the best classification accuracy and high test-retest reliability. (b–c) Exemplar group subnetworks identified by CSORD.

Qualitatively, CSORD identified all commonly found subnetworks in the literature [34]. The extracted visuospatial subnetwork and right executive control subnetwork are shown in Fig. 2(b-c) as exemplar results. CSORD also identified a subnetwork (Fig. 3) that comprises the basal ganglia, thalamus, higher visual cortex, motor areas, and part of the cerebellum. These regions constitute the visual corticostriatal loop [35], striato-thalamo-cortical (STC) loop, and cerebello-thalamo-cortical (CTC) loop [36], which are rarely identified as a single subnetwork. Instead, state-of-the-art techniques typically declare the basal ganglia and cerebellum as separate subnetworks [32, 37], failing to capture cortical projections from subcortical regions.

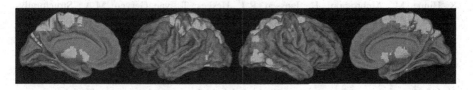

Fig. 3. A group subnetwork identified by CSORD that comprises the visual corticostriatal, CTC, and STC loops. Note that the cerebellum is outside the presented views.

5   Conclusions

We proposed CSORD to combine information from fMRI and dMRI data in identi-fying overlapping brain subnetworks. On synthetic data covering a diverse set of network configurations, we showed that CSORD provides significantly higher sub-network identification accuracy than a number of state-of-the-art techniques. On real data, we illustrated that CSORD is not only more robust to inter-session variability than most of the contrasted techniques, but it also achieved the highest classification accuracy. Importantly, standard techniques typically declare the basal ganglia, cere-bellum, and motor cortex as separate subnetworks, despite their known joint involvements in various motor loops. In contrast, CSORD was able to extract a single subnetwork comprising these well-known interacting motor regions.

Acknowledgments. Bernard Ng is supported by the Lucile Packard Foundation for Children's Health, Stanford NIH-NCATS-CTSA UL1 TR001085 and Child Health Research Institute of Stanford University.

References

1. Biswal, B., Yetkin, F.Z., Haughton, V.M., Hyde, J.S.: Functional connectivity in the motor cortex of resting human brain using echoplanar MRI. Magn. Reson. Med. **34**, 537–541 (1995)
2. McKeown, M.J., Makeig, S., Brown, G.G., Jung, T.-P., Kindermann, S.S., Bell, A.J., Sejnowski, T.J.: Analysis of fMRI data by blind separation into independent spatial components. Hum. Brain Mapp. **6**, 160–188 (1998)
3. Fortunato, S.: Community detection in graphs. Phys. Rep. **486**, 75–174 (2010)
4. Wu, K., Taki, Y., Sato, K., Sassa, Y., Inoue, K., Goto, R., Okada, K., Kawashima, R., He, Y., Evans, A.C., Fukuda, H.: The overlapping community structure of structural brain network in young healthy individuals. PLoS ONE **6**, e19608 (2011)
5. Damoiseaux, J.S., Greicius, M.D.: Greater than the sum of its parts: a review of studies combining structural connectivity and resting-state functional connectivity. Brain Struct. Funct. **213**, 525–533 (2009)
6. Ng, B., Varoquaux, G., Poline, J.B., Thirion, B.: Implications of inconsistencies between fMRI and dMRI on multimodal connectivity estimation. In: Mori, K., Sakuma, I., Sato, Y., Barillot, C., Navab, N. (eds.) MICCAI 2013. LNCS, vol. 8151, pp. 652–659. Springer, Heidelberg (2013)
7. Ng, B., Varoquaux, G., Poline, J.B., Thirion, B.: A novel sparse graphical approach for multimodal brain connectivity inference. In: Ayache, N., Delingette, H., Golland, P., Mori, K. (eds.) MICCAI 2012. LNCS, vol. 7510, pp. 707–714. Springer, Heidelberg (2012)
8. Hinne, M., Ambrogioni, L., Janssen, R.J., Heskes, T., van Gerven, M.A.: Structurally-informed bayesian functional connectivity analysis. NeuroImage **86**, 294–305 (2014)
9. Venkataraman, A., Rathi, Y., Kubicki, M., Westin, C.F., Golland, P.: Joint modeling of anatomical and functional connectivity for population studies. IEEE Trans. Med. Imaging **31**, 164–182 (2012)
10. Chen, H., Li, K., Zhu, D., Jiang, X., Yuan, Y., Lv, P., Zhang, T., Guo, L., Shen, D., Liu, T.: Inferring group-wise consistent multimodal brain networks via multi-view spectral clustering. IEEE Trans. Med. Imaging **32**, 1576–1586 (2013)
11. Dodero, L., Gozzi, A., Liska, A., Murino, V., Sona, D.: Group-Wise functional community detection through joint laplacian diagonalization. In: Golland, P., Hata, N., Barillot, C., Hornegger, J., Howe, R. (eds.) MICCAI 2014. LNCS, vol. 8674, pp. 708–715. Springer, Heidelberg (2014)
12. Yoldemir, B., Ng, B., Abugharbieh, R.: Overlapping replicator dynamics for functional subnetwork identification. In: Mori, K., Sakuma, I., Sato, Y., Barillot, C., Navab, N. (eds.) MICCAI 2013. LNCS, vol. 8150, pp. 682–689. Springer, Heidelberg (2013)
13. Schuster, P., Sigmund, K.: Replicator dynamics. J. Theor. Biol. **100**, 533–538 (1983)
14. Karlin, S.: Mathematical models, problems, and controversies of evolutionary theory. Bulletin Ame. Math. Soc. **10**, 221–273 (1984)
15. Ng, B., Yoldemir, B., Abugharbieh, R.: Stable overlapping replicator dynamics for subnetwork identification. In: NIPS Workshop on Networks, pp. 461–473 (2014)
16. Meinshausen, N., Bühlmann, P.: Stability selection. J. Roy. Statist. Soc. Ser. B **72**, 417–473 (2010)

17. Ng, B., McKeown, M.J., Abugharbieh, R.: Group replicator dynamics: a novel group-wise evolutionary approach for sparse brain network detection. IEEE Trans. Med. Imaging **31**, 576–585 (2012)
18. Lohmann, G., Bohn, S.: Using replicator dynamics for analyzing fMRI data of human brain. IEEE Trans. Med. Imaging **21**, 485–492 (2002)
19. Thirion, B., Pinel, P., Tucholka, A., Roche, A., Ciuciu, P., Mangin, J.-F., Poline, J.B.: Structural analysis of fMRI data revisited: improving the sensitivity and reliability of fMRI group studies. IEEE Trans. Med. Imaging **26**, 1256–1269 (2007)
20. Torsello, A., Bulò, S.R., Pelillo, M.: Beyond partitions: allowing overlapping groups in pairwise clustering. In: Proceedings of International Conference Pattern Recognition, pp. 1–4 (2008)
21. Efron, B.: The jackknife, the bootstrap, and other resampling plans. Society of Industrial and Applied Mathematics CBMS-NSF Monographs (1982)
22. Lazar, M., Alexander, A.L.: Bootstrap white matter tractography (BOOT-TRAC). NeuroImage **24**, 524–532 (2005)
23. Van Essen, D.C., Smith, S.M., Barch, D.M., Behrens, T.E.J., Yacoub, E., Ugurbil, K.: The wu-minn human connectome project: an overview. NeuroImage **80**, 62–79 (2013)
24. Glasser, M.F., Sotiropoulos, S.N., Wilson, J.A., Coalson, T.S., Fischl, B., Andersson, J.L., Xu, J., Jbabdi, S., Webster, M., Polimeni, J.R., Van Essen, D.C., Jenkinson, M.: The minimal preprocessing pipelines for the human connectome project. NeuroImage **80**, 105–124 (2013)
25. Behzadi, Y., Restom, K., Liau, J., Liu, T.T.: A component based noise correction method (CompCor) for BOLD and perfusion based fMRI. NeuroImage **37**, 90–101 (2007)
26. Michel, V., Gramfort, A., Varoquaux, G., Eger, E., Keribin, C., Thirion, B.: A supervised clustering approach for fmri-based inference of brain states. Pattern Recogn. **45**, 2041–2049 (2012)
27. Neher, P., Stieltjes, B., Reisert, M., Reicht, I., Meinzer, H., Fritzsche, K.: MITK global tractography. In: Proceeding of SPIE Medical Imaging, p. 83144D (2012)
28. Van Den Heuvel, M., Mandl, R., Hulshoff Pol, H.: Normalized cut group clustering of resting-state fMRI data. PLoS ONE **3**, e2001 (2008)
29. Kuhn, H.W.: The hungarian method for the assignment problem. Nav. Res. Logist. Q. **2**, 83–97 (1955)
30. Rubinov, M., Sporns, O.: Complex network measures of brain connectivity: uses and interpretations. NeuroImage **52**, 1059–1069 (2010)
31. Wang, Q., Fleury, E.: Overlapping community structure and modular overlaps in complex networks. In: Ozyer, T., Erdem, Z., Rokne, J., Khoury, S. (eds.) LNSN, pp. 15–40. Springer, Netherlands (2013)
32. Smith, S.M., Fox, P.T., Miller, K.L., Glahn, D.C., Fox, P.M., Mackay, C.E., Filippini, N., Watkins, K.E., Toro, R., Laird, A.R., Beckmann, C.F.: Correspondence of the brain's functional architecture during activation and rest. In: Proceedings National Academy of Sciences, U.S.A. 106, pp. 13040–13045 (2009)
33. Fox, M.D., Raichle, M.E.: Spontaneous fluctuations in brain activity observed with functional magnetic resonance imaging. Nat. Rev. Neurosci. **8**, 700–711 (2007)
34. Van Den Heuvel, M., Hulshoff Pol, H.: Exploring the brain network: a review on resting-state fMRI functional connectivity. Eur. Neuropsychopharm. **20**, 519–534 (2010)
35. Seger, C.A.: The visual corticostriatal loop through the tail of the caudate: circuitry and function. Front. Syst. Neurosci. **7**, 104 (2013)
36. Palmer, S.J., Li, J., Wang, Z.J., McKeown, M.J.: Joint amplitude and connectivity compensatory mechanisms in parkinson's disease. Neuroscience **166**, 1110–1118 (2010)
37. Wen, X., Yao, L., Fan, T., Wu, X., Liu, J.: The spatial pattern of basal ganglia network: a resting state fMRI study. In: Proceedings of Complex Medical Engineering, pp. 43–46 (2012)

Joint 6D k-q Space Compressed Sensing for Accelerated High Angular Resolution Diffusion MRI

Jian Cheng[1,2]([✉]), Dinggang Shen[1], Peter J. Basser[2], and Pew-Thian Yap[1]

[1] Department of Radiology and BRIC, University of North Carolina at Chapel Hill,
Chapel Hill, USA
jian.cheng.1983@gmail.com
[2] Section on Tissue Biophysics and Biomimetics (STBB), PPITS, NICHD, NIBIB,
Bethesda, USA
ptyap@med.unc.edu

Abstract. High Angular Resolution Diffusion Imaging (HARDI) avoids the Gaussian diffusion assumption that is inherent in Diffusion Tensor Imaging (DTI), and is capable of characterizing complex white matter micro-structure with greater precision. However, HARDI methods such as Diffusion Spectrum Imaging (DSI) typically require significantly more signal measurements than DTI, resulting in prohibitively long scanning times. One of the goals in HARDI research is therefore to improve estimation of quantities such as the Ensemble Average Propagator (EAP) and the Orientation Distribution Function (ODF) with a limited number of diffusion-weighted measurements. A popular approach to this problem, Compressed Sensing (CS), affords highly accurate signal reconstruction using significantly fewer (sub-Nyquist) data points than required traditionally. Existing approaches to CS diffusion MRI (CS-dMRI) mainly focus on applying CS in the **q**-space of diffusion signal measurements and fail to take into consideration information redundancy in the **k**-space. In this paper, we propose a framework, called 6-Dimensional Compressed Sensing diffusion MRI (6D-CS-dMRI), for reconstruction of the diffusion signal and the EAP from data sub-sampled in both 3D **k**-space and 3D **q**-space. To our knowledge, 6D-CS-dMRI is the first work that applies compressed sensing in the full 6D **k-q** space and reconstructs the diffusion signal in the full continuous **q**-space and the EAP in continuous displacement space. Experimental results on synthetic and real data demonstrate that, compared with full DSI sampling in **k-q** space, 6D-CS-dMRI yields excellent diffusion signal and EAP reconstruction with low root-mean-square error (RMSE) using 11 times less samples (3-fold reduction in **k**-space and 3.7-fold reduction in **q**-space).

1 Introduction

Diffusion MRI (dMRI) is a unique non-invasive technique to investigate the white matter in brain. In dMRI, MR signal attenuation $E(\mathbf{q}) = S(\mathbf{q})/S(0)$ is a continuous function that depends on the diffusion weighting vector $\mathbf{q} \in \mathbb{R}^3$, where

© Springer International Publishing Switzerland 2015
S. Ourselin et al. (Eds.): IPMI 2015, LNCS 9123, pp. 782–793, 2015.
DOI: 10.1007/978-3-319-19992-4_62

$S(\mathbf{q})$ is a diffusion-weighted measurement at $\mathbf{q}$, and $S(0)$ is the measurement without diffusion weighting at $\mathbf{q} = 0$. A central problem in dMRI is to reconstruct the MR signal attenuation $E(\mathbf{q})$ from a limited number of noisy measurements in the $\mathbf{q}$-space and to estimate some meaningful quantities such as the Ensemble Average Propagator (EAP) and the Orientation Distribution Function (ODF). The EAP $P(\mathbf{R})$, which is the Fourier transform of $E(\mathbf{q})$ under the narrow pulse assumption [1], fully describes the Probability Density Function (PDF) of water molecule displacements in a voxel. The radial integral of EAP results in the ODF [1], a PDF defined on $\mathbf{S}^2$. By assuming a Gaussian EAP, Diffusion Tensor Imaging (DTI) requires only a dozen of measurements for estimating the diffusion tensor for the EAP or the diffusion signal. However, it is well reported that DTI cannot fully characterize complex micro-structure such as crossing fibers [1]. On the other hand, Diffusion Spectrum Imaging (DSI) is a model-free technique for EAP estimation. However, DSI normally requires about 515 signal measurements in $\mathbf{q}$-space, causing a scan time as long as an hour, thus limiting its clinical utility.

Compressed Sensing (CS) [2] is known for its effectiveness in signal reconstruction from a very limited number of samples by leveraging signal compressibility or sparsity. In general, the stronger the assumption is used in reconstruction, the less number of samples is needed. Note that the assumption in CS is always true if the dictionary is devised appropriately to sparsely represent signals. $\mathbf{k}$-space CS techniques, such as Sparse MRI [3,4], have been proposed to reconstruct MR images from a sub-sampled $\mathbf{k}$-space, where the sparsity dictionaries are the wavelet basis and the total variation operator. In dMRI, existing techniques mainly focus on applying CS to the $\mathbf{q}$-space [5–7]. References [5,6,8] represented diffusion signal and EAP discretely, which suffers from numerical errors in regridding and numerical integration. References [7,9,10] represented diffusion signal and EAP continuously, which have closed form expressions of Fourier transform and ODF/EAP calculation. However, this line of work fails to harness information redundancy in the k-space. The correlation of the $\mathbf{k}$-space and the $\mathbf{q}$-space can be employed for even greater sub-sampling, thus further reducing scanning while retaining good reconstruction accuracy. To our knowledge, [11,12] are the only works on signal and ODF reconstruction in joint $\mathbf{k}$-$\mathbf{q}$ space by using single-shell data (single b value), i.e., $\mathbb{R}^3 \times \mathbb{S}^2$. However, reconstruction of continuous diffusion signal and EAP in whole $\mathbf{q}$-space $\mathbb{R}^3$ is much more challenging than single shell $\mathbb{S}^2$. In this paper, we propose a framework, called 6-Dimensional Compressed Sensing diffusion MRI (6D-CS-dMRI), for reconstruction of the diffusion signal and the EAP from data sub-sampled in both 3D $\mathbf{k}$-space and 3D $\mathbf{q}$-space. To our knowledge, 6D-CS-dMRI is the first work that applies compressed sensing in the full 6D $\mathbf{k}$-$\mathbf{q}$ space and reconstructs the diffusion signal in the full continuous $\mathbf{q}$-space and the EAP in full continuous displacement $\mathbf{R}$-space. A preliminary abstract of this work was published in [13].

2   Compressed Sensing dMRI in Joint k-q Space

2.1   Sampling and Reconstruction in the 6D Joint k-q Space

Considering the diffusion-attenuated signal $S(\boldsymbol{x}, \mathbf{q})$ as a complex function in a 6-dimensional (6D) space, i.e. 3D voxel x-space and 3D diffusion q-space, for a fixed $\mathbf{q}$ value, the magnitude of $S(\boldsymbol{x}, \mathbf{q})$, denoted as $|S(\boldsymbol{x}, \mathbf{q})|$, is a 3D diffusion weighted image volume. Then the k-space measurements $\widehat{S}(\mathbf{k}, \mathbf{q})$ and the EAP are related by [14]

$$P(\boldsymbol{x}, \mathbf{R}) = \int_{\boldsymbol{x} \in \mathbb{R}^3} \frac{1}{S(\boldsymbol{x}, 0)} \underbrace{\left| \int_{\mathbf{k} \in \mathbb{R}^3} \widehat{S}(\mathbf{k}, \mathbf{q}) \exp(-2\pi j \boldsymbol{x}^T \mathbf{k}) d\mathbf{k} \right|}_{|S(\boldsymbol{x}, \mathbf{q})|} \exp(-2\pi j \mathbf{q}^T \mathbf{R}) d\mathbf{q}$$

(1)

where $\widehat{S}(\mathbf{k}, \mathbf{q})$ is the 3D Fourier transform of $S(\boldsymbol{x}, \mathbf{q})$ over $\boldsymbol{x}$, and $S(\boldsymbol{x}, 0)$ is the image volume with $\mathbf{q} = 0$. Two Fourier transforms are involved: the Fourier transform between $\widehat{S}(\mathbf{k}, \mathbf{q})$ in scanning k-space and $S(\boldsymbol{x}, \mathbf{q})$ in voxel x-space for

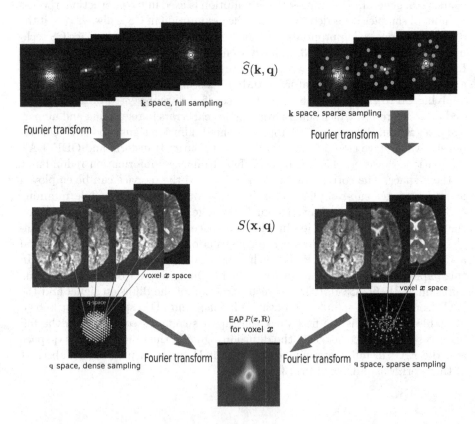

Fig. 1. Overview of reconstruction in 6D k-q space. Dense sampling (left) and sparse sampling (right) in both **k** and **q** spaces.

any fixed $\mathbf{q}$, and the Fourier transform between $E(\boldsymbol{x},\mathbf{q}) = |S(\boldsymbol{x},\mathbf{q})|/S(\boldsymbol{x},0)$ in diffusion $\mathbf{q}$-space and EAP $P(\boldsymbol{x},\mathbf{R})$ in displacement $\mathbf{R}$-space for a voxel $\boldsymbol{x}$. Instead of dense sampling in $\mathbf{k}$-space and $\mathbf{q}$-space, sparse sampling in both spaces can significantly reduce the scanning time. Figure 1 is an overview of the 6D space sampling and reconstruction framework that will be discussed in this paper. The goal is to reconstruct continuous functions $E(\boldsymbol{x},\mathbf{q})$ and $P(\boldsymbol{x},\mathbf{R})$ from a small number of samples of $\widehat{S}(\mathbf{k},\mathbf{q})$ in the joint 6D $\mathbf{k}$-$\mathbf{q}$ space.

A naive approach to 6D-CS-dMRI is to perform two CS reconstructions in association with the two Fourier transforms in Eq. (1). For a fixed $\mathbf{q}$, Sparse MRI can be used to reconstruct the 3D diffusion weighted (DW) images $S(\boldsymbol{x},\mathbf{q})$ from samples in $\mathbf{k}$-space [3]. Then all these 3D DW images can be used in a CS-dMRI technique to reconstruct the EAP [6,7]. This approach separates the estimation into two independent steps. However, the first step fails to take into consideration the diffusion signal in the same voxel across different $\mathbf{q}$ values, and in the second step, information of different voxels in the same DW images is not used.

2.2 6D-CS-dMRI Using Joint Optimization

We propose a novel reconstruction framework to jointly reconstruct the diffusion signal and EAP from the 6D space. For simplicity, we assume in the following that the baseline image $S(\boldsymbol{x},0)$ is known or pre-reconstructed by Sparse MRI [3]. The goal here is to estimate $S(\boldsymbol{x},\mathbf{q})$ and $P(\boldsymbol{x},\mathbf{R})$ from a number of samples of $\widehat{S}(\mathbf{k},\mathbf{q})$ in Eq. (1).

We use $\widehat{\boldsymbol{s}}_v$ to denote the partial Fourier sample vector of the v-th volume $S(\boldsymbol{x},\mathbf{q}_v)$ and $\boldsymbol{s}_i$ to denote the vector of the diffusion weighted signals $S(\boldsymbol{x}_i,\mathbf{q})$ at voxel i with different $\mathbf{q}$ values. We assume that the magnitude of the diffusion signal vector $\boldsymbol{s}_i$ can be sparsely represented by a real basis set $\mathbf{M}$ and coefficient vector $\boldsymbol{c}_i$, i.e. $\boldsymbol{s}_i = \mathbf{M}\boldsymbol{c}_i \odot \psi_i$, where ψ_i is the complex vector with unit magnitude that contains phase information, and $\odot$ means element-wise multiplication. Then we estimate coefficients $\{\boldsymbol{c}_i\}$ by solving

$$\min_{\{\boldsymbol{c}_i\},\{\boldsymbol{s}_v\},\{\psi_i\}} \sum_{v=1}^{N_q} \left\{ \|\mathscr{F}_p \boldsymbol{s}_v - \widehat{\boldsymbol{s}}_v\|_2^2 + \lambda_1 \mathrm{TV}(\boldsymbol{s}_v) + \lambda_2 \|\Phi \boldsymbol{s}_v\|_1 \right\} + \lambda_3 \sum_{i=1}^{N_s} \|\boldsymbol{c}_i\|_1 \quad (2)$$
$$\text{s.t.}\quad \mathbf{M}\boldsymbol{c}_i \odot \psi_i = \boldsymbol{s}_i \;\; \forall i,$$

where N_q is the number of DW images, N_s is the number of spatial voxels, $\mathscr{F}_p$ is the partial Fourier transform operator [3], $\mathrm{TV}(\cdot)$ denotes the total variation operator, Φ is a chosen wavelet dictionary. Note that $\boldsymbol{s}_i$ is a complex vector because $\widehat{\boldsymbol{s}}_v$ is complex, thus the signal representation $\mathbf{M}\boldsymbol{c}_i = |\boldsymbol{s}_i|$ is only applied to the magnitude of $\boldsymbol{s}_i$ when $\mathbf{M}$ is a real basis set. The first three terms in Eq. (2) originate from Sparse MRI [3]. The sparsity term of $\{\boldsymbol{c}_i\}$ and the equality constraint are from sparse representation in CS-dMRI [6,7]. Equation (2) is essentially a non-convex optimization problem for variable $(\{\boldsymbol{c}_i\},\{\psi_i\})$, because of the constraints $\mathbf{M}\boldsymbol{c}_i \odot \psi_i = \boldsymbol{s}_i, \forall i$.

We solve Eq. (2) using Alternating Direction Method of Multipliers (ADMM) [15]. ADMM is typically used for convex optimization, but it can also obtain a local minimum for some non-convex optimization problems [15]. The augmented Lagrangian cost function in ADMM is

$$\min_{\{c_i\},\{s_v\},\{\psi_i\},\{U_i\}} \sum_{v=1}^{N_q} \left\{ \|\mathscr{F}_p s_v - \widehat{s}_v\|_2^2 + \lambda_1 \mathrm{TV}(s_v) + \lambda_2 \|\varPhi s_v\|_1 \right\} + \lambda_3 \sum_{i=1}^{N_s} \|c_i\|_1$$

$$+ \frac{\rho}{2} \sum_{i=1}^{N_s} \|\mathbf{M} c_i \odot \psi_i - s_i + U_i\|_2^2, \tag{3}$$

where U_i is the complex Lagrangian variable U for voxel i, and ρ is the augmented Lagrangian parameter. Note that

$$\sum_{i=1}^{N_s} \|\mathbf{M} c_i \odot \psi_i - s_i + U_i\|_2^2 = \sum_{v=1}^{N_q} \|s_v(\{c_i, \psi_i\}) - s_v + U_v\|_2^2 \tag{4}$$

where U_v denotes the complex Lagrangian variables for DW images $\{s_v\}$ with q_v, and $s_v(\{c_i, \psi_i\})$ means complex DW images calculated by $\{c_i\}$ and $\{\psi_i\}$ based on the basis representation $s_i = \mathbf{M} c_i \odot \psi_i, \forall i$. Then the optimization can be separated into a sequence of three subproblems that can be solved iteratively:

$$(c_i^{(k+1)}, \psi_i^{(k+1)}) := \arg\min_{c,\psi} \|\mathbf{M} c \odot \psi - (s_i^{(k)} - U_i^{(k)})\|_2^2 + \frac{2}{\rho}\lambda_3 \|c\|_1 \tag{5a}$$

$$s_v^{(k+1)} := \arg\min_s \|\mathscr{F}_p s - \widehat{s}_v\|_2^2 + \lambda_1 \mathrm{TV}(s) + \lambda_2 \|\varPhi s\|_1 + 0.5\rho \left\| s_v^k(\{c_i, \psi_i\}) - s + U_v^{(k)} \right\|_2^2 \tag{5b}$$

$$U_i^{(k+1)} := U_i^{(k)} + \mathbf{M} c_i^{(k)} - s_i^{(k)} \tag{5c}$$

Note: (1) for complex vector $f = (f_1, f_2, \dots, f_n)^T$, $\|f\|_2^2 = \sum_{m=1}^n |f_m|^2$. (2) If $\|f\| \ge \|g\|$, then $\|f - g\|_2 \ge \|f\| - \|g\|$, and the equality holds if and only if f_m and g_m have the same phase, $\forall m$. Thus c and ψ in Eq. (5a) can be solved separately by

$$\psi_i^{(k+1)} := \mathrm{Ph}\left(s_i^{(k)} - U_i^{(k)} \right) \tag{6a}$$

$$c_i^{(k+1)} := \arg\min_c \left\| \mathbf{M} c - |s_i^{(k)} - U_i^{(k)}| \right\|_2^2 + \frac{2}{\rho}\lambda_3 \|c\|_1 \tag{6b}$$

where for a complex vector f, $\mathrm{Ph}(f) := (f_1/|f_1|, \dots, f_m/|f_m|)^T$ is the complex vector f divided by the magnitude values in each dimension, i.e., $f = |f| \odot \mathrm{Ph}(f)$.

Note that (1) The initialization of $\{s_v^{(0)}\}$ are set as the DW images $\{s_v\}$ estimated by Sparse MRI [3,16], and $\{U_v^{(0)}\}$ are set as zero. Thus the naive 6D-CS-dMRI result is actually $\{c_i^{(1)}\}$ after the initialization and the subproblem Eq. (5a) when $k = 1$; (2) Eq. (6b) is performed for each tissue voxel using CS-dMRI technique [6,7], and Eq. (5b) is performed for each DW image volume

---

Algorithm 1. 6D-CS-dMRI via ADMM

Input: Sub-sampled $\widehat{S}(\mathbf{k}, \mathbf{q})$

Output: Estimated coefficients $\{c_i\}$.

Estimate $S(\boldsymbol{x}, \mathbf{q})$ with the sub-sampled $\mathbf{q}$ values via sparse MRI [3, 16];

Estimate the brain tissue mask via $S(\boldsymbol{x}, 0)$;

Set $k = 0$; Initialize $\{U_i\}$ as 0;

repeat

$\quad$ Update $\{\psi_i^{(k+1)}\}$ voxel by voxel within the brain mask via Eq. (6a);

$\quad$ Update $\{c_i^{(k+1)}\}$ voxel by voxel within the brain mask via Eq. (6b); Set
$\quad$ $c_i^{(k+1)} = 0$ if i is outside of the mask;

$\quad$ Update $\{s_v^{(k+1)}\}$ volume by volume via Eq. (5b) and a variation of [16]; Set
$\quad$ $s_i^{(k+1)}$ as zero if voxel i is outside of the mask;

$\quad$ Update $\{U_i^{(k+1)}\}$ via Eq. (5c);

$\quad$ $k \leftarrow k + 1$;

until *The change of $\{c_i\}$ is small enough;*

---

using a variation, which considers the last term with $s_v^{(k)}(\{c_i, \psi_i\})$, of the efficient method in [16]. Since Eqs. (6a), (6b) and (5b) are iteratively updated, the information in voxel level and volume level are jointly used in each subproblem.

2.3 6D-CS-dMRI Using Learned Continuous Dictionary in SPFI

6D-CS-dMRI in Eq. (2) requires a dictionary for sparsely representing the magnitude of the diffusion signal. We choose the dictionary via Dictionary Learning Spherical Polar Fourier Imaging (DL-SPFI) [7] which learns the DL-SPF dictionary from Gaussian signals, and allows a continuous closed form expression for the EAP and diffusion signal. In SPFI [17,18], the signal in each voxel is represented by SPF basis, and after estimating the SPF coefficients, the EAP is analytically represented by dual SPF basis, i.e.,

$$E(\boldsymbol{x}_i, \mathbf{q}) = \sum_{n=0}^{N} \sum_{l=0}^{L} \sum_{m=-l}^{l} a_{i,nlm} B_{nlm}(\mathbf{q}|\zeta)$$

$$P(\boldsymbol{x}_i, \mathbf{R}) = \sum_{n=0}^{N} \sum_{l=0}^{L} \sum_{m=-l}^{l} a_{i,nlm} B_{nlm}^{\text{dual}}(\mathbf{R}|\zeta) \tag{7}$$

where $\{B_{nlm}(\mathbf{q}|\zeta)\}$ are SPF basis functions with scale parameter ζ which form a continuous complete basis with Gaussian Laguerre polynomial in radial part and Spherical Harmonics in spherical part [17], $\{B_{nlm}^{\text{dual}}(\mathbf{q})\}$ are the Fourier transforms of SPF basis functions, and EAP and diffusion signal share the same coefficients [18]. For DL-SPFI [7], in voxel $\boldsymbol{x}_i$, the basis representation is

$$s_i = \mathbf{S}_i^0 \mathbf{B} \mathbf{D} c_i = \mathbf{S}_i^0 \mathbf{B} a_i, \tag{8}$$

where $\mathbf{S}_i^0$ is a diagonal scale matrix caused by the baseline image $S(\boldsymbol{x}, 0)$ with $\mathbf{q} = 0$, $\mathbf{B}$ is the SPF basis matrix with SPF basis functions in its volumes, $\boldsymbol{a}_i$ is the SPF coefficient vector, $\mathbf{D}$ is the learned parameterization matrix for the learned DL-SPF basis matrix $\mathbf{BD}$, and $\boldsymbol{c}_i$ is the coefficient vector for the learned DL-SPF basis. It is shown in [7] that the parameterization matrix $\mathbf{D}$ can be learned from single tensor model, and then adaptively applied to different voxels by adaptively setting the scale parameter ζ in $\mathbf{B}$ based on the mean diffusivity in voxels. The learned matrix $\mathbf{D}$ and the adaptive scale setting make $\boldsymbol{c}_i$ under DL-SPF basis much sparser than $\boldsymbol{a}_i$ under the original SPF basis. For 6D-CS-dMRI, we set $\mathbf{M} = \mathbf{S}_i^0 \mathbf{BD}$ in Eq. (2), and set adaptive scale ζ based on mean diffusivity in voxel $\boldsymbol{x}_i$ as done in [7].

2.4   Implementation Issues

Following [7], we use SPF basis with $N = 4$, $L = 8$ in Eq. (5a) to learn 254 DL-SPF atoms. As shown in [7], there are two implementation details which can improve the result of CS-dMRI in Eq. (5a) using DL-SPFI. (1) The prior $E(\boldsymbol{x}, 0) = 1$ can be incorporated in Eq. (5a) by removing isotropic parts from $|\boldsymbol{s}_i^{(k)} - U_i^{(k)}|$ and $\mathbf{B}$, and focusing the estimation on the independent coefficients. (2) Additional regularization can be devised as $\|\Lambda \boldsymbol{c}\|_1$ instead of $\lambda_3 \|\boldsymbol{c}\|$ to give large regularization for the learned basis functions with small energy in the space of mixture of tensors. Please refer [7] for more details about these two issues.

There is a masking issue specifically for 6D-CS-dMRI. Note that the dictionary $\mathbf{M}$ used in Eqs. (5a) and (8) was devised for the diffusion signal whose decay is known to be close to mono-/multi-exponential decay, while the noise signal in non-tissue voxels violates this property. Thus for non-tissue voxels, the representation Eq. (8) is not sparse, resulting in large representation error with the limited number of basis we used. Note that existing CS-dMRI works [5–7] in $\mathbf{q}$-space normally perform estimation voxel by voxel or only considering information from neighborhood voxels, thus failed estimation in non-tissue voxels will not affect the estimation in tissue voxels. However if the non-tissue voxels are considered in Eq. (3), the representation error and total variation caused by these non-tissue voxels will dominate the minimization, such that the estimation of the signals in tissue voxels is problematic. Thus proper masking has to be used in 6D-CS-dMRI. We first extract the brain region using $S(\boldsymbol{x}, 0)$. Then Eq. (5a) is only performed on the tissue voxels. If $\boldsymbol{x}_i$ is a non-tissue voxel, we set $\boldsymbol{c}_i = 0$ in Eq. (6b), and after Eq. (5b) we also set $\boldsymbol{s}_i = 0$. Using this strategy, U_i, ψ_i, $\boldsymbol{c}_i$ and $\boldsymbol{s}_i$ are always zero if $\boldsymbol{x}_i$ is a non-tissue voxel. See Algorithm 1 for the 6D-CS-dMRI pipeline.

3   Experiments

3.1   Evaluation Strategy for CS Reconstruction of DWI/EAP/ODF

RMSE for Data Reconstruction. Once the coefficient vectors $\{\boldsymbol{c}_i\}$ are estimated, ODF, DWI and EAP fields all can be analytically obtained by SPF basis [7,18,19]. With a given set of samples of ODF/DWI/EAP, the Root-Mean-Square Error (RMSE) is defined as

$$\text{RMSE}(\theta) = \sqrt{\frac{1}{N}\sum_{i=1}^{N}(\hat{\theta}_i - \theta_i)^2} \tag{9}$$

where $\hat{\theta}_i$ is the estimated value for the ground truth θ_i. The RMSE is calculated for each voxel, then the mean RMSE is calculated for an estimated field of DWI/EAP/ODF.

- For DWI signal, we use two sets of samples, where one is the set of 321 uniform samples with $b = 1200\,\text{s/mm}^2$, and the other one is the DSI sampling scheme in 3D q-space. These two sample sets determine two RMSEs, which can be used to evaluate the DWI signal reconstruction respectively in a single shell and the whole q-space.
- For EAP, we use the 321 uniform orientations for EAP profile with radius $0.015\,\mu\text{m}$ as the samples in displacement space.
- For ODF defined on S^2, we use 321 uniform orientations from sphere tessellation as the samples.

Sampling Schemes in the Joint k-q Space. Conventional DSI requires 514 diffusion-weighted images and one baseline image $S(\boldsymbol{x}, 0)$ [1]. Denoting the spatial size in k-space as $N_x \times N_y \times N_z$, the size of the fully sampled data is then $N_x \times N_y \times N_z \times 514$. A 3-fold acceleration was considered in [6,7] by using only 170 samples with maximal b-value of $8000\,\text{s/mm}^2$[1]. Considering $E(\boldsymbol{x}, \mathbf{q}) = E(\boldsymbol{x}, -\mathbf{q})$, we remove antipodal symmetric samples from these 170 samples to obtain finally 138 samples, resulting in a 3.7-fold q-space acceleration. In k-space, we follow the Sparse MRI approach to perform a 3-fold sub-sampling using a polynomial distribution [3]. Thus we have a sub-sampling scheme in k-q space with the total acceleration of approximately 11-fold compared with the full DSI scheme.

Evaluation Strategy. 6D-CS-dMRI was evaluated using synthetic and real data. For synthetic data with known ground truth, the RMSE can be calculated by comparing the estimated DWI/ODF/EAP using sub-sampled data and the ground truth. For real data without ground truth, the RMSE is calculated by comparing the results of DL-SPFI using the full DSI samples with the results of 6D-CS-dMRI and naive 6D-CS-dMRI using sub-sampled data.

3.2 Synthetic Data Experiments

We generated a slice of synthetic data with size $20 \times 20 \times 1 \times 514$ using mixture of tensor model with eigenvalues $[1.5, 0.3, 0.3] \times 10^{-3}\,\text{mm}^2/\text{s}$, $S(\boldsymbol{x}, 0) = 1$ for all voxels. The generated signal is real in the $\boldsymbol{x}$-q space. By considering its imaginary part as zero, Fourier transform was performed to obtain the synthetic ground-truth Fourier samples in k-q space. Then we performed 6D-CS-dMRI and naive

---

[1] https://www.martinos.org/~berkin/DSI_Dictionary_Toolbox.zip.

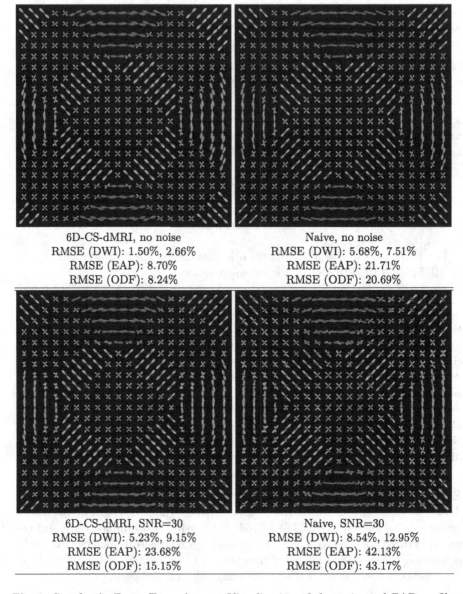

6D-CS-dMRI, no noise	Naive, no noise
RMSE (DWI): 1.50%, 2.66%	RMSE (DWI): 5.68%, 7.51%
RMSE (EAP): 8.70%	RMSE (EAP): 21.71%
RMSE (ODF): 8.24%	RMSE (ODF): 20.69%
6D-CS-dMRI, SNR=30	Naive, SNR=30
RMSE (DWI): 5.23%, 9.15%	RMSE (DWI): 8.54%, 12.95%
RMSE (EAP): 23.68%	RMSE (EAP): 42.13%
RMSE (ODF): 15.15%	RMSE (ODF): 43.17%

Fig. 2. Synthetic Data Experiment. Visualization of the estimated EAP profiles with 15 μm by 6D-CS-dMRI and naive 6D-CS-dMRI using 11-fold sub-sampling of the raw data, without and with complex Gaussian noise. Also shown are the RMSEs for ODFs and EAPs, and two RMSEs for DWI signal, where the first one is calculated for a single shell and the second one for the 3D space.

6D-CS-dMRI to 11-fold sub-sampled data in $\mathbf{k}$-$\mathbf{q}$ space. Note that although we generated data with $\psi_i = 1$, $\forall i$, 6D-CS-dMRI still estimates the unknown variables $\{\psi_i\}$ in reconstruction. To evaluate the robustness to noise, we added some complex Gaussian noise in subsamples in k-space with SNR = 30 which is defined as $S(\boldsymbol{x}, 0)/\sigma$ [7], where σ is the variance of the complex Gaussian noise, then we performed 6D-CS-dMRI and naive 6D-CS-dMRI on the noisy samples in k-q space and re-calculated the RMSE. We tuned the parameters $(\lambda_1, \lambda_2, \lambda_3, \rho)$ in reconstruction to obtain the best results in terms of RMSE of DWI signal in 3D space. Figure 2 shows the estimated EAP profiles with radius 15 μm and the mean RMSE calculated respectively for the estimated DWI, ODF and EAP fields. It demonstrates that (1) Compared with the naive approach, which introduces some small spurious lobes, 6D-CS-dMRI is more robust and obtains sharper EAP profiles which are similar to the ground truth as indicated by the lower RMSE for all DWIs, ODFs, EAPs. (2) EAP is more difficult to reconstruct, giving larger RMSE than DWI and ODF. (3) Although EAP reconstruction RMSEs are larger, the fiber directions shown in EAP profiles are close to the ground truth fiber directions. (4) DWI signal in single shell has the lowest RMSE, and it is normally easier to be estimated than DWI signal in whole 3D space.

3.3   Real Data Experiments

We evaluated 6D-CS-dMRI using the real DSI data used in [6,7] (see Footnote 1). There is no ground truth for real data, thus direct comparison between the estimated DW images and the raw DWI data is not appropriate due to noise. Following [7], the coefficients $\{c_i\}$ were first estimated by DL-SPFI from full samples in k-q space, and DWIs, ODFs, and EAP profiles were generated from these estimated coefficients as golden standards. Then we estimated the coefficients by 6D-CS-dMRI and naive 6D-CS-dMRI using 11-fold sub-sampling, and calculated RMSE by comparing the estimated DWIs/ODFs/EAPs with the golden standards reconstructed from full sampled data. Mean RMSEs for DWIs, ODFs and EAPs shown in Fig. 3 are consistent with the observations in synthetic data experiments, i.e., DWI signal in a single shell is the easiest quantity to be reconstructed, while EAP profile is the most difficult quantity. From Fig. 3, the small RMSE (3.99 % for DWIs, 13.44 % for EAPs) given by 6D-CS-dMRI using 11-fold sub-sampled data indicates that reconstruction using sub-sampled data gives results similar to reconstruction using the full samples. Since acquiring the full DSI samples requires nearly one hour, the 11-fold subsampled data only need less than 6 min. Similar to the synthetic data experiments, we also added complex Gaussian noise with SNR=30 to the sub-sampled k-space data. After adding noise, $\sqrt{\frac{\sum_{\mathbf{k},\mathbf{q}} |\widehat{S}(\mathbf{k},\mathbf{q}) - \widehat{S}^*(\mathbf{k},\mathbf{q})|^2}{\sum_{\mathbf{k},\mathbf{q}} |\widehat{S}^*(\mathbf{k},\mathbf{q})|^2}} = 0.279$, where $\widehat{S}^*(\mathbf{k}, \mathbf{q})$ is the golden standard DWI samples in k-q space. We then performed 6D-CS-dMRI and naive 6D-CS-dMRI on the noisy samples in k-q space and re-calculated the RMSEs. It can be seen from Fig. 3 that, compared with naive 6D-CS-dMRI, 6D-CS-dMRI is more robust to noise.

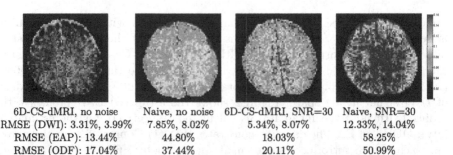

6D-CS-dMRI, no noise	Naive, no noise	6D-CS-dMRI, SNR=30	Naive, SNR=30
RMSE (DWI): 3.31%, 3.99%	7.85%, 8.02%	5.34%, 8.07%	12.33%, 14.04%
RMSE (EAP): 13.44%	44.80%	18.03%	58.25%
RMSE (ODF): 17.04%	37.44%	20.11%	50.99%

Fig. 3. Real Data Experiment. RMSE images (defined by DWI signal in 3D space) for 6D-CS-dMRI and naive 6D-CS-dMRI using 11-fold sub-sampling of the raw data, without or with complex Gaussian noise. Also shown are the mean RMSEs for DWIs, EAPs and ODFs. The first RMSE of DWI is calculated for a single shell and the second RMSE of DWI is for 3D space.

4   Conclusion

In this paper, we have proposed a novel compressed sensing framework, called 6D-CS-dMRI, for reconstruction of the continuous diffusion signal and EAP in the joint 6D $\mathbf{k}$-$\mathbf{q}$ space. To our knowledge, 6D-CS-dMRI is the first work that applies compressed sensing in the full 6D $\mathbf{k}$-$\mathbf{q}$ space and reconstructs simultaneously the diffusion signal in the full continuous $\mathbf{q}$-space and the EAP in full continuous displacement $\mathbf{R}$-space. The experiments on synthetic data and real data demonstrate that (1) compared with the reconstruction using full DSI sampling in $\mathbf{k}$-$\mathbf{q}$ space, 6D-CS-dMRI using 11-fold sub-sampling data obtains similar results with low RMSE (less than 5 % for DWI signal in synthetic data and real data), indicating that the scanning time can be reduced from nearly 1 h to less than 6 min; (2) compared with naive 6D-CS-dMRI, which performs two CS reconstruction respectively in the $\mathbf{k}$ space and the $\mathbf{q}$ space, 6D-CS-dMRI generally obtains lower RMSE and is more robust to noise. Our future work is to incorporate the proposed 6D-CS-dMRI method with existing imaging techniques in $\mathbf{k}$ space, such that 6D-CS-dMRI can be used in clinical scanners.

Acknowledgement. This work was performed at UNC with support in part by a UNC BRIC-Radiology start-up fund and NIH grants (EB006733, EB009634, AG041721, MH100217, and 1UL1TR001111).

References

1. Wedeen, V.J., Hagmann, P., Tseng, W.Y.I., Reese, T.G., Weisskoff, R.M.: Mapping complex tissue architecture with diffusion spectrum magnetic resonance imaging. Magn. Reson. Med. **54**, 1377–1386 (2005)
2. Donoho, D.L.: Compressed sensing. IEEE Trans. Inf. Theory **52**(4), 1289–1306 (2006)

3. Lustig, M., Donoho, D., Pauly, J.: Sparse MRI: the application of compressed sensing for rapid MR imaging. Magn. Reson. Med. **58**(6), 1182–1195 (2007)
4. Yang, J., Zhang, Y., Yin, W.: A fast alternating direction method for TVL1-L2 signal reconstruction from partial fourier data. IEEE J. Sel. Top. Signal Process. **4**(2), 288–297 (2010)
5. Menzel, M.I., Tan, E.T., Khare, K., Sperl, J.I., King, K.F., Tao, X., Hardy, C.J., Marinelli, L.: Accelerated diffusion spectrum imaging in the human brain using compressed sensing. Magn. Reson. Med. **66**(5), 1226–1233 (2011)
6. Bilgic, B., Setsompop, K., Cohen-Adad, J., Yendiki, A., Wald, L.L., Adalsteinsson, E.: Accelerated diffusion spectrum imaging with compressed sensing using adaptive dictionaries. Magn. Reson. Med. **68**, 1747–1754 (2012)
7. Cheng, J., Jiang, T., Deriche, R., Shen, D., Yap, P.-T.: Regularized spherical polar fourier diffusion MRI with optimal dictionary learning. In: Mori, K., Sakuma, I., Sato, Y., Barillot, C., Navab, N. (eds.) MICCAI 2013, Part I. LNCS, vol. 8149, pp. 639–646. Springer, Heidelberg (2013)
8. Merlet, S., Deriche, R.: Compressed sensing for accelerated EAP recovery in diffusion MRI. In: Computational Diffusion MRI - MICCAI Workshop (2010)
9. Cheng, J., Merlet, S., Caruyer, E., Ghosh, A., Jiang, T., Deriche, R., et al.: Compressive sensing ensemble average propagator estimation via L1 spherical polar fourier imaging. In: Computational Diffusion MRI - MICCAI Workshop (2011)
10. Merlet, S., Cheng, J., Ghosh, A., Deriche, R.: Spherical polar fourier EAP and ODF reconstruction via compressed sensing in diffusion MRI. In: ISBI (2011)
11. Mani, M., Jacob, M., Guidon, A., Liu, C., Song, A., Magnotta, V., Zhong, J.: Acceleration of high angular and spatial resolution diffusion imaging using compressed sensing. In: 2012 9th IEEE International Symposium on Biomedical Imaging (ISBI), pp. 326–329. IEEE (2012)
12. Awate, S.P., DiBella, E.V.: Compressed sensing HARDI via rotation-invariant concise dictionaries, flexible K-space undersampling, and multiscale spatial regularity. In: 2013 IEEE 10th International Symposium on Biomedical Imaging (ISBI), pp. 9–12. IEEE (2013)
13. Cheng, J., Shen, D., Yap, P.T.: Joint kq space compressed sensing for accelerated multi-shell acquisition and reconstruction of the diffusion signal and ensemble average propagator. In: ISMRM, p. 664 (2014)
14. Callaghan, P.T.: Principles of Nuclear Magnetic Resonance Microscopy. Oxford University Press, Oxford (1991)
15. Boyd, S., Parikh, N., Chu, E., Peleato, B., Eckstein, J.: Distributed optimization and statistical learning via the alternating direction method of multipliers. Found. Trends Mach. Learn. **3**(1), 1–122 (2011)
16. Yang, J., Zhang, Y.: Alternating direction algorithms for ell_1-problems in compressive sensing. SIAM J. Sci. Comput. **33**(1), 250–278 (2011)
17. Assemlal, H.E., Tschumperlé, D., Brun, L.: Efficient and robust computation of PDF features from diffusion MR signal. Med. Image Anal. **13**, 715–729 (2009)
18. Cheng, J., Ghosh, A., Jiang, T., Deriche, R.: Model-free and analytical EAP reconstruction via spherical polar fourier diffusion MRI. In: Jiang, T., Navab, N., Pluim, J.P.W., Viergever, M.A. (eds.) MICCAI 2010, Part I. LNCS, vol. 6361, pp. 590–597. Springer, Heidelberg (2010)
19. Cheng, J., Ghosh, A., Deriche, R., Jiang, T.: Model-free, regularized, fast, and robust analytical orientation distribution function estimation. In: Jiang, T., Navab, N., Pluim, J.P.W., Viergever, M.A. (eds.) MICCAI 2010, Part I. LNCS, vol. 6361, pp. 648–656. Springer, Heidelberg (2010)

Functional Nonlinear Mixed Effects Models for Longitudinal Image Data

Xinchao Luo[1,2], Lixing Zhu[3], Linglong Kong[4], and Hongtu Zhu[1](✉)

[1] Department of Biostatistics and Biomedical Research Imaging Center,
University of North Carolina at Chapel Hill, Chapel Hill, USA
`htzhu@email.unc.edu`
[2] School of Finance and Statistics, East China Normal University, Shanghai, China
[3] Department of Mathematics, Hong Kong Baptist University, Hong Kong, China
[4] Department of Mathematical and Statistical Sciences, University of Alberta,
Edmonton, Canada

Abstract. Motivated by studying large-scale longitudinal image data, we propose a novel functional nonlinear mixed effects modeling (FNMEM) framework to model the nonlinear spatial-temporal growth patterns of brain structure and function and their association with covariates of interest (e.g., time or diagnostic status). Our FNMEM explicitly quantifies a random nonlinear association map of individual trajectories. We develop an efficient estimation method to estimate the nonlinear growth function and the covariance operator of the spatial-temporal process. We propose a global test and a simultaneous confidence band for some specific growth patterns. We conduct Monte Carlo simulation to examine the finite-sample performance of the proposed procedures. We apply FNMEM to investigate the spatial-temporal dynamics of white-matter fiber skeletons in a national database for autism research. Our FNMEM may provide a valuable tool for charting the developmental trajectories of various neuropsychiatric and neurodegenerative disorders.

Keywords: Functional nonlinear mixed effects model · Functional response · Global test statistic · Simultaneous confidence band · Spatial-temporal pattern

1 Introduction

Improving understanding of brain structure and function (e.g., brain circuits) can be translated to the study of various neuropsychiatric and neurodegenerative disorders [2,3,5,9,10,14]. In effect, it is common to collect big data with great complexity and diversity in order to understand how changes in the brain

Lixing Zhu was supported by a grant from the University Grants Council of Hong Kong, China.
Hongtu Zhu was partially supported by NIH grants MH086633, RR025747, and MH092335 and NSF grants SES-1357666 and DMS-1407655.

S. Ourselin et al. (Eds.): IPMI 2015, LNCS 9123, pp. 794–805, 2015.
DOI: 10.1007/978-3-319-19992-4_63

can lead to these brain-related disorders and to understand their trajectories across the lifespan and across diverse populations. By learning more about such trajectories, one hopes to improve existing approaches and devise new ones for the prevention, treatment, and cure of such disorders. To accomplish these objectives, development of novel statistical methods and their software platforms are critically important to deal with difficulties and challenges inherent in imaging data and associated data obtained from large-scale biomedical studies.

The aim of this paper is to develop a FNMEM framework to delineate dynamic changes of longitudinal image data and their association with a set of covariates of interest and to characterize their large spatial-temporal variations. The FMPM framework is motivated by the emerging demand to analyze massive image data collected in large-scale longitudinal biomedical studies, such as the Alzeimer's disease neuroimaging initiative [12]. In those studies, longitudinal functional data from different subjects, denoted by $\{y_{ij}(s) = y_i(t_{ij}, s) : i = 1, \cdots, n\}$, are usually observed and/or normalized in a large number of locations of a common space, denoted by $\mathcal{S}$, across multiple time points $\{t_{ij} : j = 1, \cdots, T_i\}_{i \geq 1}$. Also, $\mathcal{S}$ is often a compact subset of Euclidean space.

Methodology to handle longitudinal image data is still in its infancy, and further theoretical and practical development is much needed. Most existing methods focus on the analysis of univariate (or multivariate) variables measured longitudinally [4]. Many parametric mixed effects models including both fixed and random effects are the predominant approach for characterizing both the temporal correlations and random individual variations. Although there is a great interest in the analysis of functional data with various levels of hierarchical structures [7,11,18], only a handful of them [6,17,21] focused on the development of linear mixed models for longitudinal image data. Recently, there was some attempt on the development of hierarchical geodesic models on diffeomorphism for longitudinal shape analysis [15].

Specifically, FNMEM contains two major components including a random nonlinear association map for characterizing dynamic association between image data and covariates, and a spatial-temporal process for capturing large subject variation across both spatial and temporal domains. Because of its greater flexibility, FNMEM is generally more interpretable and parsimonious, and the predictions obtained from FNMEM extend more reliably outside the observed range of the data. We explicitly incorporate the spatial-temporal smoothness into our estimation procedure in order to accurately estimate the nonlinear association map and the spatial-temporal covariance operator. We also propose a global test statistic for testing the association map and construct its asymptotic simultaneous confidence band.

2   Method

2.1   Functional Nonlinear Mixed Effects Model

A functional nonlinear mixed effects model consists of two major components. The first one is a pointwise nonlinear mixed effects model given by

$$y_{ij}(s) = f(\phi_i(s), \mathbf{x}_{ij}) + \varepsilon_{ij}(s) \quad \text{for} \quad i = 1, \ldots, n, \tag{1}$$

where $f(\cdots)$ is a real-valued, differentiable nonlinear association map, $\phi_i(s)$ is a $p \times 1$ vector of subject-specific functions, $\mathbf{x}_{ij}$ is p-dimensional covariate of interest, and $\varepsilon_i(s)$ is the corresponding random error process. It is assumed that f has continuous second-order derivative with respect to $\phi_i(s)$. For image data, it is typical that after normalization, $y_{ij}(s)$ are measured at the same location for all subjects and exhibit both the within curve and between-curve dependence structure. Thus, without loss of generality, it is assumed that $y_{ij}(s)$ are observed on the M same grid points $\mathcal{S}_0 = [0,1] = \{s_m, 0 = s_1 \leq s_2 \cdots \leq s_M = 1\}$ for all subjects and time points.

The second one is a spatial-temporal process for modeling large variations across subject-specific functions $\phi_i(s)$. Specifically, $\phi_i(s)$ is modeled as

$$\phi_i(s) = \beta(s) + b_i(s), \tag{2}$$

where $\beta(\cdot) = (\beta_1(\cdot), \cdots, \beta_p(\cdot))^T$ is a $p \times 1$ vector of fixed effect functions and $b_i(s) = (b_{i1}(s), \cdots, b_{ip}(s))^T$ is a $p \times 1$ vector of random effect functions. In addition, $\{b_i(s)\}$ and $\{\varepsilon_i(s)\}$ are independent and identical copies of $\mathrm{SP}(0, \Sigma_b(s,t))$ and $\mathrm{SP}(0, \sigma_\varepsilon^2(s)1(s = t))$ respectively, where $\mathrm{SP}(\mu(s), \Sigma(s,t))$ is a stochastic process (e.g., Gaussian process) with mean function $\mu(s)$ and covariance function $\Sigma(s,t)$.

2.2 An Example

Recently, nonlinear mixed effects models based on the Gompertz function have been used to characterize longitudinal white matter development during early childhood [3,9,14] The Gompertz function can be written as

$$y = f(\phi, t) = \textbf{asymptote} \ \exp(-\textbf{delay} \ \exp(-\textbf{speed} \ t)) = \phi_1 \exp\{-\phi_2 \phi_3^t\},$$

where ϕ_1 is asymptote, ϕ_2 is delay, and ϕ_3 is $\exp(-\textbf{speed})$. Specifically, in [14], a nonlinear mixed effects model based on the Gompertz function is given by

$$y_{ij} = \phi_{1i} \exp\{-\phi_{2i} \phi_{3i}^{t_{ij}}\} + \varepsilon_{ij} \ \text{ and } \ \phi_i = (\phi_{1i}, \phi_{2i}, \phi_{3i})^T = \beta + b_i, \tag{3}$$

where $\beta = (\beta_1, \beta_2, \beta_3)^T$ are fixed effects and b_i are random effects. For image data, an extension of model (3) is to consider a FNMEM as

$$y_{ij}(s) = \phi_{1i}(s) \exp\{-\phi_{2i}(s)\phi_{3i}(s)^{t_{ij}}\} + \varepsilon_{ij}(s) \ \text{ and } \ \phi_i(s) = \beta(s) + b_i(s). \tag{4}$$

We will use model (4) to characterize the spatial-temporal dynamics of white-matter fiber tracts.

2.3 Estimation Procedure

The next interesting question is how to estimate the fixed effect and random effect functions of FNMEM. It should be noted that the estimation procedures used in [6,17,21] are not directly applicable here due to the nonlinear association map in (1).

Estimating the Fixed Effect Functions. At each grid point $s_m \in \mathcal{S}_0$, we treat model (1) as a traditional nonlinear mixed effects model as

$$y_{ij}(s_m) = f(\beta(s_m) + b_i(s_m), \mathbf{x}_{ij}) + \varepsilon_{ij}(s_m), \tag{5}$$

where $b_i(s_m) \sim N(0, \Sigma_b(s_m, s_m))$ and $\varepsilon_{ij}(s_m) \sim N(0, \sigma^2(s_m))$. Then, we calculate the maximum likelihood estimator of $\beta(s_m)$, denoted by $\hat{\beta}(s_m)$, across all s_m. Define $K_h(t - s) = K((t - s)/h)/h$ as the kernel function, where K is the Epanechnikov kernel, and $\tilde{K}_h(s_m - s) = K_h(s_m - s)/\{\sum_{m=1}^{M} K_h(s_m - s)\}$. We calculate a kernel estimator of $\beta(s)$ as:

$$\tilde{\beta}(s) = \sum_{m=1}^{M} \tilde{K}_{h_1}(s_m - s)\hat{\beta}(s_m) \quad \text{for all} \quad s \in \mathcal{S}. \tag{6}$$

The bandwidth $\hat{h}_1$ is selected using a leave-one-out cross-validation method.

Estimating the Covariance Operators. Under certain smoothness conditions on $b_i(s)$, we use local linear regression technique to estimate all $b_i(s)$. Specifically, by using Taylor expansion for $b_i(s_m)$ at $b_i(s)$, we have

$$b_i(s_m) \approx b_i(s) + \dot{b}_i(s)(s_m - s) = B_i(s)Z(s_m - s),$$

where $B_i(s) = (b_i(s), \dot{b}_i(s))$ is a $p \times 2$ matrix and $Z(s_m - s) = (1, (s_m - s))^T$ is a p dimensional vector, in which $\dot{b}_i(s) = (\dot{b}_{i1}(s), \cdots, \dot{b}_{ip}(s))^T$ and $\dot{b}_{il}(s) = \partial b_{il}(s)/\partial s$ for $l = 1, \cdots, p$. For each i and s, we estimate $B_i(s)$ by minimizing the weighted nonlinear least squares [19]:

$$S_M(B_i(s)) \stackrel{\text{def}}{=} \sum_{j=1}^{n_i} \sum_{m=1}^{M} \left\{ y_{ij}(s_m) - f(\hat{\beta}(s_m) + B_i(s)Z(s_m - s), \mathbf{x}_{ij}) \right\}^2 K_{h_2}(s_m - s).$$

The optimal bandwidth $\hat{h}_2$ is selected using a leave-one-out cross-validation method, and an iteration algorithm is proposed to get the estimators. Finally, let $N = \sum_{i=1}^{n} n_i$, we estimate $\Sigma_b(s, t)$ by using

$$\hat{\Sigma}_b(s, t) = N^{-1} \sum_{i=1}^{n} n_i \tilde{b}_i(s)\tilde{b}_i(t)^T.$$

Functional Principal Component Analysis. With the empirical covariance $\hat{\Sigma}_b(s, t)$, we follow [13] and calculate the spectral decomposition as

$$\hat{\Sigma}_b(s, t) = \sum_{k=1}^{\infty} \hat{\lambda}_k \hat{\psi}_k(s)\hat{\psi}_k(t)^T,$$

where $\hat{\lambda}_k$ are estimated eigenvalues and $\hat{\psi}_k(s)$ are their corresponding estimated eigenfunctions. Moreover, the k-th functional principal component scores can be computes by $\hat{\xi}_{ik} = \sum_{m=1}^{M} \tilde{b}_i(s_m)\psi_k(s_m)(s_m - s_{m-1})$ for $i = 1, \cdots, n$.

2.4   Inference Procedure

The next interesting question is how to make statistical inference on the fixed effect functions of FNMEM.

Hypothesis Test. We focus on the linear hypothesis of $\beta(s)$ as follows

$$H_0 : R\beta(s) = \mathbf{b}_0(s) \text{ for all } s \quad \text{vs.} \quad H_1 : R\beta(s) \neq \mathbf{b}_0(s),$$

where R is a $r \times p$ matrix with rank r, and b_0 is a given $r \times 1$ vector of functions. A global test statistic S_n is given by

$$S_n = \int_0^1 \mathbf{d}(s)^T [R\hat{\Sigma}(s,s)R^T]^{-1}\mathbf{d}(s)ds,$$

where $\mathbf{d}(s) = R[\tilde{\beta}(s) - \text{bias}(\tilde{\beta}(s))] - \mathbf{b}_0(s)$, $\hat{\Sigma}(s,s) = \widehat{\text{Var}(\hat{\beta}(s))}$. We just drop $\text{bias}(\tilde{\beta}(s))$ when calculate the score functions for computational efficiency since $R\tilde{\beta}(s) \approx \mathbf{b}_0(s)$ and $\text{bias}(\tilde{\beta}(s)) = o_p(h_1^2)$, so that $R\text{bias}(\tilde{\beta}(s)) \approx \mathbf{0}$. Since the asymptotic distribution of S_n is very complicated, we can hardly approximate the percentiles of S_n under H_0 directly. Instead, we propose a score bootstrap method [8] to obtain the p value.

Simultaneous Confidence Bands. Give a confidence level α, we construct simultaneous confidence bands for each $\beta_l(s), l = 1, \cdots, p$ as follows:

$$P(\hat{\beta}_l^{L,\alpha}(s) < \beta_l(s) < \hat{\beta}_l^{U,\alpha}(s) \text{ for all } s \in \mathcal{S}) = 1 - \alpha,$$

where $\hat{\beta}_l^{L,\alpha}(s)$ and $\hat{\beta}_l^{U,\alpha}(s)$ are the lower and upper limits of simultaneous confidence band, respectively. We develop a resampling method to approximate the bounds as in [19].

3   Numerical Studies

In this section, we use Monte Carlo simulations and a real example to evaluate the finite sample performance of FNMEM.

3.1   Simulations

We generated multiple data sets from a FNMEM given by

$$y_{ij}(s) = \exp\{x_{ij1}\phi_{1i}(s) + x_{ij2}\phi_{2i}(s)\} + \varepsilon_i(s) \quad \text{and} \quad \phi_{li}(s) = \beta_l(s) + b_{li}(s)$$

for $l = 1, 2$, $j = 1, \cdots, n_i$ and $i = 1, \cdots, n$. We use two sets of simulations to investigate the estimation and inference procedures.

Simulation 1. The first one is to evaluate the power of the global test statistic S_n. Let s_m be equidistant time points in $[0,1]$, where $s_1 = 0$ and $s_M = 1$. Moreover, $\varepsilon_{ij}(s) \sim N(0, 0.1)$ and $(x_{ij1}, x_{ij2})^T \sim N((0,0)^T, \Sigma)$ with $\Sigma = (\sigma_{jk})_{p \times p}$, where $\sigma_{jk} = 0.3^{|k-j|}$ for $1 \leqslant k, j \leqslant p$. Furthermore, we set $b_i(s)$ as

$$b_i(s) = \sin(2\pi s) \cdot N((0,0)^T, 0.1 \times \Sigma) + \cos(2\pi s) \cdot N((0,0)^T, 0.2 \times \Sigma).$$

The functional fixed effects functions $\beta(s)$ are given by

$$\beta_1(s) = cs^2 \text{ and } \beta_2(s) = (1-s)^2.$$

To examine the hypothesis test $H_0 : \beta_1(s) = 0$ for all s against $H_1 : \beta_1(s) \neq 0$ for at least one s, we set c at different values in order to study the Type I error rates and power. Specifically, we fixed $c = 0$ to assess the Type I error, and then set $c = 0.05, 0.1, 0.15, 0.2$ to examine the power of S_n. We set $M = 25$ and $n_i = 5$. To evaluate at different sample sizes, we set $n = 50$ and 100 for each c. We calculated the rejection rate under the significance levels $\alpha = 0.05$ and 0.01 by using the score bootstrap method with $G = 500$. 200 replications are used for each simulation setting.

Figure 1 shows the power curves at two different significance levels. It can be seen that Type I error rates based on score bootstrap are well maintained under the pre-fixed significance levels when $n = 100$. The power of rejecting the null hypothesis increases with the sample size as expected. To show that FNMEM outperforms voxel-wise NMEM, we estimated $\hat{\Sigma}(s_m, s_m)$ using the asymptotic covariance matrix without smoothing, and then calculated the global testing statistic and its p-values with the score bootstrap method as in FNMEM. Figure 1 shows that voxel-wise NMEM is much less powerful than FNMEM.

Simulation 2. The second one is to explore the finite-sample performance of simultaneous confidence band. We used the same data generation procedure as Simulation 1. We fix $c = 1$ and then set $n = 50$, $n_i = 5$, $M = 25, 50$ and 75. Based on 200 replications, we calculated simultaneous confidence bands for each component of $\beta(s)$ by using the wild bootstrap method with $G = 500$. Table 1 summarizes the empirical coverage probabilities for $\alpha = 0.05$ and 0.01. Again as expected, with the number of grid points M increasing, the coverage probabilities are improved. When $M = 75$, the results are reasonable since the coverage probabilities are quite closed to the prespecified confidence levels $1 - \alpha$. The Monte Carlo errors are of size $\sqrt{0.95 \times 0.05/200} \approx 0.015$ for $\alpha = 0.05$. Figure 2 presents typical 95% and 99% simultaneous confidence bands for $M = 75$.

3.2 Real Data Analysis

We analyzed a data set taken from a national database for autism research (NDAR) (http://ndar.nih.gov/), an NIH-funded research data repository, that aims to accelerate progress in autism spectrum disorders (ASD) research through data sharing, data harmonization, and the reporting of research results. 416 high quality MRI scans are available for 253 children (126 males and 127 females) with 45 grid points, demographic information is shown in Table 2.

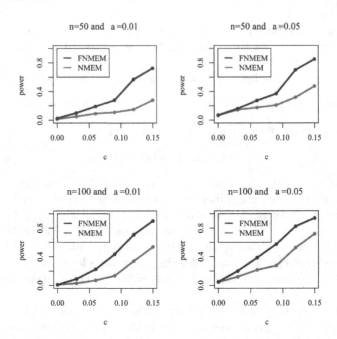

Fig. 1. Plots of power curves. Rejection rates of S_n based on score bootstrap method are calculated at six different values of c using FNMEM and NMEM, with sample size 50 and 100 at significance levels 5 % and 1 %.

Table 1. Empirical coverage probabilities of $1 - \alpha$ simultaneous confidence bands for all components of β based on 200 simulated data sets.

M	β_1	β_2	β_1	β_2
	$\alpha = 0.05$		$\alpha = 0.01$	
25	0.935	0.925	0.975	0.975
50	0.935	0.930	0.980	0.980
75	0.950	0.945	0.985	0.990

The data were processed by two key steps including a weighted least squares estimation method [1]; [20] to construct the diffusion tensors and a FSL TBSS pipeline [16] to register DTIs from multiple subjects to create a mean image and a mean skeleton. Specifically, maps of fractional anisotropy (FA) were computed for all subjects from the DTI after eddy current correction and automatic brain extraction using FMRIB software library. FA maps were then fed into the TBSS tool, which is also part of the FSL. In the TBSS analysis, the FA data of all the subjects were aligned into a common space by non-linear registration and the mean FA image were created and thinned to obtain a mean FA skeleton, which represents the centers of all WM tracts common to the group. Subsequently, each subjects aligned FA data were projected onto this skeleton.

We focus on the midsagittal corpus callosum skeleton and associated FA curves. The corpus callosum (CC) is the largest fiber tract in the human brain and is a topographically organized structure. It is responsible for much of the

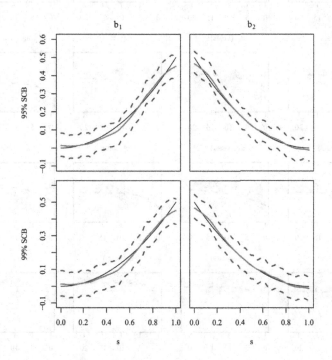

Fig. 2. Typical 95 % (the first row) and 99 % (the second row) simultaneous confidence bands for $M = 75$. The black solid, green solid, and red dash curves are, respectively, the true curves, the estimated curves and their corresponding 95 % and 99 % simultaneous confidence bands (Color figure online).

Table 2. Demographic information for participants.

Visit	Number of subjects	Age(years)	Range(years)
1	58	10.53(5.96)	[0, 18]
2	148	12.25(4.62)	[0, 21]
3	160	12.29(5.14)	[1, 22]
4	19	1.84(1.42)	[1, 6]
5	7	1.57(0.79)	[1, 3]
6	10	2.70(0.67)	[2, 4]
7	6	3.17(0.75)	[2, 4]
8	5	3.40(1.14)	[2, 5]
9	3	3.67(1.15)	[3, 5]
Gender	Male/Female		126/127

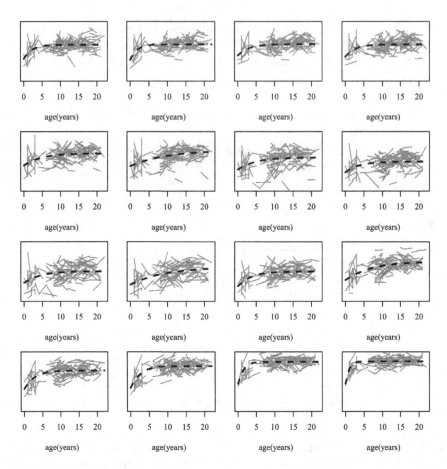

Fig. 3. Tract (red solid lines) varying as a function of age for grid points from 25 to 40, the black dash curves are estimated curves (Color figure online).

communication between the two hemispheres and connects homologous areas in the two cerebral hemispheres.

Figure 3 shows the variations of tract as age increases for grid points from 25 to 40, as well as the estimated curves at these grid points. It is observed that there are random subject-to-subject variations at each grid point along this tract as well as random subject-to-subject variations in the age effect at the selected location.

We fitted model (4) to the real data. We estimated the functional fixed effects functions $\beta(s)$ and constructed their 95 % and 99 % simultaneous confidence bands by using wild bootstrap method with $G = 500$ replications. We also constructed the global test statistic S_n to test the significance of delay and speed. The p-value of S_n is approximated by the score bootstrap method with $G = 500$ replications. Figure 5 shows the first 10 eigenvalues and 4 eigenfunctions

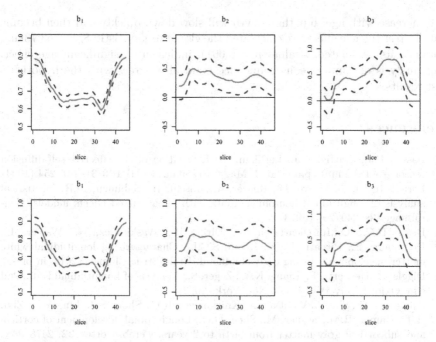

Fig. 4. The $100(1 - \alpha)\%$ simultaneous confidence bands of parameters for $\alpha = 0.05$ (the first row) and $\alpha = 0.01$ (the second row). The green solid and red dash curves are, respectively, the estimated curves and their corresponding 95 % and 99 % simultaneous confidence bands (Color figure online).

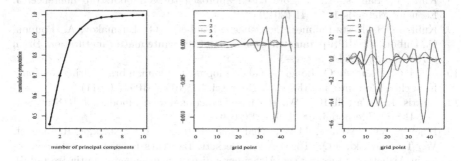

Fig. 5. The $100(1 - \alpha)\%$ cumulative proportion of the first 10 eigenvalues (left). The first 4 eigenfunctions corresponding to $b_{i1}(s)$ (middle) and $b_{i2}(s)$ (right).

of $\hat{\Sigma}_b(s, t)$. We can observe that the first four eigenvalues contribute more than 90 % (93.04 %) of the total while the rest quickly vanish to zero.

Figure 4 presents the uncertainty in the estimated coefficient functions, the horizontal line crossing $(0, 0)$ is contained. It can be seen that the horizontal lines are under the 95 % simultaneous confidence band of delay coefficients and exp($-$speed) coefficients at most of the grid points. In addition, exp($-$speed) coefficients are significantly less than 1. These may indicate that the **measures** will increase with age, but the growth will slow down quickly and then become flat. To test the age effect, we calculated the global test statistic $S_n = 763.73$ and obtained its associated p-value ($p < 0.001$), indicating a significant age effect. Our analysis of simultaneous confidence band also agrees with the hypothesis test results.

References

1. Basser, P.J., Mattiello, J., LeBihan, D.: Estimation of the effective self-diffusion tensor from the nmr spin echo. J. Magn. Resonan. Ser. B **103**(3), 247–254 (1994)
2. Bernal-Rusiel, J., Greve, D., Reuter, M., Fischl, B., Sabuncu, M.R.: Statistical analysis of longitudinal neuroimage data with linear mixed effects models. NeuroImage **66**, 249–260 (2013)
3. Dean, D.C., O'Muircheartaigh, J., Dirks, H., Waskiewicz, N., Walker, L., Doernberg, E., Piryatinsky, I., Deoni, S.C.L.: Characterizing longitudinal white matter development during early childhood. Brain Struct. Funct. (2014, in press)
4. Diggle, P., Heagerty, P., Liang, K.Y., Zeger, S.: Analysis of Longitudinal Data, 2nd edn. Oxford University Press, New York (2002)
5. Gilmore, J.H., Shi, F., Woolson, S., Knickmeyer, R.C., Short, S.J., Lin, W.L., Zhu, H.T., Hamer, R.M., Styner, M., Shen, D.G.: Longitudinal development of cortical and subcortical gray matter from birth to 2 years. Cereb. Cortex **22**, 2478–2485 (2011)
6. Greven, S., Crainiceanu, S., Caffo, B.S., Reich, D.: Longitudinal functional principal component analysis. Electron. J. Stat. **4**, 1022–1054 (2010)
7. Guo, W.: Functional mixed effects models. Biometrics **58**, 121–128 (2002)
8. Kline, P., Santos, A.: A score based approach to wild bootstrap inference. J. Econom. Methods **1**, 23–41 (2012)
9. Kulikova, S., Hertz-Pannier, L., Dehaene-Lambertz, G., Buzmakov, A., Poupon, C., Dubois, J.: Multi-parametric evaluation of the white matter maturation. Brain Struct. Funct. (2014, in press)
10. Lebel, C., Beaulieu, C.: Longitudinal development of human brain wiring continues from childhood into adulthood. J. Neurosci. **31**, 10937–10947 (2011)
11. Morris, J.S., Carroll, R.J.: Wavelet-based functional mixed models. J. R. Stat. Soc. Ser. B Stat. Methodol. **68**, 179–199 (2006)
12. Mueller, S.G., Weiner, M.W., Thal, L.J., Petersen, R.C., Jack, C.R., Jagust, W., Trojanowski, J.Q., Toga, A.W., Beckett, L.: Ways toward an early diagnosis in Alzheimer's disease: the Alzheimer's disease neuroimaging initiative (adni). Alzheimer's Dement. **1**(1), 55–66 (2005)
13. Rice, J.A., Silverman, B.W.: Estimating the mean and covariance structure nonparametrically when the data are curves. J. R. Stat. Soc. Ser. B (Methodol.) **53**, 233–243 (1991)
14. Sadeghi, N., Prastawa, M., Fletcher, P.T., Wolff, J., Gilmore, J.H., Gerig, G.: Regional characterization of longitudinal DT-MRI to study white matter maturation of the early developing brain. NeuroImage **68**, 236–247 (2013)
15. Singh, N., Hinkle, J., Joshi, S., Fletcher, P.T.: A hierarchical geodesic model for diffeomorphic longitudinal shape analysis. In: Gee, J.C., Joshi, S., Pohl, K.M., Wells, W.M., Zöllei, L. (eds.) IPMI 2013. LNCS, vol. 7917, pp. 560–571. Springer, Heidelberg (2013)

16. Smith, S.M., Jenkinson, M., Johansen-Berg, H., Rueckert, D., Nichols, T.E., Mackay, C.E., Watkins, K.E., Ciccarelli, O., Cader, M.Z., Matthews, P.M., et al.: Tract-based spatial statistics: voxelwise analysis of multi-subject diffusion data. Neuroimage **31**(4), 1487–1505 (2006)
17. Yuan, Y., Gilmore, J.H., Geng, X., Styner, M., Chen, K., Wang, J.L., Zhu, H.: Fmem: Functional mixed effects modeling for the analysis of longitudinal white matter tract data. NeuroImage **84**, 753–764 (2014)
18. Zhu, H., Brown, P., Morris, J.: Robust, adaptive functional regression in functional mixed model framework. J. Am. Stat. Assoc. **106**, 1167–1179 (2011)
19. Zhu, H., Li, R., Kong, L.: Multivariate varying coefficient model for functional responses. Ann. Stat. **40**, 2634–2666 (2012)
20. Zhu, H., Zhang, H., Ibrahim, J.G., Peterson, B.S.: Statistical analysis of diffusion tensors in diffusion-weighted magnetic resonance imaging data. J. Am. Stat. Assoc. **102**(480), 1085–1102 (2007)
21. Zipunnikov, V., Greven, S., Shou, H., Caffo, B., Reich, D.S., Crainiceanu, C.: Longitudinal high-dimensional principal components analysis with application to diffusion tensor imaging of multiple sclerosis. Ann. Appl. Stat. (2014, in press)

Author Index

Printed in the United States
By Bookmasters